Fraser and Paré's

Diagnosis of ————————

Diseases

———————— *of the*

CHEST

Fraser and Paré's

Diagnosis of
Diseases
of the
CHEST

Fourth Edition

Volume IV

R. S. Fraser, M.D.
Professor of Pathology
McGill University Health Centre
Royal Victoria Hospital
Montreal, Quebec

Nestor L. Müller, M.D., Ph.D.
Professor of Radiology
University of British Columbia
Vancouver Hospital and Health
  Sciences Centre
Vancouver, British Columbia

Neil Colman, M.D.
Associate Professor of Medicine
McGill University Health Centre
Montreal General Hospital
Montreal, Quebec

P. D. Paré, M.D.
Professor of Medicine
University of British Columbia
St. Paul's Hospital
Vancouver, British Columbia

W.B. SAUNDERS COMPANY
A Division of Harcourt Brace & Company
Philadelphia   London   Toronto   Montreal   Sydney   Tokyo

W.B. SAUNDERS COMPANY
A Division of Harcourt Brace & Company

The Curtis Center
Independence Square West
Philadelphia, Pennsylvania 19106

Library of Congress Cataloging-in-Publication Data

Fraser and Paré's Diagnosis of diseases of the chest / Richard S. Fraser . . . [et al.].—4th ed.

p.   cm.

ISBN 0–7216–6194–7

1. Chest—Diseases—Diagnosis.   I. Fraser, Richard S.
  [DNLM: 1. Thoracic Diseases—diagnosis.   2. Diagnostic Imaging.
  WF 975D536 1999]

RC941.D52 1999   617.5'4075—dc21

DNLM/DLC   98–36145

ISBN 0–7216–6194–7 (set)
ISBN 0–7216–6195–5 (vol. I)
ISBN 0–7216–6196–3 (vol. II)
ISBN 0–7216–6197–1 (vol. III)
ISBN 0–7216–6198–X (vol. IV)

FRASER AND PARÉ'S DIAGNOSIS OF DISEASES OF THE CHEST

Printed in the United States of America.

Last digit is the print number: 9   8   7   6   5   4   3   2   1

This book is dedicated to

ROBERT G. FRASER AND J. A. PETER PARÉ
who had the inspiration to recognize the importance of radiologic findings in
the diagnosis of chest disease, the dedication and perseverance to document
these and other findings in the initial editions of this book, and the grace to
teach us the value of both

and to

OUR WIVES AND CHILDREN
without whose encouragement and patience during our many hours of
reading, writing, and editing this edition would not have been completed.

Preface to the Fourth Edition

Previous editions of this book were based on the principle that the radiograph is the "focal point" or "first step" in the diagnosis of chest disease. We agree with the fundamental importance of the radiograph in this respect; however, we feel that it is best considered as one of two "pillars" of diagnosis, the other being the clinical history. Although it is of course possible to render an opinion about the nature of a patient's illness on the basis of only one of these pillars, this is fraught with potential error and should be avoided in most cases. Instead, it is our belief that the combination of a good clinical history and high-quality posteroanterior and lateral chest radiographs provides the respiratory physician or radiologist with sufficient information to significantly limit the differential diagnosis in the vast majority of patients who have chest disease and to enable a specific (and often correct) diagnosis in many. Additional information derived from ancillary radiologic procedures, laboratory tests, pulmonary function tests, and pathologic examination enables further refinement of differential diagnosis and a confident diagnosis in almost all patients. Of these additional tests, one that has undergone significant advance in the recent past is computed tomography (CT), particularly with the advent of high-resolution (HRCT) and spiral CT. The former has enabled much clearer delineation of the location and extent of disease in the lungs, pleura, and mediastinum, and the latter has greatly improved the ability to image the airways and vessels. The current edition of this book has changed to reflect the increased availability and diagnostic accuracy of these procedures; in addition, numerous figures have been added to illustrate the various abnormalities that they can identify.

Some might argue that a knowledge of the etiology, pathogenesis, and pathologic characteristics of disease is unnecessary for the clinician or radiologist to diagnose chest disease. It is our belief, however, that a thorough understanding of the overall nature of such disease will result in improved diagnostic skill. This potential refinement may be apparent in several areas, including better appreciation of the nature of radiologic abnormalities (e.g., via a knowledge of gross pathologic findings), improved knowledge of the potential value of new diagnostic tests (e.g., via an understanding of the molecular and genetic abnormalities associated with certain diseases and with the techniques by which these are identified), and a more thorough understanding of the associations between certain diseases or disease processes (e.g., viral infection and neoplasia). For these reasons, we have included a significant amount of material that is not directly relevant to diagnosis. We recognize the limitations of this approach, particularly with respect to a consideration of disease pathogenesis—the remarkable amount of research in chest disease, especially that related to cellular and molecular mechanisms, is difficult to summarize accurately, particularly since three of us have limited involvement in fundamental research. Moreover, it is inevitable that the progress that is currently being made in this research is such that some of the material in the text will be outdated at the time it is published. Despite these limitations, we consider an understanding of the etiology and pathogenesis of chest disease to be of sufficient importance to describe them to the best of our ability.

The organization of this book is based on a fairly consistent consideration of specific diseases under the headings of epidemiology, etiology and pathogenesis, pathologic characteristics, radiologic manifestations, clinical manifestations, laboratory findings (including pulmonary function tests), and prognosis and natural history. As with previous editions, a discussion of treatment has been omitted because of the rapidity with which therapeutic strategies may change and the implications that this may have. The scope of the book is such that it is meant primarily for specialists in chest disease, including pneumologists, thoracic surgeons, chest radiologists, and pathologists whose interest lies in this field. However, we believe that residents in training for these specialties will also find the text useful.

What will our readers find that is different from previous editions? Allusion has already been made to the extensive expansion of the discussion of HRCT and the addition of numerous new illustrations. Many new pathologic illustrations, both gross and microscopic, have also been included in an attempt to better explain the anatomic basis of disease. In addition to extensive updating of the material in previous editions, new sections have been written on CT of the normal lung, pulmonary transplantation, the effects on the chest of human immunodeficiency virus (HIV) infection, and pulmonary hemorrhage syndromes. The discussion of pulmonary neoplasia has been reorganized to conform more closely to the latest World Health Organization Classification of Lung Tumors. The Tables of Differential Diagnosis have been simplified to include primarily those diseases that are likely to be encountered by most pulmonary physicians; along with an increase in the number of illustrative examples, it is hoped that this version will provide a more simple and practical guide to differential diagnosis of the commonly enountered radiographic patterns of chest disease.

To make the text more accessible to the reader, the 21 chapters of the previous three editions have been expanded to 79. The subdivision is somewhat arbitrary and has necessitated repetition of material in some areas; for example, the inclusion of a chapter on chest disease in HIV infection necessarily involves a discussion of pulmonary infections and neoplasms that are also included in other, more comprehensive chapters on these subjects. As much as possible, we have tried to limit discussion of a particular topic to one place in the text; nevertheless, we have sometimes repeated material in order to minimize the necessity for the reader to refer to other sections of the book. We have also grouped chapters into larger categories based on anatomic location or presumed etiology and pathogenesis of disease; such grouping is again somewhat arbitrary, but hopefully will provide the reader easier access to appropriate information.

The reference list of the previous editions has been culled in an attempt to include those articles that are most relevant to the points we have chosen to emphasize; however, numerous reports published before 1990 have been retained. As might be expected, many references to articles published in the 1990s have also been added in an attempt to bring the text as up to date as possible. The resulting reference list contains a somewhat daunting total of approximately 31,000 citations! The inclusion of a list such as this might be questioned in light of the relatively easy availability of personal computers and electronic reference archives. However, we feel it is useful to have such references accessible to those who wish quick access to literature sources in book form. In addition, and perhaps more important in a book compiled by only four authors, we wish to provide a "factual" basis for our assertions as much as possible. As will be appreciated by those who publish in medical journals, it is inevitable that there are errors in our reference list, sometimes with respect to omission of an author or the spelling of his or her name and sometimes with respect to inappropriate attribution of statements or to omission of a key article. We apologize for these errors in advance and ask for our readers' understanding and the feedback to correct them. (Correspondence may be sent to [DDC@pathology.lan.mcgill.ca].)

The last edition of this book included a quotation from Ecclesiastes concerning the passage of time. We would also like to offer a quote of general philosophic interest, although one that is perhaps more directly related to the subject matter of this book. It derives from Maimonides, the great twelfth century scholar and physician:

> *Do not consider a thing as proof because you find it written in books: . . . there are fools who accept a thing as (such), because it is in writing.*

What we offer in the following pages are a concept of disease of the chest and an approach to its diagnosis based on the combined experience and knowledge of reported observations of four individuals. As in our everyday practice, we have attempted to be as open-minded to new ideas and as unbiased in our selection of material as possible. Despite this, such bias is to some extent inevitable and errors of commission or omission must be present. We do not, of course, advocate the unequivocal acceptance of Maimonides' aphorism; however, we trust that our readers will take his words to heart and consider the following pages and indeed the entire subject of chest disease with a questioning and open mind.

RSF
NLM
NC
PDP

Acknowledgments

The production of a book such as *Fraser and Paré's Diagnosis of Diseases of the Chest* is a huge task, and we have been fortunate in having the support and encouragement of many colleagues and friends in our endeavor. The availability and efficiency of modern computers have meant that much writing and editing have been performed directly by us; nevertheless, we could not have accomplished our task without secretarial help from Laura Fiorita, Stella Totilo, and Andrea Sanders at the McGill University Health Centre (MUHC); Catherine Goyette and Tamara Eigendorf at St. Paul's Hospital and the University of British Columbia; and Jenny Silver at the Vancouver Hospital and Health Sciences Centre. The diligence with which these individuals carried out their tasks shows in the final product and is deeply appreciated.

The majority of the case histories and radiologic illustrations reproduced in the text are derived from patients of staff members of the MUHC (particularly the Royal Victoria Hospital, the Montreal General Hospital, and the Montreal Chest Hospital Institute) and the Vancouver Hospital and Health Sciences Centre. Almost all illustrations of pathology are related to patients from the MUHC. We are indebted to our colleagues who cared for these patients, not only for their generosity in permitting us to publish the illustrations of various diseases but also for the benefit of their experience and guidance over the years. A number of these colleagues deserve particular mention for their comments and help on selected topics; these include Drs. Richard Menzies and John Kosiuk at the MUHC; Drs. Pearce Wilcox, John Fleetham, Brad Munt, and Hugh Chaun and Ms. Elisabeth Baile at the University of British Columbia; and Drs. A. Jean Buckley, John Aldrich, John Mayo, and Daniel Worsley at the Vancouver Hospital and Health Sciences Centre.

The photographic work throughout these volumes was the accomplishment of many individuals. Illustrations from former editions were provided by members of the Department of Visual Aids of the Royal Victoria Hospital; Susie Gray at the Department of Radiology, University of Alabama; Joseph Donohue, Anthony Graham, and Michael Paré of Montreal; and Sally Osborne at St. Paul's Hospital, Vancouver. Those involved in the production of new illustrations for this edition include Marcus Arts and Helmut Bernhard at the Montreal Neurological Institute Photography Department; Diane Minshall and Stuart Greene at St. Paul's Hospital, University of British Columbia; and Janis Franklin and Michael Robertson at the Vancouver Hospital Sciences Centre.

Throughout our writing and editing, we received support and cooperation from several individuals at W.B. Saunders, notably our Chief Editor, Lisette Bralow, our developmental editors Janice Gaillard and Melissa Messersmith, and our copy editors Sue Reilly and Lee Ann Draud, all of whom helped us overcome a number of the obstacles we encountered at various times. Finally, we acknowledge and thank our wives and children, without whose patience and encouragement this book would not have been completed.

RSF
NLM
NC
PDP

Contents

VOLUME ONE

VOLUME TWO

VOLUME THREE

VOLUME FOUR

PULMONARY DISEASE CAUSED BY INHALATION OR ASPIRATION OF PARTICULATES, SOLIDS, OR LIQUIDS

CHAPTER 59

Inhalation of Organic Dust

EXTRINSIC ALLERGIC ALVEOLITIS

General Characteristics

The term *extrinsic allergic alveolitis* (EAA; hypersensitivity pneumonitis, alveolar hypersensitivity) denotes a group of diseases characterized by an abnormal immunologic reaction in the lung to specific antigens contained in a wide variety of organic dusts. The list of diseases and the antigens associated with them has increased steadily since "farmer's lung" was first clearly described in 1932[1] and now contains a multitude of conditions ranging from this entity, which is probably the most common and the most widely recognized, to such unlikely conditions as pituitary snuff–taker's lung and hen-litter hypersensitivity (Table 59–1). Regardless of the name of the disease and the specific exposure involved, striking similarities exist among the clinical, pathologic, and radiologic features of all these diseases, suggesting that they share a common pathogenesis.

The exact criteria required to make the diagnosis of EAA are not clearly defined. However, most would probably agree that the following list, if fulfilled totally, would justify confident inclusion of a condition in this group of abnormalities:

1. Exposure to an organic dust of sufficiently small particle size to penetrate into the most distal lung parenchyma

2. Episodes of dyspnea, frequently accompanied by a dry cough, fever, malaise, and elevation of the white blood cell count, occurring some hours after exposure to the relevant antigen

3. Auscultatory evidence of bilateral crackles heard best over the lung bases bilaterally

4. Radiographic or CT evidence of diffuse ground-glass opacities or ill-defined small nodules, commonly associated in the acute stage with air-space consolidation

5. Pulmonary function tests revealing a reduction in vital capacity, carbon monoxide diffusing capacity, arterial P_{O_2}, and static compliance; evidence of airway obstruction may be present, particularly in long-term disease[2]

6. The presence in the serum of precipitins against the suspected antigen

7. The finding in fluid obtained on bronchoalveolar lavage (BAL) of an increased number of T lymphocytes, predominantly suppressor cells, and an increased level of immunoglobulin

8. The presence of bronchiolitis and interstitial pneumonitis, frequently with granuloma formation, in lung biopsy specimens

9. Resolution of systemic and respiratory symptoms after cessation of exposure to the antigen (although the persistence of exertional dyspnea, abnormal pulmonary function test values, and radiographic changes indicates irreversible interstitial pulmonary fibrosis in some cases)[3, 4]

When considering a diagnosis of EAA, it is important to remember that not all of the features listed above are necessarily found in a given patient; whether a specific organic dust deserves to be implicated as a cause of the disease depends largely on the number of criteria fulfilled.[3, 5, 6] In addition, many clinical features of the disease lack specificity.

Pathogenesis

The development of EAA is dependent on the size, immunogenicity, and number of inhaled organic particles and on the immune response of the affected individual. The small size of the antigenic particles is clearly important because particles greater than 5 to 6 μm are mostly trapped on the nasal or upper airway epithelium, where they are relatively innocuous.[7] In addition, a large amount of inhaled antigen is probably necessary to provide a strong stimulus for an immune response. Investigations of situations known to be associated with EAA have shown this to be the case.

Table 59–1. VARIETIES OF EXTRINSIC ALLERGIC ALVEOLITIS

DISEASE	PRINCIPAL RESPONSIBLE ANTIGENS	EXPOSURE SOURCE	ADDITIONAL FEATURES	SELECTED REFERENCES
Anhydride-induced lung disease	Trimollitic anhydride(?), Phthalic anhydride(?)	Polyester powder paint	Similar to isocyanate-induced lung disease	293
Bagassosis	*Thermoactinomyces sacchari*	Moldy sugar cane residue (bagasse)		294–296
Bird-fancier's (pigeon-breeder's) lung	Avian proteins contained in serum, excreta, or feathers	Pigeons, budgerigars, canaries, parakeets, chickens, ducks, turkeys, geese	With farmer's lung, the most common form of EAA	297–300
Building-associated EAA	*Thermoactinomyces* species; *Epicoccum nigrum* Various fungi: (*Serpula, Paecilomyces, Aspergillus, Leucogyrophana* species)	Decayed wood, damp walls, other materials in human habitations		217, 307, 336
Cheese-worker's lung	*Penicillium* species	Moldy cheese		301, 302
Coffee-worker's lung	?	Coffee bean roasting		303
Composter's or gardener's lung	?	Yard clippings, poorly ventilated greenhouse		304, 305
Detergent-worker's lung	*Bacillus subtilis*	Manufacture of proteolytic enzyme by *B. subtilis* for use in detergents		306
Farmer's lung	Thermophilic bacteria (*Micropolyspora faeni, Thermoactinomyces* species)		Affects males aged 40–50 yr; peak incidence during season when stored hay is used for cattle feeding; acute illness in 1/3 of patients, insidious in remainder; prevalence among farmers in different communities 1%–10%; should not be confused with organic dust toxic syndrome.	166, 308, 309
Fishmeal-worker's lung	Fish protein (?)	Preparation of meat		310
Hot-tub–bather's lung	*Mycobacterium avium–intracellulare* complex		*See also* humidifier lung	311
Humidifier lung	Bacteria: *Thermoactinomyces* species Fungi: *Penicillium* species, *Cladosporium* species Amebae: *Sphaeropsidales* species, *Acanthamoeba castellani, Naegleria gruberi*	Air conditioners, humidifiers, damp floors or walls, hot tubs	May be difficult to diagnose because of obscure exposure history; symptoms may develop in the evening of the first day back at work after a long weekend	311–315
Isocyanate-induced lung disease	Hexamethylane di-isocyanate, diphenylmethane di-isocyanate, and others	Electronics industry, autobody shops	Although caused by inorganic material, this abnormality is clinically identical to EAA caused by organic dusts	246, 247
Japanese summer-type allergic alveolitis	*Tricosporum cutaneum*	House dust	Principal form of EAA in Japan; occurs in summer months and subsides in autumn	228
Laboratory-worker's lung	Pauli's reagent, rat serum, and others			316–318
Lycoperdonosis	Mushrooms of genus *Lycoperdon*			319
Machine-operator's lung	*Pseudomonas fluorescens*(?), *Acinetobacter iwoffii*(?), nontuberculous mycobacteria(?)	Contaminated metal-working fluid		320, 337, 338
Malt-worker's lung	*Aspergillus clavatus*	Moldy malt		321
Maple bark disease	*Cryptostroma corticale*	Tree bark	Affects sawmill workers	322
Mollusk-shell–worker's lung		Mollusk-shell dust in a button factory		151
Mushroom-worker's lung	*Micropolyspora faeni, Micromonospora vulgaris, Pleurotus ostreatus, Pholiota nameko*	Compost used for mushroom culture	Steam pasteurization during culture of mushroom encourages rapid growth of thermophilic actinomycetes	202, 205

Table 59–1. VARIETIES OF EXTRINSIC ALLERGIC ALVEOLITIS *Continued*

DISEASE	PRINCIPAL RESPONSIBLE ANTIGENS	EXPOSURE SOURCE	ADDITIONAL FEATURES	SELECTED REFERENCES
New Guinea lung	*Streptomyces viridis (?)*	Thatched roofs		323
Orchid-grower's lung	*Cryptostroma corticale*			324
Peat-moss–worker's lung	*Monocillium* species(?), *Penicillium* species(?)	Processing plant		339
Pituitary snuff–taker's lung	Pig or ox pituitary extract	Extract used for treatment of diabetes insipidus		325
Polyester powder lung	Phthalic anhydride(?)			340
Polyurethane foam injection–worker's lung	1,3-*bis* (isocyanatomethyl) cyclohexane pre-polymer			326
Prawn-worker's lung	Shellfish protein (?)	Forced air used to blow meat out of tails		327
Sawmill-worker's lung	*Trichoderma konigii*			267
Sequoiosis	*Aureobasidium pullulans* (?) *Graphium* species (?)	Moldy redwood sawdust		328
Soy sauce–brewer's lung	*Aspergillus oryzae*			329
Starch-spray lung	?	Ironing clothes		330
Stipatosis	?	Esparto grass		331
Suberosis	*Penicillium frequentans*	Moldy cork	Occurs principally in cork workers in Portugal	332
Tobacco-worker's lung	?	Moldy raw tobacco		334
Wood pulp–worker's disease	*Alternaria* species	Wood pulp		335

For example, it has been estimated that as many as 750,000 particles per minute may be deposited on the air-space epithelium in a farmer working in an atmosphere of moldy hay;[8] similarly, it has been estimated that there are about 500,000,000 potentially antigenic fungal spores per gram of moldy bagasse![9]

There is substantial controversy regarding the precise mechanisms of the immune response responsible for the features of EAA. The recognition that individuals exposed to organic antigen produced immunoglobulin G (IgG) and IgM precipitating antibodies to the antigen led to the hypothesis that immune complex–mediated complement activation and neutrophil chemotaxis were responsible for the tissue injury (classic type III response).[10] Several clinical and experimental observations support this hypothesis. For example, high levels of immune complexes have been found in the BAL fluid of patients who have acute EAA, and their presence was associated with clinical symptoms and abnormalities of diffusing capacity in one small group of patients.[11] In addition, pigeon breeders who have active disease have higher levels of specific antibodies to pigeon serum and droppings than do healthy exposed workers; moreover, these antibodies appear to be produced locally, at least in part.[12] Animals sensitized by intratracheal administration of particulate antigen derived from *Micropolyspora faeni* (the agent responsible for farmer's lung) and subsequently challenged with this antigen develop lesions of EAA; if such animals are depleted of complement by cobra venom factor before antigen challenge, there is a significant reduction in the number of lesions.[13]

Despite these observations, affected patients have normal complement levels, and the vasculitis often seen in type III immune reactions is not a characteristic pathologic feature of the disease. Furthermore, the presence of serum antibodies appears to be more an indicator of antigen exposure than a marker of disease.[10, 14, 15] For example, 30% to 40% of symptom-free bird fanciers have precipitins to avian antigen,[16–18] 20% to 50% of healthy farmers exposed to moldy hay have antibodies to farmer's lung hay antigens,[19, 20] and 10% to 15% of symptom-free malt workers have positive serologic reactions to malt products.[21, 22]

A variety of cells are undoubtedly involved in the pathogenesis of EAA. Alveolar macrophages in the BAL fluid of patients who have acute EAA spontaneously secrete much higher levels of tumor necrosis factor-α and interleukin-1 (IL-1; cytokines implicated in granuloma formation)[23] and of granulocyte-macrophage colony-stimulating factor (which favors lymphocyte accumulation)[24] than do macrophages from control subjects. It also appears that both *M. faeni* and immune complexes can initiate the release of these proinflammatory cytokines from alveolar macrophages.[10] Alveolar macrophages also release a number of enzymes, such as elastase, collagenase, and lysozyme, as well as oxygen metabolites, which may contribute to early alveolar damage.[10] Animal models of EAA have demonstrated that macrophage-derived leukotrienes, released in response to IgG immune complexes, may play a role in macrophage-mediated antigen presentation to T cells; lipoxygenase inhibitors markedly inhibit granuloma formation in these models.[10]

Neutrophils are attracted to the lung by complement activation[25] and have also been implicated in the pathogenesis of the disease. Although both symptom-free farmers and farmers who have EAA develop neutrophilia after exposure to moldy hay, the neutrophils of farmers who have clinically evident disease are activated and primed to release toxic oxygen metabolites and proteinases.[26, 27] Moreover, antigen challenge in affected patients results in an alveolitis that is initially neutrophilic[28, 29] or mixed neutrophilic and lymphocytic[30] before becoming predominantly lymphocytic. These findings suggest a role for neutrophils in the production of early lung damage.

T-cell–dependent mechanisms are likely responsible for the subsequent evolution of the inflammatory process.[3, 10, 31, 32] BAL fluid from patients who have active disease generally contains more than 70% T cells; these are in an activated state[33, 34] and produce a variety of proinflammatory cytokines,[3, 10] including macrophage inflammatory protein-1α, IL-2,[34a] and IL-8.[35] The results of animal experiments have shown that disease can be transmitted to naïve animals by transfer of peripheral lymphocytes from affected animals[36, 37] and by transfer of spleen cells sensitized by culturing with antigen and concanavalin A.[38] This adoptive transfer requires intact function of CD4 cells in the recipient animal;[39] however, inhibition of these cells in the recipient animal does not interfere with an early neutrophil response to inhaled antigen.[40]

More than 40% of the lymphocytes in BAL fluid are suppressor cells;[10, 41] increased numbers of natural killer (NK) lymphocytes are also found. Both these cell types may function to down-regulate the cell-mediated inflammatory response.[10] In fact, depletion of NK cells in a murine model of EAA leads to the development of massive pulmonary fibrosis.[42] These observations may explain the finding that a high number of lymphocytes in BAL fluid does not correlate with long-term outcome, either in individuals who have a history of farmer's lung[43] or in farmers with no such history despite similar BAL findings.[44] An anti-inflammatory effect of IL-6,[10] IL-10,[10] and IL-12,[44a] released from alveolar macrophages and other cells, also has been described. Thus, as in a number of other pulmonary abnormalities, it is likely that the expression of disease depends on a balance between pro- and anti-inflammatory processes.[10]

Mast cells may also play an immunomodulatory role in EAA. They are increased in number in both tissue sections[45] and samples of BAL fluid (in which they are frequently degranulated).[46, 47] Although their exact role is not understood and their presence in human disease does not appear to correlate with outcome,[48] a model of EAA using mice deficient in mast cells has been characterized by a significant reduction in inflammatory response.[10] Plasma cells have also been found to be increased in the BAL fluid of affected patients, although the pathophysiologic significance of this is unclear.[49]

Altered surfactant metabolism might also be involved in pathogenesis. The level of surfactant protein A is elevated in the BAL fluid of affected patients;[50] despite this increase, there is evidence that it loses the immunomodulatory control it normally exerts on lymphocytes, a process that might contribute to lymphocyte infiltration of lung tissue.[51] Antigen exposure in patients who have EAA causes increased expression of intercellular adhesion molecule-1 on lymphocytes and alveolar macrophages in BAL fluid.[52, 53] This molecule is also shed into the alveolar lining fluid and the circulation, where its level appears to correlate with disease activity.

For obscure reasons, cigarette smoking appears to protect against the development of EAA. A highly significant positive correlation has been observed between lack of cigarette smoking and the development of both active EAA (farmer's and pigeon-breeder's lung)[54–56] and specific serum antibodies.[55, 57–61a] For example, in one study of Japanese families who developed summer-type EAA, 27 (66%) of 41 nonsmokers developed disease, whereas only 3 (27%) of 11 similarly exposed smokers were ill.[62] In another investigation of pigeon breeders, patients who smoked had lower levels of immunoglobulin in BAL fluid after inhalation challenge.[63] Smokers who have farmer's lung have also been found to have a higher ratio of CD4 to CD8 BAL cells than nonsmokers.[64] Despite these findings, the results of a study from Japan showed chronic disease, frequent relapse, and poor outcome to be much more prevalent in workers who smoked than in nonsmokers.[65]

Whether and to what extent genetic predisposition accounts for the variability in individual response to inhaled antigen is a matter of some controversy.[66] In some populations, a link has been strongly suggested. For example, in Mexican patients who have pigeon-breeder's disease, there is a relative risk of close to 5 for exposed patients carrying the HLA-DR7 phenotype when compared with the general population;[67] similarly, Japanese patients who have summer-type EAA have a somewhat increased prevalence of HLA-DQw3 compared with controls.[68] It has also been speculated that a "second factor," such as viral infection or insecticide exposure, is required for the disease to develop in some patients, in addition to genetic predisposition.[66] This hypothesis is supported by the results of some animal experiments.[69]

Why only some patients develop pulmonary fibrosis is also unclear. Profibrotic factors, such as fibronectin, fibroblast growth factor, and vibronectin,[70] are found in the BAL fluid of patients who have EAA and may even be identified in symptom-free farmers who have continued exposure to antigen and previous episodes of disease.[71] In one investigation, diminution of local collagenolysis appeared to play a role in the development of fibrosis.[72] In another, insidious onset of disease and a relatively large number of CD4 lymphocytes in BAL fluid correlated with the development of fibrosis.[73]

Impaired mucociliary clearance has been demonstrated in a small group of pigeon breeders.[74] The contribution of this abnormality to disease pathogenesis is unknown.

Pathologic Characteristics

The histologic features of the many different varieties of EAA are strikingly similar and, with few exceptions, do not permit differentiation. The exceptions are maple-bark disease (in which the causative fungus may be identified),[75] bagassosis (in which vegetable fibers may be seen),[76] and suberosis (in which cork dust may be identified).[77]

As might be anticipated, the pathologic characteristics depend partly on the intensity of exposure to the allergen and partly on the stage of the disease at which the biopsy is taken.[78] One study of early disease was performed in a 26-year-old farmer who had a typical clinical history of farmer's lung and who underwent biopsy 36 hours after the administration of a test exposure to moldy hay antigen.[79] Histologic examination showed capillary congestion and a polymorphic cellular infiltrate within alveoli in the vicinity of small airways and in and around the walls of medium-sized blood vessels. Although there was no mention of necrosis or thrombosis, immunofluorescent studies showed deposits of IgG, IgM, and C3 in the same vessels, and the findings were interpreted as vasculitis. In patients who have symptomatic disease, other investigators have reported morphologic changes in apparently early lesions that have also been interpreted as vasculitis.[80–82]

When biopsy is performed during the later stages of typical acute disease, the histologic appearance consists of a combination of bronchiolitis and alveolitis with granuloma formation.[81–86] The alveolitis consists of both interstitial and intra-alveolar components and is seen in virtually all cases. Within the interstitium, there is an inflammatory infiltrate that consists predominantly of lymphocytes accompanied by variable numbers of histiocytes, plasma cells, polymorphonuclear leukocytes, and eosinophils (Fig. 59–1). The infiltrate is usually patchy in distribution with a tendency to more severe involvement of peribronchiolar regions; uncommonly, it is extensive and confluent.[87] Within alveolar air spaces, a similar cellular infiltrate is frequently present; foamy macrophages are prominent in some cases, probably as a consequence of airway obstruction secondary to obliterative bronchiolitis. Evidence of alveolar epithelial and capillary endothelial damage is seen in some cases, consisting either of intra-alveolar proteinaceous material with admixed polymorphonuclear leukocytes and red blood cells (Fig. 59–2) or of plugs of intra-alveolar fibroblastic tissue.

Loosely formed granulomas composed of epithelioid histiocytes, multinucleated giant cells, or both are seen in 65% to 75% of cases[81, 82, 88] (see Fig. 59–1); single multinucleated giant cells associated with a lymphocytic infiltrate may also be seen. Unlike the granulomas typical of sarcoidosis, those of EAA are often somewhat poorly defined at their periphery and typically lack surrounding fibrosis. Most are solid, although small foci of central necrosis are occasionally seen.[84] Foreign material, sometimes birefringent, is common within the granulomas or the solitary multinucleated giant cells (Fig. 59–3); for example, in one series of 60 patients who had farmer's lung, 36 (60%) showed this feature.[85]

Bronchiolitis is also a frequent finding, being observed in about half of the patients who had farmer's lung in the series cited above,[85] and showing an incidence in different reviews of 25% to 100%.[83, 89–92] The usual pattern is that of an organizing exudate adjacent to a focus of epithelial ulceration or a plug of fibroblastic connective tissue (Fig. 59–4). In exceptional cases, alveolitis is mild and the major pathologic changes occur in the bronchioles.[93]

Depending on the severity and frequency of individual bouts of lung damage, a variable degree of interstitial fibrosis eventually supervenes.[94] As in the acute inflammatory stage, the fibrosis is at first mild and patchy in distribution at the microscopic level but eventually progresses into grossly visible scars.[85] Such fibrosis can be localized, in which case it may be most prominent in peribronchial or periseptal areas; sometimes it is more diffuse, resembling advanced idiopathic pulmonary fibrosis (IPF) with honeycombing. If exposure to the inciting antigen is discontinued, granulomas tend to disappear,[82] although mononuclear inflammatory cells and solitary multinucleated giant cells containing refractile foreign material frequently remain.[81, 83]

Electron microscopic appearances have been described by several groups of investigators;[81, 82, 96, 97] abnormalities include swelling and bleb formation of alveolar epithelial and capillary endothelial cells and alterations in the basement membrane.[96, 97] An unusual case of apparent EAA has also been reported in which there was deposition of amyloid in the alveolar septa.[98]

Radiologic Manifestations

As with the pathologic manifestations, the radiologic findings vary with the stage of the disease. Early in the course of the acute stage, the chest radiograph may show no discernible abnormality, even in patients who have florid pathologic changes on lung biopsy.[99–101] Later on, the characteristic finding consists of bilateral areas of consolidation, which may be diffuse or involve mainly the lower lung zones.[102–105] The air-space consolidation may be extensive, particularly in the lower lung zones, and may obscure the nodular pattern characteristic of the subacute stage (Fig. 59–5).

The radiographic abnormalities in subacute disease usually involve mainly the middle and lower lung zones.[103, 104, 106] The most characteristic pattern consists of poorly defined small nodular opacities (Fig. 59–6);[104] another common abnormality is a poorly defined, hazy increase in lung opacity (ground-glass opacity, Fig. 59–7).[103, 106, 107] The change in radiographic patterns between episodes of acute and subacute disease—diffuse involvement of both lungs as evidenced by a persistent nodular pattern, superimposition of consolidation with acute exacerbations, and resolution of the latter pattern within a few days of the initial acute clinical presentation (see Fig. 59–5)—should suggest the diagnosis.

Hilar lymph node enlargement has been said to be a common finding in some forms of EAA.[108] In our experience and that of others, however, evidence of lymphadenopathy is seldom seen on the chest radiograph; for example, in studies of 26 patients who had mushroom-worker's lung[109] and 27 who had farmer's lung,[110] no patients were found to have radiographic evidence of hilar or mediastinal lymph node enlargement. In a more recent investigation, lymphadenopathy was evident on the radiograph in only 1 of 13 patients.[111] By contrast, mediastinal lymph node enlargement—defined as a short-axis diameter equal to or greater than 10 mm—is seen relatively commonly on CT.[112] The enlarged nodes may measure more than 15 mm in short-axis diameter and usually involve only one or two nodal stations.[112] In one study of 17 patients, the abnormality was identified in 9 (53%);[112] however, most investigators have found a prevalence of about 5% to 15%.[106, 111, 113] The difference may be related to the underlying cause of EAA or to the stage of the disease. For example, in one study of patients who had bird-fancier's lung, enlarged nodes were identified on CT in 3 of 24 (12%) patients who had chronic EAA but in none of 21 patients who had subacute disease.[113]

Although the chest radiograph in patients who have subacute EAA is frequently abnormal—in greater than 90% of patients in some studies[114–116]—normal findings are not unusual.[116] For example, normal radiographs have been described in up to 33% of patients who have bird-fancier's lung[113, 117] or malt-worker's lung.[21] By contrast, radiographic abnormalities consistent with EAA may be present in the absence of clinical symptoms, a situation that pertained to 10 (5%) of 200 pigeon breeders in one series.[17] Although this figure may have been influenced by radiologic overreading, the association itself is not at all surprising in view

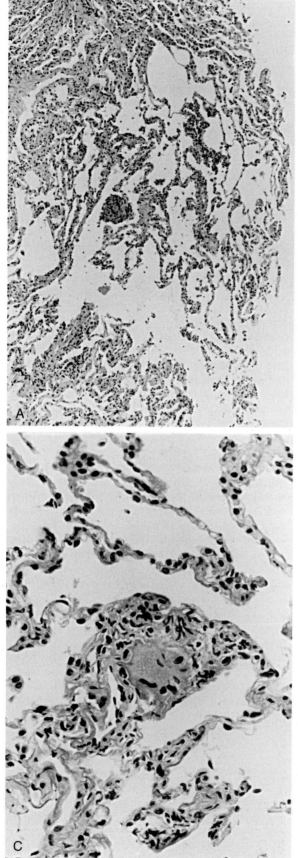

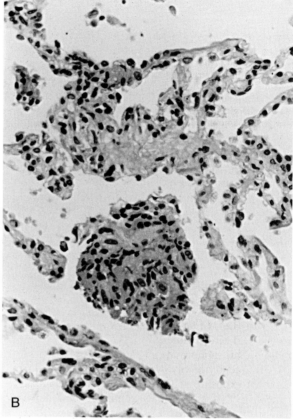

Figure 59–1. Extrinsic Allergic Alveolitis. A transbronchial biopsy specimen *(A)* shows focal mild interstitial thickening by an infiltrate of mononuclear inflammatory cells (seen to better advantage in *B*). A single granuloma is evident; although it appears to be free in the alveolar air space, further cuts showed it to be within a septum. A magnified view of another tissue fragment from the same biopsy specimen *(C)* shows a single multinucleated giant cell associated with a sparse lymphocytic infiltrate.

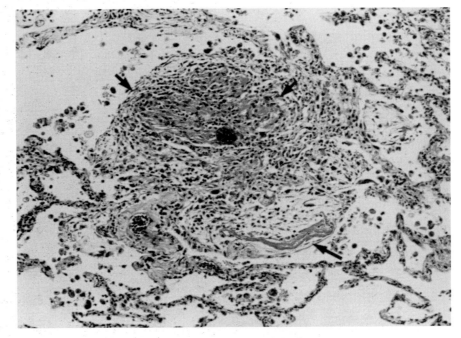

Figure 59–2. Extrinsic Allergic Alveolitis. A rather large focus of inflammation expands the alveolar interstitium and extends into adjacent air spaces. A single, poorly formed granuloma containing a multinucleated giant cell is evident *(short arrows)*. Organizing eosinophilic exudate *(long arrow)* within an air space indicates epithelial and probably endothelial damage. The patient was a 56-year-old man who had the acute onset of fever and dyspnea associated with a reticulonodular pattern on the radiograph shortly after turning on his home heater. (×100.)

of the evidence on BAL of active alveolitis in symptom-free exposed farmers and bird handlers.[118, 119]

The radiographic abnormalities in patients who have subacute EAA frequently resolve completely within 10 days to 3 months after exposure if the patient is removed from the environment.[83, 104] If exposure is continued or repeated or if the initial exposure is especially severe, the diffuse nodular pattern characteristic of the acute and subacute stages is replaced by changes characteristic of diffuse interstitial fibrosis (Fig. 59–8)—a medium to coarse reticular pattern, loss of lung volume, and (sometimes) compensatory overinflation of lung zones that are less affected. Although the fibrosis may be diffuse[120] (*see* Fig. 59–8), frequently there is a definite zonal predominance. Several investigators,

including those who used CT, have demonstrated a predominantly middle or lower lung zone involvement (Fig. 59–9).[106, 120, 121] For example, in one study of 16 patients, the fibrosis involved mainly the middle lung zones in 7 (44%), the lower lung zones in 2, and the upper lung zones in 1;[120] no zonal predominance was evident in 7 (44%) cases. In another investigation of 19 patients, the fibrosis involved mainly the lower lung zones in 8 (42%), the middle lung zones in 3 (16%), and the upper lung zones in 3 (16%) (Fig. 59–10);[121] no zonal predominance was seen in 5 patients (26%).

As might be expected, HRCT is superior to chest radiography in the demonstration of parenchymal abnormalities in patients who have EAA;[105, 106, 113] in particular, it may reveal abnormalities in patients who have clinically or bi-

Text continued on page 2372

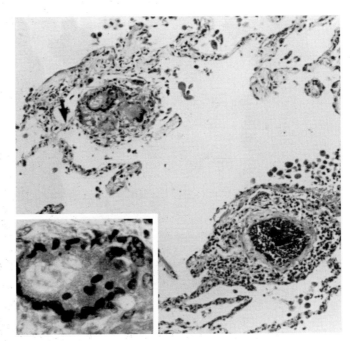

Figure 59–3. Extrinsic Allergic Alveolitis. The section shows a small focus of perivascular inflammation at the lower right and a cluster of multinucleated giant cells, apparently in an alveolar septum (the base of the septum is indicated by the *arrow*). Foreign material is present within the multinucleated giant cells (seen to better advantage in the magnified inset). (×100; inset ×480.)

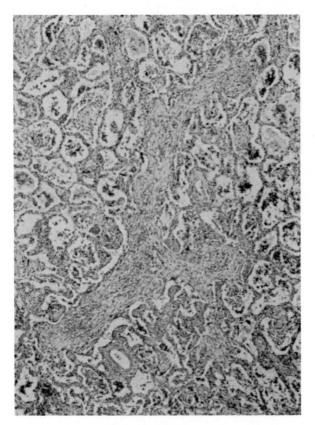

Figure 59–4. Extrinsic Allergic Alveolitis (EAA): Bronchiolitis. A magnified view of an open lung biopsy specimen shows a moderate degree of interstitial pneumonitis and a branching plug of fibroblastic tissue that occludes the lumen of several transitional airways. Granulomas were evident elsewhere in the biopsy specimen. The patient was a farmer who had typical symptoms of EAA. (×50.)

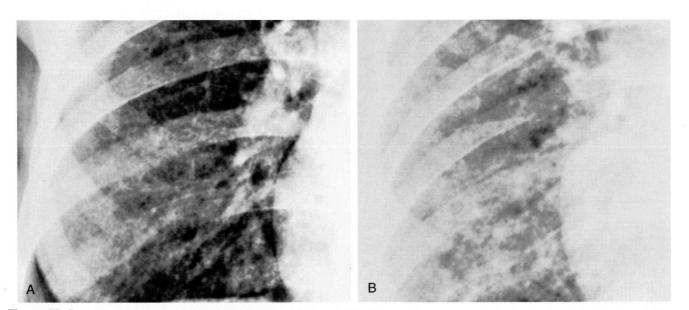

Figure 59–5. Extrinsic Allergic Alveolitis (EAA) (Farmer's Lung). This 25-year-old woman was admitted to the hospital with a 2-week history of moderate dyspnea. A detail view of the lower half of the right lung *(A)* reveals poorly defined small nodular opacities consistent with subacute EAA. Three months after her original episode, she was admitted for a second time following the acute onset of dyspnea, cough, and high fever. The chest radiograph at this time *(B)* demonstrates consolidation superimposed on the nodular opacities. This appearance is consistent with an acute exacerbation of EAA as a result of re-exposure to moldy hay.

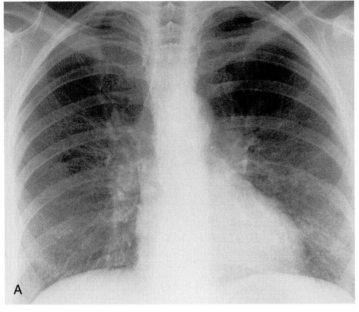

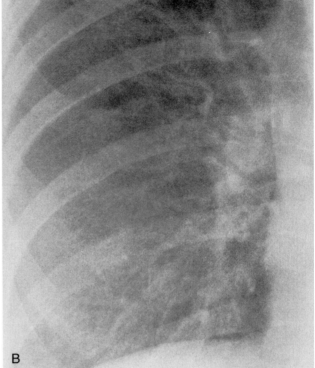

Figure 59–6. Subacute Extrinsic Allergic Alveolitis. A posteroanterior chest radiograph *(A)* demonstrates poorly defined small nodular opacities throughout both lungs (better visualized on the magnified view of the right lung *[B]*). The patient was a 47-year-old woman who had subacute farmer's lung.

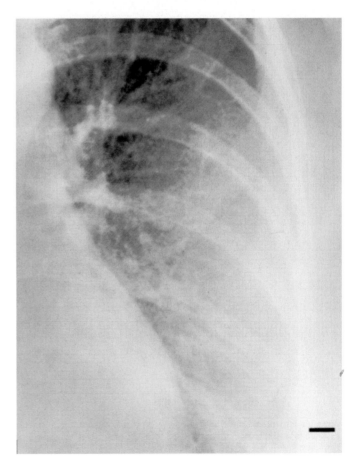

Figure 59–7. Extrinsic Allergic Alveolitis (Farmer's Lung). A detail view of the left lung from a posteroanterior chest radiograph *(A)* reveals a ground-glass opacity that shows considerable lower zonal predominance. Identical features were seen in the right lung. The bar represents 1 cm. The patient was a young woman who presented with progressive dyspnea following an unusually heavy exposure to moldy hay.

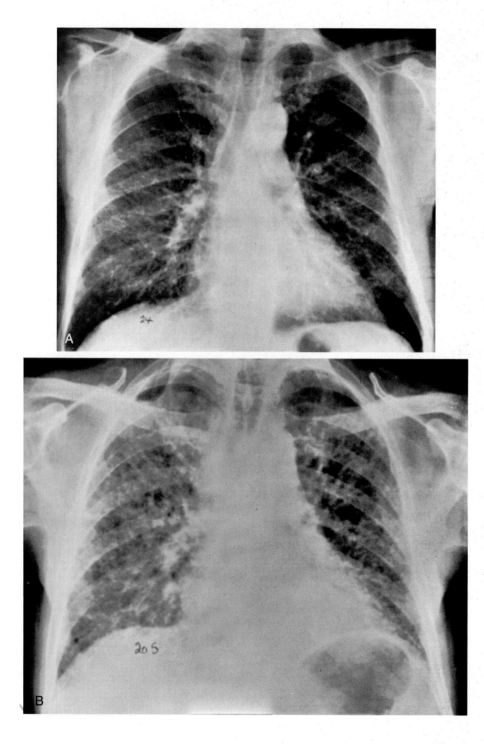

Figure 59–8. Extrinsic Allergic Alveolitis (Bird-Fancier's Lung). One year before the radiograph illustrated in *A*, this 61-year-old man acquired a budgerigar with which he spent a good deal of time. Shortly before this radiograph, he had noted the onset of shortness of breath on exertion. The radiograph revealed a diffuse, coarse, reticular pattern indicative of interstitial disease, compatible with a diagnosis of bird-fancier's lung. Approximately 1½ years later, by which time the patient was severely dyspneic at rest, the radiograph *(B)* showed severe loss of volume of both lungs and a marked worsening of the diffuse interstitial disease. In some areas, the pattern is honeycomb in type. A marked loss of volume has occurred in the 1½-year interval as a result of fibrosis. The patient's serum was positive for budgerigar precipitins.

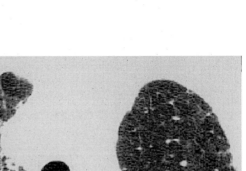

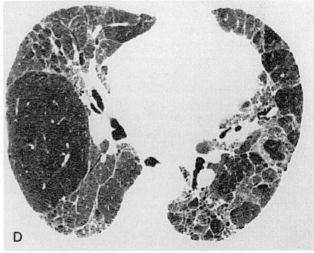

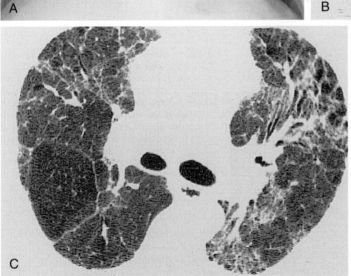

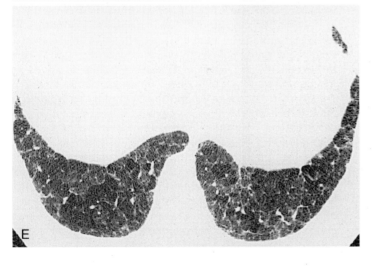

Figure 59–9. Chronic Extrinsic Allergic Alveolitis (EAA).
A posteroanterior chest radiograph *(A)* demonstrates irregular linear opacities involving mainly the middle lung zones. Lung volumes are decreased. High-resolution CT (1-mm collimation) at the level of the aortic arch *(B)* shows mild fibrosis. Much more extensive fibrosis is present at the level of the bronchus intermedius *(C)* and the right middle lobe bronchus *(D)*. The fibrosis has a random distribution in the transverse plane and is characterized by the presence of irregular lines of attenuation and distortion of the lung architecture. Mild honeycombing is evident in the posterior basal segments of the lower lobes. HRCT through the lung bases *(E)* shows relative sparing. This distribution of disease is characteristic of chronic EAA. The diagnosis was proved by open lung biopsy.

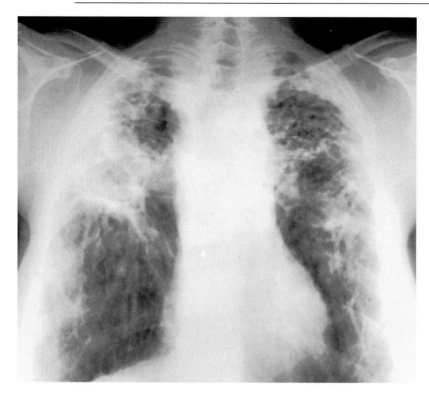

Figure 59–10. Extrinsic Allergic Alveolitis (Bird-Fancier's Lung). A posteroanterior chest radiograph in a 61-year-old woman shows coarse reticulation with marked upper and midzonal predominance. Emphysematous changes are present in the lower lobes. The patient had a long history of exposure to household birds.

opsy-proven disease and normal chest radiographs (Fig. 59–11).[113, 115, 122] For example, in one study of 21 patients who had subacute disease and abnormal HRCT scans, 7 (33%) had normal chest radiographs.[113] However, the sensitivity of HRCT is not 100%,[106] as exemplified by a study of swimming pool employees in which the diagnosis of EAA was based on two or more work-related signs or symptoms, abnormal results on transbronchial biopsies, or abnormal lymphocytosis in BAL fluid[115]—only 1 of 11 subjects (9%) had abnormal findings on the chest radiograph, whereas 5 (45%) had abnormal HRCT findings. (Note, however, that the HRCT scans in this study were performed at 4-cm slice intervals; because optimal assessment of infiltrative lung disease requires scans at 1-cm intervals, mild localized abnormalities might have been missed.) The improved visualization of parenchymal abnormalities on HRCT in the appropriate clinical context may allow confident diagnosis in patients who have normal or questionable abnormalities on chest radiograph. For example, in one study of 208 patients with various chronic interstitial lung diseases, including 13 who had subacute or chronic disease, a confident correct diagnosis of EAA was made on a combination of clinical and radiographic findings in 6 and on a combination of clinical, radiographic, and HRCT findings in 10.[111]

The HRCT findings of acute EAA consist of bilateral areas of consolidation superimposed on small centrilobular nodular opacities.[105, 122] The consolidation may be diffuse or involve mainly the lower lung zones. The findings in subacute EAA consist most often of diffuse bilateral areas of ground-glass attenuation (*see* Fig. 59–11), centrilobular nodular opacities (Fig. 59–12), or both.[105, 106, 113, 115] In one review of 15 patients who had subacute disease, diffuse ground-glass attenuation was present in 11 (73%) and centrilobular nodular opacities in 6 (40%).[106] In another review of 21 patients who had subacute bird-breeder's EAA, the most

common finding (seen in 16 patients [76%]) was the presence of centrilobular nodules.[113] In this study, 11 of the patients (52%) had bilateral areas of ground-glass attenuation. Although the areas of ground-glass attenuation and the centrilobular opacities are usually diffuse, they are often most marked in the middle and lower lung zones.[106] Another frequent finding in patients who have subacute EAA is a pattern of mosaic attenuation caused by areas of ground-glass attenuation and focal areas of air-trapping[123] (Fig. 59–13). In one review of 22 patients, this was found in 19 (86%). Such areas frequently have a striking lobular distribution and are associated with evidence of air-trapping on expiratory HRCT scans. Their extent correlates with an increase in RV and RV-to-TLC ratio.[123]

The chronic stage of EAA is manifested on HRCT by evidence of fibrosis, frequently associated with features of subacute disease.[105, 113, 120] In one review of the HRCT scans in 16 patients, the areas of fibrosis were characterized by the presence of irregular linear opacities and architectural distortion.[120] The irregular lines had a random distribution in the transverse plane in 44% of patients, were predominantly subpleural in 37%, and were peribronchovascular in 19%. Honeycombing was identified in 11 (69%) patients. In 44% of patients, the irregular linear opacities and honeycombing involved mainly the middle lung zones (*see* Fig. 59–9), and in 38% they were distributed evenly throughout the three lung zones. Upper lobe predominance was only present in 1 of the 16 patients (6%). Extensive areas of ground-glass attenuation and small centrilobular opacities were also present in 15 (94%) and 10 (62%) patients, respectively; these abnormalities were again present mainly in the middle and lower lung zones.

In the appropriate clinical context, the HRCT findings in EAA are characteristic enough to be highly suggestive of the diagnosis.[111] However, similar HRCT abnormalities may

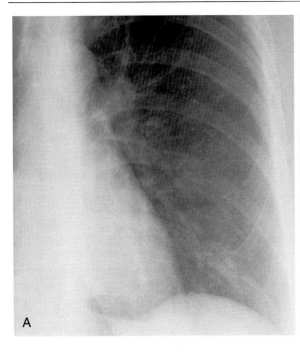

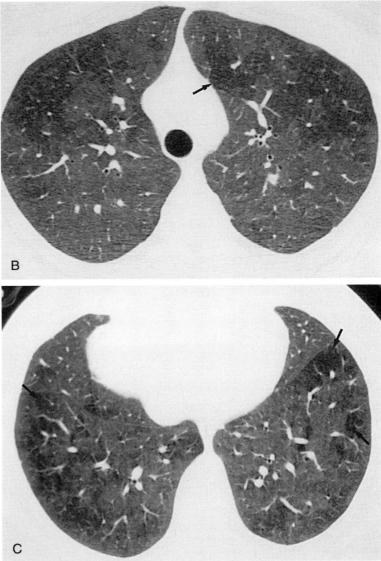

Figure 59–11. Subacute Extrinsic Allergic Alveolitis (EAA). A 42-year-old woman presented with progressive shortness of breath over several months. Chest radiographs before admission and at admission were interpreted as normal. Even in retrospect it is difficult to appreciate the mild hazy increased opacity on the magnified view of the left lung from the admission chest radiograph *(A)*. HRCT scans *(B* and *C)* demonstrate extensive areas of ground-glass attenuation and focal areas of low attenuation and decreased perfusion *(arrows)*. The findings are most suggestive of subacute EAA. The diagnosis was proved by open lung biopsy.

be seen in other interstitial lung diseases. In clinical practice, the main alternative diagnostic considerations are IPF and desquamative interstitial pneumonitis (DIP). The accuracy of HRCT in differential diagnosis was assessed in a study of 33 patients who had IPF, 3 who had DIP, and 27 who had EAA.[121] In all patients, the diagnosis was proved by open-lung biopsy. In 19 of the patients who had EAA, the disease was chronic (symptoms lasting more than 1 year); 8 had acute or subacute symptoms. The HRCT findings in subacute EAA—particularly the presence and distribution of areas of ground-glass attenuation—were often indistinguishable from those of DIP. In 8 of 19 patients who had chronic EAA (42%), the fibrosis involved mainly the lower lung zones, compared with 27 of 33 patients (81%) who had IPF. In 26% of patients who had chronic EAA, the fibrosis had no zonal predominance, whereas in 16% it involved mainly the upper zones, and in another 16% mainly the middle lung zones. In comparison, the fibrosis showed no zonal predominance in 9% of patients who had IPF and involved mainly the middle lung zones in 6%. Thus, although there is an overlap of the distribution of fibrosis in patients who

have chronic EAA and IPF, the two conditions can often be distinguished by the relative sparing of the lower half of the lower lung zone, the lack of peripheral predominance of the fibrosis, and the frequent presence of centrilobular nodules in EAA. These findings permitted a high level of confidence in diagnosis in 39 (62%) patients; in these, the diagnosis was correct in 23 of 26 patients who had IPF and in 12 of 13 patients who had EAA. The authors concluded that CT allows distinction of EAA from IPF in most cases; however, subacute EAA may resemble DIP, and chronic EAA may resemble IPF.[121]

Clinical Manifestations

As more cases of EAA are reported, involving an ever-increasing variety of organic antigens, it has become clear that the diagnosis must be based primarily on the clinical history and that meticulous inquiry may be required to uncover an exposure coincident with the development of acute respiratory symptoms. A history of exposure to any organic dust, either animal or vegetable, of small enough size and in

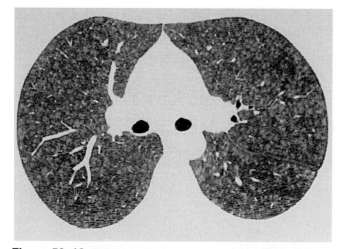

Figure 59–12. Subacute Extrinsic Allergic Alveolitis. HRCT scan (1-mm collimation) demonstrates bilateral, poorly defined small nodular opacities. Note that these are a few millimeters away from the pleura, including interlobar fissures, and a few millimeters away from major vessels, a characteristic distribution of centrilobular nodules. The patient had proven subacute bird fancier's lung.

sufficient concentration should lead to consideration of the diagnosis. In our experience, a history of recurrent "colds" or fever in the context of interstitial lung disease should raise suspicion of the abnormality. Episodic symptoms may occur in the absence of demonstrable abnormalities on the chest radiograph, which has been found to be normal in as many as 20% of patients who have farmer's lung,[36] including those who have dramatic symptoms.[124] Clearly, the most important first step in diagnosis is to think of its possibility, thereby avoiding the attribution of the clinical findings to infection. Careful inquiry about exposure to potential offending antigens should follow. If the clinical picture appears compatible with EAA, it is important to continue to consider the diagnosis, even when there is no obvious exposure to an offending antigen.

Intermittent exposure of susceptible individuals to a high concentration of antigen is accompanied by recurrent episodes of fever, chills, dry cough, and dyspnea, whereas continuous exposure to a lower concentration characteristically results in gradually progressive dyspnea in the absence of systemic symptoms.[19, 66, 125, 126] For example, pigeon breeders who intermittently visit coops outside the home usually suffer acute symptoms 4 to 6 hours after exposure to the offending birds,[92] whereas budgerigar fanciers, whose exposure to antigen in the home tends to be continuous and in low concentrations, develop the insidious form of the disease.[127]

The diagnosis of farmer's lung is easily made when a patient presents with a history of recurrent systemic and respiratory symptoms that appear several hours after he or she has entered a barn containing moldy hay. In many cases, however, patients may experience no more than slowly increasing dyspnea, cough, and weight loss, which they may attribute in part to cigarette smoking; in such circumstances, they may delay seeking medical advice until the disease has progressed to irreversible fibrosis.[125, 128]

Clinical evidence specifically suggestive of airway disease may also be present in patients who have acute EAA. In a small number of patients, usually those who have a history of allergy, the presentation is confounded by clinical features consistent with asthma;[19, 129] in these individuals, an acute asthmatic episode develops within a few minutes of exposure, subsides slowly, and may be repeated as a "late" response some 4 to 6 hours after the initial episode of bronchospasm.[130] Clinical features of chronic bronchitis are not uncommon in nonsmoking bird fanciers, being found in 30% in one study[131] and 15% in another.[18] Although the abnormality was much more common in patients who also had typical symptoms of EAA, it was the only finding in 8%; however, it was not determined whether this prevalence was greater than that in a suitable control population. The prevalence of chronic bronchitis increases as the serum antibody level rises,[18, 131, 132] perhaps indicating a link with

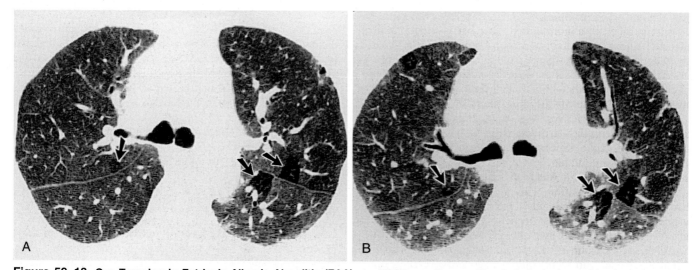

Figure 59–13. Gas Trapping in Extrinsic Allergic Alveolitis (EAA). An HRCT scan (1-mm collimation) obtained at end inspiration *(A)* shows bilateral areas of ground-glass attenuation. Focal areas of low attenuation and decreased vascularity are evident in both right and left lungs *(arrows)*. A scan obtained at end expiration *(B)* demonstrates expected loss of volume and increased attenuation of both lungs. However, note that the focal areas of decreased attenuation have not changed in volume *(arrows)*, a characteristic finding of gas trapping. The patient had open lung biopsy–proven subacute EAA superimposed on chronic EAA (bird-breeder's lung).

greater exposure. In one study of 5,703 French farmers, a strong positive relationship was found between the typical syndrome of farmer's lung and chronic bronchitis.[133] On the basis of these observations, it appears reasonable to consider chronic cough and sputum production as clinical features of recurrent or chronic EAA; despite this, bronchitis related to dust exposure may occur in the absence of EAA.

No physical findings are specific for the diagnosis of EAA. Auscultatory examination of the chest may or may not reveal crackles[134] or a peculiar inspiratory "squawk,"[135] findings that have been attributed to the opening up of airways of various sizes. These are common to many pulmonary interstitial and bronchiolar diseases. In one study, crackles persisted in patients who continued to be exposed to antigen but disappeared in those in whom exposure ceased.[136] Clubbing is common in chronic (fibrotic) disease.[66]

For all intents and purposes, EAA is a disease that is confined to the lungs, a characteristic that aids in distinguishing it from interstitial lung diseases associated with systemic manifestations. However, a possible relationship has been noted between EAA and celiac disease.[137, 138] In a study of 14 patients who had bird-fancier's lung and had jejunal biopsies performed because of symptoms and results of special investigations that suggested malabsorption, villous atrophy was found in 5.[139] In a second study of 18 biopsy-proven cases of celiac disease, however, there was no evidence of interstitial lung disease by either chest radiography or pulmonary function tests.[140]

Pulmonary Function Tests

Pulmonary function tests are useful in the assessment of functional impairment in the naturally occurring disease and in the determination of the response to antigen challenge. The overall pattern is restrictive, with a slight to moderate reduction in FEV_1 that is proportional to the decrease in vital capacity. Both static compliance and diffusing capacity are frequently reduced, reflecting the interstitial thickening seen histologically.[114, 141–143] In addition, at least some patients have evidence of small airway obstruction as reflected by the finding of air-trapping[144] and decreased midexpiratory flow rates.[3] These abnormalities have been documented in affected pigeon breeders[145] and would presumably be present in patients who have other variants of EAA if looked for assiduously enough. After acute exposure, measurements should be carried out within 4 to 8 hours because function may return to normal by 12 to 14 hours.[142]

Although restrictive lung function is the most commonly described long-term outcome in patients who have chronic EAA, some patients develop airflow obstruction. In fact, in one remarkable investigation of 33 nonsmoking farmers who had lung function studies performed 6 years after an initial evaluation, 13 had an obstructive profile, 1 had restrictive change, 3 had isolated reductions in diffusing capacity, and 13 had normal tests;[2] 9 of the patients who had airflow obstruction had evidence of emphysema on HRCT. Similarly, in a group of 22 nonsmoking patients who had avian EAA and who were followed sequentially, lung function became normal in 13;[146] however, a restrictive pattern was seen in 7 (32%) and an obstructive pattern in 4 (18%). In another study of 88 patients who had farmer's lung and 83 control farmers, emphysema was found in 23% of the

former and only 7% of the latter.[95] Among the patients who had farmer's lung, emphysema was seen in 18% of the nonsmokers and 44% of the smokers; corresponding figures for the control individuals were 4% and 20%.

Laboratory Findings and Diagnosis

Generally speaking, laboratory tests are not particularly useful in establishing a diagnosis of EAA. Neutrophilia with a shift to the left may be seen in acute disease or after antigen provocation testing; eosinophilia is rare. Serum angiotensin-converting enzyme levels have been found to be normal in studies of patients who had farmer's[147] and pigeon-breeder's lung.[148] In one survey, levels of both lysozyme and angiotensin-converting enzyme were higher in patients who had a history of farmer's lung than in healthy farmers and controls, although the levels showed considerable overlap.[149] Some investigators have suggested that enhanced clearance of technetium 99m–DTPA is a more sensitive early EAA marker than abnormalities of lung function;[150] however, the clinical relevance of this finding remains to be determined.

Although the presence of serum precipitins serves as a marker of exposure to a specific antigen, serologic testing generally lacks sufficient specificity to be of diagnostic value.[6, 66] For the same reasons, as well as the lack of reliable commercially available antigen, skin testing is also not useful in diagnosis.[3, 61]

The clinical and radiologic features often suggest the diagnosis of EAA when they develop in the context of a recognized sensitizing exposure. Improvement after avoidance of the offending antigen strengthens the diagnostic presumption. Although the precise role of various biopsy procedures has not been well defined, biopsy may be indicated when the clinical diagnosis seems uncertain, especially when other diseases requiring different therapy are considered.[6, 66] In acute EAA, the differential diagnosis includes organic toxic dust syndrome and viral and other forms of "atypical" pneumonia; the differential diagnosis in chronic disease includes sarcoidosis, IPF, and other forms of interstitial lung disease. Transbronchial biopsy may yield specimens that are interpreted as compatible with EAA. In an appropriate context, we and others think that this finding is sufficient for confirmation of the diagnosis.[151, 152] When results of transbronchial biopsy are nonspecific, or when suggestive results are discrepant with other clinical observations, open-lung biopsy may be indicated. The latter is usually definitive in making the diagnosis, although distinction from acute fungal disease may require a careful search for organisms.[6] Provocational challenge with specific antigens has been useful in confirming the diagnosis of some variants, such as bird-fancier's lung;[162] however, sensitivity and specificity are only about 80%.

Prognosis and Natural History

The prognosis is good for patients whose disease is recognized at an early stage and who are removed from exposure to antigen. In the more insidious cases in which the disease is not initially recognized, considerable fibrosis and a variable degree of pulmonary insufficiency can develop before the cause is detected. In one long-term follow-up of 101 patients who had farmer's lung, the FVC improved over the first year, and the Dco continued to improve over a 2-year period;[153] the PaO_2 improved over the first month and remained stable thereafter. Persistent exposure to antigen in a small group of pigeon breeders who had recurrent attacks of EAA resulted in an accelerated decline in lung function compared with those whose exposure had ceased.[154] In a study of 22 pigeon breeders, complete recovery of normal lung function or significant improvement occurred in all those who were exposed for less than 2 years before withdrawal from exposure, whereas only 6 of 10 patients who had longer exposures had this outcome.[146] In a national survey of bird fanciers in Britain, the restrictive ventilatory defects tended to diminish after avian withdrawal only in patients younger than 45 years of age whose symptoms had been present for less than 2 years.[56] In a study of 92 patients who had farmer's lung followed for a mean of about 15 years (range, 2.25 to 40 years), 36 (39%) were found to have radiographic evidence of interstitial disease and 39 (42%) to have a PaO_2 of less than 70 mm Hg;[155] 10 of 59 nonsmokers had FEV_1-to-FVC ratios below 70%. Farmers with a history of five or more symptomatic recurrences had the worst function, and the authors concluded that such patients should leave the farm for good.

In another survey of 86 patients who had farmer's lung and were followed for a period of 5 years, most of the clinical improvement occurred during the first month, and little occurred after 6 months.[156] After 5 years, 65% of patients still had respiratory symptoms, 40% had impaired pulmonary function, and 32% showed persistent diffuse radiographic opacities. Similar findings have been reported by other investigators.[157] With regard to prognosis, it did not appear to make much difference in either study whether patients left or continued working on the farm (presumably while limiting further exposure). In summary, a better outcome is associated with early disease and antigen avoidance after diagnosis; chronic symptoms before diagnosis and persistent exposure lead to progressive decline in lung function.

The overall mortality in patients who have EAA appears to be low. In one investigation of Finnish farmers, only 0.7% died of the disease between 1980 and 1990;[158] most deaths occurred in patients who had chronic symptoms and radiographic abnormalities. On the other hand, mortality in a group of Mexican patients who had chronic pigeon breeder's disease was similar to that of patients who had IPF, when correction was made for the degree of fibrosis at presentation.[159] These very different prognoses can be understood by recognizing the differences in presentation of the Finnish and Mexican patients: most of the former had episodic EAA, whereas most of the latter had a clinical course of indolently progressive breathlessness associated with radiographic manifestations and functional indices of fibrotic lung disease.[158, 159]

Specific Forms of Allergic Alveolitis

Farmer's Lung

Farmer's lung is the earliest described and most thoroughly investigated of the many forms of EAA. In Japan, it has been shown to be one of the more common variants,[160] an observation that likely holds true for other countries.

Although it may have been recognized for centuries, the earliest clear description in English is generally accredited to Campbell in 1932.[161] Many of the early reports originated in Great Britain and Scandinavia, the disease being known by names such as thresher's lung, harvester's lung, bronchomycosis feniseciorum (mycosis of hay-makers or harvesters), and Norwegian hemp disease.

Original descriptions reflected the type of patient who is likely to be seen in a large medical center;[94] however, other more recent studies have shown that many farmers have the clinical syndrome without exhibiting all the immunologic and radiologic manifestations commonly associated with the disease.[163–165] For example, in one investigation of 471 farmers from Wyoming, 14 (4%) were considered likely to have EAA;[165] only three of these had a reticulonodular pattern radiographically, and only two had precipitating antibodies to *M. faeni* in their serum. In a group of 77 farmers with probable farmer's lung culled from a larger group of 1,763 active farmers, about 22% had crackles on physical examination, 10% had restrictive lung function, and only 9% had radiographic abnormalities.[166] Only two of 381 farmers from Northern Ireland had a combination of antibody to *M. faeni*, delayed onset of symptoms after exposure, and restrictive lung function, in contrast to 5% who had the diagnosis previously made by a physician and 10% who recounted a typical history. The prevalence of the syndrome among farmers in different communities has ranged from less than 1%[164] to 10%.[55, 163, 165, 167, 168] It is difficult to reconcile these data; however, it is likely that estimates of the prevalence of farmer's lung that are based solely on the patients' symptoms or on incomplete evaluation are exaggerated.

Some investigators have found that about 90% of patients who have farmer's lung have precipitating antibodies to thermophilic actinomycetes (85% to 90% to *M. faeni*).[19, 125] Others have found positive precipitins to actinomycete species in about 50% of patients who have chronic disease and in as many as 100% of those who have acute disease.[94, 163, 164, 169, 170] In fact, a significant number of patients have serum precipitins to thermophilic actinomycetes other than *M. faeni*, and it has been recommended that screening material for serologic testing should include antigens from the following thermophilic organisms:[171] *M. faeni* and *Thermoactinomyces vulgaris* (three strains), *Thermoactinomyces viridis*, *Thermoactinomyces sacchari*, *Thermoactinomyces candidus*, *Thermoactinomyces lisko*, and *Thermoactinomyces koski*. Some patients also appear to react to fungi (most commonly *Aspergillus fumigatus*[164, 165, 172–174] and, rarely, other organisms, such as *Candida albicans*[175]). Immunofluorescent studies of lung biopsy specimens of patients who have acute farmer's lung have revealed antibodies to thermophilic actinomycetes in bronchiolar walls and alveolar septa;[89, 176] this finding has been absent in patients with chronic disease.[176]

Farmer's lung typically affects men between 40 and 50 years of age and has a peak incidence during the season when stored hay is used for feeding cattle. The clinical picture varies according to the degree of exposure to antigens in the moldy hay and to the degree of sensitivity of the farmer. The classic acute-onset type of disease occurs in perhaps no more than a third of cases.[125] More commonly, patients complain of gradual progression of dyspnea, cough, and weight loss, accompanied by fever, chills, malaise, and aches and pains.[125, 128, 164] A number of other occupation-related diseases (including asthma, organic dust toxic inhalation syndrome [see page 2379], and chronic bronchitis) also occur in farmers; because these can cause some of the symptoms of EAA, clinical confusion may ensue. In addition to the usual history of the disease occurring in farmers exposed to moldy hay, there have been reports of EAA associated with the handling of moldy lichen[177] and with exposure to the gram-negative bacterium *Erwinia herbicola* in grain workers.[178]

As discussed previously, the prognosis is not clearly linked to a decision to leave the farm. In fact, patients who are careful to prevent recurrent attacks appear to do as well as those farmers who avoid all exposure.[36] Interestingly, patients who choose to quit farming have derangements of pulmonary function very similar to those who continue the occupation; one group of investigators found the decision to quit is based more on the farmer's perception of his ability to continue farming rather than the degree of objectively determined disability.[179] Elevated levels of two markers of collagen synthesis—galactosylhydroxylysyl glucosyltransferase and procollagen type III amino-terminal propeptide—have been found in BAL fluid of some affected patients[180, 181] and have been correlated with irreversible pulmonary impairment.[181]

Bird-Fancier's Lung

Bird-fancier's lung was originally described in a breeder of parakeets and is commonly associated with budgerigars and pigeons; as a result, it has often been termed *pigeon-breeder's lung*. However, because it has also been shown to occur in people coming in contact with many other species, including parrots, hens, ducks, turkeys, geese, and even wild birds such as owls or Moluccan cockatoos,[183, 184] the all-inclusive term *bird-fancier's lung* is now favored.

The prevalence in specific settings varies considerably. For example, although well-documented cases have been reported following exposure to chickens and turkeys,[107, 185–188] surveys of poultry workers have indicated that this occupation is not especially hazardous;[188] in fact, two groups failed to uncover a single case.[58, 189] These observations may be related to the finding that antibodies to avian antigens in poultry workers are not elevated to the same degree as has been reported in pigeon breeders.[118, 190] Although well-documented cases of disease have been described only rarely in canary fanciers,[191] this variety may be more common than is generally recognized because specific antibodies cannot be detected with the standard avian antigens, which contain only sera from pigeons, budgerigars, and hens.

The antigen responsible for the disease in pigeon breeders consists of protein contained in bird serum that is secreted into the lumen of the gut, excreted, and inhaled from droppings.[182, 192] In one study of pigeon fanciers, there was a positive correlation between antibody level and active disease, acute episodes occurring during the late summer months corresponding to the period of maximal avian contact in the sporting season.[193] An association between disease activity and IgG3[194] and IgG1[182] antibodies to pigeon intestinal mucin has been found by some investigators.

Most patients give a history of direct contact with birds; however, second-hand exposure has occasionally been implicated. For example, two cases have been described in wives of pigeon breeders, one of whom was exposed only to her husband's coveralls.[92] Moreover, even after removal of birds from the home environment, antigen can persist at a significant level for a prolonged period, despite apparently adequate cleaning.[195] In one patient, it was apparently caused by exposure to a feather wreath[196] and in another to goose feathers in a duvet.[227]

Histologically, numerous foamy macrophages in both intra-alveolar and interstitial locations have been identified in several cases of bird-fancier's lung.[87, 88] Although this finding has been said to be characteristic of this variety of disease, the extent to which it is simply a manifestation of obstructive pneumonitis secondary to bronchiolitis is not clear.

Many patients appear reluctant to abandon their hobby, and despite their efforts to reduce exposure, antibody titers remain high. The clinical course in these patients may be benign; however, some have loss of lung function and persisting troubling symptoms.[197] When disease is chronic and associated with fibrotic lung disease, mortality can be significant; for example, in a group of 78 such patients from Mexico, the 5-year survival rate was only 71%.[159]

Mushroom-Worker's Lung

The specific agents responsible for this form of disease are usually the same as those in farmer's lung (i.e., *M. faeni* and *Micromonospora vulgaris*);[109, 198–200] however, a variety of other related organisms have also been implicated.[201] In addition, there are a number of reports of EAA implicating the spores of the mushroom species *Pholiota nameko* in Japan[202–204] and *Pleurotos ostreatus* (in workers involved in the production of oyster mushrooms).[205]

The culture of mushrooms requires a process of steam pasteurization to destroy microorganisms; temperatures during this process rise to 60° C at 100% humidity, which encourages the rapid growth of thermophilic actinomycetes. Subsequently, the compost is spread on trays and mixed with mushroom mycelia grown on manure and grain. This process, which is called spawning, gives rise to clouds of dust that may be inhaled by unprotected workers. The clinical and immunologic features of the ensuing disease are similar to those of farmer's lung. Although radiographically visible hilar lymph node enlargement has been said to be common,[108] no enlargement was seen in one study of 26 patients.[109]

Bagassosis

Bagasse is a fibrous material composed almost entirely of cellulose and other complex plant carbohydrates that remains after the sugar-containing juice has been extracted from sugar cane. It has a wide variety of uses, including the production of charcoal, animal food, particleboard and fiberboard, lacquerware, and paper;[206, 207] EAA can be seen in workers in any of these industries. The disease occurs as a result of inhaling bagasse fibers contaminated by the microorganism *T. sacchari*;[208, 209] in one study of 22 patients judged on clinical grounds to have the disease, 14 possessed serum precipitins to this organism.[210] It is more likely to occur as a result of exposure to freshly produced bagasse or bagasse fibers stored indoors than to moldy bagasse stored outside.[211]

A curious feature of this disease noted by some patients is an aversion to cigarette smoking.[212] Pathologic characteristics have been described in several patients;[76, 213] particulate matter resembling bagasse fibers can be identified on histologic examination in some cases.[76]

Building-Associated Extrinsic Allergic Alveolitis

The comprehensive term *building-associated EAA* is used to include all cases of EAA caused by antigenic material contained in human habitations, usually within contaminated equipment used to heat, humidify, or cool air,[214–218] and sometimes on damp floors or walls.[219, 220] In most cases, the causative agents are thermophilic actinomycetes[176, 215, 221] and *Penicillium* species;[215, 219, 220, 222] thermotolerant bacteria (rod-shaped bacilli resembling *Bacillus cereus*),[223] *Cladosporium* (from an enclosed hot-tub room and ultrasonic humidifier),[217, 224] amebae,[225, 226] and other fungi[218] have also been incriminated.

Because the disease is acquired in the office or home, it may be difficult to diagnose, particularly if the clinical presentation is insidious rather than intermittent and acute. Supporting evidence for the diagnosis may be provided by the demonstration of serum precipitins, abnormal chest radiographs or CT scans, the presence of appropriate pulmonary function test abnormalities, and positive results from histologic studies. However, it may be necessary to confirm the diagnosis by demonstrating pulmonary function abnormalities after inhalation challenge with the suspected antigen or clinical remission coincidental to removal of the patient from the site of suspected contamination.

Japanese Summer-Type Extrinsic Allergic Alveolitis

Summer-type EAA is the most common form of EAA seen in Japan; of 835 cases of the disease reported in one series, 621 (almost 75%) were of this type.[228] The disorder occurs in the summer months and subsides spontaneously in midautumn, only to reappear in sensitized patients the following summer. Several reports indicate that the causative agent is *Trichosporon cutaneum*, an arthrospore-forming yeast that belongs to the same family of *Cryptococcaceae* as *Cryptococcus neoformans* and *C. albicans*.[228–230] High levels of specific IgA and secretory IgA antibodies are found in both serum and BAL fluid of affected patients.[231] Although most cases are seen in the home, one patient apparently became sensitized to *T. cutaneum* while working at a plant growing the mushroom *P. nameko*.[232]

Malt-Worker's Lung

Heavy exposure to the fungus *Aspergillus clavatus* has been shown to result in the typical clinical picture of EAA in a small percentage of malt workers.[21, 233] A survey of 711 of these workers in Scotland revealed a clinical history compatible with the disease in 37 (about 5%);[22] 30 (81%) of these had antibodies to *A. clavatus* mycelial antigens in their sera, compared with only 11% of symptom-free malt workers. In this study, there was no serologic evidence to implicate actinomycetes or fungi other than *A. clavatus* in the production of pulmonary disease. As with other variations of EAA, precipitating antibodies may be present in the serum in the absence of symptoms of the disease.[21]

Maple Bark–Worker's Lung

Maple bark–worker's lung is a rare disease that was originally described in 36 sawmill workers.[234] The responsible antigen appears to be the spore of the fungus *Cryptostroma corticale* (*Coniosporium corticale*), which resides deep in the bark of the maple tree. Spores have been identified in lung biopsy specimens, and precipitating antibodies have been found in patients' sera.[75, 235, 236]

Pituitary Snuff–Taker's Lung

Powdered extract of pig or ox pituitary glands was formerly administered by nasal insufflation in the treatment of diabetes insipidus; several cases of lung disease consistent with EAA resulting from this treatment have been reported.[237–239] In one of these, the responsible antigenic material was identified as the hormone constituents of the pituitary rather than species-specific antigens of the animal from which the pituitary originated.[239]

Suberosis

Suberosis is a variant of EAA that occurs in cork workers and has been reported mostly from Portugal.[77, 240, 241] The serum of affected patients contains a high level of precipitins to moldy cork dust, but not to extracts of clean cork dust.[240] *Penicillium frequentans* has been implicated as the likely antigenic source.[241]

Isocyanate-Associated Extrinsic Allergic Alveolitis

Isocyantes are molecules used commercially to polymerize polyhydroxyl and polyglycol compounds to form polyurethanes. They also react with water to produce carbon dioxide, a process exploited in the production of flexible polyurethane foam. Their application is widespread and includes the manufacturing of flexible and rigid polyurethane foam, the application of two-part polyurethane paints by brush or spray painting, and in flexible packaging, in which they are used in inks and laminating adhesives.[242] Although these agents are not organic dusts, the pneumonitis they cause is identical clinically, radiologically, and pathologically to that of the organic dust–related EAA.

Isolated case reports of EAA had been reported since the early 1970s after exposure to diphenylmethane di-isocyanate (MDI),[243, 244] toluene di-isocyanate (TDI),[244a, b] and hexamethylene di-isocyanate (HDI).[244c, d] Interstitial pneumonitis similar to that seen in EAA has also been produced in experimental animals.[245] Diagnostic criteria include the presence of fever and dyspnea several hours after beginning work with the chemical, neutrophilia, restrictive lung function, a reticular or reticulonodular pattern on chest radiography, the presence of antibodies to albumen–isocyanate conjugates, lymphocytosis in BAL fluid, and compatible pathology.[246, 247] Careful evaluation of exposed workers revealed a response consistent with EAA in 8 (4.7%) of 167 workers exposed to MDI in one series[246] and in about 1% of 1,780 workers exposed to a variety of isocyanates, mainly MDI, in a second.[247]

Detergent-Worker's Lung

Detergent-worker's lung is presumed to be caused by a hypersensitivity reaction to *Bacillus subtilis*, a spore-forming organism that produces large quantities of proteolytic enzyme used in the manufacture of detergent products. The development of sensitization is well recognized in the industry. There is also an account of an entire family becoming sensitized following exposure in their home to wood dust contaminated by *B. subtilis*; confirmation of the cause was obtained by provocation challenge testing.[248] Depite the evidence implicating *B. subtilis*, immunodiffusion studies have failed to demonstrate specific precipitins to extracts of the organism.[249–251]

Cases have been reported in which a diffuse, transient reticulonodular pattern developed on the chest radiograph.[252, 253] Both restrictive and obstructive patterns have been described on lung function testing,[254] the former associated with a reduction in diffusing capacity. Follow-up of exposed workers has been associated with persistence of impaired function in one survey[255] but with no residual functional abnormalities in another.[256]

SWINE CONFINEMENT AND THE LUNG

About 700,000 Americans are exposed to livestock and poultry in confined areas. Swine-confinement workers account for the largest group of exposed individuals who have frequent and severe health problems,[257] nearly 70% experiencing one or more respiratory symptoms. A variety of disorders can result from exposure to the "organic soup" of the swine confinement areas, including bronchitis, asthma, organic dust toxic syndrome (*see* farther on), chronic sinusitis, and hydrogen sulfide intoxication.[257]

Workers are exposed to high concentrations of many organic dusts (including molds, pollens, swine hair, animal foods, corn flour, grain mites, and aerosolized fecal matter), endotoxin, hydrogen sulfide, methane, carbon dioxide, carbon monoxide, ammonia, various microorganisms, and a wide variety of volatile compounds produced by anaerobic microorganisms in hog manure pits.[257–261] Which of these substances is responsible for a specific clinical disorder is not always clear. Some investigators have suggested that the total dust or ammonia levels are most closely linked to a decline in lung function,[258] whereas others have postulated that the level of endotoxin or other microbial substances in the bioaerosol is the major determinant.[259, 262, 263]

The response of a given worker to inhalation of material from a swine confinement area must depend on the precise nature of the exposure and on individual susceptibility; however, cough, sputum production, throat, nose and eye irritation, chest tightness, breathlessness, wheezing, and myalgia are each seen in at least 25% of workers.[257] Workers are more likely to be affected with increasing duration and intensity of exposure. Symptoms are also more severe and frequent among cigarette smokers and in patients who

are atopic or who have pre-existing respiratory tract disease.[257, 264] In one study, 14 nonsmoking, healthy individuals were placed in a swine-confinement building for a period of 3 to 5 hours;[265] all but one of the subjects had previously been unexposed to swine dust. In the building used for the study, dust and endotoxin levels were high, and concentrations of ammonia, carbon dioxide, and hydrogen sulfide were low. Comparison of BAL fluid obtained before and 24 hours after the exposure revealed an intense inflammatory response, consisting largely of neutrophils with a lesser number of eosinophils. When the same experiment was repeated with another group of subjects, activated T lymphocytes were also found to be increased in BAL fluid (albeit to a much lesser extent than neutrophils).[266] These observations are consistent with the observation that asthma accounts for only a small percentage of the symptoms in these workers; instead, most appear to be the result of a nonallergic inflammatory reaction.[260] However, this does not preclude an important role for allergy and asthma in specific workers.[260] Elevations in serum levels of IL-6 and tumor necrosis factor-α have also been demonstrated in a group of 14 previously unexposed individuals following swine dust exposure; it is possible that these cytokines have a role in the pathogenesis of the systemic effects.[268]

In one investigation, swine-confinement workers were found to have about a threefold increase in the prevalence of chronic bronchitis compared with a control group of nonfarming men.[268] This abnormality is associated with a small degree of chronic airflow obstruction, a development that has been correlated with the finding of a reduction in lung function over the course of a workshift in these individuals.[262] Workers also have an excess annual decline in FEV_1 and FVC compared with nonfarming individuals after controlling for age, height, smoking, and baseline lung function.[269] Symptomatic patients with[270] and without[271–273] abnormal baseline lung function are more likely to have airway hyper-responsiveness as assessed by methacholine provocation testing, compared with controls.

ORGANIC DUST TOXIC SYNDROME

Organic dust toxic syndrome (ODTS) can be defined as a febrile illness following exposure to organic dust in individuals who do not have evidence of EAA;[274] despite this, some investigators believe that the two abnormalities represent a spectrum of findings in one disease, rather than two separate entities.[275] Typically, fever and influenza-like symptoms occur 4 to 8 hours after dust exposure; symptoms of dry cough, chest tightness, mild dyspnea, and wheezing may also be present.[283] The syndrome encompasses diseases previously described by a variety of names, including humidifier fever (in office and hospital workers),[277–282] pulmonary mycotoxicosis, grain fever, pig fever, cotton fever, and woodchip fever.[274, 283, 284] (Bronchitis and asthma, both of which are common in farmers[285–288] and are the result of inhalation of a variety of organic compounds, are discussed separately on pages 2174 and 2120.)

The disorder is probably common; up to 10% of exposed farmers[274] and 35% of swine-confinement workers[257] develop the characteristic fever. In fact, it has been estimated that the disorder may be 50 times more common than EAA in farmers.[289]

The cause and pathogenesis of ODTS are obscure, and the name of the syndrome may be a misnomer; however, the findings in one animal model suggest that symptoms are the result of combined exposure to fungal organisms and endotoxin.[290] In one study of a small group of farmers, ODTS appeared to occur after exposure to extraordinarily high levels of fungal spores.[291] Some cases have been associated with evidence of bronchiolitis and release of IL-1 from alveolar macrophages.[283] In an investigation of a small group of healthy individuals, exposure to wood-chip mulch was found to be associated with the presence of proinflammatory cytokines and an increased number of neutrophils in BAL fluid.[284] Pulmonary function changes are minimal.[257, 292] In three patients who were exposed to massive amounts of dust in a silo, histologic findings in open lung biopsy specimens included acute and organizing diffuse alveolar damage (in two patients) and acute bronchopneumonia (in the other).[276]

The disorder shares some features with EAA: both frequently occur after exposure to moldy vegetable matter and improve rapidly without therapy.[274, 283] However, it is important to distinguish the two because ODTS causes no permanent impairment of lung function.

REFERENCES

1. Campbell JM: Acute symptoms following work with hay. BMJ 2:1143, 1932.
2. Lalancette M, Carrier G, Laviolette M, et al: Farmer's lung: Long-term outcome and lack of predictive value of bronchoalveolar lavage fibrosing factors. Am Rev Respir Dis 148:216, 1993.
3. Sharma OP, Fujimura N: Hypersensitivity pneumonitis: A noninfectious granulomatosis. Semin Respir Infect 10(2):96, 1995.
4. Rose C, King TE Jr: Controversies in hypersensitivity pneumonitis (editorial). Am Rev Resp Dis. 145(1):1, 1992.
5. Fink JN: Hypersensitivity pneumonitis. Clin Chest Med 13(2):303, 1992.
6. Richerson HB, Bernstein IL, Fink JN, et al: Guidelines for the clinical evaluation of hypersensitivity pneumonitis: Report of the Subcommittee on Hypersensitivity Pneumonitis. J Allergy Clin Immun 84(5 Pt 2):839, 1989.
7. Hargreave FE: Extrinsic allergic alveolitis (review article). Can Med Assoc J 108:1150, 1973.
8. Lacey J, Lacey ME: Spore concentrations in the air of farm buildings: Extrinsic allergic alveolitis. Trans Br Mycol Soc 47:547, 1964.
9. Salvaggio JE: Hypersensitivity pneumonitis: Pandora's box. N Engl J Med 283:314, 1970.
10. Salvaggio JE, Millhollon BW: Allergic alveolitis: New insights into old mysteries. Respir Med 87:495, 1993.
11. Soda K, Ando M, Sakata T, et al: C1q and C3 in bronchoalveolar lavage fluid from patients with summer-type hypersensitivity pneumonitis. Chest 93:76, 1988.
12. Reynolds SP, Edwards JH, Jones KP, et al: Immunoglobulin and antibody levels in bronchoalveolar lavage fluid from symptomatic and asymptomatic pigeon breeders. Clin Exp Immunol 86:278, 1991.
13. Wilson MR, Schuyler MR, Cashner F, et al: The effect of complement depletion on hypersensitivity pneumonitis lesions induced by *Micropolyspora faeni* antigen. Clin Allergy 11:131, 1981.
14. Cormier Y, Bélanger J: The fluctuant nature of precipitating antibodies in dairy farmers. Thorax 44:469, 1989.
15. Salvaggio J: Diagnostic significance of serum precipitins in hypersensitivity pneumonitis. Chest 62:242, 1972.
16. Hargreave FE, Pepys J: Allergic respiratory reactions in bird fanciers provoked by allergen inhalation provocation test. J Allergy Clin Immunol 50:157, 1972.
17. Fink JN, Schlueter DP, Sosman AJ, et al: Clinical survey of pigeon breeders. Chest 62:277, 1972.
18. Rodriguez de Castro F, Carrillo T, Castillo R, et al: Relationship between characteristics of exposure to pigeon antigens. Chest 103:1059, 1993.
19. Pepys J, Jenkins PA: Precipitin (FLH) test in farmer's lung. Thorax 20:21, 1965.
20. Marx JJ Jr, Gray RL: Comparison of the enzyme-linked immunosorbent assay and double immunodiffusion test for the detection and quantitation of antibodies in farmer's lung disease. J Allergy Clin Immunol 70:109, 1982.
21. Channell S, Blyth W, Lloyd M, et al: Allergic alveolitis in maltworkers: A clinical, mycological, and immunological study. Q J Med 38:351, 1969.
22. Grant IWB, Blackadder ES, Greenberg M, et al: Extrinsic allergic alveolitis in Scottish maltworkers. Br Med J 1:490, 1976.
23. Denis M, Bedard M, Laviolette M, et al: A study of monokine release and natural killer activity in the bronchoalveolar lavage of subjects with farmer's lung. Am Rev Respir Dis 147:934, 1993.
24. Dakhama A, Israel-Assayag E, Cormier Y: Altered immunosuppressive activity of alveolar macrophages in farmer's lung disease. Eur Respir J 9:1456, 1996.
25. Pesci A, Bertorelli G, Dall'Aglio PP, et al: Evidence in bronchoalveolar lavage for third type immune reactions in hypersensitivity pneumonitis. Eur Respir J 3:359, 1990.
26. Vogelmeier C, Krombach F, Münzing, et al: Activation of blood neutrophils in acute episodes of farmer's lung. Am Rev Respir Dis 148:396, 1993.
27. Tremblay GM, Sallenave J-M, Israel-Assayag E, et al: Elafin/elastase specific inhibitor in bronchoalveolar lavage of normal subjects and farmer's lung. Am J Respir Crit Care Med 154:1092, 1996.
28. Fournier E, Tonnel AB, Gosset P, et al: Early neutrophil alveolitis after antigen inhalation in hypersensitivity pneumonitis. Chest 88:563, 1985.
29. van den Bosch JM, Heye C, Wagenaar SS, et al: Bronchoalveolar lavage in extrinsic allergic alveolitis. Respiration 49:45, 1986.
30. Reynolds SP, Jones KP, Edwards JH, et al: Inhalation challenge in pigeon breeder's disease: BAL fluid changes after 6 hours. Eur Respir J 6:467, 1993.
31. Wahlstrom J, Berlin M, Lundgren R, et al: Lung and blood T-cell receptor repertoire in extrinsic allergic alveolitis. Eur Respir J 10:772, 1997.
32. Trentin L, Zambello R, Facco M, et al: Selection of T lymphocytes bearing limited TCR-Vb regions n the lung of hypersensitivity pneumonitis and sarcoidosis. Am J Respir Crit Care Med 155:587, 1997.
33. Johnson MA, Nemeth A, Condez A, et al: Cell-mediated immunity in pigeon breeders' lung: The effect of removal from antigen exposure. Eur Respir J 2:444, 1989.
34. Satake N, Nagai S, Kawatani A, et al: Density of phenotypic markers on BAL T-lymphocytes in hypersensitivity pneumonitis, pulmonary sarcoidosis and bronchiolitis obliterans with organizing pneumonia. Eur Respir J 6:477, 1993.
34a. Dakhama A, Israel-Assayag E, Cormier Y: Role of interleukin-2 in the development and persistence of lymphocytic alveolitis in farmer's lung. Eur Respir J 11:1281, 1998.
35. Denis M: Proinflammatory cytokines in hypersensitivity pneumonitis. Am J Respir Crit Care Med 151:164, 1995.
36. Cormier Y, Laviolette M: Farmer's Lung. Semin Respir Med 14:31, 1993.
37. Schuyler M, Cook C, Listrom M, et al: Blast cells transfer experimental hypersensitivity pneumonitis in guinea pigs. Am Rev Respir Dis 137:1449, 1988.
38. Richerson HB, Coon JD, Lubaroff D: Adoptive transfer of experimental hypersensitivity pneumonitis in the LEW rat. Am J Respir Crit Care Med 151:1205, 1995.
39. Schuyler M, Gott K, Edwards B, et al: Experimental hypersensitivity pneumonitis. Am J Respir Crit Care Med 149:1286, 1994.
40. Schuyler M, Gott K, Edwards B, et al: Experimental hypersensitivity pneumonitis: Effect of Thy1.2+ and CD8+ cell depletion. Am J Respir Crit Care Med 151:1834, 1995.
41. Hamagami S, Miyagawa T, Ochi T, et al: A raised level of soluble CD8 in bronchoalveolar lavage fluid in summer-type hypersensitivity pneumonitis in Japan. Chest 101:1044, 1992.
42. Denis M: Mouse hypersensitivity pneumonitis: Depletion of NK cells abrogates the spontaneous regression phase and leads to massive fibrosis. Exp Lung Res 18:761, 1992.
43. Cormier Y, Bélanger J, Laviolette M: Prognostic significance of bronchoalveolar lymphocytosis in farmer's lung. Am Rev Respir Dis 135:692, 1987.
44. Gariépy L, Cormier Y, Laviolette M, et al: Predictive value of bronchoalveolar lavage cells and serum precipitins in asymptomatic dairy farmers. Am Rev Respir Dis 140:1386, 1989.
44a. Gudmundsson G, Monick MM, Hunninghake GW: IL-12 modulates expression of hypersensitivity pneumonitis. J Immunol 161:991, 1998.
45. Pesci A, Bertorelli G, Olivieri D: Mast cells in bronchoalveolar lavage fluid and in transbronchial biopsy specimens of patients with farmer's lung disease. Chest 100:1197, 1991.
46. Haslam PL, Dewar A, Butchers P, et al: Mast cells, atypical lymphocytes and neutrophils in bronchoalveolar lavage in extrinsic allergic alveolitis. Am Rev Respir Dis 135:35, 1987.
47. Miadonna A, Pesci A, Tedeschi A, et al: Mast cell and histamine involvement in farmer's lung disease. Chest 105:1184, 1994.
48. Laviolette M, Cormier Y, Loiseau A, et al: Bronchoalveolar mast cells in normal farmers and subjects with farmer's lung. Am Rev Respir Dis 144:855, 1991.
49. Drent M, van Velzen-Blad H, Diamant M, et al: Differential diagnostic value of plasma cells in bronchoalveolar lavage fluid. Chest 103:1720, 1993.
50. Hamm H, Lührs J, Guzman y Rotaeche J, et al: Elevated surfactant protein A in bronchoalveolar lavage fluids from sarcoidosis and hypersensitivity pneumonitis patients. Chest 106:1766, 1994.
51. Lesur O, Mancinin NM, Janot C, et al: Loss of lymphocyte modulatory control by surfactant lipid extracts from acute hypersensitivity pneumonitis: Comparison with sarcoidosis and idiopathic pulmonary fibrosis. Eur Respir J 7:1944, 1994.
52. Shijubo N, Imai K, Shigehara K, et al: Soluble intercellular adhesion molecule-1 (ICAM-1) in sera and bronchoalveolar lavage (BAL) fluids of extrinsic allergic alveolitis. Clin Exp Immunol 102:91, 1995.
53. Pforte A, Schiessler A, Gais P, et al: Expression of the adhesion molecule ICAM-1 on alveolar macrophages and in serum in extrinsic allergic alveolitis. Respiration 60:221, 1993.
54. Warren CPW: Extrinsic allergic alveolitis: A disease commoner in nonsmokers. Thorax 32:567, 1977.
55. Gruchow HW, Hoffmann RG, Marx JJ Jr, et al: Precipitating antibodies to farmer's lung antigens in a Wisconsin farming population. Am Rev Resp Dis 124:411, 1981.
56. A national survey of bird fancier's lung including its possible association with jejunal villous atrophy. (A report to the Research Committee of the British Thoracic Society.) Br J Dis Chest 78:75, 1984.
57. Andersen P, Christensen KM: Serum antibodies to pigeon antigens in smokers and nonsmokers. Acta Med Scand 213:191, 1983.
58. Andersen P, Schonheyder H: Antibodies to hen and duck antigens in poultry workers. Clin Allergy 14:421, 1984.
59. Cormier Y, Belanger J, Durand P: Factors influencing the development of serum precipitins to farmer's lung antigen in Quebec dairy farmers. Pediatr Radiol 15:123, 1985.
60. Homma Y, Terai T, Matsuzaki M: Incidence of serum-precipitating antibodies to farmer's lung antigens in Hokkaido. Respiration 49:300, 1986.
61. Carrillo T, Rodriguez de Castro F, Cuevas M, et al: Effect of cigarette smoking on the humoral immune response in pigeon fanciers. Allergy 46:241, 1991.
61a. Baldwin CI, Todd A, Bourke S, et al: Pigeon fanciers' lung: Effects of smoking on serum and salivary antibody responses to pigeon antigens. Clin Exp Immunol 113:166, 1998.
62. Arima K, Ando M, Ito K, et al: Effect of cigarette smoking on prevalence of summer-type hypersensitivity pneumonitis caused by *Trichosporon cutaneum*. Arch Environ Health 47:274, 1992.
63. Reynolds SP, Edwards JH, Jones KP, et al: Immunoglobulin and antibody levels in bronchoalveolar lavage fluid from symptomatic and asymptomatic pigeon breeders. Clin Exp Immunol 86:278, 1991.
64. Ando M, Konishi K, Yoneda R, et al: Difference in the phenotypes of bronchoalveolar lavage lymphocytes in patients with summer-type hypersensitivity pneumonitis, farmer's lung, ventilation pneumonitis, and bird fancier's lung: Report of a nationwide epidemiologic study in Japan. J Allergy Clin Immunol 87:1002, 1991.

65. Ohtsuka Y, Munakata M, Tanimura K, et al: Smoking promotes insidious and chronic farmer's lung disease, and deteriorates the clinical outcome. Intern Med 34:966, 1995.
66. Selman M, Chapela R, Raghu G: Hypersensitivity pneumonitis: Clinical manifestations, pathogenesis, diagnosis and therapeutic strategies. Semin Respir Med 14:353, 1993.
67. Selman M, Teran L, Mendoza A, et al: Increase of HLA-DR7 in pigeon breeder's lung in a Mexican population. Clin Immunol Immunopathol 44:63, 1987.
68. Ano M, Hirayama K, Soda K, et al: HLA-DQw3 in Japanese summer-type hypersensitivity pneumonitis induced by *Trichosporon cutaneum*. Am Rev Respir Dis 140:948, 1989.
69. Cormier Y, Israel-Assayag E, Fournier M, et al: Modulation of experimental hypersensitivity pneumonitis by Sendai virus. J Lab Clin Med 121:683, 1993.
70. Teschler H, Pohl WR, Thompson AB, et al: Elevated levels of bronchoalveolar lavage vitronectin in hypersensitivity pneumonitis. Am Rev Respir Dis 147:332, 1993.
71. Cormier Y, Laviolette M, Cantin A, et al: Fibrogenic activities in bronchoalveolar lavage fluid of farmer's lung. Chest 104:1038, 1993.
72. Selman M, Montaño M, Ramos C, et al: Lung collagen metabolism and the clinical course of hypersensitivity pneumonitis. Chest 94:347, 1988.
73. Murayama J, Yoshizawa Y, Ohtsuka M., et al: Lung fibrosis in hypersensitivity pneumonitis: Association with CD4 + but not CD8 + cell dominant alveolitis and insidious onset. Chest 104:38, 1993.
74. Hasani A, Johnson M, Pavia D, et al: Impairment of lung mucociliary clearance in pigeon fanciers. Chest 102:887, 1992.
75. Emanuel DA, Wenzel FJ, Lawton BR: Pneumonitis due to *Cryptostroma corticale* (maple-bark disease). N Engl J Med 274:1413, 1966.
76. Sodeman WA, Pullen RL: Bagasse disease of the lungs. Arch Intern Med 73:365, 1944.
77. Pimentel JC, Alvila R: Respiratory disease in cork workers (suberosis). Thorax 28:409, 1973.
78. Totten RS, Reid DHS, Davis HD, et al: Farmer's lung: Report of two cases in which lung biopsies were performed. Am J Med 25:803, 1958.
79. Ghose T, Landrigan P, Killeen R, et al: Immunopathological studies in patients with farmer's lung. Clin Allergy 4:119, 1974.
80. Barrowcliff DF, Arblaster PG: Farmer's lung: A study of an early acute fatal case. Thorax 23:490, 1968.
81. Kawanami O, Basset F, Barrios R, et al: Hypersensitivity pneumonitis in man: Light- and electron-microscopic studies of 18 lung biopsies. Am J Pathol 110:275, 1983.
82. Tukiainen P, Taskinen E, Korhola O, et al: Farmer's lung: Needle biopsy findings and pulmonary function. Eur J Respir Dis 61:3, 1980.
83. Seal RME, Hapke EJ, Thomas GO, et al: The pathology of the acute and chronic stages of farmer's lung. Thorax 23:469, 1968.
84. Sutinen S, Reijula K, Huhti E, et al: Extrinsic allergic bronchiolo-alveolitis: Serology and biopsy findings. Eur J Respir Dis 64:271, 1983.
85. Reyes CN, Wenzel FJ, Lawton BR, et al: The pulmonary pathology of farmers' lung disease. Chest 81:142, 1982.
86. Hogg JC: The histologic appearance of farmer's lung. Chest 81:133, 1982.
87. Eyckmans L, Gyselen A, Lauwerijns J, et al: Pigeon breeder's lung: Report of three cases. Dis Chest 53:358, 1968.
88. Hensley GT, Garancis JC, Cherayil GD, et al: Lung biopsies of pigeon breeders' disease. Arch Pathol 87:572, 1969.
89. Wenzel FJ, Emanuel DA, Gray RL: Immunofluorescent studies in patients with farmer's lung. J Allergy 48:224, 1971.
90. Schlueter DP, Fink JN, Hensley GT: Wood-pulp workers' disease: A hypersensitivity pneumonitis caused by Alternaria. Ann Intern Med 77:907, 1972.
91. Emanuel DA, Wenzel FJ, Bowerman CI, et al: Farmer's lung: Clinical, pathologic and immunologic study of twenty-four patients. Am J Med 37:392, 1964.
92. Riley DJ, Saldana M: Pigeon breeder's lung: Subacute course and the importance of indirect exposure. Am Rev Respir Dis 107:456, 1973.
93. Harries MG, Heard B, Geddes D: Extrinsic allergic bronchiolitis in a bird fancier. Br J Ind Med 41:220, 1984.
94. Bankin J, Kobayashi M, Barbee RA, et al: Pulmonary granulomatoses due to inhaled organic antigens. Med Clin North Am 51:459, 1967.
95. Erkinjuntti-Pekkanen R, Rytkonen H, Kokkarinen JI, et al: Long-term risk of emphysema in patients with farmer's lung and matched control farmers. Am J Respir Crit Care Med 158:662, 1998.
96. Takemura T, Hiraga Y, Oomichi M, et al: Ultrastructural features of alveolitis in sarcoidosis. Am J Respir Crit Care Med 152:360, 1995.
97. Planes C, Valeyre D, Loiseau A, et al: Ultrastructural alterations of the air-blood barrier in sarcoidosis and hypersensitivity pneumonitis and their relation to lung histopathology. Am J Respir Crit Care Med 150:1067, 1994.
98. Orriols R, Aliaga JL, Rodrigo MJ, et al: Localised alveolar-septal amyloidosis with hypersensitivity pneumonitis. Lancet 339:1261, 1992.
99. Hargreave F, Hinson KF, Reid L,, et al: The radiologic appearances of allergic alveolitis due to bird sensitivity (bird fancier's lung). Clin Radiol 23:1, 1972.
100. Mindell HJ: Roentgen findings in farmer's lung. Radiology 97:341, 1970.
101. Arshad M, Braum SR, Sunderrajan EV: Severe hypoxemia in farmer's lung disease with normal findings on chest roentgenogram. Chest 91:274, 1987.
102. Zylak CJ: Hypersensitive lung disease due to avian antigens. Radiology 114:45, 1975.
103. Mönkäre S, Ikonen M, Haahtela T: Radiologic findings in farmer's lung: Prognosis and correlation to lung function. Chest 87:460, 1985.
104. Cook PG, Wells IP, McGavin CR: The distribution of pulmonary shadowing in farmer's lung. Clin Radiol 39:21, 1988.
105. Silver SF, Müller NL, Miller RR, Lefcoe MS: Hypersensitivity pneumonitis: Evaluation with CT. Radiology 173:441, 1989.
106. Hansell DM, Moskovic E: High-resolution computed tomography in extrinsic allergic alveolitis. Clin Radiol 43:8, 1991.
107. Hargreave F, Hinson KF, Reid L, et al: The radiological appearances of allergic alveolitis due to bird sensitivity (bird fancier's lung). Clin Radiol 23:1, 1972.
108. Sakula A: Mushroom-worker's lung. Br Med J 3:708, 1967.
109. Stoltz JL, Arger PH, Benson JM: Mushroom worker's lung disease. Radiology 119:61, 1976.
110. Frank RC: Farmer's lung: A form of pneumoconiosis due to organic dusts. Am J Roentgenol 79:189, 1958.
111. Grenier P, Chevret S, Beigelman C, et al: Chronic diffuse infiltrative lung disease: Determination of the diagnostic value of clinical data, chest radiography, and CT with Bayesian analysis. Radiology 191:383, 1994.
112. Niimi H, Kang EY, Kwong JS,, et al: CT of chronic infiltrative lung disease: Prevalence of mediastinal lymphadenopathy. J Comput Assist Tomogr 20:305, 1996.
113. Remy-Jardin M, Remy J, Wallaert B, Müller NL: Subacute and chronic bird breeder hypersensitivity pneumonitis: Sequential evaluation with CT and correlation with lung function tests and bronchoalveolar lavage. Radiology 189:111, 1993.
114. Monkare S: Clinical aspects of farmer's lung: Airway reactivity, treatment and prognosis. Eur J Respir Dis 137(Suppl):1, 1984.
115. Lynch DA, Rose CS, Way D, King TE Jr: Hypersensitivity pneumonitis: Sensitivity of high-resolution CT in a population-based study. Am J Roentgenol 159:469, 1992.
116. Gaensler EA, Carrington CB: Open biopsy for chronic diffuse infiltrative lung disease: Clinical, roentgenographic, and physiological correlations in 502 patients. Ann Thorac Surg 30:411, 1980.
117. Dinda P, Chatterjee SS, Riding WD: Pulmonary function studies in bird breeder's lung. Thorax 24:374, 1969.
118. Moore VL, Pedersen GM, Hauser WC, et al: A study of lung lavage materials in patients with hypersensitivity pneumonitis: In vitro response to mitogen and antigen in pigeon breeders' disease. J Allergy Clin Immunol 65:365, 1980.
119. Cormier Y, Belanger J, Beaudoin J, et al: Abnormal bronchoalveolar lavage in asymptomatic dairy farmers: Study of lymphocytes. Am Rev Respir Dis 130:1046, 1984.
120. Adler BD, Padley SP, Müller NL, Remy-Jardin M, Remy J: Chronic hypersensitivity pneumonitis: High-resolution CT and radiographic features in 16 patients. Radiology 185:91, 1992.
121. Lynch DA, Newell JD, Logan PM, King TE Jr, Müller NL. Can CT distinguish hypersensitivity pneumonitis from idiopathic pulmonary fibrosis? Am J Roentgenol 165:807, 1995.
122. Akira M, Kita N, Higashihara T, Sakatani M, Kozuka T: Summer-type hypersensitivity pneumonitis: Comparison of high-resolution CT and plain radiographic findings. Am J Roentgenol 158:1223, 1992.
123. Hansell DM, Wells AU, Padley SPG, Müller NL: Hypersensitivity pneumonitis: Correlation of individual CT patterns with functional abnormalities. Radiology 199:123, 1996.
124. Arshad M, Braun SR, Sunderrajan EV: Severe hypoxemia in farmer's lung disease with normal findings on chest roentgenogram. Chest 91:274, 1987.
125. Pepys J: Pulmonary hypersensitivity disease due to inhaled organic antigens. Ann Intern Med 64:943, 1966.
126. Fink JN: Clinical features of hypersensitivity pneumonitis. Chest 89:193S, 1986.
127. Warren WP: Hypersensitivity pneumonitis due to exposure to budgerigars. Chest 62:170, 1972.
128. Allergic alveolitis (editorial). BMJ 3:691, 1967.
129. Staines FH, Forman JA: A survey of "farmer's lung." J Coll Gen Pract 4:351, 1961.
130. Pelikan Z, Schot JDL, Koedijk FHJ: The late bronchus-obstructive response to bronchial challenge with pigeon faeces and its correlation with precipitating antibodies (IgG) in the serum of patients having long-term contact with pigeons. Clin Allergy 13:203, 1983.
131. Bourke S, Anderson K, Lynch P, et al: Chronic simple bronchitis in pigeon fanciers. Chest 95:598, 1989.
132. Carrillo T, Rodriguez de Castro F, Cuevas M, et al: Chronic bronchitis in pigeon fanciers (letter). Chest 98:508, 1990.
133. Dalphin JC, Debieuvre D, Pernet D, et al: Prevalence and risk factors for chronic bronchitis and farmer's lung in French dairy farmers. Br J Industr Med 50:941, 1993.
134. Davies D: Bird fancier's disease (editorial). BMJ 287:1239, 1983.
135. Earis JE, Marsh K, Pearson MG, et al: The inspiratory "squawk" in extrinsic allergic alveolitis and other pulmonary fibroses. Thorax 37:923, 1982.
136. Leblanc P, Belanger J, Laviolette M, et al: Relationship among antigen contact, alveolitis, and clinical status in farmer's lung disease. Arch Intern Med 146:153, 1986.
137. Berrill WT, Eade OE, Fitzpatrick PF, et al: Bird-fancier's lung and jejunal villous atrophy. Lancet 2:1006, 1975.
138. Robinson TJ: Coeliac disease with farmer's lung. BMJ 1:745, 1976.
139. A national survey of bird fancier's lung including its possible association with jejunal villous atrophy. (A report to the Research Committee of the British Thoracic Society.) Br J Dis Chest 78:75, 1984.
140. Tarlo SM, Broder I, Prokipchuk EJ, et al: Association between celiac disease and lung disease. Chest 80:715, 1981.
141. Petro W, Muller E, Bergmann K-C, et al: Impaired CO transfer factors in bird fancier's lung. Lung 155:269, 1978.

142. Boyd G, McSharry CP, Banham SW, et al: A current view of pigeon fancier's lung: A model for pulmonary extrinsic allergic alveolitis. Clin Allergy 12(Suppl):53, 1982.

143. Warren CPW, Tse KS, Cherniack RM: Mechanical properties of the lung in extrinsic allergic alveolitis. Thorax 33:315, 1978.

144. Sovijarvi ARA, Kuusisto P, Muittari A, et al: Trapped air in extrinsic allergic alveolitis. Respiration 40:57, 1980.

145. Boyd G: Pulmonary function changes in pigeon fancier's lung. Respir Med 84:5, 1990.

146. De Gracia J, Morell F, Bofill JM, et al: Time of exposure as a prognostic factor in avian hypersensitivity pneumonitis. Respir Med 83:139, 1989.

147. Tewksbury DA, Marx JJ Jr, Roberts RC, et al: Angiotensin-converting enzyme in farmer's lung. Chest 79:102, 1981.

148. McCormick JR, Thrall RS, Ward PA, et al: Serum angiotensin-converting enzyme levels in patients with pigeon-breeder's disease. Chest 80:431, 1981.

149. Turton CWG, Firth G, Grundy E, et al: Raised enzyme markers of chronic inflammation in asymptomatic farmer's lung. Thorax 36:122, 1981.

150. Bourke SJ, Banham SW, McKillop JH, et al: Clearance of Tc-DTPA in pigeon fancier's hypersensitivity pneumonitis. Am Rev Respir Dis 142:1168, 1990.

151. Orriols R, Aliaga JL, Anto JM: High prevalence of mollusc shell hypersensitivity in nacre factory workers. Eur Respir J 10:780, 1997.

152. Lacasse Y, Fraser RS, Fournier M, et al: Diagnostic accuracy of transbronchial biopsy in acute farmer's lung disease. Chest 112:1459, 1997.

153. Kokkarinen JI, Tukiainen HO, Terho EO: Recovery of pulmonary function in farmer's lung. Am Rev Respir Dis 147:793, 1993.

154. Schmidt CDW, Jensen RL, Christensen LT, et al: Longitudinal pulmonary function changes in pigeon breeders. Chest 93:359, 1988

155. Braun SR, doPico GA, Tsiatis A, et al: Farmer's lung disease: Long-term clinical and physiologic outcome. Am Rev Respir Dis 119:185, 1979.

156. Monkare S, Haahtela T: Farmer's lung: A 5-year follow-up of eighty-six patients. Clin Allergy 17:143, 1987.

157. Cormier Y, Belanger J: Long-term physiologic outcome after acute farmer's lung. Chest 87:796, 1985.

158. Kokkarinen J, Tukiainen H, Terho EO: Mortality due to farmer's lung in Finland. Chest 106:509, 1994.

159. Pérez-Padilla R, Salas J, Chapela R, et al: Mortality in Mexican patients with chronic pigeon breeder's lung compared with those with usual interstitial pneumonia. Am Rev Respir Dis 148:49, 1993.

160. Yoshida K, Suga M, Nishiura Y, et al: Occupational hypersensitivity pneumonitis in Japan: Data on a nationwide epidemiological study. Occup Environ Med 52:570, 1995.

161. Campbell JM: Acute symptoms following work with hay. Br Med J 2:1143, 1932.

162. Ramirez-Venegas A, Sansores RH, Perez-Padilla R, et al: Utility of a provocation test for diagnosis of chronic pigeon breeder's disease. Am J Respir Crit Care Med 158:862, 1998.

163. Grant IWB, Blyth W, Wardrop VE, et al: Prevalence of farmer's lung in Scotland: A pilot survey. BMJ 1:530, 1972.

164. Smyth JT, Adkins GE, Lloyd M, et al: Farmer's lung in Devon. Thorax 30:197, 1975.

165. Matsen D, Klock LE, Wensel FJ, et al: The prevalence of farmer's lung in an agricultural population. Am Rev Respir Dis 113:171, 1976.

166. Depierre A, Dalphin JC, Pernet D, et al: Epidemiological study of farmer's lung in five districts of the French Doubs province. Thorax 43:429, 1988.

167. Morgan DC, Smyth JT, Lister RW, et al: Chest symptoms and farmer's lung: A community survey. Br J Ind Med 30:259, 1973.

168. Gump DW, Babbott FL, Holly C, et al: Farmer's lung disease in Vermont. Respiration 37:52, 1979.

169. Boyd G, Parratt D: Improved diagnosis of farmer's lung using the fluorescent antibody technique. Thorax 29:417, 1974.

170. Hapke EJ, Seal RME, Thomas GO, et al: Farmer's lung: A clinical, radiographic, functional, and serological correlation of acute and chronic stages. Thorax 23:451, 1968.

171. Wenzel FJ, Gray RL, Roberts RC, et al: Serologic studies in farmer's lung: Precipitins to the thermophilic actinomycetes. Am Rev Respir Dis 109:464, 1974.

172. Farmer's lung (leading article). BMJ 3:189, 1975.

173. Baur X, Dexheimer E: Hypersensitivity pneumonitis concomitant with acute airway obstruction after exposure to hay dust. Respiration 46:354, 1984.

174. Meeker DP, Gephardt GN, Cordasco EM, et al: Hypersensitivity pneumonitis versus invasive pulmonary aspergillosis: Two cases with unusual pathologic findings and review of the literature. Am Rev Respir Dis 143:431, 1991.

175. Ando M, Yoshida K, Nakashima K, et al: Role of Candida albicans in chronic hypersensitivity pneumonitis. Chest 105:317, 1994.

176. Fink JN, Banaszak EF, Barboriak JJ, et al: Interstitial lung disease due to contamination of forced air systems. Ann Intern Med 84:406, 1976.

177. Reijula K, Sutinen S, Tuuponen T, et al: Pulmonary fibrosis, with sarcoid granulomas and angiitis, associated with handling of mouldy lichen. Eur J Respir Dis 64:625, 1983.

178. Dutkiewicz J, Kus L, Dutkiewicz E, et al: Hypersensitivity pneumonitis in grain farmers due to sensitization to Erwinia herbicola. Ann Allergy 54:65, 1985.

179. Bouchard S, Morin F, Bédard G, et al: Farmer's lung and variables related to the decision to quit farming. Am J Respir Crit Care Med 152:997, 1995.

180. Teschler H, Thompson AB, Pohl WR, et al: Bronchoalveolar lavage procollagen-III-peptide in recent onset hypersensitivity pneumonitis: Correlation with extracellular matrix components. Eur Respir J 6:709, 1993.

181. Anttinen H, Terho EO, Myllyla R, et al: Two serum markers of collagen biosynthesis as possible indicators of irreversible pulmonary impairment in farmer's lung. Am Rev Respir Dis 133:88, 1986.

182. Baldwin CI, Todd A, Bourke SJ, et al: IgG subclass responses to pigeon intestinal mucin are related to development of pigeon fanciers' lung. Clin Exp Allergy 28:349, 1998.

183. Choy AC, Patterson R, Ray AH, et al: Hypersensitivity pneumonitis in a raptor handler and a wild bird fancier. Ann Allergy Asthma Immunol 74:437, 1995.

184. Kokkarinen J, Tukiainen H, Seppä A, et al: Hypersensitivity pneumonitis due to native birds in a bird ringer. Chest 106:1269, 1994.

185. Warren CPW, Tse KS: Extrinsic allergic alveolitis owing to hypersensitivity to chickens: Significance of sputum precipitins. Am Rev Respir Dis 109:672, 1974.

186. Korn DS, Florman AL, Gribetz I: Recurrent pneumonitis with hypersensitivity to hen litter. JAMA 205:44, 1968.

187. Bütikofer E, de Weck AL: Poultry keeper's lung. Ger Med Monthly 15:245, 1970.

188. Boyer RS, Klock LE, Schmidt CD, et al: Hypersensitivity lung disease in the turkey raising industry. Am Rev Respir Dis 109:630, 1974.

189. Elman AJ, Tebo T, Fink JN, et al: Reactions of poultry farmers against chicken antigens. Arch Environ Health (Chicago) 17:98, 1968.

190. Andersen P, Christensen KM, Jensen BE, et al: Antibodies to pigeon antigens in pigeon breeders: Detection of antibodies by an enzyme-linked immunosorbent assay. Eur J Respir Dis 63:113, 1982.

191. Sutton PP, Pearson A, DuBois RM: Canary fancier's lung. Clin Allergy 14:429, 1984.

192. Faux JA, Wells ID, Pepys J: Specificity of avian serum proteins in tests against the sera of bird fanciers. Clin Allergy 1:159, 1971.

193. McSharry C, Lynch PP, Banham SW, et al: Seasonal variation of antibody levels among pigeon fanciers. Clin Allergy 13:293, 1983.

194. Todd A, Coan R, Allen A: Pigeon breeders' lung: IgG subclasses to pigeon intestinal mucin and IgA antigens. Clin Exp Immunol 92:494, 1993.

195. Craig TJ, Hershey J, Engler RJM, et al: Bird antigen persistence in the home environment after removal of the bird. Ann Allergy 69:510, 1992.

196. Meyer FJ, Bauer PC, Costabel U: Feather wreath lung: Chasing a dead bird. Eur Respir J 9:1323, 1996.

197. Bourke SJ, Banham SW, Carter R, et al: Longitudinal course of extrinsic allergic alveolitis in pigeon breeders. Thorax 44:415, 1989.

198. Jackson E, Welch KMA: Mushroom worker's lung. Thorax 25:25, 1970.

199. Craig DB, Donevan RE: Mushroom-worker's lung. Can Med Assoc J 102:1289, 1970.

200. Chan-Yeung M, Grzybowski S, Schonell ME: Mushroom worker's lung. Am Rev Respir Dis 105:819, 1972.

201. Van den Bogart HG, Van den Ende G, Van Loon PC, et al: Mushroom worker's lung: Serologic reactions to thermophilic actinomycetes present in the air of compost tunnels. Mycopathologia 122:21, 1993.

202. Ishii M, Kikuchi A, Kudoh K, et al: Hypersensitivity pneumonitis induced by inhalation of mushroom (Pholiota nameko) spores. Intern Med 33:683, 1994.

203. Konishi K, Mouri T, Kojima Y, et al: Three cases of hypersensitivity pneumonitis caused by inhalation of spores of Pholiota nameko and the background of the disease. Nippon Kyobu Shikkan Gakkai Zasshi 32:655, 1994.

204. Nakazawa T, Tochigi T: Hypersensitivity pneumonitis due to mushroom (Pholiota nameko) spores. Chest 95:1149, 1989.

205. Cox A, Folgering HT, van Griensven LJ: Extrinsic allergic alveolitis caused by spores of the oyster mushroom Pleurotus ostreatus. Eur Respir J 1:466, 1988.

206. Hur T, Cheng KC, Yang GY: Hypersensitivity pneumonitis: Bagassosis. Kao Hsiung I Hsueh Ko Hsueh Tsa Chih 10:558, 1994.

207. Ueda A, Aoyama KM, Ueda T, et al: Recent trends in bagassosis in Japan. Br J Ind Med 49:499, 1992.

208. Salvaggio JE, Seabury JH, Buechner HA, et al: Bagassosis: Demonstration of precipitins against extracts of thermophilic actinomycetes in the sera of affected individuals. J Allergy 39:106, 1967.

209. Hargreave FE, Pepys J, Holford-Strevens V: Bagassosis. Lancet 1:619, 1968.

210. Salvaggio J, Arquembourg P, Seabury J, et al: Bagassosis. IV. Precipitins against extracts of thermophilic actinomycetes in patients with bagassosis. Am J Med 46:538, 544, 1969.

211. Salvaggio JE, Buechner HA, Seabury JH, et al: Bagassosis. I. Precipitins against extracts of crude bagasse in the serum of patients. Ann Intern Med 64:748, 1966.

212. Weill H, Buechner HA, Gonzales E, et al: Bagassosis: A study of pulmonary function in 20 cases. Ann Intern Med 64:737, 1966.

213. Boonpucknavig V, Bhamarapravati N, Kamtorn P, et al: Bagassosis: A histopathologic study of pulmonary biopsies from six cases. Am J Clin Pathol 59:461, 1973.

214. Patterson R, Fink JN, Miles WB, et al: Hypersensitivity lung disease presumptively due to Cephalosporium in homes contaminated by sewage flooding or by humidifier water. J Allergy Clin Immunol 68:128, 1981.

215. Arnow PM, Fink JN, Schlueter DP, et al: Early detection of hypersensitivity pneumonitis in office workers. Am J Med 64:236, 1978.

216. Muittari A, Kuusisto P, Virtanen P, et al: An epidemic of extrinsic allergic alveolitis caused by tap water. Clin Allergy 10:77, 1980.

217. Suda T, Sato A, Ida M, et al: Hypersensitivity pneumonitis associated with home ultrasonic humidifiers. Chest 107(3):711, 1995.

218. Woodard ED, Friedlander B, Lesher RJ, et al: Outbreak of hypersensitivity pneumonitis in an industrial setting. JAMA 259(13):1965, 1988.

219. Saltos N, Saunders NA, Bhagwandeen SB, et al: Hypersensitivity pneumonitis in a mouldy house. Med J Aust 2:244, 1982.

220. Fergusson RJ, Milne LJR, Crompton G: Penicillin allergic alveolitis: Faulty installation of central heating. Thorax 39:294, 1984.

221. Kurup VP, Barboriak JJ, Fink JN, et al: *Thermoactinomyces candidus*, a new species of thermophilic actinomycetes. Int J Systemic Bacteriol 25:150, 1975.

222. Park HS, Jung KS, Kim SO, et al: Hypersensitivity pneumonitis induced by *Penicillium expansum* in a home environment. Clin Exp Allergy 24:383, 1994.

223. Kohler PF, Gross G, Salvaggio J, et al: Humidifier lung: Hypersensitivity pneumonitis related to thermotolerant bacterial aerosols. Chest 69(Suppl):294, 1976.

224. Jacobs RL, Thorner RE, Holcomb JR, et al: Hypersensitivity pneumonitis caused by *Cladosporium* in an enclosed hot-tub area. Ann Intern Med 105:204, 1986.

225. van Assendelft A, Forsen K-O, Keskinen H, et al: Humidifier-associated extrinsic allergic alveolitis. Scand J Work Environ Health 5:35, 1979.

226. Edwards JH, Griffiths AJ, Mullins J: Protozoa as sources of antigen in "humidifier fever." Nature 264:438, 1976.

227. Haitjema T, van Velzen-Blad H, van den Bosch JM. Extrinsic allergic alveolitis caused by goose feathers in a duvet. Thorax 47(11):990, 1992.

228. Ando M, Arima K, Yoneda R, et al: Japanese summer-type hypersensitivity pneumonitis. Am Rev Respir Dis 144:765, 1991.

229. Shimazu K, Ando M, Sakata T, et al: Hypersensitivity pneumonitis induced by *Trichosporon cutaneum*. Am Rev Respir Dis 130:407, 1984.

230. Yoshida K, Ando M, Sakata T, et al: Environmental mycological studies on the causative agent of summer-type hypersensitivity pneumonitis. J Allergy Clin Immunol 81:475, 1988.

231. Ando M, Yoshida K, Soda K, et al: Specific bronchoalveolar lavage IgA antibody in patients with summer-type hypersensitivity pneumonitis induced by *Trichosporon cutaneum*. Am Rev Respir Dis 134:177, 1986.

232. Kishimoto N, Mouri M, Sakurai S, et al: A case of hypersensitivity pneumonitis in *Pholiota nameko's* manufacturer. Nippon Kyobu Shikkan Gakkai Zasshi 31:275, 1993.

233. Riddle HFV, Chanell S, Blyth W, et al: Allergic alveolitis in a maltworker. Thorax 23:271, 1968.

234. Towey JW, Sweany HC, Huron WH: Severe bronchial asthma apparently due to fungus spores in maple bark. JAMA 99:453, 1932.

235. Parish WE: Farmer's lung. Part I. An immunological study of some antigenic components of mouldy foodstuffs. Thorax 18:83, 1963.

236. Emanuel DA, Lawton BR, Wenzel FJ: Maple-bark disease: Pneumonitis due to *Coniosporium corticale*. N Engl J Med 26:333, 1962.

237. Mahon WE, Scott DJ, Ansell G, et al: Hypersensitivity to pituitary snuff with miliary shadowing in the lungs. Thorax 22:13, 1967.

238. Pepys J, Jenkins PA, Lachmann PJ, et al: An iatrogenic autoantibody: Immunological responses to "pituitary snuff" in patients with diabetes insipidus. Clin Exp Immunol 1:377, 1966.

239. Harper LO, Burrell RG, Lapp NL, et al: Allergic alveolitis due to pituitary snuff. Ann Intern Med 73:581, 1070.

240. Avila R, Villar TG: Suberosis: Respiratory disease in cork workers. Lancet 1:620, 1968.

241. Moral AJ, Arias J, Garcia MA, et al: Extrinsic allergic alveolitis caused by *Penicillium frequentans*. Arch Bronconeumol 30:462, 1994.

242. Newman Taylor AJ: Occupational asthma and byssinosis. *In* Parkes WR (ed): Occupational Lung Disorders. 3rd ed. Oxford, Butterworth Heinemann, 1994.

243. Malo J-L, Zeiss CR: Occupational hypersensitivity pneumonitis after exposure to diphenylmethane diisocyanate. Am Rev Respir Dis 125:113, 1982.

244. Baur X, Dewair M, Rommelt H: Acute airway obstruction followed by hypersensitivity pneumonitis in an isocyanate (MDI) worker. J Occup Med 26:285, 1984.

244a. Fink JN, Schlueter DP: Bathtub refinisher's lung: An unusual response to toluene diisocyanate. Am Rev Respir Dis 118:955, 1978.

244b. Yoshizawa Y, Ohtsuka M, Noguchi K, et al: Hypersensitivity pneumonitis induced by toluene diisocyanate: Sequelae of continuous exposure. Ann Intern Med 110:31, 1989.

244c. Malo JL, Ouimet G, Cartier A, et al: Combined alveolitis and asthma due to hexamethylene diisocyanate (HDI), with demonstration of crossed respiratory and immunologic reactivities to diphenylmethane diisocyanate (MDI). J Allergy Clin Immunol 72:413, 1983.

244d. Selden A, Belin L, Wass U: Isocyanate exposure and hypersensitivity pneumonitis—report of a probable case and prevalence of specific immunoglobulin G antibodies among exposed individuals. Scand J Work Environ Health 15:234, 1989.

245. Yamada K, Amitani R, Niimi A, et al: Interstitial pneumonitis-like lesions in guinea-pigs following repeated exposure to toluene diisocyanate. Eur Respir J 8:1300, 1995.

246. Vandenplas O, Malo JL, Dugas M, et al: Hypersensitivity pneumonitis-like reaction among workers exposed to piphenylmethane diiocyanate (MDI). Am Rev Respir Dis 147:338, 1993.

247. Baur X: Hypersensitivity pneumonitis (extrinsic allergic alveolitis) induced by isocyanates. J Allergy Clin Immunol 95:1004, 1995.

248. Johnson CL, Bernstein IL, Gallagher JS, et al: Familial hypersensitivity pneumonitis induced by *Bacillus subtilis*. Am Rev Respir Dis 122:339, 1980.

249. Pepys J, Hargreaves FE, Longbottom JL, et al: Allergic reactions of the lungs to enzymes of *Bacillus subtilis*. Lancet 1:1181, 1969.

250. Dijkman JH, Borghans JGA, Savelberg PJ, et al: Allergic bronchial reactions to inhalation of enzymes of *Bacillus subtilis*. Am Rev Respir Dis 107:387, 1973.

251. Webster JR, Cugell DW, Cunningham L, et al: Detergent worker lung: A hypertensive pulmonary disease? Chest 61:174, 1972.

252. Little DC, Dolovich J: Respiratory disease in industry due to *B. subtilis* enzyme preparations. Can Med Assoc J 108:1120, 1973.

253. Flindt MLH: Pulmonary disease due to inhalation of derivatives of *Bacillus subtilis* containing proteolytic enzyme. Lancet 1:1177, 1969.

254. Lichtenstein LM: Human experimentation by industry: The case of "enzyme" detergents. Ann Intern Med 75:964, 1971.

255. Greenberg M, Milne JF, Watt A: Survey of workers exposed to dust containing derivatives of *Bacillus subtilus*. Br Med J 2:629, 1970.

256. Flood DF, Blofeld RE, Bruce CF, et al: Lung function, atopy, specific hypersensitivity, and smoking of workers in the enzyme detergent industry over 11 years. Br J Ind Med 42:43, 1985.

257. Donham KJ: Respiratory disease hazards to workers in livestock and poultry confinement structures. Semin Respir Med 14:49, 1993.

258. Donham KJ, Reynolds SJ, Whitten P, et al: Respiratory dysfunction in swine production facility workers: Dose-response relationships of environmental exposures and pulmonary function. Am J Ind Med 27:405, 1995.

259. Zejda JE, Barber E, Dosman JA, et al: Respiratory health status in swine producers relates to endotoxin exposure in the presence of low dust levels. J Occup Med 36:49, 1994.

260. Zuskin E, Kanceljak B, Schacter EN, et al: Immunological and respiratory findings in swine farmers. Environ Res 56:120, 1991.

261. Quinn TJ, Donham KJ, Merchant JA, et al: Peak flow as a measure of airway dysfunction in swine confinement operators. Chest 107:1303, 1995.

262. Schwartz DA, Donham KJ, Olenchock SA, et al: Determinants of longitudinal changes in spirometric function among swine confinement operators and farmers. Am J Respir Crit Care Med 151:47, 1995.

263. Wang Z, Malmberg P, Larsson B-M, et al: Exposure to bacteria in swine-house dust and acute inflammatory reactions in humans. Am J Respir Crit Care Med 154:1261, 1996.

264. Zuskin E, Zagar Z, Schacter EN, et al: Respiratory symptoms and ventilatory capacity in swine confinement workers. Br J Ind Med 49:435, 1992.

265. Larsson KA, Eklund AG, Hansson LO, et al: Swine dust causes intense airways inflammation in healthy subjects. Am J Respir Crit Care Med 150:973, 1994.

266. Muller-Suur C, Larsson K, Malmberg P, et al: Increased number of activated lymphocytes in human lung following swine dust inhalation. Eur Respir J 10:376, 1997.

267. Halpin DM, Graneek BJ, Turner-Warwick M, et al: Extrinsic allergic alveolitis and asthma in a sawmill worker: Case report and review of the literature. Occup Environ Med 51:160, 1994.

268. Zejda JE, Hurst TS, Rhodes CS, et al: Respiratory health of swine producers. Chest 103:702, 1993.

269. Senthilselvan A, Dosman JA, Kirychuk SP, et al: Accelerated lung function decline in swine confinement workers. Chest 111:1733, 1997.

270. Bessette L, Boulet LP, Tremblay G, et al: Bronchial responsiveness to methacholine in swine confinement building workers. Arch Environ Health 48:73, 1993.

271. Schwartz DA, Landas SK, Lassise DL, et al: Airway injury in swine confinement workers. Ann Intern Med 116:630, 1992.

272. Choudat D, Goehen M, Korobaeff M, et al: Respiratory symptoms and bronchial reactivity among pig and dairy farmers. Scand J Work Environ Health 20:48, 1994.

273. Carvalheiro MF, Peterson Y, Rubenowitz E, et al: Bronchial reactivity and work-related symptoms in farmers. Am J Ind Med 27:65, 1995.

274. Rask-Andersen A: Organic dust toxic syndrome among farmers. Br J Ind Med 46:233, 1989.

275. Weber S, Kullman G, Petsonk E, et al: Organic dust exposures from compost handling: Case presentation and respiratory exposure assessment. Am J Ind Med 24:365, 1993.

276. Perry LP, Iwata M, Tazelaar HD, et al: Pulmonary mycotoxicosis: A clinicopathologic study of three cases. Mod Pathol 11:432, 1998.

277. Anderson K, Watt AD, Sinclair D, et al: Climate, intermittent humidification and humidifier fever. Br J Industr Med 46:671, 1989.

278. Mamolen M, Lewis DM, Blanchet MA, et al: Investigation of an outbreak of "humidifier fever" in a print shop. Am J Ind Med 23:483, 1993.

279. Taylor AN, Pickering CAC, Turner-Warwick M, et al: Respiratory allergy to a factory humidifier contaminant presenting as pyrexia of undetermined origin. Br Med J 2:94, 1978.

280. Cockcroft A, Edwards J, Campbell I: Investigation of an outbreak of humidifier fever in a hospital operating theatre. Br J Dis Chest 74:317, 1980.

281. Edwards JH, Cockcroft A: Inhalation challenge in humidifier fever. Clin Allergy 11:227, 1981.

282. Banaszak EF, Thiede WH, Fink JN: Hypersensitivity pneumonitis due to contamination of an air conditioner. N Engl J Med 283:271, 1970.

283. do Pico GA: Hazardous exposure and lung disease among farm workers. Clin Chest Med 13(2):311, 1992.

284. Wintermeyer SF, Kuschner WG, Wong H, et al: Pulmonary responses after wood chip mulch exposure. J Occup Environ Med 39:308, 1997.

285. Dalphin JC, Bildstein F, Pernet D, et al: Prevalence of chronic bronchitis and respiratory function in a group of dairy farmers in the French Doubs province. Chest 95:1244, 1989.

286. Dalphin JCH, Pernet D, Dubiez A, et al: Etiologic factors of chronic bronchitis in dairy farmers. Chest 103:417, 1993.

287. Blainey AD, Topping MD, Ollier S, et al: Respiratory symptoms in arable farmworkers: Role of storage mites. Thorax 43:697, 1988.

288. Cuthbert OD, Jeffrey IG: Barn allergy: An allergic respiratory disease of farmers. Semin Respir Med 14:73, 1993.

289. Wright JL: Inhalational lung injury causing bronchiolitis. Clin Chest Med 14(4):635, 1993.

290. Shahan TA, Sorenseon WG, Lewis DM: Superoxide anion production in response to bacterial lipopolysaccharide and fungal spores implicated in organic dust toxic syndrome. Environ Res 67:98, 1994.

291. Malmberg P, Rask-Andersen A, Rosenhall L: Exposure to microorganisms associated with allergic alveolitis and febrile reactions to mold dust in farmers. Chest 103:1202, 1993.
292. Malmberg P, Rask-Andersen A: Organic dust toxic syndrome. Semin Respir Med 14:38, 1993.
293. Piirila P, Keskinen H, Anttila S, et al: Allergic alveolitis following exposure to epoxy polyester powder paint containing low amounts (<1%) of acid anhydrides. Eur Respir J 10:948, 1997.
294. Salvaggio JE, Buechner HA, Seabury JH, et al: Bagassosis. I. Precipitins against extracts of crude bagasse in the serum of patients. Ann Intern Med 64:748, 1966.
295. Salvaggio JE, Seabury JH, Buechner HA, et al: Bagassosis: Demonstration of precipitins against extracts of thermophilic actinomycetes in the sera of affected individuals. J Allergy 39:106, 1967.
296. Salvaggio JE, Arquembourg P, Seabury J, et al: Bagassosis. IV. Precipitins against extracts of thermophilic actinomycetes in patients with bagassosis. Am J Med 46:538, 544, 1969.
297. Hendrick DJ, Faux JA, Marshall R: Budgerigar fancier's lung: The commonest variety of allergic alveolitis in Britain. Br Med J 2:81, 1978.
298. Boyer RS, Klock LE, Schmidt DC, et al: Hypersensitivity lung disease in the turkey raising industry. Am Rev Respir Dis 109:630, 1974.
299. Warren CPW, Tse KS: Extrinsic allergic alveolitis owing to hypersensitivity to chickens: Significance of sputum precipitins. Am Rev Respir Dis 109:672, 1974.
300. Sutton PP, Pearson A, DuBois RM: Canary fancier's lung. Clin Allergy 14:429, 1984.
301. Campbell JA, Kryda JF, Truehaft MW, et al: Cheese worker's hypersensitivity pneumonitis. Am Rev Respir Dis 127:495, 1983.
302. Galland C, Reynaud C, De Haller R, et al: Cheese-washer's disease: A current stable form of extrinsic allergic alveolitis in a rural setting. Rev Mal Respir 8:381, 1991.
303. Van Toorn DW: Coffee worker's lung: A new example of extrinsic allergic alveolitis. Thorax 25:399, 1970.
304. Brown JE, Masood D, Couser JI, et al: Hypersensitivity pneumonitis from residential composting: Residential composter's lung. Ann Allergy Asthma Immunol 74:45, 1995.
305. Yoshida K, Ueda A, Yamasaki H, et al: Hypersensitivity pneumonitis resulting from *Aspergillus fumigatus* in a greenhouse. Arch Environ Health 48:260, 1993.
306. Flood DF, Blofeld RE, Bruce CF, et al: Lung function, atopy, specific hypersensitivity, and smoking of workers in the enzyme detergent industry over 11 years. Br J Ind Med 42:43, 1985.
307. Bryant DH, Rogers P: Allergic alveolitis due to wood-rot fungi. Allergy Proc 12:89, 1991.
308. Smyth JT, Adkins GE, Lloyd M, et al: Farmer's lung in Devon. Thorax 30:197, 1975.
309. Gump DW, Babbott FL, Holly C, et al: Farmer's lung disease in Vermont. Respiration 37:52, 1979.
310. Avila R: Extrinsic allergic alveolitis in workers exposed to fish meal and poultry. Clin Allergy 1:343, 1971.
311. Cockroft A, Edwards J, Campbell I: Investigation of an outbreak of humidifier fever in a hospital operating theatre. Br J Dis Chest 74:317, 1980.
312. Fergusson RJ, Milne LJR, Crompton G: Penicillium-allergic alveolitis: Faulty installation of central heating. Thorax 39:294, 1984.
313. Edwards JH, Griffiths AJ, Mullins J: Protozoa as sources of antigen in "humidifier fever." Nature 264:438, 1976.
314. Jacobs RL, Thorner RE, Holcomb JR, et al: Hypersensitivity pneumonitis caused by *Cladosporium* in an enclosed hot-tub area. Ann Intern Med 105:204, 1986.
315. Pal TM, de Monchy JG, Groothoff JW, et al: The clinical spectrum of humidifier disease in synthetic fiber plants. Am J Ind Med 31:682, 1997.
316. Lunn JA, Hughes DTD: Pulmonary hypersensitivity to the grain weevil. Br J Industr Med 24:158, 1967.
317. Carroll KB, Pepys J, Longbottom JL, et al: Extrinsic allergic alveolitis due to rat serum proteins. Clin Allergy 5:44, 1975.
318. Evans WV, Seaton A: Hypersensitivity pneumonitis in a technician using Pauli's reagent. Thorax 34:767, 1979.
319. Strand RD, Neuhauser EBD, Sornberger CF: Lycoperdonosis. N Engl J Med 277:89, 1967.
320. Bernstein DI, Lummus ZL, Santilli G, et al: Machine operator's lung: A hypersensitivity pneumonitis disorder associated with exposure to metalworking fluid aerosols. Chest 108:636, 1995.
321. Emanuel DA, Wenzel FJ, Lawton BR: Pneumonia due to *Cryptostroma corticale* maple-bark disease. N Engl J Med 274:1413, 1966.
322. Grant IWB, Blackadder ES, Greenberg M, et al: Extrinsic allergic alveolitis in Scottish maltworkers. Br Med J 1:490, 1976.
323. Blackburn CRB, Green W: Precipitins against extracts of thatched roofs in the sera of New Guinea natives with chronic lung disease. Lancet 2:1396, 1966.
324. Shepherd GM, Michelis MA, Macris NT, et al: Hypersensitivity pneumonitis in an orchid grower associated with sensitivity to the fungus *Cryptostroma corticale.* Ann Allergy Chest 103:522, 1989.
325. Harper LO, Burrell RG, Lapp NL, et al: Allergic alveolitis due to pituitary snuff. Ann Intern Med 73:581, 1970.
326. Simpson C, Garabrant D, Torrey S, et al: Hypersensitivity pneumonitis-like reaction and occupational asthma associated with 1,3-bis (isocyanatomethyl) cyclohexane pre-polymer. Am J Ind Med 30:48, 1996.
327. Gaddie J, Legge JS, Friend JAR: Pulmonary hypersensitivity in prawn workers. Lancet 2:1350, 1980.
328. Cohen HI, Merigan TC, Kosek JC, et al: Sequoiosis: A granulomatous pneumonitis associated with redwood sawdust inhalation. Am J Med 43:785, 1967.
329. Tsuchiya Y, Shimokata K, Ohara H, et al: Hypersensitivity pneumonitis in a soy sauce brewer caused by *Aspergillus orzae.* J Allergy Clin Immunol 91:688, 1993.
330. DoPico GA, Layton CR Jr, Clayton JW, et al: Acute pulmonary reaction to spray starch with soil repellent. Am Rev Respir Dis 108:1212, 1973.
331. Zamarron C, del Campo F, Paredes C: Extrinsic allergic alveolitis due to exposure to esparto dust. J Intern Med 232:177, 1992.
332. Avila R, Villar TG: Suberosis: Respiratory disease in cork workers. Lancet 1:620, 1968.
333. Alegre J, Morell F, Cobo E: Respiratory symptoms and pulmonary function of workers exposed to cork dust, toluene diisocyanate, and conidia. Scand J Work Environ Health 16:175, 1990.
334. Nefedov VB, Popova LA, Zhalolov ZZH: Lung function in tobacco growers suffering from exogenous allergic alveolitis. Ter Arkh 63:124, 1991.
335. Schlueter DP, Fink JN, Hensley GT: Wood-pulp worker's disease: A hypersensitivity pneumonitis caused by *Alternaria.* Ann Intern Med 77:907, 1972.
336. Hogan MB, Patterson R, Pore RS, et al: Basement shower hypersensitivity secondary to *Epicoccum nigrum.* Chest 110:855, 1996.
337. Zacharisen MC, Kadambi AR, Schleuter DP, et al: The spectrum of respiratory disease associated with exposure to metal working fluids. J Occup Environ Med 40:640, 1998.
338. Kreiss K, Cox-Ganser J: Metalworking fluid–associated hypersensitivity pneumonitis: A workshop summary. Am J Ind Med 32:423, 1997.
339. Cormier Y, Israel-Assayag E, Bedard G, et al: Hypersensitivity pneumonitis in peat moss processing plant workers. Am J Respir Crit Care Med 158:412, 1998.
340. Piirila P, Keskinen H, Anttila S, et al: Allergic alveolitis following exposure to epoxy polyester powder paint containing low amounts (< 1%) of acid anhydrides. Eur Respir J 10:948, 1997.

CHAPTER *60*

Inhalation of Inorganic Dust (Pneumoconiosis)

At the Fourth International Pneumoconiosis Conference held in Bucharest in 1971, pneumoconiosis was defined as "the accumulation of dust in the lungs and the tissue reactions to its presence."[1] Such reactions generally take one or both of two clinicopathologic forms.

1. *Fibrosis*, which can be focal and nodular (as in silicosis) or diffuse (as in asbestosis). This process is proba-

bly related to a toxic effect of the inhaled substance on pulmonary epithelial and/or inflammatory cells;[2] it often results in radiographic abnormalities and, if extensive enough, may lead to significant functional impairment.

2. *Aggregates of particle-laden macrophages* with minimal or no accompanying fibrosis, a reaction that is typically seen with inert dusts, such as iron, tin, and barium. Although sometimes associated with chronic radiographic abnormalities, this reaction usually results in few, if any, functional or clinical manifestations.

In addition to these two well-defined pathologic manifestations of disease, there is also evidence that inhaled particles in polluted air may have an important effect on the overall health of the general population,[3] by increasing both the mortality and the morbidity from respiratory disease.[4–7]

To establish a causal relationship between an inhaled dust and an adverse biologic effect in a particular individual or occupational group, demonstration of a history of significant dust exposure as well as abnormalities in pulmonary function, chest radiographs, CT images, or lung structure is required. Analysis of the concentration and particle size of the dust in the workers' "breathing zone" can be useful, and the results should be taken into consideration whenever available. Analysis of inorganic material in the lungs themselves, obtained from either tissue specimens or bronchoalveolar lavage (BAL) fluid samples,[8, 9] can also be helpful. Such analysis ranges from simple examination by standard light microscopy to tissue digestion and particle quantification to energy-dispersive x-ray analysis (*see* page 355).[9a] A detailed occupational history is also important, not only in helping to determine a direct relationship between occupation and disease, but also because certain jobs not usually regarded as harmful can become so if carried out in proximity to other, potentially hazardous occupations, such as welding and sandblasting.[10]

Even when all investigations show convincing evidence for the presence of a pneumoconiosis, the precise cause may not be evident. This uncertainty is related, in part, to the fact that individuals in many occupations are exposed to more than one type of dust; an analysis of lung tissue can reflect this multiplicity, and it is sometimes difficult to attribute pathologic changes to one specific substance. For example, shale miners sometimes develop progressive massive fibrosis similar to that seen in coal miners; their lungs have been shown to contain dust composed of a combination of kaolinite, mica, and silica,[11] each of which can itself cause pulmonary disease. Individuals in numerous other occupations, such as locomotive drivers and stokers, plastics manufacturers,[12] dental technicians,[13–15] foundry workers,[16, 17] welders,[18] and miners and millers of many minerals,[19] are also at risk for the development of pneumoconiosis caused by inhalation of more than one dust; in fact, the term *mixed dust pneumoconiosis* is sometimes used to refer to the ensuing disease.[20] Pathologically, such disease is typically localized to the peribronchiolovascular interstitium and is characterized by the accumulation of numerous dust-containing macrophages and a variable amount of fibrous tissue (Fig. 60–1).

Because pneumoconiosis is by definition related to dust exposure, the disease is strongly associated with the workplace, particularly with jobs that lead to the production of abundant airborne particles. Recognition of the relationship

between such particles and pulmonary disease has led to the imposition of government regulations to control the amount of respirable dust in the workplace. Although such regulations have had an effect in reducing both the prevalence and the severity of disease, exposure continues to be poorly controlled in many industries,[21, 22] particularly in "developing" countries.[23] Current surveillance systems for pneumoconiosis probably underestimate the prevalence of disease in the latter regions; however, it is likely that their extent will become more evident in the future as a result of dissemination of knowledge and thorough epidemiologic studies.[24]

Although the inorganic dust pneumoconioses are predominantly occupational diseases, there is no question that they can also develop in individuals who live in the vicinity of industrial plants (particularly those handling asbestos or beryllium) but who do not work there. Such "para-occupational" disease can occur in spouses and children of workers who transport hazardous material on clothing from the workplace into the home[25] or in individuals who simply breathe air contaminated by the nearby mine or industry. Therefore, in any patient in whom the presence of a dust-related disease is suspected, an occupational history should also be obtained from family members. In addition, the site of the patient's residence in relation to industrial plants should be considered. It is also important to remember that inhalation of potentially toxic particles can occur in the house unassociated with their occupational use[26, 27] and in an environment in which there are no hazardous industries (e.g., in association with dust storms[27] or soil that has a high content of a specific mineral[28]).

The reaction of the lung to inhaled inorganic dust depends on many factors, each of which is important by itself but all of which must be considered in combination because they are to a certain extent interdependent. These factors include the chemical nature of the dust, the size and shape of dust particles, the concentration of dust particles in the ambient air, the duration of an individual's exposure to the dust, the rate and pattern of breathing as the dust is inhaled, the distribution and clearance of inhaled dust in the lungs, and individual variations in immune and inflammatory response. These factors are discussed in greater detail on page 126.

INTERNATIONAL CLASSIFICATION OF RADIOGRAPHS OF THE PNEUMOCONIOSES

The chest radiograph is an important tool in detecting the effects of dust particle deposition in the lungs and in measuring disease progression.[29] For it to be useful in epidemiologic studies, however, it is essential that an acceptable classification of extent of involvement be followed and a standard nomenclature be employed. Several such classifications have been developed over the years, all of which have evolved from the first International Labour Office (ILO) classification contained in the "Report of the International Conference on Silicosis," Johannesburg, 1930.[30] The most widely used schema is the ILO 1980 International Classification of Radiographs of the Pneumoconioses.[30a]

The object of this classification is to codify the radiographic changes of the pneumoconioses in a simple, reproducible manner. Although it does not define pathologic enti-

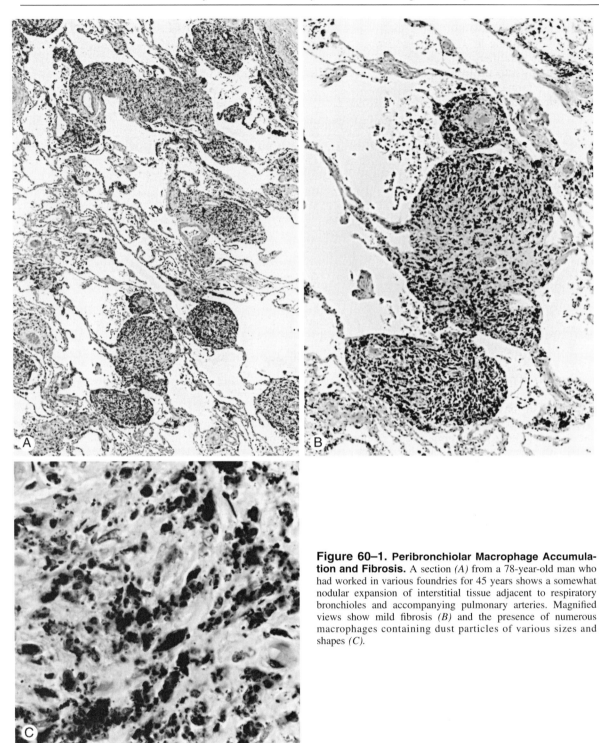

Figure 60–1. Peribronchiolar Macrophage Accumulation and Fibrosis. A section *(A)* from a 78-year-old man who had worked in various foundries for 45 years shows a somewhat nodular expansion of interstitial tissue adjacent to respiratory bronchioles and accompanying pulmonary arteries. Magnified views show mild fibrosis *(B)* and the presence of numerous macrophages containing dust particles of various sizes and shapes *(C).*

ties, it possesses the considerable advantage of providing a uniform, semiquantitative method of reporting the type and extent of disease, thus leading to international comparability of pneumoconiosis statistics. The classification provides a means of systematically recording the radiographic changes in the chest caused by the inhalation of all types of mineral dusts, including coal, silica, carbon, asbestos, and beryllium. It is particularly valuable for epidemiologic studies but is also useful in the evaluation of patients for compensation purposes. Standard reference radiographs have been selected to illustrate the ILO 1980 classification and can be purchased

from the ILO office. Because the schema employs radiographic descriptors that are somewhat different from those generally used throughout this book, a short glossary of terms follows.

International Labour Office Radiographic Terms

Terms requiring explanation are discussed here. All other terms used in the classification are self-explanatory and identical in context to those used elsewhere in this book.

Small Rounded Opacities. These are well-circumscribed opacities or nodules ranging in diameter from barely visible up to 10 mm. The qualifiers *p*, *q*, and *r* subdivide the predominant opacities into three diameter ranges—p, up to 1.5 mm; q, 1.5 to 3 mm; and r, 3 to 10 mm.

Small Irregular Opacities. This term is employed to describe a pattern that, elsewhere in this book, has been designated *linear, reticular,* or *reticulonodular*—in other words, a netlike pattern. Although the nature of these opacities is such that the establishment of quantitative dimensions is considerably more difficult than with rounded opacities, the ILO has seen fit to establish three categories—s, width up to about 1.5 mm; t, width exceeding 1.5 mm and up to about 3 mm; and u, width exceeding 3 mm and up to about 10 mm.

To record shape and size, two letters must be used. Thus, if the reader considers that all or virtually all opacities are one shape and size, this is noted by recording the symbol twice, separated by an oblique stroke (e.g., *q/q*). If another shape or size is seen, this is recorded as the second letter (e.g., *q/t*). The designation *q/t* means that the predominant small opacity is round and of size q but that there are, in addition, a significant number of small irregular opacities of size t. In this way, any combination of small opacities can be recorded.

Profusion. This term refers to the number of small rounded or small irregular opacities per unit area or zone of lung. There are four basic categories: category 0, small opacities absent or less profuse than in category 1; category 1, small opacities definitely present but few in number (normal lung markings are usually visible); category 2, numerous small opacities (normal lung markings are usually partly obscured); and category 3, very numerous small opacities (normal lung markings are usually totally obscured). These categories can be further subdivided by employing a 12-point scale, in which there is a continuum of changes from complete normality to the most advanced category or grade:[31, 32]

0/−	0/0	0/1
1/0	1/1	1/2
2/1	2/2	2/3
3/2	3/3	3/+

Employing this scale, the radiograph is first classified in the usual way into one of the four categories—0, 1, 2, or 3. If the category above or below is considered as a serious alternative during the process, it is recorded (e.g., a radiograph in which profusion is considered to be category 2 but for which category 1 was seriously considered as an alternative would be graded category 2/1). If no alternative is considered (i.e., the profusion was definitely category 2), it would be classified *2/2*.

A subdivision is also possible within categories 0 and 3. Category 0/1 is profusion of category 0 with category 1 seriously considered as an alternative. Category 0/0 is a radiograph in which there are no small opacities or one in which a few opacities are thought to be present but are not sufficiently definite or numerous for category 1 to be considered. If the absence of small opacities is particularly obvious, profusion should be recorded as 0/−. Such a category might be seen in a healthy nonsmoking adolescent. A radiograph that shows profusion markedly higher than that classifiable as 3/3 would be recorded as 3/+. The ILO standard films are the final arbitrators of opacity profusion and take precedence over any application of a verbal description of profusion. A film is placed in category 1 if it resembles the ILO standard film of the same category and opacity type. Thus, this type of reading should always be done side by side with the ILO standard films.

Large Opacities. This term is used for opacities that are larger than the maximum permitted for small rounded opacities (i.e., > 10 mm). Three categories are recognized: category A, an opacity having a greatest diameter exceeding 1 cm up to and including 5 cm or several opacities each greater than 1 cm, the sum of whose greatest diameters does not exceed 5 cm; category B, comprising one or more opacities larger or more numerous than those in category A whose combined area does not exceed the equivalent of the right upper lung zone; and category C, consisting of one or more opacities whose combined area exceeds the equivalent of the right upper lung zone.

Extent. Each lung is divided into three zones—upper, middle, and lower—by horizontal lines drawn at one third and two thirds of the vertical distance between the apex of the lung and the dome of the diaphragm.

Radiographic Interpretation

Since enactment in 1969 of the U.S. Federal Coal Miners' Health and Safety Act, which provided certain benefits to coal miners who have pneumoconiosis, much attention has been directed toward decision-making processes and observer error in the radiographic diagnosis of pneumoconiosis.[33–35] A common feature of all published reports has been an exceptionally high degree of interreader variability and observer error, which has been attributed to a combination of lack of experience with the classification systems employed, lack of familiarity with the radiographic manifestations of pneumoconiosis, and poor film quality.

As a result of these deficiencies, the National Institute of Occupational Safety and Health (NIOSH) has established an examination that is administered to physicians who wish to be certified as interpreters of chest radiographs in pneumoconiosis programs; the examination is preceded by a weekend course administered by the American College of Radiology. Completion of the course establishes the physician as an *A reader*; successful completion of the examination results in the designation *B reader*. To maintain B reader status, a candidate must undergo a recertification examination every 4 years. Nonexpert readings of films compare poorly with ILO readings when this methodology is used as a screening tool for exposed workers.[36] Expert readers are also unlikely to "overread" films as positive, as illustrated in a large study of nonexposed blue-collar workers.[37] There is little doubt, however, that there is a background level of opacities consistent with the radiographic appearance of pneumoconiosis in populations who do not have occupational exposure to dust.[38, 39] In one meta-analysis in which this issue was addressed, a population prevalence of 5.3% was identified for small densities of profusion greater than or equal to 1/0.[38] The prevalence was significantly greater in Europe (11.3%) than in North America (1.6%), in men (5.5%) than in women (3.5%), and in older than in younger individuals.

In North America, the age-specific pooled prevalence was 2.3% in studies in which the mean patient age was greater than or equal to 50 years and only 0.6% in those in which it was less than 50.

When assessing radiographic progression of simple pneumoconiosis in individual miners, it is recommended that all films be viewed together in known temporal order.[29, 35, 40] Side-by-side reading has been shown to lead to substantially lower observer error and variability than independent reading. The manner of application of the ILO system to epidemiologic studies has been variable,[41] however, making it difficult to compare the findings of all studies in an ideal fashion.

SILICA

Silica is a ubiquitous, abundant mineral composed of regularly arranged molecules of silicon dioxide (SiO_2). It occurs in three forms: (1) *crystalline*, which exists primarily as quartz, tridymite, or cristobalite, depending on the temperature of formation; (2) *microcrystalline*, consisting of minute crystals of quartz bonded together by amorphous silica and exemplified by flint and chert; and (3) *amorphous* (noncrystalline), consisting of kieselguhr (composed of the skeletal remains of diatoms) or vitreous forms (derived by heating and rapid cooling of crystalline material). Occupational exposure to and the fibrogenic potential of these substances vary, a feature that is important in understanding the development of disease in different individuals and different situations. Pure ("free") silica is composed predominantly of SiO_2 and must be distinguished from other substances in which SiO_2 is combined with an appreciable proportion of cations ("combined" silica, silicates); the latter include asbestos, talc, and mica and are associated with different clinicopathologic forms of disease (*see* farther on).

Epidemiology

Exposure to a concentration of silica high enough to result in radiographic and pathologic manifestations of silicosis occurs predominantly in occupational settings. Numerous occupations have been associated with such exposure; examples include sandblasting; stonecutting, engraving, and polishing; work with gemstones;[42, 43] the use of clay dye by Japanese rush matting workers;[44] foundry work involving the production of molds, knocking out of castings, and cleaning and polishing (fettling) of the final product;[45] the manufacture of grinding wheels,[46] glass and silica bricks, and crucibles; slate pencil manufacturing;[47, 48] the use of potter's clay and powdered flint in the ceramic industry;[49, 50] and the use of ochre,[51] bentonite,[52] and enamel.[53] The reader is referred to more comprehensive sources for further details of these and other forms of work;[54-59] however, several deserve specific comment.

Because of the ubiquity of silica in the earth's crust, mining, tunneling, and quarrying almost inevitably lead to some exposure to the mineral, unless it involves pure limestone or marble.[57] Thus, the mining of such varied substances as gold, tin, iron, copper, nickel, silver, granite,[51, 60-62] and uranium[57] is a particularly common cause of silicosis.

Moreover, the mining of other minerals recognized as causes of pneumoconiosis—such as coal, tungsten,[63] and barium[64, 65]—can also be accompanied by silica exposure, and there is no doubt that the lung disease that appears in some individuals who work with these minerals results from "contaminating" silica, at least in part.

Diatomaceous earth is used in the manufacture of paints, varnishes, and insecticides and in filtration and other processes.[66-69] Although generally considered to be relatively inert in its amorphous form, the substance is converted into cristobalite and tridymite when heated,[57] and exposure to these substances has been associated with a rare but apparently virulent form of disease. Silica flour is a finely ground form of the mineral composed of 99% SiO_2; it has been employed as an abrasive, paint extender, and filler for cosmetics and other manufactured items.[70] Its use as an abrasive scouring powder was among the earliest recognized causes of the acute variety of silicosis (*see* farther on);[71, 72] more recently, its use as a polisher or buffer has been reported to be responsible for cases of silicosis in gemstone[73] and jade[74] workers in Hong Kong and in furniture workers in Japan.[75] In one study of 1,809 workers involved in mining and processing of diatomaceous earth in a California facility, evidence of silicosis was identified in 81 (4.5%).[75a]

Although the nature of the occupations involved in exposure to silica dust limits the disease mainly to men, roughly half the individuals at risk in the pottery industry are women, many of whom exhibit typical features of pneumoconiosis.[76] One form of environmental lung disease characterized by increased silica deposition is seen predominantly in women. This variety is associated with the inhalation of fine sand particles and is thus encountered principally in deserts, such as the Negev in Israel.[77] Histologic examination of the lungs of a number of affected individuals has revealed only increased silica deposition without the usual silicotic reaction, leading to the designation *simple siliceous pneumoconiosis* rather than silicosis. This disease is both environmental and occupational because it may involve increased dust inhalation in the tents during the making of cloth from sheep's wool. It is analogous to the Transkei silicosis that is restricted to Bantu women who grind their food with sandstone, thus freeing large amounts of silica particles into the air.[78] Other environmental, nonoccupational exposure to silica causing disease has occurred in some Himalayan populations[79, 80] and in individuals who have perversely inhaled domestic scouring powder.[81-83]

Although the precise incidence and prevalence of silicosis are difficult to assess, there can be little doubt that the disease is one of the most frequent of the pneumoconioses. It has been estimated that as many as 3 million workers in 238,000 processing plants in the United States are potentially exposed to silica dust.[84] Although government regulations in some countries limit the severity of such exposure, current surveillance systems for silicosis likely underestimate the prevalence of the disease because exposure continues to be poorly controlled in many industries.[21, 22, 85-88] In one investigation of 577 people who had silicosis and were reported to the Michigan Department of Public Health between 1987 and 1995, more than half were from hospital identification of disease;[89] most had advanced silicosis, and less than half had applied for compensation. Although most patients had begun working in iron foundries in the 1930s or 1940s and had been exposed to silica dust for more than 20 years, about 15% had exposure to dust beginning in the 1960s or later, including three whose first exposure was in the 1980s. In the United States, silicosis was listed on death certificates as a primary or contributing cause of death in more than 4,000 workers between 1979 and 1990;[90] some of them have been young adults.[90a]

In "developing" countries, the situation is much worse. For example, in a study of 1,520 black South African gold miners who died from "unnatural" causes in 1990–1991, approximately 13% were found to have evidence of silicosis at autopsy.[91] In China, almost 75,000 cases of silicosis were identified between 1949 and 1986;[92] among the pneumoconioses, it accounted for the greatest potential years of life and work lost.

Pathogenesis

In addition to clinical and pathologic observations, numerous investigations of experimental animals and cell cultures have resulted in the recognition of a variety of factors that may be important in the pathogenesis of silica-induced pulmonary disease. Such factors must attempt to explain the two fundamental histologic reactions to inhaled silica: (1) the *silicotic nodule*, which is characterized by dense, often concentric lamellae of collagen and which when multiple and conglomerated result in a lesion termed *progressive massive fibrosis* (PMF)*; and (2) *silicoproteinosis*, which typically occurs in individuals or animals exposed to high concentrations of silica and which is characterized by alveolar filling by lipoproteinaceous material similar to that seen in idiopathic alveolar proteinosis. The majority of experimental studies have focused on the first of these reactions because it is by far the more common.[56, 93–96a]

As might be expected, the likelihood of disease and its severity are determined to a large extent by the intensity of exposure to crystalline silica dust. The U.S. Public Health Service statements of concentration of dust particles in the atmosphere describe primary and secondary thresholds. The *primary threshold* consists of 5×10^6 particles less than 10 μm in size per cubic foot; exposure to concentrations below this level does not result in silicosis. The *secondary threshold* consists of 100×10^6 particles of the same size per cubic foot; all persons exposed at or above this level acquire silicosis. Although the risk for silicosis is thus related to total exposure, the latent period for its development appears to be largely independent of dose.[97] In addition, because of the typical long latency for the development of silicosis after exposure, because disease may progress after exposure has ceased, and because silicosis may be diagnosed only after the worker has left the workforce, estimates of risk after any given exposure may be flawed.[90] The appreciation of this uncertainty has called into question the appropriateness of certain safety standards and has led to the proposal of the more stringent exposure standard of 0.05 mg/m³ by NIOSH.

*Although some lesions do not appear to be progressive and, according to the size definition, many are clearly not massive, the term "progressive massive fibrosis" is firmly entrenched in the literature and is used throughout this text.

The interaction of silica with the pulmonary macrophage is a key factor in the pathogenesis of silicosis. Shortly after deposition of dust in alveolar ducts, pulmonary alveolar macrophages become concentrated in the area,[98] an event possibly initiated by activation of complement present in the alveolar lining fluid.[99] Such activation releases C5a, a powerful macrophage chemoattractant.[100] The inhaled particles are ingested by alveolar macrophages or penetrate to the interstitium, where they may be engulfed by tissue macrophages.[56] There is evidence that the latter react differently to silica than alveolar macrophages[101] and that this reaction is more important in the pathogenesis of ensuing fibrosis.[102, 103]

The fundamental physicochemical characteristic of silica responsible for its toxicity is uncertain. It appears likely to be related to its surface properties, perhaps surface charge,[104] and is unassociated with solubility and surface area.[93] Although early *in vitro* studies suggested that silica ingestion resulted in macrophage death and the release of a variety of toxic products,[105–107] it now appears that alveolar macrophages that have ingested silica have normal viability and basal function *in vivo*.[108, 109] The results of both human[110–112] and animal[113, 114] studies have shown that such silica-exposed macrophages release a variety of fibroblast growth factors, including tumor necrosis factor (TNF),[113] macrophage-derived growth factor,[115] transforming growth factor-β,[112] interferon,[116] fibronectin,[111, 117] and interleukin-1 (IL-1).[118, 119] These substances appear to be associated with the subsequent accumulation of fibroblasts and fibroblast products.[93] Although macrophages may also release products that inhibit fibroblast activation, such as prostaglandin E_2,[121] there is evidence that that this is relatively unimportant in the pathogenesis of the disease.[110] An increased amount of IL-10 has been found to be produced by cells in BAL fluid after silica exposure in a murine model of silicosis;[122] although this was associated with an anti-inflammatory effect, the fibrotic response to silica in the lung was unexpectedly amplified in the long term. In humans exposed to inorganic dusts, oxidant release from macrophages is also enhanced;[123, 124] these toxic chemicals may act by causing epithelial cell damage, thereby facilitating the exposure of interstitial cells, such as fibroblasts, to the products of macrophage and lymphocyte secretion.[96]

The interaction of macrophages with other inflammatory or immune cells is also likely to be important in the pathogenesis of silicosis.[120, 125] Lymphocytes—particularly T-helper cells—are increased in number in BAL fluid from both patients and experimental animals that have silicosis.[126, 127] Inflammatory mediators, such as IL-1, induce T lymphocytes to release IL-2,[118, 119] which creates an expanded population of activated helper T lymphocytes. These, in turn, may secrete mediators that activate and amplify macrophage function.[93]

Several observations support the hypothesis that immune-related tissue damage is involved in the pathogenesis of silicosis, including the presence of a variety of serologic abnormalities—such as rheumatoid factor, antinuclear antibodies,[128] immune complexes,[129, 130] and polyclonal gamma globulin[130, 131]—and, occasionally, clinical evidence of immune disturbance,[132–138] particularly kidney disease.[132, 133, 139, 140] Protein adsorbed onto silica crystals can theoretically act as an antigen, and it has been speculated that the silicotic nodule contains antigen-antibody precipitates.[131] BAL fluid from patients who have silicosis also contains an increased quantity of immunoglobulin that appears to be produced locally.[141] It is possible that collagen itself serves as the antigen for these reactions,[142-144] resulting in a cycle in which antibodies stimulate macrophages to enhance fibrosis, thereby increasing antibody response in a positive feedback fashion.

Polymorphonuclear leukocytes are an important source of proteolytic enzymes and reactive oxygen species and could theoretically be responsible for some tissue damage in silicosis.[145] These cells have been shown to accumulate in the lungs of silica-exposed individuals, with or without evidence of silicosis.[108] Leukotriene B$_4$ released from macrophages has been implicated as a chemoattractant in the process.[113] There is also experimental evidence that mast cells are involved.[146] Because BAL fluid in patients who have silicosis contains significant amounts of protease and elastase inhibitors,[147] the quantitative effect of neutrophils in the pathogenesis of silicosis is uncertain.[94]

The reasons for the development of PMF in some individuals and not others are unclear. In general, it is associated with a high lung content of silica,[148] a history of tuberculosis,[149, 150] or a background of increased profusion of small opacities.[149] It is possible that genetic differences may explain variations in disease severity among workers who have similar dust exposures; for example, workers who have PMF have a higher prevalence of HLA-AW19,[151] and an excess prevalence of HLA A29 and B44 has been described in workers with simple silicosis.[152] Environmental factors, such as cigarette smoke or inhaled fibrogenic particles in addition to silica, may also be involved. For example, there is evidence that cigarette smoke increases epithelial permeability to silica;[153] because the severity of fibrosis may be related to the amount of silica reaching the interstitial tissue,[102, 103] this may be important in explaining individual reactions.

In contrast to the fibrosis associated with chronic, relatively low-dose exposure to silica, it is perhaps surprising that acute exposure to large amounts of dust results in little collagen deposition in both animals[154] and humans.[155, 156] Instead, it is associated with the production of abundant intra-alveolar proteinaceous material, virtually identical histologically and ultrastructurally to that seen in alveolar proteinosis.[156] The pathogenesis of this reaction is unclear. Experimentally, instillation of silica into the lungs is followed by type I alveolar cell injury and type II cell hyperplasia and hypertrophy,[157, 158] suggesting that an increase in surfactant-producing cells might be a factor. Although it is theoretically possible that silica also directly stimulates type II cells to manufacture and secrete excessive alveolar lining material, experimental findings suggest that this does not occur.[159, 160]

It has also been hypothesized that silica may disturb the ability of macrophages to clear normally produced surfactant from the alveolar air space, thus resulting in its increase at this site.[161] Freshly fractured silica possesses a greater biologic reactivity than the aged form;[162] for example, oxidant production has been found to be enhanced and antioxidant production depressed when silica is freshly fractured rather than aged.[163] Because acute silicoproteinosis is associated with occupations in which fractured silica is likely to be generated, it is possible that these or other related effects are important in the pathogenesis of the disease. The reason for

the lack of fibrosis in acute silicoproteinosis is also unclear; however, it has been shown that coating silica particles with alveolar lining material results in significantly less cytotoxicity for ingesting macrophages,[164] a finding that may result in decreased production of fibrogenic mediators relative to classic silicosis. Altered macrophage function probably underlies the greater susceptibility to tuberculosis of patients who have both silicosis and acute silicoproteinosis; *Mycobacterium tuberculosis* grows much more rapidly in cultures of macrophages exposed to sublethal doses of quartz than in those without such exposure.[165]

Pathologic Characteristics

The pathologic features of silicosis have been reviewed in detail in a report by the Silicosis and Silicate Disease Committee of NIOSH.[166] Grossly, silicotic nodules range from 1 to 10 mm in diameter and typically are more numerous in the upper lobes and parahilar regions than elsewhere (Fig. 60–2). Cut sections show the nodules to be more or less well defined, spherical or irregularly shaped, and firm to hard in texture; calcification or ossification is occasionally present. Depending on the admixture of other dusts, the nodules range in color from slate gray to dense black. Coalescence of nodules results in larger masses that can occupy virtually an entire lobe (PMF) (Fig. 60–3). Such masses are usually associated with adjacent (irregular) emphysema and may be cavitated as a result of ischemia, tuberculosis, or infection by anaerobic organisms.[167] Bronchopulmonary lymph nodes are often somewhat enlarged and rubbery in consistency as a result of fibrosis; the latter may extend beyond the nodal capsule into the adjacent bronchial wall and may be associated with distortion of the underlying bronchial anatomy (Fig. 60–4) and, rarely, significant airway stenosis.[167a]

Microscopically, the earliest lesions are characteristically located in the peribronchiolar, interlobular septal, and pleural interstitial tissues. Initially, they consist predominantly of macrophages with scattered reticulin fibers. As the lesions enlarge, the central portions become hypocellular and composed of mature collagen, sometimes arranged in more or less concentric lamellae; a peripheral zone of macrophages and lesser numbers of plasma cells and lymphocytes surrounds this central portion (Fig. 60–5). Occasionally, the inflammation is granulomatous in nature, similar to that seen in Caplan's lesions of coal workers' pneumoconiosis (CWP) (*see* farther on). Type II cells adjacent to the fibrotic region may be hyperplastic and presumably are the source from which these cells have been identified in BAL specimens.[168] A variable number of birefringent silicate crystals 1 to 3 μm in length can usually be identified by polarization microscopy in the cellular areas of the fibrotic nodules (*see* Fig. 60–5); these can also be identified by their metachromatic staining with toluidine blue.[169] Occasionally, crystals are not apparent with polarization microscopy, and more sophisticated techniques, such as scanning electron microscopy, are required to reveal their presence.[170]

The larger conglomerate lesions of PMF are also composed of hyalinized collagen admixed with variable numbers of pigmented macrophages. The concentric lamellar appearance of the collagen seen in silicotic nodules is frequently

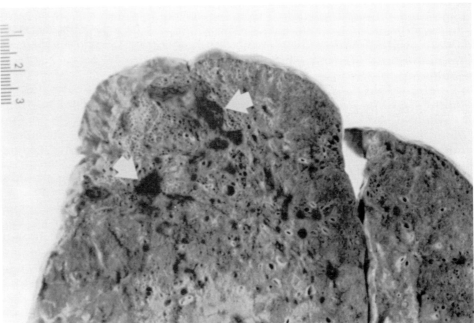

Figure 60–2. Silicosis: Silicotic Nodules. A slice of an upper lobe and superior segment of the lower lobe shows multiple well-defined, somewhat irregularly shaped nodules within the lung parenchyma *(arrows)*. The nodules are black as a result of the presence of abundant anthracotic pigment.

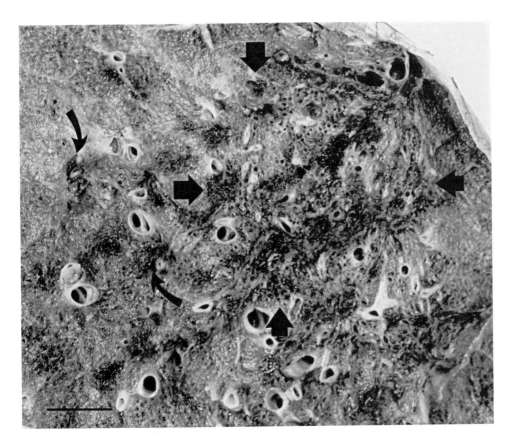

Figure 60–3. Silicosis: Progressive Massive Fibrosis. A magnified view of the posterior segment of the right upper lobe shows several small discrete silicotic nodules *(curved arrows)*. In addition, confluence of nodules has resulted in an irregularly shaped area of fibrosis approximately 3 × 4 cm in extent *(indicated by large arrows)*. (Bar = 1 cm.)

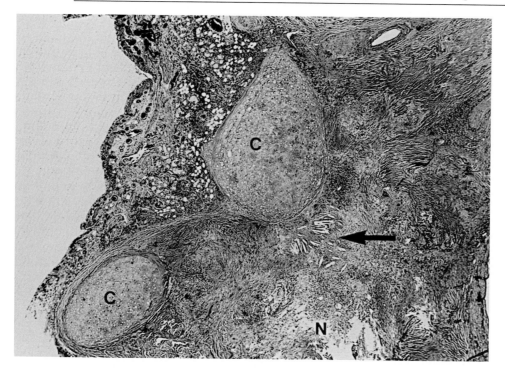

Figure 60–4. Silicosis: Bronchial Wall Fibrosis. A focus of fibrosis caused by silicosis has extended outside a peribronchial lymph node into the adjacent bronchial wall (the node itself is not visible in the illustration). The fibrous tissue and pigment-laden macrophages extend into the submucosa; the bronchial cartilage plates (C) are somewhat distorted. Note the cholesterol clefts *(arrow)* and focal necrosis (N) indicating the histologic changes of progressive massive fibrosis. (×15.)

not evident. Focal necrosis is common in the central portions (Fig. 60–6) and is occasionally associated with granulomatous inflammation, in which case the presence of tuberculous infection should be considered.

Fibrotic nodules identical to those found in the lungs can also be identified elsewhere in the body (sometimes in individuals with no history of significant occupational dust exposure,[171] in which case their origin is unclear). As might be expected, they are most frequent in the hilar and mediastinal lymph nodes; in fact, in our experience, this is the most common pathologic manifestation of silica exposure, presumably reflecting relatively greater concentration of dust at these sites than in the lungs and decreased exposure of the worker population as a result of government regulations. As in peribronchial lymph nodes, the fibrous reaction may extend outside the nodal capsule into adjacent mediastinal tissue; because of this spread and the firmness of the nodes, there may be confusion with metastatic carcinoma at mediastinoscopy or intraoperative mediastinal exploration. Fibrotic nodules caused by silica are also occasionally found in the liver, spleen, intra-abdominal lymph nodes, and bone marrow.[139, 171a]

The pathologic findings in acute heavy silica exposure differ significantly from those described previously. Although there may be mild interstitial fibrosis and focal small nodular lesions, well-defined collagenous nodules are typically absent. Instead, alveolar air spaces are more or less diffusely filled by somewhat granular, periodic acid–Schiff (PAS)–positive proteinaceous material identical to that seen in idiopathic alveolar proteinosis (Fig. 60–7). Macrophages are present in increased numbers, and alveolar type II cells show a varying degree of hyperplasia and hypertrophy. Ultrastructurally, the intra-alveolar material contains macrophages and desquamated type II cells as well as membranous material resembling that seen in the normal alveolar lining layer.[156]

Radiologic Manifestations

The classic radiographic pattern of silicosis consists of multiple nodular opacities ranging from 1 to 10 mm in diameter (Figs. 60–8 and 60–9). The nodules are usually well circumscribed and of uniform density. Although profusion can be fairly even throughout both lungs, there is commonly considerable upper lobe predominance. The nodules also tend to involve mainly the posterior portion of the lungs (*see* Fig. 60–8).[172] Nodules have been identified on pathologic examination that were not seen on premortem chest radiographs in many cases.[173] Calcification of nodules is evident on the radiograph in 10% to 20% of cases (Fig. 60–10). A reticular pattern may be seen when silicosis is caused by diatomaceous earth[66, 67] but is distinctly uncommon in other settings.

The radiographic pattern of small round or irregular opacities is commonly referred to as *simple* silicosis, in contrast to *complicated* silicosis (PMF). The latter is characterized by large opacities (conglomerate shadows) (Fig. 60–11) usually in the upper lobes (Fig. 60–12). By definition, the opacities measure greater than 1 cm in diameter; they may become very large (Fig. 60–13), exceeding the volume of an upper lobe in aggregate. The shadow margins may be irregular and somewhat ill-defined or smooth,[174] creating an interface that parallels the lateral chest wall (*see* Fig. 60–13). The opacities commonly develop in the midzone or periphery of the lung; with time, they tend to migrate toward the hilum, leaving emphysematous lung between the fibrotic tissue and the pleural surface.[175] Although usually bilateral, unilateral opacities may occur and may be confused with carcinoma (Fig. 60–14). Cavitation develops occasionally. The more extensive the conglomerate fibrosis, the less apparent is nodularity in the remainder of the lungs (*see* Fig. 60–14).[175] There is seldom any radiographic evidence of pleural abnormality.

Text continued on page 2402

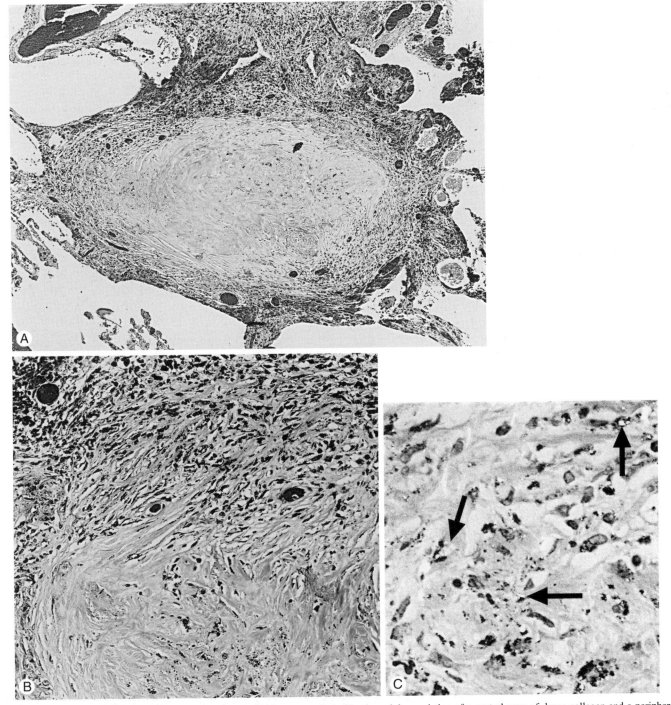

Figure 60–5. Silicotic Nodule. A histologic section *(A)* shows a typical silicotic nodule consisting of a central zone of dense collagen and a peripheral rim of macrophages in which abundant foreign particulate material is situated. A section at higher magnification *(B)* shows these characteristics to better advantage. *(A, ×40; B, ×150.)* Magnified view *(C)* of macrophages with polarization microscopy shows multiple variably sized and shaped refractile (white) particles *(arrows)* consistent with silicates.

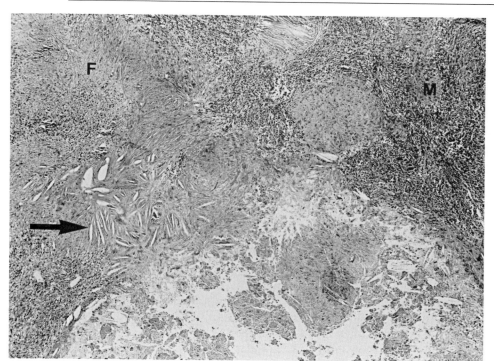

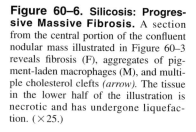

Figure 60–6. Silicosis: Progressive Massive Fibrosis. A section from the central portion of the confluent nodular mass illustrated in Figure 60–3 reveals fibrosis (F), aggregates of pigment-laden macrophages (M), and multiple cholesterol clefts *(arrow)*. The tissue in the lower half of the illustration is necrotic and has undergone liquefaction. (×25.)

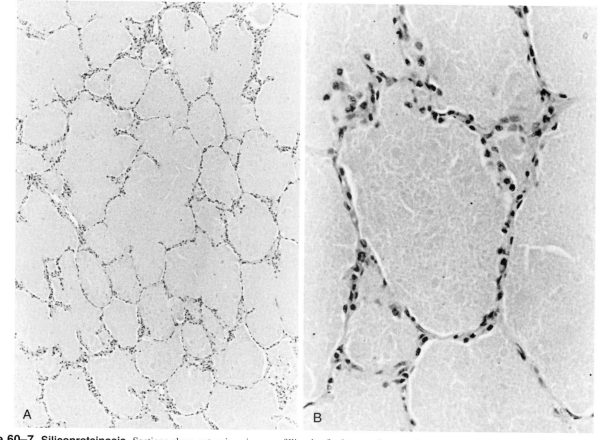

Figure 60–7. Silicoproteinosis. Sections show extensive air-space filling by finely granular proteinaceous material identical to that seen in idiopathic alveolar proteinosis. Alveolar septa are essentially unremarkable. The patient was a 25-year-old dental technician who was exposed to a large quantity of silica dust while manufacturing dental prostheses. (Courtesy of Dr. Joachim Majo, Barcelona, Spain.)

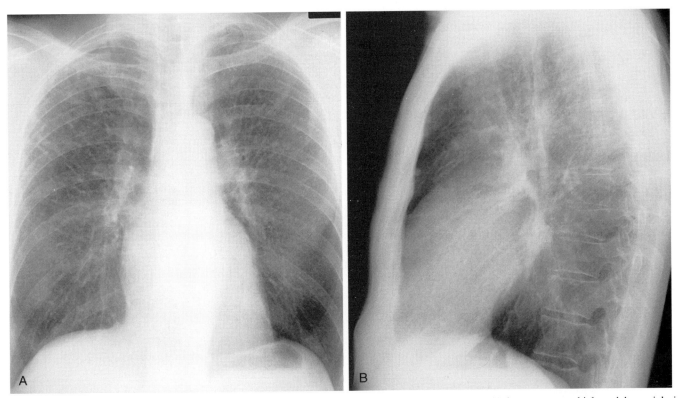

Figure 60–8. Silicosis: Characteristic Radiographic Findings. A posteroanterior chest radiograph *(A)* demonstrates multiple nodules mainly in the middle and upper lung zones. A lateral radiograph *(B)* reveals that most of the nodules are situated in the posterior half of the lungs. The nodules measure more than 3 mm in diameter (International Labour Office [ILO] r shape). Their profusion is 2/1, slightly less than the ILO standard radiograph for a profusion of 2/2 but considerably more than that with a score of 1/1. The patient was a 60-year-old miner.

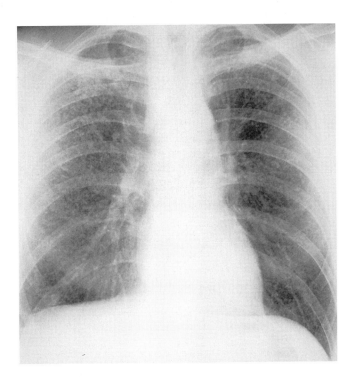

Figure 60–9. Silicosis: Characteristic Radiographic Findings. A posteroanterior chest radiograph demonstrates numerous well-defined small nodules mainly in the upper and middle lung zones. The nodules measure 1.5 to 3 mm in diameter (International Labour Office [ILO] q size nodules), and the profusion is 2/3 (slightly greater than the ILO standard radiograph for profusion 2/2 but considerably less than the standard for profusion 3/3). Early conglomeration is present near the lung apices.

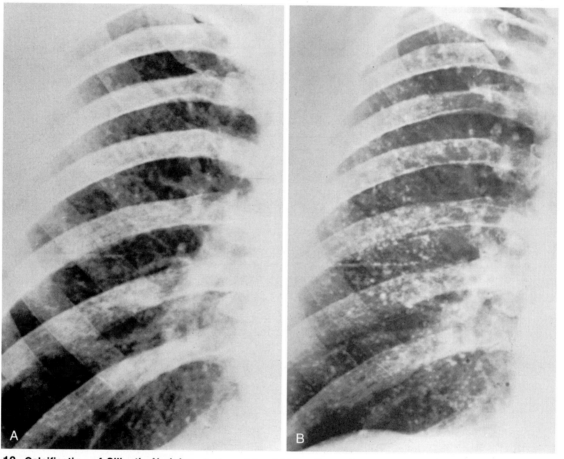

Figure 60–10. Calcification of Silicotic Nodules. A view of the right hemithorax from a posteroanterior radiograph of a 32-year-old man *(A)* reveals involvement of all lung zones by small irregular opacities of unit density. Eighteen years later *(B),* multiple punctate calcifications had developed throughout the right lung, representing calcification of the silicotic nodules. The patient had a history of 26 years' work in South African gold mines. (Courtesy of Dr. Raymond Glynn-Thomas, Medical Bureau for Occupational Diseases, Johannesburg, South Africa.)

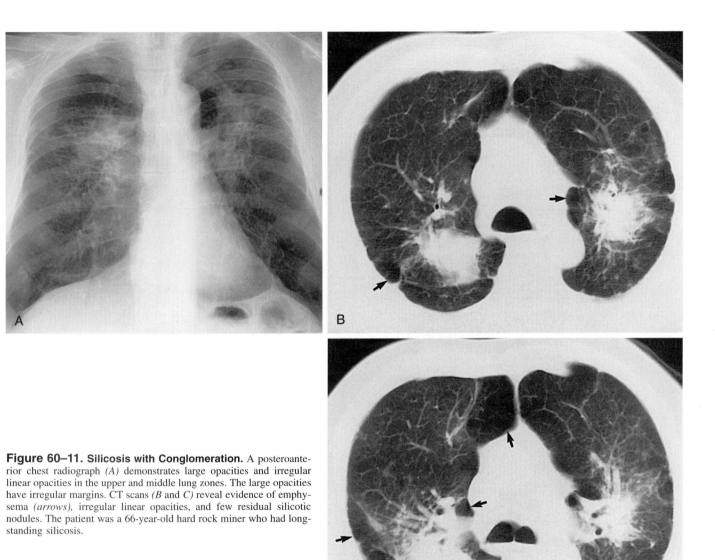

Figure 60–11. Silicosis with Conglomeration. A posteroante-rior chest radiograph *(A)* demonstrates large opacities and irregular linear opacities in the upper and middle lung zones. The large opacities have irregular margins. CT scans *(B* and *C)* reveal evidence of emphy-sema *(arrows),* irregular linear opacities, and few residual silicotic nodules. The patient was a 66-year-old hard rock miner who had long-standing silicosis.

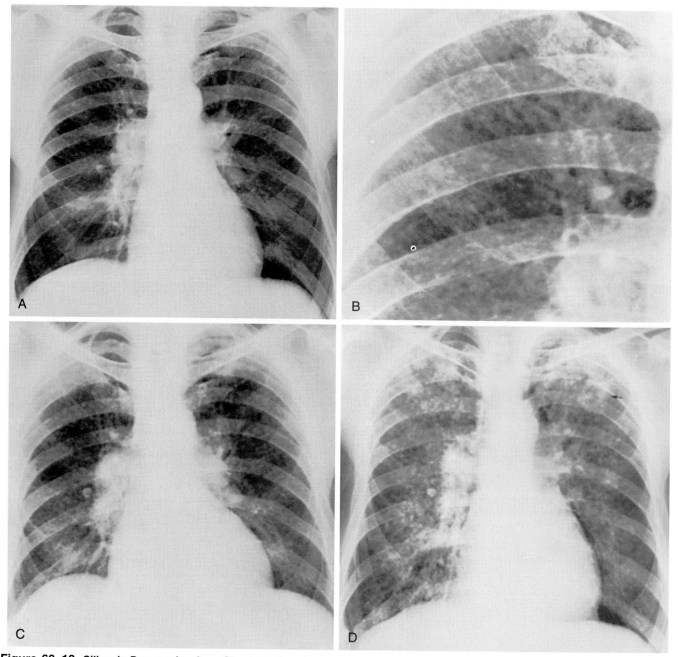

Figure 60–12. Silicosis Progressing from Simple to Conglomerate. A 54-year-old foundry worker was asymptomatic at the time of the first radiograph *(A)*. The opacities throughout both lungs are predominantly small and rounded and are more evident in the upper and mid zones than in the bases. The nodules are relatively discrete, as revealed in a magnified view of the right upper lung *(B)*. An exceptional degree of hilar lymph node enlargement is present bilaterally. Four years later *(C)*, the nodules are more numerous and have become confluent in the subapical zones bilaterally so as to form shadows of homogeneous density (conglomeration). A radiograph *(D)* taken 7 years after *C* reveals marked progression of the disease; not only are the nodules more numerous, but their density is considerably greater than had been observed earlier. By this time, confluence of shadows in the subapical zones had progressed considerably; one on the left had undergone cavitation *(arrow)*.

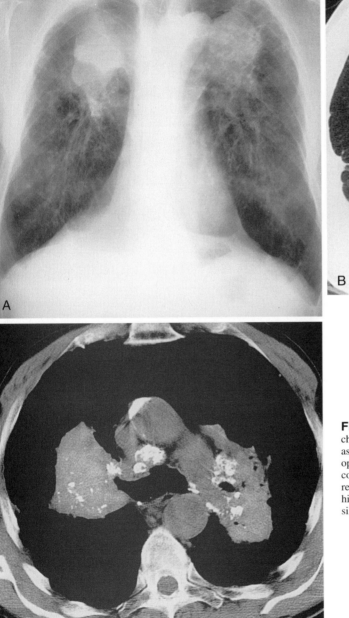

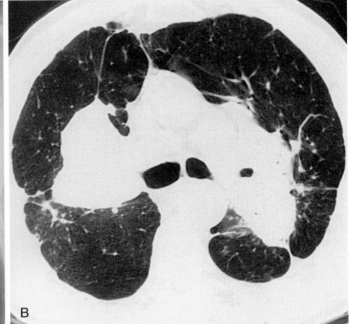

Figure 60–13. Silicosis with Conglomeration. A posteroanterior chest radiograph *(A)* demonstrates large opacities in the upper lung zones associated with marked retraction of the hila superiorly. Several nodular opacities can be seen, mainly in the midlung zones. HRCT *(B)* demonstrates conglomerate masses and extensive emphysema. Soft tissue windows *(C)* reveal calcification within the lung parenchyma and within mediastinal and hilar lymph nodes. The patient was a 70-year-old man with long-standing silicosis related to hard rock mining.

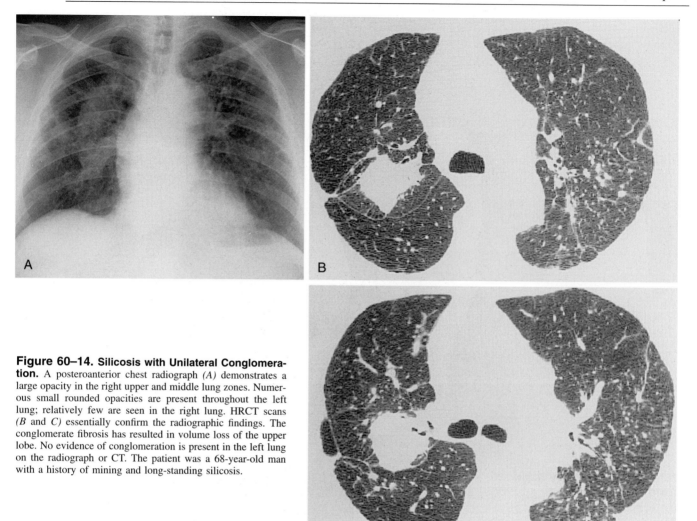

Figure 60–14. Silicosis with Unilateral Conglomeration. A posteroanterior chest radiograph *(A)* demonstrates a large opacity in the right upper and middle lung zones. Numerous small rounded opacities are present throughout the left lung; relatively few are seen in the right lung. HRCT scans *(B* and *C)* essentially confirm the radiographic findings. The conglomerate fibrosis has resulted in volume loss of the upper lobe. No evidence of conglomeration is present in the left lung on the radiograph or CT. The patient was a 68-year-old man with a history of mining and long-standing silicosis.

Hilar lymph node enlargement is common and may occur with or without associated silicosis (Fig. 60–15).[175, 176] Calcification is not uncommon—in one series of 1,905 cases, it was identified in 4.7%[177]—and characteristically tends to involve mainly the periphery of the nodes, a finding referred to as *eggshell calcification.* Although occasionally seen in other conditions (Fig. 60–16),[178, 178a] this pattern is almost pathognomonic of silicosis; its occurrence in coal and metal miners has been attributed to concomitant exposure to silica.[176] Although most common in the hilar lymph nodes, eggshell calcification also develops rarely in lymph nodes in the mediastinum[177] and the intra-abdominal and retroperitoneal areas.[178]

The enlarged lymph nodes may lead to problems in diagnosis in some patients. For example, enlarged silicotic nodes in the retroperitoneum have been confused with metastatic pancreatic carcinoma.[179] In one patient who had *Mycobacterium avium-intracellulare* infection, bronchial obstruction developed from broncholithiasis as a result of eroding infected silicotic nodes.[180] Mediastinal nodes may encroach on the phrenic nerve, resulting in unilateral diaphragmatic paralysis.[181] We have also seen one patient in whom enlarged hilar lymph nodes were associated with fibrosing mediastinitis resulting in obstruction of the right interlobar pulmonary artery (Fig. 60–17).

Ten to 20 years' exposure usually is necessary before the appearance of radiographic abnormalities.[182] The onset of disease is sometimes accelerated, however, particularly in patients exposed to high concentrations of dust in a relatively confined area.[183] Such disease has radiographic features similar to those of the classic form except that they develop over a period of only a few years (Fig. 60–18). As indicated previously, particularly large exposure to silica dust, such as may occur in sandblasters, can result in silicoproteinosis. This variant is characterized by bilateral parenchymal consolidation similar to alveolar proteinosis that progresses rapidly over a period of months or 1 or 2 years.[184, 185]

Another variant of classic silicosis is Caplan's syndrome, which consists of the presence of large necrobiotic nodules superimposed on a background of simple silicosis. It is a manifestation of rheumatoid lung disease and is seen more commonly in coal workers' pneumoconiosis than in silicosis (*see* page 2416). In a controlled study of patients who had silicosis with and without rheumatoid arthritis, the rate of progression of the silicosis was found to be greater in the former, as was the probability that the silicosis was

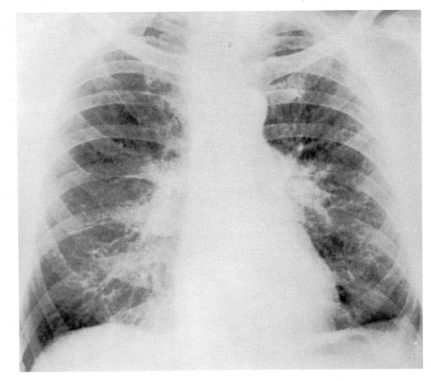

Figure 60–15. Silicosis with Hilar Lymph Node Enlargement. A posteroanterior radiograph reveals a rather coarse reticular pattern evenly distributed throughout both lungs. Hilar lymph nodes are enlarged bilaterally. This patient, a 57-year-old man, had worked underground in a gold mine for many years.

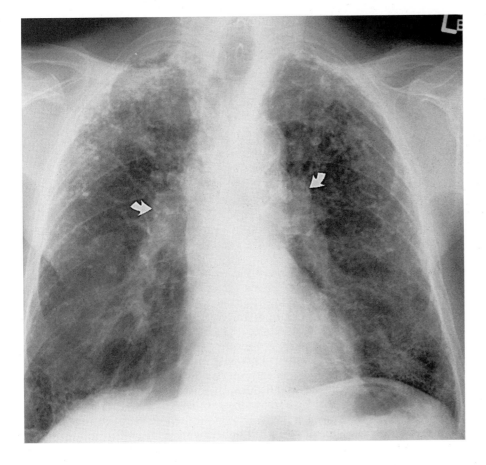

Figure 60–16. Eggshell Calcification of Lymph Nodes in Silicosis. A posteroanterior chest radiograph demonstrates numerous calcified silicotic nodules mainly in the upper lung and midlung zones. Several enlarged hilar and mediastinal lymph nodes are present with peripheral (eggshell) calcification *(arrows)*. The patient was a 78-year-old man who had been a miner for more than 20 years.

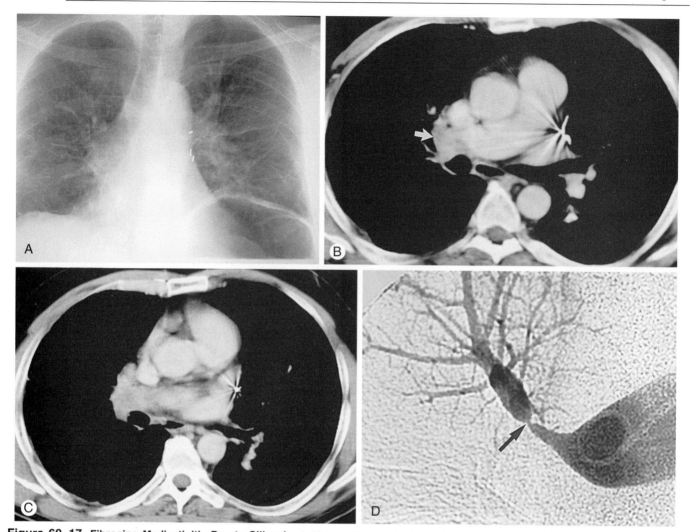

Figure 60–17. Fibrosing Mediastinitis Due to Silicosis. A 43-year-old man who had emigrated recently from India presented with progressive dyspnea. He had undergone previous left lower lobectomy for silicotuberculosis. He had no history of exposure to dust. A posteroanterior chest radiograph *(A)* demonstrates localized irregular linear opacities in both lungs and postoperative changes related to the previous lobectomy. The vascularity of the right lung is decreased. Contrast-enhanced CT scans *(B and C)* demonstrate nonenhancing soft tissue density in the region of the right interlobar pulmonary artery *(arrow)* causing obstruction to blood flow. A view from a selective right pulmonary angiogram *(D)* demonstrates complete obstruction of the right interlobar pulmonary artery and marked focal narrowing *(arrow)* of the artery to the right upper lobe. At surgery the patient was shown to have unresectable fibrosing mediastinitis. Pathologic assessment from surgical biopsy specimens demonstrated silicotic nodules in lymph nodes and surrounding tissue.

manifested by larger nodules (type r) at the time of presentation.[186]

Radiographic progression of silicosis after removal from exposure has been well established. For example, in one study of 1,902 workers who had no radiographic evidence of PMF a maximum of 4 years before leaving the occupation, 172 subsequently developed PMF on follow-up examination.[187] Despite the development of conglomerate lesions after leaving employment, this cohort of workers showed no overall progression or regression of the grades of simple pneumoconiosis.

The CT findings of silicosis have been described by several investigators.[172, 188–190] The characteristic abnormalities are similar to those on the radiograph: sharply defined small nodules that may be diffuse throughout the lungs but frequently are most numerous in the upper lung zones (Fig. 60–19). In patients who have relatively mild disease, the nodules may be seen only in the posterior aspect of the upper lobes.[172, 191] Nodules adjacent to the visceral pleura

may appear as rounded or triangular areas of attenuation, which, when confluent, may simulate pleural plaques ("pseudoplaques") (Figs. 60–19 and 60–20). Confluent nodules (PMF) usually have irregular margins and may contain areas of calcification (*see* Fig. 60–13); surrounding emphysema is usually present. Hilar or mediastinal lymph node enlargement is also apparent in approximately 40% of patients.[191]

Distinction of small nodules from vessels is easier on conventional or spiral CT (*see* Fig. 60–19) than on HRCT (*see* Fig. 60–20).[192] The last-named technique, however, allows better assessment of fine parenchymal detail and of emphysema. Furthermore, HRCT may allow detection of nodules in patients who have normal radiographic and conventional CT findings[189] and is particularly helpful in the assessment of patients who have nodules less than 1.5 mm in diameter.[190] In one investigation of 49 patients exposed to silica dust in mines and foundries, 13 (40%) of 32 patients who had normal radiographs had evidence of silicosis on CT;[189] in three of these cases (10%), the abnormality was

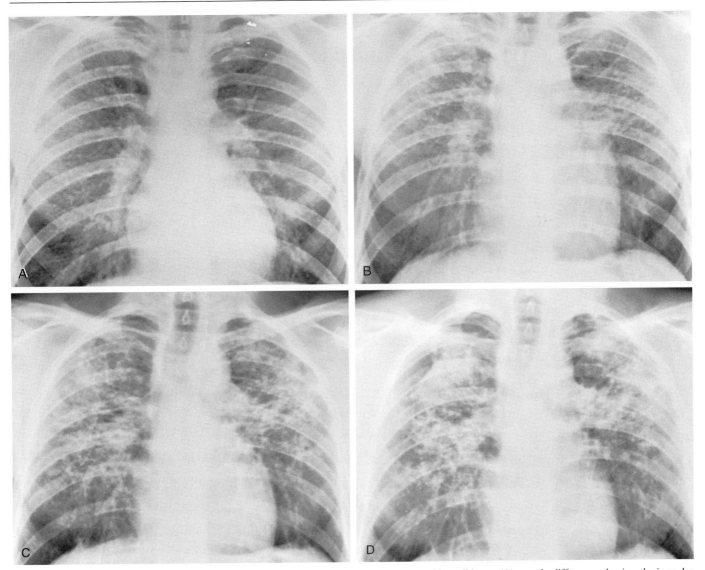

Figure 60–18. Silicosis Showing Rapid Progression. A radiograph of a 27-year-old sandblaster *(A)* reveals diffuse, predominantly irregular opacities more prominent in the upper lung zones; hilar lymph nodes are enlarged. Two years later *(B)*, lung volume had reduced somewhat, particularly in the upper lung zones (note the upward displacement of both hila). The opacities in the upper lungs were showing early coalescence. Three years later *(C)*, large opacities had developed in the upper lung zones, and 7 years after he was originally seen *(D)*, the large opacities had become much larger. Note the sharply defined lateral margin of the large opacity on the right.

visible only on HRCT. Conventional CT and HRCT may also allow detection of early confluence of nodules not apparent on the radiograph.[172, 189] Therefore in the assessment of patients who have possible silicosis, it is recommended that conventional or spiral CT scans be obtained and be supplemented by HRCT scans obtained at three to five levels through the upper lung and midlung zones.[192, 193]

The characteristic CT findings of PMF consist of focal soft tissue masses often with irregular margins and surrounded by areas of emphysema.[188, 189, 194] On magnetic resonance imaging (MRI), confluent nodules usually have signal intensity similar to that of muscle on T1-weighted images and lower signal intensity on T2-weighted images.[194a] Central areas of increased signal intensity on T2-weighted MR images may be seen; these have been shown to correspond to low attenuation on CT and are suggestive of necrosis.[194a]

In one study of 17 patients who had silicosis and 6 controls, the qualitative and quantitative assessment of sili-cosis on chest radiographs and CT scans was compared with the results of pulmonary function tests.[172] The extent of silicosis as assessed on CT was also compared with the extent estimated from chest radiographs using the ILO 1980 classification. Good correlation was found between the CT visual scores and the chest radiographic ILO profusion score ($r = 0.84$); however, there was poor correlation between the nodular profusion on the chest radiograph and CT with the functional impairment. A significant positive correlation was seen between the extent of emphysema on CT and the functional impairment as assessed by the FEV_1 per cent predicted ($r = 0.66$) and the diffusing capacity ($r = 0.71$). Emphysema associated with silicosis was easily detected on CT but not on the radiographs.

Emphysema in silicosis may be secondary to PMF or to other causes, particularly cigarette smoking. To distinguish these factors, one group of investigators compared the CT findings and pulmonary function tests in 18 patients who

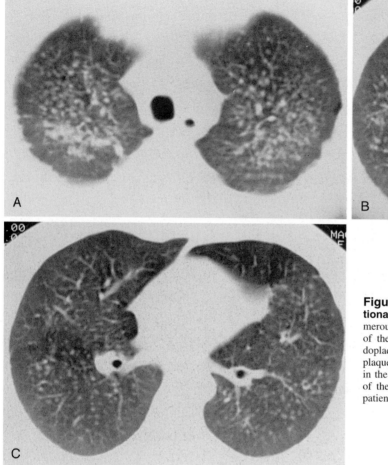

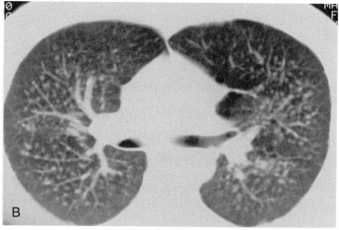

Figure 60–19. Silicosis: Characteristic Findings on Conventional CT. Conventional 10-mm collimation CT scans demonstrate numerous well-defined small nodules, most abundant in the posterior half of the upper lung zones *(A)*. CT at this level also demonstrates pseudoplaques (i.e., subpleural nodules resulting in an appearance resembling plaques). The nodules also have a perivascular distribution, most evident in the scan obtained through the midlung zones *(B)*. CT scan at the level of the inferior pulmonary veins *(C)* shows relatively few nodules. The patient was a 50-year-old miner.

had silicosis and who were ex-smokers or current smokers and 12 patients who had silicosis and were lifetime non-smokers.[194] The extent of emphysema on CT correlated with airway obstruction as assessed by the FEV$_1$ and the decrease in carbon monoxide diffusing capacity (D$_{LCO}$), independent of its association with either cigarette smoking or grade of silicosis. The severity of silicosis was associated with a decrease in D$_{LCO}$ independent of its association with either cigarette smoking or per cent emphysema but did not correlate with the FEV$_1$. Among the patients who did not have PMF, smokers had worse emphysema than nonsmokers; however, there was no such difference among patients who had PMF. One of the nonsmoking subjects who had silicosis but did not have PMF had evidence of emphysema on CT.

Clinical Manifestations

The diagnosis of silicosis usually is based on the identification of a diffuse nodular or reticulonodular pattern on the chest radiograph of a patient who has an occupational history compatible with exposure to dust containing high concentrations of SiO$_2$. In contrast to many other inhalation diseases caused by inorganic and organic dusts, the fibrosis and associated disability in silicosis frequently are progressive, even after removal of the patient from the dusty environment.[195] Thus, it is not uncommon for a patient to present

with symptoms many years after leaving the occupation responsible for the dust exposure. This is an important point to remember because only a complete occupational history, ranging over a patient's entire working life, may provide the clue to the diagnosis.

Many patients are asymptomatic when first seen. Some complain of shortness of breath, initially on exertion only but becoming increasingly severe as the radiographic abnormalities worsen. As might be expected, dyspnea has been found to be more common in patients who have radiographic evidence of silicosis than in individuals who have silica exposure and normal chest radiographs.[196] In one series of hospitalized patients who had silicosis, crackles and wheezes were evident in the majority;[197] however, in our experience, asymptomatic ambulatory patients who have silicosis usually have no adventitious sounds on auscultation. With progressive destruction of pulmonary tissue, pulmonary hypertension, cor pulmonale, and, eventually, right-sided heart failure develop. The major pulmonary abnormality associated with the development of cor pulmonale appears to be the severity of associated emphysema, the extent of fibrosis being of lesser importance.[198]

In contrast to classic silicosis, in which the great majority of patients are asymptomatic and an exposure of 10 to 20 years is required before the disease becomes evident radiographically, a small number of patients develop symptomatic disease within 5 to 10 years of exposure (so-called

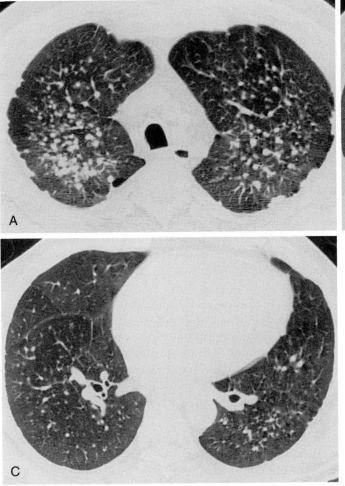

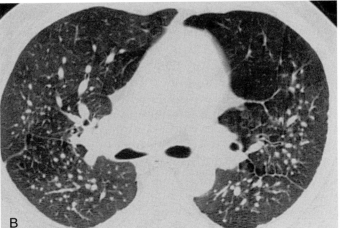

Figure 60–20. Silicosis: Characteristic Findings on HRCT. HRCT scan performed in the same patient as Figure 60–19 demonstrates well-defined nodules mainly involving the upper lung zones *(A)*. The margins of the nodules are better defined on HRCT than on the corresponding conventional CT scan, and the pseudoplaques resulting from subpleural nodules are better seen. Because of the thinner section (1.5 mm compared to 10 mm), the profusion of nodules appears to be smaller, and the nodules are more difficult to distinguish from vessels. This is particularly evident on the images through the midlung *(B)* and lower lung zones *(C)*.

accelerated silicosis). Apart from its relatively early onset and rapid progression, the radiographic, clinical, and pathologic features of this variant are identical to those of more classic disease. Although this form is probably less common today than previously as a result of dust control in the workplace, cases are still observed in conditions of environmental neglect.[85]

Silicoproteinosis is another relatively acute and even more rapidly progressive form of disease. This variant was reported initially in quartzite millers[199] and workers in the scouring powder industry;[71, 72] it has also been described in tunnel workers, silica flour workers,[199] and sandblasters.[155, 200, 201] The last-named often remove their masks after sandblasting and then proceed to paint in the dusty atmosphere; when disease develops, it often leads to death as a result of respiratory failure, not uncommonly with a complicating pneumothorax.[200]

The combination of an occupational history and typical radiographic changes usually suffices to permit confident diagnosis of silicosis. Occasionally, it is necessary to confirm the diagnosis with tissue samples. In some instances, histologic features of biopsy specimens are sufficient for diagnosis. Although transbronchial or open biopsy specimens are probably the most efficacious in this regard, the diagnosis has also been made by needle biopsy; in one study, the core of tissue was considered to be compatible with silicosis in almost two thirds of patients in whom the final diagnosis

was confirmed.[202] In other cases, chemical analysis of lung ash content, scanning electron microscopy, and x-ray energy spectrometry of tissue specimens have been used.[203, 204] X-ray microanalysis has also been used to examine BAL fluid obtained from patients who have a history of exposure to silica, either with or without silicosis;[205] somewhat surprisingly, quantification was unable to distinguish between exposed and affected workers. The false-negative rate was almost 15% and the false-positive rate 5%, using unexposed individuals who did or did not have intestinal lung disease as controls.

Bronchoscopy may show evidence of airway stenosis, sometimes resembling carcinoma.[167a] The mucosa may have a gray or even black appearance as a result of the extension of arthracotic-pigment containing macrophages from adjacent lymph nodes (however, a similar appearance can be seen in association with tuberculous bronchostenosis).

Laboratory Findings

Silicosis is accompanied by a rise in angiotensin-converting enzyme;[206–209] in fact, high serum levels of the enzyme have been found to correlate with progression of the disease.[208] As mentioned previously, serologic abnormalities, including the presence of rheumatoid factor, antinuclear antibodies,[128] and immune complexes,[129, 130] are common. A polyclonal increase in gammaglobulin is also seen in some patients.[130, 131]

Pulmonary Function Tests

Quantification of clinical disability is often necessary for compensation purposes; pulmonary function tests are essential in this regard. (When interpreting these tests, it is important to remember that the effects of silicosis and dust exposure on lung function may be confounded by those of cigarette smoking.) Function may be normal in the early stages of disease,[210, 211] and exercise testing is not more sensitive than routine lung function in demonstrating early impairment.[212] Higher degrees of profusion of simple nodular silicosis may be associated with significant loss of lung function,[213] however, as well as a greater loss of function over time than is seen in workers who have lesser degrees of profusion, after correction for smoking history, age, and initial lung function values.[214] When dyspnea is present, impairment of function may be obstructive, restrictive, or a combination of both.[213, 215, 216] Diffusing capacity may be decreased;[210, 215, 217] the combination of this finding with hyperinflation and decrease in flow rates constitutes a pattern of functional impairment identical to that of uncomplicated pulmonary emphysema. Although arterial oxygen saturation may be normal at rest, exercise gives rise to hypoxemia, particularly in patients who have PMF.[215, 218] In the late stages of the disease, carbon dioxide retention may develop.[219] Conglomeration of nodules is associated with a significant reduction in lung compliance, lung volumes, and diffusing capacity.[220]

The observation that significant emphysema in non-smoking silica-exposed workers is relatively rare[203, 210, 211, 215] has been used by many clinicians to argue against a relationship between dust exposure and the development of chronic air-flow obstruction. This argument, however, does not allow for the potential synergistic effects of dust and tobacco smoke;[221] moreover, it ignores the results of studies that demonstrate functionally important airway damage in both experimental animals[222] and nonsmoking workers who have been exposed heavily to dust (*see* page 2174).[223–226] Several examples suffice to illustrate this relationship. The risk of developing significant emphysema has been shown in one investigation to be 3.5 times greater in miners heavily exposed to dust compared with miners who have lighter dust exposures.[227] In one autopsy study of 242 nonsmoking South African gold miners who had undergone pulmonary function testing within a few years of death, advanced silicosis was associated with a significant degree of both air-flow obstruction and restriction.[228] Investigations of Vermont granite workers in which there was appropriate control for the effects of age and smoking have revealed excessive loss of FEV_1 with time in the dust-exposed individuals in the absence of radiologic evidence of silicosis[226] as well as more rapid development of small airway abnormalities with increasing dust exposure in both smokers and nonsmokers.[229] These results have been confirmed in a French study of silica-exposed workers;[230] similar effects on the FEV_1 have been documented in granite quarry workers from Singapore[231] and retired miners from Colorado.[232] In another study in which emphysema grade was determined by HRCT, a

significant excess of emphysema and pulmonary function abnormalities was found in workers who had silicosis and in dust-exposed workers who did not have the disease, after controlling for age and smoking history.[233] The evidence supports the hypothesis that the dusty environment of silica-exposed workers can contribute to the development of chronic air-flow obstruction and emphysema.

Prognosis and Natural History

Symptomatic patients who have silicosis have a poorer prognosis than asymptomatic patients; in fact, asymptomatic patients who have simple nodular silicosis have a life expectancy similar to that of the general population.[234] In patients with silicosis, older age is associated with increased mortality.[234, 235] The prognosis and natural history of silicosis are also related to two serious potential complications—carcinoma and tuberculosis.

Relationship to Neoplasia

In 1996, silica was recognized as an occupational carcinogen by the International Agency for Research on Cancer.[236] The strength of the association is much greater for workers who have silicosis[237–243, 274, 274a] than for those who have been exposed to silica but have no evidence of the disease.[227, 244–247] The relative risk for pulmonary carcinoma among the former patients often exceeds 3.0 and has been found to be as high as 6.0 in some studies;[241, 248] by contrast, the relative risk of carcinoma in the absence of silicosis has been estimated to be 1.3.[249] The excess risk has been reported in workers in industries unassociated with exposure to other occupational carcinogens, such as stone cutters,[250–252] and has been shown to be independent of cigarette smoking.[227, 241, 242, 246, 248, 253–255] These relationships are discussed in detail in Chapter 31 (*see* page 1077).

Relationship to Pulmonary Tuberculosis

There is little question that silicosis predisposes to tuberculosis;[256] however, the prevalence of this complication in workers who have silicosis depends to a large extent on the prevalence of tuberculosis in the population from which the workers come.[257] Although it is customary to associate the development of tuberculosis with the presence of PMF, there is evidence that its risk increases with increasing profusion of simple nodular shadows;[258] the likelihood of developing tuberculosis is greater in workers who have any degree of silicosis compared with similarly exposed workers without silicosis.[258] In patients who have silicosis, the development of tuberculosis is a strong independent predictor of mortality.[235] It may be extremely difficult to isolate tubercle bacilli during life in patients who have tuberculosis and silicosis, particularly those who have PMF, despite postmortem demonstration of active tuberculous infection;[259] identification of organisms by polymerase chain reaction might prove to be useful in this setting.[260]

Relationship to Connective Tissue Disease

The association of progressive systemic sclerosis with silicosis and with exposure to high concentrations of silica dust is well established.[90] The evidence for a similar association of silicosis and rheumatoid arthritis is less clear; however, if real, it is unlikely to be strong.[90] A causal association between systemic lupus erythematosus and silica exposure should be suspected only in the presence of acute or accelerated silicosis.[90]

COAL AND CARBON

The inhalation and retention in the lung of dust composed predominantly of carbon (often termed *anthracosis*) is seen in many individuals,[261] particularly those who smoke or live in a city or industrial environment. Microscopically, such material is easily recognized as dense black particles, mostly 1 to 2 μm in size, within macrophages adjacent to terminal or proximal respiratory bronchioles and in the pleura. The material is also commonly present in bronchopulmonary, hilar, and mediastinal lymph nodes to which it characteristically imparts a distinct blackness on gross examination. Although predominantly composed of carbon, the particles also contain traces of other substances, such as silica and iron. Nevertheless, associated fibrosis or emphysema is invariably minimal or absent (except when associated with cigarette smoking), and it is generally believed that the presence of such particles is of no pathologic or functional significance.

Such innocuous environmental anthracosis is caused by the inhalation of relatively small amounts of dust. Inhalation of large amounts of carbonaceous material, however, either in the form of coal dust or as substances derived from coal or petroleum products, can be associated with significant pulmonary disease. Because quantity is important in this effect, such disease occurs almost exclusively in the workplace, where the concentration of these materials is much greater than that in nonoccupational settings. The most important occupation in terms of the number of individuals affected is coal mining, the resulting disease being appropriately called *coal workers' pneumoconiosis*. Workers involved in the production or use of graphite,[262–266] carbon black,[267] and carbon electrodes[268] are affected less often. The possibility that pulmonary disease is occasionally caused by inhalation of fly ash has also been suggested.[269, 270]

Epidemiology

Coal

Coal is a sedimentary rock formed by the action of pressure, temperature, and chemical reactions on vegetable material. The percentage of pure carbon varies with different types, brown coal and lignite containing the least and anthracite the most.[271] The degree of exposure to carbon dust thus depends to some extent on the type of coal being mined, a feature that may partly explain the variability in incidence of CWP from colliery to colliery. Perhaps more important in this regard are local geologic variations;[272] some coal seams are thick (up to 100 feet), whereas others are much thinner and are separated by seams of silica-containing rock.[271] Mining in the latter situation can result in significant concomitant exposure to silica and other substances, a feature that probably explains the occurrence of classic silicosis in a small percentage of coal miners.[272, 273, 275]

Certain occupations within the coal mine are also associated with different likelihoods of developing disease and the form that such disease takes. For example, because the majority of dust is produced at the coal face,[275] workers of cutting and loading machines are at greater risk than those involved in transportation or maintenance at the mine surface. Similarly, miners drilling through quartz and workers involved in the maintenance or construction of underground roadways or the transportation of coal to the surface by railway (during which time sand has been put on the rails to increase traction) are more likely to come in contact with silica and to develop classic silicosis.[271, 273]

The impact of U.S. federal legislation in 1969, in which substantially lower dust levels were mandated for American coal mines, is now being felt, and the prevalence of CWP in the United States is less than it used to be.[276] Because current allowable dust levels of 2 mg/M^3 are sufficient to result in pneumoconiosis and because workers who have had previous, more intense dust exposures may still be in the workforce, new cases of the disease will undoubtedly continue to be identified.

With current environmental standards, it is estimated that 2% to 12% of American coal miners will develop category 2 or greater disease after a 40-year working life, whereas approximately 1% to 7% will develop PMF.[277, 278] These estimates are slightly in excess of those calculated for British underground miners, in whom simple pneumoconiosis has been predicted to develop in 9% and PMF in 0.7%.[279] Although these figures are comparable to those 30 years ago, they would represent a distinct improvement in disease prevalence compared to earlier in the century: surveys carried out in the early 1970s in the Appalachian region of the United States showed that approximately 10% of active coal miners had pneumoconiosis, about a third of whom had PMF;[280, 281] by contrast, an earlier review of a similar population showed that almost 50% of miners had simple pneumoconiosis, and 15% had complicated disease.[282] Most of these latter workers likely retired from the workforce as a result of their disease with resulting improvement in prevalence statistics in the later studies.[283]

Other Carbonaceous Substances

Fly ash is the solid residue that remains after the combustion of coal; the particles so formed are composed of a variety of elements, including silica, aluminum, and iron.[269] Because of these substances, workers in occupations associated with a high concentration of fly ash are theoretically at risk for developing pneumoconiosis; in fact, a high content of such particles has been demonstrated in the lungs of some individuals who have pulmonary fibrosis.[269, 270] Nevertheless, the majority of clinical and experimental evidence suggests that this material is not fibrogenic.[284]

Graphite (crystalline carbon) occurs both naturally as a mineral and as an artificial substance derived from heated coal or coke. It is used in the manufacture of steel, lubricants, lead pencils, nuclear reactors, and electrodes.[285] Pulmonary disease identical to CWP has been described occasionally in individuals engaged in these occupations.[262–266]

Carbon black is produced from the flames of natural

gas and various petroleum products. It has been used as a filler in rubber, plastics, phonographic records, and inks[267] and in the manufacture of carbon paper and carbon electrodes. The importance of carbon black as a cause of pulmonary disease is unclear. Although examples of pneumoconiosis attributed to heavy exposure during the manufacture of such products had been reported rarely before 1990,[267, 268, 286] a 1993 survey of carbon black workers in seven European countries, including more than 1,000 for whom chest radiographs were available, revealed the presence of reticular abnormalities in 25%.[287] The likelihood of identifying these abnormalities was related to total cumulative dust exposure. By contrast, in a report of the results of a survey of process workers in a factory producing continuous filament carbon fiber, no evidence of ill effects on the lungs was found by radiographic, spirometric, or clinical assessments.[288] Similar results were demonstrated in a factory in which activated charcoal was manufactured, in which workers had been exposed to pure carbon dust for up to 11 years.[289]

Pathologic, radiographic, and clinical findings in workers exposed to large amounts of carbon in whatever form are similar; however, because the vast majority of such individuals are involved in coal mining, most of the reported literature and much of the following description relate to CWP.

Pathogenesis

The precise pathogenetic factors involved in the development of simple CWP and complicating PMF are unclear, and several agents or processes, either alone or in combination, may be responsible. As might be expected, the most important factor may be the quantity of inhaled coal. The prevalence of CWP and the risk of progressing to a higher category of simple pneumoconiosis are both related to cumulative dust exposure.[283, 290, 291] Similarly, PMF is more likely to occur in workers who have had heavy dust exposure and who have large amounts of dust in their lungs at autopsy.[291–296] Although the major effect of dust is its influence on the development of CWP, even workers who do not have radiologic evidence of CWP have an increased risk of developing PMF with increasing dust exposure.[291] Associated tuberculosis may be important in determining progression to PMF in China, where the infection is particularly prevalent;[297] however, it appears to play little role in other regions. The results of more recent studies have confirmed the importance of higher profusion category[298, 299] and younger age at diagnosis of CWP[298] as risk factors for the subsequent development of PMF. One group of investigators found patients who were lighter in weight for their height to be at increased risk for PMF.[298] A high degree of correlation between the presence of PMF and the degree and type of pathologic abnormality in perihilar lymph nodes has also been described.[300]

Because PMF in patients with silicosis is similar both pathologically and radiologically to that in patients who have CWP, it has been suggested that contamination of coal dust by silica may be responsible for the lesion in the latter individuals.[301] A number of findings argue against this hypothesis, however, including (1) the observation that there is a wide variation in the amount of silica in the lungs of coal workers who have PMF;[271] (2) the finding in at least some studies that the severity of CWP is more closely related to total carbon content of the lung than to the concentration of silica;[302] and (3) the observation that workers who are exposed almost exclusively to carbon, such as those involved with carbon black or carbon electrodes, can develop lesions identical to those that occur in underground coal workers.[263, 266–268, 286]

These observations have, in turn, been challenged. For example, it has been speculated that there may be differential clearance and enhanced retention of silica in mixed dust exposures, allowing for an effect disproportionate to its inhaled concentration.[303] In addition, critical analysis of many of the articles claiming to report pure carbon exposure has shown that their determinations of the composition of inhaled dust can be faulted. In fact, silica as well as other minerals mixed with inhaled coal dust may influence the body's response to this dust mixture in a complex and as yet ill-defined fashion. For example, in one study of the lungs of 490 British coal miners, investigators found evidence for two distinct histologic varieties of PMF, one apparently formed by conglomeration of several nodular lesions and the other by enlargement of a single lesion.[301] The two patterns were associated with different degrees of lung dust content and colliery rank, and the authors suggested that the effect of silica (perhaps itself affected by the presence of other inhaled substances, such as kaolinite and mica) might be important in pathogenesis.

An understanding of the cellular and molecular basis of CWP is also incomplete, in part because of a failure to distinguish between the effects of carbon and the effects of contaminating silica and other elements present in coal dust. Similar to silicosis, CWP is associated with the production of oxidants,[304, 305] probably derived predominantly from alveolar macrophages.[306] Compared with that from healthy individuals, BAL fluid from patients who have CWP has revealed lymphocytosis; evidence of increased alveolar permeability; increased IL-6, TNF-α,[307] type I insulin-like growth factor (IGF-1), fibronectin,[93] and platelet-derived growth factor (PDGF);[308] and decreased interferon-γ.[309] As in other diseases, the functions of these cytokines are varied and their interaction complex; for example, the overall role of IL-6 may be an antifibrotic one,[309] whereas IGF-1 and PDGF appear to promote fibrosis.[308] Other cytokines are also likely to be important in pathogenesis; for example, peripheral monocytes of miners who have CWP have been shown to have enhanced release of TNF-α, which can stimulate the adhesion of polymorphonuclear neutrophils to endothelium, stimulate fibroblast growth, and induce production and release of IL-1 and reactive oxygen species from mononuclear phagocytes.[310, 311]

The presence in coal miners of hypergammaglobulinemia,[312] rheumatoid factor, and antinuclear or antilung antibodies has also raised the possibility of an immunologic mechanism in the pathogenesis of CWP. Although some investigators have found titers of rheumatoid factor and autoantibodies to be higher than those in control subjects before the development of radiographic abnormalities,[313] most have shown them to rise with increasing severity of radiographically determined category of disease.[313–318] In one study, the prevalence of antilung antibodies and lymphocyte-mediated cellular cytotoxicity was found to be higher in smoking than in nonsmoking miners.[319]

Caplan[320] originally reported the association between rheumatoid arthritis and CWP. In addition, Caplan and colleagues[316] described an increased incidence of rheumatoid factor in miners who had the r type of small rounded opacities as well as in patients who had irregular, large opacities unassociated with overt rheumatoid arthritis. Other workers have confirmed and extended these observations. For example, in one investigation of 109 coal workers who had pneumoconiosis, circulating antinuclear antibody and rheumatoid factor were found in almost 15% of miners who had simple pneumoconiosis and 45% of those who had category C PMF.[314] Other workers have shown positive test results for rheumatoid factor in 30% to 40%[315] and for antinuclear antibodies in 75%[317] of patients who have PMF. One group also demonstrated the presence of rheumatoid factor to be a marker for more rapid progression of pneumoconiosis.[321] In addition, lung-reactive antibodies have been identified in the serum of miners[322] and in rats and mice exposed to coal dust.[323] Although positive titers of all these serum antibodies are not in the same range as those found in connective tissue diseases, in most cases their level has been recorded as at least 1/10, a finding observed in only 2% to 3% of the normal male population.[314]

Three groups of investigators have failed to reveal an association between either simple or complicated CWP and any specific histocompatibility antigen;[324–326] however, another group showed the more rapid development of CWP in miners who had HLA DRB8 and resistance to the development of CWP in those who had DRB1 and DRB2.[327] Despite this abundant evidence suggesting a role for immunologic factors in the development of PMF, the details of possible pathogenetic mechanisms are not understood.

Pathologic Characteristics

The two morphologic findings characteristic of CWP are the coal macule and PMF.[271, 328, 329] The former is characterized by deposits of anthracotic pigment unassociated with fibrosis, a finding sometimes referred to as *simple* pneumoconiosis. PMF is defined as a focus of fibrosis and pigment deposition larger than 1 cm in diameter and is sometimes designated *complicated* pneumoconiosis. In addition, smaller foci of fibrous tissue (so-called nodular lesions) can be found in many cases, either with or without features of PMF.[271, 329]

Grossly, coal macules are stellate or round, nonpalpable foci that are black and range in size from 1 to 5 mm (Fig. 60–21). They are scattered fairly uniformly throughout the lung parenchyma, although they tend to be more numerous at the apex than at the base. In uncomplicated disease, lung

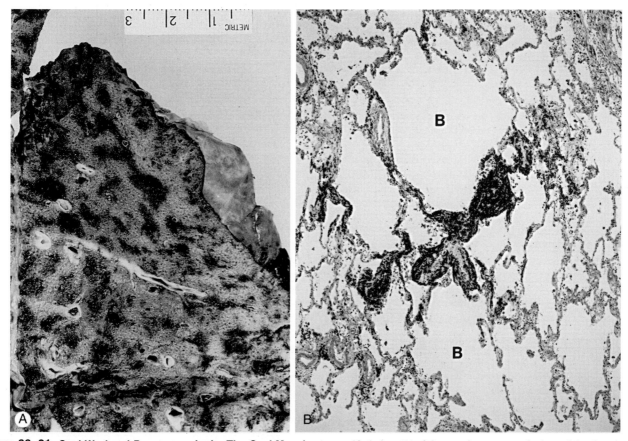

Figure 60–21. Coal Workers' Pneumoconiosis: The Coal Macule. A magnified view *(A)* of the superior segment of a lower lobe shows multiple foci of dense black pigmentation that are of irregular shape but are fairly evenly spaced. Emphysema is present but is difficult to appreciate in this thick, formalin-fixed section. Note also the dense zone of subpleural pigment deposition. A histologic section *(B)* shows numerous alveolar macrophages containing abundant anthracotic pigment situated in the interstitial tissue adjacent to respiratory bronchioles (B). No fibrosis is evident. The bronchioles are moderately dilated. (×40.)

tissue between the macules is typically normal in structure and color, although interlobular septa and peribronchial connective tissue and lymph nodes are also usually heavily pigmented. Microscopically, the macule consists of numerous pigment-laden macrophages in the interstitial tissue adjacent to respiratory bronchioles (*see* Fig. 60–21); reticulin fibers can be identified between the macrophages, but mature collagen is minimal or absent. Aggregates of pigment-laden macrophages can also be seen in adjacent alveolar air spaces, especially in lung tissue derived from active miners. Bronchioles within the macules are frequently distended (*see* Fig. 60–21), a finding often designated *focal emphysema*.[281, 330] Depending on the type of coal or form of carbon dust that has been inhaled,[271] the particulate material within the

macrophages differs somewhat in shape, size, color, and translucency. Ferruginous bodies composed of coal can be identified occasionally (Fig. 60–22); they are similar to those that occur with asbestos exposure except for the presence of relatively large, black cores.

Although the coal macule is characteristic of CWP, identical lesions can be found in individuals from other environments,[261] and the simple presence of a macule does not constitute definite evidence of occupational dust exposure. Microscopic foci of macrophage aggregates similar to those in the coal macule can also be identified in regional lymph nodes and occasionally outside the thorax in tissues such as bone marrow.[331]

Palpable gray or black nodules smaller than 1 cm in

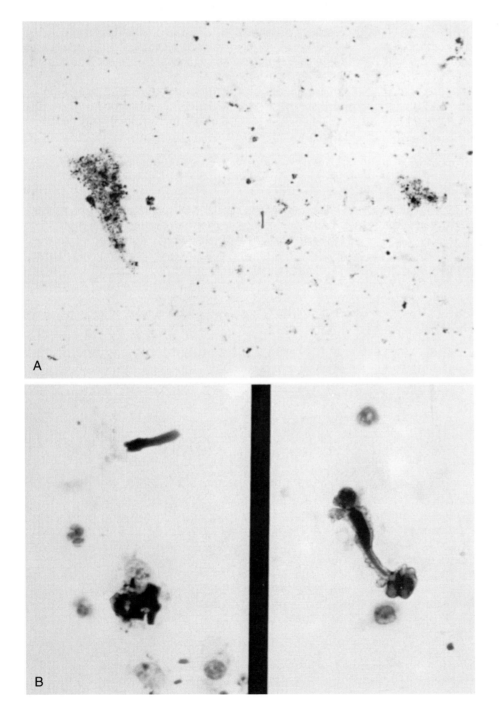

Figure 60–22. Coal Workers' Pneumoconiosis: Transthoracic Needle Aspirate. A filter preparation from a transthoracic needle aspirate *(A)* shows single and clustered cells, many of which appear to contain foreign material. Magnified views of two foci *(B)* show this material to be black, irregular in shape, and localized both within macrophages (on the left) and free (on the right). The latter particle is a ferruginous body, consisting of a central black core (representing the coal particle) and a transparent somewhat nodular iron-protein coat. This material was aspirated from a patient who had an upper lobe mass that resembled a carcinoma. (*A*, ×100; *B*, ×800; Papanicolaou stain.)

diameter can also be found in the lungs of many coal workers. Although these are described separately, they blend imperceptibly with the macule on the one hand and with PMF on the other,[301] and it is likely that they represent part of a spectrum of changes rather than pathogenetically distinct lesions. The nodules can be stellate or round and are fairly well delimited from adjacent lung. They have a variable histologic composition, some consisting of a haphazard mixture of pigment-laden macrophages, free dust, and reticulin and collagen fibers (Fig. 60–23) and others possessing a relatively discrete central zone of pigment-free collagen surrounded by pigment-laden macrophages resembling small silicotic nodules. Degenerative changes identical to those seen in PMF are present occasionally.[271] Other palpable nodules, such as rheumatoid nodules of Caplan's syndrome (*see* page 2416) and infectious granulomas, are seen less frequently.

The lesions of PMF are firm or somewhat rubbery in consistency and either round or irregular in shape. They may be unilateral or bilateral and develop most often in the posterior segment of an upper lobe or superior segment of a lower lobe,[268, 332, 333] a localization that is thought by some to be related to poor lymphatic drainage.[334] A lesion can extend across the pleura into an adjacent lobe or mediastinum. Adjacent emphysema is not uncommon. Cut sections often reveal a necrotic center containing black fluid that can be washed away, leaving a cavity. In most cases, the pathogenesis of the necrosis is ischemia;[335, 336] vascular obliteration both within and adjacent to the region of PMF is a common histologic finding (*see* farther on), and avascular zones can be demonstrated by lung perfusion scanning.[337] Occasionally, cavitation is caused by tuberculous infection.

The microscopic features of PMF are similar to those of the smaller palpable nodules already described. Bundles of haphazardly arranged, sometimes hyalinized bands of collagen are interspersed with numerous pigment-laden macrophages and abundant free pigment; the latter tends to be more evident in the central regions.[338] Foci of degenerated and frankly necrotic tissue, cholesterol clefts, and mononuclear inflammatory cells are often present. Although the hyalinized tissue is usually assumed to be collagen, biochemical analysis has shown a high proportion of a noncollagenous, insoluble protein,[339] at least some of which is probably fibronectin.[340] Airways and blood vessels can be incorporated within and destroyed by the expanding fibrotic process (Fig. 60–24), and vessels at the periphery of the lesion frequently show endarteritis obliterans.

Cor pulmonale is common at autopsy of patients who have complicated CWP and is occasionally seen in those who have the simple form of the disease.[341–343] In most patients in the latter group, this complication can be explained on the basis of associated chronic obstructive pulmonary disease or silicosis.

Pathologic features of pneumoconiosis associated with graphite and carbon black exposure are similar to those of CWP except that the complicating effects of silica that may be seen with the latter are typically absent. Graphite crystals may be coated with deposits of iron and protein (ferruginous bodies) and can be identified in tissue sections and by digestion techniques.[344, 345]

Radiologic Manifestations

The radiographic pattern of simple pneumoconiosis is typically one of small, round opacities (nodular).[346–348] Occasionally—particularly in the early stages—it is predominantly reticular (small irregular opacities) or reticulonodular (Fig. 60–25).[349] The nodules range from 1 to 5 mm in diameter, tend to be somewhat less well defined than those of silicosis, and have a "granular" density in contrast to the homogeneous density of silicotic nodules. Radiographic-

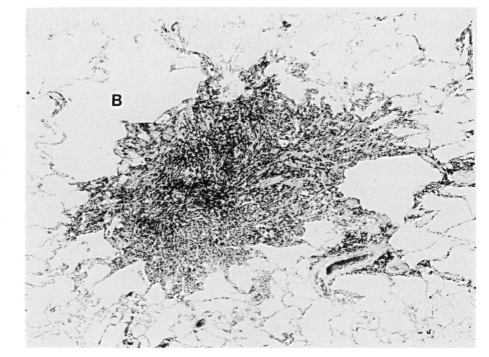

Figure 60–23. Coal Workers' Pneumoconiosis: Nodular Lesion. A histologic section shows a stellate focus of pigmented macrophages adjacent to two respiratory bronchioles, one of which is mildly dilated (B). Connective tissue stains showed abundant reticulin fibers but only mild collagen deposition. In contrast to the typical coal macule, this lesion was palpable. (×40.)

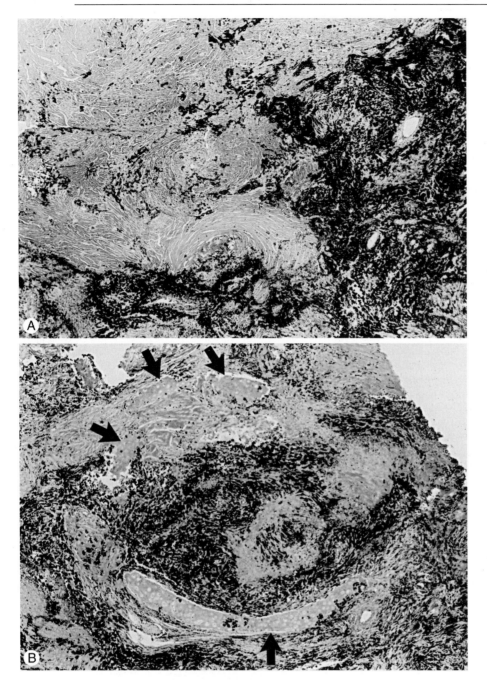

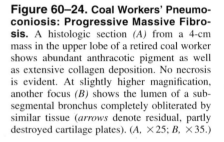

Figure 60–24. Coal Workers' Pneumoconiosis: Progressive Massive Fibrosis. A histologic section *(A)* from a 4-cm mass in the upper lobe of a retired coal worker shows abundant anthracotic pigment as well as extensive collagen deposition. No necrosis is evident. At slightly higher magnification, another focus *(B)* shows the lumen of a subsegmental bronchus completely obliterated by similar tissue (*arrows* denote residual, partly destroyed cartilage plates). (*A,* ×25; *B,* ×35.)

pathologic correlative studies suggest that the opacity of individual nodules cannot be entirely attributed to the coal dust, whose density is only slightly greater than unity.[350] Despite these observations, it is generally agreed that the radiographic manifestations of CWP cannot be distinguished from those of silicosis with any degree of confidence.

Calcification of pulmonary nodules is identified radiographically in 10% to 20% of older coal miners, particularly anthracite workers.[351, 352] The calcification begins as a central dot, thus helping to differentiate these nodules from those of silicosis, in which the calcification tends to be diffuse. Eggshell calcification is uncommon; for example, in one study of 1,063 coal miners whose chest radiographs showed evidence of pneumoconiosis, it was evident in only 1.3%, all of whom had worked 20 or more years in the mines.[351]

The appearance of large opacities indicates the development of complicated pneumoconiosis (PMF). These lesions range from 1 cm in diameter to the volume of a whole lobe in aggregate. Although most commonly restricted to the upper half of the lungs, they may also occur in the lower lung zones (Fig. 60–26). They are usually observed on a background of simple pneumoconiosis but have been found to develop in miners whose initial chest radiographs 4 to 5 years earlier were considered to be within normal limits.[353] The complication is said to occur in about 30% of patients who have diffuse bilateral opacities.[280, 354] It typically starts near the periphery of the lung and is manifested as a mass that has a well-defined lateral border that parallels the rib cage and projects 1 to 3 cm from it.[351] The medial margin of the mass is often ill-defined in contrast to its sharp lateral

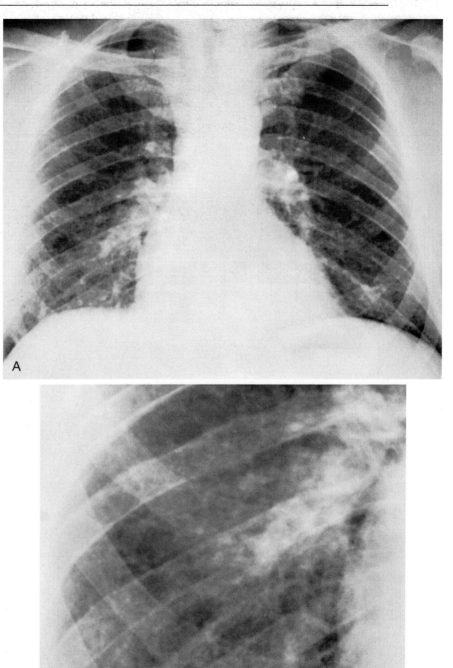

Figure 60–25. Coal Workers' Pneumoconiosis. This posteroanterior radiograph *(A)* and magnified view of the lower half of the right lung *(B)* reveal a coarse reticulonodular pattern throughout both lungs, affecting the upper lung zones least. Both hila are enlarged and possess a contour suggestive of lymph node enlargement. The patient, a 45-year-old miner, was admitted to the hospital complaining of increasing shortness of breath. Approximately 15 years previously, he had worked underground in a Belgian coal mine for 7 years and had been exposed to heavy concentrations of dust but had never worn a mask. At the time of admission, he stated that he was short of breath after walking 100 yards on level ground or climbing 7 to 10 steps. Pulmonary function studies were within normal limits except for a slight reduction in functional residual capacity; studies of lung mechanics revealed normal compliance and airway resistance.

border, a configuration that was observed in 22 of 50 coal miners in one study.[351] The masses of PMF tend to be thicker in one dimension than the other; for example, they tend to produce a broad face on a posteroanterior radiograph and a thin shape on a lateral radiograph, frequently paralleling the major fissure.[351] As might be expected, this spindle-shaped configuration creates a radiographic opacity that is considerably less dense in one projection than in the other. PMF is usually homogeneous in density, unless cavitation has developed. This complication occurs only occasionally; it may develop after exposure to coal dust has ceased and, in

contrast to simple pneumoconiosis, may progress in the absence of further exposure.[280, 347, 355]

As with the conglomerate shadows of silicosis, PMF usually originates in the lung periphery and gradually migrates toward the hilum, leaving a zone of emphysematous lung between it and the chest wall. Particularly when unilateral, a large mass may closely simulate pulmonary carcinoma. Because PMF is occasionally unassociated with radiographic evidence of nodularity,[351] the correct diagnosis in these cases may not be suspected in the absence of an appropriate occupational history. The smooth, sharply de-

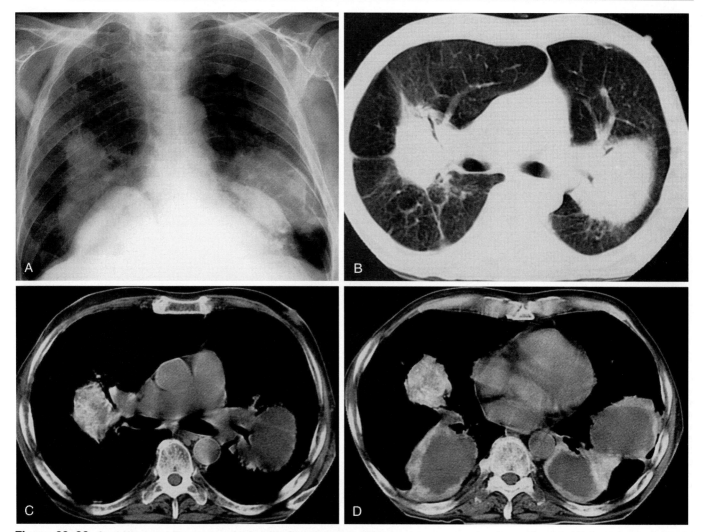

Figure 60–26. Coal Workers' Pneumoconiosis with Conglomerate Masses. An anteroposterior chest radiograph *(A)* shows large opacities in the middle and lower lung zones. A 10-mm collimation CT scan at the level of the right upper lobe bronchus *(B)* demonstrates bilateral perihilar conglomerate masses. Irregular linear opacities and distortion of lung architecture indicative of fibrosis and emphysema are also evident. Soft tissue windows *(C and D)* demonstrate that three of the conglomerate masses have large central areas of decreased attenuation suggestive of necrosis. The patient was a 65-year-old man with a 30-year history of exposure to coal dust. (Courtesy of Dr. Martine Remy-Jardin, Centre Hospitalier Regional et Universitaire de Lille, Lille, France.)

fined lateral border and the somewhat flattened configuration characteristic of these lesions are useful clues in differentiation from a pulmonary carcinoma, whose borders tend to be less well defined and whose configuration is typically spherical. Occasionally, a lesion of PMF contains foci of calcification, an obvious additional aid in radiographic differential diagnosis. Linear calcification may also be seen along the border of an area of PMF, invariably along the lateral margin.[351]

Caplan's syndrome consists of the presence of necrobiotic nodules associated with rheumatoid arthritis superimposed on a background of inorganic dust exposure (*see* page 1438).[320] The nodules are more regular in contour and more peripherally located than the masses of PMF (Fig. 60–27). They range in size from 0.5 to 5 cm in diameter and are seen most often in workers who have subcutaneous rheumatoid nodules and whose chest radiographs are classified as category 0 or 1 simple pneumoconiosis.

In contrast to similar comparisons in silicosis, the radio-

graphic findings correlate well with pathologic abnormalities in CWP.[350, 356] The effects of film quality and other factors on the radiographic categorization of the disease have been analyzed in several studies.[357–359]

The CT findings of CWP are similar to those of silicosis and consist of small nodules that may be seen diffusely throughout both lungs but are most numerous in the upper lung zones.[190, 360, 361] In patients who have mild disease, the nodules may involve only the upper lung zones and show a posterior predominance.[360] A random distribution is typical, although in some cases HRCT may demonstrate a centrilobular predominance.[193, 360] Subpleural nodules are seen in approximately 80% of patients who have other parenchymal nodules. Confluence of such nodules may result in linear areas of increased attenuation a few millimeters wide (pseudoplaques).[193] Correlation of HRCT with pathologic specimens has demonstrated that these subpleural micronodules may also be associated with localized thickening of the visceral pleura as a result of fibrosis.[362] Calcification of

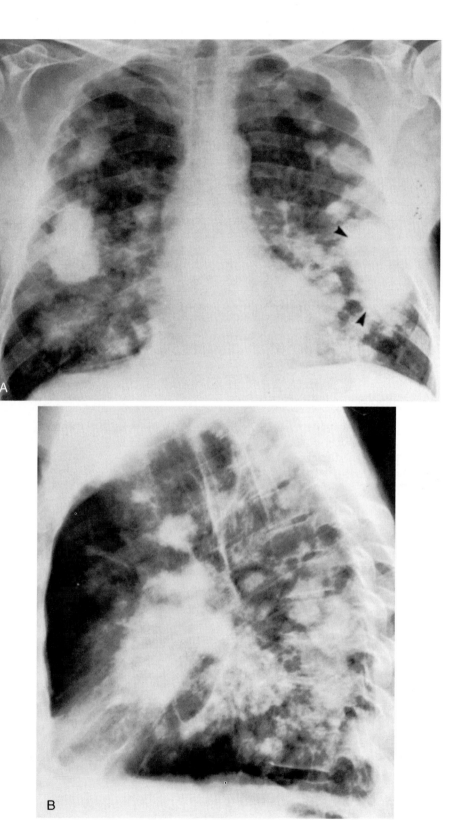

Figure 60–27. Caplan's Syndrome. Posteroanterior *(A)* and lateral *(B)* radiographs reveal a multitude of fairly well-circumscribed nodules ranging in diameter from 1 to 5 cm, scattered randomly throughout both lungs with no notable anatomic predilection. No cavitation is apparent, and there is no evidence of calcification. This patient, a 56-year-old man, had been a coal miner for many years and in recent years had developed arthralgia, which proved to be due to rheumatoid arthritis. As a means of establishing the nature of the pulmonary nodules, a percutaneous needle aspiration was carried out on the large mass situated in the lower portion of the left lung *(arrowheads in A):* Several milliliters of inky black fluid were aspirated.

nodules can be identified in approximately 30% of patients. Hilar or mediastinal lymphadenopathy is also seen in about 30% of cases; the majority of enlarged nodes are calcified.[360]

Large opacities (PMF) in patients who have CWP usually have irregular borders associated with distortion of the surrounding lung architecture and emphysema.[193, 360] Less commonly, they have regular borders and are unassociated with emphysema.[360] The large opacities occur most commonly in the upper lung zones and, although frequently bilateral, may be unilateral (most commonly in the right upper lung zone).[360]

CT has been shown by several investigators to be superior to chest radiography in the detection of small nodules.[190, 360, 361] Conventional CT and HRCT are considered to be complementary in assessment (Fig. 60–28).[193, 360] In one prospective study of 170 coal dust–exposed workers, posteroanterior and lateral chest radiographs, contiguous conventional (10-mm-thick sections) CT scans, and HRCT scans (2-mm-thick sections) at five selected levels were compared.[360] Findings consistent with CWP were detected on CT in 11 of 48 (23%) workers who had no evidence of pneumoconiosis on chest radiographs (ILO profusion score < 1/0); in some patients whose radiographs were interpreted as showing findings consistent with pneumoconiosis, CT showed the abnormalities to consist of bronchiectasis or emphysema, rather than the macules of CWP.

Clinical Manifestations

Symptoms of cough, sputum production, and dyspnea are more common in miners who have early CWP than in miners who have similar smoking and dust exposure histories but no radiographic evidence of disease.[363] These symptoms are even more frequent and severe in workers who have PMF, who also suffer from recurrent attacks of purulent bronchitis. Copious amounts of black sputum may be produced when an ischemic lesion of PMF liquefies and ruptures into a bronchus ("melanoptysis"), in which circumstance a cavity should be visible radiographically.[364–366] With progression of the disease, dyspnea usually worsens; cor pulmonale and right-sided heart failure may ensue.

The degree of breathlessness appears to be directly related to the stage of the disease. In patients who have simple pneumoconiosis, there is usually no breathlessness on exertion despite increasing radiographic abnormality, unless there is associated emphysema. By contrast, in those who have complicated disease, breathlessness is nearly always severe and increases with progression of radiographic changes.[367] Physical examination may reveal decreased breath sounds and a few crackles. A patient has been described who developed vocal cord paralysis as a result of impingement of PMF on the recurrent laryngeal nerve.[368] As in silicosis, the risk of developing tuberculosis is increased in workers who have CWP;[271, 369] for example, a survey of Spanish coal miners, both with and without pneumoconiosis, revealed a risk of developing the infection three times that of the general surrounding population.[256]

There is little doubt that coal dust inhalation is related to the development of emphysema and chronic air-flow obstruction;[370] in addition, coal workers appear to be susceptible to chronic bronchitis.[371–374] In several investigations, emphysema has been shown to be present more often and to be more severe in patients who have CWP than in those who do not;[375, 376] emphysema also correlates with the degree of exposure to coal dust[377] and is additive to the effects of cigarette smoking.[294, 378, 379] In one investigation, nonsmokers who had experienced intermediate and high dust exposure levels had the same prevalence of abnormal lung function as smokers who had no dust exposure.[374] In one autopsy

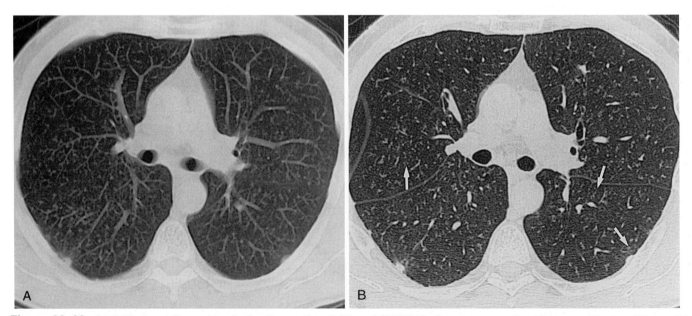

Figure 60–28. Coal Workers' Pneumoconiosis: Conventional CT and HRCT Findings. A conventional 10-mm collimation CT scan *(A)* demonstrates small nodules in both lungs. Subpleural nodules mimicking pleural plaques are also evident posteriorly. On HRCT *(B)*, the nodules are more difficult to distinguish from vessels. The nodular and branching opacities, however, clearly have a centrilobular distribution *(arrows)*. The subpleural pseudoplaques are also better defined on the HRCT image. (Courtesy of Dr. Martine Remy-Jardin, Centre Hospitalier Regional et Universitaire de Lille, Lille, France.)

study, the prevalence of emphysema was found to be greater in patients who had an increased severity of pneumoconiosis.[380] In a second such study, a strong association was also identified between dust content and emphysema in both nonsmokers and smokers.[381] Dust exposure and impairment of lung function were also linked in two large groups of American coal miners,[382, 383] although these results have been criticized because of poor validation of dust exposures.[384]

Laboratory Findings

Gallium scanning and labeled diethylenetriamine pentaacetate (DTPA) uptake are both abnormal in workers who have CWP,[385] reflecting the presence of lung injury and inflammation. The acute phase reactants C-reactive protein and fibrinogen are also elevated;[386] whether monitoring their levels serves any useful purpose remains to be determined. In one investigation, measurement of serum procollagen III was not found to be helpful in predicting progression of disease.[387] As indicated previously, hypergammaglobulinemia[312] and elevated serum levels of rheumatoid factor and antinuclear antibodies are common.[313–318]

Pulmonary Function Tests

Published results of pulmonary function testing in coal workers are variable, largely because of differences in population groups studied. Retired miners generally show more impairment than those who are working, an apparent paradox that is presumably explained by the observation that the former tend to leave their job because of disability (the appreciation of good lung function in working miners being an example of the "healthy worker" effect). Other variables that influence results include cigarette smoking and the particle size of coal dust inhaled.

One often cited study of pulmonary function published in 1955 involved patients who had simple pneumoconiosis and a control group of the same age; apart from minor disturbances in gas distribution, no significant differences in function were identified.[388] The results of a more recent long-term follow-up study of coal miners who did not have PMF but who were suspected of having suffered greater than average effects from dust exposure showed a relationship between exposure and FEV_1;[295] this suggests that even moderate exposure to dust can cause severe impairment of lung function in some miners. This hypothesis has been supported by the results of other studies in which a deterioration in FEV_1 has been shown to be related to cumulative dust exposure in coal workers whose chest radiographs were normal.[294, 389] In another investigation, patients who had radiographic changes suggestive of early disease (ILO classification 0/1 or 1/0) and CT scans that confirmed the presence of such disease, had lower $FEV_{1.0}/FVC$ ratios than similarly exposed individuals who had normal radiographs.[414]

Diffusing capacity can be reduced in miners who smoke but is usually normal in nonsmoking miners who have simple pneumoconiosis.[390, 391] Focal impairment of $\dot{V}/\dot{Q}$ ratios resulting in impaired gas exchange has been described in nonsmoking coal miners despite normal spirometric findings.[392] One assessment of lung mechanics in the early stages

of simple CWP has shown a loss of elastic recoil, implying the presence of emphysema.[393] Reduced diffusion, impaired gas exchange, and pulmonary hypertension have been described in coal workers who manifest category p micronodular disease.[280, 394–396] In a correlative radiographic, physiologic, pathologic, and clinical study of 247 coal miners, extensive emphysema was more common in patients who had this micronodular pattern than in those who had larger nodules, whether the pneumoconiosis was simple or complicated.[375] Other investigators have related the development of physiologic obstruction and emphysema to the late appearance of small irregular opacities (type s or t).[347, 348, 397]

In contrast to simple CWP, PMF is frequently associated with physiologic evidence of airway obstruction, reduced diffusing capacity, abnormal blood gases, and increased pulmonary arterial pressures.[398, 399] In one investigation, changes in function were attributed not only to PMF and the extent of emphysema, but also to small airway disease and interstitial fibrosis.[400] A comparison of pulmonary function in coal workers who had Caplan's syndrome and those who had PMF showed significantly less obstruction in the former patients but no significant difference in DLCO.[401]

Prognosis and Natural History

Mortality studies in coal miners[402] and coke oven workers[403] have shown no increase in the standardized mortality rate, despite an increase in the incidence of death from respiratory disease; in both these studies, this apparent paradox was explained on the basis of a significant decrease in the incidence of death from heart disease. Other investigators, however, have shown modest reductions in survival of men who have simple CWP,[404, 405] partly as a result of chronic obstructive pulmonary disease. Workers who have higher degrees of PMF, both smokers and nonsmokers, have significantly increased mortality rates.[406] In one investigation, miners who developed PMF when young had one third the survival rate of those who do not have CWP after a 22-year period of observation.[404] In contrast to patients who have silicosis, coal workers who have simple pneumoconiosis seldom show progression of disease if removed from the dust-ridden environment.[407, 408]

ASBESTOS

Asbestos is the general term given to a group of fibrous minerals composed of combinations of silicic acid with magnesium, calcium, sodium, and iron. The word is derived from the Greek, meaning *inextinguishable*,[409] reflecting the resistance of the substance to heat and acid as well as its strength, durability, and flexibility.

Mineralogically, asbestos can be divided into two major groups: the *serpentines*, of which the only member of commercial importance is chrysotile, and the *amphiboles*, which include amosite (brown asbestos), crocidolite (blue asbestos), anthophyllite, tremolite, and actinolite. Chrysotile, tremolite, and crocidolite are responsible for the vast majority of pleuropulmonary disease, the form and severity of which vary with the different fiber types. Crocidolite and, to a lesser extent, amosite are considered the most dangerous because of their carcinogenic potential.[410] Tremolite is a contaminant in most chrysotile mines and has been the subject of some debate concerning its pathogenicity;[411] however, most experts now agree that the substance can cause disease identical to that of the other forms of asbestos.[411-413] Anthophyllite was mined and used in Finland until 1970, but commercial production has now ceased, and it is usually identified in small amounts in lung fiber analyses.

Chrysotile fibers are curved, whereas the amphiboles are straight (Fig. 60–29). These physical properties as well as chemical differences are responsible for the varying uses of asbestos; for example, chrysotile fibers are particularly suitable for textile manufacture because they are long and pliable, whereas crocidolite and amosite are of greater value for marine insulation because they are more acid resistant. Different physiochemical properties between chrysotile and the amphiboles are also likely to have an influence on deposition patterns and clearance in the lung and on pathogenicity.

Epidemiology

The use of asbestos in industry increased enormously during the first three quarters of the twentieth century; world production jumped from 500 tons in 1900 to 3 million tons in 1968[415] to an estimated 6 million tons in 1981.[416] As a result of concerns about asbestos exposure and cancer, more recent production has stabilized at about 4 million tons per year.[409] Although recognition of the harmful effects of asbestos exposure has resulted in better control of dust levels and an overall decrease in total exposure, the potential for the development of serious disease still exists.[417-421] For example, it has been estimated that in the United States 8 to 9 million people have had occupational exposure to asbestos[422, 423] and that such exposure will eventually result in 300,000 deaths.[424]

The major producers of asbestos are Russia, Canada (principally Quebec), Zimbabwe, and South Africa; virtually all amosite and crocidolite is produced in South Africa, and most chrysotile comes from Russia and Quebec. Chrysotile is the most important form commercially, accounting for about 95% of the total asbestos marketed in the United States and elsewhere, mainly as asbestos cement.[409] In mining and milling, exposure occurs predominantly to only one type of fiber, although small amounts of other types may be present, even in commercially "pure" preparations.[425] By contrast, mixtures of fibers are commonly employed in construction and in the manufacture of textiles, and exposure to several fiber types is routine in these situations.

The three major sources of exposure to asbestos are (1) the primary occupations of asbestos mining and its processing in a mill, (2) numerous secondary occupations involving its use in a variety of industrial and commercial products, and (3) nonoccupational (environmental or paraoc-

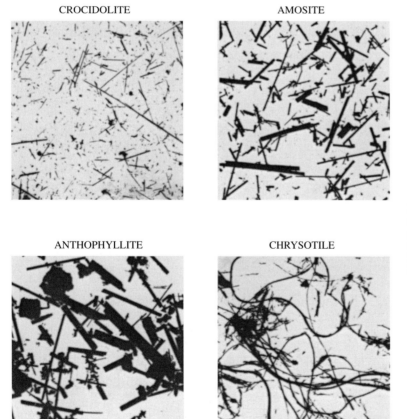

Figure 60–29. Types of Asbestos Fiber. Electron microscopic views of four different types of asbestos fiber show the amphiboles (crocidolite, amosite, and anthophyllite) to be straight and chrysotile to be distinctly curved. (From Timbrell B: Physical factors as etiologic mechanisms. IARC Sci Pub 8: 295, 1973.)

10 μm

cupational) exposure to contaminated air. In some individuals, such as those living adjacent to asbestos mines, such nonoccupational exposure can be substantial; however, in the majority, it is minimal and is evidenced only by the presence of asbestos fibers in digests of lung tissue.

The secondary uses of asbestos are numerous (Table 60–1). The most important are in the construction industry, in which asbestos is extensively incorporated in cement, pipes, tiles, mouldings, and paneling; shipbuilding and repair;[426-428] boiler making and repair;[429] railroad occupations;[430] the manufacture of textiles and plastics;[431] the manufacture and repair of gaskets and brake linings (although most insulation and friction materials are now made with nonasbestos fibers[409]); dentistry (affecting both dentists and dental technicians);[432] and the jewelry industry.[433] Although the risk of asbestos exposure applies during the manufacturing process, it is greater during demolition, such as occurs in construction[418] and elevator servicing.[434] Although the fiber is generally assumed to be well bound and harmless once it is incorporated into manufactured products,[435] reports of significant levels of airborne asbestos in buildings with deteriorating insulation leaves even this assumption in

doubt.[436, 437] Such potential exposure may be the cause of the increased prevalence of asbestos-related disease that has been reported in groups such as public school custodians.[438]

Environmental exposure to asbestos dust also occurs in individuals not directly involved in asbestos-related occupations.[439] The wide distribution of this mineral throughout the world is indicated by the frequency with which asbestos bodies can be found in routine autopsies, the prevalence ranging from 1% in rural Italy[440] to as high as 60% in New York City.[441] In urban areas such as Miami,[442] Glasgow,[441] London,[443] Pittsburgh,[444] Melbourne,[445] and Montreal,[446] the prevalence has ranged from 25% to 50%.

Although the identification of asbestos bodies in the lungs in routine autopsies indicates that exposure to the mineral is almost universal, there is no evidence that this is associated with a significant risk for the development of pleuropulmonary disease in most individuals.[447, 448] However, there is a substantial amount of evidence that individuals who live in the vicinity of a mine, mill, or factory that engenders heavy asbestos dust pollution have a greater incidence of pleural plaques and mesothelioma.[449-452] In fact, these abnormalities can develop in persons whose only expo-

Table 60–1. OCCUPATIONS AT RISK FOR ASBESTOS EXPOSURE: MINING, MILLING, MANUFACTURING, AND SECONDARY USES

PROCESS	PRODUCTS MADE OR USED	JOBS POTENTIALLY AT RISK
Production		
Mining		Rock mining, loading, trucking
Milling		Crushing, milling
Handling		Transport workers, dockers, loaders, those who unpack jute sacks (replaced with sacks that do not permit fibers to escape)
Primary Uses		
Spray insulation	Spray of fiber mixed with oil	Spray insulators (construction, shipbuilding)
Filler and grouting		
Manufacturing of textiles	Cloth, curtains, lagging, protective clothing, mailbags, padding, conveyor belts	Blending, carding, spinning, twisting, winding, braiding, weaving, slurry mixing, laminating, molding, drying
Manufacturing of cement products	Sheets, pipes, roofing shingles, gutters, ventilation shafts, flower pots	Blending, slurry preparation, rolling, pressing, pipe cutting
Manufacturing of paper products	Millboard, roofing felt, fine-quality electrical papers, flooring felt, fillers	
Manufacturing of friction materials	Automotive products: gaskets, clutch plates, brake linings	
Manufacturing of insulation products	Pipe and boiler insulation, bulkhead linings for ships	
Applications		
Construction		
New construction	Boards and tiles; putties, caulk, paints, joint fillers; cement products (tiles, pipes, siding, shingles)	Direct: carpenters, laggers, painters, tile layers, insulation workers, sheet metal and heating equipment workers, masons Indirectly: all other workers on construction sites, such as plumbers, welders, electricians
Repair, demolition		Demolition workers for all of these
Shipbuilding		
Construction	Insulation materials (boards, mattresses, cloth) for engines, hull, decks, lagging of ventilation and water pipes, cables	Laggers, refitters, strippers, steam fitters, sailmakers, joiners, shipwrights, engine fitters, masons, painters, welders, caulkers
Repair, refits	Insulation materials, as described for Construction	Directly: all above jobs on refits, dry dock, and other repair operations Indirectly: maintenance fitters and repairers, electricians, plumbers, welders, carpenters
Automotive industry		
Manufacture	Gaskets, brake linings, undercoating	Installation of brake linings, gaskets, and so on
Repair	Gaskets, brake linings, undercoating	Service people, brake repairers, body repairers, auto mechanics

Modified from Becklake MR: Am Rev Respir Dis 114:187, 1976.

sure is the repeated handling of the clothes of asbestos workers.[453–456] In addition, a particularly high prevalence of nonoccupational asbestos-related disease has been reported in some areas of Corsica[28] (where houses have been built on asbestos surface deposits) and from the Metsovo area of northwest Greece[457, 458] and isolated villages in Turkey[434, 459–461] (where the soil, which contains tremolite, has been used as a whitewash for buildings); although the manifestations of disease in these situations have been largely pleural—many of the inhabitants have pleural plaques and some mesothelioma—the possibility of an association with pulmonary carcinoma has also been raised.[462]

In clinical practice, a history of environmental or paraoccupational asbestos exposure may not be readily apparent from a cursory inquiry because the exposure may have occurred many years before the recognition of disease and may have been of short duration. An example of how remote nonoccupational exposure may be is illustrated by the story of two brothers aged 27 and 33 years who presented with chest wall and diaphragmatic pleural calcification and whose only exposure was playing in childhood in the cellar of their home, which was also used by their father in a muffler repair business.[454] Although disease caused by asbestos exposure, particularly mesothelioma, has been well described in workers who manufacture friction materials, such as brake and clutch linings,[463] the fear that there may be significant environmental contamination by asbestos dust from automobile brakes has been eliminated by studies showing that the high heat of friction on application of brakes converts asbestos to an inert nonfibrous silicate known as fosterite.[285, 464]

Pathogenesis

The pathogenesis of asbestos-related pleuropulmonary disease is complex and incompletely understood.[465, 466] The toxicity of the mineral itself appears to be related to its fibrous nature because pulverized asbestos does not cause disease.[409] Fiber dose, dimension, and durability may all influence both fibrogenicity and carcinogenicity, with longer, thinner, more durable fibers being the most biologically important.[465] Factors related to the host, including pulmonary clearance and immunologic status, and the presence of other noxious substances, such as cigarette smoke, are also undoubtedly important in determining the nature and severity of the final reaction to inhaled fibers. This section briefly outlines the factors involved in the development of asbestosis; those related to carcinogenesis of the lung and pleura are discussed on pages 1074 and 2810.

The development of asbestosis depends on the intensity and duration of exposure to asbestos fibers. Exposure has usually been accepted as a surrogate for dose in determining dose-response relationships for asbestos-related diseases; however, determinations of lung burden of asbestos fiber have enhanced the appreciation of the biology and epidemiology of these disorders.[467] It is intuitively apparent that the quantity of fiber retained in the lung is a function of both the amount of fiber that is inhaled and the amount that is subsequently cleared; both are important determinants of disease. For example, the results of an autopsy analysis of a group of Quebec chrysotile miners and millers suggest that the pathogenesis of both mesothelioma and asbestosis is

linked to tremolite, a contaminant of chrysotile that is more rapidly cleared by the lung.[468] In this study, there appeared to be no correlation between the severity of pulmonary fibrosis and total fiber length, surface area, or mass.[468, 469] The same authors performed a similar study of a group of shipyard workers from the Pacific Northwest, who had been exposed to both chrysotile and amosite fibers.[470] In this group, the concentration of lung amosite, the major residual fiber, most closely correlated with asbestosis. Although these investigations have included only small numbers of control subjects (exposed workers who did not have disease), studies in a sheep model suggest that the development of disease is linked to fiber retention.[471] Although dose-response relationships exist for all pleuropulmonary manifestations of asbestos exposure, the heaviest fiber burdens are associated with asbestosis.[467, 472–474]

Although the majority of inhaled asbestos is transported out of the lung via the mucociliary escalator,[475] a variable proportion enters the interstitium, the amount depending on the efficiency of fiber clearance and the asbestos dose itself. Passage from the air-space lumen to the interstitium may be accomplished by transport within macrophages, by direct penetration across the epithelium (either within or between epithelial cells),[475] or by the organization of an intraluminal exudate after epithelial injury.[476] The initial inflammatory reaction to retained fibers is an accumulation of macrophages, particularly at transitional airway bifurcations and to a lesser extent in alveoli.[93, 409] This accumulation occurs both by recruitment of peripheral blood monocytes and by replication of macrophages at the site of fiber deposition.[477] Activated complement may be the initial chemoattractant.[478] It is also likely that alveolar interstitial macrophages increase in number and secrete potentially harmful cytokines after asbestos transfer across the epithelium.[479] Evidence of airway epithelial injury (such as increased incorporation of tritiated thymidine) can be seen as soon as 24 hours after fiber inhalation in experimental animals.[480] Such epithelial damage may facilitate the passage of fibers from the air spaces into the interstitial tissue, a process that is undoubtedly important in the development of fibrosis.

Animal and human studies have shown that the activated macrophages that accumulate at the sites of asbestos deposition secrete a variety of proinflammatory and profibrotic cytokines—including fibronectin, PDGF, IGF-1, fibroblast growth factor, IL-1β and IL-6, TNF-α, granulocyte macrophage colony-stimulating factor, and neutrophil chemotactic factor—and inflammatory mediators such as leukotriene B_4 and prostaglandin E_2.[93, 409, 482–486] These substances are clearly important as mediators of the ensuing disease. For example, in the sheep model of asbestosis, fibronectin, neutrophil chemotactic factors, and fibroblast growth factors are required both to initiate and to sustain fibrosis.[93] Persistent BAL neutrophilia in asbestos-exposed men has also been associated with progressive deterioration in lung function,[487–489] the presence of crackles on physical examination,[490, 491] and abnormal gas exchange.[491] Higher concentrations of fibronectin and PGE_2 released from cultured alveolar macrophages from asbestos-exposed workers are associated with restrictive lung function, and a neutrophilic and eosinophilic alveolitis is seen in workers who have asbestosis, independent of cigarette smoking.[485, 491] As is the case for the finding of BAL neutrophilia, increased BAL eosinophils and fibronectin also predict worsening lung function with time.[489]

Asbestos-related tissue damage may occur by several mechanisms, one of the most important being direct damage by free radicals and other reactive oxygen species.[493–495] Endothelial injury produced by these substances may lead to the elaboration of prostacyclin, resulting in increased vascular permeability and other manifestations of inflammation.[496] The observation that genes involved in antioxidant defense are up-regulated in rats exposed to asbestos fiber is additional evidence that oxidants have a pathogenetic role.[497] In the sheep model of asbestosis, alveolar macrophages also release plasminogen activator, a protease that can cause tissue destruction, early in the course of disease.[498] Patients who have asbestosis demonstrate increased procoagulant activity in BAL fluid, which likely derives from both endothelial cells and alveolar macrophages.[499] This imbalance in the coagulation cascade might account for the enhanced fibrin deposition seen pathologically and may play a role in development of fibrosis. Deficiency of the enzyme glutathione-S-transferase does not appear to be related to tissue damage.[500]

Not everyone exposed to heavy concentrations of asbestos develops asbestosis; in fact, the dose-response relationship is weaker in this condition than in pneumoconioses such as CWP. This observation has raised the possibility that other extrinsic agents or intrinsic host factors may be important in the pathogenesis of disease. The most extensively studied extrinsic agent has been tobacco smoke. There is good epidemiologic evidence that cigarette smoking is associated with an increase in the prevalence of radiographically detectable small irregular opacities compatible with asbestosis in asbestos-exposed populations.[501, 502, 504–508] The mechanism behind this association is unclear. Animal models of asbestosis suggest that it may be related to enhanced retention of short fibers[509–511] (although the results of some studies have suggested that longer fibers are more fibrogenic than shorter ones[512–514]). Cigarette smoking also increases the number of macrophages and neutrophils in BAL fluid of patients who have asbestosis,[515] augments the release of reactive oxygen species and of the profibrotic cytokine TNF from alveolar macrophages,[493, 516] and enhances fiber transport across the airway epithelium.[517, 518] There is evidence that asbestos increases the levels of Clara cell protein (CC16) and surfactant-associated protein (SP-A) in distal air spaces;[519] by inhibiting phospholipase A_2, these molecules can potentially have an effect on local inflammatory and profibrotic events. However, because levels of CC-16 are reduced in the BAL fluid of asbestos-exposed smokers compared with asbestos-exposed nonsmokers, the importance of this effect in enhancing cigarette smoke-asbestos interaction is unclear. Lastly, a greatly enhanced asbestos-fiber burden has been demonstrated in the airways of asbestos workers who smoke compared with similarly exposed nonsmokers.[520] Any or all of these effects may be related to the the development of tissue damage and fibrosis.

Intrinsic host factors that might be important in determining individual susceptibility to the harmful effects of asbestos include the efficiency of alveolar and tracheobronchial clearance, variation in underlying lung structure,[521] and immunologic status. The last-named has been the most thoroughly studied, both in animal models and in affected workers. Some patients who have asbestos exposure demonstrate a predominantly lymphocytic alveolitis,[522] a form of inflammation that seems to protect against the development of pulmonary fibrosis[488, 522] but to promote the development of pleural plaques.[523] This observation has been supported by experiments in mice with severe combined immunodeficiency, who have been shown to develop a more severe inflammatory and fibrotic response to asbestos than control animals.[524] This protective effect may be related to the elaboration of γ-interferon, which has antifibrotic properties.[522, 525] There is also evidence that the presence of a lymphocytic alveolitis may be associated with a decreased risk for the development of mesothelioma.[526] In a large study of asbestos-exposed workers, most of whom did not have asbestosis, an increased helper-to-suppressor T cell ratio was found in peripheral blood associated with an increase in suppressor CD8 cells in BAL fluid, suggesting a redistribution of these cells from blood to lung.[527] Workers who had pleural plaques had an increased helper-to-suppressor ratio of T lymphocytes in BAL fluid; similar changes were seen in the peripheral blood of the few workers who had asbestosis.

As in some other pneumoconioses, evidence of altered immunologic activity is not uncommon in asbestos-exposed individuals. Circulating rheumatoid and antinuclear factors have been identified in 25% to 30% of asbestos workers who have abnormal chest radiographs, albeit in titers considerably lower than those usually identified in connective tissue diseases.[528] In workers exposed to asbestos, some investigators have found hypergammaglobulinemia, a variety of additional autoantibodies, and even immune complexes.[529–531] Although such B-cell hyperactivity appears to correlate with radiographic progression of asbestosis,[531] there is as yet no clear-cut evidence that it is directly involved in the pathogenesis of the disease.[529, 530] In contrast to B-cell function, cell-mediated immunity, as measured by either delayed hypersensitivity skin tests or *in vitro* methods, is reduced in patients who have relatively advanced asbestosis;[532–534] the results of one investigation suggest that this abnormality may antedate the radiographic appearance of fibrosis.[534]

Although the studies just cited raise the possibility of an immunologic factor in the pathogenesis of asbestosis, not all investigators have confirmed this. For example, in an investigation of anthophyllite asbestos workers in Finland, the prevalence of rheumatoid factor was found to be similar to that in healthy control groups.[535] In another study of long-term asbestos workers from Quebec (more than half of whom had asbestosis) and a reference population of local residents, no significant difference in the frequency of HLA phenotypes was found between the two groups.[536] These results have been confirmed in more recent studies.[537, 538]

Pathologic Characteristics

Pathologic abnormalities in the chest caused by asbestos inhalation can occur in the pleura, lung parenchyma, airways, and lymph nodes. Pleural disease is the most common and usually takes the form of parietal pleural plaques; localized visceral pleural fibrosis, more or less diffuse pleural fibrosis, and mesothelioma (each of which can be associated with pleural effusion) also occur. Pulmonary manifestations include diffuse interstitial fibrosis (asbestosis), round atelectasis, peribronchiolar fibrosis, and pulmonary carcinoma.

In addition to these pathologic abnormalities, evidence of asbestos exposure can also be seen in tissue sections by the identification of iron-coated asbestos fibers. These asbestos bodies are most often found in lung parenchyma but also occur in airway walls and intrathoracic lymph nodes. The discovery of such bodies in tissue sections, pulmonary secretions, or BAL fluid does not by itself signify the presence of asbestos-related pleuropulmonary disease; however, it strongly suggests that the patient has been exposed to a significant quantity of the mineral, usually in an occupational setting.

Pleural Manifestations

Pleural Plaques

As indicated, pleural plaques are the most common form of asbestos-related pleuropulmonary disease and are frequently unassociated with any other pathologic abnormality.[539–542] Grossly, they typically consist of well-demarcated, pearly white foci of hard fibrous tissue, 2 to 5 mm thick and several centimeters in diameter.[543] They can have a smooth or nodular surface and be round, elliptical, or irregular in shape (Fig. 60–30).[544] Foci of calcification are not uncommon and are occasionally extensive. Characteristically, the plaques are located on the parietal pleura overlying the ribs and on the dome of a hemidiaphragm. They are generally absent from the apices, costophrenic angles, and anterior chest wall and are almost always bilateral. Although plaques identical to those on the parietal pleura can also occur on the visceral surface, they are distinctly uncommon in this location; in our experience, such plaques are small and tend to be located in the interlobar fissures. Plaques can also be found on the peritoneal surface.[545]

Histologically, plaques are composed of dense bands of collagen often arranged in a "basket-weave" configuration (Fig. 60–31); inflammation, characterized by lymphocytes, is usually mild and focal.[541, 543, 544] Rarely, the fibrous tissue has an active (fibroblastic) appearance, suggesting a stage in plaque development (*see* Fig. 60–31); such "presumptive" plaques are seen most often in biopsy specimens taken during the investigation of benign asbestos effusion. Asbestos bodies are invariably absent in the plaques, although uncoated fibers may be demonstrated when the tissue is dissolved or ashed and examined under polarized light or by electron microscopy.[539, 546, 547]

Parietal pleural plaques are common, the incidence in consecutive routine autopsies ranging from about 5% to 10%.[541, 543] In most cases, there is evidence of prior asbestos exposure, as indicated by either an appropriate occupational history or the presence of a substantial number of asbestos bodies or uncoated asbestos fibers within the lungs.[540, 541, 548–550] In some patients, however, asbestos bodies are not demonstrable, and an exposure history is lacking;[539, 540, 551] as a result, plaques cannot be regarded as absolute evidence of an asbestos etiology, although they are certainly highly suggestive. Whether non–asbestos-related plaques are caused by trauma, infection, or inhalation of other mineral fibers usually cannot be established.

The pathogenesis of pleural plaques is unclear, and several mechanical, chemical, and immunologic mechanisms have been invoked to explain their formation.[459] It is known that inhaled asbestos fibers can be deposited in the periphery of the lung, from which they can be transported to the pleura. Mesothelial cells are able to phagocytose foreign particles, including asbestos, and have been shown to secrete the fibroblast chemoattractant, fibronectin.[552] Direct stimulation of pleural connective tissue cells by the asbestos fibers is also theoretically possible. Why the plaques preferentially develop in the parietal pleura is not apparent.

Focal Visceral Pleural Fibrosis

Relatively discrete foci of visceral pleural fibrosis morphologically distinct from pleural plaques are also not uncommon after asbestos exposure. They are most frequently located on the lateral aspect of a lower lobe and consist of ill-defined areas of fibrous tissue that usually measure only 0.5 to 1 mm in thickness. In fact, the fibrosis may be manifested by no more than a creamy white "cloudiness" that is barely perceptible as thickening (Fig. 60–32). More advanced lesions may appear to radiate from a central focus of relatively thicker fibrous tissue (*see* Fig. 60–32). The underlying lung may be normal or may show partial or complete collapse (round atelectasis; *see* farther on). Histologically, the lesion consists of mature fibrous tissue that contains a variable number of chronic inflammatory cells. Unless associated with round atelectasis or located in a fissure, the abnormality is unlikely to be detected on chest radiographs or CT.

Diffuse Pleural Fibrosis

In contrast to the relatively discrete foci of visceral and parietal pleural fibrosis described previously, some patients show more diffuse pleural thickening.[423] Although this thickening can be restricted to either the parietal[423] or visceral[553] pleura, it usually involves both and is accompanied by interpleural adhesions. The fibrosis can extend to adjacent interlobar fissures and interlobular septa[423] and even into the mediastinum;[554] however, because the lung parenchyma itself is not affected, asbestosis is by definition not present. Histologically, the lesions are composed of mature collagen and a variable number of chronic inflammatory cells. Acute fibrinous pleuritis[423] and interstitial fibrosis limited to the adjacent pulmonary parenchyma[553] are sometimes present.

It is not clear whether this form of pleural disease represents an exaggeration of one or both of the other two forms of fibrosis or is a pathogenetically separate process. In one study of seven patients who had diffuse pleural fibrosis, one or more episodes of prior pleural effusion were identified, suggesting that organization of the effusion might have been responsible for the chronic changes.[423] The presence of numerous inflammatory cells within the fibrous tissue in some cases has also raised the possibility of an immunologic contribution to the pathogenesis.[554]

Pleural Effusion

Histologic examination of the pleura from patients who have benign asbestos effusion may show fibrosis and nonspecific chronic inflammation;[555, 556] however, in our experience, an organizing fibrinous exudate is more common. In many cases, the fibrosis is a microscopic finding only, although in

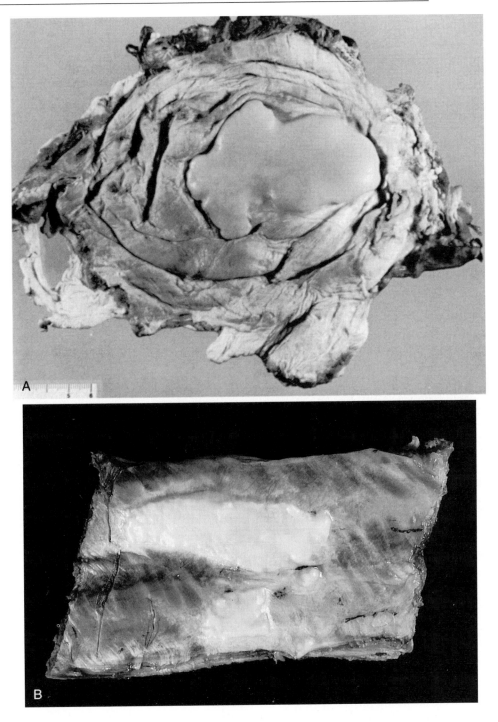

Figure 60–30. Parietal Pleural Plaques: Gross Appearance. A specimen of a hemidiaphragm *(A)* shows a smooth, pearly white, well-circumscribed area of fibrosis on the tendinous portion. A segment of two ribs *(B)* shows similar foci of fibrosis, one of which is elongated and roughly parallel to the long axis of the rib.

some it has also been associated with grossly identifiable diffuse pleural fibrosis.[423] Mesothelial hyperplasia may be present and must be distinguished from mesothelioma. As with other forms of asbestos-related pleural disease, the pathogenesis of nonneoplastic effusion is unclear. On the basis of experimental studies in rabbits, it has been suggested that interaction between asbestos fibers and pleural tissue results in the release of non–complement-related chemotactic factors that cause the effusion.[557] This hypothesis has been supported by the results of a study of rabbit mesothelial cells in which incubation with asbestos fibers was followed by the release of a substance that possessed chemotactic activity for neutrophils.[558]

Mesothelioma

There is no doubt of the association between asbestos exposure and the development of mesothelioma. The pathologic features and pathogenesis of this tumor are discussed in greater detail on page 2810.

Pulmonary Manifestations

Asbestos Body

Asbestos bodies are seen commonly in tissue sections in association with asbestos pleuropulmonary disease. They consist of a central transparent asbestos fiber surrounded by

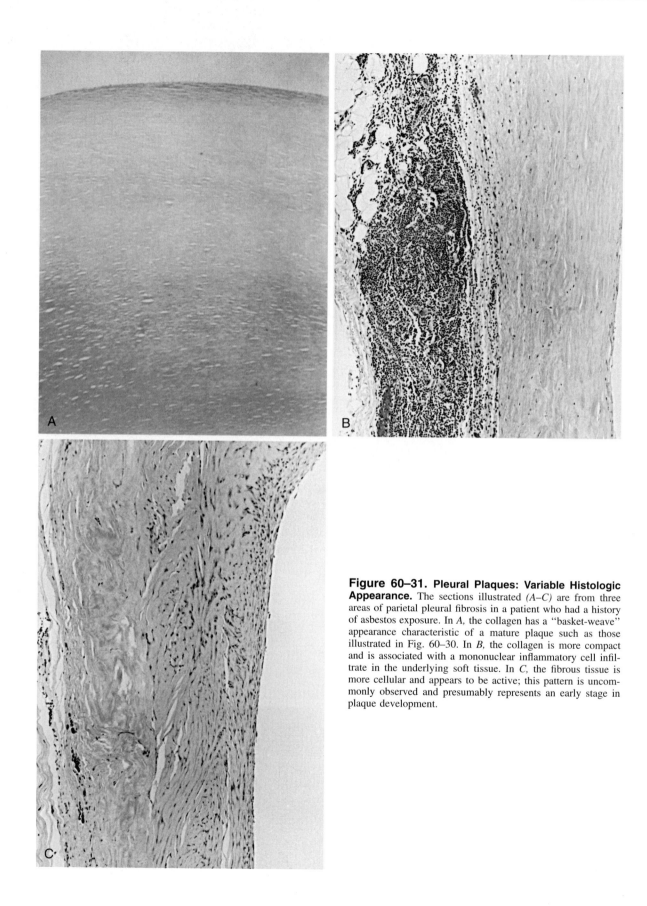

Figure 60–31. Pleural Plaques: Variable Histologic Appearance. The sections illustrated *(A–C)* are from three areas of parietal pleural fibrosis in a patient who had a history of asbestos exposure. In *A*, the collagen has a "basket-weave" appearance characteristic of a mature plaque such as those illustrated in Fig. 60–30. In *B*, the collagen is more compact and is associated with a mononuclear inflammatory cell infiltrate in the underlying soft tissue. In *C*, the fibrous tissue is more cellular and appears to be active; this pattern is uncommonly observed and presumably represents an early stage in plaque development.

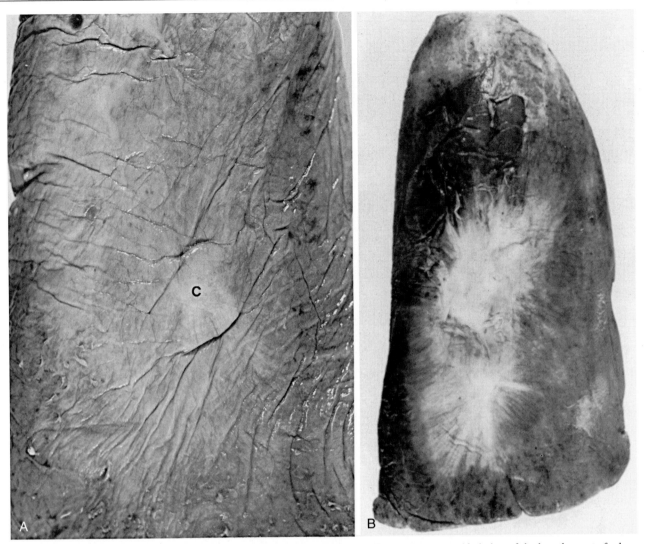

Figure 60–32. Localized Visceral Pleural Fibrosis Secondary to Asbestos Exposure. A magnified view of the lateral aspect of a lower lobe *(A)* shows a large portion of the pleura to have a creamy white appearance (compare with the normal pleura at the edge of the specimen). Except for the central region (C), the actual thickening of the pleura is barely perceptible. The lateral surface of another lower lobe *(B)* shows a more obvious but still rather poorly demarcated area of fibrosis that appears to radiate from two central foci. The underlying lung was unremarkable. (A fibrinous exudate related to premortem pneumonia is evident on the superior segment.) Both patients had a history of asbestos exposure.

a variably thick coat of iron and protein (Fig. 60–33). Most bodies measure 2 to 5 μm in width and 20 to 50 μm in length; the asbestos fibers themselves usually range from 0.1 to 1.5 μm in diameter.[559] The shape is quite variable depending on the length of the asbestos fiber, the amount and pattern of deposition of the protein-iron coat, and whether the body is whole or fragmented. The coat is often segmented over the length of the fiber and sometimes forms bulbous projections at both ends, resulting in a drumstick appearance (*see* Fig. 60–33). The majority are straight, although curved and angulated forms can be seen. The core of most asbestos bodies consists of amphiboles, especially amosite and crocidolite.[559, 560] The relative paucity of chrysotile cores probably results from the tendency of this substance to dissolve and fragment into forms that are too short to form bodies.[561]

In tissue sections, asbestos bodies are usually found in macrophages and may be in the interstitial tissue or air spaces; as indicated previously, they are rarely identified in pleural plaques. They can also be present in hilar and mediastinal lymph nodes[562] and even in extrathoracic visceral organs,[563, 564] where they have been reported to cause fibrosis.[565] Their presence in airway secretions, such as sputum, has been well documented in individuals who have occupational exposure,[566–568] and they are sometimes seen in specimens obtained by transthoracic needle aspiration.[569] They are usually not evident in specimens of pleural fluid.[568] Staining for iron can be helpful for identification, especially when few bodies are present.

Light microscopic examination of fluid obtained by BAL has also been employed as a means of identifying asbestos bodies. Using this technique, evidence of previous exposure to asbestos can be readily documented,[570] the number of asbestos bodies found in the fluid specimens generally correlating with the number in lung tissue sections.[571, 572] Although significant exposure has been considered to be excluded by either the complete absence of asbestos bodies[490, 573] or the presence of a small number,[574] there are some

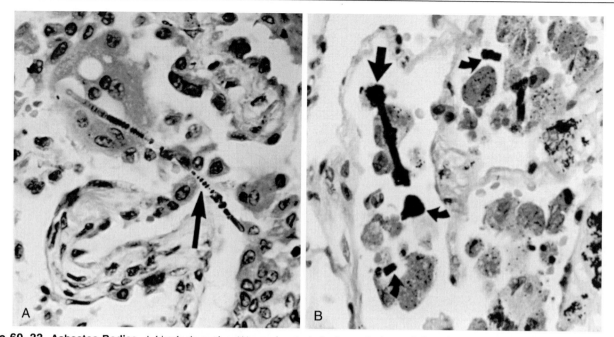

Figure 60–33. Asbestos Bodies. A histologic section *(A)* reveals a typical asbestos body consisting of a slightly curved, elongated structure with a finely beaded iron-protein coat. The asbestos fiber itself can be identified as a thin line in the center of the coat near one end of the body *(arrow).* In another section *(B),* other asbestos bodies show a more prominent iron-protein coat obscuring the enclosed asbestos fiber; some bodies appear to be fragmented *(curved arrows):* A characteristic drumstick form is taken by one *(straight arrow).* (A and B, ×400.)

exposed workers whose fluid contains no bodies.[575] In one study, the highest asbestos body counts were found in patients who had clinical evidence of asbestosis;[574] however, in two others, quantitative analysis did not serve to distinguish asbestos workers who had disease from those who did not,[490] and no association of body number with radiographic or functional abnormalities could be documented.[575]

It is widely believed that asbestos bodies are formed within an alveolar macrophage by deposition of a glycoprotein matrix and iron around a phagocytosed asbestos fiber.[559, 576] There is some evidence, however, that iron-protein deposition may also take place in the extracellular tissue adjacent to the macrophage.[577] The source of the iron may be red blood cells released as a result of asbestos-related tissue injury or circulating iron stores.[559] The encasement of foreign material by an iron-glycoprotein coat is not unique to asbestos; it has been shown to occur in experimental animals around fiberglass or synthetic aluminum silicate particles[578] and in humans around a variety of particles, including talc, mica, carbon *(see* Figs. 60–22 and 60–65), diatomaceous earth, rutile (a form of titanium dioxide), fly ash, zeolite, silicon carbide, and even iron itself.[579–582] With the exception of zeolite, such nonasbestos ferruginous bodies can usually be distinguished from true asbestos bodies by the appearance of the fiber core, which is thin and translucent with asbestos and black or colored and often thick with other particles.[579, 580]

Although for practical reasons, asbestos bodies are most often identified in tissue sections, their true number is best estimated by examining concentrates of digested lung tissue;[583] for example, it has been estimated that microscopic examination of 30 to 40 fields at a magnification of 400 would be necessary to find a single asbestos body in a tissue section from lung that contains 5,000 bodies per gram.[584] Because of its sensitivity, the use of a digestion technique

permits identification of asbestos bodies in virtually all individuals in the general population,[585, 586] whereas microscopic examination of tissue sections reveals them only rarely in the absence of occupational exposure.

Attempts have been made to correlate the number of asbestos bodies seen in tissue sections with the number identified in tissue digests. In one study of six individuals who had asbestosis or asbestos-related neoplasia, an average of two asbestos bodies on 2 × 2 cm iron-stained tissue sections 5 μm thick was found to be equivalent to approximately 200 asbestos bodies per gram of wet-fixed lung tissue.[587] In another investigation of seven patients who had asbestosis, one asbestos body in a 4-μm tissue section of average area 3.25 cm^2 was found to be equivalent to 1,000 per gram of wet tissue.[588] A mathematical model has been developed that has been claimed to be even more accurate in predicting total lung asbestos body concentration from the number of asbestos bodies in tissue sections.[584] Even in the presence of fibrosis and a high asbestos fiber burden, however, asbestos bodies may be scarce or absent in tissue sections of some subjects.[589]

Although the presence of a substantial number of asbestos bodies in digested lung samples examined by ordinary light or phase contrast microscopy is a reliable indicator of significant asbestos exposure, it is clear that the absolute number of asbestos *bodies* identified by these means is a gross underestimation of the total number of uncoated asbestos *fibers* as determined by electron microscopic examination.[559, 585, 590] Thus, the ratio of uncoated to coated fibers in lung digests ranges from approximately 7:1 to 5,000:1 in different series.[585] Because it is likely that the fibers rather than the coated asbestos bodies are involved in the pathogenesis of disease, this discrepancy in number is clearly important. In individuals who do not have occupational exposure, most uncoated fibers are short (< 5 μm in length) and consist of chrysotile or noncommercial amphiboles, such as tremolite and anthophyllite.[591]

The number of asbestos bodies and fibers per gram of digested lung tissue is roughly proportional to both the presence and severity of disease and the degree of occupational exposure.[559, 585, 586, 592] Thus, individuals who have well-documented high exposure generally have a 20-fold to 100-fold increase in the total number of fibers within the lung compared to controls;[585] individuals who have asbestosis or mesothelioma often have a 100-fold to 1,000-fold relative increase.[585] As might be expected, individuals who have environmental (nonoccupational) asbestos exposure generally have levels between those of individuals who have an occupational history and those of the general population.[593] Analysis of specific fibers may be helpful in distinguishing background exposure to asbestos from that related to occupational exposure, the finding of chrysotile or tremolite fibers longer than 8 μm being highly suggestive of the latter.[594]

Asbestosis

Asbestosis can be defined as diffuse pulmonary parenchymal interstitial fibrosis secondary to the inhalation of asbestos fibers. The condition is usually associated with a history of prolonged occupational exposure to asbestos and with a large number of asbestos bodies and fibers in samples of lung tissue treated by digestion techniques.[585] Frequently, asbestos bodies are also visible in tissue sections, where they may also be present in great numbers.

Grossly, the fibrosis is most prominent in the subpleural regions, particularly of the lower lobes, and varies from a slightly coarsened appearance of the parenchyma to obvious honeycomb change (Fig. 60–34).[544, 592] As might be expected from this gross description, the microscopic appearance varies from a mild increase in interstitial collagen to complete obliteration of normal lung architecture associated with the formation of thick fibrous bands and cystic spaces (Fig. 60–35). An inflammatory cellular reaction is usually mild; if prominent, the possibility of idiopathic pulmonary fibrosis should be considered. It is important to remember that parenchymal fibrosis limited to the immediate subpleural region may represent a reaction to adjacent pleural fibrosis, rather than asbestosis; thus, to diagnose the latter condition, fibrosis should also be documented at a distance from the subpleural region when the pleura is fibrotic.

The cystic spaces formed as a result of the parenchymal fibrosis may be lined by metaplastic bronchiolar cells or by hyperplastic type II cells, the latter sometimes containing well-demarcated eosinophilic inclusions within their cytoplasm that are identical histochemically and ultrastructurally to those seen in the liver secondary to alcohol toxicity (Mallory's hyaline) (Fig. 60–36).[595, 596] (When first described, these inclusions were thought to be specifically related to injury by asbestos;[595] however, it is now apparent that they can be caused by a variety of pulmonary insults.[596] Thus, from a diagnostic point of view, their principal significance is that they not be confused with viral inclusions.) A grading system to assess the severity of interstitial fibrosis on a systematic basis has been proposed.[544]

The earliest histologic change in asbestosis is considered by some authorities to consist of fibrosis in the walls of respiratory bronchioles.[425, 544, 597] According to this view,

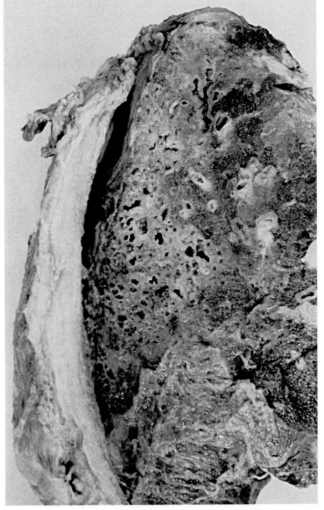

Figure 60–34. Diffuse Pleural Fibrosis and Asbestosis. A slice through the midportion of a lower lobe shows marked pleural thickening and parenchymal interstitial fibrosis. The pleural lesion consists of fibrous tissue, which extends over most of the costal surface; although focally it appears to be related predominantly to the parietal pleura, interpleural adhesions are present in many areas. The pulmonary fibrosis is most evident in the subpleural region and has a distinctive honeycomb appearance.

the process begins in the most proximal of such airways and extends in time to involve membranous and other respiratory bronchioles and eventually the adjacent alveolar interstitium; as the disease progresses, greater portions of lung parenchyma are affected in a centrifugal fashion. Although there is no doubt that peribronchiolar fibrosis occurs in association with asbestos exposure (Fig. 60–37), some investigators have suggested that it may represent a process pathogenetically distinct from pulmonary parenchymal fibrosis and should thus be termed *mineral dust airway disease* rather than asbestosis.[598–601] This view is based on the observation that airway abnormalities similar to those in asbestos workers can be identified in patients who have a history of exposure to mineral dust other than asbestos,[600] implying that the airway changes represent a nonspecific reaction. The results of experimental studies in sheep have also provided evidence for two distinct pulmonary reactions, one related to small airways and the other to the parenchymal interstitium.[598] Whatever its relationship to interstitial fibrosis, the peri-

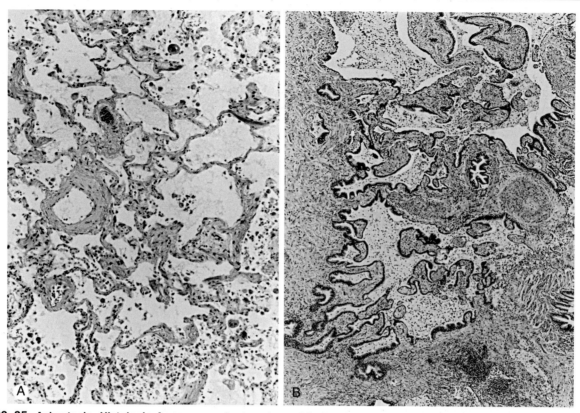

Figure 60–35. Asbestosis: Histologic Appearance. Sections show mild *(A)* and severe *(B)* interstitial fibrosis. In *A*, collagen is present in the walls of several transitional airways and alveolar septa. In *B*, there is marked distortion of lung architecture associated with the presence of broad bands of fibrous tissue and cystic spaces focally lined by metaplastic bronchiolar epithelium (corresponding to honeycomb lung). (*A*, ×100; *B*, ×30.)

bronchiolar and alveolar duct fibrosis seems likely to be related to the air-flow obstruction that is observed in both patients[602–606] and experimental animals.[598, 607, 608]

Round Atelectasis

Round atelectasis consists of a focus of collapsed lung parenchyma partly surrounded by thickened, invaginated pleura.[609–613] Although the area of collapse is usually only several centimeters in diameter and located in the periphery of the lung, involvement of a whole lobe can be seen.[614] The majority of cases are associated with asbestos-related visceral pleural fibrosis;[615–618] other causes, such as tuberculosis, are evident occasionally. Grossly, the atelectatic lung is poorly defined and appears to blend imperceptibly with the adjacent normal lung parenchyma (Fig. 60–38).[610] The overlying pleura is invariably fibrotic and shows one or more invaginations that may measure as much as 0.5 cm in thickness and extend several centimeters into the adjacent lung (Fig. 60–39). Pleural wrinkling and folding and a variable degree of alveolar collapse and fibrosis are seen microscopically (*see* Fig. 60–38). The pathogenesis of the disorder is discussed on page 522.

Other Forms of Pulmonary Parenchymal Disease

The histologic pattern of bronchiolitis obliterans with organizing pneumonia (BOOP) has been described in biopsy specimens from some patients whose radiographs have shown a localized opacity.[32, 619] It is not clear whether these cases represent an unusual reaction to inhaled asbestos or simply idiopathic BOOP in patients who happen to have been exposed to asbestos. Both lymphocytic interstitial pneumonitis[620] and idiopathic pulmonary fibrosis[621] have been reported in asbestos-exposed individuals. Distinction of these abnormalities from asbestosis can be difficult; histologic features that favor idiopathic pulmonary fibrosis include the presence of a prominent interstitial inflammatory reaction, a predominance of parenchymal compared to peribronchiolar fibrosis, a varied pattern with foci of apparently active disease (inflammation, fibroblastic tissue) adjacent to foci of mature interstitial fibrous tissue, and an absence of asbestos bodies. Rarely, the lungs of asbestos-exposed individuals have also been reported to show granulomatous inflammation similar to sarcoidosis;[619] again, it is unclear whether this represents an unusual reaction to asbestos or an entirely different disease process.

Pulmonary Carcinoma

As with mesothelioma, there is no doubt about the significant relationship between asbestos exposure and pulmonary carcinoma, particularly in cigarette smokers; the issue is discussed in Chapter 31 (*see* page 1074).

Radiologic Manifestations

Radiologic manifestations of asbestos-related disease are much more common in the pleura than in the paren-

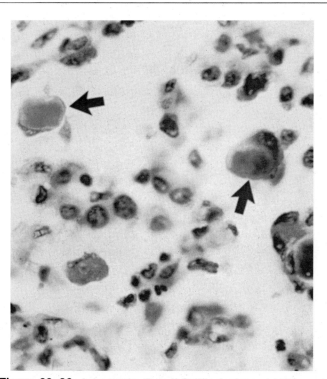

Figure 60–36. Asbestosis: Type II Cell Inclusions. A highly magnified view of lung parenchyma with asbestosis shows macrophages and hyperplastic type II cells, some of which contain smudged, densely eosinophilic cytoplasmic inclusions *(arrows);* they are similar to those seen in hepatocytes secondary to alcohol toxicity (Mallory's hyaline). (×600.)

chyma.[622-625] For example, in one study of 40 patients, only 5 had parenchymal changes; pleural plaques were the sole manifestation of disease in the other 35.[625] In another study of 56 patients, 48% showed asbestos pleural disease alone; 41%, combined pleural and parenchymal manifestations; and

11%, parenchymal changes alone.[623] Radiographic evidence of pleural abnormalities is present in the majority of patients who have asbestosis; in one investigation of 133 such patients, 88 (66%) had pleural changes, including 78 (59%) who had pleural calcification.[626] Overall, it has been estimated that there may be as many as 1.3 million people in the United States who have radiographically detectable asbestos-related pleural thickening.[422]

CT, in particular HRCT, has a higher sensitivity than chest radiography in the detection of both pleural and parenchymal abnormalities.[627-629] In a prospective analysis of 100 asbestos-exposed workers, pleural abnormalities were evident on the chest radiograph in 53 and on HRCT in 93;[628] parenchymal abnormalities consistent with asbestosis were present on the radiograph in 35 and on HRCT in 73. Asbestos-related pleural thickening can be seen in 95% to 100% of patients who have evidence of asbestosis on HRCT.[627, 628, 630]

Pleural Manifestations

Four types of radiologic abnormality occur in the pleura: focal plaque formation, diffuse thickening, calcification, and effusion. Each type may occur alone or in combination with the others.

Pleural Plaques

Radiographically, pleural plaques usually are more prominent in the lower half of the thorax and tend to follow the ribs when seen *en face*.[546, 631, 632] They may be smooth or nodular in contour and can measure up to 1 cm in thickness, although they are usually thinner (Fig. 60–40). They are seen most commonly on the domes of the diaphragm, on the posterolateral chest wall between the seventh and tenth ribs, and on the lateral chest wall between the sixth and ninth

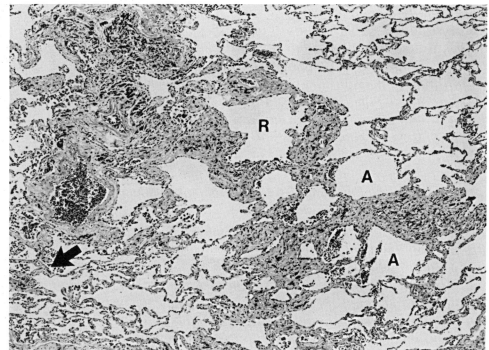

Figure 60–37. Peribronchiolar Fibrosis Associated with Asbestos Exposure. In this histologic section, the wall of a respiratory bronchiole (R) and its daughter alveolar ducts (A) are substantially thickened by fibrous tissue, pigmented macrophages, and a mild lymphocytic infiltrate. The adjacent parenchyma shows focal mild interstitial fibrosis *(arrow).* The pattern is consistent with early asbestosis (asbestos bodies were easily identified in the fibrotic areas and the adjacent lung parenchyma). The patient was a 55-year-old man employed as an insulator. (×40.)

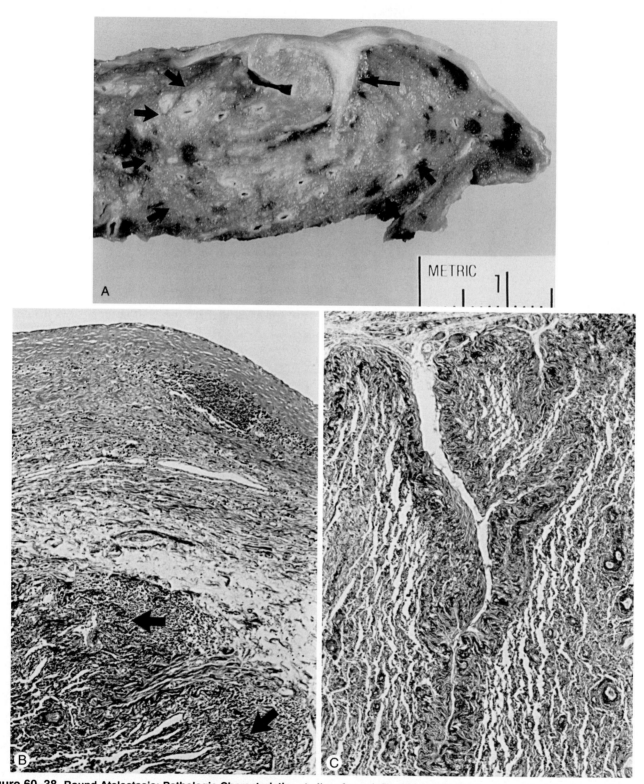

Figure 60–38. Round Atelectasis: Pathologic Characteristics. A slice of an uninflated lower lobe *(A)* shows a poorly defined, somewhat rounded focus of atelectasis *(short arrows)* that blends almost imperceptibly with normal lung. The overlying visceral pleura is fibrotic and focally invaginates into the underlying parenchyma *(long arrow)*. A histologic section *(B)* shows pleural fibrosis and wrinkling of the pleural elastic lamina *(arrows)*. A section through one of the deep pleural invaginations *(C)* reveals more extensive wrinkling. The adjacent lung is atelectatic and shows mild fibrosis. (*B,* ×60; *C,* ×40; both Verhoeff–van Gieson.) (From Menzies R, Fraser R: Round atelectasis. Am J Surg Pathol 11:674, 1987.)

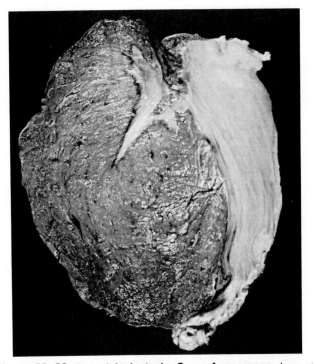

Figure 60–39. Round Atelectasis: Gross Appearance. A resected segment of lower lobe shows marked pleural fibrosis that is continuous with a somewhat triangular invagination that extends approximately 2 cm into the adjacent lung. The latter appears dense in the region of the invagination, reflecting the presence of atelectasis.

ribs.[449, 624, 633-635] The earliest manifestation is a thin line of unit density visible under a rib in the axillary region. Although usually multiple, occasionally only a single plaque is visible.

Because they frequently occur along the posterolateral

and anterolateral portion of the thorax, plaques may be difficult to identify on posteroanterior and lateral radiographs, particularly when viewed *en face*. Sometimes, they are more readily detected on a tangential 45-degree oblique view.[624, 636, 637] Plaques may be bilateral and symmetric, bilateral and asymmetric or, less commonly, unilateral.[503, 638-640] For unexplained reasons, unilateral plaques are identified more commonly on the left (Fig. 60–41).[641] For example, in one review of radiographs of 105,064 civilian and military employees of the U.S. Navy, 1,914 were considered to have plaques, bilateral in 81% and unilateral in 19%;[639] in workers who had unilateral plaques, the left-to-right ratio was 3.5:1. In patients who have bilateral disease, the width and extent of plaques as well as the extent of calcification, are also frequently greater on the left than on the right, at least on radiographs.[640] In one study of CT scans from 40 patients who had asbestos-related plaques, there was no significant predominance in either hemithorax.[641a]

Although plaques usually involve the parietal pleura, they may also be seen in the visceral pleura, including the interlobar fissures (Fig. 60–42).[642] Thickening of fissures not related to plaques is also common. In a radiographic study of an asbestos-exposed population and a control group, thickening of the interlobar fissures was seen in 54% of asbestos workers compared with 16% in the unexposed control group.[642] Fissural thickening was present in 85% of workers who had parietal pleural plaques and in 36% of those without plaques; it was particularly common in patients who had pulmonary fibrosis (affecting 85%) but was also identified in 45% of those who did not have evidence of asbestosis.

Although the detection of plaques radiographically is highly specific for a history of asbestos exposure, the sensitivity is relatively poor. Depending on the criteria for diagnosis, the frequency with which plaques are recognized on the chest radiograph ranges from only 8% to 40% of cases in

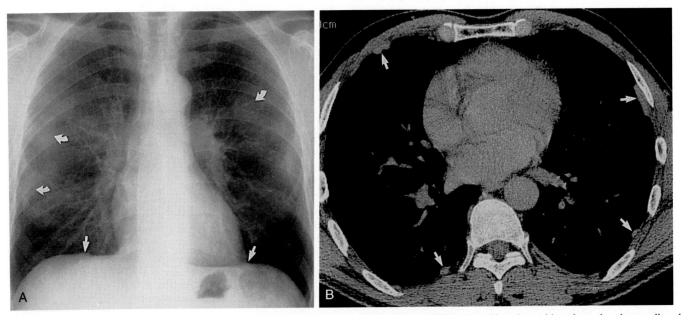

Figure 60–40. Pleural Plaques. A posteroanterior chest radiograph *(A)* demonstrates multiple pleural-based opacities along the chest wall and diaphragm. Several are viewed tangentially *(straight arrows)*, whereas others are ill-defined because they are viewed *en face (curved arrows)*, indicating their origin from the posterolateral or anterolateral chest wall. HRCT *(B)* confirms the presence of bilateral plaques *(arrows)*. The patient was a 51-year-old shipyard worker.

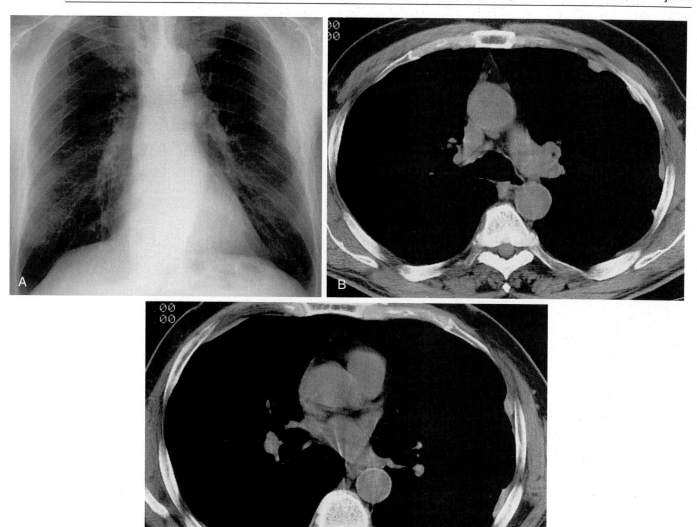

Figure 60–41. Markedly Asymmetric Pleural Plaques. A posteroanterior chest radiograph *(A)* in a 74-year-old shipyard worker shows evidence of pleural plaques only on the left side. HRCT at the level of the tracheal carina *(B)* also demonstrates only plaques on the left side. HRCT through the lower lung zones demonstrates prominent plaques on the left and thin plaques on the right.

which they are demonstrable at autopsy.[541] In one study, the combination of bilateral posterolateral plaques at least 5 mm thick or bilateral calcified diaphragmatic plaques was shown to have a 100% positive predictive value for the diagnosis of autopsy-proven asbestos-related pleural disease;[643] however, these criteria allowed detection of only 12% of plaques. Use of less strict criteria resulted in a considerable number of false-positive diagnoses.

The greatest problem in the radiographic diagnosis of pleural plaques (as well as diffuse pleural thickening) lies in distinguishing them from normal companion shadows of the chest wall—not those that are associated with the first three ribs (because this area is rarely involved in asbestos-related pleural disease), but those muscle and fat shadows that can be identified in as many as 75% of normal posteroanterior radiographs along the inferior convexity of the thorax. In fact, it is sometimes impossible to differentiate pleural plaques from companion shadows on the radiograph.

HRCT has a greater sensitivity than either conventional CT or chest radiography in the detection of these abnormalities.[627, 628, 644] With this technique, plaques can be identified as circumscribed areas of pleural thickening separated from the underlying rib and extrapleural soft tissues by a thin layer of fat (*see* Figs. 60–40 and 60–41). Normally, a 1- to 2-mm-thick stripe of soft tissue attenuation is visible on HRCT scans in the intercostal spaces at the point of contact between the lung and chest wall.[645] This stripe, called the *intercostal stripe*, consists of visceral and parietal pleura, endothoracic fascia, and the innermost portion of intercostal muscle. Most of the thickness of the stripe is related to the intercostal muscle because the endothoracic fascia is thin and the combined thickness of visceral and parietal pleura and normal fluid is only 0.2 to 0.4 mm.[645] The stripe can be seen because a layer of intercostal fat separates the innermost intercostal muscle from the internal intercostal muscles. Normally, no soft tissue attenuation is seen adjacent to a rib or

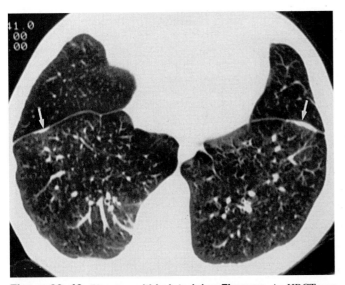

Figure 60–42. Plaques within Interlobar Fissures. An HRCT scan demonstrates pleural plaques in the right and left major fissures *(arrows).* Also noted are curvilinear opacities in the right paravertebral region extending to an area of pleural thickening. The patient was a 71-year-old man who had previously worked in a shipyard.

in the paravertebral regions because the intercostal muscles do not pass internally to the ribs or vertebrae and because the pleura and endothoracic fascia are not thick enough to be seen in these locations. Therefore, any distinct stripe of soft tissue attenuation internal to a rib or in the paravertebral region is abnormal.[645]

In one study of 30 patients in whom conventional and oblique radiographs revealed pleural shadows of uncertain origin, CT demonstrated that the opacities were the result of subpleural fat accumulation in 14 (47%);[644] of the remaining 16 patients, 10 had definite pleural plaques, 4 had no evidence of either plaques or fat, and 2 demonstrated shadows that could not be attributed with certainty to either plaques or fat.

Calcification

Although noncalcified pleural plaques are the most common radiographic manifestation of asbestos-related disease, they are clearly more striking when calcified (Fig. 60–43). The frequency of calcification is quite variable, ranging from 0% to 50% in different series;[449, 623, 625, 646] these differences in prevalence are probably related to differences in the type of inhaled asbestos. As might be expected, the complication is seen more commonly on CT than on the radiograph. In a study of 100 asbestos-exposed American workers, it was detected on chest radiography in 13, on conventional CT in 16, and on HRCT in 20.[628]

Calcified plaques vary from small linear or circular shadows to shadows that completely encircle the lower portion of the lungs.[647] When calcification is minimal, a radiograph overexposed at maximal inspiration facilitates visibility.[648] The most common site is the diaphragm, although it may be seen at any location.[649] The complication generally does not develop until at least 20 years after the first exposure to asbestos,[624, 649] although the occupational exposure can be relatively short; for example, two patients have been

described in whom isolated calcified diaphragmatic plaques developed approximately 20 years after occupational exposure of only 8 and 11 months.[650]

Diffuse Pleural Thickening

In contrast to a pleural plaque, diffuse thickening is manifested as a generalized, more or less uniform increase in pleural width. Although the term is not precisely defined in the 1980 ILO classification, diffuse pleural thickening is generally considered to be present radiologically when there is a smooth uninterrupted pleural density extending over at least one fourth of the chest wall with or without obliteration of the costophrenic angles.[651] It is diagnosed on CT when a continuous area of pleural thickening greater than 3 mm extends for more than 8 cm craniocaudally and 5 cm around the perimeter of the hemithorax.[652]

On HRCT, the margin between an area of diffuse pleural thickening and the adjacent lung is frequently irregular as a result of parenchymal fibrosis, in contrast to the usually sharply circumscribed margins of pleural plaques.[653] The abnormality is usually associated with contralateral pleural abnormalities, either diffuse pleural thickening or plaques.[654, 655] Although calcification may be present, it is seldom extensive.[655, 656] As with other causes of fibrothorax, asbestos-related pleural thickening seldom involves the mediastinal pleura (although it frequently affects the parietal pleura abutting the paravertebral gutters [Fig. 60–44]).[655, 657] The absence of involvement of the mediastinal pleura can be readily assessed at CT and is often helpful in distinguishing benign from malignant pleural thickening; for example, in one study of 19 patients, only 1 of 8 who had fibrothorax had thickening of the mediastinal pleura as compared with 8 of 11 who had mesothelioma.[655]

Pleural Effusion

Asbestos-associated pleural effusion is often not appreciated (Fig. 60–45).[658–660] The most comprehensive report of its prevalence and incidence was a study of 1,135 exposed workers and 717 control subjects in which benign asbestos effusion was defined by[660] (1) a history of exposure to asbestos; (2) confirmation of the presence of effusion by radiographs, thoracentesis, or both; (3) absence of other disease related to pleural effusion; and (4) absence of malignant tumor within 3 years. According to these criteria, 34 benign effusions (3%) were identified in the exposed workers compared to none in the control subjects. The likelihood of the presence of effusion was dose related. The latency period was shorter than for other asbestos-related disorders, being the most common abnormality during the first 20 years after exposure. Most effusions were small, 28% recurred, and 66% were unassociated with symptoms.

The major differential diagnoses are tuberculosis and mesothelioma. Of 12 patients in one series, mesothelioma was recognized in one patient 9 years after the first documented effusion.[658] Of four patients in another series, two eventually developed mesothelioma.[661] Differentiation from a tuberculous effusion can be made with confidence only if biopsy and culture specimens are negative. The subject of asbestos-related effusion is discussed in greater detail on page 2754.

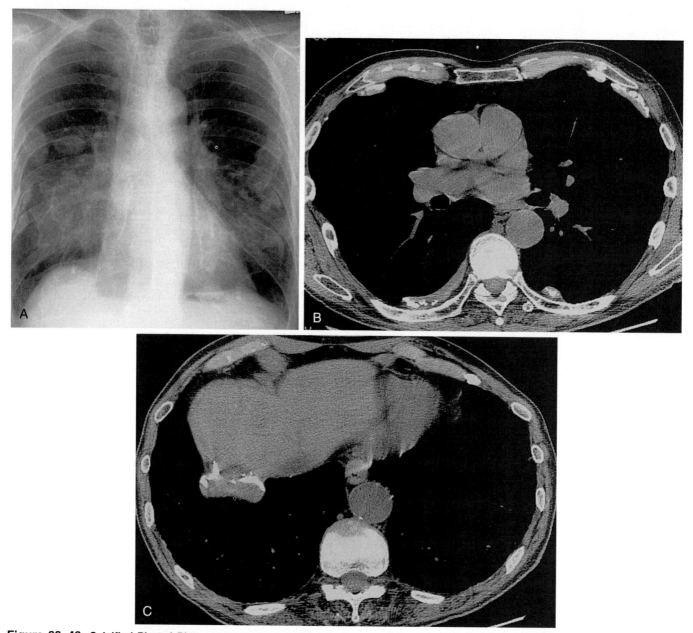

Figure 60–43. Calcified Pleural Plaques. A posteroanterior chest radiograph *(A)* in an 82-year-old man demonstrates numerous bilateral calcified pleural plaques. The patient had worked for many years in a shipyard. HRCT *(B and C)* demonstrates calcified plaques along the posteromedial and anterolateral chest wall and right hemidiaphragm.

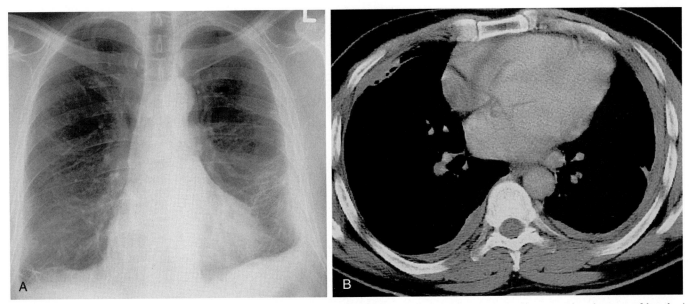

Figure 60–44. Diffuse Asbestos-Related Pleural Thickening. A 47-year-old cement worker presented with progressive shortness of breath. A posteroanterior chest radiograph *(A)* demonstrates diffuse bilateral pleural thickening as well as blunting of the costophrenic sulci. Curvilinear opacities extending to the thickened pleura are present in the left lung. An HRCT scan *(B)* confirms the presence of marked pleural thickening. The inner margin of the thickened pleura is irregular because of areas of fibrosis or atelectasis in the adjacent lung. Despite the extensive pleural thickening in the paravertebral portion of the pleura and lateral chest wall, there is no evidence of involvement of the mediastinal pleura.

Mesothelioma

The most characteristic radiologic manifestation of mesothelioma consists of diffuse pleural thickening (pleural rind) with associated loss of volume of the ipsilateral hemithorax (Fig. 60–46) (*see* also page 2820).[662–666] Pleural effusion is frequently present and is characteristically not associated with contralateral shift of the mediastinum because of the restrictive action of the pleural tumor. Occasionally, the thickening is focal and simulates a pleural plaque.[665, 666] Features that favor mesothelioma include nodular pleural thickening, mediastinal pleural thickening, involvement of the interlobar fissures, and presence of pleural effusion.[655, 657, 665, 666] Pleural plaques are identified on CT in about 30% to 70% of patients who have mesothelioma and pleural calcification in 20% to 50%.[655, 665, 666] The latter is almost invariably within pleural plaques and only rarely within the tumor itself.[667, 668]

In the vast majority of cases, mesothelioma can be readily distinguished from benign asbestos-related pleural plaques on the radiograph and on CT. It may be more difficult, however, to distinguish the tumor from diffuse asbestos-related pleural thickening or other causes of benign or malignant pleural disease.[655, 657] In one review of the CT findings in 74 consecutive patients who had diffuse pleural disease, of whom 39 had malignant disease and 35 benign, features that were most suggestive of malignant disease included circumferential pleural thickening, nodular pleural thickening, parietal pleural thickening of more than 1 cm, and mediastinal pleural involvement (Fig. 60–47).[655] The sensitivities of these findings in detecting malignant pleural involvement were 41%, 51%, 36%, and 56%, with specificities ranging from 88% to 100%; 28 of the 39 malignant cases (sensitivity 72%, specificity 83%) were identified correctly by the presence of one or more of these criteria.

Pulmonary Manifestations

Asbestosis

Asbestosis is typically manifested on the chest radiograph by the presence of irregular small linear opacities (Fig. 60–48). The development of these abnormalities may be divided into three stages:[669] (1) an early stage of fine reticulation occupying predominantly the lower lung zones and associated with a ground-glass appearance that is probably the result of both pleural thickening and interstitial fibrosis; (2) a stage in which irregular small opacities become more marked, creating a prominent interstitial reticulation; during this stage, the combination of parenchymal and pleural abnormalities leads to partial obscuration of the heart border—the so-called shaggy heart sign—and of the diaphragm; and (3) a late stage in which reticulation becomes visible in the midlung and upper lung zones and the cardiac and diaphragmatic contours become more obscured.[175, 669]

Hilar lymph node enlargement is seldom if ever evident on the radiograph;[648] however, mediastinal lymph nodes greater than 1 cm in diameter are frequently seen on CT.[670] Although asbestosis characteristically exhibits considerable mid- and lower zonal predominance, a small number of patients have been reported in whom slowly progressive pleural and parenchymal fibrosis occurred in the lung apices.[671] Large opacities measuring 1 cm or more in diameter have also been described in occasional patients who have asbestosis;[672] however, these patients have also been exposed to quartz, and it is likely that the latter was responsible for the conglomerate shadows.

Although the radiographic findings of asbestosis are not specific, the diagnosis should be strongly suspected when irregular linear opacities are associated with pleural plaques or diffuse pleural thickening. In approximately 20% of patients who have radiographic findings of asbestosis, however,

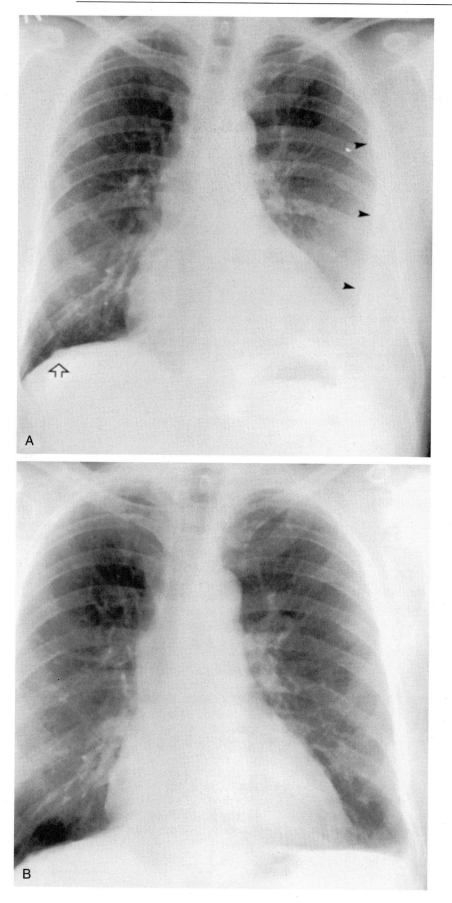

Figure 60–45. Asbestos-Induced Pleural Effusion, Plaque Formation, and Round Atelectasis. A posteroanterior chest radiograph *(A)* shows a left pleural effusion of moderate size *(arrowheads).* A small plaque *(open arrow)* is present on the right hemidiaphragm. A vague opacity is visible behind the right atrial shadow. A posteroanterior radiograph taken 6 months later *(B)* reveals regression of the pleural effusion, although there is residual pleural fibrosis.

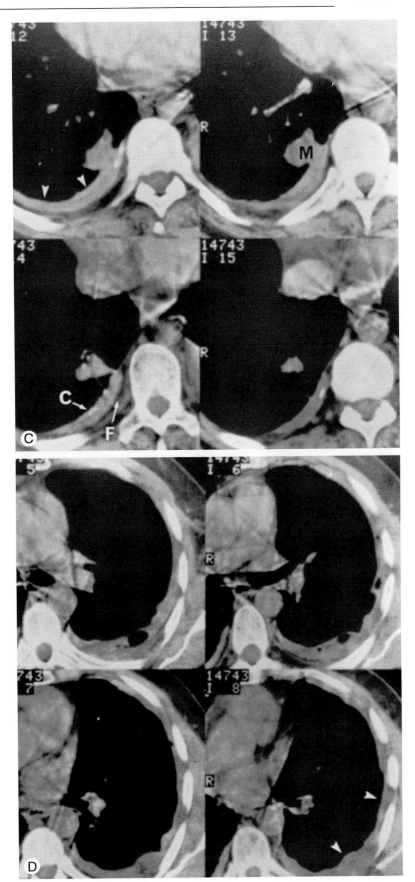

Figure 60–45 *Continued.* Contiguous 10-mm-thick CT scans (obtained on the same day as the radiograph in *B)* through the right *(C)* and left *(D)* lower lobes demonstrate extensive bilateral posteromedial pleural thickening *(arrowheads)*. Note the linear calcifications (C) and increased fat (F) in relation to the thickened pleura on the right. A mass (M) is present adjacent to the thickened pleura.

Illustration continued on following page

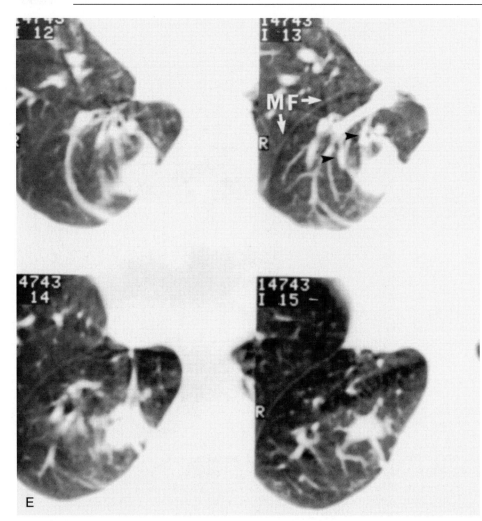

Figure 60–45 *Continued.* CT scans with lung window technique *(E)* through the mass demonstrate the typical features of round atelectasis: Note the curvilinear displacement of the nearby bronchovascular bundles (*comet tail* sign) *(arrowheads)*. The major fissure (MF) is displaced posteromedially, indicting loss of volume of the right lower lobe. The patient was a 55-year-old man.

there is no radiographic evidence of asbestos pleural disease.[673] Moreover, radiographs fail to demonstrate any parenchymal abnormalities in 10% to 20% of patients who have pathologically proven asbestosis.[674, 675]

As with other conditions, CT—particularly HRCT—allows detection of parenchymal abnormalities not evident on the chest radiograph.[627–629, 663] In one prospective study of 100 asbestos-exposed workers, HRCT findings suggestive of asbestosis were present in 43 of 45 (96%) workers who satisfied clinical criteria of asbestosis, compared to 35 (78%) individuals who had radiographic abnormalities.[628] Another investigation of 60 asbestos workers demonstrated characteristic features of asbestosis in 100% of patients examined by HRCT, compared to 90% for chest radiography.[627] In a review of the HRCT findings and pulmonary function tests in 169 asbestos-exposed workers who had normal chest radiographs (ILO profusion score < 1/0), CT abnormalities consistent with asbestosis were found in 57;[629] this group of patients had significantly lower vital capacity and DLco than the workers who had normal CT scans.

The most common HRCT manifestations of asbestosis are intralobular linear opacities, irregular thickening of interlobular septa, subpleural curvilinear opacities, subpleural small rounded or branching opacities, and parenchymal bands.[627, 628, 676, 677] Small, round (dotlike), and branching subpleural opacities are considered to be the earliest manifes-

tation of disease.[676] These are typically visible a few millimeters from the pleural surface in a centrilobular distribution. HRCT-pathologic correlation has shown the opacities to reflect the presence of peribronchiolar fibrosis.[676] Subpleural curvilinear opacities are linear areas of increased attenuation of variable length located within 1 cm of the pleura and parallel to the inner chest wall (Fig. 60–49).[677] The majority measure between 5 and 10 cm in length. They are seen most commonly in early disease, although they may reflect honeycombing; they may also represent atelectasis adjacent to pleural plaques.[656, 676, 678]

Another common HRCT feature seen in asbestos-exposed workers is the presence of parenchymal bands, defined as linear opacities measuring 2 to 5 cm in length coursing through the lung, usually to abut an area of pleural thickening.[628] Pathologic correlation has shown these bands to correspond to fibrosis along the bronchovascular sheath or interlobular septa with associated distortion of parenchymal architecture.[678] The bands are more common in asbestosis than in other causes of pulmonary fibrosis; for example, in one study, they were present in 79% of patients who had asbestosis compared with 11% of patients who had idiopathic pulmonary fibrosis.[679] As in other causes of interstitial pulmonary fibrosis, architectural distortion of the secondary lobules and irregular thickening of the interlobular septa are commonly seen in asbestosis (Fig. 60–50). With progression

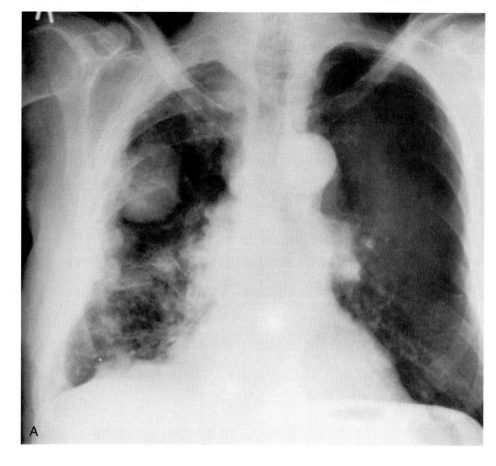

Figure 60–46. Diffuse Mesothelioma. An overpenetrated posteroanterior chest radiograph *(A)* shows a reduction in volume of the right hemithorax. There is marked thickening of the pleura over the whole of the right lung, including its mediastinal surface. The thickening is nodular and is associated with a large pleural-based mass in the upper axillary region.

Illustration continued on following page

of fibrosis, irregular linear opacities and honeycombing predominate (Fig. 60–51).[630, 680] At all stages, the abnormalities involve predominantly the subpleural regions of the lower lung zones.[654, 678, 680]

These HRCT findings, similar to those on the radiograph, are nonspecific, and no single sign can be considered diagnostic of asbestosis.[681] The likelihood of asbestos-related interstitial fibrosis, however, increases with the number of abnormalities identified.[630] The accuracy of HRCT in predicting the presence of asbestosis was assessed in a group of 24 patients and 6 lungs obtained at autopsy;[630] histologic evidence of asbestosis was present in 25 of the 30 patients or lungs. The most common HRCT findings consisted of intralobular lines or thickened interlobular septa, parenchymal bands, architectural distortion of the secondary lobules, subpleural lines, and honeycombing. To confidently identify the cases as asbestosis, three of these abnormalities had to be identified on CT; although a positive interpretation based on one or two abnormalities increased the sensitivity, it resulted in a substantial decrease in specificity. The procedure was considered to identify insufficient abnormalities to diagnose asbestosis in 5 of the 25 (20%) cases, whereas 10 radiographs (40%) were nondiagnostic.

Because the abnormalities in patients who have mild asbestosis are often limited to the posterior aspects of the lower lung zones, it is recommended that CT scans in these patients be obtained in both supine and prone positions or only in the prone position.[628, 630, 682] Scans with the patient prone are important to distinguish the normal increased opacity in the dependent lung regions from mild fibrosis. In fact,

it has been shown that taking a small number of prone images at selected levels in the lower lung zones has a high sensitivity in the detection of asbestos-related pulmonary and pleural abnormalities.[682] This procedure, combined with low radiation dose scans, may become a cost-effective method of screening for asbestosis in high-risk populations.[682, 683]

Gallium-67 lung scans have been shown to be positive in patients who have asbestosis and in sheep exposed to asbestos, a feature possibly attributable to increased transepithelial leakage of serum proteins bound to the isotope as well as to its uptake by intra-alveolar macrophages.[716] Increased epithelial protein permeability, as assessed by DTPA scanning, has also been demonstrated in individuals who have asbestosis.[488, 717]

Round Atelectasis

The characteristic radiologic manifestation of round atelectasis is a rounded or oval, pleural-based opacity associated with loss of volume and with curving of adjacent pulmonary vessels and bronchi (the comet-tail sign).[684, 685] The opacity typically abuts an area of pleural thickening or a pleural effusion. The comet-tail sign of pulmonary vessels and bronchi as they are swept around and into the focus of atelectasis is easier to identify on CT than on the radiograph (Fig. 60–52). The abnormality may occur anywhere in the lungs but is most commonly found in the posterior aspect of the lower lobes.[686–689] It may be unilateral or bilateral (Fig. 60–53) and may measure from 2 to 7 cm in diameter.

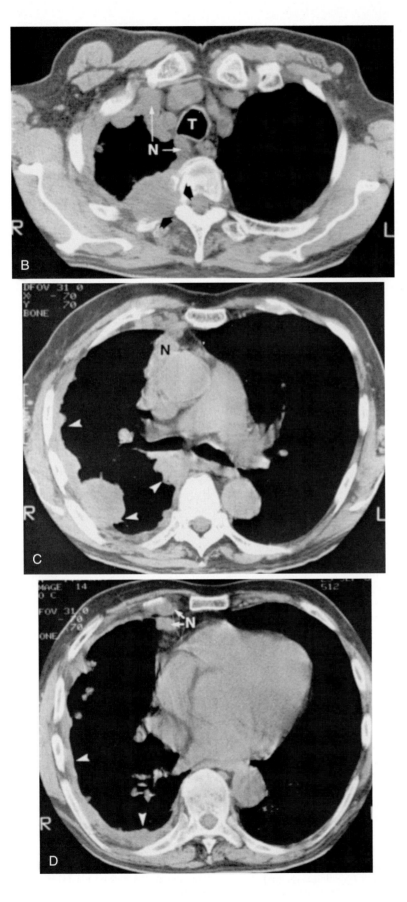

Figure 60–46 *Continued.* CT scans through the upper *(B)*, middle *(C)*, and lower *(D)* thorax confirm the extensive right pleural thickening *(arrowheads)* and demonstrate extrapleural extension of the neoplasm in and around the ribs and vertebra *(closed arrows)* and within some of the mediastinal lymph nodes (N). The diagnosis of mesothelioma was confirmed at autopsy several months later.

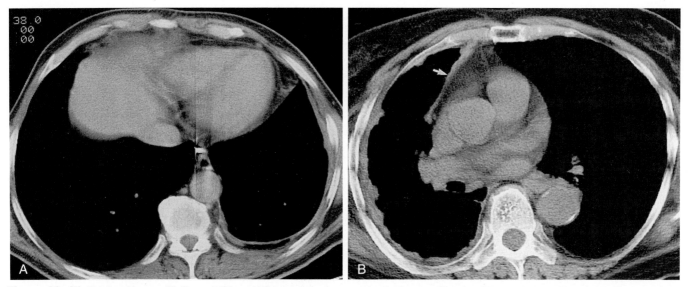

Figure 60–47. Benign Versus Malignant Pleural Thickening. A conventional 10-mm collimation CT scan *(A)* in a 59-year-old man demonstrates extensive thickening of the posteromedial, lateral, and anterior aspects of the left pleura; the mediastinal pleura is uninvolved. The patient had been exposed to asbestos many years before as a carpenter. Pleural biopsy specimens demonstrated only fibrosis. A CT scan in an 80-year-old woman *(B)* demonstrates extensive right pleural thickening. Involvement of the mediastinal pleura *(arrows)* as well as nodular appearance of the pleural thickening is evident. Biopsy demonstrated mesothelioma.

Significant enhancement may occur with intravenous contrast administration.[690, 691]

As indicated previously, the majority of cases follow asbestos exposure; however, some have been described in association with other causes of pleural thickening or effusion.[689, 692] The lesion may develop and progress over a few months or several years. In one series of 74 patients, it occurred on a background of benign asbestos pleurisy in 9 and slowly increasing pleural thickening in 13;[692] in the remaining 39 patients, it was a new finding, earlier radiographs showing only plaques or being normal. The magnetic resonance appearance has been described in one patient.[693] Similar to CT, it demonstrated the abnormality as a peripheral mass abutting an area of pleural thickening with associated vessels curving into the area of atelectasis. Curved low-signal lines within the atelectatic lung were postulated to be caused by indentations of the visceral pleura.[693] Round atelectasis is not metabolically active on 2-[18F] fluoro-2-deoxy-D-glucose (FDG) positron emission tomography (PET).[693a] FDG-PET imaging therefore can be helpful in differentiating the abnormality from pulmonary carcinoma.[693a]

Clinical Manifestations

The great majority of patients who have pleuropulmonary asbestos-related disease have no symptoms.[449, 669] Benign pleural effusions may or may not be associated with pleural pain.[556, 694–696] They are recurrent in 15% to 30% of cases,[696, 697] are usually smaller than 500 ml, are often serosanguineous,[556, 696, 697] and persist from 2 weeks to 6 months.[696, 697] Although they can occur in the absence of pleural plaques, more often these are present at the time of effusion.[697] In one study of 22 patients who had benign pleural effusion attributed to asbestos exposure, the mean duration of exposure was 5.5 years (in one case, it was said

to occur after only 2 weeks), and the mean interval between exposure and presentation was about 16 years.[696] Persistent pleuritic pain with intermittent pleural friction rubs has been described in some patients.[696]

In the absence of underlying chronic obstructive pulmonary disease, breathlessness is usually associated with pulmonary interstitial fibrosis; occasionally, it is caused partly or entirely by diffuse pleural fibrosis.[423, 508, 699–702] In patients who have asbestosis, shortness of breath seldom develops sooner than 20 to 30 years after initial exposure.[703, 704] It is usually progressive, despite discontinuation of asbestos exposure. Prolonged asbestos exposure can also cause cough, either dry or productive of mucopurulent sputum; this symptom can be present with or without dyspnea on exertion and in the absence of radiographic or physiologic evidence of asbestosis.[705] In one cohort study of asbestos workers, wheeze and dyspnea were associated with a significant risk for restrictive lung function impairment;[706] smaller but similar functional deficits were associated with a history of cough, sputum production, and chronic bronchitis.

Physical examination may reveal evidence of deformity of the thoracic cage caused by underlying pleural disease, even in asymptomatic patients. Pleural effusion may be suggested by unilateral or bilateral dullness on percussion and decreased breath sounds. Crackles are common at the lung bases in workers who have had prolonged exposure to asbestos;[707] in two studies, they were present in about one third of workers compared with only 5% of control subjects.[708, 709] They are particularly common in patients in whom the diagnosis of asbestosis has been made radiographically,[710] being found in 58% in one series[711] and in 64% in another.[712] In one study in which time-expanded waveform analysis was employed, fine crackles were detected in all 12 patients who had asbestosis;[713] differences in the timing and nature of the crackles could be discerned between patients who had left ventricular failure and those who had asbestos-related pleural disease. The presence of crackles also correlates with derangement of pulmonary function.[710]

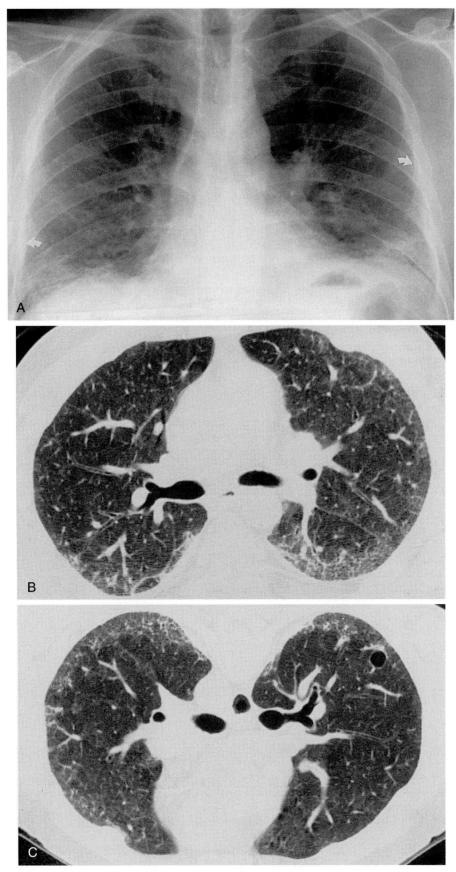

Figure 60–48. Asbestosis. A posteroanterior chest radiograph *(A)* in a 54-year-old shipyard worker demonstrates irregular linear opacities in the lower lung zones. Note associated low lung volumes and bilateral pleural plaques *(arrows)*. HRCT scans in the supine *(B)* and prone *(C)* positions demonstrate irregular linear opacities involving predominantly the subpleural lung regions. The opacities represent both intralobular lines and thickening of interlobular septa. Localized areas of ground-glass attenuation in the subpleural lung regions are also evident.

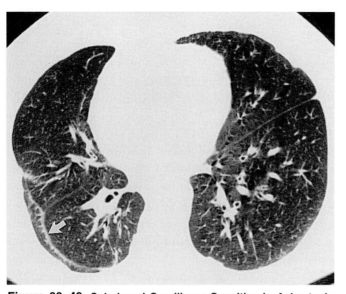

Figure 60–49. Subpleural Curvilinear Opacities in Asbestosis. An HRCT scan demonstrates a subpleural curvilinear opacity in the right lung running parallel to the pleura *(arrow)*. Bilateral pleural plaques and evidence of early fibrosis in the posterior aspect of the left lung are also present. The parenchymal abnormalities did not change in the prone position. The patient was a 58-year-old shipyard worker.

Finger clubbing is also a frequent sign in asbestosis,[704] having been observed in 32% of patients in one series[711] and in 42% in another.[712] The prognostic significance of the finding was evaluated in 167 patients who had asbestosis certified by the London Pneumoconiosis Medical Panel from 1958 to 1975.[714] In the individuals who had clubbing, it was found to develop early in the clinical course of the disease and to be associated with a lower diffusing capacity, a higher mortality rate, and a greater likelihood of progression of pulmonary fibrosis than in those who did not. Thus, its presence is an indication of a more severe form of disease; however, finger clubbing was not associated with heavier

asbestos exposure. If the patient lives long enough and survives complicating mesothelioma or pulmonary carcinoma, signs of cor pulmonale may develop. Rarely, patients who have asbestosis develop chronic constrictive pericarditis.[715]

Pulmonary Function Tests

Patients who have asbestosis usually show a restrictive pattern of pulmonary function, with decreased vital capacity, residual volume, and diffusion capacity and preservation of relatively good ventilatory function.[718, 719] Many patients, however, show some degree of airway obstruction as well as a result of asbestos-induced bronchiolar fibrosis and narrowing[720–722] or enhancement of the effects of cigarette smoking.[723] In addition, the prevalence of CT-diagnosed emphysema in workers who have early asbestosis (54%) has been found to be double that of those who do not;[233] such emphysema undoubtedly contributes to the air-flow obstruction. Because many asbestos workers smoke cigarettes, the measurement of total lung capacity (TLC) by itself is an insensitive means of assessing functional impairment in asbestosis.[724] Many workers who have significant asbestosis have normal or increased TLC as a result of the presence of associated air-flow obstruction.[724, 725] Therefore, helium dilution methods are particularly unsuitable for assessing lung volumes in these patients.[727] An accelerated decline in lung function has been noted in dust-exposed workers in the absence of a clinical and radiographic diagnosis of asbestosis.[721, 728, 729] Pulmonary compliance characteristically is greatly reduced[215, 704, 707, 730–732] and may be an early marker of pulmonary fibrosis when the chest radiograph is normal.[733]

Hypoxemia may be observed on exercise, but the P_{CO_2} is usually normal or low. One group of investigators found a ratio of $P(A-a)O_2/\dot{V}O_2$ greater than 35 during exercise to be quite specific for asbestosis in a group of workers who had a spectrum of asbestos-related disorders, including air-

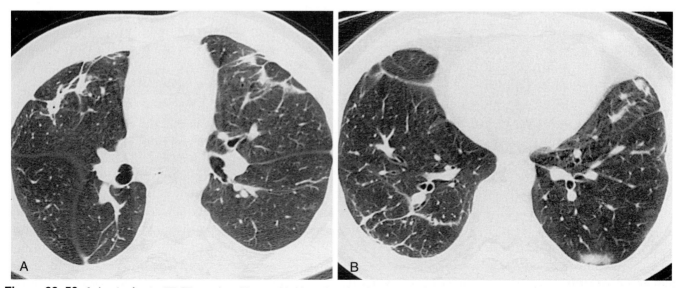

Figure 60–50. Asbestosis. An HRCT scan in a 45-year-old shipyard worker demonstrates irregular linear opacities, interlobular septal thickening, and evidence of architectural distortion in the anterior aspect of the midlung zones *(A)*. Irregular thickening of interlobular septa in the right lower lobe *(B)* is also evident.

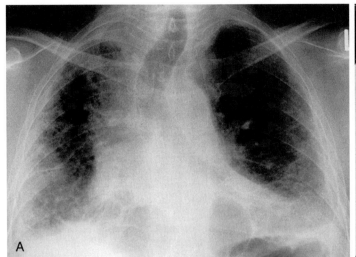

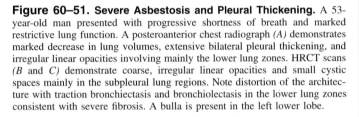

Figure 60–51. Severe Asbestosis and Pleural Thickening. A 53-year-old man presented with progressive shortness of breath and marked restrictive lung function. A posteroanterior chest radiograph *(A)* demonstrates marked decrease in lung volumes, extensive bilateral pleural thickening, and irregular linear opacities involving mainly the lower lung zones. HRCT scans *(B* and *C)* demonstrate coarse, irregular linear opacities and small cystic spaces mainly in the subpleural lung regions. Note distortion of the architecture with traction bronchiectasis and bronchiolectasis in the lower lung zones consistent with severe fibrosis. A bulla is present in the left lower lobe.

flow obstruction and pleural disease;[734] however, the measurement lacked sensitivity. Employing electron microscopic and stereologic techniques, another group concluded that measurable diffusion abnormalities were caused chiefly by ventilation-perfusion imbalance rather than increased thickness of the alveolar septa.[734a]

In one investigation in which the radiographic and functional characteristics of patients who had asbestosis were compared with those of patients who had idiopathic pulmonary fibrosis, pulmonary function was found to be better in patients who had asbestosis than in those who had idiopathic pulmonary fibrosis with the same degree of radiographic parenchymal abnormality.[735] Patients who have idiopathic pulmonary fibrosis also have worse gas exchange on exercise than do those who have asbestosis,[736] the former having greater falls in arterial oxygen saturation and higher levels of dead space ventilation.

It has become clear that asbestos-related pleural disease can also affect lung function adversely.[718, 721, 737, 738] Both pleural plaques and diffuse pleural thickening cause decreases in vital capacity, although the effects of diffuse thickening are more marked.[719, 739–741] Some investigators have linked the presence of asbestos pleural disease to the finding of air-flow obstruction greater than that expected for

the degree of cigarette smoking;[742–744] this finding might be explained by concomitant asbestos-related airway disease. When restriction is the result of diffuse pleural thickening, correction of the diffusing capacity for alveolar volume gives a higher coefficient of diffusion that may not accurately reflect the severity of any accompanying parenchymal fibrosis.[745, 746]

Exercise testing is often used to evaluate asbestos-exposed workers as part of compensation assessment. In one group of 120 asbestos-exposed workers who were seeking compensation, a large number were limited by cardiac function.[747] This finding contrasts with those of later studies, in which patients who had diffuse pleural thickening alone or pleural plaques had ventilatory abnormalities on exercise, with normal cardiovascular responses;[748, 749] in these patients, there was excessive ventilation, high dead space ventilation, and (sometimes) oxygen desaturation, the last-named suggesting the presence of underlying occult pulmonary fibrosis.

Diagnosis

In the presence of characteristic radiographic findings, the diagnosis of asbestos-related disease should be based

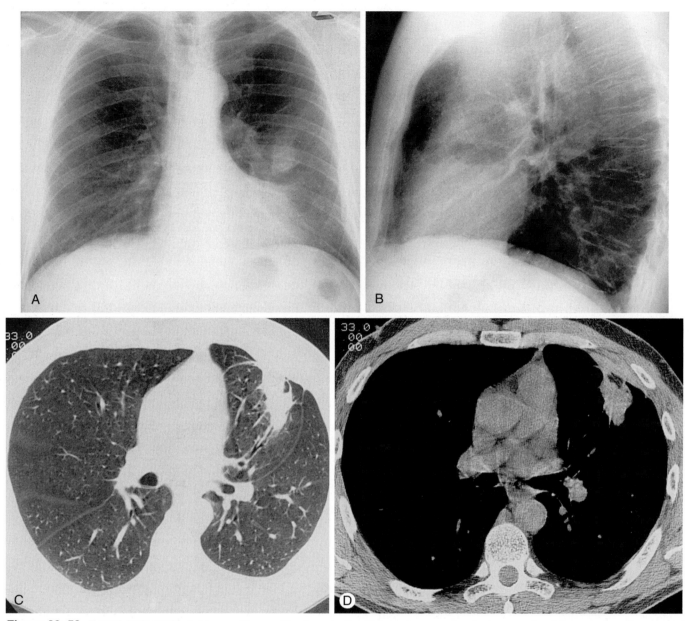

Figure 60–52. Round Atelectasis. A 54-year-old man with a long-standing history of exposure to asbestos was referred for evaluation of a suspected left lung mass. Posteroanterior *(A)* and lateral *(B)* chest radiographs demonstrate evidence of left pleural thickening and a 3-cm mass in the left lung. The margins of the mass are poorly defined, indicating that it is pleural based. An HRCT scan *(C)* demonstrates an oval soft tissue mass in the lingula associated with loss of volume and anterior displacement of the major fissure. Vessels and bronchi can be seen curving into and sweeping around the area of atelectasis. Soft tissue windows *(D)* demonstrate that the area of atelectasis abuts a focal area of pleural thickening. The size of the mass was stable over a 3-year follow-up period.

primarily on a complete occupational history;[750] if this is not forthcoming, inquiry should be directed toward the possibility of nonoccupational exposure. This approach applies to women as well as to men, not only because of the potential for significant asbestos exposure from the cleaning of clothes of occupationally exposed male members of the family, but also because women may have been occupationally exposed as well, sometimes remotely.[454, 751, 752] The combination of a history of exposure, positive radiographic findings, bibasilar fine crackles, clubbing, and impaired pulmonary function (including significant reductions in vital capacity, diffusing capacity, and compliance) is virtually diagnostic of asbestosis.[426]

As indicated previously, BAL can be useful in establishing asbestos exposure,[753–755] although the absence of asbestos bodies by this technique does not exclude the diagnosis of asbestos-associated disease.[756] The yield of asbestos bodies at bronchoscopy can be increased by performing lavage in the lower lobes.[757] In comparison with BAL, sputum examination is an insensitive method of assessing lung asbestos burden; however, when asbestos bodies are identified in these specimens, a high lung asbestos burden is likely.[758] Lung biopsy can confirm a suspected diagnosis but is seldom indicated; in fact, in the presence of advanced disease, it can be a hazardous procedure.[759] Electron microscopic examination of transbronchial biopsy specimens has been reported

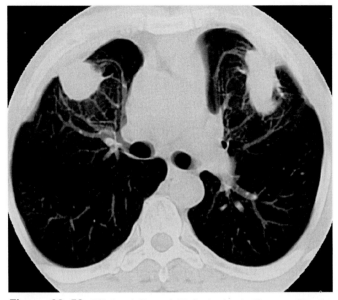

Figure 60–53. Bilateral Round Atelectasis. A 10-mm collimation CT scan in a 58-year-old patient demonstrates bilateral round atelectasis. Vessels and bronchi can be seen sweeping around and into the focal area of atelectasis. There is evidence of volume loss with anterior displacement of the right upper lobe bronchi. The bilateral areas of atelectasis abut calcified pleural plaques. (Courtesy of Dr. Louise Samson, Hotel Dieu de Montréal, Quebec.)

to be useful in establishing low-level occupational exposure.[760] The procedure also may be useful in determining unsuspected asbestos exposure in open-lung biopsy specimens, thus avoiding an inappropriate diagnosis of idiopathic pulmonary fibrosis.[761]

The chest radiograph is normal in 10% to 20% of patients in whom there is histologic evidence of fibrosis.[762] This situation raises the question as to what the minimal diagnostic criteria for asbestosis should be and how the diagnosis can be made in workers who have normal chest radiographs. As discussed previously, HRCT is clearly a more sensitive tool for the appreciation of early pulmonary fibrosis than radiography.[763–769] In workers who have an appropriate exposure history, latency from first exposure to dust, and pulmonary function disturbance, the diagnosis of asbestosis can be confirmed by HRCT, even if the radiograph is normal. Many patients who have a normal or equivocal chest radiograph and a history of significant asbestos exposure have an abnormal gallium scan;[770] the majority of these go on to develop radiologic evidence of asbestosis.[409] HRCT, however, has largely supplanted this test in the investigation of patients who have equivocal evidence of asbestosis after other investigations.

A poorly defined opacity in the periphery of a lung of a patient who has asbestos-related pleural disease often represents round atelectasis; although the radiologic appearance is characteristic, particularly on CT, transthoracic needle aspiration may be required to rule out carcinoma.[612, 613, 771, 772]

Prognosis and Natural History

The two most important complications of asbestos inhalation are pulmonary fibrosis and pleuropulmonary malig-

nancy. The likelihood of developing clinically evident asbestosis depends (at least in part) on cumulative dust exposure and time from first contact with the mineral. Disabling respiratory disease and cor pulmonale usually develop only in those individuals who have a history of heavy dust exposure and then typically 30 or more years after initial contact. The mortality related to asbestosis increased in the United States between 1970 and 1990, from 0.49 per million persons to 3.06 per million.[773] Because dust control measures have been in place in the United States and most other "developed" countries since the 1960s, the number of patients who have such severe disease can be expected to peak in the 1990s and to fall thereafter. The 10-year risk of death as a result of asbestosis increases significantly with increasing severity of baseline fibrosis, as assessed clinically, functionally, and radiographically.[773]

Of all nonneoplastic pulmonary diseases, those related to asbestos have the highest incidence of associated neoplasia, especially pulmonary carcinoma and pleural mesothelioma.[774, 775] In a cohort study of 11,000 Quebec chrysotile workers, the standardized mortality rates for pulmonary carcinoma and mesothelioma were 1.4 and 25, respectively;[776, 777] of the 5,350 individuals who died between 1975 and 1992, approximately 320 died of pulmonary carcinoma, 48 of asbestosis, and 25 of mesothelioma. There has been vigorous debate in the literature about when the cancer risk of asbestos was first recognized;[778] however, since the mid-1950s, the relationship has been documented in numerous pathologic and epidemiologic studies.[774, 779, 780] A latent period of at least 20 years from the time of first exposure to the development of malignancy is characteristic.[781] The degree of exposure, as indicated by occupational history and the number of asbestos bodies or fibers in lung tissue, is usually high.[431, 782–787] Most,[750, 788, 789] albeit not all,[782] investigators have found that the relationship between malignancy and asbestos exposure is linear. These issues are discussed in greater detail on pages 1074 and 2807.

A variety of extrathoracic neoplasms have also been reported to have an increased frequency after asbestos exposure, the one with the closest association probably being peritoneal mesothelioma.[790, 791] A number of workers have also found evidence for an increased incidence of gastrointestinal,[447, 792, 793] renal,[794] oropharyngeal,[794] and laryngeal[795–798] carcinoma as well as leukemia[793, 799] and lymphoma.[800] In addition to malignancy, excess mortality of asbestos-exposed workers is seen from nonmalignant respiratory disease.[801] In one intriguing study, a relative risk of death from ischemic heart disease of 3.5 was reported in a group of workers who had asbestosis compared with a similarly exposed group without lung function abnormalities.[802] Other investigators have not shown an excess risk of deaths from ischemic heart disease in asbestos-exposed populations,[802] even in workers most heavily exposed to dust;[803] however, this failure could be related to the "healthy worker" effect.

In contrast to patients who have silicosis, those who have asbestosis do not appear to be at greater risk for tuberculosis than the general population;[804] however, in one large study of causes of death among miners and millers of crocidolite in Western Australia, an excess mortality from the infection was found.[805]

OTHER SILICATES

As discussed previously, it is important to make a distinction between silica (i.e., SiO_2) and silicates (which consist of SiO_2 combined with one or more cations). Silica is clearly a highly toxic substance that is the cause of many cases of pulmonary disease. Although silicates are also generally toxic to cells in tissue culture, with the exception of asbestos this capacity appears to be poorly expressed *in vivo*, and pulmonary disease is uncommon or rare after their inhalation. In fact, the pathogenicity of some of the minerals is open to question even when disease is present because other substances that are clearly toxic, such as asbestos or silica itself, are commonly inhaled at the same time as the silicate.

Because silicates are crystalline, they can be identified as birefringent, needle-shaped or platelike particles on polarization light microscopy. Although the size and shape of such particles may suggest their nature, definitive identification of the specific mineral usually requires the use of energy-dispersive x-ray spectroscopy or analysis of tissue digests.

Talc

Talc is a hydrated magnesium silicate that usually occurs in the form of sheetlike crystals that are easily cleaved into thin plates.[807] It is used in the manufacture of such diverse products as leather, rubber, paper, textiles, ceramic tiles, and roofing material. It is also used as an additive in paint, food, many pharmaceuticals, cosmetics, insecticides, and herbicides. Individuals in any of these occupational settings may be exposed to potentially harmful levels of dust. Others at risk include workers involved in talc mining and milling,[808–810] individuals who work with soapstone,[811, 812] and workers exposed to commercial talcum powder.[813–815] Pulmonary disease related to talc can also develop in nonoccupational settings by several mechanisms, including (1) accidental inhalation of talcum powder in small children, a process that may be associated with acute fatal respiratory insufficiency as a result of tracheobronchial obstruction;[816, 817] (2) intravenous injection of oral medications containing talc as a filler, a form of microembolization discussed in detail in Chapter 49 (*see* page 1857); (3) obsessional inhalation of commercial talcum powder;[813] and (4) rarely, following talc pleurodesis, as in one patient who developed bilateral interstitial disease and pleural effusion.[818] (Despite the common contamination of talc with asbestos, there appears to be little, if any, risk for the development of mesothelioma after talc pleurodesis.[819])

Because other elements, such as iron and nickel, are usually incorporated within the talc crystal and because the substance is often found in association with other minerals, such as quartz, mica, kaolin, and various types of asbestos, the composition of commercially available talc is quite variable from region to region and from industry to industry.[807, 810, 820, 821] As a result, the pattern of pulmonary disease associated with its inhalation is variable, leading to the use of such terms as *talco-asbestosis*, *talco-silicosis*, and *pure talcosis*.[822] Although there is no doubt that talc itself can induce a foreign body giant cell reaction, its ability in pure form to induce fibrosis has been put into question by the

results of both epidemiologic and animal studies;[807] in fact, it has even been suggested that the majority, if not all, of the functionally and radiologically significant pulmonary abnormalities associated with talc are caused by other substances. It seems likely, however, that true inhalational talcosis does occur, as evidenced by reported cases in which significant pulmonary disease has been caused by exposure to dust apparently uncontaminated by asbestos or silica.[812, 822–824] As might be expected, there appears to be an association between the degree of exposure and the risk of development of pleuropulmonary disease.[810]

Pathologic findings are variable and, as indicated, may be caused in some cases by asbestos or silica rather than talc alone.[812, 822] Abnormalities include pleural fibrosis (sometimes with calcification and plaque formation identical to that seen in asbestos-related pleural disease), foci of nodular or stellate parenchymal fibrosis, more or less diffuse interstitial fibrosis (Fig. 60–54), and peribronchiolar and perivascular macrophage infiltrates.[823] Nonnecrotizing granulomatous inflammation has been identified in some cases.[823, 825] Macrophages and multinucleated giant cells containing irregularly shaped birefringent plates or needle-like crystals, representing ingested talc, are common (*see* Fig. 60–54). Talc-associated ferruginous bodies are also frequent.[823] Occasionally, talc is minimal or absent on routine histologic examination, its presence being identified only with the use of scanning electron microscopy.[825] In suspected cases, optical and electron microscopy may reveal talc particles in BAL fluid.[818, 820]

The principal radiologic abnormality is pleural plaques similar to those of asbestos-related disease. They may be massive and extend over much of the surface of both lungs.[809, 810, 826, 827] Occasionally, they involve the pericardium. In one study of 221 workers exposed to tremolite talc, pleural plaques were seen in 14 (6%).[646] Parenchymal involvement is said to be similar to that in asbestosis,[827–829] the radiographic pattern being one of general haziness, nodulation, and reticulation, with sparing of the apices and costophrenic sulci.[809, 829] Some cases may show confluence of lesions, creating large opacities (Fig. 60–55).[830]

When present, symptoms are similar to those of other pneumoconioses and include dyspnea and productive cough. Decreased breath sounds (presumably related to pleural thickening), crackles at the lung bases, limited chest expansion, and finger clubbing may be found on physical examination.[827, 831] As with other minerals, disease may become manifest many years after exposure has ceased, and careful occupational history taking may be necessary to reveal its presence.[806] Serum angiotensin-converting enzyme is increased in some patients.[832]

Compared with other minerals, such as asbestos and silica, talc appears to be a relatively innocuous substance. For example, in one study of 110 men employed in the mining and processing of soapstone in Sweden, only 5 individuals (all who had at least 20 years' exposure) showed radiographic evidence of pneumoconiosis;[811] in all 5, this was minimal and was unassociated with clinical impairment. Epidemiologic studies of individuals exposed to talc have shown increased mortality from nonmalignant respiratory disease and an increased risk of pulmonary carcinoma.[833, 834] With respect to malignancy, it is likely that other agents, such as radon and asbestos, are more important than talc

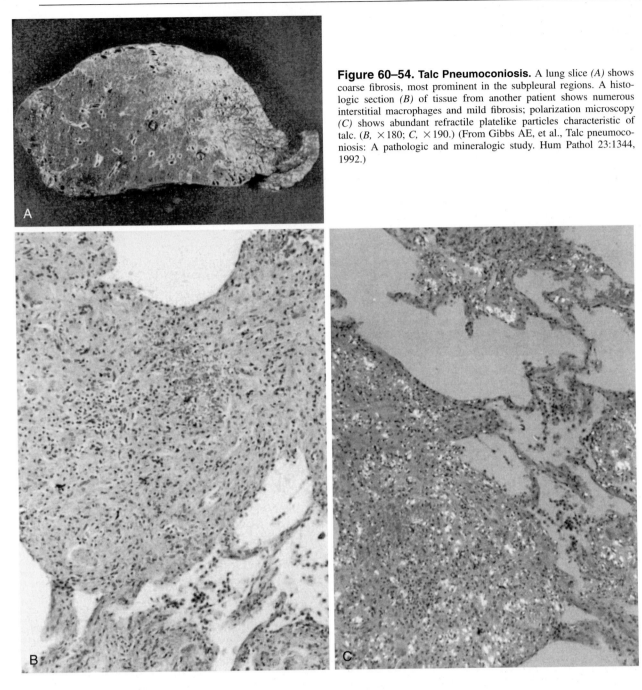

Figure 60–54. Talc Pneumoconiosis. A lung slice *(A)* shows coarse fibrosis, most prominent in the subpleural regions. A histologic section *(B)* of tissue from another patient shows numerous interstitial macrophages and mild fibrosis; polarization microscopy *(C)* shows abundant refractile platelike particles characteristic of talc. (*B*, ×180; *C*, ×190.) (From Gibbs AE, et al., Talc pneumoconiosis: A pathologic and mineralogic study. Hum Pathol 23:1344, 1992.)

itself.[833–835] A possible association with nontuberculous mycobacterial infection has been hypothesized.[835a]

Decreases in vital capacity, TLC, and DLCO have been reported in many exposed workers.[836, 837] DLCO is said to correlate with the extent of parenchymal involvement seen radiographically. Restrictive pulmonary function impairment has been described in patients who have pleural disease only.[810, 838]

Mica

Micas are complex aluminum silicates, of which three forms are commercially available:

1. *Muscovite*, a potassium compound that, because of its transparency and resistance to heat and electricity, is used in the manufacture of windows for stoves and furnaces; the substance is also an important constituent of slate (along with quartz), and workers involved in the mining and use of this substance (e.g., in roofing, highway construction, and tiling) have been reported to develop a distinctive pneumoconiosis.[839]

2. *Phlogopite*, a magnesium compound that is used in the electrical industry.

3. *Vermiculite*, another magnesium compound whose uses relate primarily to its fire resistance and its insulation and ion-exchange properties; it is also used as a filler in many substances (such as soil, animal feed, adhesives, cements, and enamels) and a carrier for various chemicals, including herbicides, insecticides, fungicides, and fertilizers.[840]

Similar to talc, micas are often associated with other minerals, particularly tremolite asbestos,[840] and the possibility that

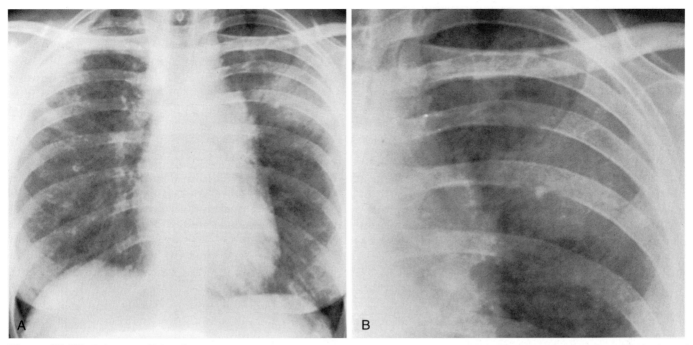

Figure 60–55. Pulmonary Talcosis. A 31-year-old woman had noted the onset of dyspnea on exertion several months previously and at the time of this radiograph could climb only 10 stairs without stopping. She had to use two pillows to sleep, and on occasion she awoke during the night gasping for breath. There was no cough or recent hemoptysis. A posteroanterior radiograph *(A)* reveals extensive involvement of both lungs by a rather coarse reticular pattern. In the upper axillary zone on the right and in the left midlung *(B)* are two areas of homogeneous consolidation possessing poorly defined margins. Paratracheal lymph node enlargement is present bilaterally, more marked on the left. At thoracotomy, biopsy specimens obtained from lung and lymph node revealed multiple foci of dense fibrosis lying in close proximity to blood vessels and containing extremely numerous, doubly refractile crystals. In view of these findings, the patient was questioned further and finally admitted to an extraordinary history of excessive inhalation of lavender-scented talcum powder during a 3-month period when she was pregnant 2 years previously. She was in the habit of spreading the talcum powder liberally over the pillow and blankets at night and actually inhaled it in large amounts from her cupped hands. Subsequent assay of the particles observed histologically proved them to be talc.

they can cause disease by themselves has been questioned.[841] For example, workers exposed to vermiculite contaminated with fibrous tremolite have been found to have a high incidence of benign pleural effusion, plaques, and pleural thickening,[840] abnormalities well known to be caused by asbestos alone. In addition, although there have been many reports of possible pneumoconiosis caused by micas,[840, 842–844] the documentation of the relationship between occupational exposure and pathologic findings has not always excluded other causative agents. Thus, although a literature review in 1985 documented 66 cases reported as mica pneumoconiosis, the evidence that it was caused by mica exposure alone was considered by the authors to be reasonably convincing in only 26.[845] Animal experiments have demonstrated the substance to have little or no fibrogenic activity,[846] although the validity of these studies has, in turn, been questioned.[845] Despite these uncertainties, occasional cases have been reported in which apparently pure mica exposure has been associated with pulmonary fibrosis,[841, 847] and it seems reasonable to conclude that the risk of developing pulmonary disease from mica inhalation is present but slight. Radiographic and clinical manifestations are indistinguishable from those associated with exposure to asbestos or talc.[646]

Fuller's Earth

The term *Fuller's earth* refers to a variety of clays with different chemical compositions that were formerly used in the process of fulling (removing grease from wool) and are now employed in the refining of oils, in filtering and purification, in the bonding of molding sands in foundry work, and as a filler in cosmetics and pharmaceuticals. Prolonged exposure to the substance in these occupations or during its mining or milling has been associated with simple pneumoconiosis and, occasionally, PMF.[835, 848] Although it is likely that some of these cases are the result of concomitant silica exposure,[848] the possibility of a toxic action of the clays has not been excluded.

Pathologic changes associated with exposure to Fuller's earth occur mainly in the upper lobes and consist of an increase in reticulin surrounding dust particles, with little fibrosis or cellular reaction.[849, 850] Radiographic changes are said to consist of a prominence of bronchovascular markings and, in some cases, PMF.[851]

Kaolin

The term *kaolin* (china clay, ball clay, fire clay) derives from the Chinese *Kauling* or high ridge, the name given a hill near Jauchau Fu, China, where the clay was first mined.[852] It actually designates a group of clays, of which kaolinite, a hydrated aluminum silicate, is the most important member. This substance is used industrially as a filler in plastics, rubber, paints, textiles, pharmaceuticals, and adhesives; as a coating for paper; as an absorbent;[853] and in the manufacture of firebricks.[854] Although water is usually employed in quarrying or strip mining to minimize the risk of dust exposure, subsequent drying, bagging, and transporting can result in high concentrations of aerosolized kaolin and the potential for pulmonary disease. For example, in a study of 65 workers in a Georgia kaolin mine, pneumoconiosis occurred only in workers exposed in the processing area, where the mean respirable dust level was greater than 12 times that in the mine itself.[855] Exposure to kaolinite can also occur in workers involved in the mining, crushing, or grinding of china stone,[856] in which quartz is likely to be an important contaminant, and in the mining of shale.[11] Pulmonary disease has also been reported after the use of a liquid kaolin suspension for pleural poudrage in the treatment of recurrent spontaneous pneumothorax.[857]

Although it seems likely that kaolinite alone can cause pulmonary disease,[853, 858] it is probable that some cases are complicated by the inhalation of other particulates,[856] partly because the purity of raw clay varies considerably. For example, in some regions, such as Georgia in the United States, kaolin is relatively silica-free,[853] whereas in others, there is a substantial amount of admixed quartz and other minerals.

The incidence of chest disease varies in reported series. In one investigation, it was concluded that the general state of health in kaolin workers differed little from that of the regional general population of corresponding age and race.[859] By contrast, in a study of 553 Cornish china clay workers exposed to kaolin dust for periods exceeding 5 years, 48 (9%) showed clinical and radiographic evidence of pulmonary disease;[861] abnormalities were present in almost 25% of those exposed for more than 15 years. In another study of china clay workers from the same area, approximately three quarters were judged to have radiographs of category 0, 20% of category 1, and 5% of categories 2 and 3;[861] 19 workers (1%) were considered to have PMF. The prevalence of pneumoconiosis in Georgia kaolin workers has been estimated to be about 10%.[862] Although disabling pneumoconiosis is generally believed to develop in only a small proportion of affected individuals,[863–865] in one investigation of workers who processed kaolin in a Georgia mine, a significant degree of restrictive pulmonary dysfunction was found that correlated with the number of years of exposure.[866]

Pathologic features have been described in workers from Georgia[853] and Cornwall.[856] In the former, the features were similar to those of CWP, consisting of peribronchiolar macules containing numerous pigment-laden macrophages and interspersed reticulin fibers and of larger masses without definite anatomic localization that measured up to 12 cm in diameter. The latter were composed almost entirely of macrophages and only small amounts of collagen; coagulation necrosis and obliterative vascular changes similar to those seen in complicated CWP were also present. In the Cornish workers, variable degrees of interstitial and nodular fibrosis were seen, the latter correlating with the pulmonary quartz content.

The radiographic pattern varies. In some cases, there may be no more than a general increase in lung markings. With prolonged and severe exposure, a diffuse nodular and miliary mottling is present; when it develops, the appearance of PMF is identical to that seen in silicosis and CWP.[867, 868] Clinical findings are nonspecific. Complicating tuberculosis has been reported,[869] possibly in patients who have associated silicosis.

Zeolites (Erionite)

Zeolites are a group of more than 30 naturally occurring minerals composed of hydrated aluminum silicates that are found in deposits of volcanic ash.[870] They are widely used as absorbents and for filtration. Most do not have a fibrous form and are not considered toxic; erionite, however, is fibrous and has been associated with a variety of pulmonary abnormalities. The richest deposits of this material are in Turkey and the western United States, particularly Nevada and Utah. The initial indication that the substance might be harmful came from Turkey, where epidemiologic studies revealed a high prevalence of pleural plaques, mesothelioma, and pulmonary carcinoma, apparently unassociated with asbestos exposure.[871–874] Subsequent investigators have also documented the presence of interstitial fibrosis.[870, 871, 874]

Miscellaneous Silicates

An association between *mullite* (an artificial aluminum silicate used in the preparation of cat litter) and the presence of pulmonary disease has been documented in one report.[875] Affected patients complained of dyspnea and cough; some showed radiographic abnormalities consistent with fibrosis.

Nepheline is a mineral composed of sodium, potassium, and aluminum silicates that occurs in crystalline form in many igneous rocks; SiO_2 is bound to it in a complex crystal lattice. The rock is milled to a fine powder, which is used in the production of pottery glazes. At least three cases have been reported in which pneumoconiosis occurred as a result of exposure to the dust.[876, 877] The radiographic changes consist of diffuse interstitial disease, bilateral lymph node enlargement, and focal areas of atelectasis (presumably the result of airway compression by enlarged nodes).[877]

Wollastonite is a naturally occurring acicular or fibrous metasilicate used in ceramics and as a substitute for asbestos in some applications; it is similar in form, length, and diameter to the amphiboles.[878] There is fairly convincing radiographic and functional evidence that this substance can cause interstitial fibrosis,[878–880] although we are unaware of any pathologic studies confirming it.

Taconite is a low-grade ore consisting of iron, quartz, and numerous silicates, including cummingtonite-grunerite, a relative of amosite asbestos. Although there is some evidence that the substance may be fibrinogenic or carcinogenic, definite proof is lacking.[881, 882]

INERT RADIOPAQUE DUSTS

Iron

Workers in many occupations are exposed to dust containing a high content of iron, usually in the form of iron oxide (Fe_2O_3). When this substance is inhaled in sufficient quantity, it causes *siderosis*, a condition generally believed to be unassociated with fibrosis or functional impairment.

When the iron is admixed with a substantial quantity of silica, however, the resulting *silicosiderosis* (mixed-dust pneumoconiosis) can lead to appreciable pulmonary fibrosis and disability. This abnormality is potentially of some importance; for example, it was estimated in the early 1980s that approximately 4 million workers in the United States had had possible exposure.

The majority of affected individuals are electric arc or oxyacetylene torch workers, who are exposed to Fe_2O_3 in fumes derived from melted iron emitted during the welding process. Other cases of siderosis or silicosiderosis are found in individuals involved in the mining and processing of iron ores (such as hematite, magnetite, siderite,[884] and metallic pigments such as ochre), in workers in iron and steel rolling mills, in foundry workers (particularly those involved with cleaning steel castings[16, 17] and boiler scalers), and in silver polishers (*see* farther on).

As indicated previously, Fe_2O_3 inhaled in relatively pure form is believed to cause no significant inflammatory reaction or pulmonary fibrosis.[885] This belief is supported by the results of experimental studies in animals in which various iron compounds inhaled or injected intratracheally have not caused fibrosis.[886, 887] In addition, workers exposed for many years to Fe_2O_3 in high concentration are usually not disabled and show little evidence of fibrosis at autopsy, even when the iron content of their lungs is high.[17, 885, 888, 889]

Despite the relative benignity of pure siderosis, occupations associated with iron dust or fume production frequently generate other noxious materials. In fact, the mineral content of fumes derived from the welding process may be quite variable, depending on the composition of the metal being welded or of the welding electrode itself, or both. Among the additional materials that may be present are carbon, manganese, titanium, aluminum, various silicates (including asbestos), and free silica.[890] As the proportion of these substances in the fumes or dusts increases, the propensity for

pulmonary damage and fibrosis also increases, resulting in the clinical, radiographic, and pathologic features characteristic of silicosiderosis. Although free silica is probably the most important agent responsible for the development of pulmonary disease in these circumstances, analyses of tissue and BAL fluid specimens have suggested that the fibrogenic reaction in some cases of welder's pneumoconiosis is also related to other substances.[891–893] Workers can also develop pulmonary disease as a result of a direct effect of toxic gases or fumes created during welding, resulting in several clinicopathologic syndromes (e.g., metal fume fever, chemical pneumonitis, hypersensitivity pneumonitis, and chronic bronchitis [*see* page 2174]).[890]

Pathologically, pure siderosis is characterized by the presence of Fe_2O_3 predominantly in macrophages in the peribronchovascular interstitium.[18, 895, 896] Iron-containing macrophages can also be seen within alveolar air spaces, particularly in individuals who were active welders at the time of death or biopsy (Fig. 60–56); these macrophages can frequently be detected in sputum specimens.[897] The iron may appear as an amorphous, tan-colored particle or may have a central black core. Although Fe_2O_3 does not react with Prussian blue, with time, many aggregates become associated with endogenous iron and thus stain with this dye. Fibrosis is usually absent or minimal in cases of pure Fe_2O_3 inhalation but is present to a variable degree if fibrogenic substances are also present;[896] in this situation, the appearance is similar to that of silicosis and is characterized by solitary or conglomerate nodules, the latter occasionally being large enough to be designated PMF (Fig. 60–57). In contrast to pure silicosis, however, the nodules are usually rather poorly defined and stellate. Aggregates of Fe_2O_3, either free or within macrophages, can often be found admixed within the fibrous tissue.

The radiographic pattern in pure siderosis is reticulonodular and widely disseminated (Fig. 60–58). In one evalua-

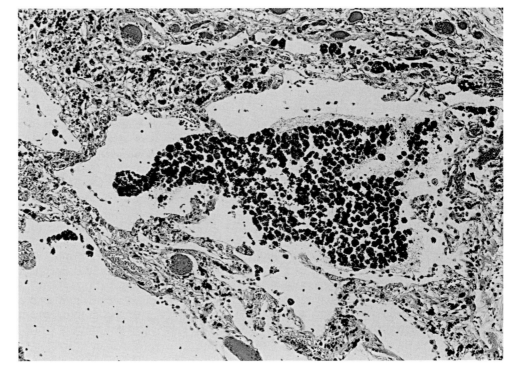

Figure 60–56. Pulmonary Siderosis. The section shows a large cluster of iron-containing macrophages within pulmonary air spaces. A smaller amount of iron is also present in the adjacent bronchiolar wall. Although there is some fibrosis in both airway wall and lung parenchyma, in this illustration, overall it was mild and present only focally. The patient was an electric arc welder who died accidentally. (×100.)

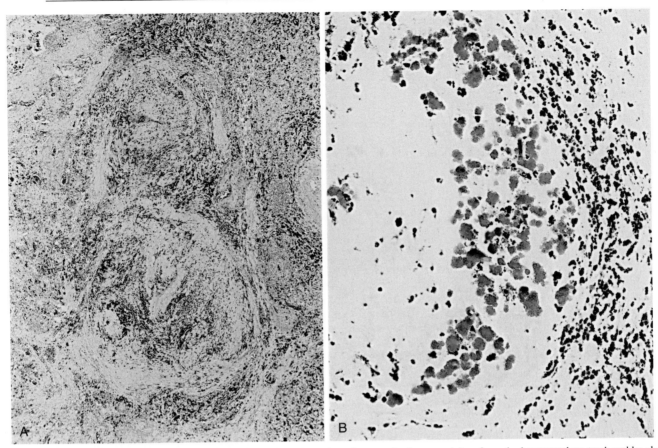

Figure 60–57. Silicosiderosis. A histologic section *(A)* from a 3-cm irregular mass in the upper lobe of a retired oxyacetylene torch welder shows extensive fibrosis with abundant interspersed pigment. Note the two rounded areas in the central portion that suggest that the mass was formed by confluence of multiple nodules. A magnified view of the pigmented material *(B)* shows it to consist of small black particles (predominantly anthracotic pigment) and larger, rather amorphous granules representing iron dioxide. *(A,* ×25; *B,* ×250.)

tion of 661 British electric arc welders, 7% showed small rounded opacities of 0/1 category or higher, there being a clear association between prevalence and years of exposure;[898] only 10 workers showed changes greater than 2/2. Opacities have been shown experimentally to correlate with localized aggregates of Fe_2O_3-laden macrophages[887] and are caused by the density of the Fe_2O_3 itself.[899] Individual shadows appear to be of lesser density than the nodules of silicosis. In contrast to the majority of cases of pneumoconiosis, the radiographic abnormalities can disappear partly or completely when patients are removed from dust exposure.[900] In silicosiderosis, the pattern depends somewhat on the concentration of free silica in the inhaled dust: When it is relatively low, the appearance is similar to that of pure siderosis or CWP;[16] when it is high, the pattern is identical to that of silicosis.[888]

Patients who have siderosis have no symptoms of chest disease; those who have siderosilicosis may complain of cough and dyspnea. In some patients, symptoms tend to be worse after the Monday work shift, suggesting that they are caused by fumes and vapors derived from the molding process. Even in the absence of radiographic abnormality, arc welders[901] and foundry workers[902] have been found to have a higher prevalence of bronchitis than control subjects. Pulmonary function studies of welders may show values considered to be within normal limits;[865] however, evidence of mild air-flow obstruction, even in nonsmokers, has been demonstrated by some investigators.[903–905]

The incidence of pulmonary carcinoma is significantly higher in patients who have siderosis or silicosiderosis than in the general population.[906–908] It is also higher in iron miners, although they are also exposed to other potential carcinogens.[909–911] In addition, squamous metaplasia, in many cases with atypical features, has been reported in a substantial number of iron foundry workers.[897] In one epidemiologic study in Scotland, higher standardized mortality rates for pulmonary carcinoma were grouped in residential areas most exposed to pollution from the foundries.[912] Despite these findings, there is no direct evidence linking Fe_2O_3 per se with the development of carcinoma.

Iron and Silver

Argyrosiderosis results from the use of jeweler's rouge—which is composed in part of Fe_2O_3—as a polishing agent in the finishing of silver products. When it is applied with a buffer, small particles of Fe_2O_3 and silver are generated that may be inhaled. The radiographic manifestation in affected patients is rather characteristic, consisting of a fine stippled pattern in contrast to the reticulonodular pattern of siderosis. Pathologic examination shows the presence of

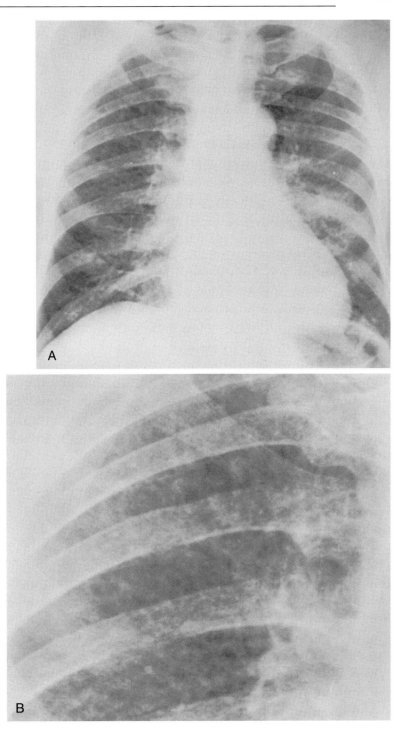

Figure 60–58. Pulmonary Siderosis. A 63-year-old man had worked as an electric arc welder for a railway company for 20 years. He was asymptomatic, this radiograph being part of a screening examination. Pulmonary function tests revealed lung volumes, ventilation, and diffusing capacity all to be in the low-normal range (the patient had been a heavy smoker for many years). The posteroanterior radiograph *(A)* and magnified view of the upper lung *(B)* reveal a diffuse reticulonodular pattern throughout both lungs, the opacities being of "low" density and thus rather poorly visualized. Hilar lymph nodes are not enlarged.

iron-laden macrophages in a distribution similar to that of pure siderosis; in addition, silver can be identified in the alveolar walls and the walls of small arteries and veins, particularly in relation to the internal elastic laminae.[913] Patients are typically asymptomatic.

Tin

Pneumoconiosis caused by inhalation of tin (*stannosis*) occurs predominantly in individuals employed in the handling of the ore after it has been mined, especially in indus-

tries in which tin oxide fumes are created. Pathologic findings simulate the macule of CWP: Pigment-laden macrophages are found in alveoli, interlobular septa, and (most prominently) in aggregates adjacent to terminal bronchioles and proximal respiratory bronchioles; fibrosis is minimal or absent.[914] In contrast to CWP, focal emphysema is not a prominent feature.[914]

The high density of tin (atomic number 50) results in a dramatic radiographic appearance, consisting of multiple tiny shadows of high density, about 1 mm in diameter, distributed evenly throughout the lungs.[915] Linear opacities may be present in the paramediastinal zone, in the vicinity of the diaphragm, and in the costophrenic angles. Lymph node enlargement has not been observed. A second pattern, seen chiefly in furnace workers in the tin ore industry, consists of larger, somewhat less numerous nodules.[916]

Even in the presence of significant radiographic abnormalities, clinical manifestations are typically absent. For example, in one study of 215 individuals exposed to tin oxide fumes, 95% of whom had worked in the environment for at least 3 years, 121 (56%) showed an abnormality on the chest radiograph;[915] none had symptoms or signs referable to the chest.

Barium

Barium and its salts, particularly barium sulfate, have a wide variety of industrial uses as coloring or weighting agents, as fillers in numerous products, and in the manufacture of glass. Workers in many of these occupations as well as those who mine the ore can develop pulmonary disease (*baritosis*). Originally described in Italian workers,[888, 917] the abnormality has also been reported in the German,[918] French,[919] American,[920] and British[921] literature. Pulmonary disease caused by barium can also be seen after its aspiration or embolization in the hospital (*see* pages 2513 and 1865).

Radiographic abnormalities may develop after minimal exposure. As a result of the high radiopacity of barium (atomic number 56), the discrete shadows in the chest radiograph are extremely dense, creating an awesome appearance. The apices and bases usually are spared, and massive shadows do not occur.[921] The lesions characteristically regress after the patient is removed from the dust-filled environment.[888, 918, 921] Microscopic examination shows particles of barium in macrophages in air spaces and interstitial tissue, unassociated with fibrosis.

In one study of 118 Algerian workers exposed to dust containing a high content of barium sulfate, approximately 50% had abnormal chest radiographs.[919] Some of the affected individuals complained of chronic cough, expectoration, and asthma-like attacks; the degree of pulmonary function impairment was similar in those who had and who did not have radiographic abnormality.

Antimony

Antimony is procured mainly from the mineral stibnite and is handled either as unrefined ore or as a fine white powder.[922] The main exposures are to antimony trioxide and, to a lesser extent, antimony pentoxide.[923] The substance is used in cosmetics; in the manufacture of batteries, pewter, printing type, and electrodes; in the compounding of rubber; in textiles, paints, and plastics as a flame retardant; and in ceramics as an opacifier.[922]

There has been little pathologic description of the effects of antimony on the lungs; in one brief report, dust-laden macrophages were identified in alveolar septa and perivascular tissue unaccompanied by fibrosis.[922] There is also experimental evidence confirming the lack of fibrogenic potential.[924]

The chest radiograph of affected individuals reveals minute dense opacities scattered widely throughout both lungs.[924] In one report of 51 workers exposed for at least 10 years to dust containing a high concentration of the mineral, radiographs were described as showing numerous *p* and occasional *q* opacities;[923] PMF was not seen. Respiratory symptoms were judged to be similar to those found in other pneumoconioses. Approximately 50% of workers had pustular skin lesions. There is no evidence that the dust causes significant disturbances in pulmonary function.

Rare Earths

The rare earth elements include cerium (quantitatively the most important), scandium, yttrium, lanthanum, and 14 other minerals. Their atomic numbers range from 51 to 71, explaining the remarkable density of the radiographic shadows with which they may be associated. The elements are used in reactor control rods; in the manufacturing and polishing of colored glass; in the manufacture of flints; and as part of an alloy in cast iron, light metals, and heating conductors. Industrial exposure and reported cases of pneumoconiosis occur chiefly in workers in the graphic arts who are exposed to fumes from carbon arc lamps.[925]

There are few pathologic descriptions of the effects of rare earths on the lung. In animal experiments, they appear to be practically inert,[926] inducing only small collections of macrophages and, in one model of intratracheally administered lanthanum, an eosinophil response.[927] Some investigators, however, have described granulomatous inflammation and parenchymal fibrosis in exposed humans;[928, 929] there is evidence that the extent and progression of disease in these individuals depends to some extent on the thorium content of the dust.[928] As a result of these observations, earlier views that lanthanum causes benign pneumoconiosis only have been supplanted by the belief that it can result in pulmonary fibrosis, even in the absence of radioactive contaminants.[930]

The typical radiographic pattern consists of widely disseminated punctate opacities of great density, in one patient categorized as *q* opacities of 2/3 severity;[931] similar to some others described in the literature,[932] this patient was asymptomatic despite the spirometric demonstration of a restrictive impairment. Pulmonary "fibrosis" has also been described in some cases.[929]

MISCELLANEOUS INORGANIC DUSTS

Beryllium

Beryllium is a light, highly conductive mineral whose major commercial source is the aluminum silicate beryl, from which it is extracted at high temperature. Potentially important environmental exposure can occur to beryllium oxides during the extraction process and to a variety of beryllium alloys; beryl itself appears to be nontoxic.

Immediately before and during the 1940s, when its toxicity was first appreciated, the majority of cases of berylliosis resulted from exposure to beryllium in refineries, to beryllium alloys in metal working, and to fluorescent phosphor production for use in lamps. In 1949, dust control measures were introduced, which resulted in a dramatic decrease in the incidence of disease. It was not totally eradicated, however, and many new cases have been reported since.[933] In a 1973 survey of workers in a beryllium extraction and processing plant that had been in operation for 14 years, 31 of 214 workers had radiographic changes compatible with interstitial disease;[934] it was determined that they had been exposed to dust concentrations well above the recommended level. It appears that beryllium sensitization does not occur in workers who are exposed to levels less than 0.01 μg/m³;[935] however, it has occurred in workers exposed to a level of 0.9 μg/m³,[936] a value that is well below the Occupational Safety and Health Administration safety standard of 2.0 μg/m³.

The current major sources of exposure to beryllium have been outlined in reviews[937, 938] and include the processing and handling of beryllium compounds in the aerospace and electronics industry, the manufacture of gyroscopes and nuclear reactors,[939] the development of nuclear weapons,[940] the processing of ceramics, and the development or handling of beryllium metal alloys.[937, 941] Many components of automobiles and computers are composed of beryllium metal alloys;[937] disease has also been described in individuals involved in the manufacturing of dental prostheses.[942] Although significant exposure is still theoretically possible from breaking fluorescent lights, this is rarely seen today. Nonoccupational exposure causing disease has also been well described; it is invariably the chronic type (*see* farther on) and tends to occur in the household (e.g., a wife exposed to her husband's work clothes[943]) or in proximity to a site of beryllium use (e.g., secretaries and security guards working in a nuclear weapons facility).[939]

Berylliosis may occur in an acute or chronic form; as a result of improved industrial hygiene, the latter is now by far the more common.[938]

Acute Berylliosis

The majority of patients affected with acute berylliosis have been exposed to a high level of dust, nowadays usually accidentally while working in beryllium refineries. Depending on the intensity of exposure, the clinical presentation may be either fulminating or insidious. In both situations, the pathologic changes are identical to those seen in other forms of acute chemical pneumonitis, consisting of bronchitis, bronchiolitis, and various stages of diffuse alveolar damage (interstitial and air-space edema, hyaline membranes, and fibrosis).[944, 945] Granulomatous inflammation does not occur.

The fulminating variety develops rapidly after an overwhelming exposure and may be rapidly fatal.[946] Clinical and radiographic manifestations are those of acute pulmonary edema.

The insidious variety produces symptoms weeks or even months after the initial exposure.[947] The onset is heralded by a dry cough, substernal pain, shortness of breath on exertion, anorexia, weakness, and weight loss. Auscultatory findings include crackles and, in some cases, wheezes suggestive of asthma.[948] Various nonpulmonary manifestations, including rhinitis, pharyngitis, conjunctivitis, and dermatitis, may occur with or without clinical and radiologic evidence of pulmonary involvement.[948] The chest radiograph usually does not become abnormal until 1 to 4 weeks after the onset of symptoms. Diffuse, symmetric, and bilateral "haziness"

is seen in the earliest stage of the disease followed by the development of irregular patchy opacities scattered rather widely throughout the lungs. Subsequently, discrete or confluent mottling may be observed.[946, 948] Complete radiographic clearing may take 2 to 3 months.[948, 949] Pulmonary function studies have shown abnormal gas exchange at rest and on exercise, reduction in vital capacity, normal residual volume, and normal maximal breathing capacity (suggesting the absence of air-flow limitation).[947] Removal from exposure to the dust results in gradual return to normal function.

Chronic Berylliosis

As indicated previously, chronic berylliosis is much more common than the acute variety and takes the form of a systemic granulomatous disease involving the lungs, pleura, lymph nodes, skin, and many visceral organs.

Pathogenesis

The frequent delay in onset of disease from the time of exposure, the decrease in beryllium content of the lungs of affected individuals with time (*see* farther on), the common presence of granulomatous inflammation, and the poor correlation between the degree of exposure and the development of disease all suggest that the pathogenesis of chronic berylliosis has an immunologic basis. Several specific clinical and experimental findings support this conclusion. Assuming an immunologic pathogenesis, it would be expected that the severity of exposure, including both dust and fume concentration, would not be a major factor in predicting the development of disease; reports of berylliosis associated with an air concentration of beryllium below the permissible exposure limit of 2 μg/m³ appear to bear out this hypothesis.[941, 950] Cutaneous granulomatous inflammation develops in approximately 70% of affected patients on patch testing with a solution of beryllium sulfate. Similarly, blast transformation and the production of macrophage inhibition factor are common when lymphocytes of affected patients are cultured in the presence of beryllium.[951–955] This lymphocyte sensitization appears to be reversible with decreased beryllium exposure,[956] a finding that may be related to the reversibility of lung function abnormalities (*see* farther on).

Either by itself or acting as a hapten, beryllium appears to act as an antigen in invoking a delayed-type hypersensitivity response.[957] In this respect, the pathogenesis of berylliosis is remarkably similar to sarcoidosis, the disorder it imitates both clinically and pathologically. Pulmonary injury is an early event in the disease process. Markers of epithelial cell damage (e.g., serum KL-6) and alveolar-capillary permeability (e.g., BAL fluid/serum albumin) are elevated in patients who have chronic berylliosis and are able to distinguish between disease and sensitization.[958] The pattern of cytokine release from lymphocytes suggests that Th1 cells are activated after beryllium exposure;[959] levels of TNF-α, IL-6,[960, 961] interferon-γ, and IL-2 are typically elevated, whereas those of IL-4 and IL-7 are not.[954, 962] The expansion of certain T-cell subsets in BAL fluid is also consistent with a local response to an antigen that includes beryllium.[894] Finally, levels of soluble TNF receptor I and II in serum and soluble IL-6 receptors and TNF receptor II in BAL fluid correlate with pulmonary lymphocytosis and clinical measures of disease severity.[961]

A genetic marker for beryllium susceptibility has been identified in the HLA-DP allele in a position involved in susceptibility to autoimmune disorders. In one study, 97% of patients who had chronic berylliosis expressed the HLA-DPB1*0201 allele with glutamic acid present at residue 69, compared with only 30% of controls.[963] In another study of workers who were machining beryllium, 25% of those who were positive for this marker developed berylliosis compared with only 3.2% of those who were negative.[964]

Pathologic Characteristics

The characteristic pulmonary abnormality in chronic berylliosis is interstitial pneumonitis,[945] which may have one or more of three histologic patterns: (1) a more or less diffuse mononuclear cell infiltrate unassociated with granulomatous inflammation (Fig. 60–59); (2) a similar infiltrate containing loose epithelioid cell aggregates and scattered multinucleated giant cells, frequently associated with calcified intracellular inclusions (Schaumann's bodies); or (3) well-formed, discrete, nonnecrotizing granulomas indistinguishable from those of sarcoidosis (*see* Fig. 60–59). Interstitial fibrosis is also common, occurring either diffusely within the parenchymal interstitium or in the form of well-defined nodules, often with central hyalinization, necrosis, or both.

In contrast to most other dusts that cause pneumoconiosis, beryllium is largely removed from the lungs with time and excreted in the urine (although it may be stored in bone and liver for many years); as a result, quantitative studies show significantly less tissue content of beryllium in chronic than in acute disease.[945] Despite this, the substance can be detected within affected tissues by laser probe and emission spectroscopy[965] and by laser ion mass analysis.[966] Measurements are most often made on tissue samples or urine, in which case there can be quantitative assessment; however, semiquantitative analysis can also be performed on frozen or formalin-fixed tissue sections.[967] Although there is overlap, in most patients the beryllium content of the lung and mediastinal lymph nodes is greater than that of normal individuals and of patients who have sarcoidosis.[968]

Radiologic Manifestations

The radiographic pattern is neither specific nor diagnostic.[969] When the degree of involvement is relatively minor, the pattern has been described as a diffuse, finely granular "haziness" with a tendency to sparing of the apices and bases.[970] With more severe involvement, ill-defined nodules of moderate size are scattered diffusely throughout the lungs, sometimes associated with lymph node enlargement (Fig. 60–60). Calcification of nodules may occur.[971] In a group of 17 patients in whom the presence of chronic berylliosis was established by means of a positive lymphocyte proliferation

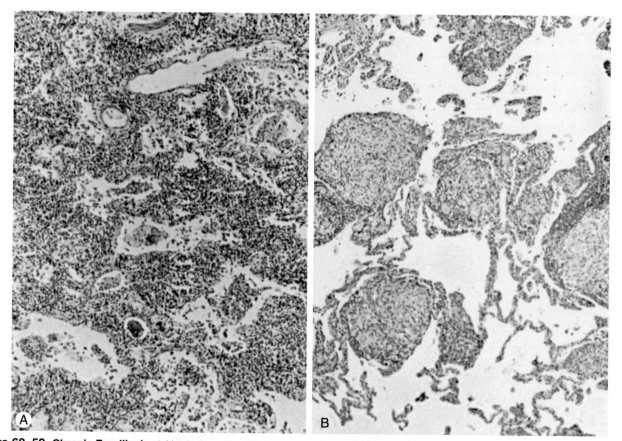

Figure 60–59. Chronic Berylliosis. A histologic section *(A)* shows severe interstitial infiltration by mononuclear inflammatory cells unassociated with granuloma formation. A different histologic pattern is shown in *B*, consisting of patchy, nonnecrotizing granulomatous inflammation within the pulmonary interstitium, similar to that seen in sarcoidosis. (From Freiman DG, Hardy HL: Beryllium disease. Hum Pathol 1:30, 1970.)

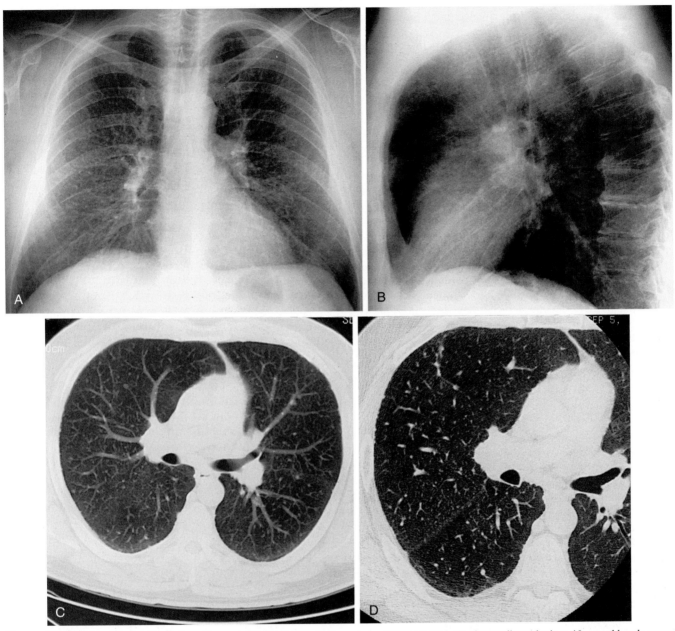

Figure 60–60. Berylliosis: Radiographic and CT Findings. Posteroanterior *(A)* and lateral *(B)* chest radiographs in a 46-year-old male ceramic plant worker show bilateral hilar adenopathy and fine nodules. The profuse fine nodules are confirmed on conventional CT *(C)* and HRCT *(D)* images. They are more evident on the 10-mm conventional CT image because more of them are contained within the imaging volume. The HRCT image, however, better demonstrates the tendency of the nodules to cluster along the visceral pleura, a distribution similar to that seen in patients with sarcoidosis. (Courtesy of Dr. David Lynch, University of Colorado Health Sciences Center, Denver, CO.)

test on BAL fluid, the most common radiographic abnormality consisted of diffuse, small, round and irregular opacities that involved all lung zones;[972] hilar node enlargement, linear scars, lung distortion, bullae, and pleural thickening were found less commonly. These changes did not correlate with pulmonary function abnormalities.

The findings on HRCT were compared with those on radiography in one study of 28 patients who had biopsy-proven disease.[973] Abnormalities related to beryllium were found in 21 (75%) patients by HRCT and in 15 (54%) by chest radiography. The most common findings seen with the former procedure were thickened interlobular septa and small nodular opacities (*see* Fig. 60–60). The nodules were

well-defined and were seen mainly along the bronchovascular bundles or interlobular septa, a distribution similar to that in sarcoidosis.[974, 975] Other findings included pleural irregularities—presumably related to coalescence of subpleural nodules—in 7 (25%) patients and hilar or mediastinal lymph node enlargement in 11 (39%). Lymph node enlargement was seen only in patients who had an associated parenchymal abnormality.

In advanced cases, the pattern may be chiefly reticular and associated with a marked decrease in volume. CT scans in these patients demonstrate a predominantly reticular pattern frequently associated with honeycombing.[973, 976] Conglomeration of nodules may result in the formation of large opacities similar to those seen in silicosis.[973, 977] Spontaneous pneumothorax occurs in slightly more than 10% of cases.[971] Rare complications include fungus ball formation[978] and extensive calcification of the nodules.[977]

Clinical Manifestations

The majority of patients reported to have chronic berylliosis have been exposed to the dust for more than 2 years. Typically, symptoms develop insidiously after a latent period that may be as long as 15 years after the last exposure to dust.[948, 979, 980] Occasionally, patients have minimal symptoms and radiographic manifestations.[883] Some investigators believe that the disease can be precipitated by certain trigger factors, such as pregnancy, withdrawal from exposure, and even the performance of a beryllium patch test.[950, 981]

Early symptoms include cough, fatigue, weight loss, increasing dyspnea on exertion, and, sometimes, migratory arthralgia. Crackles may be heard on auscultation, and the liver and spleen may be palpable. With progression of disease, cyanosis may become evident, and in approximately 30% of patients, clubbing of the fingers and toes develops; cor pulmonale is frequent at this stage. Symptoms of systemic disease may be related to myocarditis, gout, and neprolithiasis. Dermal lesions similar to those seen in sarcoidosis may occur.

Laboratory Findings and Diagnosis

Hypergammaglobulinemia, hypercalciuria, hyperuricemia, and polycythemia are not uncommon findings;[948, 979, 980, 982] up to 10% of patients develop renal calculi. The serum angiotensin-converting enzyme level may be elevated, although this may also be seen in healthy beryllium-exposed workers.[983] The total number of cells obtained by BAL is increased, principally owing to larger numbers of lymphocytes;[954] most are CD4 + T cells,[957] and there is consequently an increased helper-to-suppressor ratio. In nonsmokers, the intensity of this "lymphocytic alveolitis" correlates with the clinical severity of the berylliosis.[984]

Confirmation of the diagnosis may be obtained by a patch test showing hypersensitivity to beryllium.[985, 986] The proliferative response to beryllium of lymphocytes in specimens obtained by BAL has also been proposed as a useful diagnostic test,[941, 987–989] although its expense and time-consuming nature may preclude its use as a screening tool.[990] A positive test may precede the development of clinically evident disease or abnormalities of pulmonary function.[991, 992] Abnormal peripheral blood lymphocyte proliferation on exposure to beryllium is seen in most patients;[951, 955, 991] this test may be useful in differential diagnosis of other granulomatous disorders[989] because beryllium-exposed workers who do not have disease or sensitization do not demonstrate this response. In one study of a small number of patients who had chronic berylliosis, one group of workers found this test to show 100% sensitivity and specificity.[988] In one study, a serum neopterin value of 1.27 ng/ml in workers who had an abnormal beryllium lymphocyte proliferation test was 88% specific and had a positive predictive value of 92% for the diagnosis of chronic beryllium disease.[993]

For obvious reasons, the disease may be confused with sarcoidosis.[941, 994] Careful elucidation of any history of possible exposure to beryllium helps prevent diagnostic error. As indicated previously, although there is overlap between healthy individuals and patients who have sarcoidosis or berylliosis, the tissue level of beryllium is generally higher in berylliosis, and its measurement may be helpful in some cases in which exposure history is unclear.[968]

Pulmonary Function Tests

Abnormalities of pulmonary function are common.[996] In one investigation of 41 patients, they were apparent in 39;[997] 16 manifested an obstructive pattern, 8 manifested a restrictive one, and 15 had diminished diffusing capacity without evidence of either obstruction or restriction. Patients who had obstructive lung disease were not necessarily smokers. Similar findings were reported in a more recent study.[998] Evidence of functional derangement may precede radiographic evidence of disease;[999] the first measurable abnormality is likely an elevation of dead space ventilation on exercise.[998] In more advanced disease, PaO_2 is decreased, even at rest. Diffusing capacity may be reduced, and alveolar-arterial oxygen difference may be increased. A few patients have functional impairment suggestive of emphysema.

Prognosis and Natural History

The prognosis of patients who have symptomatic, chronic berylliosis is poor,[997, 998] particularly when there is complicating cor pulmonale. There is evidence that the presence of a granulomatous reaction in the lung parenchyma as opposed to simple mononuclear inflammatory cell infiltration is associated with a better prognosis.[945] Despite these findings, there is evidence that a reduction in the concentration of beryllium in the air can result in a significant improvement in lung function. For example, in one study of 20 men who had hypoxemia at the time air pollution was reduced, 13 showed improvement in arterial blood gases and lower alveolar-arterial gradients in a follow-up study 3 years later;[1000] some of these patients also showed an improvement in the severity of radiographic abnormalities.

Beryllium is a well-known carcinogen that is capable of causing pulmonary carcinoma in animals.[1001] Large cohort studies support the hypothesis that it is a carcinogen for humans as well,[1002, 1003] particularly for those individuals who have suffered from acute berylliosis.

Aluminum

Because of its versatility and metallic properties, occupational contact with aluminum is common: in the United States, approximately 2 million individuals are exposed directly to aluminum oxide, and almost the same number have contact with base or coated metal.[1004] Exposure can occur in several situations, including the following:

1. In the reduction of alumina to metallic aluminum during the process of smelting.[1005] This occurs in large rooms (pot rooms) that contain many potentially toxic gases and fumes in addition to aluminum dust. Although bauxite itself is generally believed to be innocuous, the results of one pathologic study suggested that it may cause pulmonary

fibrosis.[1007] In addition, workers involved in the mining and refining of bauxite have been found to have an increasing prevalence of low-profusion reticular densities radiologically with increasing dust exposure, an effect enhanced by smoking but unexplained by age.[1008]

2. During the preparation or use of aluminum powder derived either from stamping of cold metal (flake type) or directly from molten metal (granular type).[1009–1013]

3. During aluminum arc welding.[1014–1016]

4. During the grinding or polishing of aluminum products[1017, 1018] or in the manufacture or use of aluminum-based abrasive grinding tools.[1004]

Although each of these situations has been associated with pulmonary disease, it is not certain that aluminum is the pathogenetic agent in every instance because there is often concomitant exposure to other potentially toxic substances.[1005, 1019] This pathogenetic uncertainty is supported by experimental animal studies in which there has been minimal or no pulmonary reaction to inhaled aluminum.[1020, 1021] In addition, after the observation that silicosis does not develop in rabbits that inhale dust containing 1 part of aluminum to 100 parts of freshly fractured quartz,[1022] aluminum was added prophylactically to dust inhaled by miners exposed to silica;

such addition apparently has had no untoward effects.[1023] Despite these findings, other animal experiments have been associated with a significant fibrotic reaction to inhaled aluminum,[1024, 1025] implying that true toxicity may occur in some situations. Although differences in the species, method of aluminum administration, or form of aluminum employed (e.g., fibrous versus nonfibrous[1004]) may underlie the discrepant findings in the experimental studies, it has been hypothesized that host factors, perhaps mediated by immunologic mechanisms, may also be responsible.[1013, 1016]

Pathologic findings in the lungs of individuals exposed to aluminum are variable and, as indicated, may be caused in some cases by substances other than aluminum itself. Diffuse interstitial fibrosis has been described in workers engaged in smelting[1026, 1027] and in the production of grinding wheels[1004] and abrasives.[1010] Other histologic reactions that have been reported include desquamative interstitial pneumonitis,[1014] alveolar proteinosis,[1017] and diffuse granulomatous inflammation.[1013, 1016]

Radiographic abnormalities may become apparent after a few months or several years of exposure.[215, 1011] Fully developed changes consist of a fine-to-coarse reticular pattern widely distributed throughout the lungs (Fig. 60–61), sometimes with a nodular component.[1011] The fibrosis fre-

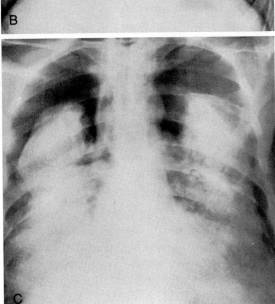

Figure 60–61. Bauxite Pneumoconiosis (Shaver's Disease). A 29-year-old man had been exposed for a number of years to bauxite in the manufacture of corundum. The first posteroanterior radiograph *(A)* revealed a coarse reticulonodular pattern throughout both lungs involving predominantly the upper and middle lung zones. Slightly more than 1 year later *(B)*, the disease had extended to a remarkable degree, the reticulonodular shadows being confluent in many areas. Shortly after this second radiograph was obtained, the patient suffered bilateral pneumothorax *(C)* associated with marked collapse of both lungs. This was one of several similar episodes of pneumothorax, some of which were unilateral and others bilateral.

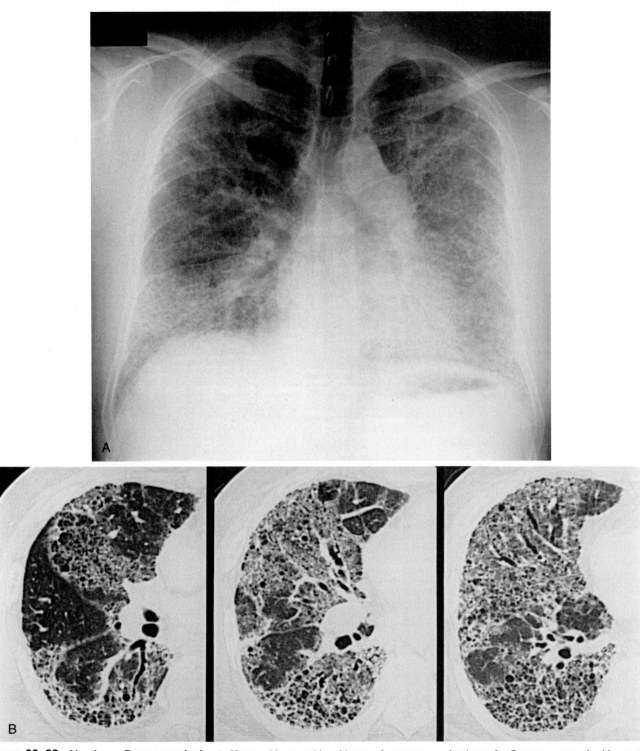

Figure 60–62. Aluminum Pneumoconiosis. A 52-year-old man with a history of exposure to aluminum for 7 years presented with exertional dyspnea. A posteroanterior chest radiograph *(A)* demonstrates a diffuse, bilateral reticular pattern. HRCT images targeted to the right lung *(B)* better demonstrate the reticular pattern and the presence of honeycombing. (Courtesy of Dr. Masanori Akira, Department of Radiology, National Kinki Chuo Hospital Chest Disease, Osaka, Japan.)

quently involves the upper lobes.[1004] HRCT findings have been described in one study of six workers, in whom the abnormalities consisted of predominantly small nodular opacities in two and a reticular pattern in four;[1029] honeycombing was also present in two patients (Fig. 60–62). In five of the six patients, the abnormalities involved mainly the upper lung zones. Lung volume may be greatly decreased, and the pleura may become thickened; spontaneous pneumothorax is a frequent complication (*see* Fig. 60–61).

Breathlessness is the chief symptom; in severe cases, it may be disabling and lead to death from pulmonary insufficiency.[1010, 1011] Work in aluminum smelters has been associated with the development of both asthma and chronic air-flow obstruction.[1030–1039] Pulmonary function studies have shown both restrictive and obstructive disease with reduction in diffusing capacity.[215, 1004] No association with the development of carcinoma was found in one cohort study.[1006]

Cobalt and Tungsten Carbide

The term *hard metal* is usually used to refer to an alloy of tungsten, carbon, and cobalt, occasionally with the addition of small amounts of other metals, such as titanium, tantalum, nickel, and chromium.[1040, 1041] The resulting product is extremely hard and resistant to heat and is used extensively in the drilling and polishing of other metals. Exposure to dust can occur during either the manufacture or the use of the metal and is well recognized as a cause of interstitial pneumonitis and fibrosis.[1042–1046]

The etiology and pathogenesis of disease are unclear. The results of experimental studies in animals suggest that cobalt is the causative agent,[1041, 1047] a hypothesis supported by the observation that diamond polishers—who are exposed to high concentrations of cobalt alone—develop pulmonary disease virtually identical to that seen in hard metal workers.[1048] There is evidence, however, that the effects of cobalt are enhanced by the presence of tungsten carbide;[1041] moreover, in some autopsy studies of patients who have interstitial fibrosis and a history of exposure to hard metals, cobalt has not been found in the lung tissue.[1049, 1050] It has thus been suggested that the disease may result in some workers from a hypersensitivity reaction analogous to that seen in berylliosis.[1044, 1049] Some cases of asthma have also been associated with cobalt exposure;[1051, 1052] there is evidence that this may be caused by an immunologically mediated hypersensitivity reaction,[1053, 1054] possibly enhanced by cigarette smoking.[1055]

Pathologic findings are predominantly those of interstitial pneumonitis and fibrosis.[1040, 1047] Characteristically, numerous macrophages are present in alveolar air spaces, creating a pattern simulating desquamative interstitial pneumonitis. In many cases, multinucleated giant cells are prominent, both in the air spaces and lining alveolar walls, resulting in a pattern of giant cell interstitial pneumonitis (Fig. 60–63);[1040, 1044, 1056, 1057] the giant cells can also be seen in cytology specimens obtained by bronchial washing.[1058] Obliterative bronchiolitis has been noted occasionally.[1040, 1056] Particulate material may or may not be identified within the macrophages or giant cells by light microscopy; spectroscopic analysis reveals predominantly tungsten with little evidence of cobalt.[1040]

The radiographic findings consist of a diffuse micronodular and reticular pattern, sometimes associated with lymph node enlargement; the reticulation may be coarse[1059] and in advanced disease may be accompanied by small cystic spaces.[1047, 1060] In one study of two hard metal workers, the HRCT findings consisted of bilateral areas of ground-glass attenuation, areas of consolidation, and extensive reticular opacities and traction bronchiectasis indicative of fibrosis (Fig. 60–64);[1029] autopsy correlation in one case showed the areas of ground-glass attenuation and consolidation to correspond to aggregates of mononuclear and multinucleated giant cells.

Symptoms include cough, sometimes productive,[1043]

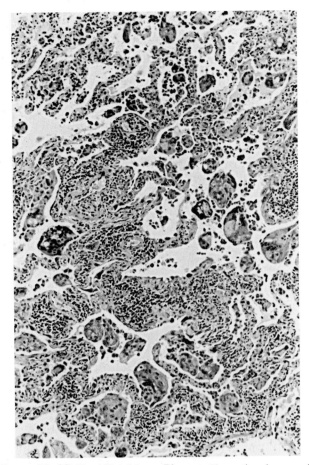

Figure 60–63. Hard Metal Lung Disease. The section shows moderately severe interstitial pneumonitis and fibrosis and the presence of a large number of irregular multinucleated giant cells in the alveolar air spaces. (×80.)

and dyspnea on exertion; severe respiratory insufficiency sometimes develops and can prove fatal.[1059, 1061, 1062] Weight loss out of proportion to the degree of respiratory impairment is frequently seen, possibly related to the elaboration of TNF-α by lung inflammatory cells.[1063]

In the appropriate clinical setting, the identification of multinucleated giant cells in BAL fluid supports the diagnosis. Eosinophilia was noted in the BAL fluid of one worker who had combined heavy metal and aluminum dust exposure.[1064] Pulmonary function tests reveal both restrictive[1043, 1065] and obstructive patterns,[1066] and diffusing capacity may be reduced.[1043, 1047, 1065] Minor alterations in spirometry without radiologic abnormalities were described in a group of diamond polishers[1066a] and in a group of saw filers[1067] exposed to "high" cobalt exposure, which nevertheless respected the industry threshold limit value for cobalt.

Silicon Carbide

Silicon carbide (carborundum) is produced by fusion at high temperature of high-grade sand, finely ground carbon (coke), salt, and wood dust.[1068] The resulting product is extremely hard and is used as an abrasive. Although the findings of experimental animal studies have suggested that

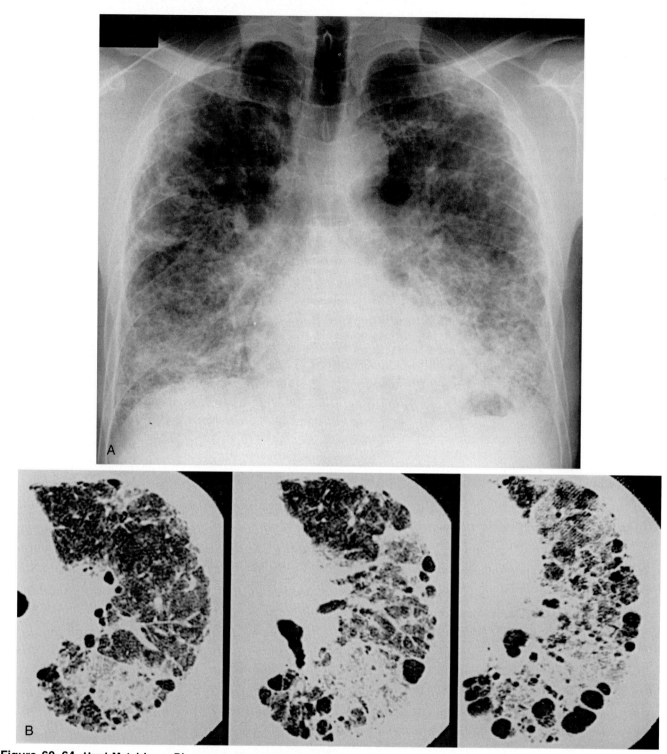

Figure 60–64. Hard Metal Lung Disease. A 45-year-old Japanese man presented with exertional dyspnea. He had a history of exposure to hard metal for 5 years. A chest radiograph *(A)* demonstrates a coarse reticular pattern involving mainly the peripheral lung regions and the lower lung zones. HRCT images targeted to the left lung *(B)* demonstrate extensive areas of ground-glass attenuation. Irregular linear opacities and traction bronchiectasis consistent with fibrosis are also evident. Several cystic spaces consistent with end-stage honeycombing are present in the subpleural lung regions. (Courtesy of Dr. Masanori Akira, Department of Radiology, National Kinki Chuo Hospital Chest Disease, Osaka, Japan.)

the substance is inert,[1068–1070] workers in the carborundum industry have had pathologic evidence of interstitial fibrosis and macrophage accumulation[1071] accompanied by radiographic and pulmonary function abnormalities.[1069, 1072–1075] It is not certain to what extent these changes are caused by silica derived from the sand, by other contaminants in the dust such as cristobalite or tridymite, or by silicon carbide fibers produced during the manufacturing process.[1069, 1076, 1077]

Silicon carbide can be identified in tissue sections as thin black fibers often associated with an iron-protein coat (ferruginous bodies) (Fig. 60–65). Some investigators have suggested a possible association of exposure with pulmonary carcinoma;[1071] however, in one large epidemiologic study, no evidence of excess deaths from this cause was found.[1078] Radiographic findings include nodular, reticulonodular, or reticular opacities with or without hilar lymphadenopathy (Fig. 60–66).[1079, 1081] Pleural plaques similar to those seen in asbestos-exposed individuals have also been described.[1075]

Polyvinyl Chloride

In its pure form, polyvinyl chloride is a white powder that is produced by polymerization under pressure of the gas vinyl chloride;[1082] it is used in the manufacture of plastics, synthetic fibers, and numerous other commercial products. There is evidence that inhalation of the substance, either during its production or its use in the manufacture of other materials, may be associated with chronic pulmonary disease. Epidemiologic studies have shown the presence of radiographic abnormalities consistent with pneumoconiosis in 3% to 20% of workers.[1083–1085] Evidence of obstructive pulmonary function was identified in almost half of workers in one investigation. Occasional case reports in humans and experimental studies in animals have also documented a possible association between exposure and the presence of interstitial pneumonitis and fibrosis or the accumulation of interstitial and intra-alveolar macrophages.[1082, 1086–1089] An immunologically-mediated multisystem disorder manifested by Raynaud's phenomenon, acro-osteolysis, thrombocytopenia, portal fibrosis, and hepatic and pulmonary dysfunction has also been ascribed to both polyvinyl chloride and vinyl chloride.[1089a, b, c]

Titanium Dioxide

Titanium dioxide (rutile, anatase) is derived from the ore ilmenite and is used chiefly as a pigment in paints, paper, and other products; as a mordant in dyeing; as a food additive; and as an alloy in some hard metals. Pathologic examination of the lungs of workers who have been in contact with the substance has generally shown alveolar and interstitial accumulation of pigment-laden macrophages but

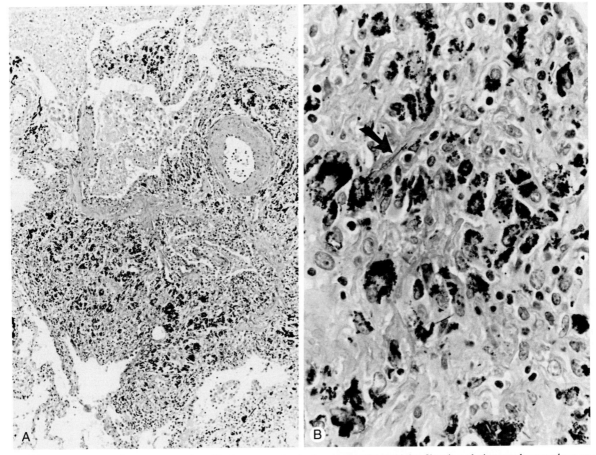

Figure 60–65. Carborundum Lung. The section *(A)* shows a moderate degree of peribronchiolar fibrosis and pigmented macrophage accumulation. Higher magnification *(B)* shows macrophages to contain abundant "anthracotic" pigment and scattered ferruginous bodies *(arrow)* that have a black fibrous core, representing carborundum. *(A, ×60; B, ×250.)*

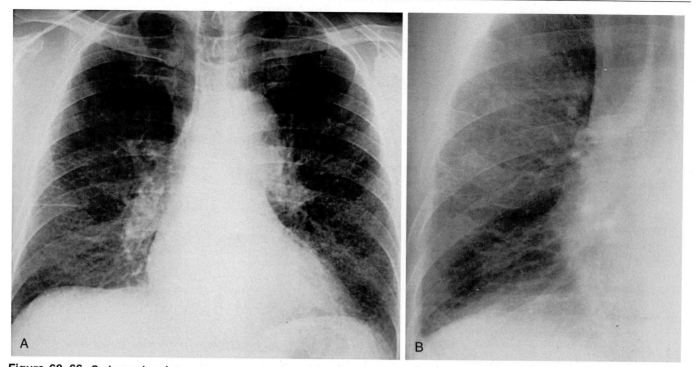

Figure 60–66. Carborundum Lung. A posteroanterior chest radiograph *(A)* demonstrates bilateral hilar lymphadenopathy as well as small nodular and irregular linear opacities involving mainly the lower lung zones. A magnified view of the right lower lung *(B)* better demonstrates the fine reticulonodular pattern and interlobular septal thickening. The patient had been exposed to carborundum for 33 years in a factory manufacturing abrasives. (Courtesy of Dr. Gaston Ostiguy, Maisonneuve-Rosemont Hospital, Montreal.)

no[1090] or minimal[1091] fibrosis. The apparent innocuity of the material has been corroborated by experimental studies in animals.[1091] Despite these observations, clinical and radiographic disease and histologically evident interstitial fibrosis have been documented in some patients,[1093] and the inertness of the substance has been questioned.

Nonnecrotizing granulomatous inflammation was identified in a biopsy specimen from one patient;[1094] because of a positive lymphocyte transformation test on exposure to titanium, the authors considered the possibility of a hypersensitivity reaction similar to that proposed for berylliosis. In macrophages, titanium dioxide appears as small black granules similar to "anthracotic" pigment (Fig. 60–67); however, in contrast to the latter, they are strongly birefringent.[1091, 1092] Radiographic changes considered consistent with pneumoconiosis have been reported in workers involved in pigment production.[1090–1092] A cross-sectional survey of 209 titanium metal production workers showed a reduction in ventilatory capacity and radiographic evidence of pleural plaques and thickening not clearly attributable to asbestos exposure.[1095] In another investigation of 67 workers in a paint factory in Nigeria, almost 50% were found to have pulmonary symptoms (chest pain, cough) and about 40% to have functional evidence of restrictive lung disease.[1080]

Volcanic Dust

Volcanic eruption occurs when magma (liquid rock) is extruded from the depths of the earth to its surface. Although

the magma may simply flow over the rim of the volcano onto the adjacent earth (where it is known as lava), violent eruption into the atmosphere can also occur and can produce large amounts of ash (tephra). Depending on the severity and nature of the eruption (e.g., whether it is vertical or at an angle to the earth's surface) and on the composition of the magma itself, significant quantities of potentially harmful ash may be spewed into the atmosphere.

The best-studied volcanic eruption from the point of view of human health occurred at Mount Saint Helens in 1980.[1096] As of 1981, 35 individuals were known to have died directly as a result of the eruption;[1097] among the 25 who underwent autopsy, the majority were considered to have asphyxiated as a result of major airway plugging by mucus and inhaled volcanic ash.[1098] In individuals outside the areas of most severe damage, there was a mild increase in the number of acute respiratory complaints, such as cough, wheezing, and dyspnea, probably secondary to airway irritation.[1096] A considerable increase in emergency department attendance by patients who had asthma and bronchitis was also recorded at local hospitals.[1099]

The long-term consequences, if any, of volcanic ash inhalation are unclear. It has been estimated that free crystalline silicates formed about 3% to 7% of the ash of the Mount Saint Helens eruption,[1096] and it is conceivable that persons who suffered heavy exposure might develop chronic pulmonary disease, presumptively and rather remarkably designated *pneumonoultramicroscopicsilicovolcanoconiosis*![1100] Whether individuals exposed to ash derived from other volcanic sites also have a risk for the development of disease is unclear.

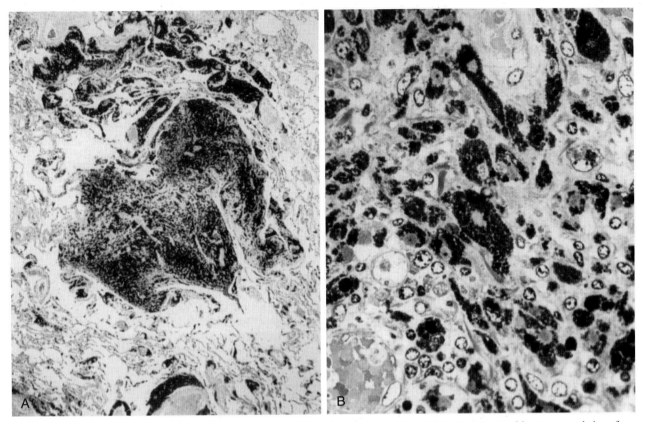

Figure 60–67. Titanium Lung. A section of lung shows patchy, moderately severe interstitial thickening *(A)* caused by an accumulation of numerous macrophages *(B)* containing finely granular black pigment; there is minimal fibrosis. (*A,* ×25; *B,* ×630.) (From Moran CA, Mullick FG, Ishak KG, et al: Identification of titanium in human tissues. Hum Pathol 22:450, 1991.)

Synthetic Mineral Fibers

Synthetic mineral fibers are amorphous silicates derived from industrial slag, volcanic rock, ceramic, or glass. Their diameter and length vary considerably, depending on the specific use to which they are put;[1101] for example, fibers used in textiles and as reinforcement in plastics and other materials are mostly between 9 and 25 μm in diameter, whereas those employed in insulation are generally smaller (3 to 6 μm). In contrast to natural silicates, such as asbestos, synthetic fibers break transversely rather than longitudinally when traumatized, resulting in small fragments whose diameter is the same as that of their parents.[1101] Because the potential for causing disease is related to a high length-to-diameter ratio, at least in part,[467, 1101, 1102] this effect may be important in explaining the relative lack of toxicity of these substances.

The bulk of evidence suggests that inhaled synthetic mineral fibers have little, if any, harmful effects on the lungs.[1101] In one autopsy study, no gross or microscopic abnormality was found in the lungs of workers exposed to fiberglass;[1101] in addition, the total number of fibers per gram of dry lung was similar to that of a control group, implying adequate clearance of inhaled particles.[1103] Inhalation of synthetic mineral fibers by rats, hamsters, and monkeys has failed to cause significant fibrosis or neoplasia;[1101, 1104] no alteration of pulmonary structure or inflammatory reaction has been observed except for the presence of alveolar macrophages during the early stages and the development of pro-

teinosis in some animals after 90 days of inhalation.[1105] In addition to these pathologic studies, most epidemiologic investigations, radiographic surveys, and tests of pulmonary function of workers exposed to synthetic mineral fibers have shown no differences from those of appropriate controls.[1101, 1104, 1106, 1107]

Despite the abundant evidence implying lack of pathogenicity of these fibers, the possibility that toxicity might occur in some situations cannot be entirely excluded. It has been suggested, for example, that the results cited previously may simply reflect a relatively low dust exposure.[1107, 1108] In addition, the results of some studies have raised the possibility that the fibers can cause significant tissue damage.[1109] For example, in one investigation of 1,448 fiberglass workers, a statistically significant increase in the number of deaths caused by respiratory disease other than cancer and pneumonia was identified compared with controls.[1110] In another survey of workers involved in the manufacture of refractory ceramic fibers, a type of man-made vitreous fiber, pleural plaques were identified in 5 of 19 workers (26%) who had more than 20 years' exposure, a finding that was not explained by asbestos exposure.[1111] In addition, in a murine model of intense fiberglass exposure, the pulmonary response to fiberglass was found to be similar to that described for crocidolite asbestos.[1112]

The results of several investigations of pulmonary function have also raised questions about the lack of toxicity of synthetic mineral fibers.[1113] For example, in one group of appliance manufacturing workers who had little or no asbestos exposure and who had more than 20 years' exposure to fiberglass, pleural and parenchymal changes as well as alterations in lung function similar to those of asbestos-exposed workers were described in 13%.[1114] However, this study has been criticized for its failure to include control radiographs in the interpretation of the films,[1115] for its failure to adjust for smoking intensity,[1115] and for inadequate consideration of the effects of associated asbestos exposure.[1116] In another study of insulation workers exposed to rock and glass wool, the presence of obstructive lung function and a faster rate of decline in FEV_1 compared to a control group of non–dust-exposed bus drivers were identified.[1117] In a third investigation of workers involved in the manufacture of refractory ceramic fibers, a significant decrease in FVC was found in those individuals who had at least 7 years exposure.[995]

On the basis of the results of these various studies, it seems reasonable to conclude that there is a possible, albeit quantitatively uncertain, risk for the development of pulmonary disease after exposure to man-made mineral fibers.

In contrast to the relative benignity of inhaled synthetic mineral fibers, their instillation directly into the pleural or peritoneal cavities of experimental animals has been shown to be associated with the development of mesothelioma.[1102] Some man-made mineral fibers have been shown to cause hydroxyl radical mediated DNA base modification *in vitro*, possibly explaining the fibers' carcinogenicity.[1118] Despite these observations, no association between mineral fiber inhalation and human mesothelioma has been documented. Some investigators have argued that fibrous glass materials are carcinogenic and that they may be as potent in this respect as asbestos on a fiber-per-fiber basis.[1119] However, when cigarette smoking is taken into account, no increase in the prevalence of pulmonary carcinoma has been found in exposed workers.[1120–1124]

Dust Exposure in Dental Technicians

Although the radiographic abnormalities that sometimes develop in dental technicians have been attributed to SiO_2, it is probable that other agents are involved as well: Air concentration exposure studies and mineralogic analyses of BAL fluid and lung tissue of affected patients have disclosed a variety of substances in addition to silica, including chromium, nickel, aluminum, cobalt, molybdenum, beryllium, acrylic resin, and alginate impression powder.[14, 15, 1125–1128] The prevalence of pulmonary disease in this occupation may be significant; in one study of dental technicians who had more than 30 years' exposure, 22% were found to have radiologic evidence of pneumoconiosis.[1129]

Cement Dust

The results of several studies, some epidemiologic and others single case reports, have implicated cement as a cause of pneumoconiosis.[1130] In a radiographic survey of 195 cement workers, many years' exposure to a high concentration of raw and mixed cement dust was found to be associated with the accentuation of linear markings and ill-defined micronodulation;[1131] however, little or no evidence of radiographic abnormality has been found in other studies.[1131, 1132] Although an increased incidence of carcinoma of the stomach was described in cement workers in one study,[1133] no increase in mortality was observed from respiratory disease. It has been speculated that cement dust may be involved in the pathogenesis of chronic air-flow obstruction in tunnelers using the shotcrete method (in which the tunnel is excavated by shooting a mixture of cement, water, and sand under high pressure).[1134] A case of alveolar proteinosis arising in a cement truck driver has also been reported.[1135] It is possible that these abnormalities may have been caused by the quartz and asbestos that are present in varying amounts in some cement.

Zirconium

Zirconium is a heavy metal used as an alloy in the nuclear industry and in the glazing of ceramic tiles. A single case of pulmonary fibrosis has been reported in association with its use.[1136] Granulomatous interstitial disease imitating sarcoidosis or acute hypersensitivity pneumonitis has also been described in some individuals.[1137–1139] Such effects are unusual, however; in one long-term study of 178 men followed from 1975 to 1988, no evidence of radiographic or functional abnormalities related to the mineral was identified.[1140]

Nylon Flock

Flock is finely cut nylon that is used in upholstery, clothing, and automobiles. An excess incidence of chronic diffuse interstitial lung disease has been described in two North American nylon flock production/flocking plants;[1028, 1141] in one study of 165 workers in a plant in Rhode Island, 7 (4%) were affected. Tissue obtained from transbronchial and wedge lung biopsy specimens has demonstrated nonspecific interstitial pneumonitis or (rarely) bronchiolitis obliterans organizing pneumonia;[1028] nodular lymphoid infiltrates with germinal centers have been seen in most patients, particularly in a peribronchovascular distribution. No granulomatous inflammation has been noted, and the precise cause of the abnormalities has not been identified.

In one investigation of eight patients, four had diffuse reticulonodular opacities, one had patchy consolidation, and three had normal chest radiographs.[1028] HRCT demonstrated bilateral patchy areas of ground-glass attenuation in six patients and peripheral honeycombing in the other two patients;[1028] two patients had focal areas of consolidation and one had diffuse micronodularity associated with the areas of ground-glass attenuation. Symptoms of dry cough and dyspnea occur with a mean latency of 6 years after initial exposure. Improvement has been noted after cessation of exposure and with the use of corticosteroids; however, no workers have recovered completely during the reported follow-up period.[1141]

REFERENCES

1. The Fourth International Pneumoconiosis Conference: Working Party on the Definition of Pneumoconiosis Report. Geneva, 1971.
2. Vallyathan V, Mega JF, Shi X, et al: Enhanced generation of free radicals from phagocytes induced by mineral dusts. Am J Respir Cell Mol Biol 6:404, 1992.
3. Utell MJ, Samet JM: Particulate air pollution and health: New evidence on an old problem. Am Rev Respir Dis 147:1334, 1993.
4. Pope CA III, Dockery DW: Acute health effects of PM_{10} pollution on symptomatic and asymptomatic children. Am Rev Respir Dis 145:1123, 1992.
5. Schwartz J, Dockery DW: Increased mortality in Philadelphia associated with daily air pollution concentrations. Am Rev Respir Dis 145:600, 1992.
6. Dockery DW, Schwartz K, Spengler JD: Air pollution and daily mortality: Associations with particulates and acid aerosols. Environ Res 59:362, 1992.
7. Pope CA III: Respiratory hospital admissions associated with PM_{10} pollution in Utah, Salt Lake, and Cache Valleys. Arch Environ Health 46:90, 1991.
8. Chariot P, Couste B, Guillon F, et al: Nonfibrous mineral particles in bronchoalveolar lavage fluid and lung parenchyma from the general population. Am Rev Respir Dis 146:61, 1992.
9. Dumortier P, De Vuyst P, Yernault JC: Comparative analysis of inhaled particles contained in human bronchoalveolar lavage fluids, lung parenchyma and lymph nodes. Environ Health Perspect 102:257, 1994.
9a. Brady AR, Vallyathan NV, Craighead JE: Use of scanning electron microscopy and x-ray energy spectrometry to determine the elemental content of inclusions in human tissue lesions. *In* Becker RP, Johari O (eds): Scanning Electron Microscopy/1978/II. AMF O'Hare, IL, Scanning Electron Microscopy, Inc, 1978, pp 615–621.
10. Weill H: Epidemiologic methods in the investigation of occupational lung disease. Am Rev Respir Dis 112:1, 1975.
11. Seaton A, Lamb D, Brown WR, et al: Pneumoconiosis of shale miners. Thorax 36:412, 1981.
12. Harris DK: Some hazards in the manufacture and use of plastics. Br J Ind Med 16:221, 1959.
13. Morgenroth K, Kronenberger H, Michalke G, et al: Morphology and pathogenesis of pneumoconiosis in dental technicians. Pathol Respir Pract 179:528, 1985.
14. Rom WN, Lockey JE, Lee JS, et al: Pneumoconiosis and exposures of dental laboratory technicians. Am J Public Health 74:1252, 1984.
15. De Vuyst P, Vande Weyer R, De Coster A, et al: Dental technician's pneumoconiosis: A report of two cases. Am Rev Respir Dis 133:316, 1986.
16. McLaughlin AIG: Pneumoconiosis in foundry workers. Br J Tuberc 51:297, 1957.
17. McLaughlin AIG, Harding HE: Pneumoconiosis and other causes of death in iron and steel foundry workers. AMA Arch Ind Health 14:350, 1956.
18. Morgan WKC, Kerr HD: Pathologic and physiologic studies of welders' siderosis. Ann Intern Med 58:293, 1963.
19. Edstrom HW, Rice DMD: "Labrador lung": An unusual mixed dust pneumoconiosis. CMAJ 126:27, 1982.
20. Mark GJ, Monroe CB, Kazemi H: Mixed pneumoconiosis: Silicosis, asbestosis, talcosis, and berylliosis. Chest 75:726, 1979.
21. Reilly MJ, Rosenman KD, Watt FC, et al: Silicosis surveillance—Michigan, New Jersey, Ohio and Wisconsin, 1987–1990. MMWR CDC Surveillance Summaries 42:23, 1993.
22. Huang J, Shibita E, Takeuchi Y, et al: Comprehensive health evaluation of workers in the ceramics industry. Br J Ind Med 50:112, 1993.
23. Van Sprundel MP: Pneumoconiosis: The situation in developing countries. Exp Lung Res 15:5, 1990.
24. Petrova E, Tsacheva N, Marinova B: Pneumoconioses in Bulgaria—prevalence, development, prognosis and prevention. Cent Eur J Public Health 2:47, 1994.
25. Knishkowy B, Baker EL: Transmission of occupational disease to family contacts. Am J Ind Med 9:543, 1986.
26. Salvi S, Joshi DR, Tayade BO: Hut lung—a domestically acquired pneumoconiosis. J Assoc Physicians India 42:746, 1994.
27. Saiyed HN, Sharma YK, Sadhu HG, et al: Non-occupational pneumoconiosis at high altitude villages in central Ladakh. Br J Ind Med 48:825, 1991.
28. Rey F, Boutin C, Viallat JR, et al: Environmental asbestotic pleural plaques in northeast Corsica: Correlations with airborne and pleural mineralogic analysis. Environ Health Perspect 102:251, 1994.
29. Amandus HE, Reger RB, Pendergrass EP, et al: The pneumoconioses: Methods of measuring progression. Chest 63:736, 1973.
30. International Labor Office (League of Nations): Silicosis. Records of the international conference held at Johannesburg 13–27 August 1930. International Labour Office, Studies and Reports, Series F (Industrial Hygiene), No. 13. Geneva, International Labour Office, 1930, pp 86–93.
30a. International Labor Office: Guidelines for the use of ILO International classification of radiographs of pneumoconioses. Geneva, 1980, pp 1–48.
31. Liddell FDK: An experiment in film reading. Br J Ind Med 20:300, 1963.
32. Liddell FDK, Lindars DC: An elaboration of the I.L.O. classification of simple pneumoconiosis. Br J Ind Med 26:89, 1969.
33. Felson B, Morgan WKC, Bristol LJ, et al: Observations on the results of multiple readings of chest films on coal miners' pneumoconiosis. Radiology 109:19, 1973.
34. Morgan RH, Donner MW, Gayler BW, et al: Decision processes and observer error in the diagnosis of pneumoconiosis by chest roentgenography. Am J Roentgenol 117:757, 1973.
35. Amandus HE, Pendergrass EP, Dennis JM, et al: Pneumoconiosis: Inter-reader variability in the classification of the type of small opacities in the chest roentgenogram. Am J Roentgenol 122:740, 1974.
36. Albin M, Engholm G, Fröström K, et al: Chest x ray films from construction workers: International Labour Office (ILO 1980) classification compared with routine readings. Br J Ind Med 49:862, 1992.
37. Castellan RM, Sanderson WT, Petersen MR: Prevalence of radiographic appearance of pneumoconiosis in an unexposed blue collar population. Am Rev Respir Dis 131:684, 1985.
38. Meyer JD, Islam SS, Ducatman AM, et al: Prevalence of small lung opacities in populations unexposed to dusts. Chest 111:404, 1997.
39. Zitting AJ: Prevalence of radiographic small lung opacities and pleural abnormalities in a representative adult population sample. Chest 107:126, 1995.
40. Liddell FDK: Assessment of radiological progression of simple pneumoconiosis in individual miners. Br J Ind Med 31:185, 1974.
41. Mulloy KB, Coultas DB, Samet JM: Use of chest radiographs in epidemiological investigations of pneumoconioses. Br J Ind Med 50:273, 1993.
42. White NW, Chetty R, Bateman ED: Silicosis among gemstone workers in South Africa: Tiger's-eye pneumoconiosis. Am J Ind Med 19:205, 1991.
43. Rastogi SK, Gupta BN, Chandra H, et al: A study of the prevalence of respiratory morbidity among agate workers. Int Arch Occup Environ Health 63:21, 1991.
44. Hosoda Y, Ueda A, Fujii T: Clay dye pneumoconiosis among rush mat workers. Semin Respir Med 12:55, 1991.
45. Landrigan PJ, Cherniack MG, Lewis FA, et al: Silicosis in a grey iron foundry: The persistence of an ancient disease. Scand J Work Environ Health 12:32, 1986.
46. Posner E: Pneumoconiosis in makers of artificial grinding wheels, including a case of Caplan's syndrome. Br J Ind Med 17:109, 1960.
47. Saiyed HN, Parikh DJ, Ghodasara NB, et al: Silicosis in slate pencil workers: I. An environmental and medical study. Am J Ind Med 8:127, 1985.
48. Saiyed HN, Chatterjee BB: Rapid progression of silicosis in slate pencil workers: II. A follow-up study. Am J Ind Med 8:135, 1985.
49. Rees D, Cronje R, du Toit RS: Dust exposure and pneumoconiosis in a South African pottery: 1. Study objectives and dust exposure. Br J Ind Med 49:459, 1992.
50. Gerhardsson L, Ahlmark A: Silicosis in women: Experience from the Swedish Pneumoconiosis Register. J Occup Med 27:347, 1985.
51. Roche AD, Picard D, Vernhes A: Silicosis of ocher workers: A clinical and anatomopathologic study. Am Rev Tuberc 77:839, 1958.
52. Phibbs BP, Sundin RE, Mitchell RS: Silicosis in Wyoming bentonite workers. Am Rev Respir Dis 103:1, 1971.
53. Erdélyi J, Ökrös A: Über die durch emaileinatmung bewirkten erkrankungen. [Enamel pneumoconiosis.] Fortschr Röntgenstr 92:235, 1960.
54. Parkes WR: Occupational Lung Disease. 3rd ed. Oxford, Butterworth-Heinemann, 1994.
55. Balaan MR, Weber SL, Banks DE: Clinical aspects of coal worker's pneumoconiosis and silicosis. Occup Med 8:19, 1993.
56. Graham WG: Silicosis. Clin Chest Med 13:253, 1992.
57. Morgan WKC, Seaton A: Occupational Lung Diseases. Philadelphia, WB Saunders, 1995.
58. Lapp NL: Lung disease secondary to inhalation of nonfibrous minerals. Clin Chest Med 2:219, 1981.
59. Ziskind M, Jones RN, Weill H: Silicosis. Am Rev Respir Dis 113:643, 1976.
60. Graham WGB, Ashikaga T, Hemenway D, et al: Radiographic abnormalities in Vermont granite workers exposed to low levels of granite dust. Chest 100:1507, 1991.
61. Ng TP, Phoon WH, Lee HS, et al: An epidemiological survey of respiratory morbidity among granite quarry workers in Singapore: Radiological abnormalities. Ann Acad Med Singapore 21:305, 1992.
62. Costello J, Graham WG: Vermont granite workers' mortality study. Am J Ind Med 13:483, 1988.
63. Pang D, Fu SC, Yang GC: Relation between exposure to respirable silica dust and silicosis in a tungsten mine in China. Br J Ind Med 49:38, 1992
64. Seaton A, Ruckley VA, Addison J, et al: Silicosis in barium miners. Thorax 41:591, 1986.
65. Trapp E, Renzetti AD Jr, Kobayashi T, et al: Cardiopulmonary function in uranium miners. Am Rev Respir Dis 101:27, 1970.
66. Oechsli WR, Jacobson G, Brodeur AE: Diatomite pneumoconiosis: Roentgen characteristics and classification. Am J Roentgentol 85:263, 1961.
67. Caldwell DM: The coalescent lesion of diatomaceous earth pneumoconiosis. Am Rev Tuberc 77:644, 1958
68. Beskow R: Silicosis in diatomaceous earth factory workers in Sweden. Scand J Respir Dis 59:216, 1978.
69. Cooper WC, Sargent EN: A 26-year radiographic follow-up of workers in a diatomite mine and mill. J Occup Med 26:456, 1984.
70. Banks DE, Morring KL, Boehlecke BA, et al: Silicosis in silica flour workers. Am Rev Respir Dis 124:445, 1981.
71. Middleton EL: The present position of silicosis in industry in Britain. BMJ 2:485, 1929.
72. Gong H Jr, Tashkin DP: Silicosis due to intentional inhalation of abrasive

scouring powder: Case report with long-term survival and vasculitic sequelae. Am J Med 67:358, 1979.

73. Ng TP, Tsin TW, O'Kelly FJ, et al: A survey of the respiratory health of silica-exposed gemstone workers in Hong Kong. Am Rev Respir Dis 135:1249, 1987.

74. Ng TP, Allan WG, Tsin TW, et al: Silicosis in jade workers. Br J Ind Med 42:761, 1985.

75. Kawakami M, Sato S, Takishima T: Silicosis in workers dealing with tonoko: Case reports and analyses of tonoko. Chest 72:635, 1977.

75a. Hughes JM, Weill H, Checkoway H, et al: Radiographic evidence of silicosis risk in the diatomaceous earth industry. Am J Respir Crit Care Med 158:807, 1998.

76. Prowse K, Allen MB, Bradbury SP: Respiratory symptoms and pulmonary impairment in male and female subjects with pottery workers' silicosis. Ann Occup Hyg 33:375, 1989.

77. Hirsch M, Bar-Ziv J, Lehmann E, et al: Simple siliceous pneumoconiosis of Bedouin females in the Negev desert. Clin Radiol 25:507, 1974.

78. Palmer PES, Daynes G: Transkei silicosis. S Afr Med J 41:1182, 1967.

79. Norboo T, Angchuk PT, Yahya M, et al: Silicosis in a Himalayan village population: Role of environmental dust. Thorax 46:341, 1991.

80. Saiyed HN, Sharma YK, Sadhu HG, et al: Non-occupational pneumoconiosis at high altitude villages in central Ladakh. Br J Ind Med 48:825, 1991.

81. Dumontet C, Biron F, Vitrey D, et al: Acute silicosis due to inhalation of a domestic product. Am Rev Respir Dis 143:880, 1991.

82. Gong H, Tashkin DP: Silicosis due to intentional inhalation of abrasive scouring powder. Am J Med 67:358, 1979.

83. Daize E, Marti-Flich J, Palmier B, et al: Acute silicosis caused by intentional inhalation of scouring powder. Ann Fr Anesth Reanim 13:251, 1994.

84. International Agency for Research on Cancer: Silica and some silicates. IARC Monogr Eval Carcinog Risks Hum vol 42, 1986.

85. Seaton A, Legge JS, Henderson J, et al: Accelerated silicosis in Scottish stonemasons. Lancet 337:341, 1991.

86. Valiante DJ, Rosenman KD: Does silicosis still occur? JAMA 262:3003, 1989.

87. Carel RS, Salman H, Bar-Ziv J: "Souvenir" casting silicosis. Chest 106:1272, 1994.

88. Banks DE, Balaan M, Wang M: Silicosis in the 1990s revisited. Chest 111:837, 1997.

89. Rosenman KD, Reilly MJ, Kalinowski DJ, et al: Silicosis in the 1990s. Chest 111:779, 1997.

90. Beckett W, Abraham J, Becklake M, et al: Adverse effects of crystalline silica exposure. Am J Respir Crit Care Med 155:761, 1997.

90a. Silicosis deaths among young adults—United States, 1968–1994. MMWR 47:331, 1998.

91. Murray J, Kielkowski D, Reid P: Occupational disease trends in black South African gold miners. Am Rev Respir Crit Care Med 153:706, 1996.

92. Zhong Y, Li D: Potential years of life lost and work tenure lost when silicosis is compared with other pneumoconioses. Scand J Work Environ Health. 21(Suppl 2):91, 1995.

93. Bégin R, Cantin A, Massé S: Recent advances in the pathogenesis and clinical assessment of mineral dust pneumoconioses: Asbestosis, silicosis and coal pneumoconiosis. Eur Respir J 2:988, 1989.

94. Davis GS: The pathogenesis of silicosis. Chest 3:166, 1986.

95. Lapp NL, Castranova V: How silicosis and coal workers' pneumoconiosis develop—a cellular assessment. Occup Med 8:35, 1993.

96. Heppleston AG: Pathogenesis of mineral pneumoconiosis. In Parkes WR (ed): Occupational Lung Disease. 3rd ed. Oxford, Butterworth-Heinemann, 1994.

96a. Mossman BT, Churg A: Mechanisms in the pathogenesis of asbestosis and silicosis. Am J Respir Crit Care Med 157:1666, 1998.

97. Hnizdo E, Sluis-Cremer GK: Risk of silicosis in a cohort of white South African gold miners. Am J Ind Med 24:447, 1993.

98. Brody AR, Roe MW, Evans JN, et al: Deposition and translocation of inhaled silica in rats: Quantification of particle distribution, macrophage participation, and function. Lab Invest 47:533, 1982.

99. Warheit DB, Overly LA, George G, et al: Pulmonary macrophages are attracted to inhaled particles through complement activation. Exp Lung Res 14:51, 1988.

100. Reynolds HY: Lung inflammation: Role of endogenous chemotactic factors in attracting polymorphonuclear granulocytes. Am Rev Respir Dis 127:16, 1983.

101. Sjöstrand M, Absher PM, Hemenway DR, et al: Comparison of lung alveolar and tissue cells in silica-induced inflammation. Am Rev Respir Dis 143:47, 1991.

102. Bowden DH, Hedgecock C, Adamson IYR: Silica-induced pulmonary fibrosis involves the reaction of particles with interstitial rather than alveolar macrophages. J Pathol 158:73, 1989.

103. Adamson IYR, Prieditis H, Bowden DH: Instillation of chemotactic factor to silica-injected lungs lowers interstitial particle content and reduces pulmonary fibrosis. Am J Pathol 1421:319, 1992.

104. Bagchi N: What makes silica toxic? Br J Ind Med 49:163, 1992.

105. Allison AC, Harington JS, Birbeck M: An examination of the cytotoxic effects of silica on macrophages. J Exp Med 124:141, 1966.

106. Kane AB, Stanton RP, Raymond EG, et al: Dissociation of intracellular lysosomal rupture from the cell death caused by silica. J Cell Biol 87:643, 1980.

107. Gee JBL: Cellular mechanisms in occupational lung disease. Chest 78(Suppl):384, 1980.

108. Bégin RO, Cantin AM, Boileau RD, et al: Spectrum of alveolitis in quartz-exposed human subjects. Chest 92:1061, 1987.

109. Christman JW, Emerson RJ, Graham WGB, et al: Mineral dust and cell recovery from the bronchoalveolar lavage of healthy Vermont granite workers. Am Rev Respir Dis 132:393, 1985.

110. Brown GP, Monicj M, Hunninghake GW: Fibroblast proliferation induced by silica-exposed human alveolar macrophages. Am Rev Respir Dis 138:85, 1988.

111. Bégin R, Martel M, Desmarais Y, et al: Fibronectin and procollagen 3 levels in bronchoalveolar lavage of asbestos-exposed human subjects and sheep. Chest 89:237, 1986.

112. Jagirdar J, Bégin R, Dufresne A, et al: Transforming growth factor-β (TGF-β) in silicosis. Am J Respir Crit Care Med 154:1076, 1996.

113. Dubois CM, Bissonnette E, Rola-Pleszczynski M: Asbestos fibers and silica particles stimulate rat alveolar macrophages to release tumour necrosis factor. Am Rev Respir Dis 139:1257, 1989.

114. Lugano EM, Dauber JH, Elias JA, et al: The regulation of lung fibroblast proliferation by alveolar macrophages in experimental silicosis. Am Rev Respir Dis 129:767, 1984.

115. Kovacs EJ, Kelley J: Release of macrophage-derived growth factor during acute lung injury induced by bleomycin. J Leukoc Biol 37:1, 1985.

116. Hunninghake GW, Hemken C, Brady M, et al: Immune interferon is a growth factor for human lung fibroblasts. Am Rev Respir Dis 134:1025, 1986.

117. Bitterman PB, Rennard SI, Adelberg S, et al: Role of fibronectin as a growth factor for fibroblasts. J Cell Biol 97:1925, 1983.

118. Schmidt JA, Oliver CN, Lepe-Zuniga JL, et al: Silica-stimulated monocytes release fibroblast proliferation factors identical to interleukin. Int J Clin Invest 73:1462, 1984.

119. Kampschmidt RF, Worthington ML III, Mesecher MI: Release of interleukin-1 (IL-1) and IL-1-like factors from rabbit macrophages with silica. J Leukoc Biol 39:123, 1986.

120. Mohr C, Davis GS, Graebner C, et al: Reduced release of leukotrienes B₄ and C₄ from alveolar macrophages of rats with silicosis. Am J Respir Cell Mol Biol 7:542, 1992.

121. Gritter HL, Adamson IYR, King GM: Modulation of fibroblast activity by normal and silica-exposed alveolar macrophages. J Pathol 148:263, 1986.

122. Huaux F, Jouahed J, Hudspith B, et al: Role of interleukin-10 in the lung response to silica in mice. Am J Respir Cell Mol Biol 18:51, 1998.

123. Wallaert B, Lassalle P, Fortin F, et al: Superoxide anion generation by alveolar inflammatory cells in simple pneumoconiosis and in PMF of nonsmoking coal workers. Am Rev Respir Dis 141:129, 1990.

124. Brown GM, Donaldson K: Degradation of connective tissue components by lung derived leucocytes in vitro: Role of proteases and oxidants. Thorax 43:132, 1988.

125. Davis GS: Pathogenesis of silicosis: Current concepts and hypotheses. Lung 164:139, 1986.

126. Struhar D, Harbeck RJ, Mason RJ: Lymphocyte populations in lung tissue, bronchoalveolar lavage fluid, and peripheral blood in rats at various times during the development of silicosis. Am Rev Respir Dis 139:28, 1989.

127. Hubbard AK: Role for T lymphocytes in silica-induced pulmonary inflammation. Lab Invest 61:46, 1989.

128. Rom WN, Turner WG, Kanner RE, et al: Antinuclear antibodies in Utah coal miners. Chest 3:515, 1983.

129. Jones RN, Turner-Warwick M, Ziskind M, et al: High prevalance of antinuclear antibodies in sandblasters' silicosis. Am Rev Respir Dis 113:393, 1976.

130. Doll NJ, Stankus RP, Hughes J, et al: Immune complexes and autoantibodies in silicosis. J Allergy Clin Immunol 68:281, 1981.

131. Vigliani EC, Pernis B: Immunological factors in the pathogenesis of the hyaline tissue of silicosis. Br J Ind Med 15:8, 1958.

132. Giles RD, Sturgill BC, Suratt PM, et al: Massive proteinuria and acute renal failure in a patient with acute silicoproteinosis. Am J Med 64:336, 1978.

133. Banks DE, Milutinovic J, Desnick RJ, et al: Silicon nephropathy mimicking Fabry's disease. Am J Nephrol 3:279, 1983.

134. Sluis-Cremer GK, Hessel PA, Hnizdo E, et al: Relationship between silicosis and rheumatoid arthritis. Thorax 41:596, 1986.

135. Neyer U, Woss E, Neuweiler J: Wegener's granulomatosis associated with silicosis. Nephrol Dial Transplant 9:559, 1994.

136. McHigh NJ, Whyte J, Harvey G, et al: Anti-topoisomerase I antibodies in silica-associated systemic sclerosis: A model for autoimmunity. Arthritis Rheum 37:1198, 1994.

137. Dionisio M, Cozzoline G, Matarazzo M, et al: A case of silicosis associated with Crohn's disease: Diagnostic and pathogenetic considerations. Panminerva Med 35:173, 1993.

138. Puisieux F, Hachulla E, Brouillard M, et al: Silicosis and primary Gougerot-Sjogren syndrome. Rev Med Int 15:575, 1994.

139. Slavin RE, Swedo JL, Brandes D, et al: Extrapulmonary silicosis: A clinical, morphologic, and ultrastructural study. Hum Pathol 16:393, 1985.

140. Boujemaa W, Lauwerys R, Bernard A: Early indicators of renal dysfunction in silicotic workers. Scand J Work Environ Health 20:180, 1994.

141. Calhoun WJ, Christman JW, Ershler WB, et al: Raised immunoglobulin concentrations in bronchoalveolar lavage fluid in healthy granite workers. Thorax 41:266, 1986.

142. Burrell R, Esber HJ, Hagadorn JE, et al: Specificity of lung reactive antibodies in human serum. Am Rev Respir Dis 94:743, 1966.

143. Lewis DM, Burrell R: Induction of fibrogenesis by lung antibody-treated macrophages. Br J Ind Med 33:35, 1976.

144. Nagaoka T, Tabata M, Kobayashi K, et al: Studies on production of anticollagen antibodies in silicosis. Environ Res 60:12, 1993.

145. Gusev VA, Danilovskaja YV, Vatolkina OY, et al: Effect of quartz and alumina

dust on generation of superoxide radicals and hydrogen peroxide by alveolar macrophages, granulocytes and monocytes. Br J Ind Med 50:732, 1993.

146. Suzuki N, Horiuchi T, Ohta K, et al: Mast cells are essential for the full development of silica-induced pulmonary inflammation: A study with mast cell-deficient mice. Am J Respir Cell Mol Biol 9:475, 1993.

147. Scharfman A, Hayem A, Davril M, et al: Special neutrophil elastase inhibitory activity in BAL fluid from patients with silicosis and asbestosis. Eur Respir J 2:751, 1989.

148. Leibowitz MC, Goldstein B: Some investigations into the nature and cause of massive fibrosis (MF) in the lungs of South African gold, coal, and asbestos mine workers. Am J Ind Med 12:129, 1987.

149. Ng TP, Chan SL: Factors associated with massive fibrosis in silicosis. Thorax 46:229, 1991.

150. Chiappino G, Vigliani EC: Role of infective, immunological and chronic irritative factors in the development of silicosis. Br J Ind Med 39:253, 1982.

151. Koskinen H, Tiilikainen A, Nordman H: Increased prevalence of HLA-Aw19 and of phenogroup Aw19,B18 in advanced silicosis. Chest 83:848, 1983.

152. Kreiss K, Danilovs JA, Newman LS: Histocompatibility antigens in a population based silicosis series. Br J Ind Med 46:364, 1989.

153. Nery LE, Florencio RT, Sandoval PRM, et al: Additive effects of exposure to silica dust and smoking on pulmonary epithelial permeability: A radioaerosol study with technetium-99m labelled DTPA. Thorax 48:264, 1993.

154. Heppleston AG, Wright MA, Stewart JA: Experimental alveolar lipo-proteinosis following the inhalation of silica. J Pathol 101:293, 1970.

155. Buechner HA, Ansari A: Acute silicoproteinosis: A new pathologic variant of acute silicosis in sandblasters, characterized by histologic features resembling alveolar proteinosis. Dis Chest 55:274, 1969.

156. Hoffman EO, Lamberty J, Pizzolato P, et al: The ultrastructure of acute silicosis. Arch Pathol 96:104, 1973.

157. Bowden DH, Adamson IYR: The role of cell injury and the continuing inflammatory response in the generation of silicotic pulmonary fibrosis. J Pathol 144:149, 1984.

158. Miller BE, Dethloff LA, Gladen BC, et al: Progression of type II cell hypertrophy and hyperplasia during silica-induced pulmonary inflammation. Lab Invest 57:546, 1987.

159. Suwabe A, Panos RJ, Voelker DR: Alveolar type II cells isolated after silica-induced lung injury in rats have increased surfactant protein A (SP-A) receptor activity. Am J Respir Cell Mol Biol 4:264, 1991.

160. Kawada H, Horiuchi T, Shannon JM, et al: Alveolar type II cells, surfactant protein A (SP-A), and the phospholipid components of surfactant in acute silicosis in the rat. Am Rev Respir Dis 140:460, 1989.

161. Miller BE, Hook GER: Isolation and characterization of hypertrophic Type II cells from the lungs of silica-treated rats. Lab Invest 58:565, 1988.

162. Vallyathan V, Shi X, Dalal NS, et al: Generation of free radicals from freshly fractured silica dust: Potential role in acute silica-induced lung injury. Am Rev Respir Dis 138:1213, 1988.

163. Vallyathan V, Castranova D, Pack D, et al: Freshly fractured quartz inhalation leads to enhanced lung injury and inflammation. Am J Respir Crit Care Med 152:1003, 1995.

164. Emerson RJ, Davis GS: Effect of alveolar lining material-coated silica on rat alveolar macrophages. Environ Health Perspect 51:81, 1983.

165. Allison AC, Hart PD: Potentiation by silica of the growth of *Mycobacterium tuberculosis* in macrophage cultures. Br J Exp Pathol 49:465, 1968.

166. Craighead JE, Kleinerman J, Abraham JL, et al: Diseases associated with exposure to silica and nonfibrous silicate minerals. Arch Pathol Lab Med 112:673, 1988.

167. del Campo JM, Hitado J, Gea G, et al: Anaerobes: A new aetiology in cavitary pneumoconiosis. Br J Ind Med 39:392, 1982.

167a. Kampalath BN, McMahon JT, Cohen A, et al: Obliterative central bronchitis due to mineral dust in patients with pneumoconiosis. Arch Pathol Lab Med 122:56, 1998.

168. Schuyler MR, Gaumer HR, Stankus RP, et al: Bronchoalveolar lavage in silicosis: Evidence of type II cell hyperplasia. Lung 157:95, 1980.

169. Curran RC: Observations on the formation of collagen in quartz lesions. J Pathol Bacteriol 66:271, 1953.

170. Craighead JE, Vallyathan MV: Cryptic pulmonary lesions in workers occupationally exposed to dust containing silica. JAMA 244:1939, 1980.

171. Tosi P, Franzinelli A, Miracco C, et al: Silicotic lymph node lesions in nonoccupationally exposed lung carcinoma patients. Eur J Respir Dis 68:362, 1986.

171a. Eide J, Gylseth B, Skaug V: Silicotic lesions of the bone marrow: Histopathology and microanalysis. Histopathology 8:693, 1984.

172. Bergin CJ, Müller NL, Vedall S, et al: CT in silicosis: Correlation with plain films and pulmonary function tests. Am J Roentgenol 146:477, 1986.

173. Theron CP, Walters LG, Webster I: The international classification of radiographs of the pneumoconioses: Based on the findings in 100 deceased white South African gold miners: An evaluation. Med Proc (Johannesburg) 10:352, 1964.

174. Greening RR, Heslep JH: The roentgenology of silicosis. Semin Roentgenol 2:265, 1967.

175. Pendergrass EP: Caldwell Lecture 1957—Silicosis and a few of the other pneumoconioses: Observations on certain aspects of the problem, with emphasis on the role of the radiologist. Am J Roentgenol 80:1, 1958.

176. Jacobson G, Felson B, Pendergrass EP, et al: Eggshell calcifications in coal and metal workers. Semin Roentgenol 2:276, 1967.

177. Bellini F, Ghislandi E: "Egg-shell" calcifications at extrahilar sites in a silico-tuberculotic patient. Med Lav 51:600, 1960.

178. Jacobs LG, Gerstl B, Hollander AG, et al: Intra-abdominal egg-shell calcifications due to silicosis. Radiology 67:527, 1956.

178a. Gross BH, Schneider HJ, Proto AV: Eggshell calcification of lymph nodes: An update. Am J Roentgenol 135:1265, 1980.

179. Tschopp JM, Rossini MJ, Richon CA, et al: Retroperitoneal silicosis mimicking pancreatic carcinoma in an Alpine miner with chronic lung silicosis. Thorax 47:480, 1992.

180. Cahill BC, Harmon KR, Shumway SJ, et al: Tracheobronchial obstruction due to silicosis. Am Rev Respir Dis 145:719, 1992.

181. Nicod J-L, Gardiol D: Silicose et paralysie du diaphragme. [Silicosis and paralysis of the diaphragm.] Schweiz Med Wochenschr 94:1461, 1964.

182. Paterson JF: Silicosis in hardrock miners in Ontario: The problem and its prevention. Can Med Assoc J 84:594, 1961.

183. Michel RD, Morris JF: Acute silicosis. Arch Intern Med 113:850, 1964.

184. Dee PM, Suratt P, Winn W: The radiographic findings in acute silicosis. Radiology 126:359, 1978.

185. Buechner HA, Ansari A: Acute silicoproteinosis: A new pathologic variant of acute silicosis in sandblasters, characterized by histologic features resembling alveolar proteinosis. Dis Chest 55:274, 1969.

186. Sluis-Cremer GK, Hessel PA, Hnizdo E, et al: Relationship between silicosis and rheumatoid arthritis. Thorax 41:596, 1986.

187. Maclaren WM, Soutar CA: Progressive massive fibrosis and simple pneumoconiosis in ex-miners. Br J Ind Med 42:734, 1985.

188. Bégin R, Bergeron D, Samson R, et al: CT assessment of silicosis in exposed workers. Am J Roentgenol 148:509, 1987.

189. Bégin R, Ostiguy G, Fillion R, Colman N: Computed tomography scan in the early detection of silicosis. Am Rev Respir Dis 144:697, 1991.

190. Akira M, Higashihara T, Yokoyama K, et al: Radiographic type p pneumoconiosis: High-resolution CT. Radiology 171:117, 1989.

191. Grenier P, Chevret S, Beigelman C, et al: Chronic diffuse infiltrative lung disease: Determination of the diagnostic value of clinical data, chest radiography, and CT with Bayesian analysis. Radiology 191:383, 1994.

192. Mathieson JR, Mayo JR, Staples CA, Müller NL: Chronic diffuse infiltrative lung disease: Comparison of diagnostic accuracy of CT and chest radiography. Radiology 171:111, 1989.

193. Remy-Jardin M, Remy J, Farre I, Marquette CH: Computed tomographic evaluation of silicosis and coal worker's pneumoconiosis. Radiol Clin North Am 30:1155, 1992.

194. Kinsella M, Müller N, Vedal S, et al: Emphysema in silicosis. Am Rev Respir Dis 141:1497, 1990.

194a. Matsumoto S, Mori H, Miyake H, et al: MRI signal characteristics of progressive massive fibrosis in silicosis. Clin Radiol 53:510, 1998.

195. Nozaki S, Sawada Y: Progress of simple pulmonary silicosis in retired miners. Jpn J Clin Tuberc 18:154, 1959.

196. Koskinen H: Symptoms and clinical findings in patients with silicosis. Scand J Work Environ Health 11:101, 1985.

197. Munakata M, Homma Y, Matsuzaki M, et al: Rales in silicosis: A correlative study with physiological and radiological abnormalities. Respiration 48:140, 1985.

198. Murray J, Reid G, Kielkowski D, et al: Cor pulmonale and silicosis: A necropsy based case-control study. Br J Ind Med 50:544, 1993.

199. Oleru UG: Respiratory and nonrespiratory morbidity in a titanium oxide paint factory in Nigeria. Am J Ind Med 12:173, 1987.

200. Bailey WC, Brown M, Buechner HA, et al: Silico-mycobacterial disease in sandblasters. Am Rev Respir Dis 110:115, 1974.

201. Hughes JM, Jones RN, Gilson JC, et al: Determinants of progression in sandblasters' silicosis. Ann Occup Hyg 26:701, 1982.

202. Tukiainen P, Taskinen E, Korhola O, et al: TruCut needle biopsy in asbestosis and silicosis: Correlation of histological changes with radiographic changes and pulmonary function in 41 patients. Br J Ind Med 35:292, 1978.

203. Funahashi A, Schlueter DP, Pintar K, et al: Value of in situ elemental microanalysis in the histologic diagnosis of silicosis. Chest 85:506, 1984.

204. Nugent KM, Dodson RF, Idell S, et al: The utility of bronchoalveolar lavage and transbronchial lung biopsy combined with energy-dispersive x-ray analysis in the diagnosis of silicosis. Am Rev Respir Dis 140:1438, 1989.

205. Lusuardi M, Capelli A, Donner CF, et al: Semi-quantitative x-ray microanalysis of bronchoalveolar lavage samples from silica-exposed and nonexposed subjects. Eur Respir J 5:798, 1992.

206. Gronhagen-Riska C, Kurppa K, Fyhrquist F, et al: Angiotensin-converting enzyme and lysozyme in silicosis and asbestosis. Scand J Respir Dis 59:228, 1978.

207. Bucca C, Veglio F, Rolla G, et al: Serum angiotensin converting enzyme (ACE) in silicosis. Eur J Respir Dis 65:477, 1984.

208. Nordman H, Koskinen H, Froseth B: Increased activity of angiotensin-converting enzyme in progressive silicosis. Chest 86:203, 1984.

209. Serbescu A, Paunescu E: The importance of assessing angiotensin-converting activity on silicosis patients. Pneumoftiziologia 41:17, 1992.

210. Teculescu DR, Stanescu DC: Carbon monoxide transfer factor for the lung in silicosis. Scand J Respir Dis 51:150, 1970.

211. Renzetti AD Jr, Kobayashi T, Bigler A, et al: Regional ventilation and perfusion in silicosis and in the alveolar-capillary block syndrome. Am J Med 49:5, 1970.

212. Violante B, Brusasco V, Buccheri G: Exercise testing in radiologically-limited simple pulmonary silicosis. Chest 3:411, 1986.

213. Ng TP, Chan SL: Lung function in relation to silicosis and silica exposure in granite workers. Eur Respir J 5:986, 1992.

214. Cowie RL: The influence of silicosis on deteriorating lung function in gold miners. Chest 113:340, 1998.
215. Becklake MR: Pneumoconioses. *In* Fenn WO, Rahn H (eds): Handbook of Physiology, Section III, Vol 2. Baltimore, Waverly Press, 1965, pp 1601–1614.
216. Cowie RL, Mabena SK: Silicosis, chronic airflow limitation and chronic bronchitis in South African gold miners. Am Rev Respir Dis 143:80, 1991.
217. Wang X, Yano E, Nonaka K, et al: Respiratory impairments due to dust exposure: A comparative study among workers exposed to silica, asbestos, and coalmine dust. Am J Ind Med 31:495, 1997.
218. Bégin R, Ostiguy G, Cantin A, et al: Lung function in silica-exposed workers: A relationship to disease severity assessed by CT scan. Chest 94:539, 1988.
219. Bates DV, Macklem PT, Christie RV: Respiratory Function in Disease: An Introduction to the Integrated Study of the Lung. 2nd ed. Philadelphia, WB Saunders, 1971.
220. Bégin R, Ostiguy G, Cantin A, Bergeron D: Lung function in silica-exposed workers: A relationship to disease severity assessed by CT scan. Chest 94:539, 1988.
221. Hnizdo E: Combined effects of silica dust and tobacco smoking on mortality from chronic obstructive lung disease in gold miners. Br J Ind Med 47:656, 1990.
222. Wright JL, Harrison N, Wiggs B, et al: Quartz but not iron oxide causes airflow obstruction, emphysema, and small airways lesions in the rat. Am Rev Respir Dis 138:129, 1988.
223. Soutar C, Campbell S, Gurr D, et al: Important deficits of lung function in three modern colliery populations. Am Rev Respir Dis 147:797, 1993.
224. Musk AW, Rouse IL, Rivera B,et al: Respiratory disease in nonsmoking Western Australian goldminers. Br J Ind Med 49:750, 1992.
225. Oxman AD, Muir DC, Shannon HS, et al: Occupational dust exposure and chronic obstructive pulmonary disease: A systematic overview of the evidence. Am Rev Respir Dis 148:38, 1993.
226. Graham WG, Weaver S, Ashikaga T, et al: Longitudinal pulmonary function losses in Vermont granite workers—a re-evaluation. Chest 106:125, 1994.
227. Hnizdo E, Sluis-Cremer GK, Abramowitz JA: Emphysema type in relations to silica dust exposure in South African gold miners. Am Rev Respir Dis 143:1241, 1991.
228. Hnizdo E, Sluis-Cremer GK, Baskind E, et al: Emphysema and airway obstruction in nonsmoking South African gold miners with long exposure to silica dust. Occup Environ Med 51:557, 1994.
229. Chia KS, Ng TP, Jeyaratnam J: Small airways function of silica-exposed workers. Am J Ind Med 22:155, 1992.
230. Choudat D, Frisch C, Barrat G, et al: Occupational exposure to amorphous silica dust and pulmonary function. Br J Ind Med 47:763, 1990.
231. Ng TP, Phoon WH, Lee HS, et al: An epidemiological survey of respiratory morbidity among granite quarry workers in Singapore: Chronic bronchitis and lung function impairment. Ann Acad Med Singapore 21:312, 1992.
232. Kreiss K, Greenberg LM, Kogut SJH, et al: Hard-rock mining exposures affect smokers and nonsmokers differently. Am Rev Respir Dis 139:1487, 1989.
233. Bégin R, Filion R, Ostiguy G: Emphysema in silica- and asbestos-exposed workers seeking compensation. Chest 108:647, 1995.
234. Infante-Rivard C, Armstrong B, Ernst P, et al: Descriptive study of prognostic factors influencing survival of compensated silicotic patients. Am Rev Respir Dis 144:1070, 1991.
235. Ng TP, Chan SL, Lee J: Predictors of mortality in silicosis. Respir Med 86:115, 1992.
236. International Agency for Research on Cancer: Silica, some silicates, coal dust and para-aramid fibrils. IARC Monogr Eval Carcinog Risks Hum vol 68, 1996.
237. Finkelstein M, Liss GM, Krammer F, et al: Mortality among workers receiving compensation awards for silicosis in Ontario 1940–85. Br J Ind Med 44:588, 1987.
238. Carta P, Cocco PL, Casula D: Mortality from lung cancer among Sardinian patients with silicosis. Br J Ind Med 48:122, 1991.
239. Amandus HE, Castellan RM, Shy C, et al: Reevaluation of silicosis and lung cancer in North Carolina dusty trades workers. Am J Ind Med 22:147, 1992.
240. Amandus H, Costello J: Silicosis and lung cancer in U.S. metal miners. Arch Environ Health 46:82, 1991.
241. Chiyotani K, Saito K, Okubo T, et al: Lung cancer risk among pneumoconiosis patients in Japan, with special reference to silicotics. IARC Sci Publ 97:95, 1990.
242. Infante-Rivard C, Armstrong B, Petitclerc M, et al: Lung cancer mortality and silicosis in Quebec, 1938–85. Lancet 2:1504, 1989.
243. Hnizdo E, Murray J, Klempman S: Lung cancer in relation to exposure to silica dust, silicosis and uranium production in South African gold miners. Thorax 52:271, 1997.
244. Neuberger M, Kundi M: Occupational dust exposure and cancer mortality—results of a prospective cohort study. IARC Sci Publ 97:65, 1990.
245. Siemiatycki J, Gerin M, Dewar R, et al: Silica and cancer associations from a multicancer occupational exposure case-referent study. IARC Sci Publ 97:29, 1990.
246. Checkoway H, Heyer NJ, Demers PA, et al: Mortality among workers in the diatomaceous earth industry. Br J Ind Med 50:586, 1993.
247. Steenland K, Brown D: Mortality study of gold miners exposed to silica and nonasbestiform amphibole minerals: An update with 14 more years of follow-up. Am J Ind Med 27:217, 1995.
248. Smith AH, Lopipero PA, Barroga VR: Meta-analysis of studies of lung cancer among silicotics. Epidemiology 6:617, 1995.

249. Steenland K, Loomis D, Shy C, et al: Review of occupational lung carcinogens. Am J Ind Med 29:474, 1996.
250. Lynge E, Kurppa K, Kristofersen L, et al: Occupational groups potentially exposed to silica dust: A comparative analysis of cancer mortality and incidence based on the Nordic occupational mortality and cancer incidence registers. IARC Sci Publ 97:7, 1990.
251. Mehnert WH, Staneczek W, Mohner M, et al: A mortality study of a cohort of slate quarry workers in the German Democratic Republic. IARC Sci Publ 97:55, 1990.
252. Guenel P, Hojberg G, Lynge E: Cancer incidence among Danish stone workers. Scand J Work Environ Health 15:265, 1989.
253. Forastiere F, Lagorio S, Michelozzi P, et al: Silica, silicosis and lung cancer among ceramic workers: A case-referent study. Am J Ind Med 10:363, 1986.
254. Axelson O: Editorial—Confounding from smoking in occupational epidemiology. Br J Ind Med 46:505, 1989.
255. Wang Z, Dong D, Liang X, et al: Cancer mortality among silicotics in China's metallurgical industry. Int J Epidemiol 25:913, 1996.
256. Mosquera JA, Rodrigo L, Gonzalvez F: The evolution of pulmonary tuberculosis in coal miners in Asturias, northern Spain. Eur J Epidemiol 10:291, 1994.
257. Becklake MR: The mineral dust diseases. Tuber Lung Dis 73:13, 1992.
258. Cowie RL: The epidemiology of tuberculosis in gold miners with silicosis. Am J Respir Crit Care Med 150:1460, 1994.
259. Brink GC, Grzybowski S, Lane GB: Silicotuberculosis. Can Med Assoc J 82:959, 1960.
260. Cheng SJ, Ma Y, Pan YX: A study on the diagnosis of pulmonary tuberculosis and silicotuberculosis by PCR. Chung Hua Chieh Ho Ho Hu Hsi Tsa Chih 16:221, 1993.
261. Fisher ER, Watkins G, Lam NV, et al: Objective pathological diagnosis of coal workers' pneumoconiosis. JAMA 245:1829, 1981.
262. Lister WB: Carbon pneumoconiosis in a synthetic graphite worker. Br J Ind Med 18:114, 1961.
263. Miller AA, Ramsden F: Carbon pneumoconiosis. Br J Ind Med 18:103, 1961.
264. Pendergrass EP, Vorwald AJ, Mishkin MM, et al: Observations on workers in the graphite industry: Part I. Med Radiogr Photogr 43:70, 1967.
265. Pendergrass EP, Vorwald AJ, Mishkin MM, et al: Observations on workers in the graphite industry: Part II. Med Radiogr Photogr 44:2, 1968.
266. Gaensler EA, Cadigan JB, Sasahara AA, et al: Graphite pneumoconiosis of electrotypers. Am J Med 41:864, 1966.
267. Miller AA, Ramsden F: Carbon pneumoconiosis. Br J Ind Med 18:103, 1961.
268. Watson AJ, Black J, Doig AT, et al: Pneumoconiosis in carbon electrode makers. Br J Ind Med 16:274, 1959.
269. Golden EB, Varnock ML, Hulett LD Jr, et al: Fly ash lung: A new pneumoconiosis? Am Rev Respir Dis 125:108, 1982.
270. Shrivastava DK, Kapre SS, Cho K, et al: Acute lung disease after exposure to flay ash. Chest 106:309, 1994.
271. Green FHY, Laqueur WA: Coal workers' pneumoconiosis. Pathol Ann 15:333, 1980.
272. Naeye RL, Mahon JK, Dellinger WS: Rank of coal and coal workers' pneumoconiosis. Am Rev Respir Dis 103:350, 1971.
273. Seaton A, Dodgson J, Dick JA, et al: Quartz and pneumoconiosis in coalminers. Lancet 2:1272, 1981.
274. Finkelstein MM: Radiographic silicosis and lung cancer risk among workers in Ontario. Am J Ind Med 34:244, 1998.
274a. de Klerk NH, Musk AW: Silica, compensated silicosis, and lung cancer in Western Australian goldminers. Occup Environ Med 55:243, 1998.
275. Banks DE, Bauer MA, Castellan RM, et al: Silicosis in surface coalmine drillers. Thorax 38:275, 1983.
276. Attfield MD, Castellan RM: Epidemiological data on US coal miners' pneumoconiosis. Am J Public Health 82:964, 1992.
277. Arrfield MD, Morring K: An investigation into the relationship between coal workers' pneumoconiosis and dust exposure in U.S. coal miners. Am Ind Hyg Assoc J 53:486, 1992.
278. Attfield MD, Seixas NS: Prevalence of pneumoconiosis and its relationship to dust exposure in a cohort of U.S. bituminous coal miners and ex-miners. Am J Ind Med 27:137, 1995.
279. Attfield MD: British data on coal miners' pneumoconiosis and relevance to US conditions. Am J Public Health 82:978, 1992.
280. Morgan WKC: Respiratory disease in coal miners. JAMA 231:1347, 1975.
281. Penman RW: Conference on pneumoconiosis: A summary of the conclusions from an international conference on coal workers' pneumoconiosis. Am Rev Respir Dis 102:243, 1970.
282. Morgan WKC, Burgess DB, Jacobsen G, et al: The prevalence of coal workers' pneumoconiosis in U.S. coal miners. Arch Environ Health 27:221, 1973.
283. Lapp NL, Parker JE: Coal workers' pneumoconiosis. Clin Chest Med 13:243, 1992.
284. Bonnell JA, Schilling CJ, Massey PMO: Clinical and experimental studies of the effects of pulverized fuel ash: A review. Ann Occup Hyg 23:159, 1980.
285. Morgan WKC, Seaton A: Occupational Lung Disease. Philadelphia, WB Saunders, 1975, p 241.
286. Crosbie WA: The respiratory health of carbon black workers. Arch Environ Health 41:346, 1986.
287. Gardiner K, Trethowan NW, Harrington JM, et al: Respiratory health effects of carbon black: A survey of European carbon black workers. Br J Ind Med 50:1082, 1993.
288. Jones HD, Jones TR, Lyle WH: Carbon fibre: Results of a survey of process

workers and their environment in a factory producing continuous filament. Ann Occup Hyg 26:861, 1982.

289. Uragoda CG: Clinical and radiographic study of activated carbon workers. Thorax 44:303, 1989.

290. Arrfield MD, Morring K: The derivation of estimated dust exposures for U.S coal miners working before 1970. Am Ind Hyg Assoc J 53:248, 1992.

291. Hurley JF, Alexander WP, Hazledine DJ, et al: Exposure to respirable coalmine dust and incidence of PMF. Br J Ind Med 444:661, 1987.

292. Douglas AN, Robertson A, Chapman JS, et al: Dust exposure, dust recovered from the lung, and associated pathology in a group of British coalminers. Br J Ind Med 43:795, 1986.

293. King EJ, Maguire BA, Nagelschmidt G: Further studies of the dust in lungs of coal-miners. Br J Ind Med 13:9, 1956.

294. Love RG, Miller BG: Longitudinal study of lung function in coal-miners. Thorax 37:193, 1982.

295. Hurley JF, Soutar CA: Can exposure to coalmine dust cause a severe impairment of lung function? Br J Ind Med 43:150, 1986.

296. Soutar CA, Collins HP: Classification of PMF of coalminers by type of radiographic appearance. Br J Ind Med 41:334, 1984.

297. Liu L: Logistic regression analysis of risk factors influencing the occurrence of category III pneumoconiosis in the coal mine. Chung Hua Liu Hsing Ping Hsueh Tsa Chih 12:277, 1991.

298. Maclaren WM, Hurley JF, Collins HPR, et al: Factors associated with the development of PMF in British coalminers: A case-control study. Br J Ind Med 46:597, 1989.

299. Gautrin D, Auburtin G, Alluin F, et al: Recognition and progression of coal workers' pneumoconiosis in the collieries of northern France. Exp Lung Res 20:395, 1994.

300. Seal RME, Cockcroft A, Kung I, et al: Central lymph node changes and PMF in coalworkers. Thorax 41:531, 1986.

301. Davis JMG, Chapman J, Collings P, et al: Variations in the histological patterns of the lesions of coal workers' pneumoconiosis in Britain and their relationship to lung dust content. Am Rev Respir Dis 128:118, 1983.

302. Seaton A: Coalworkers pneumoconiosis in Britain today and tomorrow. BMJ 284:1507, 1982.

303. Parkes WR: Pneumoconiosis associated with coal and other carbonaceous materials. In Parkes WR (ed): Occupational Lung Disorders. 3rd ed. Oxford, Butterworth-Heinemann, 1994.

304. Ghio AJ, Quigley DR: Complexation of iron by humic-like substances in lung tissue: Role in coal workers' pneumoconiosis. Am J Physiol 267:L173, 1994.

305. Evelop CT, Bos RP, Borm PJ: Decreased glutathione content and glutathione S-transferase activity in red blood cells of coal miners with early stages of pneumoconiosis. Br J Ind Med 50:633, 1993.

306. Wallaert B, Lassalle P, Fortin F, et al: Superoxide anion generation by alveolar inflammatory cells in simple pneumoconiosis and in PMF of nonsmoking coal workers. Am Rev Respir Dis 141:129, 1990.

307. Vanhée D, Gosset P, Marquette CH, et al: Secretion and mRNA expression of TNFa and IL-6 in the lungs of pneumoconiosis patients. Am J Respir Crit Care Med 152:298, 1995.

308. Vanhee D, Gosset P, Wallaert B, et al: Mechanisms of fibrosis in coal worker's pneumoconiosis. Am J Respir Crit Care Med 150:1049, 1994.

309. Lesur OJ, Mancine NM, Humbert JC, et al: Interleukin-6, interferon-gamma and phospholipid levels in the alveolar lining fluid of human lungs. Chest 106:407, 1994.

310. Borm PJA, Palmen N, Engelen JJM, et al: Spontaneous and stimulated release of tumour necrosis factor-alpha (TNF) from blood monocytes of miners with coal workers pneumoconiosis. Am Rev Respir Dis 138:1589, 1988.

311. Porcher JM, Oberson D, Viseux N, et al: Evaluation of tumour necrosis factor-alpha (TNF) as an exposure or risk marker in three French coal mining regions. Exp Lung Res 20:433, 1994.

312. Robertson MD, Boyd JE, Collins HP, et al: Serum immunoglobulin levels and humoral immune competence in coalworkers. Am J Ind Med 6:387, 1984.

313. Rom WN, Turner WG, Kanner RE, et al: Antinuclear antibodies in Utah coal miners. Chest 83:515, 1983.

314. Soutar CA, Turner-Warwick M, Parkes WR: Circulating antinuclear antibody and rheumatoid factor in coal pneumoconiosis. BMJ 3:145, 1974.

315. Wagner JC, McCormick JN: Immunological investigations of coal workers' disease. J R Coll Physicians Lond 2:49, 1967.

316. Caplan A, Payne RB, Withey JL: A broader concept of Caplan's syndrome related to rheumatoid factors. Thorax 17:205, 1962.

317. Lippman M, Eckert HL, Hahon N, et al: Circulating antinuclear and rheumatoid factors in coal miners: A prevalence study in Pennsylvania and West Virginia. Ann Intern Med 79:807, 1973.

318. Pearson DJ, Mentnech MS, Elliot JA, et al: Serologic changes in pneumoconiosis and PMF of coal workers. Am Rev Respir Dis 124:696, 1981.

319. Robertson MD, Boyd JE, Fernie JM, et al: Some immunological studies on coalworkers with and without pneumoconiosis. Am J Ind Med 4:467, 1983.

320. Caplan A: Certain unusual radiological appearances in the chest of coal-miners suffering from rheumatoid arthritis. Thorax 8:29, 1953.

321. Yeh Y, Lai Y: Influence of rheumatoid factor in coalminers' pneumoconiosis in the Fujian Shaowu colliery, South China. Br J Ind Med 47:143, 1990.

322. Burrell R: Immunological aspects of coal workers' pneumoconiosis. Ann N Y Acad Sci 200:94, 1972.

323. Burrell R, Flaherty DK, Schreiber JK: Immunological studies of experimental coal workers' pneumoconiosis. Presented at the Fourth International Conference on Inhaled Particles, Edinburgh, September 1975.

324. Heise ER, Mentnech MS, Olenchock SA, et al: HLA-A1 and coalworkers' pneumoconiosis. Am Rev Respir Dis 119:903, 1979.

325. Rasche B, Reisner MTR, Islam MS, et al: Individual factors in the development of coal miners' pneumoconiosis. Ann Occup Hyg 26:713, 1982.

326. Soutar CA, Coutts I, Parkes WR, et al: Histocompatibility antigens in coal miners with pneumoconiosis. Br J Ind Med 40:34, 1983.

327. Rihs HP, Lips P, May-Taube K, et al: Immunogenetic studies on HLA-DR in German coal miners with and without coal worker's pneumoconiosis. Lung 172:347, 1994.

328. Heppleston AG: The essential lesion of pneumokoniosis in Welsh coal workers. J Pathol Bacteriol 59:453, 1947.

329. Kleinerman J, Green F, Harley RA, et al: Pathology standards for coal workers' pneumoconiosis. Arch Pathol Lab Med 103:375, 1979.

330. Morgan WKC, Lapp NL: Respiratory disease in coal miners. Am Rev Respir Dis 113:531, 1976.

331. Pelstring RJ, Kim CK, Lower EE, et al: Marrow granulomas in coal workers' pneumoconiosis: A histological study with elemental analysis. Am J Clin Pathol 89:553, 1988.

332. Gough J, Heppleston AG: The pathology of the pneumoconioses. In King EJ, Fletcher CM (eds): Industrial Pulmonary Diseases: A Symposium Held at the Postgraduate Medical School of London, 18–20 September 1957 and 25–27 March 1958. London, J & A Churchill, 1960, pp 23–26.

333. Lyons JP, Campbell H: Relation between PMF, emphysema, and pulmonary dysfunction in coalworkers' pneumoconiosis. Br J Ind Med 38:125, 1981.

334. Goodwin RA, Des Prez RM: Apical localization of pulmonary tuberculosis, chronic pulmonary histoplasmosis, and PMF of the lung. Chest 83:801, 1983.

335. Prignot J, Van de Velde R: La cavitation aseptique des pseudo-tumeurs dans l'anthraco-silicose. Etude clinique et radiologique. [Aseptic cavitation of pseudotumors in anthracosilicosis: Clinical and radiological study.] J Fr Med Chir Thorac 12:623, 1958.

336. Theodos PA, Cathcart RT, Fraimow W: Ischemic necrosis in anthracosilicosis. Arch Environ Health 2:609, 1961.

337. Seaton A, Lapp NL, Chang CEJ: Lung perfusion scanning in coal workers' pneumoconiosis. Am Rev Respir Dis 103:338, 1971.

338. Gross P, Detreville RTP: The lung as an embattled domain against inanimate pollutants: A precis of mechanisms. Am Rev Respir Dis 106:684, 1972.

339. Wagner JC, Wusteman FS, Edwards JH, et al: The composition of massive lesions in coal miners. Thorax 30:382, 1975.

340. Wagner JC, Burns J, De Munday JM: Presence of fibronectin in pneumoconiotic lesions. Thorax 37:54, 1982.

341. Lapp NL, Seaton A, Kaplan KC, et al: Pulmonary hemodynamics in symptomatic coal miners. Am Rev Respir Dis 104:418, 1971.

342. Naeye RL, Laqueur WA: Chronic cor pulmonale: Its pathogenesis in Appalachian bituminous coal workers. Arch Pathol 90:487, 1970.

343. Fernie JM, Douglas AN, Lamb D, et al: Right ventricular hypertrophy in a group of coalworkers. Thorax 38:436, 1983.

344. Town JD: Pseudoasbestos bodies and asteroid giant cells in a patient with graphite pneumoconiosis. Can Med Assoc J 98:100, 1968.

345. Johnson FB: Identification of graphite in tissue sections. Arch Pathol Lab Med 104:491, 1980.

346. Cockcroft AE, Wagner JC, Seal EM, et al: Irregular opacities in coalworkers' pneumoconiosis: Correlation with pulmonary function and pathology. Ann Occup Hyg 26:767, 1982.

347. Musk AW, Cotes JE, Bevan C, et al: Relationship between type of simple coalworkers pneumoconiosis and lung function: A 9-year follow-up study of subjects with small rounded opacities. Br J Ind Med 38:313, 1981.

348. Cockcroft A, Lyons JP, Andersson N, et al: Prevalence and relation to underground exposure of radiological irregular opacities in South Wales coal workers with pneumoconiosis. Br J Ind Med 40:169, 1983.

349. Trapnell DH: Septal lines in pneumoconiosis. Br J Radiol 37:805, 1964.

350. Gough J, James WRL, Wentworth JE: A comparison of the radiological and pathological changes in coalworkers' pneumoconiosis. J Fac Radiol 1:28, 1949.

351. Williams JL, Moller GA: Solitary mass in the lungs of coal miners. Am J Roentgenol 117:765, 1973.

352. Young RC Jr, Rachel RE, Carr PG, Press HC: Patterns of coal workers' pneumoconiosis in Appalachian former coalminers. J Natl Med Assoc 84:41, 1992.

353. Shennan DH, Washington JS, Thomas DJ, et al: Factors predisposing to the development of PMF in coal miners. Br J Ind Med 38:321, 1981.

354. Davies D: Disability and coal workers' pneumoconiosis. BMJ 2:652, 1974.

355. Seaton A, Soutar CA, Melville AWT: Radiological changes in coalminers on leaving the industry. Br J Dis Chest 74:310, 1980.

356. Caplan A: Correlation of radiological category with lung pathology in coal workers' pneumoconiosis. Br J Ind Med 19:171, 1962.

357. Pendergrass EP: An evaluation of some of the radiologic patterns of small opacities in coal workers' pneumoconiosis. Am J Roentgenol 115:457, 1972.

358. Reger RB, Smith CA, Kibelstis JA, et al: The effect of film quality and other factors on the roentgenographic categorization of coal workers' pneumoconiosis. Am J Roentgenol 115:462, 1972.

359. Reger RB, Amandus HE, Morgan WKC: On the diagnosis of coal workers' pneumoconiosis: Anglo-American disharmony. Am Rev Respir Dis 108:1186, 1973.

360. Remy-Jardin M, Degreef JM, Beuscart R, et al: Coal worker's pneumoconiosis: CT assessment in exposed workers and correlation with radiographic findings. Radiology 177:363, 1990.

361. Gevenois PA, Pichot E, Dargent S, et al: Low grade coal worker's pneumoconiosis: Comparison of CT and chest radiography. Acta Radiol 35:351, 1994.

362. Remy-Jardin M, Beuscart R, Sault MC, et al: Subpleural micronodules in diffuse infiltrative lung diseases: Evaluation with thin-section CT scans. Radiology 177:133, 1990.

363. Rebstock-Bourgkard E, Chau N, Caillier I, et al: Respiratory symptoms of coal miners presenting radiological pulmonary abnormalities. Rev Epidemiol Sante Publique 42:533, 1994.

364. Ball J: The natural history and management of coal workers' pneumoconiosis. *In* King EJ, Fletcher CM (eds): Industrial Pulmonary Diseases: A Symposium held at the Postgraduate Medical School of London, 18–20 September 1957 and 25–27 March 1958. London, J & A Churchill, 1960, pp 241–254.

365. Cathcart RT, Theodos PA, Fraimow W: Anthracosilicosis. Selected aspects related to the evaluation of disability, cavitation, and the unusual x-ray. Arch Intern Med 106:368, 1960.

366. Mosquera JA: Massive melanoptysis: A serious unrecognized complication of coal worker's pneumoconiosis. Eur Respir J 1:766, 1988.

367. Pendergrass EP: The Pneumoconiosis Problem, with Emphasis on the Role of the Radiologist. Springfield, IL, Charles C Thomas, 1958, pp 16–17.

368. Sherani TM, Angelini GD, Passani SP, et al: Vocal cord paralysis associated with coalworkers' pneumoconiosis and PMF. Thorax 39:683, 1984.

369. James WRL: The relationship of tuberculosis to the development of massive pneumokoniosis in coal workers. Br J Tuberc 48:89, 1954.

370. Seaton A: Editorial: Coalmining, emphysema and compensation. Br J Ind Med 47:433, 1990.

371. Rom WN, Kanner RE, Renzetti AD Jr, et al: Respiratory disease in Utah coal miners. Am Rev Respir Dis 123:372, 1981.

372. Douglas AN, Lamb D, Ruckley VA: Bronchial gland dimensions in coalminers: Influence of smoking and dust exposure. Thorax 37:760, 1982.

373. Leigh J, Wiles AN, Glick M: Total population study of factors affecting chronic bronchitis prevalence in the coal mining industry of New South Wales, Australia. Br J Ind Med 43:263, 1986.

374. Marine WM, Gurr D, Jacobsen M: Clinically important respiratory effects of dust exposure and smoking in British coal miners. Am Rev Respir Dis 137:106, 1988.

375. Ryder R, Lyons JP, Campbell H, et al: Emphysema in coal workers' pneumoconiosis. BMJ 3:481, 1970.

376. Cockcroft A, Seal RME, Wagner JC, et al: Postmortem study of emphysema in coalworkers and noncoalworkers. Lancet 2:600, 1982.

377. Leigh J, Outhred KG, McKenzie HI, et al: Quantified pathology of emphysema, pneumoconiosis, and chronic bronchitis in coal workers. Br J Ind Med 40:258, 1983.

378. Rogan JM, Attfield MD, Jacobsen M, et al: Role of dust in the working environment in development of chronic bronchitis in British coal miners. Br J Ind Med 30:217, 1973.

379. Soutar CA, Hurley JF: Relationship between dust exposure and lung function in miners and ex-miners. Br J Ind Med 43:150, 1986.

380. Ruckley VA, Gauld SJ, Chapman JS, et al: Emphysema and dust exposure in a group of coal workers. Am Rev Respir Dis 129:528, 1984.

381. Leigh J, Driscoll TR, Cole BD, et al: Quantitative relation between emphysema and lung mineral content in coalworkers. Occup Environ Med 51:400, 1994.

382. Attfield MD, Hodous TK: Pulmonary function of U.S coal miners related to dust exposure estimates. Am Rev Respir Dis 145:605, 1992.

383. Seixas NS, Robins TG, Attfield MD, et al: Longitudinal and cross sectional analyses of exposure to coal mine dust and pulmonary function in new miners. Br J Ind Med 50:929, 1993.

384. Morgan WKC: Coal mining, emphysema, and compensation revisited. Br J Ind Med 50:1051, 1993.

385. Sussking H, Rom WN: Lung inflammation in coal miners assessed by uptake of ^{67}GA-citrate and clearance of inhaled ^{99m}Tc-labelled diethylenetriamine pentaacetate aerosol. Am Rev Respir Dis 146:47, 1992.

386. Rego GF, Achaerandio GO, Cuervo VG, et al: Presence of acute phase response in coal workers' pneumoconiosis. Br J Ind Med 48:193, 1991.

387. Schins RP, Borm PJ: Serum procollagen type III peptide in coal workers' pneumoconiosis: A five-year follow-up study. Exp Lung Res 20:445, 1994.

388. Gilson J, Hugh-Jones P: Lung function in coal workers' pneumoconiosis. Medical Research Council, Special Report 290, HMSO London, 1955.

389. Nemery B, Veriter C, Brasseur L, et al: Impairment of ventilatory function and pulmonary gas exchange in nonsmoking coalminers. Lancet 2:1427, 1987.

390. Kibelstis JA: Diffusing capacity in bituminous coal miners. Chest 63:501, 1973.

391. Seaton A, Lapp NL, Morgan WKC: The relationship of pulmonary impairment in simple coal workers' pneumoconiosis to type of radiologic capacity. Br J Ind Med 29:50, 1972.

392. Susskind H, Acevedo JC, Iwai J, et al: Heterogeneous ventilation and perfusion: A sensitive indicator of lung impairment in nonsmoking coalminers. Eur J Respir 1:232, 1988.

393. Legg SJ, Cotes JE, Bevan C: Lung mechanics in relation to radiographic category of coalworkers' simple pneumoconiosis. Br J Ind Med 40:28, 1983.

394. Rasmussen DL, Laquer WA, Futterman P, et al: Pulmonary impairment in Southern West Virginia coal miners. Am Rev Respir Dis 98:658, 1968.

395. Lyons JP, Clarke WG, Hall AM, et al: Transfer factor (diffusing capacity) for the lung in simple pneumoconiosis of coal workers. BMJ 4:772, 1967.

396. Rasmussen DL, Nelson CW: Respiratory function in Southern Appalachian coal miners. Am Rev Respir Dis 103:240, 1971.

397. Cockcroft A, Berry G, Cotes JE, et al: Shape of small opacities and lung function in coalworkers. Thorax 37:765, 1982.

398. Morgan WKC, Lapp NL: Respiratory disease in coal miners. Am Rev Respir Dis 113:531, 1976.

399. Musk AW, Cotes JE, Bevan C, et al: Relationship between type of simple coal workers' pneumoconiosis and lung function: A nine-year follow-up study of subjects with small rounded opacities. Br J Ind Med 38:313, 1981.

400. Lyons JP, Campbell H: Relation between PMF, emphysema, and pulmonary dysfunction in coal workers' pneumoconiosis. Br J Ind Med 38:125, 1981.

401. Constantinidis K, Musk AW, Jenkins JP, et al: Pulmonary function in coal workers with Caplan's syndrome and nonrheumatoid complicated pneumoconiosis. Thorax 33:764, 1978.

402. Cochrane AL, Moore F, Moncrieff CB: Are coalminers, with low "risk factors" for ischaemic heart disease at greater risk of developing PMF? Br J Ind Med 39:265, 1982.

403. Davies GM: A mortality study of coke oven workers in two South Wales integrated steelworks. Br J Ind Med 34:291, 1977.

404. Miller BG, Jacobson M: Dust exposure, pneumoconiosis and mortality of coalminers. Br J Ind Med 42:723, 1985.

405. Meijers JM, Swaen GM, Slangen JJ, et al: Long-term mortality in miners with coal workers' pneumoconiosis in the Netherlands: A pilot study. Am J Ind Med 19:43, 1991.

406. Sadler RL, Roy TJ: Smoking and mortality from coalworkers' pneumoconiosis. Br J Ind Med 47:141, 1990.

407. Cochrane AL, Moore F: A 20-year follow-up of men aged 55–64 including coal-miners and foundry workers in Staveley, Derbyshire. Br J Ind Med 37:226, 1980.

408. Morgan WKC, Lapp NL, Seaton D: Respiratory disability in coal miners. JAMA 243:2401, 1980.

409. Bégin R, Dufresne A, Plante F, et al: Asbestos related disorders. Can Respir J 1:167, 1994.

410. Sluis-Cremer GK, Liddell FDK, Logan WPD, et al: The mortality of amphibole miners in South Africa, 1946–80. Br J Ind Med 49:566, 1992.

411. Case BW: Health effects of tremolite now and in the future. Ann N Y Acad Sci 643:491, 1991.

412. Weill H, Abraham JL, Balmes JR, et al: Health effects of tremolite. Am Rev Respir Dis 142:1453, 1990.

413. Churg A, Wright JL, Vedal S: Fiber burden and patterns of asbestos-related disease in chrysotile miners and millers. Am Rev Respir Dis 148:25, 1993.

414. Bourgkard E, Bernadac P, Chau N, et al: Can the evolution to pneumoconiosis be suspected in coal miners? Am J Respir Crit Care Med 158:504, 1998.

415. Leading article: Asbestosis. BMJ 3:62, 1967.

416. Selikoff IJ: Household risks with inorganic fibers. Bull N Y Acad Med 57:947, 1981.

417. Henneberger PK, Stanbury MJ: Patterns of asbestosis in New Jersey. Am J Ind Med 21:689, 1992.

418. Oksa P, Koskinen H, Rinne JP, et al: Parenchymal and pleural fibrosis in construction workers. Am J Ind Med 21:561, 1992.

419. Cullen MR, Lopez-Carrillo L, Alli B, et al: Chrysotile asbestos and health in Zimbabwe: II. Health status survey of active miners and millers. Am J Ind Med 19:171, 1991.

420. Cullen MR, Baloyi RS: Chrysotile asbestos and health in Zimbabwe: I. Analysis of miners and millers compensated for asbestos-related diseases since independence. Am J Ind Med 19:161, 1991.

421. Talcott JA, Thurber WA, Kantor AF, et al: Asbestos-associated disease in a cohort of cigarette-filter workers. N Engl J Med 321:1220, 1989.

422. Rogan WJ, Gladen BC, Ragan ND, et al: U.S. prevalence of occupational pleural thickening: A look at chest x-rays from the first National Health and Nutrition Examination Survey. Am J Epidemiol 126:893, 1987.

423. Miller A, Teirstein AS, Selikoff IJ: Ventilatory failure due to asbestos pleurisy. Am J Med 75:911, 1983.

424. Landrigan PJ: Commentary: Environmental disease—a preventable epidemic. Am J Public Health 82:941, 1992.

425. Craighead JE, Mossman BT: The pathogenesis of asbestos-associated diseases. N Engl J Med 306:1446, 1982.

426. Murphy RLH Jr, Gaensler EA, Ferris BG, et al: Diagnosis of "asbestosis": Observations from a longitudinal survey of shipyard pipe coverers. Am J Med 65:488, 1978.

427. Kilburn KH, Warshaw R, Thornton JC: Asbestosis, pulmonary symptoms and functional impairment in shipyard workers. Chest 88:254, 1985.

428. Selikoff IJ, Lilis R, Levin G: Asbestotic radiological abnormalities among United States merchant marine seamen. Br J Ind Med 47:292, 1990.

429. Demers RY, Neale AV, Robins T, et al: Asbestos-related pulmonary disease in boilermakers. Am J Ind Med 17:327, 1990.

430. Oliver LC, Eisen EA, Greene RE, et al: Asbestos-related disease in railroad workers: A cross-sectional study. Am Rev Respir Dis 131:499, 1985.

431. McDonald AD, Fry JS, Woolley AJ, et al: Dust exposure and mortality in an American factory using chrysotile, amosite, and crocidolite in mainly textile manufacture. Br J Ind Med 40:368, 1983.

432. Sherson D, Maltbaek N, Olsen O: Small opacities among dental laboratory technicians in Copenhagen. Br J Ind Med 45:320, 1988.

433. Kern DG, Frumkin H: Asbestos-related disease in the jewelry industry: Report of two cases. Am J Ind Med 13:407, 1988.

434. Baris YI, Artvinli M, Sahin AA, et al: Non-occupational asbestos related chest disease in a small Anatolian village. Br J Ind Med 45:841, 1988.

435. Cordier S, Lazar P, Brochard P, et al: Epidemiologic investigation of respiratory effects related to asbestos inside insulated buildings. Arch Environ Health 42:303, 1987.

436. Sebastien P, Bignon J, Martin M: Indoor airborne asbestos pollution: From the ceiling and the floor. Science 216:1410, 1982.

437. Ganor E, Fischbein A, Brenner S, et al: Extreme airborne asbestos concentrations in a public building. Br J Ind Med 49:486, 1992.

438. Oliver LC, Sprince NL, Greene R: Asbestos-related disease in public school custodians. Am J Ind Med 19:303, 1991.

439. Young I, West S, Jackson J, et al: Prevalence of asbestos related lung disease among employees in nonasbestos industries. Med J Aust 1:464, 1981.

440. Peacock PR, Biancifiori C, Bucciarelli E: Examination of lung smears for asbestos bodies in 109 consecutive necropsies in Perugia. Eur J Cancer 5:155, 1969.

441. Roberts GH: Asbestos bodies in lungs at necropsy. J Clin Pathol 20:570, 1967.

442. Thomson JG, Graves WM Jr: Asbestos as an urban air contaminant. Arch Pathol 81:458, 1966.

443. Donisch I, Swettenham KV, Hathorn MKS: Prevalence of asbestos bodies in a necropsy series in East London: Association with disease, occupation, and domiciliary address. Br J Ind Med 32:16, 1975.

444. Cauna D, Totten RS, Gross P: Asbestos bodies in human lungs at autopsy. JAMA 192:371, 1965.

445. Xipell JM, Bhathal PS: Asbestos bodies in lungs: An Australian report. Pathology 1:327, 1969.

446. Anjilvel L, Thurlbeck WM: The incidence of asbestos bodies in the lungs in random necropsies in Montreal. Can Med Assoc J 95:1179, 1966.

447. Becklake MR: Asbestos-related diseases of the lung and other organs: Their epidemiology and implications for clinical practice. Am Rev Respir Dis 114:187, 1976.

448. Churg A: Lung asbestos content in long-term residents of a chrysotile mining town. Am Rev Respir Dis 134:125, 1986.

449. Kiviluoto R: Pleural calcification as a roentgenologic sign of nonoccupational endemic anthophyllite asbestosis. Acta Radiol 194:1, 1960.

450. Newhouse ML: A study of the mortality of workers in an asbestos factory. Br J Ind Med 26:294, 1969.

451. Bianchi C, Brollo A, Ramani L, et al: Exposure to asbestos in Monfalcone, Italy: A necropsy-based study. IARC Sci Publ 112:127, 1991.

452. Rey F, Boutin C, Viallat JR, et al: Environmental asbestotic pleural plaques in northeast Corsica: Correlations with airborne and pleural mineralogic analysis. Environ Health Perspec 5:251, 1994.

453. Champion P: Two cases of malignant mesothelioma after exposure to asbestos. Am Rev Respir Dis 103:821, 1971.

454. Epler GR, Fitzgerald MX, Gaensler EA, et al: Asbestos-related disease from household exposure. Respiration 39:229, 1980.

455. Sider L, Holland EA, Davis TM Jr, et al: Changes on radiographs of wives of workers exposed to asbestos. Radiology 164:723, 1987.

456. Magnani C, Terracini B, Ivaldi C, et al: A cohort study on mortality among wives of workers in the asbestos cement industry in Casale Monferrato, Italy. Br J Ind Med 50:779, 1993.

457. Constantopoulos SH, Goudevenos JA, Saratzis N, et al: Metsovo lung: Pleural calcification and restrictive lung function in northwestern Greece: Environmental exposure to mineral fiber as etiology. Environ Res 38:319, 1985.

458. Constantopoulos SH, Saratzis NA, Kontogiannis D, et al: Tremolite whitewashing and pleural calcifications. Chest 92:709, 1987.

459. Yazicioglu S, Ilcayto R, Balci K, et al: Pleural calcification, pleural mesotheliomas, and bronchial cancers caused by tremolite dust. Thorax 35:564, 1980.

460. Baris YI, Sahin AA, Erkan ML: Clinical and radiological study in sepiolite workers. Arch Environ Health 35:343, 1980.

461. De Vuyst P, Mairesse M, Gaudichet A, et al: Mineralogical analysis of bronchoalveolar fluid as an aid to diagnosis of "imported" pleural asbestosis. Thorax 38:628, 1983.

462. De Vuyst P, Dumortier P, Jacobovitz D, et al: Environmental asbestosis complicated by lung cancer. Chest 105:1593, 1994.

463. Berry G, Newhouse ML: Mortality of workers manufacturing friction materials using asbestos. Br J Ind Med 40:1, 1983.

464. Wright GW: Asbestos and health in 1969. Am Rev Respir Dis 100:467, 1969.

465. Donaldson K, Brown RC, Brown GM: Respirable industrial fibres: Mechanisms of pathogenicity. Thorax 48:390, 1993.

466. Mossman BT, Churg A: Mechanisms in the pathogenesis of asbestosis and silicosis. Am J Respir Crit Care Med 157:1666, 1998.

467. Becklake MR: Editorial—Fiber burden and asbestos-related lung disease: Determinants of dose-response relationships. Am J Respir Crit Care Med 150:1488, 1994.

468. Churg A, Wright JL, Vedal S: Fiber burden and patterns in millers. Am Rev Respir Dis 148:25, 1993.

469. Churg A, Wright JL, Depaoli L, et al: Mineralogic correlates of fibrosis in Chrysotile miners and millers. Am Rev Respir Dis 139:891, 1989.

470. Churg A, Vedal S: Fiber burden and patterns of asbestos-related disease in workers with heavy mixed Amosite and Chrysotile exposure. Am J Respir Crit Care Med 150:663, 1994.

471. Bégin R, Massé S, Sébastien P, et al: Asbestos exposure and retention as determinants of airway disease and asbestos alveolitis. Am Rev Respir Dis 134:1176, 1986.

472. Gibbs AR, Gardner MJ, Pooley FD, et al: Fiber levels and disease in workers from a factory predominantly using amosite. Envir Health Perspec 5:261, 1994.

473. Green FH, Harley R, Vallyathan V: Exposure and mineralogical correlates of pulmonary fibrosis in chrysotile asbestos workers. Occup Environ Med 54:549, 1997.

474. Wagner JC, Newhouse ML, Corrin B, et al: Correlation between fibre content of the lung and disease in East London asbestos factory workers. Br J Ind Med 45:305, 1988.

475. Mossman BT, Kessler JB, Ley BW, et al: Interaction of crocidolite asbestos with hamster respiratory mucosa in organ culture. Lab Invest 36:131, 1977.

476. Adamson IYR, Bowden DH: Crocidolite-induced pulmonary fibrosis in mice: Cytokinetic and biochemical studies. Am J Pathol 122:261, 1986.

477. Spurzem JR, Saltini C, Rom W, et al: Mechanisms of macrophage accumulation in the lungs of asbestos-exposed subjects. Am Rev Respir Dis 136:276, 1987.

478. Brody AR: Pulmonary cell interactions with asbestos fibers in vivo and in vitro. Chest 89:155, 1986.

479. Adamson IYR, Letourneau HL, Bowden DH: Comparison of alveolar and interstitial macrophages in fibroblast stimulation after silica and long or short asbestos. Lab Invest 64:339, 1991.

480. Brody AR, Overby LH: Incorporation of tritiated thymidine by epithelial and interstitial cells in bronchiolar-alveolar regions of asbestos-exposed rats. Am J Pathol 134:133, 1989.

481. Review of Fibre Toxicology. Sheffield, Health and Safety Executive (UK).

482. Zhang Y, Lee TC, Guillemin B, et al: Enhanced IL-1 beta and tumour necrosis factor-alpha release and messenger RNA expression in macrophages from idiopathic pulmonary fibrosis or after asbestos exposure. J Immunol 150:4188, 1993.

483. Perkins RC, Scheule RK, Hamilton R, et al: Human alveolar macrophage cytokine release in response to in vitro and in vivo asbestos exposure. Exp Lung Res 19:55, 1993.

484. Rom WN, Travis WD, Brody AR: Cellular and molecular basis of the asbestos-related diseases. Am Rev Respir Dis 143:408, 1991.

485. Garcia JGN, Friffith DE, Cohen AB, et al: Alveolar macrophages from patient with asbestos exposure release increased levels of leukotriene B$_4$. Am Rev Respir Dis 139:1494, 1989.

486. Hayes AA, Rose AH, Musk AW, et al: Neutrophil chemotactic factor release and neutrophil alveolitis in asbestos-exposed individuals. Chest 94:521, 1988.

487. Cullen MR, Merrill WW: Association between neutrophil concentration in bronchoalveolar lavage fluid and recent losses in diffusing capacity in men formerly exposed to Asbestos. Chest 102:682, 1992.

488. Al Jarad NA, Gellert AR, Rudd RM: Bronchoalveolar lavage and ^{99m}Tc-DTPA clearance as prognostic factors in asbestos workers with and without asbestosis. Respir Med 87:265, 1993.

489. Schwartz DA, Davis CS, Merchant JA, et al: Longitudinal changes in lung function among asbestos-exposed workers. Am J Respir Crit Care Med 150:1243, 1994.

490. Xaubet A, Rodriquez-Roisin R, Bombi JA, et al: Correlation of bronchoalveolar lavage and clinical and functional findings in asbestosis. Am Rev Respir Dis 133:848, 1986.

491. Robinson BW, Rose AH, James A, et al: Alveolitis of pulmonary asbestosis: Bronchoalveolar lavage studies in crocidolite- and chrysotile-exposed individuals. Chest 90:396, 1986.

492. Robinson BWS, Rose AH, James A, et al: Alveolitis of pulmonary asbestosis. Chest 90:396, 1986.

493. Kamp DW, Graceffa P, Pryor WA, et al: The role of free radicals and asbestos-induced disease. Free Radic Biol Med 12:293, 1992.

494. Goodglick LE, Pietras LA, Kane AB: Evaluation of the causal relationship between crocidolite asbestos-induced lipid peroxidation and toxicity to macrophages. Am Rev Respir Dis 139:1265, 1989.

495. Kamp DW, Weitzman SA: Asbestosis: Clinical spectrum and pathogenic mechanisms. Proc Soc Exp Biol Med 214:12, 1997.

496. Garcia JGN, Gray LD, Dodson RF, et al: Asbestos-induced endothelial cell activation and injury. Am Rev Respir Dis 138:958, 1988.

497. Quinlan TR, Marsh JP, Janssen YMW, et al: Dose-responsive increases in pulmonary fibrosis after inhalation of asbestos. Am J Respir Crit Care Med 150:200, 1994.

498. Cantin A, Allard C, Bégin R: Increased alveolar plasminogen activator in early asbestosis. Am Rev Respir Dis 139:604, 1989.

499. Callahan KS, Griffith DE, Garcia JGN: Asbestos exposure results in increased lung procoagulant activity in vivo and in vitro. Chest 98:112, 1990.

500. Jakobsson K, Rannug A, Alexandrie AK, et al: Genetic polymorphism for glutathione-S-transferase mu in asbestos cement workers. Occup Environ Med 51:812, 1994.

501. Weiss: Cigarette smoke, asbestos, and small irregular opacities. Am Rev Respir Dis 130:293, 1984.

502. Ducatman AM, Withers B, Yang WN: Smoking and roentgenographic opacities in US Navy asbestos workers. Chest 97:810, 1990.

503. Karjalainen A, Karhunen PJ, Lalu K, et al: Pleural plaques and exposure to mineral fibers in a male urban necropsy population. Occup Environ Med 51:456, 1994.

504. Blanc PD, Golden JA, Gamsu G, et al: Asbestos exposure—cigarette smoking interactions among shipyard workers. JAMA 259:370, 1988.

505. Weiss W: Cigarette smoking and small irregular opacities. Br J Ind Med 48:841, 1991.

506. Barnhart S, Thornquist M, Omenn GS, et al: The degree of roentgenographic parenchymal opacities attributable to smoking among asbestos-exposed subjects. Am Rev Respir Dis 141:1102, 1990.

507. Kilburn KH, Warshaw RH: Severity of pulmonary asbestosis as classified by international labour organisation profusion of irregular opacities in 8749 asbestos-exposed American workers. Arch Intern Med 152:325, 1992.

508. Lilis R, Miller A, Godbold J, et al: Radiographic abnormalities in asbestos insulators: Effects of duration from onset of exposure and smoking: Relationships of dyspnea with parenchymal and pleural fibrosis. Am J Ind Med 20:1, 1991.

509. Mcfadden D, Wright J, Wiggs B, et al: Cigarette smoke increases the penetration of asbestos fibers into airway walls. Am J Pathol 123:95, 1986.

510. McFadden D, Wright JL, Wiggs B, et al: Smoking inhibits asbestos clearance. Am Rev Respir Dis 133:372, 1986.

511. Churg A, Wright JL, Hobson J, et al: Effects of cigarette smoke on the clearance of short asbestos fibres from the lung and a comparison with the clearance of long asbestos fibres. Int J Exp Pathol 73:287, 1992.

512. Davis JM, Addison J, Bolton RE, et al: The pathogenicity of long versus short fibre samples of amosite asbestos administered to rats by inhalation and intraperitoneal injection. J Exp Pathol 67:415, 1986.

513. Donaldson K, Brown GM, Brown DM, et al: Inflammation generating potential of long and short fibre amosite asbestos samples. Br J Ind Med 46:271, 1989.

514. Mossman BT, Gee JBL: Asbestos-related diseases. New Engl J Med 320:1721, 1989.

515. Schwartz DA, Galvin JR, Merchant RK, et al: Influence of cigarette smoking on bronchoalveolar lavage cellularity in asbestos-induced lung disease. Am Rev Respir Dis 145:400, 1992.

516. Morimoto Y, Kido M, Tanaka I, et al: Synergistic effects of mineral fibres and cigarette smoke on the production of tumour necrosis factor by alveolar macrophages of rats. Br J Ind Med 50:955, 1993.

517. Churg A, Hobson J, Berean K, et al: Scavengers of active oxygen species prevent cigarette smoke–induced asbestos fiber penetration in rat tracheal explants. Am J Pathol 135:599, 1989.

518. Churg A, Hobson J, Wright J: Effects of cigarette smoke dose and time after smoke exposure on uptake of asbestos fibers by rat tracheal epithelial cells. Am J Respir Cell Mol Biol 3:265, 1990.

519. Lesur O, Bernard AM, Bégin RO: Clara cell protein (CC-16) and surfactant-associated protein (SP-A) in asbestos-exposed workers. Chest 109:467, 1996.

520. Churg A, Stevens B: Enhanced retention of asbestos fibers in the airways of human smokers. Am J Respir Crit Care Med 151:1409, 1995.

521. Becklake MR, Toyota B, Stewart M, et al: Lung structure as a risk factor in adverse pulmonary responses to asbestos exposure: A case-referent study in Quebec chrysotile miners and millers. Am Rev Respir Dis 128:385, 1983.

522. Rom WN, Travis WD: Lymphocyte-macrophage involvement in nonsmoking individuals occupationally exposed to asbestos. Chest 101:779, 1992.

523. Wallace JM, Oishi JS, Barbers RG, et al: Bronchoalveolar lavage cell and lymphocyte phenotype profiles in healthy asbestos-exposed shipyard workers. Am Rev Respir Dis 139:33, 1989.

524. Corsini E, Luster MI, Mahler J, et al: A protective role for T lymphocytes in asbestos-induced pulmonary inflammation and collagen deposition. Am J Respir Cell Mol Biol 11:531, 1994.

525. Robinson BW, Rose AH, Hayes A, et al: Increased pulmonary gamma interferon production in asbestosis. Am Rev Respir Dis 138:278, 1988.

526. Constantopoulos SH, Dalavanga YA, Sakellariou K, et al: Lymphocytic alveolitis and pleural calcifications in nonoccupational asbestos exposure. Am Rev Respir Dis 146:1565, 1992.

527. Sprince NL, Oliver LC, McLoud TC, et al: Asbestos exposure and asbestos-related pleural and parenchymal disease. Am Rev Respir Dis 143:822, 1991.

528. Turner-Warwick M, Parkes WR: Circulating rheumatoid and antinuclear factors in asbestos workers. BMJ 1:886, 1965.

529. Doll NJ, Diem JE, Jones RN, et al: Humoral immunologic abnormalities in workers exposed to asbestos cement dust. J Allergy Clin Immunol 72:509, 1983.

530. Deshazo RD, Hendrick DJ, Diem JE, et al: Immunologic aberrations in asbestos cement workers: Dissociation from asbestosis. J Allergy Clin Immunol 72:454, 1983.

531. Huuskonen MS, Rasanen JA, Juntunen J, et al: Immunological aspects of asbestosis: Patients' neurological signs and asbestosis progression. Am J Ind Med 5:461, 1984.

532. Haslam PL, Lukoszek A, Merchant JA, et al: Lymphocyte responses to phytohaemagglutinin in patients with asbestosis and pleural mesothelioma. Clin Exp Immunol 31:178, 1978.

533. Pierce R, Turner-Warwick M: Skin tests with tuberculin (PPD), *Candida albicans* and *Trichophyton* spp. in cryptogenic fibrosing alveolitis and asbestos related lung disease. Clin Allergy 10:229, 1980.

534. Lange A, Garncarek D, Tomeczako J, et al: Outcome of asbestos exposure (lung fibrosis and antinuclear antibodies) with respect to skin reactivity: An 8-year longitudinal study. Environ Res 41:1, 1986.

535. Toivanen A, Salmivalli M, Molnar G: Pulmonary asbestosis and autoimmunity. BMJ 1:691, 1976.

536. Bégin R, Menard H, Decarie F, et al: Immunogenetic factors as determinants of asbestosis. Lung 165:159, 1987.

537. Shih JF, Hunninghake GW, Goeken NE, et al: The relationship between HLA-A, B, DQ and Dr antigens and asbestos-induced lung disease. Chest 104:26, 1993.

538. Jarad NA, Uthayakumar S, Buckland EJ, et al: The histocompatibility antigen in asbestos related disease. Br J Ind Med 49:826, 1992.

539. Warnock ML, Prescott BT, Kuvahara TJ: Numbers and types of asbestos fibers in subjects with pleural plaques. Am J Pathol 109:37, 1982.

540. Churg A: Asbestos fibers and pleural plaques in a general autopsy population. Am J Pathol 109:88, 1982.

541. Wain SL, Roggli VL, Foster WL Jr: Parietal pleural plaques, asbestos bodies, and neoplasia. Chest 86:707, 1984.

542. Churg A, Golden J: Current problems in the pathology of asbestos-related disease. Pathol Ann 17(pt 2):33, 1982.

543. Roberts GH: The pathology of parietal pleural plaques. J Clin Pathol 24:348, 1971.

544. Craighead JE, Abraham JL, Churg A, et al: The pathology of asbestos-associated diseases of the lungs and pleural cavities: Diagnostic criteria and proposed grading schema. Arch Pathol Lab Med 106:544, 1982.

545. Mollo F, Bellis D, Magnani C, et al: Hyaline splenic and hepatic plaques: Correlation with cirrhosis, pulmonary tuberculosis, and asbestos exposure. Arch Pathol Lab Med 117:1017, 1993.

546. Hourihane DO, Lessof L, Richardson PC: Hyaline and calcified pleural plaques as an index of exposure to asbestos: A study of radiological and pathological features of 100 cases with a consideration of epidemiology. BMJ 1:1069, 1966.

547. Meurman L: Asbestos bodies and pleural plaques in a Finnish series of autopsy cases. Acta Pathol Microbiol Scand 181(Suppl):97, 1966.

548. Francis D, Jussuf A, Mortensen T, et al: Hyaline pleural plaques and asbestos bodies in 198 randomized autopsies. Scand J Respir Dis 58:193, 1977.

549. Hillerdal G: Pleural plaques in a health survey material: Frequency, development and exposure to asbestos. Scand J Respir Dis 59:257, 1978.

550. Albelda SM, Epstein DM, Gefter WB, et al: Pleural thickening: Its significance and relationship to asbestos dust exposure. Am Rev Respir Dis 126:621, 1982.

551. Sison RF, Hruban RH, Moore GW, et al: Pulmonary disease associated with pleural "asbestos" plaques. Chest 95:831, 1989.

552. Kuwahara M, Kuwahara M, Verma K, et al: Asbestos exposure stimulates pleural mesothelial cells to secrete the fibroblast chemoattractant, fibronectin. Am J Respir Cell Mol Biol 10:167, 1994.

553. Stephens M, Gibbs AR, Pooley FD, et al: Asbestos induced diffuse pleural fibrosis: Pathology and mineralogy. Thorax 42:583, 1987.

554. O'Brien CJ, Franks AJ: Paraplegia due to massive asbestos-related pleural and mediastinal fibrosis. Histopathology 11:541, 1987.

555. Sluis-Cremer GK, Webster I: Acute pleurisy in asbestos exposed persons. Environ Res 5:380, 1972.

556. Gaensler EA, Kaplan AI: Asbestos pleural effusion. Ann Intern Med 74:178, 1971.

557. Shore BL, Daughaday CC, Spilberg I: Benign asbestos pleurisy in the rabbit. Am Rev Respir Dis 128:481, 1983.

558. Antony VB, Owen CL, Hadley KJ: Pleural mesothelial cells stimulated by asbestos release chemotactic activity for neutrophils in vitro. Am Rev Respir Dis 139:199, 1989.

559. Churg AM, Warnock ML: Asbestos and other ferruginous bodies: Their formation and clinical significance. Am J Pathol 102:447, 1981.

560. Churg A, Warnock ML: Analysis of the cores of asbestos bodies from members of the general population: Patients with probable low-degree exposure to asbestos. Am Rev Respir Dis 120:781, 1979.

561. Warnock ML, Churg AM: Asbestos bodies. Chest 77:129, 1980.

562. Roggli VL, Benning TL: Asbestos bodies in pulmonary hilar lymph nodes. Mod Pathol 3:513, 1990.

563. Kobayashi H, Ming ZW, Watanabe H, et al: A quantitative study on the distribution of asbestos bodies in extrapulmonary organs. Acta Pathol Jpn 37:375, 1987.

564. Auerbach O, Conston AS, Garfinkel L, et al: Presence of asbestos bodies in organs other than the lung. Chest 77:133, 1980.

565. Kobayashi H, Okamura A, Ohnishi Y, et al: Generalized fibrosis associated with pulmonary asbestosis. Acta Pathol Jpn 33:1223, 1983.

566. Roggli VL, Greenberg SD, McLarty JV, et al: Comparison of sputum and lung asbestos body counts in former asbestos workers. Am Rev Respir Dis 122:941, 1980.

567. Wheeler TM, Johnson EH, Coughlin D, et al: The sensitivity of detection of asbestos bodies in sputa and bronchial washings. Acta Cytol 32:647, 1988.

568. Greenberg SD: Cytopathology of asbestos-associated pulmonary disease. Diagn Cytopathol 1:177, 1985.

569. Roggli VL, Johnston WW, Kaminsky DB: Asbestos bodies in fine needle aspirates of the lung. Acta Cytol 28:493, 1984.

570. Corhay JL, Delavignette JP, Bury T, et al: Occult exposure to asbestos in steel workers revealed by bronchoalveolar lavage. Arch Environ Health 45:278, 1990.

571. De Vuyst P, Dumortier P, Moulin E, et al: Asbestos bodies in bronchoalveolar lavage reflect lung asbestos body concentration. Eur Respir J 1:362, 1988.

572. Sebastien P, Armstrong B, Monchaux G, et al: Asbestos bodies in bronchoalveolar lavage fluid and in lung parenchyma. Am Rev Respir Dis 137:75, 1988.

573. Gellert AR, Kitajewska JY, Uthayakumar S, et al: Asbestos fibres in bronchoalveolar lavage fluid from asbestos workers: Examination by electron microscopy. Br J Ind Med 43:170, 1986.

574. Roggli VL, Piantadosi CA, Bell DY: Asbestos bodies in bronchoalveolar lavage fluid: A study of 20 asbestos-exposed individuals and comparison to patients with other chronic interstitial lung diseases. Acta Cytol 30:470, 1986.

575. Schwartz DA, Galvin JR, Burmeister LF, et al: The clinical utility and reliability of asbestos bodies in bronchoalveolar fluid. Am Rev Respir Dis 144:684, 1991.

576. Suzuki Y, Churg J: Structure and development of the asbestos body. Am J Pathol 55:79, 1969.

577. Koerten HK, Hazekamp J, Kroon M, et al: Asbestos body formation and iron accumulation in mouse peritoneal granulomas after the introduction of crocidolite asbestos fibers. Am J Pathol 136:141, 1990.

578. Gross P, deTreville RTP, Cralley LJ, et al: Pulmonary ferruginous bodies: Development in response to filamentous dusts and a method of isolation and concentration. Arch Pathol 85:539, 1968.

579. Crouch E, Churg A: Ferruginous bodies and the histologic evaluation of dust exposure. Am J Surg Pathol 8:109, 1984.

580. Churg A, Warnock ML, Green M: Analysis of the cores of ferruginous (asbestos) bodies from the general population. Lab Invest 40:31, 1979.

581. Sebastien P, Gaudichet A, Bignon J, et al: Zeolite bodies in human lungs from Turkey. Lab Invest 44:420, 1981.

582. Dodson RF, O'Sullivan MF, Corn CJ, et al: Ferruginous body formation on a nonasbestos mineral. Arch Pathol Lab Med 109:849, 1985.

583. Steele RH, Thomson KJ: Asbestos bodies in the lung: Southampton (U.K.) and Wellington (New Zealand). Br J Ind Med 39:349, 1982.

584. Vollmer RT, Roggli VL: Asbestos body concentrations in human lung: Predictions from asbestos body counts in tissue sections with a mathematical model. Hum Pathol 16:713, 1985.

585. Churg A: Fiber counting and analysis in the diagnosis of asbestos-related disease. Hum Pathol 13:381, 1982.

586. Roggli VL, Greenberg SD, Seitzman LW, et al: Pulmonary fibrosis, carcinoma, and ferruginous body counts in amosite asbestos workers. Am J Clin Pathol 73:496, 1980.

587. Roggli VL, Pratt PC: Numbers of asbestos bodies on iron-stained tissue sections in relation to asbestos body counts in lung tissue digests. Hum Pathol 14:355, 1983.

588. Murai Y, Kitagawa M, Yasuda M, et al: Asbestos fiber analysis in seven asbestosis cases. Arch Environ Health 49:67, 1994.

589. Warrock ML, Wolery G: Asbestos bodies and fibers and the diagnosis of asbestosis. Environ Res 44:29, 1987.

590. Dodson RF, Williams MG Jr, O'Sullivan MF, et al: A comparison of the ferruginous body and uncoated fiber content in the lungs of former asbestos workers. Am Rev Respir Dis 132:143, 1985.

591. Churg A, Warnock M: Asbestos fibers in the general population. Am Rev Respir Dis 122:669, 1980.

592. Davis JMG: The pathology of asbestos-related disease. Thorax 39:801, 1984.

593. Case BW, Sebastien P: Environmental and occupational exposures to chrysotile asbestos: A comparative microanalytic study. Arch Environ Health 42:185, 1987.

594. Churg A: Editorial: Analysis of lung asbestos content. Br J Ind Med 48:649, 1991.

595. Kuhn C III, Kuo TT: Cytoplasmic hyalin in asbestosis: A reaction of injured alveolar epithelium. Arch Pathol 95:190, 1973.

596. Warnock ML, Press M, Churg A: Further observations on cytoplasmic hyaline in the lung. Hum Pathol 11:59, 1980.

597. Bellis D, Andrion A, Delsedime L, et al: Minimal pathologic changes of the lung and asbestos exposure. Hum Pathol 20:102, 1989.

598. Bégin R, Massé S, Sébastien P, et al: Asbestos exposure and retention as determinants of airway disease and asbestos alveolitis. Am Rev Respir Dis 134:1176, 1986.

599. Wright JL, Churg A: Morphology of small-airway lesions in patients with asbestos exposure. Hum Pathol 15:68, 1984.

600. Churg A, Wright JL: Small-airway lesions in patients exposed to nonasbestos mineral dusts. Hum Pathol 14:688, 1983.

601. Churg A: Asbestos fiber content of the lungs in patients with and without asbestos airways disease. Am Rev Respir Dis 127:470, 1983.

602. Churg A, Wright JL, Wiggs B, et al: Small airways disease and mineral dust exposure. Am Rev Respir Dis 131:139, 1985.

603. Cohen BM, Adasczik A, Cohen EM: Small airways changes in workers exposed to asbestos. Respiration 45:296, 1984.

604. Bégin R, Cantin A, Berthiaume Y, et al: Airway function in lifetime-nonsmoking older asbestos population. Am J Med 75:631, 1983.

605. Rodrigues-Roisin R, Merchant JEM, Cochrane GM, et al: Maximal expiratory flow volume curves in workers exposed to asbestos. Respiration 39:158, 1980.

606. Secker-Walker RH, Ho JE: Regional lung function in asbestos workers: Observations and speculations. Respiration 43:8, 1982.

607. Bégin R, Masse S, Bureau MA: Morphologic features and function of the airways in early asbestosis in the sheep model. Am Rev Respir Dis 126:870, 1982.

608. Wright JL, Tron V, Filipenko D, et al: Pathophysiologic correlations in asbestos-induced airway disease in the guinea pig. Exp Lung Res 11:307, 1986.

609. Blesovsky A: The folded lung. Br J Dis Chest 60:19, 1966.

610. Menzies R, Fraser R: Round atelectasis: Pathologic and pathogenetic features. Am J Surg Pathol 11:674, 1987.

611. Dernevik L, Garzinsky P, Hultman E, et al: Shrinking pleuritis with atelectasis. Thorax 37:252, 1982.

612. Doyle TC, Lawler GA: CT features of rounded atelectasis of the lung. Am J Roentgenol 143:225, 1984.

613. Tallroth K, Kiviranta K: Round atelectasis. Respiration 45:71, 1984.

614. Chung-Park M, Tomashefski JF Jr, Cohen AM, et al: Shrinking pleuritis with lobar atelectasis, a morphologic variant of "round atelectasis." Hum Pathol 20:382, 1989.

615. Mintzer RA, Gore RM, Vogelzang RL, et al: Rounded atelectasis and its association with asbestos-induced pleural disease. Radiology 139:567, 1981.

616. Hillerdal G, Hemmingsson A: Pulmonary pseudotumours and asbestos. Acta Radiol Diagn 21:615, 1980.

617. Mintzer RA, Cugell DW: The association of asbestos-induced pleural disease and rounded atelectasis. Chest 81:457, 1982.

618. Hillerdal G: Rounded atelectasis: Clinical experience with 74 patients. Chest 95:836, 1989.

619. Hammar SP: Controversies and uncertainties concerning the pathologic features and pathologic diagnosis of asbestosis. Semin Diagn Pathol 9:102, 1992.

620. Rom WN, Travis WD: Lymphocyte-macrophage alveolitis in nonsmoking individuals occupationally exposed to asbestos. Chest 101:779, 1992.

621. Gaensler EA, Jederlinic PJ, Churg A: Idiopathic pulmonary fibrosis in asbestos-exposed workers. Am Rev Respir Dis 144:689, 1991.

622. Hurwitz M: Roentgenologic aspects of asbestosis. Am J Roentgenol 85:256, 1961.

623. Freundlich IM, Greening RR: Asbestosis and associated medical problems. Radiology 89:224, 1967.

624. Fletcher DE, Edge JR: The early radiological changes in pulmonary and pleural asbestosis. Clin Radiol 21:355, 1970.

625. Anton HC: Multiple pleural plaques, part II. Br J Radiol 41:341, 1968.

626. Zitting A, Huuskonen MS, Alanko K, et al: Radiographic and physiological findings in patients with asbestosis. Scand J Work Environ Health 4:275, 1978.

627. Friedman AC, Fiel SB, Fisher MS, et al: Asbestos-related pleural disease and asbestosis: A comparison of CT and chest radiography. Am J Roentgenol 150:269, 1988.

628. Aberle DR, Gamsu G, Ray CS, et al: Asbestos-related pleural and parenchymal fibrosis: Detection with high-resolution CT. Radiology 166:729, 1988.

629. Staples CA, Gamsu G, Ray CS, et al: High-resolution computed tomography and lung function in asbestos-exposed workers with normal chest radiographs. Am Rev Respir Dis 139:1502, 1989.

630. Gamsu G, Salmon CJ, Warnock ML, Blanc PD: CT quantification of interstitial fibrosis in patients with asbestosis: A comparison of two methods. Am J Roentgenol 164:63, 1995.

631. Sargent EN, Gordonson J, Jacobson G, et al: Bilateral pleural thickening: A manifestation of asbestos dust exposure. Am J Roentgenol 131:579, 1978.

632. Sprince NL, Oliver LC, McLoud TC: Asbestos-related disease in plumbers and pipefitters employed in building construction. J Occup Med 27:771, 1985.

633. Lawson JP: Pleural calcification as a sign of asbestosis: A report of three cases. Clin Radiol 14:414, 1963.

634. Schneider L, Wimpfheimer F: Multiple progressive calcific pleural plaque formation: A sign of silicatosis. JAMA 189:328, 1964.

635. Oosthuizen SF, Theron CP, Sluis-Cremer GK: Calcified pleural plaques in asbestosis: An investigation into their significance. Med Proc (Johannesburg) 10:496, 1964.

636. Mackenzie FAF: The radiological investigation of the early manifestations of exposure to asbestos dust. Proc R Soc Med 64:834, 1971.

637. Bégin R, Boctor M, Bergeron D, et al: Radiographic assessment of pleuropulmonary disease in asbestos workers: Posteroanterior, four view films, and computed tomograms of the thorax. Br J Ind Med 41:373, 1984.

638. Fisher MS: Asymmetrical changes in asbestos-related disease. J Can Assoc Radiol 36:110, 1985.

639. Withers BF, Ducatman AM, Yang WN: Roentgenographic evidence for predominant left-sided location of unilateral pleural plaques. Chest 95:1262, 1984.

640. Hu H, Beckett L, Kelsey K, Christiani D: The left-sided predominance of asbestos-related pleural disease. Am Rev Respir Dis 148:981, 1993.

641. Sargent EN, Gordonson T, Jacobson G, et al: Bilateral pleural thickening: A manifestation of asbestos dust exposure. Am J Roentgenol 131:579, 1978.

641a. Gallego JC: Absence of left-sided predominance in asbestos-related pleural plaques: A CT study. Chest 113:1034, 1998.

642. Rockoff SD, Kagan E, Schwartz A, et al: Visceral pleural thickening in asbestos exposure: The occurrence and implications of thickened interlobar fissures. J Thorac Imaging 2:58, 1987.

643. Hillerdal G, Lindgren A: Pleural plaques: Correlation of autopsy findings to radiographic findings and occupational history. Eur J Respir Dis 61:315, 1980.

644. Sargent EN, Boswell WD Jr, Ralls PW, et al: Subpleural fat pads in patients exposed to asbestos: Distinction from noncalcified pleural plaques. Radiology 152:273, 1984.

645. Im JG, Webb WR, Rosen A, Gamsu G: Costal pleural: Appearance at high-resolution CT. Radiology 171:125, 1989.

646. Smith AR: Pleural calcification resulting from exposure to certain dusts. Am J Roentgenol 67:375, 1952.

647. Kleinfeld M: Pleural calcification as a sign of silicatosis. Am J Med Sci 251:215, 1966.

648. Krige L: Asbestosis—with special reference to the radiological diagnosis. S Afr J Radiol 4:13, 1966.

649. Solomon A: Radiology of asbestosis. Environ Res 3:320, 1970.

650. Sargent EN, Jacobson G, Wilkinson EE: Diaphragmatic pleural calcification following short occupational exposure to asbestos. Am J Roentgenol 115:473, 1972.

651. McLoud TC, Woods BO, Carrington CB, et al: Diffuse pleural thickening in an asbestos-exposed population: Prevalence and causes. Am J Roentgenol 144:9, 1985.

652. Lynch DA, Gamsu G, Aberle DR: Conventional and high resolution computed tomography in the diagnosis of asbestos-related diseases. Radiographics 9:523, 1989.

653. Hillerdal G, Malmberg P, Hemmingsson A: Asbestos-related lesions of the pleura: Parietal plaques compared to diffuse thickening studied with chest roentgenography, computed tomography, lung function, and gas exchange. Am J Ind Med 18:627, 1990.

654. Aberle DR, Gamsu G, Ray CS, Feuerstein IM: Asbestos-related pleural and parenchymal fibrosis: Detection with high-resolution CT. Radiology 166:729, 1988.

655. Leung AN, Müller NL, Miller RR: CT in differential diagnosis of diffuse pleural disease. Am J Roentgenol 154:487, 1990.

656. Friedman AC, Fiel SB, Radecki PD, Lev-Toaff AS: Computed tomography of benign pleural and pulmonary parenchymal abnormalities related to asbestos exposure. Semin Ultrasound CT MR 11:393, 1990.

657. Müller NL: Imaging of the Pleura. Radiology 186:297, 1993.

658. Gaensler EA, Kaplan AI: Asbestos pleural effusion. Ann Intern Med 74:178, 1971.

659. Sluis-Cremer GK, Webster I: Acute pleurisy in asbestos exposed persons. Environ Res 5:380, 1972.

660. Epler GR, McLoud TC, Gaensler EA: Prevalence and incidence of benign asbestos pleural effusion in working population. JAMA 247:617, 1982.

661. Eisenstadt HB: Benign asbestos pleurisy. JAMA 192:419, 1965.

662. Rabinowitz JG, Efremidis SC, Cohen B, et al: A comparative study of mesothelioma and asbestosis using computed tomography and conventional chest radiography. Radiology 144:453, 1982.

663. Katz D, Kreel L: Computed tomography in pulmonary asbestosis. Clin Radiol 30:207, 1979.

664. Adams VI, Unni KK, Muhm JR, et al: Diffuse malignant mesothelioma of pleura: Diagnosis and survival in 92 cases. Cancer 58:1540, 1986.

665. Grant DC, Seltzer SE, Antman KH, et al: Computed tomography of malignant pleural mesothelioma. J Comput Assist Tomogr 7:626, 1983.

666. Kawashima A, Libshitz HI: Malignant pleural mesothelioma: CT manifestations in 50 cases. Am J Roentgenol 155:965, 1990.

667. Goldstein B: Two malignant pleural mesotheliomas with unusual histological features. Thorax 34:375, 1979.

668. Nichols DM, Johnson MA: Calcification in a pleural mesothelioma. J Can Assoc Radiol 34:311, 1983.

669. Smith KW: Pulmonary disability in asbestos workers. AMA Arch Ind Health 12:198, 1955.

670. Sampson C, Hansell DM: The prevalence of enlarged mediastinal lymph nodes in asbestos-exposed individuals: A CT study. Clin Radiol 45:340, 1992.

671. Hillerdal G: Asbestos exposure and upper lobe involvement. Am J Roentgenol 139:1163, 1982.

672. Solomon A, Goldstein B, Webster I, et al: Massive fibrosis in asbestosis. Environ Res 4:430, 1971.

673. Gefter WB, Conant EF: Issues and controversies in the plain-film diagnosis of asbestos-related disorders in the chest. J Thorac Imaging 3:11, 1988.

674. Epler GR, McLoud TC, Gaensler EA, et al: Normal chest roentgenograms in chronic diffuse infiltrative lung disease. N Engl J Med 298:934, 1978.

675. Kipen HM, Lilis R, Suzuki Y, et al: Pulmonary fibrosis in asbestos insulation workers with lung cancer: A radiological and histopathological evaluation. Br J Ind Med 44:96, 1987.

676. Akira M, Yokoyama K, Yamamoto S, et al: Early asbestosis: Evaluation with high-resolution CT. Radiology 178:409, 1991.

677. Yoshimura H, Hatakeyama M, Otsuji H, et al: Pulmonary asbestosis: CT study of subpleural curvilinear shadow. Radiology 158:653, 1986.

678. Akira M, Yamamoto S, Yokoyama K, et al: Asbestosis: High-resolution CT-pathologic correlation. Radiology 176:389, 1990.

679. Al-Jarad N, Strickland B, Pearson MC, et al: High-resolution computed tomographic assessment of asbestosis and cryptogenic fibrosing alveolitis: A comparative study. Thorax 47:645, 1992.

680. Primack SL, Hartman TE, Hansell DM, Müller NL: End-stage lung disease: CT findings in 61 patients. Radiology 189:681, 1993.

681. Bergin CJ, Castellino RA, Blank N, Moses L: Specificity of high-resolution CT findings in pulmonary asbestosis: Do patients scanned for other indications have similar findings? Am J Roentgenol 163:551, 1994.

682. Murray KA, Gamsu G, Webb WR, et al: High-resolution computed tomography sampling for detection of asbestos-related lung disease. Acad Radiol 2:111, 1995.

683. Majurin ML, Varpula M, Kurki T, Pakkala L: High-resolution CT of the lung in asbestos-exposed subjects: Comparison of low-dose and high-dose HRCT. Acta Radiol 35:473, 1994.

684. Mintzer RA, Gore RM, Vogelzang RL, et al: Rounded atelectasis and its association with asbestos-induced pleural disease. Radiology 139:567, 1981.

685. Schneider HJ, Felson B, Gonzalez LL: Rounded atelectasis. Am J Roentgenol 134:225, 1980.

686. Franzblau A: Asbestos-associated round atelectasis: A case report and review of the literature. Mt Sinai J Med 56:321, 1989.

687. Lynch DA, Gamsu G, Ray CS, Aberle DR: Asbestos-related focal lung masses: Manifestations on conventional and high-resolution CT scans. Radiology 169:603, 1988.

688. McHugh K, Blaquiere RM: CT features of rounded atelectasis. Am J Roentgenol 153:257, 1989.

689. Carvalho PM, Carr DH: Computed tomography of folded lung. Clin Radiol 41:86, 1990.

690. Taylor PM: Dynamic contrast enhancement of asbestos-related pulmonary pseudotumours. Br J Radiol 61:1070, 1988.

691. Westcott JL, Hllisey MJ, Volpe JP: Dynamic CT of round atelectasis. Radiology 181:182, 1991.

692. Hillerdal G: Rounded atelectasis: Clinical experience with 74 patients. Chest 95:836, 1989.

693. Verschakelen JA, Demaerel P, Coolen J, et al: Rounded atelectasis of the lung: MR appearance. Am J Roentgenol 152:965, 1989.

693a. McAdams HP, Erasmus JJ, Patz EF, et al: Evaluation of patients with round atelectasis using 2-[¹⁸F]fluoro-2-deoxy-D-glucose PET. J Comput Assist Tomogr 22:601, 1998.

694. Smyth MDP, Goodman NG, Basu AP, et al: Pulmonary asbestosis. Chest 60:270, 1971.

695. Eisenstadt HB: Asbestos pleurisy. Dis Chest 46:78, 1964.

696. Robinson BWS, Musk AW: Benign asbestos pleural effusion: Diagnosis and course. Thorax 36:896, 1981.

697. Hillerdal G: Non-malignant asbestos pleural disease. Thorax 36:669, 1981.

698. Miller A: Chronic pleuritic pain in four patients with asbestos induced pleural fibrosis. Br J Ind Med 47:147, 1990.

699. Rosenstock L, Barnhart S, Heyer NJ, et al: The relation among pulmonary function, chest roentgenographic abnormalities and smoking status in an asbestos-exposed cohort. Am Rev Respir Dis 138:272, 1988.

700. McGavin CR, Sheers G: Diffuse pleural thickening in asbestos workers: Disability and lung function abnormalities. Thorax 39:604, 1984.

701. Britton MG: Asbestos pleural disease. Br J Dis Chest 76:1, 1982.

702. Hilt B, Lien JT, Lund-Larsen PG: Lung function and respiratory symptoms in subjects with asbestos-related disorders: A cross-sectional study. Am J Ind Med 11:517, 1987.

703. Schüler P, Maturana V, Cruz E, et al: Pulmonary asbestosis. Rev Chil Enferm Torax 25:37, 1959.

704. Kleinfeld M, Messite J, Shapiro J: Clinical, radiological, and physiological findings in asbestosis. Arch Intern Med 117:813, 1966.

705. Enarson DA, Embree V, MacLean L, et al: Respiratory health in chrysotile asbestos miners in British Columbia: A longitudinal study. Br J Ind Med 45:459, 1988.

706. Brodken CA, Barnhart S, Anderson G, et al: Correlation between respiratory symptoms and pulmonary function in asbestos-exposed workers. Am Rev Respir Dis 148:32, 1993.

707. Murphy RLH Jr, Ferris BG Jr, Burgess WA, et al: Effects of low concentrations of asbestos: Clinical, environmental, radiologic and epidemiologic observations in shipyard pipe coverers and controls. N Engl J Med 285:1271, 1971.

708. Mitchell CA, Charney M, Schoenberg JB: Early lung disease in asbestos-product workers. Lung 154:261, 1978.

709. Shirai F, Kudoh S, Shibuya A, et al: Crackles in asbestos workers: Auscultation and lung sound analysis. Br J Dis Chest 75:386, 1981.

710. Begin R, Cantin A, Berthiaume Y, et al: Clinical features to stage alveolitis in asbestos workers. Am J Ind Med 8:521, 1985.

711. Huuskonen MS: Clinical features, mortality and survival of patients with asbestosis. Scand J Work Environ Health 4:265, 1978.

712. Picado C, Roisin RR, Sala H, et al: Diagnosis of asbestosis: Clinical, radiological and lung function data in 42 patients. Lung 162:325, 1984.

713. Al Jarad N, Davies SW, Logan-Sinclair R, et al: Lung crackle characteristics in patients with asbestosis. Respir Med 88:37, 1994.

714. Coutts II, Gilson JC, Kerr IH, et al: Significance of finger clubbing in asbestosis. Thorax 42:117, 1987.

715. Fischbein L, Namade M, Sach RN, et al: Chronic constrictive pericarditis associated with asbestosis. Chest 94:646, 1988.

716. Bégin R, Cantin A, Drapeau G, et al: Pulmonary uptake of gallium-67 in asbestos-exposed humans and sheep. Am Rev Respir Dis 127:623, 1983.

717. Gellert AR, Perry D, Langford JA, et al: Asbestosis: Bronchoalveolar lavage fluid proteins and their relationship to pulmonary epithelial permeability. Chest 88:730, 1985.

718. Miller A: Pulmonary function in asbestosis and asbestos-related pleural disease. Environ Res 61:1, 1993.

719. Miller A, Lilis R, Godbold J, et al: Relationship of pulmonary function to radiographic interstitial fibrosis in 2,611 long-term asbestos insulators. Am Rev Respir Dis 145:263, 1992.

720. Griffith DE, Garcia JG, Dodson RF, et al: Airflow obstruction in nonsmoking, asbestos and mixed dust-exposed workers. Lung 171:213, 1993.

721. Miller A, Lilis R, Godbold J, et al: Spirometric impairments in long-term insulators. Chest 105:175, 1994.

722. Fournier-Massey G, Becklake MR: Pulmonary function profiles in Quebec asbestos workers. Bull Physiopathol Respir (Nancy) 11:429, 1975.

723. Kilburn KH, Warshaw RH: Airways obstruction from asbestos exposure. Chest 106:1061, 1994.

724. Barnhart S, Hudson LD, Mason SE, et al: Total lung capacity: An insensitive measure of impairment in patients with asbestosis and chronic obstructive pulmonary disease? Chest 93:299, 1988.

725. Kilburn KH, Warshar RH: Total lung capacity in asbestosis: A comparison of radiographic and body plethysmographic methods. Am J Med Sci 305:84, 1993.

726. Barnhart S, Hudson LD, Mason SE, et al: Total lung capacity—an insensitive measure of impairment in patients with asbestosis and chronic onstructive pulmonary disease? Chest 93:299, 1988.

727. Kilburn KH, Miller A, Warshaw RH: Measuring lung volumes in advanced asbestosis: Comparability of plethysmographic and radiographic versus helium rebreathing and single breath methods. Respir Med 87:115, 1993.

728. Chen CR, Chang HY, Suo J, et al: Occupational exposure and respiratory morbidity among asbestos workers in Taiwan. J Formos Med Assoc 91:1138, 1992.

729. Osim EE, Esin RA, Fossung FE, et al: Ventilatory function in Nigerian asbestos factory workers. East Afr Med J 69:254, 1992.

730. Bader ME, Bader RA, Selikoff IJ: Pulmonary function in asbestosis of the lung: An alveolar-capillary block syndrome. Am J Med 30:235, 1961.

731. Leathart GL: Clinical, bronchographic, radiological and physiological observations in ten cases of asbestosis. Br J Ind Med 17:213, 1960.

732. Wang ML, Lu PL: Lung function studies of asbestos workers. Scand J Work Environ Health 11(Suppl 4):34, 1985.

733. Jodoin G, Gibbs GW, Macklem PT, et al: Early effects of asbestos exposure on lung function. Am Rev Respir Dis 104:525, 1971.

734. Smith DD, Agostoni PG: The discriminatory value of the P(A-a) O_2 during exercise in the detection of asbestosis in asbestos exposed workers. Chest 95:52, 1989.

734a. Divertie MB, Cassan SM, Brown AL Jr: Ultrastructural morphometry of the diffusion surface in a case of pulmonary asbestosis. Mayo Clin Proc 50:193, 1975.

735. Cookson WO, Musk AW, Glancy JJ: Asbestosis and cryptogenic fibrosing alveolitis: A radiological and functional comparison. Aust N Z J Med 14:626, 1984.

736. Agust AGN, Roca J, Rodriguez-Roisin R, et al: Different patterns of gas exchange response to exercise in asbestosis and idiopathic pulmonary fibrosis. Eur Respir J 1:510, 1988.

737. Al Jarad N, Poulakis N, Pearson MC, et al: Assessment of asbestos-induced pleural disease by computed tomography—correlation with chest radiograph and lung function. Respir Med 85:203, 1991.

738. Broderick A, Fuortes L, Merchant JA, et al: Pleural determinants of restrictive lung function and respiratory symptoms in an asbestos-exposed population. Chest 101:684, 1992.

739. Schwartz DA, Fuortes LJ, Galvin JR, et al: Asbestos-induced pleural fibrosis and impaired lung function. Am Rev Respir Dis 141:321, 1990.

740. Bourbeau J, Ernst P, Chrome J, et al: The relationship between respiratory impairment and asbestos-related pleural abnormality in an active work force. Am Rev Respir Dis 142:837, 1990.

741. Cotes JE, King B: Relationship of lung function to radiographic reading (ILO) in patients with asbestos related lung disease. Thorax 43:777, 1988.

742. Kilburn KH, Warshaw RH: Abnormal lung function associated with asbestos disease of the pleura, the lung, and both: A comparative analysis. Thorax 46:33, 1991.

743. Kilburn KH, Warshaw R: Pulmonary functional impairment associated with pleural asbestos disease. Chest 98:965, 1990.

744. Kilburn KH, Warshaw RH: Abnormal pulmonary function associated with diaphragmatic pleural plaques due to exposure to asbestos. Br J Ind Med 47:611, 1990.

745. Wright PH, Hanson A, Kreel L, et al: Respiratory function changes after asbestos pleurisy. Thorax 35:31, 1980.

746. Cookson WO, Musk AW, Glancy JJ: Pleural thickening and gas transfer in asbestosis. Thorax 38:657, 1983.

747. Agostoni P, Smith DD, Schoene RB, et al: Evaluation of breathlessness in asbestos workers: Results of exercise testing. Am Rev Respir Dis 135:812, 1987.

748. Miller A, Bhuptsani A, Sloane MF, et al: Cardiorespiratory responses to incremental exercise in patients with asbestos-related pleural thickening and normal or slightly abnormal lung function. Chest 103:1045, 1993.

749. Shih JF, Wilson JS, Broderick A, et al: Asbestos-induced pleural fibrosis and impaired exercise physiology. Chest 105:1370, 1994.

750. Becklake MR: Asbestos-related diseases of the lungs and pleura: Current clinical issues. Am Rev Respir Dis 126:187, 1982.

751. Vianna NJ, Polan AK: Non-occupational exposure to asbestos and malignant mesothelioma in females. Lancet 1:1061, 1978

752. Stoeckle JD, Oliver LC, Hardy HL: Women with asbestosis in a medical clinic: Under reported women workers, delayed diagnosis and smoking. Women Health 7:31, 1982.

753. Dumortier P, De Vuyst P, Strauss P, et al: Asbestos bodies in bronchoalveolar lavage fluids of brake lining and asbestos cement workers. Br J Ind Med 47:91, 1990.

754. Dodson RF, O'Sullivan M, Corn CJ, et al: Analysis of ferruginous bodies in bronchoalveolar lavage from foundry workers. Br J Ind Med 50:1032, 1993.

755. Tuomi T, Oksa P, Anttila S, et al: Fibres and asbestos bodies in bronchoalveolar lavage fluids of asbestos sprayers. Br J Ind Med 49:480, 1992.

756. Schwartz DA, Galvin JR, Burmeister LF, et al: The clinical utility and reliability of asbestos bodies in bronchoalveolar fluid. Am Rev Respir Dis 144:684, 1991.

757. Teschler H, Konietzko N, Schoenfeld B, et al: Distribution of asbestos bodies in the human lung as determined by bronchoalveolar lavage. Am Rev Respir Dis 147:1211, 1993.

758. Teschler H, Thompson AB, Dollenkamp R, et al: Relevance of asbestos bodies in sputum. Eur Respir J 9:680, 1996.

759. Lerman Y, Ribak J, Selikoff IJ: Hazards of lung biopsy in asbestos workers. Br J Ind Med 43:165, 1986.

760. Kohyama N, Kyono H, Yokoyama K, et al: Evaluation of low-level asbestos exposure by transbronchial lung biopsy with analytical electron microscopy. J Electron Microsc 42:315, 1993.

761. Monso E, Tura JM, Pujadas J, et al: Lung dust content in idiopathic pulmonary fibrosis: A study with scanning electron microscopy and energy dispersive x-rays and analysis. Br J Ind Med 48:327, 1991.

762. Rockoff SD, Schwartz A: Roentgenographic underestimation of early asbestosis by international radiation classification. Chest 93:1089, 1988.

763. Staples CA, Gamsu G, Ray CS, et al: High resolution computed tomography and lung function in asbestos-exposed workers with normal chest radiographs. Am Rev Respir Dis 139:1502, 1989.

764. Bégin R, Ostiguy GR, Filion, et al: Computed tomography in the early detection of asbestosis. Br J Ind Med 50:689, 1993.

765. Klaas VE: A diagnostic approach to asbestosis, utilizing clinical criteria, high resolution computed tomography, and gallium scanning. Am J Ind Med 23:801, 1993.

766. Dujic Z, Tocilj J, Saric M: Early detection of interstitial lung disease in asbestos exposed nonsmoking workers by mid-expiratory flow rate and high resolution computed tomography. Br J Ind Med 48:663, 1991.

767. Akira M, Yokoyama K, Yamamoto S, et al: Early asbestosis: Evaluation with high resolution CT. Radiology 178:409, 1991.

768. Neri S, Antonelli A, Falaschi F, et al: Findings from high resolution computed tomography of the lung and pleura of symptom free workers exposed to amosite who had normal chest radiographs and pulmonary function tests. Occup Environ Med 51:239, 1994.

769. Gevenois PA, De Vuyst P, Dedeire S, et al: Conventional and high-resolution CT in asymptomatic asbestos-exposed workers. Acta Radiol 35:226, 1994.

770. Hayes AA, Mullan B, Lovegrove FT, et al: Gallium lung scanning and bronchoalveolar lavage in crocidolite-exposed workers. Chest 96:22, 1989.

771. Payne CR, Jaques P, Kerr IH: Lung folding simulating peripheral pulmonary neoplasm (Blesovsky's syndrome). Thorax 35:936, 1980.

772. Inoshita T, Boyd WJ: Rounded atelectasis shown by computerized tomography. South Med J 79:764, 1986.

773. Markoitz SB, Morabia A, Lilis R, et al: Clinical predictors of mortality from asbestosis in the North American insulator cohort, 1981 to 1991. Am J Respir Crit Care Med 156:101, 1997.

774. McDonald JC: Asbestos and lung cancer: Has the case been proven? Chest 78(Suppl):374, 1980.

775. McDonald JC, McDonald AD: Epidemiology of asbestos-related lung cancer. In Asbestos-Related Malignancy. Orlando, Grune & Stratton, 1986.

776. McDonald JC, Liddell FDK, Gibbs GW, et al: Dust exposure and mortality in chrysotile mining, 1910–75. Br J Ind Med 37:11, 1980.

777. McDonald JC, Liddell FDK, Dufresne A, et al: The 1891–1920 birth cohort of Quebec chrysotile miners and millers: Mortality 1976–88. Br J Ind Med 50:1073, 1993.

778. Castleman BI: Asbestos and cancer: History and public policy. Br J Ind Med 48:427, 1991.

779. McDonald AD, Case BW, Churg A, et al: Mesothelioma in Quebec chrysotile miners and millers: Epidemiology and aetiology. Ann Occup Hyg 41:707, 1997.

780. Sluis-Cremer GK: The relationship between asbestosis and bronchial cancer. Chest 78(Suppl):380, 1980.

781. Selikoff IJ, Bader RA, Bader ME, et al: Asbestosis and neoplasia. Am J Med 42:487, 1967.

782. Weill H, Hughes J, Waggenspack C: Influence of dose and fiber type on respiratory malignancy risk in asbestos cement manufacturing. Am Rev Respir Dis 120:345, 1979.

783. Stovin PGI, Partridge P: Pulmonary asbestos and dust content in East Africa. Thorax 37:185, 1982.

784. Baba K: Indications of an increase of occupational pleural mesothelioma in Japan. Sangyo Ika Daigaku Zasshi 5:3, 1983.

785. McDonald AD, Fry JS, Woolley AJ, et al: Dust exposure and mortality in an American chrysotile textile plant. Br J Ind Med 40:361, 1983.

786. Wagner JC, Moncrieff CB, Coles R, et al: Correlation between fibre content of the lungs and disease in naval stockyard workers. Br J Ind Med 43:391, 1986.

787. Hughes JM, Weill H, Hammad YY: Mortality of workers employed in two asbestos cement manufacturing plants. Br J Ind Med 44:161, 1987.

788. Leading article: Asbestos pollution and pleural plaques. Med J Aust 1:444, 1981.

789. Albin M, Johansson L, Pooley FD, et al: Mineral fibres, fibrosis, and asbestos bodies in lung tissue from deceased asbestos cement workers. Br J Ind Med 47:767, 1990.

790. Hourihane DO: The pathology of mesotheliomata and an analysis of their association with asbestos exposure. Thorax 19:268, 1964.

791. Enticknap JB, Smither WJ: Peritoneal tumours in asbestosis. Br J Ind Med 21:20, 1964.

792. Selikoff IJ, Churg J, Hammond EC: Asbestos exposure and neoplasia. JAMA 188:22, 1964.

793. Kishimoto T: Intensity of exposure to asbestos in metropolitan Kure City as estimated by autopsied cases. Cancer 69:2598, 1992.

794. Selikoff IJ, Hammond EC: Asbestos and smoking (editorial). JAMA 242:458, 1979.

795. Snell PM, McGill P: Asbestos and laryngeal carcinoma. Lancet 2:416, 1973.

796. Newhouse ML, Berry G: Asbestos and laryngeal carcinoma. Lancet 2:615, 1973.

797. Libshitz HI, Wershba MS, Atkinson GW, et al: Asbestosis and carcinoma of the larynx: A possible association. JAMA 228:1571, 1974.

798. Raffin E, Lynge E, Juel K, et al: Incidence of cancer and mortality among employees in the asbestos cement industry in Denmark. Br J Ind Med 46:90, 1989.

799. Kishimoto T, Ono T, Okada K: Acute myelocytic leukemia after exposure to asbestos. Cancer 62:787, 1988.

800. Gerber MA: Asbestosis and neoplastic disorders of the hematopoietic system. Am J Clin Pathol 53:204, 1970.

801. Albin M, Jakobsson K, Attewell R, et al: Mortality and cancer morbidity in cohorts of asbestos cement workers and referents. Br J Ind Med 47:602, 1990.

802. Sanden A, Järvholm B, Larsson S: The importance of lung function, nonmalignant disease associated with asbestos, and symptoms as predictors of ischaemic heart disease in shipyard workers exposed to asbestos. Br J Ind Med 50:785, 1993.

803. McDonald JC, Liddell FDK, Dufresne A, et al: The 1891–1920 birth cohort of Quebec chrysotile miners and millers: Mortality 1976–88. Br J Ind Med 50:1073, 1993.

804. Segarra-Obiol F, Lopez-Ibanez P, Perez NJ: Asbestosis and tuberculosis. Am J Ind Med 4:755, 1983.

805. Armstrong BK, de Klerk NH, Musk AW, et al: Mortality in miners and millers of crocidolite in Western Australia. Br J Ind Med 45:5, 1988.

806. Gysbrechts C, Michiels E, Verbeken E, et al: Interstitial lung disease more than 40 years after a 5 year occupational exposure to talc. Eur Respir J 11:1425, 1998.

807. Hildick-Smith GY: The biology of talc. Br J Ind Med 33:217, 1976.

808. Messite J, Reddin G, Kleinfeld M: Pulmonary talcosis, a clinical and environmental study. AMA Arch Ind Health 20:408, 1959.

809. Wegman DH, Peters JM, Boundy MG, et al: Evaluation of respiratory effects in miners and millers exposed to talc free of asbestos and silica. Br J Ind Med 39:233, 1982.

810. Gamble JF, Fellner W, Dimeo MJ: An epidemiologic study of a group of talc workers. Am Rev Respir Dis 119:741, 1979.

811. Ahlmark A, Bruce T, Nyström A: Pneumoconiosis (talcosis) in soapstone workers. Nord Med 59:287, 1958.

812. Berner A, Gylseth B, Levy F: Talc dust pneumoconiosis. Acta Pathol Microbiol Scand (A) 89:17, 1981.

813. Nam K, Gracey DR: Pulmonary talcosis from cosmetic talcum powder. JAMA 221:492, 1972.

814. Wells IP, Dubbins PA, Whimster WF: Pulmonary disease caused by the inhalation of cosmetic talcum powder. Br J Radiol 52:586, 1979.

815. Wells IP, Dubbins PA, Whimster WF: Pulmonary disease caused by the inhalation of cosmetic talcum powder. Br J Radiol 52:586, 1979.

816. Leading article: Accidental inhalation of talcum powder. BMJ 4:5, 1969.

817. Gould SR, Barnardo DE: Respiratory distress after talc inhalation. Br J Dis Chest 66:230, 1970.

818. Bouchàma A, Chastre J, Gaudichet A, et al: Acute pneumonitis with bilateral pleural effusion after talc pleurodesis. Chest 86:795, 1984.

819. Research Committee of the British Thoracic Association and the Medical Research Council Pneumoconiosis Unit: A survey of the long-term effects of talc and kaolin pleurodesis. Br J Dis Chest 73:285, 1979.

820. de Vuyst P, Dumortier P, Leophonte P, et al: Mineralogical analysis of bronchoalveolar lavage in talc pneumoconiosis. Eur J Respir Dis 70:150, 1987.

821. Gibbs AE, Pooley FD, Griffiths DM, et al: Talc pneumoconiosis: A pathologic and mineralogic study. Hum Pathol 23:1344, 1992.

822. Vallyathan NV, Craighead JE: Pulmonary pathology in workers exposed to nonasbestiform talc. Hum Pathol 12:28, 1981.

823. Gibbs AE, Pooley FD, Griffiths DM, et al: Talc pneumoconiosis: A pathologic and mineralogic study. Hum Pathol 23:1344, 1992.

824. Vallyathan NV, Green FHY, Craighead JE: Recent advances in the study of mineral pneumoconiosis. In Sommers SC, Rosen PP (eds): Pathology Annual, part II. New York, Appleton-Century-Crofts, 1980, p 15.

825. Lapenas DJ, Davis GS, Gale PN, et al: Mineral dusts as etiologic agents in pulmonary fibrosis: The diagnostic role of analytical scanning electron microscopy. Am J Clin Pathol 78:701, 1982.

826. Siegal W, Smith AR, Greenburg L: The dust inhaled in tremolite talc mining, including roentgenological findings in talc workers. Am J Roentgenol 49:11, 1943.

827. Kleinfeld M, Messite J, Tabershaw IR: Talc pneumoconiosis. AMA Arch Ind Health 12:66, 1955.

828. Seeler AO, Gryboski JS, MacMahon HE: Talc pneumoconiosis. AMA Arch Ind Health 19:392, 1959.

829. Porro FW, Patton JR, Hobbs AA Jr: Pneumoconiosis in the talc industry. Am J Roentgenol 47:507, 1942.

830. Alivisatos GP, Pontikakis AE, Terzis B: Talcosis of unusually rapid development. Br J Ind Med 12:43, 1955.

831. Kleinfeld M, Messite J, Shapiro J, et al: Effect of talc dust inhalation on lung function. Arch Environ Health 10:431, 1965.

832. Tukiainen P, Nickels J, Taskinen E, et al: Pulmonary granulomatous reaction: Talc pneumoconiosis or chronic sarcoidosis? Br J Ind Med 41:84, 1984.

833. Rubino GF, Scansetti G, Piolatto G, et al: Mortality study of talc miners and millers. J Occup Med 18:186, 1976.

834. Kleinfeld M, Messite J, Zaki MM: Mortality experience among talc workers: A followup study. J Occup Med 16:345, 1974.

835. Steele WT, Tabershaw IR: The mortality experience of upstate New York talc workers. J Occup Med 24:480, 1982.

835a. de Coster C, Verstraeten JM, Dumortier P, et al: Atypical mycobacteriosis as a complication of talc pneumoconiosis. Eur Respir J 9:1757, 1996.

836. Kleinfeld M, Messite J, Shapiro J, et al: Effect of talc dust inhalation on lung function. Arch Environ Health 10:431, 1965.

837. Kleinfeld M, Messite J, Shapiro J, et al: Lung function in talc workers, a comparative physiologic study of workers exposed to fibrous and granular talc dust. Arch Environ Health 9:559, 1964.

838. Gamble J, Greife A, Hancock J: An epidemiological-industrial hygiene study of talc workers. Ann Occup Hyg 26:841, 1982.

839. Craighead JE, Emerson RJ, Stanley DE: Slateworker's pneumoconiosis. Hum Pathol 23:1098, 1992.

840. Lockey JE, Brooks SM, Jarabek AM, et al: Pulmonary changes after exposure to vermiculite contaminated with fibrous tremolite. Am Rev Respir Dis 129:952, 1984.

841. Davies D, Cotton R: Mica pneumoconiosis. Br J Ind Med 40:22, 1983.

842. Dreesen WC, Dallavalle JM, Edwards TI, et al: Pneumoconiosis among mica and pegmatite workers. Public Health Bulletin No. 250. Washington, DC, US Public Health Service, 1940, pp 1–74.

843. Vorwald AJ, MacEwen JD, Smith RG: Mineral content of lung in certain pneumoconioses. Arch Pathol 74:267, 1962.

844. Pimentel JC, Menezes AP: Pulmonary and hepatic granulomatous disorders due to the inhalation of cement and mica dusts. Thorax 33:219, 1978.

845. Skulberg KR, Gylseth B, Skaug V, et al: Mica pneumoconiosis: A literature review. Scand J Work Environ Health 11:65, 1985.

846. Jones RN, Weill H, Parkes WR: Disease related to nonasbestos silicates. In Parkes WR (ed): Occupational Lung Disorders. 3rd ed. Oxford, Butterworth-Heinemann, 1994, p 557.

847. Landas SK, Schwartz DA: Mica-associated pulmonary interstitial fibrosis. Am Rev Respir Dis 144:718, 1991.

848. Phibbs BP, Sundin RE, Mitchell RS: Silicosis in Wyoming bentonite workers. Am Rev Respir Dis 103:1, 1971.

849. Sakula A: Pneumoconiosis due to Fuller's earth. Thorax 16:176, 1961.

850. Gibbs AR, Pooley FD: Fuller's earth (montmorillonite) pneumoconiosis. Occup Environ Med 51:644, 1994.

851. McNally WD, Trostler IS: Severe pneumoconiosis caused by inhalation of Fuller's earth. J Ind Hyg 23:118, 1941.

852. Sepulveda M-J, Vallyathan V, Attfield MO, et al: Pneumoconiosis and lung function in a group of kaolin workers. Am Rev Respir Dis 127:231, 1983.

853. Lapenas D, Gale P, Kennedy T, et al: Kaolin pneumoconiosis: Radiologic, pathologic, and mineralogic findings. Am Rev Respir Dis 130:282, 1984.

854. Lesser M, Zia M, Kilburn KH: Silicosis in kaolin workers and firebrick makers. South Med J 71:1242, 1978.

855. Altekruse EB, Chaudhary BA, Pearson MG, et al: Kaolin dust concentrations and pneumoconiosis at a kaolin mine. Thorax 39:436, 1984.

856. Wagner JC, Pooley FD, Gibbs A, et al: Inhalation of china stone and china clay dusts: Relationship between the mineralogy of dust retained in the lungs and pathological changes. Thorax 41:190, 1986.

857. Herman SJ, Olscamp GC, Weisbrod GL: Pulmonary kaolin granulomas. J Can Assoc Radiol 33:279, 1982.

858. Lapenas DJ, Gale PN: Kaolin pneumoconiosis: A case report. Arch Pathol Lab Med 107:650, 1983.

859. Edenfield RW: A clinical and roentgenological study of kaolin workers. Arch Environ Health 1:392, 1960.

860. Sheers G: Prevalence of pneumoconiosis in Cornish kaolin workers. Br J Ind Med 21:218, 1964.

861. Oldham PD: Pneumoconiosis in Cornish china clay workers. Br J Ind Med 40:131, 1983.

862. Kennedy T, Rawlings W Jr, Baser M, et al: Pneumoconiosis in Georgia kaolin workers. Am Rev Respir Dis 127:215, 1983.

863. Hale LW: Pneumoconiosis in Cornwall. In King EJ, Fletcher CM (eds): Industrial Pulmonary Diseases: A Symposium Held at the Postgraduate Medical School of London, 18–20 September 1957 and 25–27 March 1958. London, J & A Churchill, 1960, pp 139–145.

864. Morgan WKC, Donner A, Higgins ITT, et al: The effects of kaolin on the lung. Am Rev Respir Dis 138:813, 1988.

865. Rundle EM, Sugar ET, Ogle CJ: Analyses of the 1990 chest health survey of china clay workers. Br J Ind Med 50:913, 1993.

866. Baser ME, Kennedy TP, Dodson R, et al: Differences in lung function and prevalence of pneumoconiosis between two kaolin plants. Br J Ind Med 46:773, 1989.

867. Bristol LJ: Pneumoconioses caused by asbestos and by other siliceous and nonsiliceous dusts. Semin Roentgenol 2:283, 1967.

868. Hale LW, Gough J, King EJ, et al: Pneumoconiosis of kaolin workers. Br J Ind Med 13:251, 1956.

869. Lynch KM, McIver FA: Pneumoconiosis from exposure to kaolin dust: Kaolinosis. Am J Pathol 30:1117, 1954.

870. Baris YI, Artvinli M, Sahin AA, et al: Diffuse lung fibrosis due to fibrous zeolite (erionite) exposure. Eur J Respir Dis 70:122, 1987.

871. Casey KR, Shigeoka JW, Rom WM, et al: Zeolite exposure and associated pneumoconiosis. Chest 87:837, 1985.

872. Baris YI, Sahin AA, Ozesmi M, et al: An outbreak of pleural mesothelioma and chronic fibrosing pleurisy in the village of Karain/Ürgüp in Anatolia. Thorax 33:181, 1978.

873. Baris YI, Saracci R, Simonato L, et al: Malignant mesothelioma and radiological chest abnormalities in two villages in Central Turkey. Lancet 1:984, 1981.

874. Artvinli M, Baris YI: Environmental fiber-induced pleuro-pulmonary diseases in an Anatolian village: An epidemiologic study. Arch Environ Health 37:177, 1982.

875. Musk AW, Greville HW, Tribe AE: Pulmonary disease from occupational exposure to an artificial aluminum silicate used for cat litter. Br J Ind Med 37:367, 1980.

876. Barrie HJ, Gosselin L: Massive pneumoconiosis from a rock dust containing no free silica: Nepheline lung. Arch Environ Health 1:109, 1960.

877. Olscamp G, Herman SJ, Weisbrod GL: Nepheline rock dust pneumoconiosis: A report of 2 cases. Radiology 142:29, 1982.

878. Huuskonen MS, Tossavainen A, Koskinen H, et al: Wollastonite exposure and lung fibrosis. Environ Res 30:291, 1983.

879. Huuskonen MS, Jarvisalo J, Koskinen H, et al: Preliminary results from a cohort of workers exposed to wollastonite in a Finnish limestone quarry. Scand J Work Environ Health 9:169, 1983.

880. Hanke W, Sepulveda MJ, Watson A, et al: Respiratory morbidity in wollastonite workers. Br J Ind Med 41:474, 1984.
881. Clark TC, Harrington VA, Asta J, et al: Respiratory effects of exposure to dust in taconite mining and processing. Am Rev Respir Dis 121:959, 1980.
882. Gylseth B, Norseth T, Skaug V: Amphibole fibers in a taconite mine and in the lungs of the miners. Am J Ind Med 2:175, 1981.
883. Newman LS, Kreiss K, King TE Jr, et al: Pathologic and immunologic alterations in early stages of beryllium disease: Re-examination of disease definition and natural history. Am Rev Respir Dis 139:1479, 1989.
884. Morgan WKC: Magnetite pneumoconiosis. J Occup Med 20:762, 1978.
885. Harding HE, McLaughlin AIG, Doig AT: Clinical, radiographic, and pathological studies of the lungs of electric-arc and oxacetylene welders. Lancet 2:394, 1958.
886. Stacy BD, King EJ, Harrison CV, et al: Tissue changes in rats' lungs caused by hydroxides, oxides and phosphates of aluminium and iron. J Pathol Bacteriol 77:417, 1959.
887. Harding HE, Grout JLA, Davies TAL: The experimental production of x-ray shadows in the lungs by inhalation of industrial dusts: I. Iron oxide. Br J Ind Med 4:223, 1947.
888. Mclaughlin AIG: Iron and other radiopaque dusts. In King EJ, Fletcher CM (eds): Industrial Pulmonary Diseases: A Symposium Held at the Postgraduate Medical School of London, 18–20 September 1957 and 25–27 March 1958. London, J & A Churchill, 1960, pp 146–167.
889. Hunnicutt TN Jr, Cracovaner DJ, Myles JT: Spirometric measurements in welders. Arch Environ Health 8:661, 1964.
890. Sferlazza SJ, Beckett WS: The respiratory health of welders. Am Rev Respir Dis 143:1134, 1991.
891. Johnson NF, Haslam PL, Dewar A, et al: Identification of inorganic dust particles in bronchoalveolar lavage macrophages by energy dispersive x-ray microanalysis. Arch Environ Health 41:133, 1986.
892. Guidotti TL, Abraham JL, DeNee PB, et al: Arc welders' pneumoconiosis: Application of advanced scanning electron microscopy. Arch Environ Health 33:117, 1978.
893. Funahashi A, Schlueter DP, Pintar K, et al: Welders' pneumoconiosis: Tissue elemental microanalysis by energy dispersive x-ray analysis. Br J Ind Med 45:14, 1988.
894. Fontenot AP, Kotzin BL, Comment CE, et al: Expansions of T-cell subsets expressing particular T-cell receptor–variable regions in chronic beryllium disease. Am J Respir Cell Mol Biol 18:581, 1998.
895. Enzer N, Sander OA: Chronic lung changes in electric arc welders. J Ind Hyg 20:333, 1938.
896. Harding HE, McLaughlin AIG, Doig AT: Clinical, radiographic and pathological studies of the lungs of electric arc and oxyacetylene welders. Lancet 2:394, 1958.
897. Plamenac P, Nikulin A, Pikula B: Cytologic changes of the respiratory epithelium in iron foundry workers. Acta Cytol 18:34, 1974.
898. Attfield MD, Ross DS: Radiological abnormalities in electric-arc welders. Br J Ind Med 35:117, 1978.
899. McLaughlin AIG, Grout JLA, Barrie HJ, et al: Iron oxide dust and the lungs of silver finishers. Lancet 1:337, 1945.
900. Sander OA: The nonfibrogenic (benign) pneumoconioses. Semin Roentgenol 2:312, 1967.
901. Antti-Poika M, Hassi J, Pyy L: Respiratory diseases in arc welders. Int Arch Occup Environ Health 40:225, 1977.
902. Low I, Mitchell C: Respiratory disease in foundry workers. Br J Ind Med 42:101, 1985.
903. Hjortsberg U, Orbaek P, Arborelius Jr M: Small airways dysfunction among nonsmoking shipyard arc welders. Br J Ind Med 49:441, 1992.
904. Kilburn KH, Warshaw RH: Pulmonary functional impairment from years of arc welding. Am J Med 87:62, 1989.
905. Billings CG, Howard P: Occupational siderosis and welder's lung: A review. Monaldi Arch Chest Dis 48:304, 1993.
906. Faulds JS: Haematite pneumoconiosis in Cumberland miners. J Clin Pathol 10:187, 1957.
907. McLaughlin AIG, Harding HE: The causes of death in iron and steel workers (nonfoundry). Br J Ind Med 18:33, 1961.
908. Mun JM, Meyer-Bisch C, Pham QT, et al: Risk of lung cancer among iron ore miners: A proportional mortality study of 1,075 deceased miners in Lorraine, France. J Occup Med 29:762, 1987.
909. Chau N, Benamghar L, Pham QT, et al: Mortality of iron miners in Lorraine (France): Relations between lung function and respiratory symptoms and subsequent mortality. Br J Ind Med 50:1017, 1993.
910. Chen SY, Hayes RB, Liang SR, et al: Mortality experience of haematite mine workers in China. Br J Ind Med 47:175, 1990.
911. Pham QT, Teculescu D, Bruant A, et al: Iron miners—a ten year follow up. Eur J Epidemiol 8:594, 1992.
912. Smith GH, Williams FL, Lloyd OL: Respiratory cancer and air pollution from iron foundries in a Scottish town: An epidemiological and environmental study. Br J Ind Med 44:795, 1987.
913. Barrie HJ, Harding HE: Argyro-siderosis of the lungs in silver finishers. Br J Ind Med 4:225, 1947.
914. Robertson AJ, Rivers D, Nagelschmidt G, et al: Benign pneumoconiosis due to tin dioxide. Lancet 1:1089, 1961.
915. Robertson AJ, Whitaker PH: Radiological changes in pneumoconiosis due to tin oxide. J Fac Radiol 6:224, 1955.
916. Robertson AJ: Pneumoconiosis due to tin oxide. In King EJ, Fletcher CM (eds): Industrial Pulmonary Diseases: A Symposium Held at the Postgraduate Medical School of London, September 18–20, 1957, and March 25–27, 1958. London, J & A Churchill, 1960, pp 168–184.
917. Arrigoni A: La pneumoconiosi da bario. Clin Med Ital 64:299, 1933.
918. Huppertz A: Barytlunge. [Baritosis.] Fortschr Röntgenstr 89:146, 1958.
919. Lévi-Valensi P, Drif M, Dat A, et al: A propos de 57 observations de barytose pulmonaire. Résultats d'une enquète systématique dans une usine de baryte. [Observations on 57 cases of barium sulfate pneumoconiosis: Results of a systematic investigation in a barium sulfate mill.] J Fr Med Chir Thorac 20:443, 1966.
920. Pendergrass EP, Greening RR: Baritosis: Report of a case. AMA Arch Ind Hyg 7:44, 1953.
921. Doig AT: Baritosis: A benign pneumoconiosis. Thorax 31:30, 1976.
922. McCallum RI: Detection of antimony in process workers' lungs by X-radiation. Trans Soc Occup Med 17:134, 1967.
923. Potkonjak V, Pavlovich M: Antimoniosis: A particular form of pneumoconiosis: I. Etiology, clinical and X-ray findings. Int Arch Occup Environ Health 51:199, 1983.
924. Cooper DA, Pendergrass EP, Vorwald AJ, et al: Pneumoconiosis among workers in an antimony industry. Am J Roentgenol 103:495, 1968.
925. Waring PM, Watling RJ: Rare earth deposits in a deceased movie projectionist. A new case of rare earth pneumoconiosis? Med J Aust 153:726, 1990.
926. Hoschek R: Röentgenologische lungenveränderungen durch seltene erden. Vorläufige mitteilung. [Roentgenologic lung changes by rare earth elements: Preliminary communication.] Zentralbl Arbeitsmed 14:281, 1964.
927. Suzuki KT, Kobayashi E, Ito Y, et al: Localization and health effects of lanthanum chloride instilled intratracheally into rats. Tox 76:141, 1992.
928. Cain H, Egner E, Ruska J: Ablagerungen seltener erden in der menschlichen lunge und in tierexperiment. [Deposits of rare earth metals in the lungs of man, and in experimental animals]. Virchows Arch 374:249, 1977.
929. Vocaturo G, Colombo F, Zanoni M, et al: Human exposure to heavy metals: Rare earth pneumoconiosis in occupational workers. Chest 83:780, 1983.
930. Haley PJ: Pulmonary toxicity of stable and radioactive lanthanides. Health Phys 61:809, 1991.
931. Sulotto F, Romano C, Berra A, et al: Rare-earth pneumoconiosis: A new case. Am J Ind Med 9:567, 1986.
932. Heuck F, Hoschek R: Cer-pneumoconiosis. Am J Roentgenol 104:777, 1968.
933. Eisenbud M, Lisson J: Epidemiological aspects of beryllium induced nonmalignant lung disease: A 30 year update. J Occup Med 25:196, 1983.
934. Kanarek DJ, Wainer RA, Chamberlin RI, et al: Respiratory illness in a population exposed to beryllium. Am Rev Respir Dis 108:1295, 1973.
935. Yoshida T, Shima S, Nagaoka K, et al: A study on the beryllium lymphocyte transformation test and the beryllium levels in working environment. Ind Health 35:374, 1997.
936. Kreiss K, Mroz MM, Newman LS, et al: Machining risk of beryllium disease and sensitization with median exposures below 2 micrograms/m³. Am J Ind Med 30:16, 1996.
937. Meyer KC: Beryllium and lung disease. Chest 106:942, 1994.
938. Kriebel D, Brain JD, Sprince NL, et al: The pulmonary toxicity of beryllium. Am Rev Respir Dis 137:464, 1988.
939. Kreiss K, Mroz MM, Zhen B, et al: Epidemiology of beryllium sensitization and disease in nuclear workers. Am Rev Respir Dis 148:985, 1993.
940. Stange AW, Hilmas DE, Furman NJ: Possible health risks from low level exposure to beryllium. Toxicology 111:213, 1996.
941. Cullen MR, Kominsky JR, Rossman MD, et al: Chronic beryllium disease in a precious metal refinery: Clinical, epidemiologic, and immunologic evidence for continuing risk from exposure to low level beryllium fume. Am Rev Respir Dis 135:201, 1987.
942. Kotloff RM, Richman PS, Greenacre JK, et al: Chronic beryllium disease in a dental laboratory technician. Am Rev Respir Dis 147:205, 1993.
943. Newman LS, Kreiss K: Nonoccupational beryllium disease masquerading as sarcoidosis: Identification by blood lymphocyte proliferative response to beryllium. Am Rev Respir Dis 145:1212, 1992.
944. Hazard JB: Pathologic changes of beryllium disease: The acute disease. AMA Arch Ind Health 19:179, 1959.
945. Frieman DG, Hardy HL: Beryllium disease. Hum Pathol 1:25, 1970.
946. Denardi JM, Van Ordstrand HS, Curtis GH: Berylliosis: Summary and survey of all clinical types in ten year period. Cleve Clin Q 19:171, 1952.
947. Momose T, Koike S, Sakamoto A, et al: Impaired pulmonary function in acute beryllium poisoning. Nihon Rinsho 17:1229, 1959.
948. American College of Chest Physicians Report of the Section on Nature and Prevalence Committee on Occupational Diseases of the Chest: Beryllium disease. Dis Chest 48:550, 1965.
949. Shima M, Ohta K: Three cases of acute pneumonitis due to beryllium inhalation. Jpn J Chest Dis 19:707, 1960.
950. Cotes JE, Gilson JC, McKerrow CB, et al: A long-term follow-up of workers exposed to beryllium. Br J Ind Med 40:13, 1983.
951. Deodhar SD, Barna B, Van Ordstrand HS: A study of the immunologic aspects of chronic berylliosis. Chest 63:309, 1973.
952. Hanifin JM, Epstein WI, Cline MJ: In vitro studies of granulomatous hypersensitivity to beryllium. J Invest Dermatol 55:284, 1970.
953. Henderson WR, Fukuyama K, Epstein WL, et al: In vitro demonstration of delayed hypersensitivity in patients with berylliosis. J Invest Dermatol 58:5, 1972.

954. Daniele RP: Cell-mediated immunity in pulmonary disease. Hum Pathol 17:154, 1986.

955. Williams WJ, Williams WR: Value of beryllium lymphocyte transformation tests in chronic beryllium disease and in potentially exposed workers. Thorax 38:41, 1983.

956. Rom WN, Lockey JE, Bang KM, et al: Reversible beryllium sensitization in a prospective study of beryllium workers. Arch Environ Health 38:302, 1983.

957. Saltini C, Winestock K, Kirby M, et al: Maintenance of alveolitis in patients with chronic beryllium disease by beryllium-specific helper T cells. N Engl J Med 320:1103, 1989.

958. Inoue Y, Barker E, Daniloff E, et al: Pulmonary epithelial cell injury and alveolar-capillary permeability in berylliosis. Am J Respir Crit Care Med 156:109, 1997.

959. Tinkle SS, Schwitters PW, Newman LS: Cytokine production by bronchoalveolar cells in chronic beryllium disease. Environ Health Perspect 104(Suppl 5):969, 1996.

960. Bost TW, Riches DWH, Schumacher B, et al: Alveolar macrophages from patients with beryllium disease and sarcoidosis express increased levels of mRNA for tumor necrosis factor-α and interleukin-6 but not interleukin-1β. Am J Respir Cell Mol Biol 10:506, 1994.

961. Tinkle SS, Newman LS: Beryllium-stimulated release of tumor necrosis factor alpha, interleukin-6, and their soluble receptors in chronic beryllium disease. Am J Respir Crit Care Med 156:1884, 1997.

962. Tinkle SS, Kittle LA, Schumacher BA, et al: Beryllium induces IL-2 and IFN-gamma in berylliosis. J Immunol 158:518, 1997.

963. Richeldi L, Sorrentino R, Saltini C: HLA-DPB1 glutamate 69: A genetic marker of beryllium disease. Science 262:242, 1993.

964. Richeldi L, Kreiss K, Mroz MM, et al: Interaction of genetic and exposure factors in the prevalence of berylliosis. Am J Ind Med 32:337, 1997.

965. Prine JR, Brokeshoulder SF, McVean DE, et al: Demonstration of the presence of beryllium in pulmonary granulomas. Am J Clin Pathol 45:448, 1966.

966. Williams WJ, Kelland D: New aid for diagnosing chronic beryllium disease (CBD): Laser ion mass analysis (LIMA). J Clin Pathol 39:900, 1986.

967. Robinson FR, Brokeshoulder SF, Thomas AA, et al: Microemission spectrochemical analysis of human lungs for beryllium. Am J Clin Pathol 49:821, 1968.

968. Sprince ML, Kazemi H, Hardy HL: Current (1975) problem of differentiating between beryllium disease and sarcoidosis. Ann N Y Acad Sci 278:654, 1976.

969. Gary JE, Schatzki R: Radiological abnormalities in chronic pulmonary disease due to beryllium. AMA Arch Ind Health 19:117, 1959.

970. Tebrock HE: Beryllium poisoning (berylliosis): X-ray manifestations and advances in treatment. Am J Surg 90:120, 1955.

971. Weber AL, Stoeckle JD, Hardy HL: Roentgenologic patterns in long-standing beryllium disease: Report of 8 cases. Am J Roentgenol 93:879, 1965.

972. Aronchick JM, Rossman MD, Miller WT: Chronic beryllium disease: Diagnosis, radiographic findings, and correlation with pulmonary function tests. Radiology 163:677, 1987.

973. Newman LS, Buschman DL, Newell JD Jr, Lynch DA: Beryllium disease: Assessment with CT. Radiology 190:835, 1994.

974. Brauner MW, Grenier P, Mompoint D, et al: Pulmonary sarcoidosis: Evaluation with high-resolution CT. Radiology 172:467, 1989.

975. Müller NL, Kullnig P, Miller RR: The CT findings of pulmonary sarcoidosis: Analysis of 25 patients. Am J Roentgenol 152:1179, 1989.

976. Harris KM, McConnochie K, Adams H: The computed tomographic appearances in chronic berylliosis. Clin Radiol 47:26, 1993.

977. Gevenois PA, Weyer RV, De Vuyst P: Beryllium disease: Assessment with CT. Radiology 193:283, 1994.

978. O'Brien AA, Moore DP, Keogh JA: Pulmonary berylliosis on corticosteroid therapy with cavitating lung lesions and aspergillomata: Report on a fatal case. Postgrad Med J 63:797, 1987.

979. Hardy HL: Beryllium disease: A continuing diagnostic problem. Am J Med Sci 242:150, 1961.

980. Hall TC, Wood CH, Stoeckle JD, et al: Case data from the beryllium registry. AMA Arch Ind Health 19:100, 1959.

981. Kelley WN, Goldfinger SE, Hardy HL: Hyperuricemia in chronic beryllium disease. Ann Intern Med 70:977, 1969.

982. Stockle JD, Hardy HL, Webber AL: Chronic beryllium disease: Long-term follow-up of sixty cases and selective review of the literature. Am J Med 46:545, 1969.

983. Newman LS, Orton R, Kreiss K: Serum angiotensin converting enzyme activity in chronic beryllium disease. Am Rev Respir Dis 146:39, 1992.

984. Newman LS, Bobka C, Schumacher B, et al: Compartmentalized immune response reflects clinical severity of beryllium disease Am J Respir Crit Care Med 150:135, 1994.

985. Norris GF, Peard MC: Berylliosis: Report of two cases, with special reference to the patch test. BMJ 1:378, 1963.

986. Curtis GH: The diagnosis of beryllium disease, with special reference to the patch tests. AMA Arch Ind Health 19:150, 1959.

987. Aronchick JM, Rossman MD, Miller WT: Chronic beryllium disease: Diagnosis, radiographic findings, and correlation with pulmonary function tests. Radiology 163:677, 1987.

988. Rossman MD, Kern JA, Elias JA, et al: Proliferative response of bronchoalveolar lymphocytes to beryllium: A test for chronic beryllium disease. Ann Intern Med 108:687, 1988.

989. Mroz MM, Kreiss K, Lezotte DC, et al: Reexamination of the blood lymphocyte transformation test in the diagnosis of chronic beryllium disease. J Allergy Clin Immunol 88:54, 1991.

990. Stokes RF, Rosman MD: Blood cell proliferation response to beryllium: Analysis by receiver-operating characteristics. J Occup Med 33:23, 1991.

991. Newman LS, Kreiss K, King TE Jr, et al: Pathologic and immunologic alterations in early stages of beryllium disease. Am Rev Respir Dis 139:1479, 1989.

992. Newman LS: Significance of the blood beryllium lymphocyte proliferation test. Environ Health Perspect 104(Suppl 5):953, 1996.

993. Harris J, Bartelson BB, Barker E, et al: Serum neopterin in chronic beryllium disease. Am J Ind Med 32:21, 1997.

994. Beryllium disease among workers in a spacecraft-manufacturing plant—California. MMWR 32:419, 425, 1983.

995. Lockey JE, Levin LS, Lemasters GK, et al: Longitudinal estimates of pulmonary function in refractory ceramic fiber manufacturing workers. Am J Respir Crit Care Med 157:1226, 1998.

996. Gaensler EA, Verstraeten JM, Weil WB, et al: Respiratory pathophysiology in chronic beryllium disease: Review of thirty cases with some observations after long-term steroid therapy. AMA Arch Ind Health 19:32, 1959.

997. Andrews JI, Kazemi H, Hardy HL: Patterns of lung dysfunction in chronic beryllium disease. Am Rev Respir Dis 100:791, 1969.

998. Pappas GP, Newman LS: Early pulmonary physiologic abnormalities in beryllium disease. Am Rev Respir Dis 148:661, 1993.

999. Kriebel D, Sprince N, Eisen E, et al: Beryllium exposure and pulmonary function: A cross sectional study of beryllium workers. Br J Ind Med 45:167, 1988.

1000. Sprince NL, Kanarek DJ, Weber AL, et al: Reversible respiratory disease in beryllium workers. Am Rev Respir Dis 117:1011, 1978.

1001. Nickell-Brady C, Hahn FF, Finch GL, et al: Analysis of K-ras, p53 and c-raf-1 mutations in beryllium-induced rat lung tumours. Carcinogenesis 15:257, 1994.

1002. Ward E, Okun A, Ruder A, et al: A mortality study of workers at seven beryllium processing plants. Am J Ind Med 22:885, 1992.

1003. Steenland K, Ward E: Lung cancer incidence among patients with beryllium disease: A cohort mortality study. J Natl Cancer Inst 83:1380, 1991.

1004. Jederlinic PJ, Abraham JL, Churg A, et al: Pulmonary fibrosis in aluminum oxide workers: Investigation of nine workers, with pathologic examination and microanalysis in three of them. Am Rev Respir Dis 142:1179, 1990.

1005. Abramson MJ, Wlodarczyk JH, Saunders NA, et al: Does aluminum smelting cause lung disease? Am Rev Respir Dis 139:1042, 1989.

1006. Gibbs GW: Mortality of aluminum reduction plant workers, 1950 through 1977. J Occupat Med 27:761, 1985.

1007. Bellot SM, Schade van Westrum JAFM, Wagenvoort CA, et al: Deposition of bauxite dust and pulmonary fibrosis. Pathol Res Pract 179:225, 1984.

1008. Townsend MC, Sussman NB, Enterline PE, et al: Radiographic abnormalities in relation to total dust exposure at a bauxite refinery and alumina-based chemical products plant. Am Rev Respir Dis 138:90, 1988.

1009. Mitchell J: Pulmonary fibrosis in an aluminum worker. Br J Ind Med 16:123, 1959.

1010. Mitchell J, Manning GB, Molyneux M, et al: Pulmonary fibrosis in workers exposed to finely powdered aluminum. Br J Ind Med 18:10, 1961.

1011. Edling NPG: Aluminum pneumoconiosis: A roentgendiagnostic study of five cases. Acta Radiol 56:170, 1961.

1012. Mclaughlin AIG, Kazantzis G, King E, et al: Pulmonary fibrosis and encephalopathy associated with the inhalation of aluminum dust. Br J Ind Med 19:253, 1962.

1013. DeVuyst P, DuMortier P, Schandene L, et al: Sarcoidlike lung granulomatosis induced by aluminum dusts. Am Rev Respir Dis 135:493, 1987.

1014. Herbert A, Sterling G, Abraham J, et al: Desquamative interstitial pneumonia in an aluminum welder. Hum Pathol 13:694, 1982.

1015. Vallyathan V, Bergeron WN, Robichaux PA, et al: Pulmonary fibrosis in an aluminum arc welder. Chest 81:372, 1982.

1016. Chen W, Monnat RJ Jr, Chen M, et al: Aluminum induced pulmonary granulomatosis. Hum Pathol 9:705, 1978.

1017. Miller R: Pulmonary alveolar proteinosis and aluminum dust exposure. Am Rev Respir Dis 130:312, 1984.

1018. DeVuyst P, Dumortier P, Rickaert F, et al: Occupational lung fibrosis in an aluminium polisher. Eur J Respir Dis 68:131, 1986.

1019. Jederlinic PJ, Abraham JL, Churg A, et al: Pulmonary fibrosis in aluminum oxide workers. Am Rev Respir Dis 142:1179, 1990.

1020. Pigott GH, Gaskell BA, Ishmael J: Effects of long term inhalation of alumina fibres in rats. Br J Exp Pathol 62:323, 1981.

1021. Musk AW, Beck BD, Greville HW, et al: Pulmonary disease from exposure to an artificial aluminum silicate: Further observations. Br J Ind Med 45:246, 1988.

1022. Denny JJ, Robson WD, Irwin DA: The prevention of silicosis by metallic aluminum: I. A preliminary report. Can Med Assoc J 37:1, 1937.

1023. Campbell IK, Cass JS, Cholak J, et al: Aluminum in the environment of man: A review of its hygienic status. AMA Arch Ind Health 15:359, 1957.

1024. Gross P, Harley RA Jr, deTreville RTP: Pulmonary reaction to metallic aluminum powders. Arch Environ Health 26:227, 1973.

1025. King EJ, Harrison CV, Mohanty GP: The effect of various forms of alumina on the lungs of rats. J Pathol Bacteriol 69:81, 1955.

1026. Wyatt JP, Riddell ACR: The morphology of bauxite-fume pneumoconiosis. Am J Pathol 25:447, 1949.

1027. Gilks R, Churg A: Aluminum-induced pulmonary fibrosis: Do fibers play a role? Am Rev Respir Dis 136:176, 1987.

1028. Kern DG, Crausman RS, Durand KT, et al: Flock worker's lung: Chronic interstitial lung disease in the nylon flocking industry. Ann Intern Med 129:261, 1998.

1029. Akira M: Uncommon pneumoconioses: CT and pathologic findings. Radiology 197:403, 1995.

1030. Carta P, Boscaro G, Mantovano S, et al: Respiratory symptoms and pulmonary function in the Italian primary aluminum industry. Med Lav 83:438, 1992.

1031. Soyseth V, Kongerud J, Ekstrand J, et al: Relation between exposure to fluoride and bronchial responsiveness in aluminum potroom workers with work-related asthma-like symptoms. Thorax 49:984, 1994.

1032. Soyseth V, Kongerud K, Kjuus H, et al: Bronchial responsiveness and decline in FEV1 in aluminum potroom workers. Eur Respir J 7:888, 1994.

1033. Alessandri MV, Baretta L, Magarotto G: Chronic bronchitis and respiratory function in those employed in primary aluminum production. Med Lav 83:445, 1992.

1034. Carta P, Boscaro G, Mantovano S, et al: Respiratory symptoms and pulmonary function in the Italy primary aluminum industry. Med Lav 83:438, 1992.

1035. Kilburn KH, Warshaw RH: Irregular opacities in the lung, occupational asthma, and airways dysfunction in aluminum workers. Am J Ind Med 21:845, 1992.

1036. Soyseth V, Kongerud J: Prevalence of respiratory disorders among aluminum potroom workers in relation to exposure to fluoride. Br J Ind Med 49:125, 1992.

1037. Soyseth V, Boe J, Kongerud J: Relation between decline in FEV1 and exposure to dust and tobacco smoke in aluminium potroom workers. Occup Environ Med 54:27, 1997.

1038. Sorgdrager B, Pal TM, de Looff AJ, et al: Occupational asthma in aluminium potroom workers related to pre-employment eosinophil count. Eur Respir J 8:1520, 1995.

1039. Soyseth V, Kongerud J, Aalen OO, et al: Bronchial responsiveness decreases in relocated aluminum potroom workers compared with workers who continue their potroom exposure. Int Arch Occup Environ Health 67:53, 1995.

1040. Davison AG, Haslam PL, Corrin B, et al: Interstitial lung disease and asthma in hard-metal workers: Bronchoalveolar lavage, ultrastructural, and analytical findings and results of bronchial provocation tests. Thorax 38:119, 1983.

1041. Rizzato G, Lo Cicero S, Barberis M, et al: Trace of metal exposure in hard metal lung disease. Chest 90:101, 1986.

1042. Sprince NL, Oliver LC, Eisen EA, et al: Cobalt exposure and lung disease in tungsten carbide production. Am Rev Respir Dis 138:1220, 1988.

1043. Meyer-Bisch C, Pham QT, Mur JM, et al: Respiratory hazards in hard metal workers: A cross sectional study. Br J Ind Med 46:302, 1989.

1044. Cugell DW: The hard metal disease. Clin Chest Med 13:269, 1992.

1045. Auchincloss JH, Abraham JL, Gilbert R, et al: Health hazard of poorly regulated exposure during manufacture of cemented tungsten carbides and cobalt. Br J Ind Med 49:832, 1992.

1046. Migliori M, Mosconi G, Michetti G, et al: Hard metal disease: Eight workers with interstitial lung fibrosis due to cobalt exposure. Sci Total Environ 150:187, 1994.

1047. Coates EO Jr, Watson JHL: Diffuse interstitial lung disease in tungsten carbide workers. Ann Intern Med 75:709, 1971.

1048. Demedts M: Cobalt lung in diamond polishers. Am Rev Respir Dis 130:130, 1984.

1049. Kitamura H, Kitamura H, Tozawa T, et al: Cemented tungsten carbide pneumoconiosis. Acta Pathol Jpn 28:921, 1978.

1050. Ruttner JR, Spycher MA, Stolkin I: Inorganic particulates in pneumoconiotic lungs of hard metal grinders. Br J Ind Med 44:657, 1987.

1051. Sjogren I, Hillerdal G, Andersson A, et al: Hard metal lung disease: Importance of cobalt in coolants. Thorax 35:653, 1980.

1052. Van Cutsem LJ, Ceuppens JL, Lacquet LM, et al: Combined asthma and alveolitis induced by cobalt in a diamond polisher. Eur J Respir Dis 70:54, 1987.

1053. Shirakawa T, Kusaka Y, Fujimura N, et al: Occupational asthma from cobalt sensitivity in workers exposed to hard metal dust. Chest 95:29, 1989.

1054. Demedts M, Ceuppens JL: Respiratory diseases from hard metal or cobalt exposure—solving the enigma. Chest 95:2, 1989.

1055. Shirakawa T, Kusaka Y, Morimoto K: Combined effect of smoking habits and occupational exposure to hard metal on total IgE antibodies. Chest 101:569, 1992.

1056. Anttila S, Sutinen S, Paananen M, et al: Hard metal lung disease: A clinical, histological, ultrastructural and x-ray microanalytical study. Eur J Respir Dis 69:83, 1986.

1057. Loewen GM, Weiner D, McMahan U: Pneumoconiosis in an elderly dentist. Chest 93:1313, 1988.

1058. Tabatowski K, Roggli VL, Fulkerson WJ, et al: Giant cell interstitial pneumonia in a hard-metal worker: Cytologic, histologic and analytical electron microscopic investigation. Acta Cytol 32:240, 1988.

1059. Forrest ME, Skerker LB, Nemirott MJ: Hard metal pneumoconiosis: Another cause of diffuse interstitial fibrosis. Radiology 128:609, 1978.

1060. Bech AO, Kipling MD, Heather JC: Hard metal disease. Br J Ind Med 19:239, 1962.

1061. Nemery B, Nagels J, Verbeken E, et al: Rapidly fatal progression of cobalt lung in a diamond polisher. Am Rev Respir Dis 141:1373, 1990.

1062. Ratto D, Balmes J, Boylen T, et al: Pregnancy in a woman with severe pulmonary fibrosis secondary to hard metal disease. Chest 93:663, 1988.

1063. Rolfe MW, Paine R, Davenport RB, et al: Hard metal pneumoconiosis and the association of tumour necrosis factor-alpha. Am Rev Respir Dis 146:1600, 1992.

1064. Schwarz Y, Kivity S, Fischbein A, et al: Eosinophilic lung reaction to aluminum and hard metal. Chest 105:1261, 1994.

1065. Fischbein A, Lou JCJ, Solomon SJ, et al: Clinical findings among hard metal workers. Br J Ind Med 49:17, 1992.

1066. Sprince NL, Chamberlin RI, Hales CA, et al: Respiratory disease in tungsten carbide production workers. Chest 86:549, 1984.

1066a. Nemery B, Casier P, Roosels D, et al: Survey of cobalt exposure and respiratory health in diamond polishers. Am Rev Respir Dis 145:610, 1992.

1067. Kennedy SM, Chan-Yeung M, Marion S, et al: Maintenance of stellite and tungsten carbide saw tips: respiratory health and exposure-response evaluations. Occup Environ Med 52:185, 1995.

1068. Funahashi A: Pneumoconiosis in workers exposed to silicon carbide. Am Rev Respir Dis 129:635, 1984.

1069. Bégin R, Dufresne A, Cantin A, et al: Carborundum pneumoconiosis: Fibers in the mineral activate macrophages to produce fibroblast growth factors and sustain the chronic inflammatory disease. Chest 95:842, 1989.

1070. Bruch J, Rehn B, Song H, et al: Toxicological investigations on silicon carbide—inhalation studies. Br J Ind Med 50:797, 1993.

1071. Massé S, Bégin R, Cantin A: Pathology of silicon carbide pneumoconiosis. Mod Pathol 1:104, 1988.

1072. Hayashi H, Kajita A: Silicon carbide in lung tissue of a worker in the abrasive industry. Am J Ind Med 14:145, 1988.

1073. Marcer G, Bernardi G, Bartolucci GB, et al: Pulmonary impairment in workers exposed to silicon carbide. Br J Ind Med 49:489, 1992.

1074. Cukier A, Algranti E, Terra Filho M, et al: Pneumoconiosis in abrasive industry workers. Rev Hosp Clin Fac Med Sao Paulo 46:180, 1991.

1075. Durand P, Bégin R, Samson L et al: Silicon carbide pneumoconiosis: A radiographic assessment. Am J Ind Med 20:37, 1991.

1076. Bruch J, Rehn B, Song W, et al: Toxicological investigations on silicon carbide—in vitro cell tests and long term injection tests. Br J Ind Med 50:807, 1993.

1077. Dufresne A, Loosereewanich P, Harrigan M, et al: Pulmonary dust retention in a silicon carbide worker. Am Ind Hyg Assoc J 54:327, 1993.

1078. Wegman DH, Eisen EA: Causes of death among employees of a synthetic abrasive product manufacturing company. J Occup Med 23:748, 1981.

1079. Funahashi A, Schlueter DP, Pintar K, et al: Pneumoconiosis in workers exposed to silicon carbide. Am Rev Respir Dis 129:635, 1984.

1080. Oleru UG: Respiratory and nonrespiratory morbidity in a titanium oxide paint factory in Nigeria. Am J Ind Med 12:173, 1987.

1081. Marcer G, Bernardi G, Bartolucci GB, et al: Pulmonary impairment in workers exposed to silicon carbide. Br J Ind Med 49:489, 1992.

1082. Cordasco EM, Demeter SL, Kerkay J, et al: Pulmonary manifestations of vinyl and polyvinyl chloride (interstitial lung disease). Chest 78:6, 1980.

1083. Mastrangelo G, Manno M, Marcer G, et al: Polyvinyl chloride pneumoconiosis: Epidemiological study of exposed workers. J Occup Med 21:540, 1979.

1084. Lilis R, Anderson H, Miller A, et al: Pulmonary changes among vinyl chloride polymerization workers. Chest 69:299, 1976.

1085. Boutar C, Copland L, Thornley P, et al: An epidemiologic study of respiratory disease in workers exposed to polyvinylchloride dust. Chest 80:60S, 1981.

1086. Antti-Poika M, Nordman H, Nickels J, et al: Lung disease after exposure to polyvinyl chloride dust. Thorax 41:566, 1986.

1087. Arnaud A, De Santi PP, Garbe L, et al: Polyvinyl chloride pneumoconiosis. Thorax 33:19, 1978.

1088. Prodan L, Suciu I, Pislaru V, et al: Experimental chronic poisoning with vinyl chloride (monochloroethylene). Ann N Y Acad Sci 246:159, 1975.

1089. Argarwal DK, Kaw JL, Srivastava SO, et al: Some biochemical and histopathological changes induced by polyvinyl chloride dust in rat lung. Environ Res 16:333, 1978.

1089a. Ward AM, Udnoon S, Watkins J, et al: Immunological mechanisms in the pathogenesis of vinyl chloride disease. BMJ 1:936, 1976.

1089b. Suciu I, Prodan L, Ilea E, et al: Clinical manifestations in vinyl chloride poisoning. Ann N Y Acad Sci 246:53, 1975.

1089c. Martseller HJ, Lelbach WK: Unusual splenomegalic liver disease as evidenced by peritoneoscopy and guided liver biopsy among polyvinyl chloride production workers. Ann N Y Acad Sci 246:95, 1975.

1090. Rode LE, Ophus EM, Gylseth B: Massive pulmonary deposition of rutile after titanium dioxide exposure. Acta Pathol Microbiol Scand (A) 89:455, 1981.

1091. Elo R, Määttä K, Uksila E, et al: Pulmonary deposits of titanium dioxide in man. Arch Pathol 94:417, 1972.

1092. Yamadori I, Ohsumi S, Taguchi K: Titanium dioxide deposition and adenocarcinoma of the lung. Acta Pathol Jpn 36:783, 1986.

1093. Moran CA, Mullick FG, Ishak KG, et al: Identification of titanium in human tissues: Probable role in pathologic processes. Hum Pathol 22:450, 1991.

1094. Redline S, Barna BP, Tomashefski JF Jr, et al: Granulomatous disease associated with pulmonary deposition of titanium. Br J Ind Med 43:652, 1986.

1095. Garabrant DH, Fine LJ, Oliver C, et al: Abnormalities of pulmonary function and pleural disease among titanium metal production workers. Scand J Work Environ Health 13:47, 1987.

1096. Craighead JE, Adler KB, Butler GB, et al: Biology of disease: Health effects of Mount St. Helens volcanic dust. Lab Invest 48:5, 1983.

1097. Eisele JW, O'Halloran RL, Reay DT, et al: Deaths during the May 18, 1980 eruption of Mount St. Helens. Med Intell 305:931, 1981.

1098. Merchant JA, Baxter P, Bernstein R, et al: Health implications of the Mount St. Helens eruption: Epidemiological considerations. Ann Occup Hyg 26:911, 1982.

1099. Baxter PJ, Ing R, Falk H, et al: Mount St. Helen's eruptions: The acute respiratory etiology of volcanic ash in a North American community. Arch Environ Health 38:138, 1983.

1100. Buist S: Personal communication, 1989.

1101. Hill JW: Health aspects of man-made mineral fibres: A review. Ann Occup Hyg 20:161, 1977.

1102. Stanton MF, Layard M, Tegeris A, et al: Carcinogenicity of fibrous glass: Pleural response in the rat in relation to fiber dimension. J Natl Cancer Inst 58:587, 1977.
1103. Sebastien P: Biopersistence of man-made vitreous silicate fibers in the human lung. Env Health Perspec 5:225, 1994.
1104. Gross P: Man-made vitreous fibers: An overview of studies on their biologic effects. Am Ind Hyg Assoc J 47:717, 1986.
1105. Lee KP, Barras CE, Griffith FD, et al: Pulmonary response to glass fiber by inhalation exposure. Lab Invest 40:123, 1979.
1106. Morgan RW, Kaplan SD, Bratsberg JA: Mortality study of fibrous glass production workers. Arch Environ Health 36:179, 1981.
1107. Shannon HS, Hayes M, Julian JA, et al: Mortality experience of glass fibre workers. Br J Ind Med 41:35, 1984.
1108. Enterline PE, Marsh GM, Esmen NA: Respiratory disease among workers exposed to man-made mineral fibers. Am Rev Respir Dis 128:1, 1983.
1109. Goldsmith JR: Comparative epidemiology of men exposed to asbestos and man-made mineral fibers. Am J Ind Med 10:543, 1986.
1110. Bayliss DL, Dement JM, Wagoner JK, et al: Mortality patterns among fibrous glass production workers. Ann N Y Acad Sci 271:324, 1976.
1111. Lockey J, Lemasters G, Rice C, et al: Refactory ceramic fiber exposure and pleural plaques. Am J Respir Crit Care Med 154:1405, 1996.
1112. Adamson IY, Prieditis H, Hedgecock C: Pulmonary response of mice to fiberglass: Cytokinetic and biochemical studies. J Toxicol Environ Health 46:411, 1995.
1113. Sixt R, Bake B, Abrahamsson G, et al: Lung function of sheet metal workers exposed to fiber glass. Scand J Work Environ Health 9:9, 1983.
1114. Kilburn KH, Powers D, Warshaw RH: Pulmonary effects of exposure to fine fibreglass: Irregular opacities and small airways obstruction. Br J Ind Med 49:714, 1992.
1115. Weiss W: Pulmonary effects of exposure to fine fibreglass: Irregular opacities and small airways obstruction (letter; comment). Br J Ind Med 50:863, 1993.
1116. Bender JR: Pulmonary effects of exposure to fine fibreglass: Irregular opacities and small airways obstruction (letter; comment). Br J Ind Med 50:381, 1993.
1117. Clausen J, Netterstrom B, Wolff C: Lung function in insulation workers. Br J Ind Med 50:252, 1993.
1118. Leanderson P, Soderkvist P, Tragesson C: Hydroxyl radical mediated DNA base modification by manmade mineral fibres. Br J Ind Med 46:435, 1989.
1119. Infante PF, Schuman LD, Dement J, et al: Fibrous glass and cancer. Am J Ind Med 26:559, 1994.
1120. Chiazze L Jr, Watkins DK, Fryar C: A case-control study of malignant and nonmalignant respiratory disease among employees of a fibreglass manufacturing facility. Br J Ind Med 49:326, 1992.
1121. Wong O, Foliart D, Trent LS: A case-control study of lung cancer in a cohort of workers potentially exposed to slag wool fibres. Br J Ind Med 48:818, 1991.
1122. Chiazze L Jr, Watkins DK, Fryar C: Adjustment for the confounding effect of cigarette smoking in an historical cohort mortality study of workers in a fiberglass manufacturing facility. Br J Ind Med 49:326, 1992.
1123. Weiss W: Epidemiology of fibrous glass and lung cancer. Am J Ind Med 30:105, 1996.
1124. Lee IM, Hennekens CH, Trichopoulos D, et al: Man-made vitreous fibers and risk of respiratory system cancer: A review of the epidemiologic evidence. J Occup Environ Med 37:725, 1995.
1125. Barrett TE, Pietra GG, Maycock RL, et al: Case report: Acrylic resin pneumoconiosis: Report of a case in a dental student. Am Rev Respir Dis 139:841, 1989.
1126. Sherson D, Maltbaek N, Heydorn K: A dental technician with pulmonary fibrosis: A case of chromium-cobalt alloy pneumoconiosis? Eur Respir J 3:1227, 1990.
1127. Bernstein M, Pairon JC, Morabia A, et al: Non-fibrous dust load and smoking in dental technicians: A study using bronchoalveolar lavage. Occup Environ Med 51:23, 1994.
1128. Seldon A, Sahle W, Johansson L, et al: Three cases of dental technician's pneumoconosis related to cobalt-chromium-molybdenum dust exposure. Chest 109:837, 1996.
1129. Choudat D, Triem S, Weill B, et al: Respiratory symptoms, lung function, and pneumoconiosis among self employed dental technicians. Br J Ind Med 50:443, 1993.
1130. Albin M, Johansson L, Pooley FD, et al: Mineral fibres, fibrosis, and asbestos bodies in lung tissue from deceased asbestos cement workers. Br J Ind Med 47:767, 1990.
1131. Sander OA: Roentgen resurvey of cement workers. AMA Arch Ind Health 17:96, 1958.
1132. Parkes WR: Occupational Lung Disorders. 2nd ed. London, Butterworths, 1982.
1133. McDowall ME: A mortality study of cement workers. Br J Ind Med 41:179, 1984.
1134. Kessel R, Redl M, Mauermayer R, et al: Changes in lung function after working with the shotcrete lining method under compressed air conditions. Br J Ind Med 46:128, 1989.
1135. McCunney RJ, Godefroi R: Pulmonary alveolar proteinosis and cement dust: A case report. J Occup Med 31:233, 1989.
1136. Bartter T, Irwin RS, Abraham JL, et al: Zirconium compound-induced pulmonary fibrosis. Arch Intern Med 151:1197, 1991.
1137. Romeo L, Cazzadori A, Bontempini L, et al: Interstitial lung granulomas as a possible consequence of exposure to zirconium dust. Med Lav 85:219, 1994.
1138. Liippo KK, Anttila SL, Taikina-Aho O, et al: Hypersensitivity pneumonitis and exposure to zirconium silicate in a young ceramic tile worker. Am Rev Respir Dis 148:1089, 1993.
1139. Kotter JM, Zieger G: Sarcoid granulomatosis after many years of exposure to zirconium, "zirconium lung." Pathologe 13:104, 1992.
1140. Marcus RL, Turner S, Cherry NM: A study of lung function and chest radiographs in men exposed to zirconium compounds. Occup Med (Oxf) 46:109, 1996.
1141. Anonymous: Chronic interstitial lung disease in nylon flocking industry workers—Rhode Island, 1992–1996. MMWR 46:897, 1997.

CHAPTER 61

Aspiration of Solid Foreign Material and Liquids

ASPIRATION OF SOLID FOREIGN BODIES

Aspiration of solid foreign bodies into the tracheobronchial tree occurs most often in infants and small children;[1, 2] for example, 79% of 66 patients investigated in one series were younger than 10 years of age.[3] Despite this, the condition occurs occasionally in older individuals.[4–6] In these patients, aspiration of a solid foreign body may be manifested as acute obstruction of the larynx or trachea, a clinical presentation commonly designated *café coronary* because of its frequent occurrence in restaurants and its resemblance to myocardial infarction (*see* farther on). In other patients, however, the condition is more insidious, manifested only by repeated episodes of pneumonia. In these individuals, the diagnosis is sometimes difficult, particularly when the original episode of aspiration is forgotten.

In children, foreign body aspiration typically occurs in otherwise healthy individuals. By contrast, adults frequently have an underlying condition associated with impairment of airway protection, such as a neurologic disorder, trauma with loss of consciousness, or drug or alcohol abuse.[5–7] Although the aspirated foreign bodies that have been described are of fascinating variety, including pencils, rubber tubing, pins, needles, thermometers, metallic and plastic toys, and jewelry,[3, 8] the substance most commonly implicated is food, usually vegetable.[1, 3, 7, 9] For example, in one review of 160 patients, more than 85% of aspirated bodies were of this type, the peanut being by far the most common.[10] Although other investigators have also found peanut aspiration to be particularly common,[11, 12] local dietary habits are sometimes associated with other vegetable material.[13, 14] Additional relatively common forms of aspirated foreign body, usually seen in adults, are bone and fragments of dental and medical prostheses, such as tracheostomy tube segments (Fig. 61–1).[5, 6]

Several solid foreign bodies deserve specific comment. Inhalation of the flowering heads of various grasses has been reported by several investigators.[15–18] Some of these possess inflorescenses with well-developed terminal spikes that project proximally toward the larger airways, causing the spikes to travel farther and farther into the lung periphery, much like a lobster entering a trap; this migration may be so extensive that the grass spike traverses the pleural space and is eventually extruded through the skin.[17, 19] Similar movement has been described by aspirated staples.[20]

Broken fragments of teeth are occasionally aspirated after maxillofacial trauma, particularly in older children,[21] and radiographs of the chest should be obtained as a precautionary measure in all cases in which skull radiographs reveal absence or fracture of teeth after trauma. Cases have been reported of young children who inhaled candies that dissolved in the tracheobronchial secretions and caused severe respiratory obstruction;[22] the viscid fluid that formed as the candy dissolved was not expectorated, and bronchoscopy was necessary to remove it. A somewhat similar situation has been reported with an aspirated sucralfate tablet, the pill absorbing bronchial secretions and swelling to a size sufficient to obstruct the left main bronchus.[23] Aspirated tablets of ferrous sulfate have been reported to cause bronchial wall necrosis, in one case accompanied by massive hemoptysis and death.[24] This effect has been speculated to be related to the production of cytotoxic oxygen radicals;[24] iron deposition may be seen in the bronchial wall on biopsy specimens.

Rarely, airway obstruction occurs as a result of im-

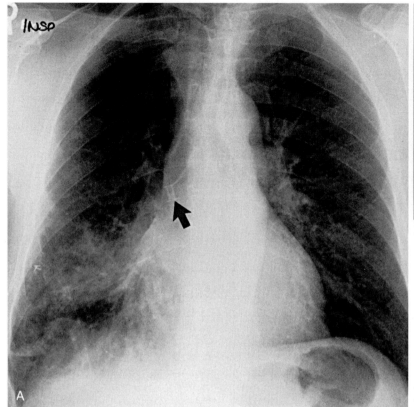

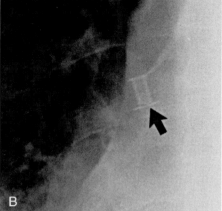

Figure 61–1. Aspiration of Esophageal Speech Device. This 59-year-old man developed areas of atelectasis and consolidation in the right middle and lower lobes after radical laryngectomy. A chest radiograph *(A)* and magnified view of the right lower chest *(B)* demonstrate an esophageal speech device *(arrows)* in the bronchus intermedius. The device was removed bronchoscopically.

paction of a foreign body in the esophagus; such was the case in a 34-year-old mentally retarded patient who swallowed a 3 × 3-cm stone, which came to rest in the upper esophagus and compressed the trachea from behind, resulting in death from asphyxiation.[25]

Pathologic Characteristics

In the early stages after aspiration, the airway wall in immediate contact with the foreign body shows edema and an acute inflammatory infiltrate or, if ulcerated, granulation tissue (Fig. 61–2); these reactions contribute directly to airway narrowing. Foreign bodies such as peanuts and other agents high in fatty acid content appear to be associated with an especially severe reaction. Occasionally, the aspirated material becomes incorporated within the granulation tissue in the bronchial wall and can appear endoscopically as a fungating "tumor," simulating carcinoma;[26] in such cases, the aspirated substance can usually be identified histologically in material obtained by biopsy (*see* Fig. 61–2).[27] Rare examples of true carcinoma associated with scarring and long-standing foreign body retention have been reported.[28] A more common result of such chronic retention is bronchial wall fibrosis and stenosis, usually accompanied by distal bronchiectasis and obstructive pneumonitis.[3, 29]

Radiologic Manifestations

Although nonreactive foreign bodies such as teeth[10] and coins[30] can be discovered incidentally on routine chest

radiography, in most cases, radiographic findings reflect the effects of partial or complete airway obstruction. Although the aspirated foreign bodies can be seen in all lobes,[30, 31] their most common site is the right lower lobe in both children[10] and adults.[30] In one series of 60 adult patients, 17 aspirated foreign bodies (28%) were located in the right lower lobe, 11 (18%) in the left lower lobe, 10 (17%) in the left main bronchus, 8 (13%) in the bronchus intermedius, 6 (10%) in the right main bronchus, 2 (3%) in the left upper lobe bronchus, 1 in the trachea, and 1 in the right upper lobe bronchus.[30]

The standard chest radiograph is helpful in locating the site of foreign body impaction in about 70% of patients;[30, 31] in the remainder, it is normal or shows nonspecific air-space opacities. In adults, the most common radiographic findings consist of atelectasis, obstructive pneumonitis (Fig. 61–3), or visualization of a radiopaque foreign body (*see* Fig. 61–1).[30, 31] Other abnormalities include air-trapping on the expiratory chest radiograph, lung abscess distal to the impacted foreign body, and occasionally, lung torsion.[30, 31] In most adults, the lung volume distal to an impacted foreign body is decreased (Fig. 61–4);[30] hyperinflation is rare.[30, 31] Although the latter finding has been said to occur in most patients in some studies of children,[10] because it can be difficult to obtain radiographs of the chest in infants and young children at the point of maximal inspiration, we suspect that the "hyperinflation" represented air-trapping on radiographs exposed at the position of slight expiration.

Pulmonary scintigraphy has been considered to be useful in the detection of endobronchial foreign bodies (*see* Fig. 61–4), particularly in infants and children or when the clinical history is suggestive and radiographic changes are equiv-

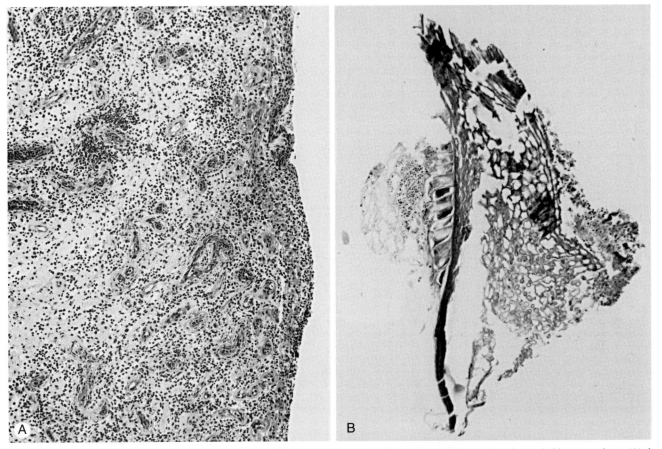

Figure 61–2. Foreign Body Aspiration: Bronchial Wall Ulceration. A section of bronchial wall from a bronchoscopic biopsy specimen *(A)* shows complete loss of surface epithelium; the subepithelial layer consists only of granulation tissue. Another section *(B)* shows a fragment of vegetable material that was removed endoscopically from the same site at the time of biopsy. The patient was a 50-year-old man with partial atelectasis of the right upper lobe; there was no history of aspiration. (*A*, ×100; *B*, ×90.)

ocal. For example, in one investigation of five children who manifested normal physical findings and only minimal radiographic abnormalities, striking perfusion deficits were noted on lung scans;[32] in all cases, the scans reverted to normal after removal of the foreign body. Despite those findings, scintigraphy has generally been supplanted by CT in the assessment of suspected aspiration.

Although computed tomography (CT) and magnetic resonance (MR) imaging are not recommended as a routine in the diagnosis of aspirated foreign bodies, each can be of value in selected cases.[33] CT usually permits demonstration of the foreign body and its precise location within the bronchial tree, even when it is radiolucent (Fig. 61–5).[34] Occasionally, MR imaging is also helpful, as in a 1½-year-old boy who had progressive wheezing and fever.[35] In this case, MR imaging showed high signal intensity in the right main bronchus; at bronchoscopy, a peanut was detected in the right main bronchus, and an attempt was made to remove it. When wheezing persisted after bronchoscopy, a second MR imaging examination again showed a high signal intensity, this time in the right lower lobe bronchus. At repeat bronchoscopy, a 5-mm fragment of peanut was removed from this site.

Bronchiectasis is an occasional complication of long-standing retention of a foreign body (*see* Fig. 61–1).[3, 30, 36] In one series of 500 patients who had this disorder, foreign bodies were considered to be the cause in 8 (four of the foreign bodies were vegetable and four mineral).[37]

Clinical Manifestations

As might be expected, the most common symptoms of foreign body aspiration are cough and choking; respiratory failure occurs rarely.[9] In children, choking is usually recognized by parents or guardians.[2, 38] Although many adult patients also give a history of choking at the time of aspiration,[10, 39, 40] it may require much persistence for the physician to elicit this when the episode is not recent. For example, in one investigation of 29 patients in whom aspiration occurred 1 month or more before disease was diagnosed, a choking history was obtained before bronchoscopy in only 15.[4] In such individuals, an asymptomatic interval may follow aspiration, especially when bronchi are not obstructed;[4, 41] such a latent period can extend to several months or even years, particularly if the aspirated material is bone or inorganic matter.[6] Eventually, disease usually becomes manifest as recurrent pneumonia, chronic cough, or hemoptysis.[6]

The café-coronary syndrome occurs in adults and is caused by lodgment of food in the upper airway, with about one third in a supraglottic location and most of the remainder at the level of the vocal cords (Fig. 61–6).[42] Risk factors

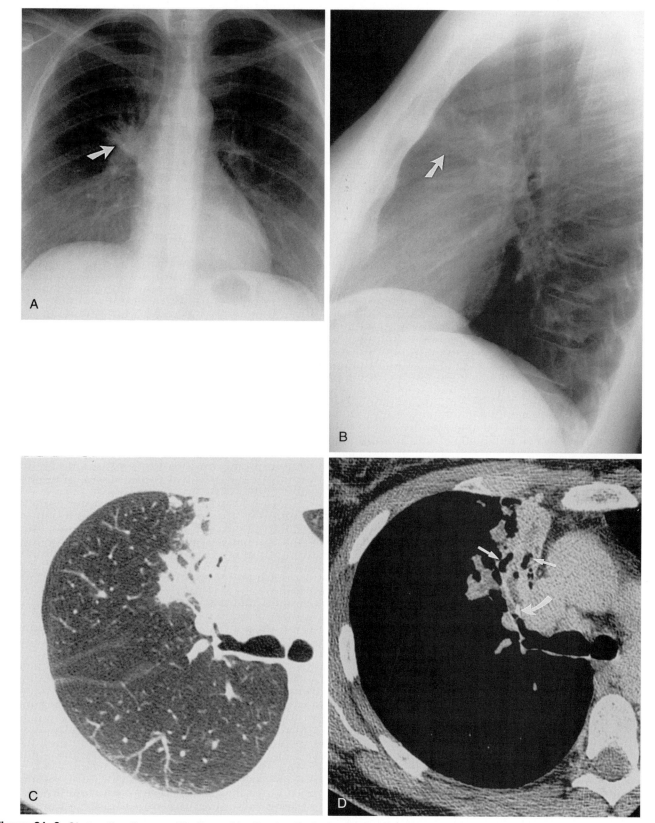

Figure 61–3. Obstructive Pneumonitis Caused by Foreign Body Aspiration. Posteroanterior *(A)* and lateral *(B)* chest radiographs in a 44-year-old woman demonstrate localized consolidation and atelectasis involving the anterior segment of the right upper lobe *(arrows)*. HRCT scans *(C* and *D)* demonstrate evidence of obstructive pneumonitis and bronchiectasis *(straight arrows)* in the anterior segment of the right upper lobe. The localized area of high attenuation *(curved arrow)* within the bronchial lumen represents an aspirated popcorn kernel.

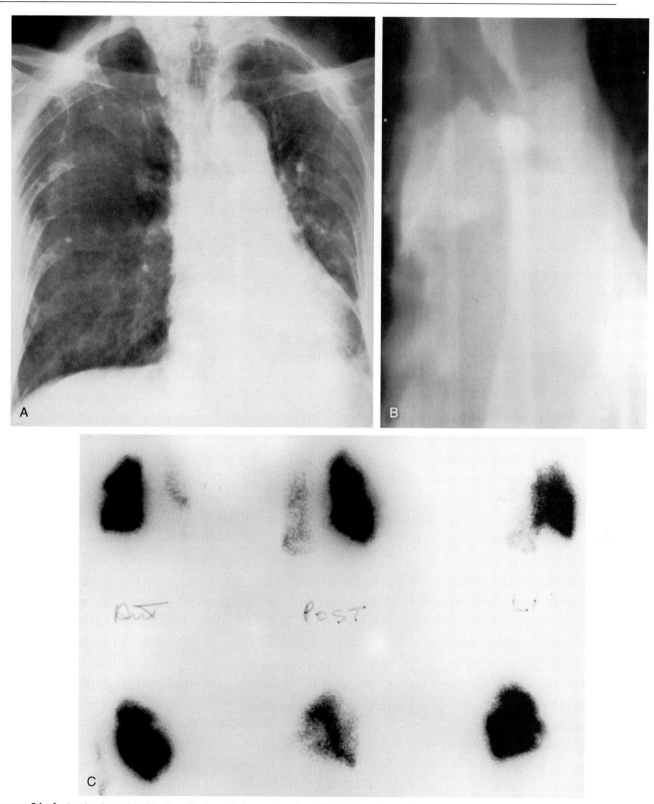

Figure 61–4. Aspiration of a Foreign Body with Impaction in a Main Bronchus. A posteroanterior radiograph *(A)* reveals moderate reduction in volume of the left lung accompanied by diffuse oligemia. A linear tomogram in anteroposterior projection *(B)* shows a circular opacity situated within and occupying the whole transverse diameter of the left main bronchus. A perfusion lung scan *(C)* confirms the marked reduction in blood flow to the left lung, the result of hypoxic vasoconstriction. At bronchoscopy, a pill was successfully removed. The patient was an elderly man.

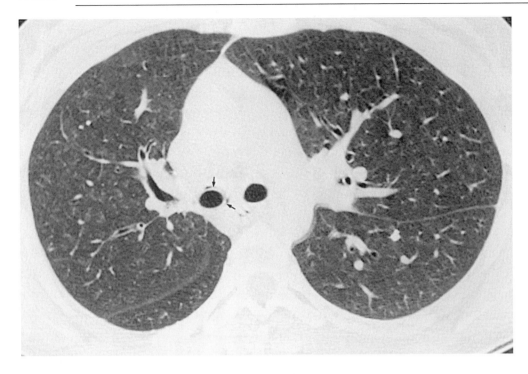

Figure 61–5. Foreign Body Aspiration. A 23-year-old drug addict presented with a 3-month history of cough productive of increasing amounts of green sputum. An HRCT scan demonstrates tubing within the lumen of the right main bronchus *(arrows)*. A small amount of secretions within the bronchial lumen and decreased attenuation, vascularity, and volume of the right lung are also evident. The plastic tube was successfully removed bronchoscopically.

include old age, alcohol consumption, sedative drugs, institutionalization in a chronic care home, neurologic diseases, parkinsonism, mental retardation, and psychiatric disorders.[42–44] The airway obstruction results in air hunger, cyanosis, and venous distention; convulsions may be a manifestation of a risk factor (epilepsy) or the result of hypoxia.[45] The sudden onset of such a catastrophic episode can lead to a misdiagnosis of myocardial infarction; however, its development during a meal, particularly when associated with an inability to speak, should suggest the true diagnosis.

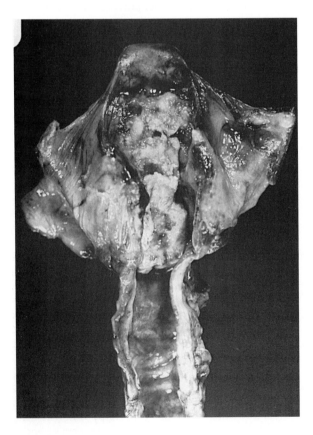

Figure 61–6. Acute Foreign Body Aspiration: Upper Airway Obstruction. The specimen consists of the larynx and upper portion of the trachea opened posteriorly. A large fragment of partially masticated meat completely occludes the laryngeal lumen. The patient was a 58-year-old man who had "passed out" while eating and died (café coronary).

ASPIRATION OF GASTRIC OR OROPHARYNGEAL SECRETIONS

The term *aspiration pneumonia* is employed by some to denote pulmonary infection caused by aspiration of bacteria-laden oropharyngeal secretions. This form of pneumonia is frequently caused by anaerobic organisms in patients who have poor oral hygiene and is commonly associated with abscess formation (*see* page 778). Although occasionally complicated by such anaerobic bacterial infection, aspiration of oropharyngeal or gastric secretions, with or without admixed food particles, can also cause significant pulmonary disease in the absence of infection. Almost invariably, this occurs in individuals who have an underlying condition predisposing to aspiration, most commonly one of the following:

- Patients with chronic debilitating disease, such as cancer
- Patients with oropharyngeal or airway instrumentation, such as those undergoing tube feeding,[46] intraoperative small bowel decompression,[47] prolonged mechanical ventilation,[48] or endoscopy for upper gastrointestinal hemorrhage[49] or those who have a tracheostomy,[50] a laryngeal mask,[51] a nasogastric tube *in situ* in the postoperative period,[52] or a feeding gastrotomy[40]
- Unconscious patients in circumstances such as general anesthesia for emergency surgery or obstetric delivery (although there is evidence from some reviews that the risk of aspiration after "routine" anesthesia is very small),[53–56] epileptic seizure, cardiopulmonary resuscitation,[57] electroconvulsive therapy, trauma, alcohol- or drug-induced stupor,[58] or cerebrovascular accident[59, 60]
- Patients who have disorders affecting swallowing,[61] such as severe developmental disabilities,[62] achalasia, esophageal or pharyngeal carcinoma, hypopharyngeal (Zenker's) diverticulum, benign esophageal stricture,[63] Chagas' disease,[64] congenital or acquired tracheoesophageal fistula (*see* page 627), pharyngeal and gastric-colon interposition,[65] and neuromuscular disease involving the esophagus or pharynx.[66–70]

Acute aspiration in these circumstances is not uncommon: in one series of 212 autopsies in which bronchopneumonia was identified, food particles associated with an inflammatory reaction were identified in the lungs in 27 (13%).[71] In another study, 41 cases of vegetable aspiration pneumonia were identified in approximately 1,500 autopsies.[72] Because the presence of aspiration is usually determined pathologically by demonstrating food particles, and because they are sometimes difficult to identify with certainty and may be sparse, the true incidence of the condition is undoubtedly higher. In addition to these postmortem investigations, evidence of aspiration, frequently subclinical, can be demonstrated in many patients who have one of the predisposing conditions listed previously.[50, 60, 73] Somewhat surprisingly, aspiration of small amounts of oropharyngeal secretions also occurs in normal individuals during sleep.[60, 74] It is possible that this is more likely to occur in older people, in whom there is evidence that the cough reflex is significantly reduced.[75]

In part because of its relatively high prevalence, gastroesophageal reflux may also be an important etiologic factor in pulmonary aspiration. In fact, this process has been implicated in a variety of pulmonary diseases, including asthma (*see* page 2113), chronic cough (with which it has been associated in about 20% of patients who have this complaint[76]), bronchitis, bronchiectasis, recurrent pneumonia, apnea, and diffuse interstitial fibrosis.[77–80] Evidence supporting these associations is derived from barium studies of the esophagus (particularly those employing cineradiography),[81] from scintigraphic investigations employing various foods labeled with radionuclides,[82, 83] and from studies using esophageal pH recordings and manometry.

Pathogenesis

The pathogenesis of pulmonary damage depends on the amount and nature of the aspirated material. The hydrochloric acid of the gastric juice appears to be an important mediator of disease. The results of some experimental studies suggest that pulmonary damage occurs predominantly when the pH of the aspirate is less than 2.5; moreover, it has been shown that prior neutralization of acid solutions instilled intratracheally reduces the severity of the pulmonary reaction.[84] In humans, it is generally assumed that the risk of pulmonary disease from gastric acid aspiration is also related to both the pH and the volume of aspirated stomach contents, being greatest when the pH is less than 2.5 and the volume more than 25 ml. There is considerable evidence, however, that pulmonary damage also occurs when the pH of aspirated fluid is greater than 2.5; for example, several experimental and clinical studies have documented the development of pulmonary disease after the aspiration of neutralized gastric acid, distilled water, and isotonic saline (*see* farther on).[85–87] In addition, it is known that antacids, modifiers of gastrointestinal tract motility, antiemetics, and H$_2$-receptor antagonists, singly or in combination, can increase pH and reduce gastric acid volume.[84, 88–90] In theory, if such medication were to be administered at the appropriate time (1 to 1.5 hours) before regurgitation and aspiration, it might be anticipated that a significant pulmonary reaction would be avoided, or at least diminished; however, despite the widespread administration of antacids to women in labor, there has been little or no change in the incidence of maternal death from aspiration.[91]

Perhaps related to these observations is the finding that aspirated acid is unlikely to cause epithelial damage directly.[92] Instead, it has been speculated that pulmonary injury is the result of recruitment and activation of neutrophils after acid-induced release of cytokines such as tumor necrosis factor-α and interleukin-8.[92] This hypothesis is supported by experiments in which neutrophils have been depleted or their action blocked, in which circumstances the severity of lung injury is considerably reduced.[93, 94]

There are several reasons for an increased risk of aspiration during pregnancy, including increased intra-abdominal pressure caused by the enlarged uterus, progesterone-related relaxation of the lower gastroesophageal sphincter, and upper airway intubation and unconsciousness as a result of anesthesia. In addition to the increased risk, the morbidity resulting from aspiration of gastric contents during labor appears to be particularly severe, and the mortality is increased.[95] It has been suggested that abnormal pulmonary water balance caused either by the pregnancy itself or by therapeutic intervention may be responsible; it has also been postulated that uterine contractions may be accompanied by failure of the stomach to empty, with resultant accumulation of a large volume of gastric contents.[95]

When aspirated gastric contents include an appreciable quantity of admixed particulates or when the aspirated material is derived from the oropharynx, the pathogenesis of pulmonary damage appears to relate to both a nonspecific reaction to the liquid and a more specific inflammatory response to the various particulates.[96, 97] As noted previously, it has been shown in several clinical and experimental studies that pulmonary disease can develop as a result of aspiration of fluid with relatively high pH: for example, aspiration of relatively neutral gastric liquid (pH 5.9) that has been filtered to remove food particles results in significant but transient hypoxemia;[85] similarly, individual case reports have been reported in which severe pulmonary edema has developed in patients who have aspirated fluid having a pH as high as 6.4.[86]

Pathologic studies have also shown evidence of lung damage caused by fluid of relatively neutral pH. Histologically, aspiration of gastric liquid at a pH higher than 4.0 has been shown to cause acute pneumonitis (characterized by edema, hemorrhage, and polymorphonuclear leukocyte infiltration) and bronchiolitis.[85, 87] In one ultrastructural investigation of the lungs of experimental animals into which solutions of varying pH and tonicity had been instilled,

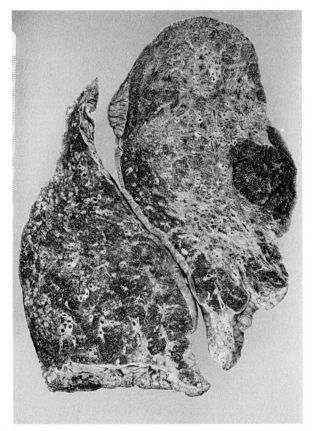

Figure 61–7. Chronic Aspiration Pneumonia. A slice of left lung shows patchy but extensive air-space fibrosis, predominantly in the upper lobe. Extensive acute bronchopneumonia is also evident in the lower lobe. The patient had an esophageal carcinoma; several episodes of aspiration had been documented clinically during the last 3 months of life.

pulmonary edema was found in all animals, including those in which distilled water was used.[98] Electron microscopic examination revealed fluid in the alveoli and separation of the vascular endothelium from the alveolar epithelium by interstitial fluid. The pH and tonicity were related to the reaction only in terms of degree and time.

Although these pathologic changes and the functional effects associated with them are less severe than when the pH of the aspirated fluid is less than 2.5,[85] they nevertheless imply that it is not acid alone that causes pulmonary damage. This has also been well illustrated in experimental studies in which pure solutions of ground-up meat and vegetable material have been aspirated, clearly resulting in a polymorphonuclear and granulomatous inflammatory response.[99] The results of some studies suggest that gastrointestinal enzymes, such as trypsin and pepsin, are unlikely to have any pathogenetic effect by themselves;[97, 100] however, some investigators have found evidence for an additive effect with gastric acid.[101] It is also possible that the osmolarity of aspirated gastric juice may be a factor in pathogenesis.[101]

Pathologic Characteristics

Pathologic changes depend on the nature and quantity of the aspirated material and on the frequency with which bouts of aspiration occur. Depending on the time after aspiration at which the lungs are examined, the gross appearance may be that of parenchymal edema and hemorrhage or an acute or organizing bronchopneumonia identical to that caused by bacteria. In the early stages, airway walls may be hyperemic and their lumens partly filled with a mucopurulent exudate. In cases of chronic repeated aspiration, there may be extensive fibrosis (Fig. 61–7); at autopsy, such cases often show evidence of remote, organizing, and acute aspiration.

The histologic reaction to aspiration of relatively pure gastric liquid of low pH reflects the usually extensive acid-induced epithelial damage. In the airways, bronchitis and bronchiolitis are accompanied by focal ulceration and an intraluminal exudate. In the early stages, the parenchyma shows only air-space edema and hemorrhage; this is followed rapidly by the appearance of necrotic debris, fibrin and, eventually, hyaline membranes. If the patient lives long enough, the exudate undergoes organization. This pattern is identical to diffuse alveolar damage of other etiologies.

The pathologic appearance differs somewhat when there is admixed particulate material in the aspirate. Edema, congestion, and hemorrhage followed by a polymorphonuclear influx are early findings in both experimental animals and patients examined at autopsy (Fig. 61–8).[72, 97, 99] Food particles are initially found free within edema fluid in airway lumens and alveolar air spaces but rapidly develop a surrounding mantle of polymorphonuclear leukocytes (*see* Fig. 61–8). Mononuclear phagocytic cells soon appear and increase in number thereafter. Foreign body giant cells, often of highly irregular shape and containing numerous nuclei, can be found as early as 24 to 48 hours after the aspiration (Fig. 61–9). Well-organized granulomas often develop and surround identifiable fragments of meat or vegetable material or necrotic debris. At this stage, foci of disease may be relatively discrete and appear both grossly and histologically as multiple nodules resembling either tuberculosis (miliary

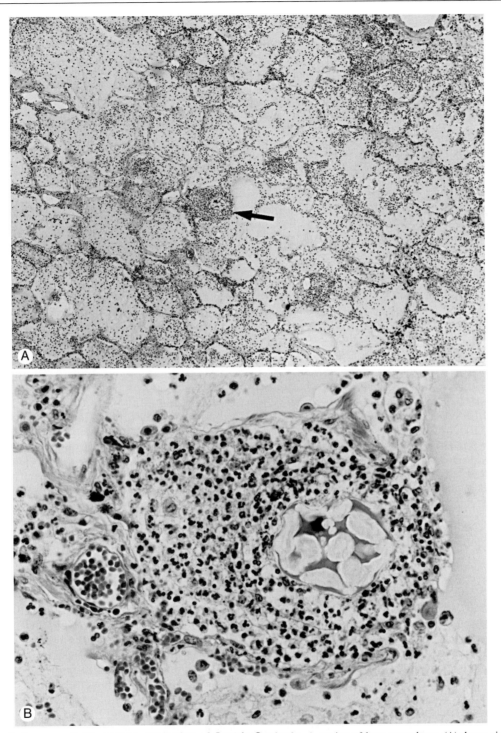

Figure 61–8. Acute Pneumonia Caused by Aspiration of Gastric Contents. A section of lung parenchyma *(A)* shows air spaces consolidated by edema and numerous polymorphonuclear leukocytes. Focally, leukocytes are aggregated around small particles of vegetable material *(arrow)*. A magnified view of the area indicated by the arrow *(B)* reveals the foreign material to good advantage; its lobulated appearance is characteristic of leguminous vegetables. The section was obtained at autopsy of a 65-year-old man with disseminated carcinoma. (*A,* ×40; *B,* ×300.)

or endobronchial pneumonic patterns) or bacterial abscesses (Fig. 61–10).[96, 102]

With the exception of the reaction to lipid (*see* farther on), little difference has been shown in experimental studies among the reactions to different types of aspirated food,[99] although granulomas appear to develop more readily and persist longer in relation to leguminous vegetable material such as peas, beans, and lentils.[72, 97] In occasional cases, it may be difficult to identify food particles within the granulomas with conviction; in these, examination of multiple sections and the use of polarization microscopy to identify the refractile cell walls found in many vegetables may help to arrive at the correct diagnosis.

Although the edema and hemorrhage of the early stage of food aspiration tend to be more or less diffuse throughout the parenchyma, the granulomatous inflammation is often

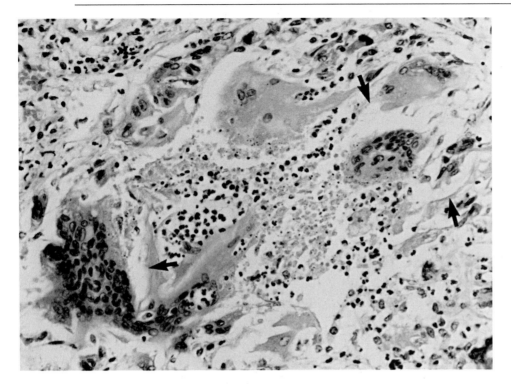

Figure 61–9. Foreign Body Giant Cell Reaction to Aspirated Gastric Contents. A section through a focus of lower lobe pneumonia shows several mutinucleated giant cells surrounding necrotic material and polymorphonuclear leukocytes. The giant cell at the lower left is irregular in shape and contains numerous nuclei, features characteristic of a reaction to aspirated foreign material, in this case vegetable. The vegetable fragments themselves are partly destroyed and are evident only as clear spaces within and adjacent to the giant cells *(arrows).* (×250.)

most severe in relation to membranous and respiratory bronchioles; thus, some degree of obliterative bronchiolitis is not uncommon (Fig. 61–11).[103] In fact, residual peribronchiolar fibrosis associated with distortion of the normal airway architecture and "bronchiolization" of the adjacent parenchyma may be the only evidence of prior aspiration (*see* Fig. 61–11).

The development of secondary bacterial pneumonia in the areas of damaged lung or of lung abscess in the case of aspirates contaminated by anaerobic or other organisms can alter the typical histologic appearance of any of the patterns described.

Radiologic Manifestations

In the patient who has aspirated a large amount of relatively pure gastric secretion at a low pH, the chest radiograph typically reveals general involvement of both lungs by patchy air-space consolidation, similar to pulmonary edema of cardiac origin or to the more diffuse permeability edema observed in the adult respiratory distress syndrome (ARDS).[104] Although discrete air-space shadows can be apparent, most opacities are confluent (Fig. 61–12). Distribution is typically bilateral and multicentric but usually favors perihilar or basal regions.[104] This perihilar distribution has been shown on CT to reflect the presence of consolidation mainly in the posterior segments of the upper lobes or superior segments of the lower lobes.[104a] In uncomplicated cases, these abnormalities often worsen for several days and thereafter improve fairly rapidly. Progression of the radiographic abnormalities after initial improvement is associated with the development of bacterial pneumonia, ARDS, or pulmonary embolism.[104] The normal size of the heart and

the absence of signs of pulmonary venous hypertension serve to differentiate the edema from that of cardiac origin.

This form of aspiration pneumonia may not show an anatomic distribution reflecting the influence of gravity. If the patient is lying in the prone or supine position at the time of aspiration, the highly irritative nature of the aspirate will result in widespread dissemination throughout the lungs (Fig. 61–13); however, predominant changes may be unilateral if the patient is lying on his or her side. If the patient survives, resolution is relatively rapid—averaging 7 to 10 days in our experience, about the same as for traumatic fat embolism but much slower than that for edema caused by acute cardiac decompensation.

In cases in which there is aspiration of oropharyngeal secretions or gastric contents containing an appreciable amount of admixed food, radiographic findings have a segmental distribution, often involving one or more of the posterior segments of the upper or lower lobes. The precise localization depends at least partly on the position of the patient at the time of aspiration.[104, 105] Some degree of atelectasis is present in almost all cases, and the picture can be typical of bacterial bronchopneumonia (Fig. 61–14). With repeated aspiration, serial radiography over a period of months or years shows much variation in the anatomic distribution of segments involved, with disease clearing in one segment and appearing anew in another (Fig. 61–15). A residuum of irregular accentuation of linear markings may remain, probably representing peribronchial scarring. Rarely, chest radiographs reveal reticulonodular[106] or miliary[107] patterns. Granulomatous pneumonitis associated with aspiration of leguminous vegetables can be manifested as 1- to 5-mm diameter nodules on the chest radiograph;[14] HRCT performed in two patients showed the nodules to have a centrilobular distribution.[14]

Text continued on page 2500

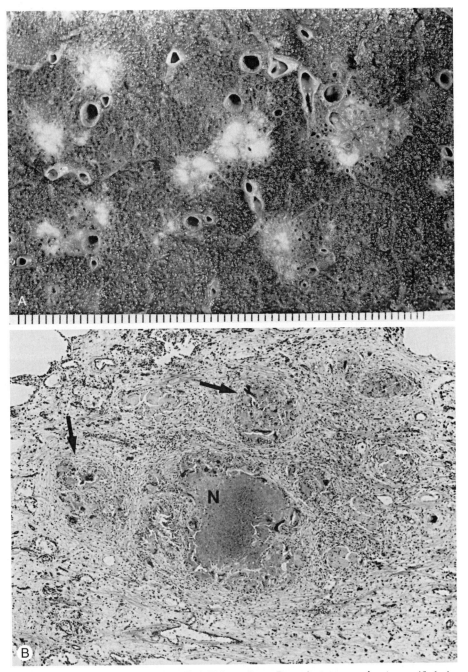

Figure 61–10. Aspiration of Gastric Contents Resembling Tuberculous Bronchopneumonia. A magnified view of lower lobe *(A)* shows multiple, fairly well-defined foci of white necrotic material surrounded by a thin rim of consolidated lung. The appearance resembles that seen in endobronchial spread of tuberculosis. A section *(B)* reveals several fairly well-defined granulomas, one of which is related to necrotic material (N); these are surrounded by fibrous tissue containing scattered lymphocytes. Again, the appearance superficially resembles tuberculosis; however, the presence of numerous multinucleated giant cells, some with irregular shapes *(arrows)*, suggests that the etiology is food aspiration rather than infection (*B*, ×40).

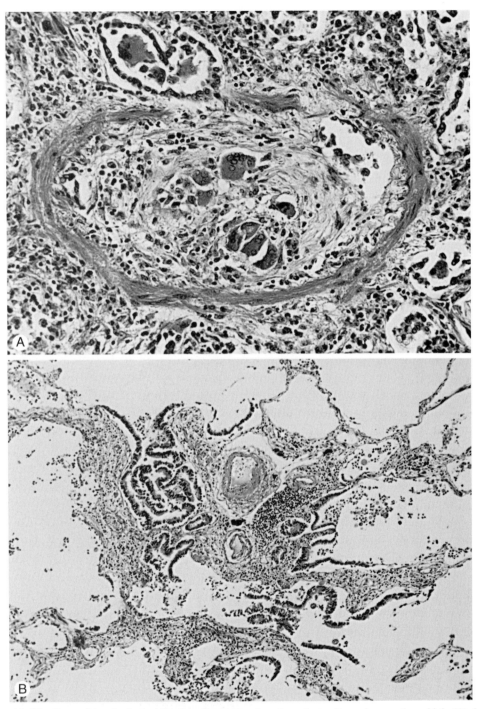

Figure 61–11. Bronchiolitis Caused by Aspirated Gastric Contents. A section of a small membranous bronchiole *(A)* shows it to be completely occluded by fibroblastic tissue containing mononuclear inflammatory cells and several multinucleated foreign body giant cells. The adjacent parenchyma is also inflamed and, although not illustrated in this photomicrograph, contained numerous fragments of vegetable material. In another patient, a section of a small membranous bronchiole *(B)* shows distortion and moderately severe fibrosis and chronic inflammation. The bronchiolar epithelium extends into the adjacent parenchyma, which is also emphysematous. Multiple foci of fibrosis and inactive granulomas, some containing foreign material, were present elsewhere in the lung parenchyma. *(A,* ×120; *B,* ×70.)

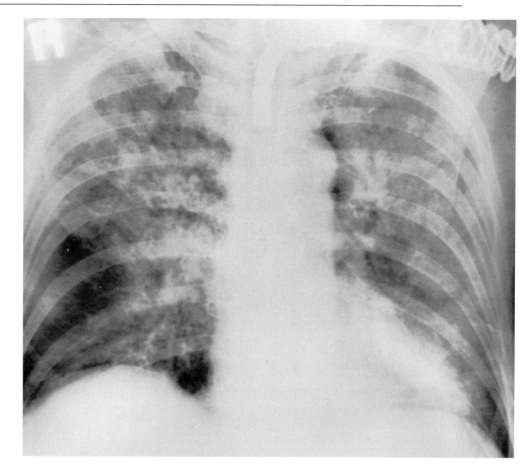

Figure 61–12. Acute Aspiration Pneumonia. While lying in a supine position after anesthesia, this 68-year-old man aspirated considerable quantities of vomitus. An anteroposterior chest radiograph performed within 2 hours reveals extensive involvement of both lungs by patchy air-space consolidation typical of acute pulmonary edema. Although a few patchy shadows are present in the lower lung zones, the predominant involvement is in the upper zones, a distribution that can be explained, at least partly, by the position of the patient at the time of aspiration.

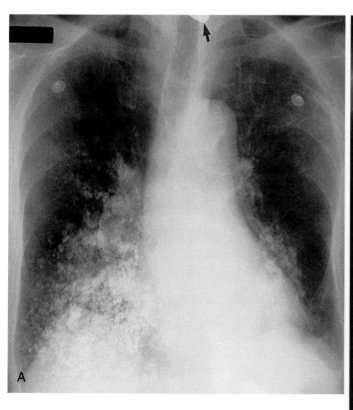

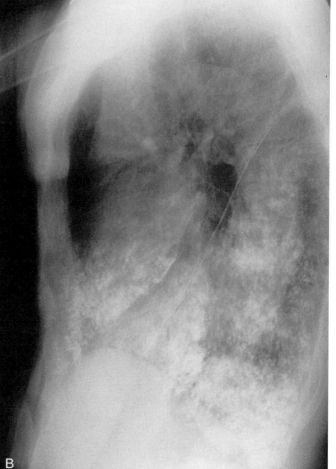

Figure 61–13. Aspiration of Oropharangeal Contents and Barium. Posteroanterior *(A)* and lateral *(B)* chest radiographs in an 88-year-old woman demonstrate barium, mainly in the right middle and lower lobes and in the left lower lobe. Barium can also be seen within the inferior margin of a Zenker's diverticulum *(arrow)*. The aspiration occurred shortly after a barium swallow.

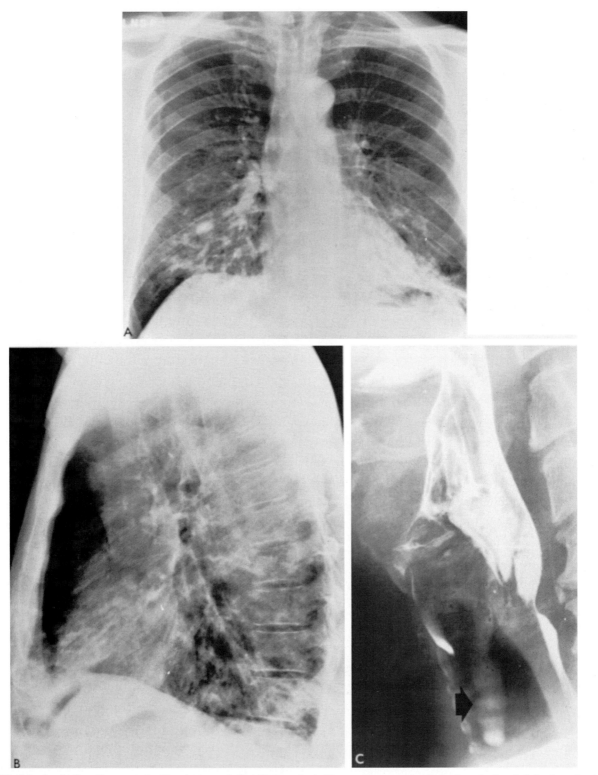

Figure 61–14. Aspiration Pneumonia (Carcinoma of the Pharynx). A 54-year-old man was admitted to the hospital for investigation of an oropharyngeal mass that proved, on biopsy, to be primary carcinoma. Chest radiographs on admission were normal. During his hospitalization, he developed cough and low-grade fever. Chest radiographs in posteroanterior *(A)* and lateral *(B)* projections reveal extensive inhomogeneous, segmental consolidation of both lower lobes, the right middle lobe, and the lingula. The possibility that this was caused by aspiration was considered, and a barium swallow was performed. A view of the hypopharynx and upper trachea in lateral projection *(C)* shows barium in the upper trachea *(arrow)*. The fact that the pulmonary disease was largely confined to the lower lung zones suggests that the aspiration occurred when the patient was erect.

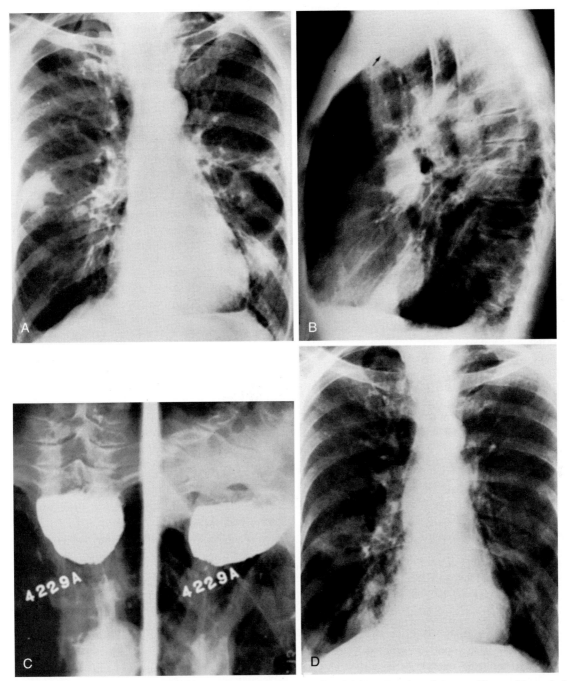

Figure 61–15. Chronic Aspiration Pneumonia Secondary to Zenker's Diverticulum. For about 2 years, a 48-year-old man had had recurrent episodes of acute lower respiratory infection associated with intermittent dysphagia. The radiographs illustrated extend over a period of 7 months. The first *(A)* reveals moderate pulmonary overinflation. Poorly defined homogeneous areas of consolidation are situated in the right midlung and in the left lower lobe, with irregular "streaking" in the axillary portion of the left lung. In lateral projection *(B)*, the several areas of pneumonia are poorly visualized; of greater significance is a homogeneous soft tissue density situated in the superior mediastinum and causing slight anterior displacement of the tracheal air column *(arrow)*. The diagnosis of hypopharyngeal (Zenker's) diverticulum was confirmed by barium studies *(C)*. About 6 months after the first radiograph, a repeat study *(D)* shows almost complete clearing of the pneumonia of the left lung and of the axillary portion of the right lung. However, there is a new area of bronchopneumonia in the posterior basal segment of the right lower lobe. The episodes of recurrent aspiration pneumonia disappeared after surgical resection of the diverticulum.

Clinical Manifestations

As indicated previously, aspiration of gastric contents of low pH occurs most commonly in patients in a comatose state, often after induction of anesthesia. Intubation does not necessarily protect the lungs, because aspirated material situated within the airway above an inflated cuff can flood the lungs when the cuff is deflated; in addition, there is sometimes leakage around an inflated cuff, a complication that has been described even with high-volume, low-pressure endotracheal cuffs.[108]

Respiratory distress may be noted before radiographic abnormalities become manifest. In this situation, fiberoptic bronchoscopy may reveal erythematous lesions of the tracheal mucosa.[109] In the early stages, diffuse crackles may be heard; once consolidation develops, patchy areas of bronchial breathing may be detected. Hypoxemia may be severe. If the patient survives the stage of acute pulmonary edema, an initially dry cough may supervene and become productive of copious purulent sputum; a variety of aerobic and anaerobic pathogens may be cultured from this material.

The presence of recurrent gastroesophageal reflux or a congenital tracheoesophageal fistula should be considered in a patient who has an unexplained cough or a history of repeated pneumonia without obvious cause. Although this applies mostly to infants and children,[110] it is also applicable to adults. The latter may also complain of choking, a symptom that is suggestive of esophageal dysfunction. Appropriate investigations include contrast studies, endoscopy, and manometry of the esophagus; prolonged pH monitoring of esophageal secretions and intragastric radioisotope instillation may also be helpful in diagnosing reflux. Methods that have been proposed to detect aspiration in patients at increased risk include pulse oximetry and radionuclide sialography.[111, 112] The results of an experimental investigation in rabbits suggest that analysis of bronchoalveolar lavage (BAL) fluid for peptic activity also may be useful.[113]

Prognosis and Natural History

As indicated previously, morbidity and mortality depend on the acidity and amount of material aspirated; the death rate of individuals who aspirate a quantity of acid gastric fluid sufficient to develop ARDS is as high as 40% to 50%.[92] In our experience, patients who survive a single bout of aspiration do not show clinical, physiologic, or radiographic sequelae. However, recovery may be prolonged: in one study of five adolescents who survived ARDS after gastric aspiration, continuing improvement in pulmonary function and gas transfer was evident 18 months after the acute episode.[114] Despite these observations, long-term follow-up has revealed persistent respiratory insufficiency in some patients.[115]

ASPIRATION OF LIPIDS

Lipid can accumulate in the lungs from either endogenous or exogenous sources.[116] The former situation is seen in such conditions as obstructive pneumonitis, pulmonary alveolar proteinosis, and hereditary errors of lipid metabolism. These conditions are entirely different in nature from the exogenous form and are considered elsewhere in this book. The term *lipid (lipoid) pneumonia* is restricted here to disease caused by the aspiration of mineral oil or of the various vegetable or animal oils present in food.

Etiology and Pathogenesis

Mineral Oil

Mineral oil is the most common agent to cause lipid pneumonia. Disease occurs most frequently when the oil is used as a lubricant in infants who have feeding difficulties, in old people who are constipated, and in patients with dysphagia caused by neurologic disease or intrinsic esophageal disease such as hypopharyngeal (Zenker's) diverticulum, carcinoma, or achalasia.[117, 118] In these situations, there are presumably repeated subclinical episodes of aspiration, eventually resulting in sufficient accumulation of lipid to cause radiologic or clinical abnormalities.

Many other settings have occasionally been associated with lipid pneumonia, and careful history taking may be necessary to elicit the appropriate source of risk. Although oil-based nose drops are not used as widely now as formerly, cases of lipid pneumonia caused by nasal medication containing liquid paraffin are still seen occasionally.[119, 120] Other substances containing mineral oil and applied to the face or nose, such as Vicks VapoRub,[121] lip gloss,[122] petroleum jelly,[123, 124] and (in one instance) an oriental folk medicine[125] have also been found to cause the disease. Experimental studies have shown that oil deposited in the nasal cavities of sleeping individuals can subsequently be identified in the lungs,[126] and it is presumably by such silent aspiration that pneumonia results in these individuals. Although not likely to be seen today, bronchopleural fistula formation and resultant lipid pneumonia have occurred secondary to oleothorax treatment of tuberculosis.[127] One remarkable case occurred in a patient who attempted suicide by immersing himself in a vat of mineral oil.[128]

Mineral oil pneumonia has also been associated with its inhalation in the form of a mist. This has been described in a variety of occupational settings, including cold reduction by water of mineral oil–coated strip steel,[129] the cleaning or lubricating of machinery such as airplane undercarriages,[130] the prevention of rust, the loosening of automobile bolts, and the handling of oil-impregnated cables.[117] It has also been reported in an individual who used the oil-containing lubricant WD-40 as a spray to relieve back pain.[131] Diffuse interstitial lipid pneumonia has been described in natives of Guyana who smoke tobacco known as *black-fat*, in which mineral oil and petroleum jelly are added to the tobacco for flavoring and as humectants; in one investigation, such disease was identified in 20% of black-fat smokers in the area under study.[132]

The pathogenesis of mineral oil–related fibrosis is not well understood. The substance is a pure hydrocarbon and is believed to be inert, a feature that may explain the lack of airway-mediated cough reflex that follows aspiration. It has been suggested that release of lysosomal enzymes by injured or dead lipid-laden macrophages may be a factor in causing fibrosis.[133] However, it is also possible that other inflammatory or immune-mediator cells are involved.[134]

Animal Lipids

The principal animal oils associated with pneumonia are those in milk or milk products[135] and in fish liver oil (most commonly from cod but also, occasionally, from shark).[136] Aspiration of these substances occurs predominantly in infants and young children during feeding. Pneumonia has also been reported to follow aspiration of ghee.[137] One unusual case of lipid pneumonia has been reported in an engineer who tested the efficiency of fire extinguishers against simulated flash fires fueled with various commercial lards, shortenings, and rancid animal renderings.[138] In contrast to mineral oils, animal fats are hydrolyzed into fatty acids, presumably by lung lipases, and their presence in the lung can cause acute hemorrhagic pneumonitis.[139]

Vegetable Lipids

Aspiration of vegetable oils occurs in a variety of circumstances and appears to possess great variability in its capacity to cause tissue damage.[139] It is likely that these substances are aspirated most commonly during eating or in association with vomiting of gastric contents, in which circumstances the oil is unlikely to be the sole offending agent; as a result, damage to the lung caused by the oil itself is difficult to assess. Only occasional instances of pure vegetable oil aspiration have been well documented; for example, an oily suspension of methenamine containing sesame and hydrogenated castor oil was implicated as the cause of pneumonia in two senile patients.[140] The custom in some parts of the world of smearing oil in babies' mouths or noses has been identified as a cause of pneumonia[74, 137] and, possibly, bronchiectasis.[141]

The pathogenesis of pulmonary disease resulting from vegetable oil aspiration is not completely understood. Some oils remain for prolonged periods in alveolar spaces without causing either fibrosis or a significant inflammatory response.[139] However, others cause tissue reactions similar to those associated with animal oils; as with the latter, hydrolysis can cause the release of fatty acids that may be important in pathogenesis.[139]

Pathologic Characteristics

As noted previously, the degree and quality of tissue reaction to aspirated oil are variable and are related to the quantity and frequency of aspiration, to the chemical characteristics of the oil, and to the complicating effects of other substances that may be aspirated at the same time. The initial reaction to many animal oils and some vegetable oils is an acute bronchopneumonia characterized by edema, intra-alveolar hemorrhage, and a mixed polymorphonuclear and mononuclear infiltrate. Macrophages become finely vacuolated as they ingest the lipid. Although most lipid is probably eliminated by metabolism in macrophages or transported up the mucociliary escalator, some enters the interstitial tissue and is transported through the lymphatics to bronchopulmonary and mediastinal lymph nodes, which can undergo hyperplasia.[142] Giant cell and granuloma formation can be absent or extensive. In the early stages of milk aspiration, amorphous, eosinophilic material resembling fibrin can

sometimes be identified within alveoli and terminal airways, representing collections of unaltered milk.[142]

The reaction to aspirated mineral oil is characterized in the early stage by an intra-alveolar infiltrate of macrophages accompanied by minimal, if any, acute inflammatory reaction. The oil is rapidly emulsified and phagocytosed, resulting in fine vacuolation of macrophages (Fig. 61–16). With time, these macrophages become predominantly interstitial in location and decrease in number. The small oil droplets in turn coalesce to form relatively large round or oval droplets situated within multinucleated giant cells (Fig. 61–17). Typically, the nuclei of these cells are compressed into a flattened rim at the edge of the oil droplet. True granulomas do not develop. Fibrous tissue containing scattered collections of lymphocytes surrounds the giant cells (*see* Fig. 61–17). In the early stages, droplets can also be identified free within interstitial tissues and the media of small arteries; endarteritis obliterans can be seen in later stages. Grossly, the area of fibrosis can form a fairly well-circumscribed, stellate tumor ("paraffinoma," Fig. 61–18), or can be more diffuse and patchy in appearance, resembling nonspecific, organized pneumonitis.

Although the staining reactions of various oils have been described,[143] the precise characterization of an oily substance within the lung can be difficult by microscopy alone. Thin-layer chromatography, chemical analysis, and infrared spectroscopy have been used for definitive identification.[120, 144–146]

Radiologic Manifestations

In the early stages, the typical pattern of disease is air-space consolidation. Depending on the quantity of oil aspirated, the resultant shadows can be confluent or discrete—in fact, isolated air-space nodules can form a distinctive feature during the early stages.[147] Although the radiographic pattern varies, its most common form is relatively homogeneous consolidation of one or more segments, often in precise segmental distribution (Fig. 61–19). In most cases, the lower lobes are predominantly affected, although in debilitated patients in a recumbent position, involvement is likely to occur in the superior segment of a lower lobe or the posterior segment of an upper lobe.[148–151] The consolidated area may be several centimeters in diameter, with poorly defined or fairly sharply defined margins. Because the oil is transported from the alveoli into the interstitium, a predominantly interstitial pattern can develop in the later stages. Rarely, chronic lipid aspiration is sufficient to result in multiple masslike opacities (Fig. 61–20). Withdrawal of the medication may be followed by slow but progressive radiographic resolution (Fig. 61–21).

Another, almost as common manifestation is a peripheral mass, sometimes with fairly well-circumscribed margins, simulating peripheral pulmonary carcinoma (Fig. 61–22).[147] This abnormality also develops chiefly in the dependent portions of the lung, although sometimes in the middle lobe or lingula. Linear shadows radiating from the periphery of such a localized mass result from the interlobular septal thickening caused by infiltration of lipid-laden macrophages and secondary chronic inflammation. Ossification is evident in some cases.[152] Rarely, the acute phase of the

Text continued on page 2506

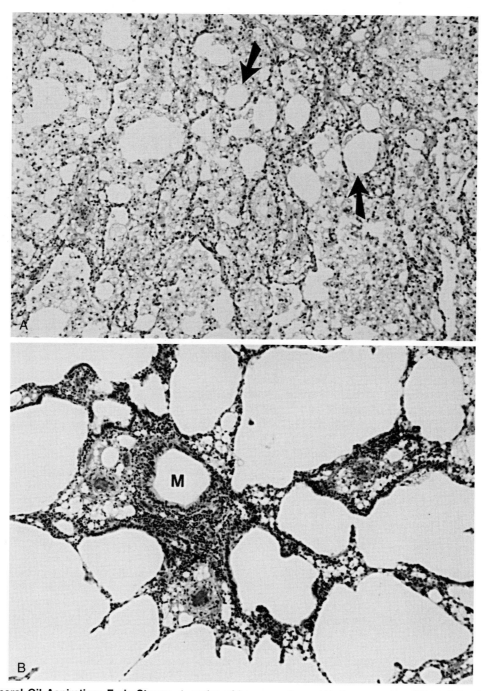

Figure 61–16. Mineral Oil Aspiration: Early Stages. A section of lung parenchyma *(A)* shows complete filling of alveolar air spaces by finely vacuolated macrophages; occasional oval clear spaces *(arrows)* probably represent free mineral oil. Note that the parenchymal interstitium is virtually normal. A somewhat later stage is revealed in a section from a different patient *(B)*, in which the air spaces are largely devoid of macrophages; instead, the interstitium (especially adjacent to a small membranous bronchiole [M]) shows a lymphocytic infiltrate and numerous lipid-laden macrophages. *(A,* ×80; *B,* ×80.)

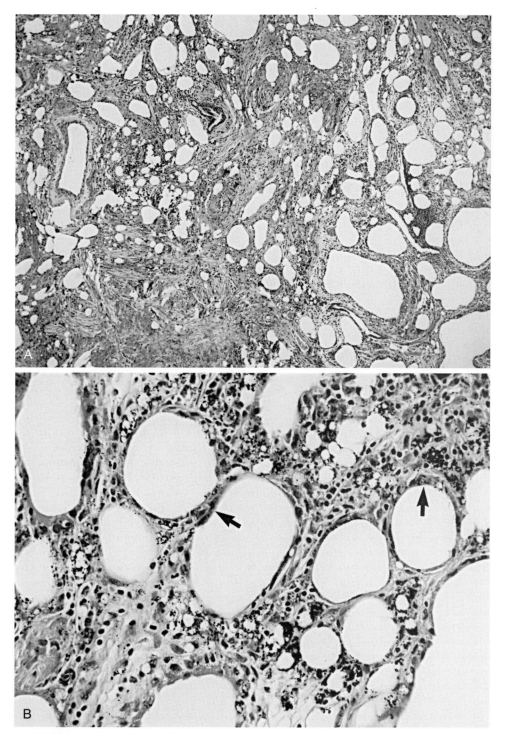

Figure 61–17. Mineral Oil Aspiration: Chronic Stage. A section from a well-circumscribed parenchymal nodule *(A)* shows fibrous tissue with admixed lymphocytes and numerous clear spaces of variable size and shape. At higher magnification *(B)*, many of the clear spaces can be seen to be surrounded by a thin rim of cytoplasm containing multiple, somewhat flattened nuclei *(arrows)*. The clear spaces represent foci of mineral oil within multinucleated giant cells. *(A,* ×40; *B,* ×250.)

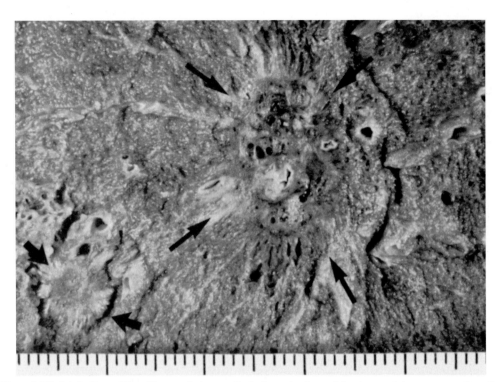

Figure 61–18. Mineral Oil Aspiration: "Paraffinoma." A magnified view of a lower lobe (resected for a presumptive diagnosis of carcinoma) shows two fairly well-defined nodules, one round *(short arrows)* and the other oval with a somewhat spiculated appearance *(long arrows)*. Histologic examination showed typical chronic lipid pneumonia.

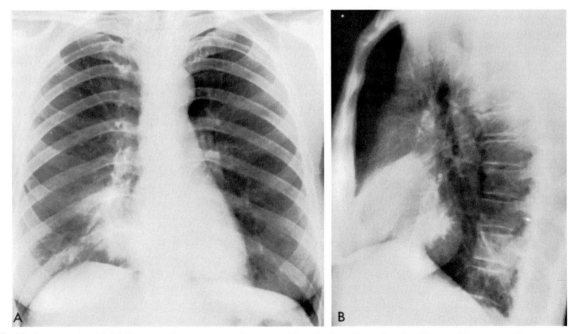

Figure 61–19. Exogenous Lipid Pneumonia. Posteroanterior *(A)* and lateral *(B)* radiographs of a 53-year-old symptom-free woman reveal poorly defined shadows of homogeneous density situated in the right middle lobe, the anterior segment of the right lower lobe, and the posterior basal segment of the left lower lobe. Thorough clinical and laboratory investigations failed to reveal the cause of these shadows. Ten years later, the patient died after rupture of a congenital berry aneurysm of the anterior cerebral artery. Autopsy revealed chronic lipid pneumonia of both lower lobes and the right middle lobe.

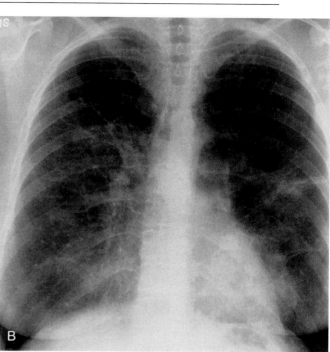

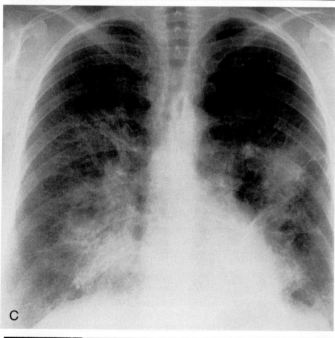

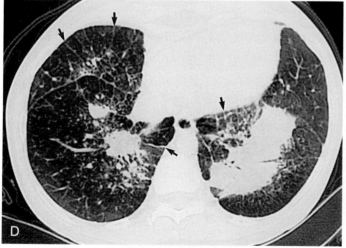

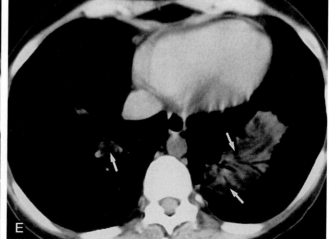

Figure 61–20. Lipid Pneumonia: Progression of Findings. A posteroanterior chest radiograph in a 27-year-old woman *(A)* demonstrates extensive bilateral parenchymal abnormalities consisting mainly of linear opacities including Kerley B lines. Small focal areas of consolidation are present in the lower lobes. A chest radiograph 6 years later *(B)* demonstrates more extensive areas of consolidation in the left lower lobe as well as focal consolidation in the lingula and right upper lobe. Linear opacities are again evident, particularly in the right lung. A chest radiograph 10 years after the initial examination *(C)* demonstrates more extensive consolidation. Irregular linear opacities are associated with these areas of consolidation, particularly in the left lung, suggesting the presence of fibrosis. A CT scan performed at this time *(D)* demonstrates focal areas of consolidation with air bronchograms in the lower lobes. Note the distortion of architecture, particularly around the consolidation in the left lower lobe, indicating the presence of fibrosis. Also note thickening of interlobular septa *(black arrows)*. Soft tissue windows *(E)* demonstrate the presence of fat within the areas of consolidation *(white arrows)*. The patient was a psychotic woman who repeatedly took mineral oil. (Courtesy of Dr. R. Levy, Vancouver General Hospital.)

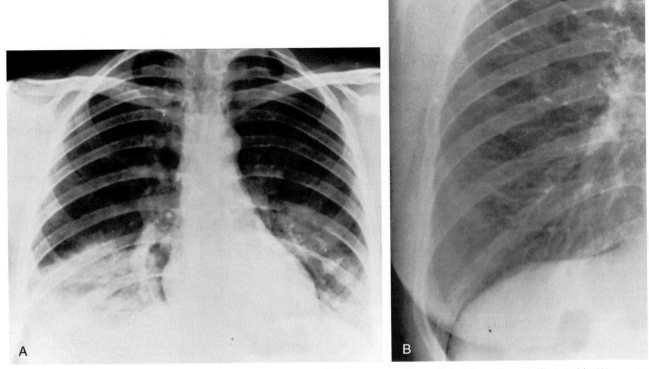

Figure 61–21. Lipid Pneumonia with Complete Radiograph Resolution. For several years before the radiograph illustrated in *(A)*, symptomatic middle-aged woman had been using oily nose drops many times a day for a stuffy nose. The radiograph reveals massive consolidation of both lower lung zones, the right more than the left. The consolidation is homogeneous except for a well-defined air bronchogram. Although the diagnosis of lipid pneumonia must be regarded as presumptive because a biopsy was not performed, the facts that the patient was asymptomatic and that oil droplets were identified in the sputum constitute reasonably convincing evidence. No treatment was given other than a change in the nose drops to a nonoily mixture. Six months later *(B)* all signs of pulmonary disease had disappeared.

process can be associated with cavitation, probably related to concomitant anaerobic infection.[116, 153]

The diagnosis of lipid pneumonia often can be made on CT by the presence of areas of low attenuation or fat attenuation (-90 Hounsfield units) within the lesion (*see* Fig. 61–22).[118, 154–157] In one investigation in which the radiographic and CT findings were compared in six patients—three who had a history of intake of shark liver oil as a restorative and three who had intake of mineral oil for constipation—chest radiography showed bilateral air-space consolidation in three, irregular masslike lesions in two, and a reticulonodular pattern in one.[157] In the three patients who had air-space consolidation, CT demonstrated attenuation lower than that of chest wall musculature but slightly higher than that of subcutaneous fat. In the two patients who had masslike lesions, there were localized areas of consolidation containing fat; irregular lines and architectural distortion suggested fibrosis around the areas of consolidation. The patient who had a reticulonodular pattern on the radiograph had no evidence of fat attenuation on CT. Occasionally, lipid pneumonia presents as multifocal areas of ground-glass attenuation associated with interlobular septal thickening, an appearance that resembles the "crazy-paving" pattern seen in alveolar proteinosis.[158]

The MR imaging findings of lipid pneumonia have been reported in a small number of patients.[159, 160] Using spin-echo imaging, areas of consolidation have high signal intensity on T1- and T2-weighted images, reflecting the lipid content of the aspirate (Fig. 61–23).[159] A specific diagnosis can also be made using chemical-shift MR imaging.[160]

Clinical Manifestations and Diagnosis

Most patients with mineral oil aspiration are asymptomatic, the abnormality being discovered on a screening chest radiograph. In fact, the diagnosis is sometimes made by histologic examination of tissue removed at thoracotomy performed on the basis of an erroneous diagnosis of pulmonary carcinoma.[151] Some patients complain of chronic, usually nonproductive cough or pleuritic pain. Rarely, aspiration of a relatively large amount of liquid oil causes an acute illness resembling infectious pneumonia.[161] Occasional patients develop hypercalcemia,[162, 163] a complication speculated to have a pathogenesis similar to that seen in sarcoidosis.

Clinical findings in cases of animal or vegetable oil aspiration are usually those of acute pneumonia. As indicated, many patients have also aspirated other material in gastric contents at the same time as the lipid, and the background and course are similar to those outlined in the section on aspiration of gastric secretions.

The diagnosis of mineral oil aspiration should be suspected in any patient with a history of exposure to oily substances, particularly if there is an underlying condition predisposing to aspiration. As indicated previously, however, the identification of an exposure history may be difficult. The finding of fat droplets in macrophages in BAL fluid supports the diagnosis;[121, 164] however, fat can sometimes be identified in the sputum of normal subjects, and its presence is not incontrovertible evidence of pulmonary disease. The value of quantification of lipid-laden alveolar macrophages in diagnosis has been stressed.[165, 166] Transthoracic needle

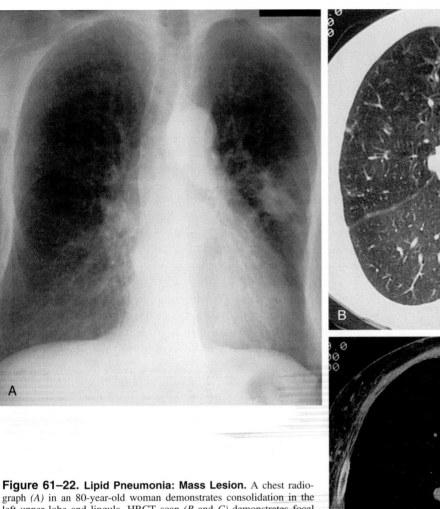

Figure 61–22. Lipid Pneumonia: Mass Lesion. A chest radiograph *(A)* in an 80-year-old woman demonstrates consolidation in the left upper lobe and lingula. HRCT scan *(B and C)* demonstrates focal area of consolidation with surrounding linear opacities and architectural distortion consistent with fibrosis. Localized areas of fat attenuation are present within the consolidation *(arrow)*, permitting the diagnosis of lipid pneumonia. The diagnosis was confirmed by fine-needle aspiration biopsy. The patient had a history of intake of mineral oil for constipation.

aspiration or transbronchial biopsy generally establishes the diagnosis in cases in which the results of BAL are uncertain.[154, 157]

Prognosis and Natural History

The natural history and long-term effects of mineral oil aspiration are variable. With small amounts, there is little, if any, clinical or functional impairment; however, if sufficient oil is aspirated over a long period, functional restrictive disease may become evident and, in severe cases, cor pulmonale may develop.[167, 168] Improvement in pulmonary function has been shown to correlate with the measured quantity of oil expectorated.[169] There is some evidence that the presence

of mineral oil in the lungs is associated with an increased risk for the development of pulmonary carcinoma[117] and infection with some species of nontuberculous mycobacteria.[170]

ASPIRATION OF WATER (DROWNING)

Drowning can be defined as death caused by asphyxia as a result of submersion in liquid (usually water), provided the victim succumbs within 24 hours of the submersion episode. *Near-drowning* is defined as survival (at least temporarily) after a submersion episode; the term has still been used if the victim dies more than 24 hours after the submersion episode. The designation *secondary near-drowning* has

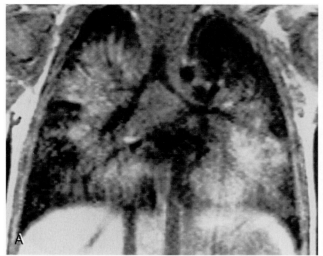

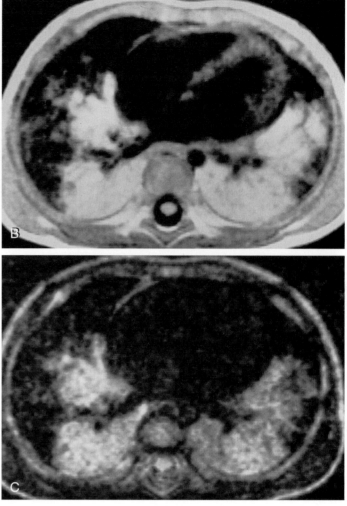

Figure 61–23. Lipid Pneumonia: MR Imaging Findings. An 8-month-old infant developed acute respiratory symptoms after oral administration of shark liver oil (Squalene) for the treatment of upper respiratory infection. A coronal *(A)* T1-weighted MR image demonstrates extensive bilateral consolidation with air bronchograms. High-signal intensity of the consolidation is apparent on both the T1-weighted *(B)* and T2-weighted *(C)* transverse images. High-signal intensity on both T1- and T2-weighted images is characteristic of fat. Note similarity of signal intensity of the areas of consolidation with the signal intensity of subcutaneous fat. The images were obtained using cardiac gated spin-echo technique with TR 500, TE 15 (T1-weighted images) and TR 2000, TE 60 (T2-weighted images). (Courtesy of Dr. Joung Sook Kim, Department of Radiology, Sanggye Paik Hospital College of Medicine, Seoul, Korea.)

been applied to those patients who die from complications of the initial submersion accident (e.g., superimposed infection). (Some authorities have suggested that this last term be abandoned because it only adds confusion to an already complicated terminology; instead, when death occurs after 24 hours, its specific cause is indicated as a complication of a near-drowning incident.[171]) The somewhat incongruous term *dry-drowning* refers to the situation in which death results from apnea secondary to laryngeal spasm, with minimal or no aspiration of water into the lungs; it has been estimated that this variety is responsible for 5% to 15% of deaths.[172, 173]

Drowning is an important cause of accidental death, particularly in children; it has been estimated that about 140,000 such deaths occur worldwide each year, of which about 7,000 to 9,000 are in the United States.[174] Of equal or greater importance is the morbidity from anoxic brain damage in patients suffering near-drowning accidents: about 25% to 35% of survivors who arrive comatose at a hospital have residual neurologic impairment.[172] Near-drowning accidents have been estimated to be from 2 to 20 times more common than drowning, indicating the magnitude of this problem.[174]

Pathogenesis

Both the tonicity and volume of aspirated water have effects on the pathogenesis of the pulmonary reaction. In experimental animals, the effects of inhaling sea water (which has about three times the tonicity of extracellular fluid) clearly differ from those of inhaling fresh water (whose salt content is negligible). The importance of tonicity was dramatically illustrated in a series of experiments on mice; those animals submerged in suitably oxygenated physiologic saline solution could survive for as long as 18 hours, whereas when this medium was replaced by sea water or tap water, the mice succumbed in less than 12 minutes.[175] The volume of water aspirated is also critical; in experimental animals, the chance of survival is very small if the volume of water inhaled exceeds 10 ml per pound body weight for sea water and 20 ml per pound for fresh water.[176] (These figures correspond to about 1.5 and 3 liters, respectively, for a 70-kg human.)

Because its tonicity is greater than that of blood, aspirated sea water draws water out of the blood into the alveoli, and ions of sodium, magnesium, calcium, and chloride pass into the blood. All of these movements result in rapid hemoconcentration, hypovolemia, and an increase in the amount of intra-alveolar fluid. The latter leads to $\dot{V}/\dot{Q}$ imbalance and significant pulmonary venous shunting. There follows a slowing of the pulse, a fall in blood pressure, and death in 4 to 5 minutes from hypoxemia and metabolic acidosis. When fresh water enters the alveoli, the situation is reversed. Because of the blood's greater tonicity, inhaled water is rapidly absorbed into the circulation, producing hemodilution and hemolysis of red blood cells.[176] The serum potassium level subsequently rises, and the serum sodium level falls; both changes may be factors in causing ventricular fibrillation. In addition, intra-alveolar water interferes with surfactant, causing some degree of alveolar collapse and $\dot{V}/\dot{Q}$ imbalance and hypoxemia.[172] It has also been speculated that neurogenic pulmonary edema may be responsible for some of the air-space consolidation seen radiographically.[177]

These experimentally observed differences between the effects of inhalation of salt and fresh water are not evident in most cases of human near-drowning; where it has been possible to carry out appropriate examinations, only occasional evidence of significant electrolyte transfer, hemoconcentration, or hemodilution have been found.[178, 179] Perhaps more important, there is little clinical difference between victims of fresh water and salt water drowning.[180]

As discussed previously, it is clear that water entering the alveoli can act as an irritant, whatever its tonicity and whichever way electrolytes flow. In one study of the ultrastructure of pulmonary alveolar capillaries in Mendelson's syndrome, pulmonary edema was present in all specimens, including those in which distilled water was the aspirated fluid;[181] changes in pH and tonicity increased the reaction only in terms of degree and time, suggesting that the pathologic process caused by fresh water aspiration is similar to that produced by acid aspiration and that the major mechanism is increased capillary permeability.

Pathologic Characteristics

Pathologic findings are somewhat variable but consist principally of air-space edema. In one study, morphologic evidence of pulmonary parenchymal damage was seen in all victims whether they survived for a few minutes or for several days;[182] hemorrhagic, desquamative, and exudative reactions developed even in those patients who survived only a few minutes. In some cases, the inhaled water contains organisms (e.g., *Aeromonas sobria*)[183] or debris such as sand, mud, fuel oil, sewage, or other pollutants, all of which can potentially increase pulmonary injury;[184] as a result, deterioration in clinical status may follow initial improvement. The presence of this foreign material, such as diatoms or green algae, can also aid in proving drowning as the cause of death.[185–187]

Radiologic Manifestations

The radiographic changes in patients who have experienced near-drowning from fresh and sea water are similar.[179] The basic finding is air-space consolidation (Fig. 61–24), the severity presumably depending on the amount

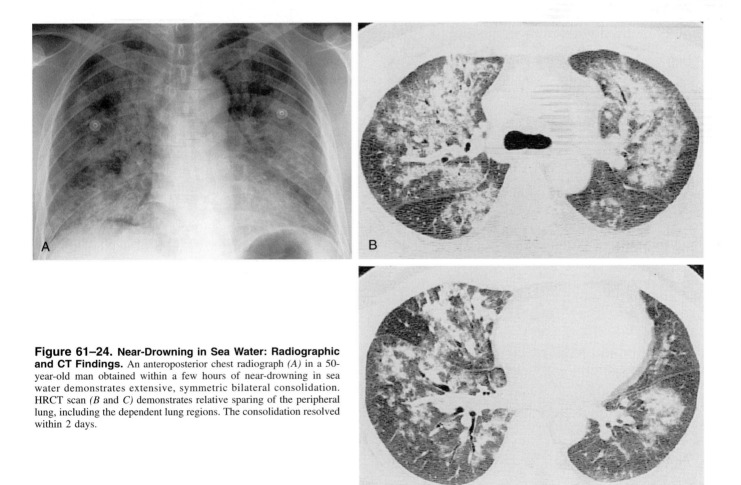

Figure 61–24. Near-Drowning in Sea Water: Radiographic and CT Findings. An anteroposterior chest radiograph *(A)* in a 50-year-old man obtained within a few hours of near-drowning in sea water demonstrates extensive, symmetric bilateral consolidation. HRCT scan *(B* and *C)* demonstrates relative sparing of the peripheral lung, including the dependent lung regions. The consolidation resolved within 2 days.

of aspirated water;[188–190] in the most severe cases, there is almost complete opacification of both lungs. Consolidation is generally bilateral and symmetric, but in relatively mild disease can be predominantly parahilar and midzonal; an asymmetric distribution can also occur (Fig. 61–25). There may be a delay in the radiographic appearance of pulmonary edema, sometimes as long as 24 to 48 hours.[190] Sand that is aspirated along with water can be radiopaque as a result of its calcium carbonate content and can cause a "sand bronchogram" on both radiographs and CT;[191, 192] sand may also be seen within the stomach. Pleural effusion occurs in some cases; in one study, it was found to be more likely in salt water than fresh water drowning and associated with a longer submersion time.[193]

The air-space consolidation generally improves over 3 to 5 days and resolves completely in 7 to 10 days.[189] In some patients, the radiographic changes persist or worsen, findings that may be the result of bacterial pneumonia or ARDS (Fig. 61–26).[179]

Clinical Manifestations

In one review of the clinical manifestations in 36 patients who experienced near-drowning (32 in salt water and 4 in chlorinated pools), 33 of the 36 survived.[179] Only 9 patients were unconscious on arrival at the hospital. Respira-

tory frequency was generally increased to between 30 and 40 breaths per minute during the initial 24 hours; thereafter, it returned to normal levels. One patient had hemoptysis. Fine inspiratory crackles were heard in all patients, and wheezing was noted in a few. In 11 patients, the electrocardiogram showed nonspecific S-T segment and T-wave changes, abnormal patterns that reverted to normal within 36 hours. Severe hypoxemia was a constant finding; the mean PaO_2 was 55 mm Hg and base excess -10 mEq/L.

Although respiratory failure is the most important pathogenetic consequence of drowning, other mechanisms may play a role in the clinical manifestations in some cases. For example, individuals who have experienced near-drowning following a dive into shallow water may have had head or cervical spine injuries.[194] In addition, a patient who has recovered consciousness and seems to be progressing favorably may, within a few hours, show increasing respiratory distress with progressive breathlessness, cyanosis, and cough. As indicated previously, it is probable that the major causes of such deterioration are ARDS and secondary bacterial infection; fungal infection is also a rare complication.[195] Disseminated intravascular coagulation has also been documented in some cases.[196]

Serum electrolyte abnormalities are uncommonly detected in near-drowning victims; nevertheless, hypermagnesemia has been measured in some salt water victims and has been advocated as a test to confirm the diagnosis.[178] As

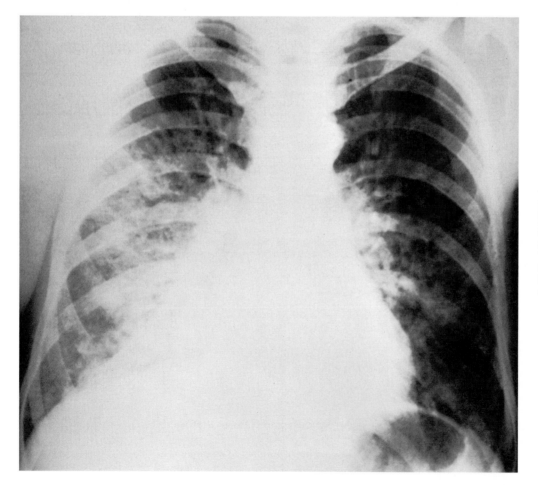

Figure 61–25. Near-Drowning in Sea Water. The man whose radiograph is shown was immersed for an indeterminate time in sea water. There is evidence of extensive bilateral air-space edema, more marked in the right than the left lung. The edema cleared in 3 days.

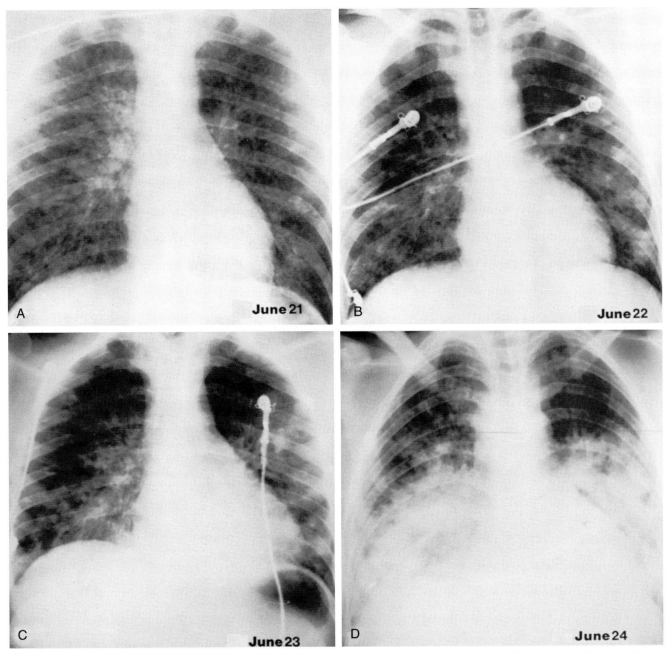

Figure 61–26. Near-Drowning in Fresh Water. A 19-year-old man was immersed in a dirty, badly polluted, fresh-water lake for a period of about 4 minutes before being rescued; he was under the influence of drugs at the time. The radiograph obtained shortly after his arrival in the emergency department *(A)* reveals widespread patchy air-space consolidation evenly distributed throughout both lungs. Heart size and configuration are normal. Twenty-four hours later *(B)*, the upper zones of both lungs had cleared considerably, although moderate edema persists in the lower zones. Forty-eight hours later *(C)*, the edema appeared to have worsened somewhat in the lower zones. Three days after the acute episode *(D)*, massive air-space consolidation had developed throughout the lower two thirds of both lungs, and the patient's clinical status had deteriorated markedly. This represents the characteristic sequence of events following near-drowning in badly polluted water and the development of acute pneumonia caused by chemicals and debris.

might be expected, such measurement is particularly likely to be abnormal following aspiration of very salty water, such as occurs in the Dead Sea;[197] sodium content there is some three times higher than ordinary sea water, whereas the potassium, calcium, and magnesium concentrations are 15, 36, and 26 times greater. In fact, one report of eight men who drowned in the Dead Sea documented hypernatremia, hypercalcemia, and hypermagnesemia sufficient to have contributed to death.[197] Hypercalcemia was also documented in

an individual who experienced near-drowning in a hot spring containing water that had a high level of calcium.[198] Hypoglycemia has been reported occasionally.[199]

Prognosis and Natural History

The prognosis in patients who have experienced near-drowning was reviewed in one retrospective study of 91

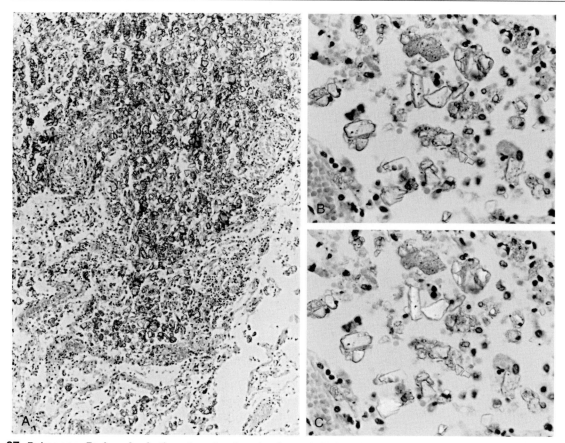

Figure 61–27. Pulmonary Barium Aspiration. A section through a focus of chalky-white parenchymal consolidation *(A)* shows filling of alveolar air spaces by macrophages and numerous irregularly shaped, platelike foreign bodies (seen to better advantage in *B*). A mild lymphocyte infiltrate is present in the adjacent alveolar septa. Polarization microscopy *(C)* confirms the refractile nature of the foreign material. The patient had aspirated during a barium meal about 1 week before death.

victims, 10 of whom died.[200] Patients who were alert on arrival in the emergency department survived; as might be expected, those who were comatose and whose pupils were fixed and dilated invariably died. As indicated previously, cerebral hypoxia may result in neuronal death that can have profound and prolonged aftereffects in those who live. It has been speculated that chances of survival are improved when submersion has occurred in cold water, possibly because the hypothermia serves to protect the brain from hypoxic injury;[201] however, the results of some investigations do not support this hypothesis.[202] A clinical staging system in which patients are divided into six groups has been reported to help predict the likelihood of survival.[193]

Although most patients recover completely from a respiratory point of view, some manifest radiographic evidence of fibrosis (linear opacities) months after recovery.[203] Few patients have had pulmonary function testing after near-drowning; in one study of two patients, an initial restrictive ventilatory pattern and abnormal gas exchange resolved completely over a 16-week follow-up period.[204] In another study, 10 symptom-free children were examined a mean of 3.3 years after submersion accidents;[205] although only mild abnormalities of peripheral airway dysfunction were detected, 7 of the 10 demonstrated bronchial hyper-responsiveness to inhaled methacholine.

ASPIRATION OF MISCELLANEOUS LIQUIDS

Aspiration of *alcohol* in various concentrations has been studied experimentally in one investigation:[206] in the early stages, there was parenchymal edema, hemorrhage, and hyaline membranes consistent with diffuse alveolar damage; in animals that survived for 1 to 4 weeks, there was prominent obliterative bronchiolitis. Pure *carbohydrate solutions*, if administered to rabbits in sufficient quantity and concentration, have been shown to cause edema, acute pneumonia, and fibrosis.[207] Experimental aspiration of *kerosene* causes pulmonary congestion and focal bronchopneumonia accompanied by a shift to the left of the static pressure-volume curve and an increase in total lung capacity.[208] Aspiration of liquid *sucralfate* has been found to cause acute upper airway obstruction in one patient and lung hemorrhage and inflammation in experimental animals.[209] Aspiration of *corrosive fluids*, such as potassium hydroxide drain cleaners, can result in severe mucosal necrosis; in one case, the sloughed mucosa caused acute bronchial obstruction and lung atelectasis.[210]

Several reports have appeared describing the development of pulmonary "edema" after aspiration of *water-soluble contrast media*,[211–213] most commonly in patients who have chronic pulmonary disease. This observation should alert radiologists to exercise caution in employing these substances in circumstances in which there is danger of aspiration. *Barium* may also be aspirated, typically following a barium meal for the investigation of dysphagia or gastrointestinal disease. Radiographs show focal dense air-space opacities (*see* Fig. 61–13, page 2497). Histologic examination may show little evidence of inflammatory reaction. The diagnosis can be confirmed by the identification of typical refractile, platelike barium crystals in tissue sections or cytologic specimens (Fig. 61–27).[214] Clinical manifestations are probably mild or absent in most cases; however, severe respiratory distress necessitating intubation has been reported.[215]

Aspiration of *metallic mercury* has been reported after accidental breakage of a thermometer or indwelling intestinal tube[216] and after a suicide attempt.[217] The material appears to incite little inflammatory reaction and is slowly removed by the mucociliary escalator and cough.[217] It can be distinguished radiographically from embolized mercury by the absence of collections of mercury within the heart chambers (*see* page 1863).

REFERENCES

1. Keith FM, Charrette EJP, Lynn RB, et al: Inhalation of foreign bodies by children: A continuing challenge in management. Can Med Assoc J 122:52, 1980.
2. Mittleman RE: Fatal choking in infants and children. Am J Forensic Med Pathol 5:201, 1984.
3. Weissberg D, Schwartz I: Foreign bodies in the tracheobronchial tree. Chest 91:730, 1987.
4. Lan RS: Non-asphyxiating tracheobronchial foreign bodies in adults. Eur Respir J 7:510, 1994.
5. Limper AH, Prakash UB: Tracheobronchial foreign bodies in adults. Ann Intern Med 112:604, 1990.
6. Chen CH, Lai CL, Tsai TT, et al: Foreign body aspiration into the lower airway in Chinese adults. Chest 112:129, 1997.
7. Wager GC, Williams JH Jr: Flexible bronchoscopic removal of radioccult polyurethane foam, with pneumonitis in a hyperventilated lobe. Am Rev Respir Dis 142:1222, 1990.
8. Jackson C: Observations on the pathology of foreign bodies in the air and food passages: Based on the analysis of 628 cases. Surg Gynecol Obstet 28:201, 1919.
9. Blazer S, Naveh Y, Friedman A: Foreign body in the airway: A review of 200 cases. Am J Dis Child 134:68, 1980.
10. Brown BS, Ma H, Dunbar JS, et al: Foreign bodies in the tracheobronchial tree in childhood. J Can Assoc Radiol 14:158, 1963.
11. Burton EM, Brick WG, Hall JD, et al: Tracheobronchial foreign body aspiration in children. South Med J 89:195, 1996.
12. Gay BB Jr: Radiologic evaluation of the nontraumatized child with respiratory distress. Radiol Clin North Am 16:91,1978.
13. Abdulmajid OA, Ebeid AM, Motaweh MM, et al: Aspirated foreign bodies in the tracheobronchial tree: Report of 250 cases. Thorax 31:635, 1976.
14. Marom EM, McAdams HP, Sporn TA, et al: Lentil aspiration pneumonia: Radiographic and CT findings. J Comput Assist Tomogr 22:598, 1998.
15. Jewett TC Jr, Butsch WL: Trials with treacherous timothy grass. J Thorac Cardiovasc Surg 50:124, 1965.
16. Merriam JC Jr, Storrs RC, Hoefnagel D: Lung disease caused by aspirated timothy-grass heads. Am Rev Respir Dis 90:947, 1964.
17. Pneumocutaneous fistula secondary to aspiration of grass (letter). J Pediatr 82:737, 1973.
18. Basok O, Yaldiz S, Kilincer L: Bronchiectasis resulting from aspirated grass inflorescences. Scand Cardiovasc J 31:157, 1997.
19. Hilman BC, Kurzweg FT, McCook WW Jr, et al: Foreign body aspiration of grass inflorescences as a cause of hemoptysis. Chest 78:306, 1980.
20. Jackson C, Jackson CL: Staples and double-pointed tacks as foreign bodies: Mechanical problems of bronchoscopic extraction. Arch Otolaryngol 22:603, 1935.
21. Pochaczevsky R, Leonidas JC, Feldman F, et al: Aspirated and ingested teeth in children. Clin Radiol 24:349, 1973.
22. Mearns AJ, England RM: Dissolving foreign bodies in the trachea and bronchus. Thorax 30:461, 1975.
23. Overdahl MC, Wewers MD: Acute occlusion of a mainstem bronchus by a rapidly expanding foreign body. Chest 105:1600, 1994.
24. Lamaze R, Trechot P, Martinet Y: Bronchial necrosis and granuloma induced by the aspiration of a tablet of ferrous sulphate. Eur Resp J 7:1710, 1994.
25. Mittleman M, Perek J, Kolkov Z, et al: Fatal aspiration pneumonia caused by an esophageal foreign body. Ann Emerg Med 14:365, 1985.
26. Chopra S, Simmons DH, Cassan SM, et al: Case reports: Bronchial obstruction by incorporation of aspirated vegetable material in the bronchial wall. Am Rev Respir Dis 112:717, 1975.
27. Ristagno RL, Kornstein MJ, Hansen-Flaschen JH: Diagnosis of occult meat aspiration by fiberoptic bronchoscopy. Am J Med 80:154, 1986.
28. Weiss E, Krusen FH: Foreign body in the lung for thirty-five years complicated by abscess and tumor formation. JAMA 78:506, 1922.
29. Tarkka M, Anttila S, Sutinen S: Bronchial stenosis after aspiration of an iron tablet. Chest 93:439, 1988.
30. Limper AH, Prakash UBS: Tracheobronchial foreign bodies in adults. Ann Intern Med 112:604, 1990.
31. Chen C-H, Lai C-L, Tsai T-T, et al: Foreign body aspiration into the lower airway in Chinese adults. Chest 112:129, 1997.
32. Rudavsky AZ, Leonidas JC, Abramson AL: Lung scanning for the detection of endobronchial foreign bodies in infants and children: Clinical and experimental studies. Radiology 108:629, 1973.
33. Berger PE, Kuhn JP, Kuhns LR: Computed tomography and the occult tracheobronchial foreign body. Radiology 134:133, 1980.
34. Ikeda M, Kitahara S, Inouye T: Large radiolucent tracheal foreign body found by CT scan caused dyspnea: An admonition on flexible fiberscopic foreign body removal. Surg Endosc 10:164, 1996.
35. O'Uchi T, Tokumaru A, Mikami I, et al: Value of MR imaging in detecting a peanut causing bronchial obstruction. Am J Roentgenol 159:481,1992.
36. Kang EY, Miller RR, Müller NL: Bronchiectasis: comparison of preoperative thin-section CT and pathologic findings in resected specimens. Radiology 195:649, 1995.
37. Kürklü EU, Williams MA, le Roux BT: Bronchiectasis consequent upon foreign body retention. Thorax 28:601, 1973.
38. Laks Y, Barzilay Z: Foreign body aspiration in childhood. Pediatr Emerg Care 4:102, 1988.
39. Miller GA, Gianturco C, Neucks HG: The asymptomatic period in retained foreign bodies of the bronchus. Am J Dis Child 95:282, 1958.
40. Cole MJ, Smith JT, Molnar C, et al: Aspiration after percutaneous gastrostomy: Assessment by Tc-99m labeling of the enteral feed. J Clin Gastroenterol 9:90, 1987.
41. Ben-Dov I, Aelony Y: Foreign body aspiration in the adult: An occult cause of chronic pulmonary symptoms. Postgrad Med J 65:299, 1989.
42. Mittleman RE: The fatal café coronary. JAMA 247:1285, 1982.
43. Irwin RS, Ashba JK, Braman SS, et al: Food asphyxiation in hospitalized patients. JAMA 237:2744, 1977.
44. Hsieh HH, Bhatia SC, Andersen JM, et al: Psychotropic medication and nonfatal cafe coronary. J Clin Psychopharmacol 6:101, 1986.
45. Northcote RJ: Pulmonary aspiration presenting with generalized convulsions. Scott Med J 28:368, 1983.
46. Strauss D, Kastner T, Ashwal S, et al: Tube feeding and mortality in children with severe disabilities and mental retardation. Pediatrics 99:358, 1997.
47. Phillips I, Jamieson CG: Pulmonary aspiration complicating intraoperative small-bowel decompression: A case report and literature review. Can J Surg 39:495, 1996.
48. Tolep K, Getch CL, Criner GJ: Swallowing dysfunction in patients receiving prolonged mechanical ventilation. Chest 109:167, 1996.
49. Lipper B, Simon D, Cerrone F: Pulmonary aspiration during emergency endoscopy in patients with upper gastrointestinal hemorrhage. Crit Care Med 19:330, 1991.
50. Elpern EH, Scott MG, Petro L, et al: Pulmonary aspiration in mechanically ventilated patients with tracheostomies. Chest 105:563, 1994.
51. Akhtar TM, Street MK: Risk of aspiration with the laryngeal mask. Br J Anaesth 72:447, 1994.
52. Miller KS, Tomlinson JR, Sahn SA: Pleuropulmonary complications of enteral tube feedings: Two reports, review of the literature, and recommendations. Chest 88:230, 1985.
53. Mellin-Olsen J, Fasting S, Gisvold SE: Routine preoperative gastric emptying is seldom indicated: A study of 85,594 anaesthetics with special focus on aspiration pneumonia. Acta Anaesthesiol Scand 40:1184, 1996.
54. Soreide E, Bjornestad E, Steen PA: An audit of perioperative aspiration pneumonitis in gynaecological and obstetric patients. Acta Anaesthesiol Scand 40:14, 1996.
55. Noble PW, Lavee AE, Jacobs MM: Respiratory diseases in pregnancy. Obstet Gynecol Clin North Am 15:391, 1988.
56. Hollingsworth HM, Pratter MR, Irwin RS: Acute respiratory failure in pregnancy. J Intensive Care Med 4:11, 1989.
57. Lawes EG, Baskett PJ: Pulmonary aspiration during unsuccessful cardiopulmonary resuscitation. Intensive Care Med 13:379, 1987.
58. Chan TY, Critchley JA: Pulmonary aspiration following Dettol poisoning: The scope for prevention. Hum Exp Toxicol 15:843, 1996.
59. Schmidt J, Holas M, Halvorson K, et al: Videofluoroscopic evidence of aspiration predicts pneumonia and death but not dehydration following stroke. Dysphagia 9:7, 1994.
60. Nakagawa T, Sekizawa K, Arai H, et al: High incidence of pneumonia in elderly patients with basal ganglia infarction. Arch Intern Med 157:321, 1997.
61. Hughes RL, Freilich RA, Bytell DE, et al: Aspiration and occult esophageal disorders: Clinical conference in pulmonary disease from Northwestern University Medical School, Chicago. Chest 80:489, 1981.
62. Rogers B, Stratton P, Msall M, et al: Long-term morbidity and management strategies of tracheal aspiration in adults with severe developmental disabilities. Am J Ment Retard 98:490, 1994.
63. McArthur MS: Pulmonary complications of benign esophageal disease. Am J Surg 151:296, 1986.
64. Camara EJ, Lima JAC, Oliveira GB, et al: Pulmonary findings in patients with chagasic megaesophagus: Study of autopsied cases. Chest 83:87, 1983.
65. Gallagher JD, Smith DS, Meranze J, et al: Aspiration during induction of anaesthesia in patients with colon interposition. Can Anaesth Soc J 32:56, 1985.
66. de Silva D, Osborne A, Simpson SA, et al: Opitz oculo-genito-laryngeal syndrome: A rare cause of recurrent aspiration pneumonia in an adult. Thorax 53:149, 1998.
67. St. Guily JL, Perie S, Willig TN, et al: Swallowing disorders in muscular diseases: Functional assessment and indications of cricopharyngeal myotomy. Ear Nose Throat J 73:34, 1994.
68. Martin BJ, Corlew MM, Wood H, et al: The association of swallowing dysfunction and aspiration pneumonia. Dysphagia 9:1, 1994.
69. Hogue CW Jr, Lappas GD, Creswell LL, et al: Swallowing dysfunction after cardiac operations: Associated adverse outcomes and risk factors including intraoperative transesophageal echocardiography. J Thorac Cardiovasc Surg 110:517, 1995.
70. Coelho CA, Ferrante R: Dysphagia in postpolio sequelae: Report of three cases. Arch Phys Med Rehabil 69:634, 1988.
71. Fetterman GH, Moran TJ: Food aspiration pneumonia. Penn Med J 45:810, 1942.
72. Knoblich R: Pulmonary granulomatosis caused by vegetable particles: So-called lentil pulse pneumonia. Am Rev Respir Dis 99:380, 1969.

73. Huxley EJ, Viroslax J, Gray WR, et al: Pharyngeal aspiration in normal adults and patients with depressed consciousness. Am J Med 64:564, 1978.

74. Annobil SH, el Tahir M, Kameswaran M, et al: Olive oil aspiration pneumonia (lipoid) in children. Trop Med Int Health 2:383, 1997.

75. Newnham DM, Hamilton SJ: Sensitivity of the cough reflex in young and elderly subjects. Age Ageing 26:185, 1997.

76. Irwin RS, Curley FJ, French CL: Chronic cough: The spectrum and frequency of causes, key components of the diagnostic evaluation, and outcome of specific therapy. Am Rev Respir Dis 141:640, 1990.

77. Barish CF, Wu WC, Castell DO: Respiratory complications of gastroesophageal reflux. Arch Intern Med 145:1882, 1985.

78. Mays EE, Dubois JJ, Hamilton GB: Pulmonary fibrosis associated with tracheo-bronchial aspiration: A study of the frequency of hiatal hernia and gastroesophageal reflux in interstitial pulmonary fibrosis of obscure etiology. Chest 69:512, 1976.

79. Stringer DA, Sprigg A, Juodis E, et al: The association of cystic fibrosis, gastroesophageal reflux, and reduced pulmonary function. J Can Assoc Radiol 39:100, 1988.

80. Ing AJ, Ngu MC, Breslin AB: Chronic persistent cough and gastroesophageal reflux. Thorax 46:479, 1991.

81. Ekberg O, Hilderfors H: Defective closure of the laryngeal vestibule: Frequency of pulmonary complications. Am J Roentgenol 145:1159, 1985.

82. McVeagh P, Howman-Giles R, Kemp A: Pulmonary aspiration studied by radio-nuclide milk scanning and barium swallow roentgenography. Am J Dis Child 141:917, 1987.

83. Crausaz FM, Favez G: Aspiration of solid food particles into lungs of patients with gastroesophageal reflux and chronic bronchial disease. Chest 93:376, 1988.

84. Chen CT, Toung TJ, Haupt HM, et al: Evaluation of the efficacy of Alka-Seltzer Effervescent in gastric acid neutralization. Anesth Analg 63:325, 1984.

85. Schwartz DJ, Wynne JW, Gibbs CP, et al: The pulmonary consequences of aspiration of gastric contents at pH values greater than 2.5. Am Rev Respir Dis 121:119, 1980.

86. Bond VK, Stoelting RK, Gupta CD: Pulmonary aspiration syndrome after inhalation of gastric fluid containing antacids. Anesthesiology 51:452, 1979.

87. Wynne JW, Reynolds JC, Hood I, et al: Steroid therapy for pneumonitis induced in rabbits by aspiration of foodstuff. Anesthesiology 51:11, 1979.

88. Gipson SL, Stovall TG, Elkins TE, et al: Pharmacologic reduction of the risk of aspiration. South Med J 79:1356, 1986.

89. Harris PW, Morison DH, Dunn GL, et al: Intramuscular cimetidine and ranitidine as prophylaxis against gastric aspiration syndrome: A randomized double-blind study. Can Anaesth Soc J 31:599, 1984.

90. Manchikanti L, Grow JB, Colliver JA, et al: Bicitra (sodium citrate) and metoclo-pramide in outpatient anesthesia for prophylaxis against aspiration pneumonitis. Anesthesiology 63:378, 1985.

91. Cimetidine and the acid-aspiration syndrome (editorial). Lancet 1:465, 1980.

92. Matthay MA, Rosen GD: Acid aspiration induced lung injury: New insights and therapeutic options. Am J Respir Crit Care Med 154:277, 1996.

93. Folkesson HG, Matthay MA, Hebert CA, et al: Acid aspiration induced lung injury in rabbits is mediated by interleukin-8–dependent mechanisms. J Clin Invest 96:107, 1995.

94. Knight PR, Druskovich G, Tait AR, et al: The role of neutrophils, oxidants, and proteases in the pathogenesis of acid induced pulmonary injury. Anesthesiology 77:772, 1992.

95. MacLennan FM: Maternal mortality from Mendelson's syndrome: An explanation? Lancet 1:587, 1986.

96. Vidyarthi SC: Diffuse miliary granulomatosis of the lungs due to aspirated vegetable cells. Arch Pathol 83:215, 1967.

97. Teabeaut JR II: Aspiration of gastric contents: An experimental study. Am J Pathol 28:51, 1952.

98. Alexander IGS: The ultrastructure of the pulmonary alveolar vessels in Mendel-son's (acid pulmonary aspiration) syndrome. Br J Anaesth 40:408, 1968.

99. Moran TJ: Experimental food-aspiration pneumonia. Arch Pathol 52:350, 1951.

100. Moran TJ: Experimental aspiration pneumonia. IV. Inflammatory and reparative changes produced by intratracheal injections of autologous gastric juice and hydrochloric acid. Arch Pathol 60:122, 1955.

101. Ohrui T, Yamaya M, Suzuki T, et al: Mechanisms of gastric juice-induced hyperpermeability of the cultured human tracheal epithelium. Chest 111:454, 1997.

102. Crome L, Valentine JC: Pulmonary nodular granulomatosis caused by inhaled vegetable particles. J Clin Pathol 15:21, 1962.

103. Matsuse T, Oka T, Kida K, et al: Importance of diffuse aspiration bronchiolitis caused by chronic occult aspiration in the elderly. Chest 110:1289, 1996.

104. Landay MJ, Christensen EE, Bynum LJ: Pulmonary manifestations of acute aspiration of gastric contents. Am J Roentgenol 131:587, 1978.

104a. Müller NL: Aspiration pneumonia. *In* Siegel BA (ed): Chest Disease (fifth series): Test Syllabus. Reston, VA, American College of Radiology, 1996, p 378.

105. Brock RC, Hodgkiss F, Jones HO: Bronchial embolism and posture in relation to lung abscess. Guy's Hosp Rep 91:131, 1948.

106. Coriat P, Labrousse J, Vilde F, et al: Diffuse interstitial pneumonitis due to aspiration of gastric contents. Anaesthesia 39:703, 1984.

107. Ros PR: Lentil aspiration pneumonia (letter). JAMA 251:1277, 1984.

108. MacRae W, Wallace P: Aspiration around high-volume, low-pressure endotra-cheal cuff. BMJ 283:1220, 1981.

109. Campinos L, Duval G, Couturier M, et al: The value of early fibreoptic bronchos-copy after aspiration of gastric contents. Br J Anaesth 55:1103, 1983.

110. Baer M, Maki M, Nurminen J, et al: Esophagitis and findings of long-term esophageal pH recording in children with repeated lower respiratory tract symp-toms. J Pediatr Gastroenterol Nutr 5:187, 1986.

111. Collins MJ, Bakheit AM: Does pulse oximetry reliably detect aspiration in dysphagic stroke patients? Stroke 28:1773, 1997.

112. Heyman S: Volume-dependent pulmonary aspiration of a swallowed radionuclide bolus. J Nucl Med 38:103, 1997.

113. Badellino MM, Buckman RF Jr, Malaspina PJ, et al: Detection of pulmonary aspiration of gastric contents in an animal model by assay of peptic activity in bronchoalveolar fluid. Crit Care Med 24:1881, 1996.

114. Brandstetter RD, Conetta R, Sander NW, et al: Adult respiratory distress syn-drome in adolescents due to aspiration of gastric contents. N Y State J Med 86:513, 1986.

115. Sladen A, Zanca P, Hadnott WH: Aspiration pneumonitis: The sequelae. Chest 59:448, 1971.

116. Genereux GP: Lipids in the lungs: Radiologic-pathologic correlation. J Can Assoc Radiol 21:2, 1970.

117. Spickard A, Hirschmann JV: Exogenous lipoid pneumonia. Arch Intern Med 154:686, 1994.

118. Gondouin A, Manzoni P, Ranfaing E, et al: Exogenous lipoid pneumonia: A retrospective multicentre study of 44 cases in France. Eur Respir J 9:1463, 1996.

119. Spatafora M, Bellia V, Ferrara G, et al: Diagnosis of a case of lipoid pneumonia by bronchoalveolar lavage. Respiration 52:154, 1987.

120. Blondal T, Hartvig P, Bengtsson A, et al: An unnecessary case of paraffin oil pneumonia. Acta Med Scand 213:227, 1983.

121. Silverman JF, Turner RC, West RL, et al: Bronchoalveolar lavage in the diagnosis of lipoid pneumonia. Diag Cytopathol 5:3, 1989.

122. Becton DL, Lowe JE, Falletta JM: Lipoid pneumonia in an adolescent girl secondary to use of lip gloss. J Pediatr 105:421, 1984.

123. Brown AC, Slocum PC, Putthoff SL, et al: Exogenous lipoid pneumonia due to nasal application of petroleum jelly. Chest 105:968, 1994.

124. Davis EW, Hampton AO, Bickham CE, et al: Lipoid pneumonia simulating tumour. J Thorac Surg 28:212, 1954.

125. Jenkins DW, Quinn DL: Lipoid pneumonia caused by an Oriental folk medicine. South Med J 77:93, 1984.

126. Quinn LH, Meyer OO: The relationship of sinusitis and bronchiectasis. Arch Otolaryngol 10:152, 1929.

127. McBurney RP, Jamplis RW, Hedberg G: Oil granuloma and lipoid pneumonitis: A complication of oleothorax. J Thorac Surg 29:271, 1955.

128. Hussain IR, Edenborough FP, Wilson RS, et al: Severe lipoid pneumonia follow-ing attempted suicide by mineral oil immersion. Thorax 51:652, 1996.

129. Cullen MR, Balmes JR, Robins JM, et al: Lipoid pneumonia caused by oil mist from a steel rolling tandem mill. Am J Ind Med 2:51, 1981.

130. Foe RB, Bigham RS Jr: Lipid pneumonia following occupational exposure to oil spray. JAMA 155:33, 1954.

131. Glynn KP, Gale NA: Exogenous lipoid pneumonia due to inhalation of spray lubricant. Chest 97:1265, 1990.

132. Miller GJ, Ashcroft MT, Beadnell HMSG, et al: The lipoid pneumonia of blackfat tobacco smokers in Guyana. Q J Med 40:457, 1971.

133. Scully RE, Galdabini JJ, McNeely BU: Case 19–1977: Lipoid pneumonia. N Eng J Med 296:1105, 1977.

134. Lauque D, Dongay G, Levade T, et al: Bronchoalveolar lavage in liquid paraffin pneumonitis. Chest 98:1149, 1990.

135. O'Hare B, Lerman J, Endo J, et al: Acute lung injury after instillation of human breast milk or infant formula into rabbits' lungs. Anesthesiology 84:1386, 1996.

136. Asnis DS, Saltzman HP, Melchert A: Shark oil pneumonia: An overlooked entity. Chest 103:976, 1993.

137. Balakrishman S: Lipoid pneumonia in infants and children in South India. BMJ 4:329, 1973.

138. Oldenberger D, Maurer WJ, Beltaos E, et al: Inhalation lipoid pneumonia from burning fats: A newly recognized industrial hazard. JAMA 222:1288, 1972.

139. Pinkerton H: The reaction to oils and fats in the lung. Arch Pathol 5:380, 1928.

140. Timmerman RJ, Schroe JA: Lipoid pneumonia caused by methenamide mande-late suspension. JAMA 225:1524, 1973.

141. Dossing M, Khan JH: Nasal or oral oil application on infants: A possible risk factor for adult bronchiectasis. Eur J Epidemiol 11:141, 1995.

142. Moran TJ: Milk-aspiration pneumonia in human and animal subjects. Arch Pathol 55:286, 1953.

143. Wagner JC, Adler DI, Fuller DN: Foreign body granulomata of the lungs due to liquid paraffin. Thorax 10:157, 1955.

144. Fox B: Liquid paraffin pneumonia—with chemical analysis and electron micros-copy. Virchows Arch 382:339, 1979.

145. Heckers H, Melcher F-W, Dittmar K, et al: Paraffin oil pneumonia: Analysis of saturated hydrocarbons in different human tissue. J Chromatogr 146:91, 1978.

146. Levade T, Salvayre R, Dongay G, et al: Chemical analysis of the bronchoalveolar washing fluid in the diagnosis of liquid paraffin pneumonia. J Clin Chem Clin Biochem 25:45, 1987.

147. Kennedy JD, Costello P, Balikian JP, et al: Exogenous lipoid pneumonia. Am J Roentgenol 136:1145, 1981.

148. Sundberg RH, Kirschner KE, Brown MJ: Evaluation of lipid pneumonia. Dis Chest 36:594, 1959.

149. Forbes G, Bradley A: Liquid paraffin as a cause of oil aspiration pneumonia. BMJ 2:1566, 1958.

150. Eyal Z, Borman JB, Milwidsky H: Solitary oil granuloma of the lung: A report of three cases. Br J Dis Chest 55:43, 1961.

151. Guidry LD, Clagett OT, McDonald JR, et al: Pulmonary resection for mineral oil granulomas. Ann Surg 150:67, 1959.

152. Salm R, Hughes EW: A case of chronic paraffin pneumonitis. Thorax 25:762, 1970.

153. Borrie J, Gwynne JF: Paraffinoma of lung: Lipoid pneumonia. Report of two cases. Thorax 28:214, 1973.

154. Wheeler PS, Stitik FP, Hutchins GM, et al: Diagnosis of lipoid pneumonia by computed tomography. JAMA 245:65, 1981.

155. Joshi RR, Cholankeril JV: Computed tomography in lipoid pneumonia. J Comput Assist Tomogr 9:211,1985.

156. Van den Plas O, Trigaux J-P, Van Beers B, et al: Gravity-dependent infiltrates in a patient with lipoid pneumonia. Chest 98:1253,1990.

157. Lee KS, Müller NL, Hale V, et al: Lipoid pneumonia: CT findings. J Comput Assist Tomogr 19:48,1995.

158. Franquet T, Giménez A, Bordes R, et al: The crazy-paving pattern in exogenous lipoid pneumonia: CT-pathologic correlation. Am J Roentgenol 170:315, 1998.

159. Seo JW, Cho EO, Kim JS, et al: MR findings of lipoid pneumonia: Report of two cases. J Korean Radiol Soc 32:265,1995.

160. Cox JE, Choplin RH, Chiles C, et al: Chemical-shift MRI of exogenous lipoid pneumonia. J Comput Assist Tomogr 20:465, 1996.

161. Beermann B, Christensson J, Moller P, et al: Lipoid pneumonia: An occupational hazard of fire eaters. BMJ 289:1728, 1984.

162. Rolla AR, Granfone A, Balogh K, et al: Granuloma-related hypercalcemia in lipoid pneumonia. Am J Med Sci 292:313, 1986.

163. Greenaway TM, Caterson ID: Hypercalcemia and lipid pneumonia. Aust N Z J Med 19:713, 1989.

164. Lauque D, Dongay G, Levade T, et al: Bronchoalveolar lavage in liquid paraffin pneumonitis. Chest 98:1149, 1990.

165. Corwin RW, Irwin RS: The lipid-laden alveolar macrophage as a marker of aspiration in parenchymal lung disease. Am Rev Respir Dis 132:576, 1985.

166. Colombo JL, Hallberg TK: Recurrent aspiration in children: Lipid-laden macrophage quantitation. Pediatr Pulmonol 3:86, 1987.

167. Steinberg I, Finby N: Lipoid (mineral oil) pneumonia and cor pulmonale due to cardiospasm: Report of a case. Am J Roentgenol 76:108, 1956.

168. Casey JF: Chronic cor pulmonale associated with lipoid pneumonia. JAMA 177:896, 1961.

169. Heckers H, Melcher F-W, Dittmar K, et al: Long-term course of mineral oil pneumonia. Lung 155:101, 1978.

170. Hutchins GM, Boitnott JK: Atypical mycobacterial infection complicating mineral oil pneumonia. JAMA 240:539, 1978.

171. Orlowski JP: Drowning, near drowning and ice water drowning. JAMA 260:390, 1988.

172. Modell JH: Drowning. N Engl J Med 328:253, 1993.

173. Orlowski JP: Drowning, near-drowning, and ice-water submersions. Pediatr Clin North Am 34:75, 1987.

174. Weinstein MD, Krieger BP: Near-drowning: Epidemiology, pathophysiology, and initial treatment. J Emerg Med 14:461, 1996.

175. Kylstra JA: Survival of submerged mammals. N Engl J Med 272:198, 1965.

176. Modell JH, Moya F: Effects of volume of aspirated fluid during chlorinated fresh water drowning. Anesthesiology 27:662, 1966.

177. Rumbak MJ: The etiology of pulmonary edema in fresh water near-drowning. Am J Emerg Med 14:176, 1996.

178. Cohen DS, Matthay MA, Cogan G, et al: Pulmonary edema associated with salt water near-drowning: New insights. Am Rev Respir Dis 146:794, 1992.

179. Hasan S, Avery WG, Fabian C, et al: Near drowning in humans: A report of 36 patients. Chest 59:191, 1971.

180. Bradley ME: Near-drowning: CPR is just the beginning. J Respir Dis 2:37, 1981.

181. Alexander IGS: The ultrastructure of the pulmonary alveolar vessels in Mendelson's (acid pulmonary aspiration) syndrome. Br J Anaesth 40:408, 1968.

182. Fuller RH: The 1962 Wellcome Prize Essay: "Drowning and the postimmersion syndrome. A clinicopathologic study." Milit Med 128:22, 1963.

183. Ender PT, Dolan MJ, Dolan D, et al: Near-drowning-associated *Aeromonas* pneumonia. J Emerg Med 14:737, 1996.

184. Noguchi M, Kimula Y, Ogata T: Muddy lung. Am J Clin Pathol 83:240, 1985.

185. Pollanen MS, Cheung C, Chiasson DA: The diagnostic value of the diatom test for drowning. I. Utility: A retrospective analysis of 771 cases of drowning in Ontario, Canada. J Forensic Sci 42:281, 1997.

186. Pollanen MS: The diagnostic value of the diatom test for drowning, II. Validity:

187. analysis of diatoms in bone marrow and drowning medium. J Forensic Sci 42:286, 1997.

187. Yoshimura S, Yoshida M, Okii Y, et al: Detection of green algae (*Chlorophyceae*) for the diagnosis of drowning. Int J Legal Med 108:39, 1995.

188. Rosenbaum HT, Thompson WL, Fuller RH: Radiographic pulmonary changes in near drowning. Radiology 83:306, 1964.

189. Hunter TB, Whitehouse WM: Freshwater near-drowning: Radiological aspects. Radiology 112:51, 1974.

190. Putman CE, Tummillo AM, Myerson DA, et al: Drowning: Another plunge. Am J Roentgenol 125:543, 1975.

191. Dunagan DP, Cox JE, Chang MC, et al: Sand aspiration with near-drowning: Radiographic and bronchoscopic findings. Am J Respir Crit Care Med 156:292, 1997.

192. Bonilla-Santiago J, Fill WL: Sand aspiration in drowning and near drowning. Radiology 128:301, 1978.

193. Szpilman D: Near-drowning and drowning classification: A proposal to stratify mortality based on the analysis of 1,831 cases. Chest 112:660, 1997.

194. Modell JH: Near drowning. Circulation 74(Suppl IV):27, 1986.

195. ter Maaten JC, Golding RP, Strack van Schijndel RJ, et al: Disseminated aspergillosis after near-drowning. Neth J Med 47:21, 1995.

196. Ports Ta, Deuel TF: Intravascular coagulation in freshwater submersion: Report of three cases. Ann Intern Med 87:60, 1977.

197. Yagil Y, Stalnikowicz R, Michaeli J, et al: Near drowning in the Dead Sea: Electrolyte imbalances and therapeutic implications. Arch Intern Med 145:50, 1985.

198. Machi T, Nakazawa T, Nakamura Y, et al: Severe hypercalcemia and polyuria in a near-drowning victim. Intern Med 34:868, 1995.

199. Boles JM, Mabille S, Scheydecker JL, et al: Hypoglycaemia in salt water near-drowning victims. Intensive Care Med 14:80, 1988.

200. Modell JH, Graves SA, Ketover A: Clinical course of 91 consecutive near-drowning victims. Chest 70:231, 1976.

201. Bolte RG, Black PG, Bowers CCP, et al: The use of extracorporeal rewarming in a child submerged for 66 minutes. JAMA 260:377, 1988.

202. Suominen PK, Korpela RE, Silfvast TG, et al: Does water temperature affect outcome of nearly drowned children? Resuscitation 35:111, 1997.

203. Glauser FL, Smith WR: Pulmonary interstitial fibrosis following near-drowning and exposure to short-term high oxygen concentrations. Chest 68(Suppl):373, 1975.

204. Jenkinson SG, George RB: Serial pulmonary function studies in survivors of near drowning. Chest 77:6, 1980.

205. Laughlin JJ, Eigen H: Pulmonary function abnormalities in survivors of near drowning. J Pediatr 100:26, 1982.

206. Moran TJ, Hellstrom HR: Experimental aspiration pneumonia. V. Acute pulmonary edema, pneumonia, and bronchiolitis obliterans produced by injection of ethyl alcohol. Am J Clin Pathol 27:300, 1957.

207. Smith RH, Moran TJ: Experimental aspiration pneumonia. III. Pneumonia produced by intratracheal injection of carbohydrate solutions. Arch Pathol 57:194, 1954.

208. Scharf SM, Heimer D, Goldstein J: Pathologic and physiologic effects of aspiration of hydrocarbons in the rat. Am Rev Respir Dis 124:625, 1981.

209. Shepherd KE, Faulkner CS, Leiter JC: Acute effects of sucralfate aspiration: Clinical and laboratory observations. J Clin Anesth 6:119, 1994.

210. Hallagan LF, Smith M: Profound atelectasis following alkaline corrosive airway injury. J Emerg Med 12:23, 1994.

211. Reich SB: Production of pulmonary edema by aspiration of water-soluble nonabsorbable contrast media. Radiology 92:367, 1969.

212. Chiu CL, Gambach RR: Hypaque pulmonary edema: A case report. Radiology 111:91, 1974.

213. Trulzch DV, Penmetsa A, Karim A, et al: Gastrograffin induced aspiration pneumonia: A lethal complication of computed tomography. South Med J 85:1255, 1992.

214. Shahar J, Mailman D, Meitzen G: Crystals in pulmonary cytologic preparations in association with aspiration of barium: A case report. Acta Cytol 38:415, 1994.

215. Penington GR: Severe complications following a "barium swallow" investigation for dysphagia. Med J Aust 159:764, 1993.

216. Tsuji HK, Tyler GC, Reddington JV, et al: Intrabronchial metallic mercury. Chest 57:322, 1970.

217. Schulze W: Röntgenologische studien nach aspiration von metallischen quecksilber. (Roentgenographic studies of metallic mercury aspiration.) Fortschr Roentgenstr 89:24, 1958.

PART XII

PULMONARY DISEASE CAUSED BY TOXINS, DRUGS, AND IRRADIATION

CHAPTER 62

Inhaled Toxic Gases, Fumes, and Aerosols

A number of gases and fumes, as well as liquids in a finely dispersed state (aerosols), can cause acute and sometimes chronic damage to the pulmonary airways and parenchyma. The reaction depends to some extent on the chemical composition of the gas or aerosol. Some substances—particularly those that are highly soluble, such as sulfur dioxide, ammonia (NH_3), and chloride—are so irritating to the nasal mucosa that individuals may stop breathing on exposure and try to run away. By contrast, less soluble gases, such as phosgene, nitrogen dioxide (NO_2), ozone, and highly concentrated oxygen, may be inhaled deeply into the lungs before the irritating effect is perceived. Other gases, particularly when inhaled in low concentration, may produce bronchitis or bronchiolitis without the chemical exposure being recognized. Despite these variable characteristics, the concentration of the gas and the duration of the exposure are the chief factors that determine the form of pulmonary damage and the clinical presentation; in appropriate circumstances, any one of these gases can cause immediate or delayed pulmonary edema and airway or alveolar epithelial necrosis.[1, 2] (Although carbon monoxide can also be considered a toxic gas, its effects are manifested primarily in the extrapulmonary tissues rather than the lungs; thus, poisoning by this substance is discussed in Chapter 79.)

The manifestation of diseases that result from inhalation of these toxic substances is variable. In many instances, the underlying abnormality is alveolocapillary damage with resultant permeability pulmonary edema (Fig. 62–1). In others, the chemical injury appears to affect the airways predominantly,[1, 2] resulting in bronchitis and bronchiolitis (*see* page 2335), sometimes complicated by atelectasis and bacterial pneumonia. Patients who survive the acute insult may feel relatively well for several weeks and then undergo abrupt or insidious clinical deterioration, with cough, shortness of breath, and fever. This delayed form of disease is reflected pathologically by obliterative bronchiolitis.[3] The complication can also occur in individuals who initially experience diffuse pulmonary edema. Acute exposure to a toxic gas of sufficient concentration may be followed by the development of persistent airway hyper-responsiveness (reactive airways dysfunction syndrome [RADS], *see* page 2123).

In addition to pulmonary disease following a single exposure to a toxic gas, it is probable that repeated exposure to a low concentration of certain gases or aerosols can cause more insidious airway irritation, contributing to the development of chronic bronchitis and chronic obstructive pulmonary disease (COPD). Because of the growth of automobile-based transport and industry throughout the world and the concentration of individuals in large urban centers, atmospheric pollution is probably the most important source of these noxious gases. The health impact of exposure to oxidants, such as ozone, sulfur dioxide, and NO_2, in polluted air is graphically demonstrated by the marked increase in hospital visits for respiratory ailments coincident with peaks of atmospheric levels of these gases.[4] In this chapter, we concentrate on the effects of acute short-term exposure to relatively high concentrations of toxic gases and fumes. The contribution of environmental exposure to the development of COPD is discussed in Chapter 55 (*see* page 2173).

GASES

Oxidants

Some inhaled gases, such as oxygen, ozone, and NO_2, have the potential to damage tissue by producing highly reactive metabolic products of oxygen that can inactivate

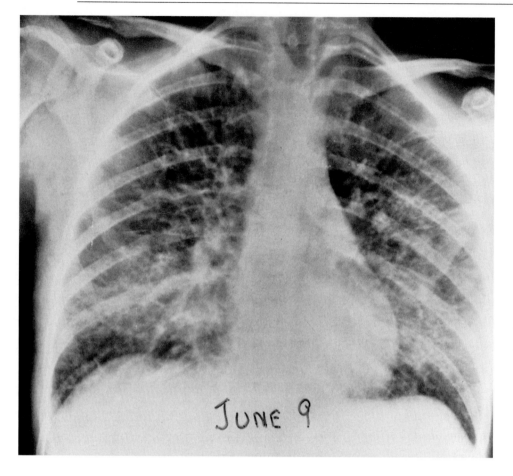

JUNE 9

Figure 62–1. Acute Pulmonary Edema Caused by Inhalation of Mixed Fumes. Four days before the radiograph illustrated, this 34-year-old woman had sprayed a lampshade with a plastic substance containing dimethylsulfate and ethylene dichloride (a paint fixative), followed by gold paint. She had experienced an abrupt onset of severe dyspnea and nonproductive cough. The radiograph shows diffuse pulmonary edema that is predominantly interstitial in location. Prominent Kerley A and B lines are visible. The heart size is normal. Her recovery was uneventful; a chest radiograph was normal 4 days later. (Courtesy of Dr. W. G. Brown, Regina Grey Nuns Hospital, Regina, Saskatchewan.)

protective enzymes in the cell, damage DNA, and destroy lipid membranes.[5-7] Reactive oxygen species also play a role in the tissue damage associated with ischemia-reperfusion and are believed to play an important role in the pathogenesis of the adult respiratory distress syndrome (ARDS).[7, 8] These agents of oxidant tissue damage are products of normal oxidation-reduction processes and include hydrogen peroxide, superoxide radical, hydroxyl radical, and singlet excited oxygen.[6, 9]

Under hyperoxic conditions and in the presence of certain poisons, intracellular production of oxygen free radicals increases markedly, resulting in chain reactions involving oxygen radicals. The latter in turn have a number of effects, including peroxidation of polyunsaturated lipids situated within the cell or on the cell membrane, depolymerization of mucopolysaccharides, protein sulfhydryl oxidation and cross-linking (resulting in enzyme inactivation), and nucleic acid damage.[6, 9, 10] In the lung, the results of the cellular damage include bronchoconstriction, increased mucus secretion, decreased surfactant function,[11] and increased microvascular permeability.[7] An additional source of oxygen radicals is the large number of neutrophils that appear in pulmonary tissue as a result of oxidant injury; it has been suggested that hyperoxia damages alveolar macrophages, resulting in the release of chemotactic factors that attract neutrophils to the lung.[12] Support for this hypothesis is provided by the results of experiments with rats treated with 95% oxygen for 6 hours, in which the chemoattractant activity of bronchoalveolar lavage (BAL) fluid has been found to increase 10-fold and to correlate with the number of neutrophils in the lavage fluid.[13]

In the presence of hyperoxia, structural abnormalities appear in the lung in as short a time as 24 hours in experimental animals.[5] These can occur throughout the lung, although involvement may be uneven and vary from animal to animal.[14] Animals exposed to a low concentration of ozone[14] or to one atmosphere of oxygen[15] show similar histologic changes: ciliated cells become vacuolated, and their mitochondria become condensed and develop an abnormal configuration of the cristae. Type I alveolar epithelial cells become swollen and may desquamate; type II cells may appear normal[14] but usually undergo proliferation, resulting in a more or less continuous cuboidal epithelium lining the alveoli.[15] Endothelial cells are also affected,[16] possibly as a result of lipid peroxidation of their cell membranes. Although alveolar macrophages may be somewhat more resistant to oxidizing substances than other cells, metabolic abnormalities can be found in them after exposure to 100% oxygen for 48 to 72 hours[17] and to NO_2 or ozone after a period of hyperoxia.[18] More prolonged administration of oxygen or ozone (5 ppm) results in structural alteration and impairment of macrophage function and in intrapulmonary antibacterial defense mechanisms.[19] Oxidant damage may also affect the efficiency of mucociliary clearance; in one experiment involving anesthetized dogs, mucus velocity fell 45% from baseline values after inhalation of 100% oxygen for 2 hours and 51% after inhalation of 50% oxygen for 30 hours.[20]

Because the lung is especially vulnerable to the effects of oxidant damage from inhaled toxins, a variety of antioxidant defenses have evolved to protect it. The enzymes responsible for maintaining low levels of oxygen radicals and thus protecting against oxidants include superoxide dismutase (SOD), catalase, glutathione and the glutathione enzymes, glutathione reductase, and glucose-6-phosphate dehydrogenase. SOD increases the dismutation rate of the superoxide radical and thus accomplishes its removal before it can react directly with cellular components.[6] Catalase acts by eliminating hydrogen peroxide, thus avoiding lipid peroxidation by hydroxyl radicals.[6, 21] Reduced glutathione serves as a scavenger of oxygen radicals in the extracellular space; levels in pulmonary epithelial lining fluid are about 100 times higher than in the extracellular fluid of most tissues.[22] Glutathione in its reduced form is a substrate that is preferred to protein sulfhydryls by oxidants, thus preventing protein sulfhydryl oxidation. Endogenous and exogenous vitamin C and vitamin E are also effective antioxidants.[23] In humans, there are three separate superoxide dismutase enzymes: manganese superoxide dismutase (Mn SOD), copper-zinc superoxide dismutase (CuZn SOD), and extracellular superoxide dismutase (EC-SOD).[24] Both Mn SOD and CuZn SOD are highly expressed in the airway epithelial cells, especially those of the small bronchioles. EC-SOD, which appears to be synthesized by alveolar type II cells, is widely distributed in the interstitial space around fibroblasts and smooth muscle cells.[25–27]

Prior exposure to inhaled oxidants, intermittently or in low concentration, exerts a protective effect that correlates with the production of antioxidants in lung tissue.[6, 15, 28, 29] Almost all adult rats die within 3 days if exposed to 100% oxygen;[28, 30] however, if they are exposed beforehand to sublethal concentrations of oxygen (in the range of 70% to 85%) for 1 week or to low concentrations of ozone (0.1 to 0.5 ppm), they can subsequently survive for long periods in 100% oxygen or in ordinarily lethal concentrations of ozone.[6, 9, 28, 30] Because sublethal exposure to ozone and oxygen is associated with a proliferation of type II pneumocytes, it has been suggested that these cells are responsible for production of SOD.[28] This hypothesis would also explain the increased tolerance to oxygen observed in rabbits whose lungs have been injured previously by the intravenous injection of oleic acid;[31] such animals have a proliferation of type II pneumocytes and simultaneously become resistant to ordinarily lethal hyperoxia.

Oxygen

Physicians first became aware of the toxic effects of oxygen therapy on the lungs and the associated pathologic and physiologic abnormalities in the 1950s and 1960s.[32–34] Studies directed at the assessment of clinical, physiologic, and pathologic alterations in the lungs of patients exposed to high concentrations of oxygen are complicated by the fact that some of the changes observed may be caused by the underlying disease, concurrent drug therapy, or artificial ventilation.[35] For example, in one review of 22 patients who had undergone prolonged mechanical ventilation with high concentrations of oxygen, the investigators concluded that oxygen could have been a contributory cause of pulmonary injury in 1 of the 6 patients who died and in 3 of the

13 survivors who showed abnormal pulmonary function 1 year later.[36]

The first description of an association of exposure to oxygen and the development of interstitial fibrosis was made in 1958.[37] In a review of the pathologic abnormalities in 70 patients who had received oxygen therapy by artificial ventilation, exudative and proliferative histologic patterns identical to those of diffuse alveolar damage of other etiology were described.[32] The exudative phase was characterized by capillary congestion, the presence of proteinaceous material and blood within alveoli, and hyaline membranes; alveolar and interlobular septal fibroblastic proliferation and hyperplasia of alveolar lining cells were observed in the proliferative phase. These two patterns are identical to those seen in animals after exposure to a high concentration of oxygen.[38, 39]

For obvious reasons, there is a paucity of studies of the effects of hyperoxia on humans who have healthy lungs. In one report, normal volunteers who inhaled pure oxygen for 6 to 12 hours failed to show hemodynamic or gas exchange abnormalities.[40] In another prospective study of patients after open heart surgery, one group was administered pure oxygen and a second group oxygen in limited concentration for periods up to 48 hours; the clinical course of the two groups was similar, and no differences were found in intrapulmonary shunting, effective compliance, or in the ratio of dead space to tidal volume. On the other hand, in another study of patients who had irreversible brain damage, patients who breathed pure oxygen for 40 hours were found to have significant changes in pulmonary function compared with those who breathed air; the former group showed an increase in wasted ventilation and intrapulmonary shunting. Small decreases in static and dynamic compliance and diffusing capacity have been detected in normal subjects breathing one atmosphere of oxygen for 30 to 48 hours.[41, 42]

Although the toxic level of oxygen is not known precisely, there is ample clinical evidence that humans can tolerate an FIO_2 of 50% for prolonged periods of time without developing irreversible pulmonary damage.[43] However, the potential deleterious effects of a combination of oxidants should be borne in mind when considering oxygen therapy; unless death from hypoxia appears imminent, high concentrations of oxygen should be avoided, especially in patients who have received cytotoxic drugs or radiation therapy or who have paraquat poisoning. The effects of various oxidants are additive, as exemplified by the increase in cell damage in animals after the addition of oxygen to NO_2.[44]

Ozone

Unlike most other gases described in this section, ozone has not produced serious acute pulmonary disease in humans. Nevertheless, there is abundant evidence that chronic inhalation of even low concentrations can cause structural changes in animal lungs and functional changes in both animal and human lungs. Ozone constitutes 90% of the measured oxidant in photochemical smog,[9] and in certain urban areas, its atmospheric concentration is equal to that known to cause structural and physiologic changes under experimental conditions. High concentrations of ozone are also found within airplanes at altitudes above 30,000 feet, in proximity to high-tension electrical discharges from welding in both air and oxygen, and in various industries in which this gas is used as an oxidizing agent.[45]

Studies of the acute effects of ozone on the lungs of a variety of animals have clearly demonstrated that the gas can induce both structural[14, 46–50] and functional[51] changes. Although the details of the pathologic abnormalities vary somewhat with the animal species, experimental techniques, and ozone concentrations, injury has been generally shown to be most prominent in small membranous and respiratory bronchioles. Depending on the stage at which the tissue is examined, this injury may take the form of either epithelial necrosis or regeneration associated with a variably intense acute inflammatory reaction. Damage to the tracheobronchial epithelium,[47, 48] bronchiolar interstitium,[50] alveolar duct epithelium,[52] and alveolar capillary endothelium[49] also has been noted by some investigators.

Morphologic changes in rat lungs exposed to low concentrations of ozone and the protective effects of vitamin E have been reported by several investigators.[10, 53] One group used scanning electron microscopy to detect the earliest changes in rat airways and alveoli after exposure to ozone at 0.3 ppm.[53] The major change occurred in the cilia, which were seen to be swollen and matted together; damage occurred earlier and was more severe in rats that were deficient in vitamin E, although even these animals appeared to acquire a tolerance to repeated ozone exposure, presumably as a result of increased production of superoxide dismutase. In another study, all rats who were exposed to 1.0-ppm ozone succumbed from pulmonary edema within 22 days;[10] the LD_{50} was 8.2 days for vitamin E–depleted animals and 18.5 days for those receiving vitamin E. In a third investigation, rats exposed to 0.8 to 1.5 ppm for 7 days were compared with a control group that breathed filtered air.[54] Analysis of lung minces showed that the net rate of collagen synthesis in the group treated with ozone was increased several-fold, in a dose-dependent manner, compared with the air-breathing rats; this increased synthesis could be prevented by the administration of methylprednisolone.

Pathologic and functional abnormalities have also been identified in several animal species after prolonged ozone exposure.[55–57] In some studies, the pathologic changes have been localized predominantly around respiratory bronchioles and have consisted of epithelial hyperplasia and hypertrophy associated with small aggregates of macrophages in adjacent alveoli.[55, 56] These abnormalities appeared to be less severe after prolonged exposure than after acute exposure, suggesting an adaptive reaction. In another investigation, the accumulation of macrophages and fibroblasts was most marked in alveolar ducts and adjacent alveoli; the abnormalities diminished dramatically after a 24-week recovery period in clean air.[57] Functional abnormalities were mild but statistically significant and included an increase in functional residual capacity and residual volume and a decrease in DLco; these findings disappeared after a 3-month recovery period.

Although these metabolic and morphologic changes have been identified predominantly in animals, it is likely that they are pertinent to ozone toxicity in humans because the concentrations of ozone in most animal studies are roughly equivalent to levels detected in smog in heavily polluted urban areas. A number of investigators have shown that acute exposure of normal volunteers to low concentrations of ozone (0.5 to 0.9 ppm) results in dry cough, chest discomfort, and impaired pulmonary function.[58–62] Considerable variation is observed among individuals in their symptomatic and functional responses, probably related to varying degrees of pre-existing airway responsiveness, smoking habits, tolerance developed from prolonged exposure, and the degree of exercise attained. In one study, symptoms, pulmonary function, and cellular and cytokine markers of inflammation in BAL fluid were measured in 56 nonsmokers and 34 smokers after exposure to ozone at a concentration of 0.22 ppm;[63] although the nonsmokers had fewer symptoms and less change in lung function, they showed an enhanced inflammatory response, suggesting an interaction of smoke and ozone.

The functional derangement that follows ozone exposure is characteristically obstructive and can be demonstrated by a variety of tests.[61, 62, 64–66] Acute ozone exposure can also cause lung restriction, predominantly by decreasing inspiratory capacity; this effect appears to be mediated by products of arachidonic acid metabolism and is related to stimulation of lung irritant receptors that inhibit full inspiration.[67, 68]

As indicated previously, the protective effect of pre-exposure to low concentrations of oxidants appears to be an important determinant of the effects of ozone.[58] A number of experiments in healthy volunteers[69–71] and in patients who have chronic bronchitis[72] have confirmed this phenomenon; it develops within 2 to 5 days of exposure but is relatively short-lived, lasting from 4 days to 3 weeks after cessation of exposure.[71] The duration of adaptation is shortest in subjects who are most sensitive to ozone.

Nitrogen Dioxide

Like ozone, NO_2 is a component of photochemical smog that can damage the lung. Considerable experimental work has been performed on animals in which the toxic effects on the lungs of relatively low concentrations of NO_2 have been documented; in addition, an abundance of clinical experience has accumulated to indicate the dire consequences of exposure to a heavy concentration of this gas in humans. Rarely, other oxides of nitrogen (e.g., dinitrogen tetroxide) have also been implicated in human disease.[73]

The results of a number of animal experiments have shown that short-term exposure to NO_2 in a concentration less than 17 ppm results in changes in bronchopulmonary epithelial and capillary endothelial cells.[74–77] As with oxygen and ozone, tolerance develops with repeated exposure coincident with regeneration of type II alveolar epithelial cells.[76] Continued exposure of rats to a low concentration of NO_2 results in interstitial fibrosis, particularly around respiratory bronchioles.[78] Destruction of pulmonary tissue may also occur at the same time: exposure to 20 ppm NO_2 for 28 days significantly accelerated the progression of the inherited emphysema that occurs in the blotchy mouse.[79] In another study of BAL fluid of adult hamsters administered 30 ppm NO_2 for 30 days, a significant increase in the number of macrophages and in elastase activity was observed.[80]

Chronic low-level exposure to NO_2 occurs mainly in indoor environments from the combustion of biofuel.[81] Experimental studies of the effects of low concentrations of NO_2 in humans have revealed few abnormalities. For example, in one investigation of nonsmoking human volunteers subjected to an atmosphere containing 0.62 ppm NO_2 while exercising for 15 to 60 minutes, no evidence of cardiopulmonary dysfunction could be detected.[82] In a second study, 22 volunteers who had COPD exercised for 1 hour in an environmental chamber containing NO_2 in concentrations ranging from 0.0 to 2.0 ppm; subsequent complete pulmonary function testing failed to reveal any impairment.[82a] Despite these results, one group of workers found a significant increase in blood levels of glutathione in 19 subjects after 2 hours of exposure to 0.2 ppm NO_2, suggesting that this low level elicited a tissue response.[83] The potential role of chronic exposure to NO_2 and other environmental pollutants in the pathogenesis of COPD is discussed in Chapter 55 (*see* page 2173).

The danger of exposure to a high concentration of NO_2 has been recognized for many years in a number of industrial settings,[84] including fuming nitric acid,[85, 86] burning shoe polish,[87] and using explosives during mining operations.[85, 88] An unusual form of exposure occurred to the Apollo astronauts during their descent from space after the Apollo-Soyuz training program in 1975:[73] at about 23,000 feet, the spacecraft cabin was filled with a yellow-brown gas consisting of monomethylhydrazine and dinitrogen tetroxide, the principal toxic irritants in rocket fuels. Toxicity has also been reported in a hockey player after exposure caused by the Zamboni used to resurface the ice in an indoor skating rink.[89]

Although these occupational settings are interesting and important in their own right, from the point of view of the number of cases, the most important condition associated with NO_2 inhalation is silo-filler's disease.[90-92] For 3 to 10 days after a silo has been filled, the fresh silage produces nitric oxide that, on contact with the air, oxidizes to form NO_2 and its polymer, nitrogen tetroxide.[93, 94] These two gases are heavier than air and can be seen as a brown-yellow "cloud" just above the silage. Anyone who enters the silo during this period inhales NO_2; the severity of subsequent toxicity is proportional to the duration and level of exposure. In a state-wide survey from New York based on hospital discharge summaries, it was estimated that the incidence of silo-filler's disease was 5 cases per 100,000 silo-associated farm-worker years.[95]

After moderate to severe exposure, the course is triphasic. During the earliest phase, pulmonary injury is manifested pathologically predominantly by bronchiolitis and peribronchiolitis, sometimes accompanied by denuding of the epithelium; diffuse alveolar damage also has been documented in some patients.[92] The clinical picture is characterized by the abrupt onset of cough, dyspnea, weakness, and a choking feeling, which usually persist. Pulmonary edema can develop within 4 to 24 hours (Fig. 62–2)[96] but usually clears without residual lung damage if the patient survives.

During the second phase, which lasts from 2 to 5 weeks, symptoms typically abate, although cough, malaise, and shortness of breath of lesser severity may persist, and weakness may worsen. The chest radiograph is normal. The third phase becomes manifest up to 5 weeks after the initial exposure and is characterized pathologically by obliterative bronchiolitis.[94, 97, 98] Radiographically, there is "miliary nodulation," the appearance of which tends to lag somewhat behind the recurrence of symptoms. Multiple discrete nodular opacities of varying size are scattered diffusely throughout the lungs (to a point of confluence in the more severe cases).[99, 100] The nodules may disappear as the clinical course progresses to a stage of chronic pulmonary insufficiency, although they usually persist for a considerable time after the acute symptoms have subsided.[100] Clinically, this stage is characterized by fever, chills, progressive shortness of

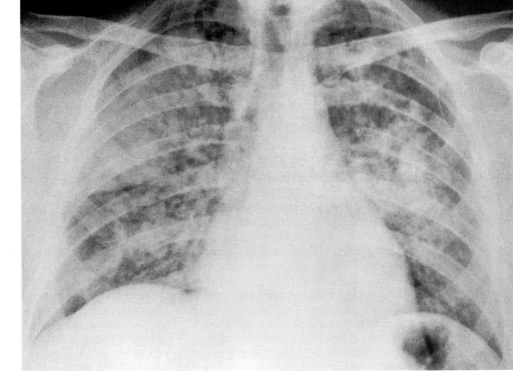

Figure 62–2. Acute Pulmonary Edema Secondary to Nitrogen Dioxide Inhalation. This 40-year-old man had spent 6 hours with several other men in an enclosed space on board ship attempting to remove a propeller with cutting torches. Such a procedure is known to be associated with accumulation of nitrogen dioxide. Toward the end of the 6 hours, the patient noted the onset of nausea, vomiting, headache, and productive cough. The posteroanterior radiograph reveals extensive bilateral air-space consolidation. The radiograph was normal 4 days later.

breath, cough, and cyanosis. Moist crackles and rhonchi may be heard on auscultation. A neutrophilic leukocytosis develops in most cases, and the $Paco_2$ may be elevated.[99]

The prognosis of acute NO_2 exposure is variable: some patients die of pulmonary insufficiency, some recover more or less completely, and others experience residual obstructive impairment of pulmonary function.[100, 101] In one report of 23 patients exposed to NO_2 in agriculture and industry, 18 developed no more than a transient upper respiratory tract syndrome, and only 5 developed pulmonary edema or obliterative bronchiolitis.[90] From their own experience and a review of the literature, the investigators concluded that most affected individuals recover completely; however, they estimated the case fatality rate to be 29% for patients who have silo-filler's disease. The case fatality ratio documented in the New York survey of silo-filler's disease mentioned previously was 20%.[95] Patients who survive often have residual functional defects, the most serious of which is RADS (*see* page 2123). Of 234 patients who had respiratory complaints after exposure to a cloud of nitrogen tetroxide that escaped from a railroad tanker car, 6 subsequently developed RADS.[102]

Other Gases

Sulfur Dioxide

Sulfur dioxide (SO_2) is a highly soluble gas whose major importance in pulmonary disease is as an atmospheric pollutant; continuous exposure to low concentrations in an urban environment may play a role in the pathogenesis of COPD (*see* page 2173). On contact with moist epithelial surfaces, SO_2 is hydrated and subsequently oxidized to form sulfuric acid (H_2SO_4), which directly causes mucosal injury; the acid may be partly neutralized, and the damage thereby diminished, by combination with endogenous NH_3 within the respiratory tract.[103] Accidental exposure to high concentrations can occur in pulp and paper factories, refrigeration plants, and oil-refining and fruit-preserving industries.[104] H_2SO_4 itself is also used in photographic developing and is capable of causing reversible obstructive disease of small airways in photographers.[105, 106] Respiratory disease among smelter workers, which has been thought to be related to SO_2, may in some instances be secondary to inhalation of mercuric sulfate.[107]

It is probable that the inhalation of SO_2 produces the same triphasic picture as does NO_2. We and others[108] have seen workers who have been accidentally exposed to H_2SO_4 suffer acute pulmonary edema that resolves within a few days and is followed months later by obstructive pulmonary disease associated with obliterative bronchiolitis and generalized bronchiectasis (Fig. 62–3). The likelihood of death or residual pulmonary damage varies considerably from victim to victim; for example, in one study of 13 men exposed to burning SO_2 in the hold of a ship, only 1 died.[109] By contrast, in another report of 5 men exposed in a paper mill, 2 men died immediately, 1 developed severe obstructive airway disease, and 2 were symptom free at follow-up (although 1 of these had abnormal pulmonary function).[110] In another investigation, 7 men accidentally exposed to SO_2 in a pyrite dust explosion were followed for 7 years.[111] The greatest

decrease in FVC, FEV_1, and maximal midexpiratory flow was observed 1 week after the accident; after about 3 months, no further decrement occurred. Four years after the accident, 3 men still manifested reversible airway obstruction, and 4 reacted positively to a histamine challenge test, suggesting the presence of RADS.

Hydrogen Sulfide

Hydrogen sulfide (H_2S) produces a characteristic rotten egg odor at 0.2 ppm and abolishes the sense of smell at levels of 150 ppm. Levels of 250 ppm cause irritation of mucous membranes with resultant keratoconjunctivitis, bronchitis, and pulmonary edema. Higher concentrations affect the central nervous system and may cause death.[112] Like cyanide, sulfide ions act as direct cytotoxins, selectively binding to cytochrome oxidase within the mitochondria and thereby disrupting the electron transport chain. H_2S also has a specific neurologic effect by causing a hyperpolarization of K^+ channels.[113]

The most common sources of exposure to H_2S are the petroleum and chemical industries[114] and decaying organic matter.[112, 115] In the latter situation, production of H_2S depends on incomplete oxidation and degradation of sulfur compounds.[114] An example of acute inhalation of such waste products can be found in the dramatic description of a patient who had "dung lung."[112] In this remarkable example, a cow kicked the lid of a large underground liquid manure storage tank into the tank and a farmer attempted to recover it; two other individuals tried to rescue him, and all three died. The risk of exposure to decaying organic matter was also evident in a study of U.S. Coast Guard records of deaths at sea among fishermen over a 10-year period:[115] in 11 incidents, 32 men died from breathing polluted air attributed to anaerobic decay of insufficiently refrigerated fish stored in an unventilated hold. Particularly in warm weather, decaying organic matter releases a variety of toxic gases, including H_2S, NH_3, methane, carbon dioxide, and carbon monoxide; H_2S is the most likely of these agents to cause death.

In one review of 5 years' experience with H_2S poisoning in the Alberta oil fields, there were 221 cases of recognized exposure with an overall mortality of 6%;[114] 5% of victims were dead on arrival at the hospital. Acute problems consisted of coma, disequilibrium, and respiratory insufficiency as a result of pulmonary edema; 74% of patients lost consciousness at the accident site. If the patient recovers, respiratory sequelae are uncommon; however, there may be long-term neurologic impairment.[116, 117]

Ammonia

NH_3 is a toxic, highly soluble alkaline gas that can play a role, along with H_2S, in causing bronchopulmonary disease on exposure to decaying organic matter.[112, 115] However, it is better known as a cause of lung damage in industry and farming, usually as a result of sudden rupture or leakage from tanks of concentrated NH_3.[118–120] Vehicular accidents involving tank transportation of this gas can result in inhalation of high concentrations by those involved, often with serious consequences.[121] For example, in one report of 47 people who were exposed to high concentrations of the gas when a container was damaged during an air raid in World

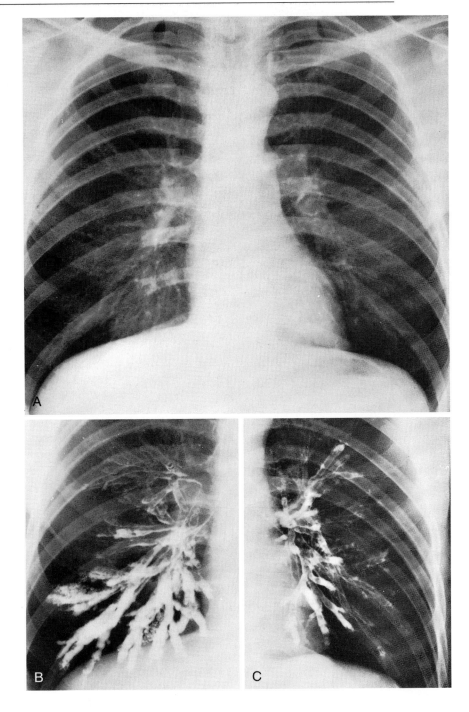

Figure 62–3. Obliterative Bronchiolitis and Bronchiectasis Secondary to Sulfur Dioxide Inhalation. Three months before these radiograph studies, this 33-year-old man was exposed to high concentrations of sulfur dioxide fumes rising from a sulfuric acid vat. Immediately after this exposure, he was said to have developed acute pulmonary edema, which gradually resolved over a period of days (this acute episode was not documented locally). Three months later, a posteroanterior radiograph *(A)* was essentially normal, although close examination revealed numerous "tram lines" in the central portions of both lungs. The lungs were somewhat overinflated. Bilateral bronchography *(B and C)* demonstrated severe cylindrical and varicose bronchiectasis of all segmental bronchi of both lungs, the dilated bronchi terminating abruptly in squared or rounded extremities. There was an almost total absence of peripheral filling. These findings are consistent with extensive obliterative bronchiolitis in addition to bronchiectasis.

War II, 13 died of pulmonary edema and purulent bronchitis.[122] Even household-strength ammonia, which has a pH of less than 12 and contains only 5% to 10% of ammonia products, can cause esophageal necrosis and ARDS when ingested in large quantity during attempted suicide.[123]

Postmortem examination often shows bronchiectasis,[118, 119] with or without obliterative bronchiolitis.[124] Conventional chest radiographs of patients who survive severe exposure can be virtually normal; bronchography was formerly necessary to detect the bronchiectasis but has been superseded by CT.[125]

In one accident at sea in which a leak developed in the refrigeration system, 14 fishermen had transient exposure to NH₃ lasting seconds to minutes;[126] clinical findings consisted of inflammation of the pharynx and conjunctiva and a few crackles and rhonchi on auscultation of the lungs. Although only one man showed a small focus of pulmonary consolidation radiographically, the mean PaO₂ for the group was only 64 mm Hg. Inhalation of a large quantity of NH₃ results in the production of copious serosanguineous and purulent tracheobronchial secretions;[122, 127] inflammation and desquamation of the mucosa of the large bronchi can be seen endoscopically.[128]

Chlorine

Exposure to chlorine gas can occur in a variety of occupational, environmental, and household settings.[129]

Heavy exposure usually occurs in industrial accidents or when the gas escapes from broken pipes or tank containers; occupational settings at particular risk are plastic and textile industries, plants for water purification, and pulp mills.[130, 131] A less common source of exposure is the use of chlorinated products for swimming pools.[132] Chlorine gas also can be generated by mixing bleach (sodium hypochlorite) and cleaning solutions containing phosphoric acid; a number of cases of pulmonary toxicity have been reported with the use of this combination.[133] Severe metabolic acidosis has been reported after the use of a combination of bleach and hydrochloric acid to clean toilets; the combination generated toxic levels of chloramine and methyl chloride, which were inhaled.[134]

Acute exposure to a high concentration of chlorine results in pulmonary edema, necrosis of airway epithelium, and bronchial inflammation (Fig. 62–4);[135] fever, conjunctivitis, nausea and vomiting, stupor, shock, and hemoptysis may be evident clinically[136, 137] and may be followed rapidly by death.[138] Cough and influenza-like symptoms, as well as throat and eye irritation, are common consequences of repeated accidental exposure to lower concentrations.[139] Postmortem examination of individuals who die from acute chlorine poisoning shows air-space edema and hemorrhage and extensive bronchial and bronchiolar epithelial necrosis;[140] evidence of epithelial damage can also be seen cytologically

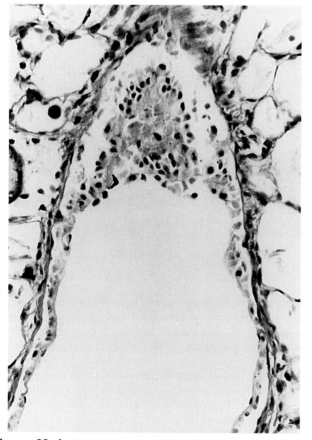

Figure 62–4. Bronchiolar Necrosis in Chlorine Toxicity. The section shows a bronchiole from a rat killed 24 hours after inhaling chlorine gas (1500 ppm) for 5 minutes as part of an experimental protocol in the investigation of reactive airways dysfunction syndrome. There is extensive epithelial necrosis and sloughing; a mild inflammatory reaction is evident.

in bronchial brush specimens taken during life.[130] Pulmonary function tests show an obstructive pattern.[141, 142] Although a number of investigators have documented complete return to normal function in a few weeks[138, 141, 142] and a maintenance of normal function over a period of several years,[138] some patients develop RADS (*see* page 2123).[131] An unusual case has been reported of a patient who was "addicted" to inhaling chlorine gas:[143] on each of three occasions when he was admitted to the hospital after indulging, he was found to have severe, partly reversible obstructive pulmonary disease, hypoxemia, cor pulmonale, and right heart failure.

Phosgene

Phosgene is the common name for carbon oxychloride ($COCl_2$), a colorless oxidizing gas that is heavier than air; the lethal exposure concentration in humans is about 500 ppm.[144] When inhaled, the gas is hydrolyzed to hydrochloric acid and carbon dioxide. Necrosis and sloughing of the airway epithelium and interstitial and alveolar edema occur as a result of the action of the acid.[145, 146]

Although phosgene is known chiefly as a highly poisonous gas used in warfare, it is also an occasional hazard in industry.[147] Cases of poisoning have been described after accidental inhalation of carbon tetrachloride from fire extinguishers[145] and in heavily exposed workers at a uranium processing plant.[148] Methylene chloride is used as a paint remover and can be converted to phosgene if heated; cases of exposure associated with pulmonary edema have been reported after its use in small, enclosed spaces heated by stoves[149, 150] RADS has been described as a long-term complication.[151] Phosgene is also a decomposition product of trichloroethylene, and toxic levels can be generated when welding is done in an atmosphere containing this substance.[152] As with NO_2 inhalation, there is a delay of several hours before the onset of dyspnea. Acute pulmonary edema can cause death, usually within 24 hours of exposure. If the patient survives the acute episode, recovery is usually complete.[145, 150]

Formaldehyde

Urea formaldehyde resins are used as adhesives in wood products (principally particleboard, fiberboard, and hardwood plywood) and as foam insulation in housing.[153, 154] Occupational exposure occurs in the manufacture of these substances, in carpentry shops,[155] and in those exposed to formalin in pathology departments[156] and funeral homes.[157] In one study of 103 medical students exposed to low concentrations of formaldehyde during a 7-month anatomy course, no abnormalities of pulmonary function could be demonstrated, even in the 12 students who had pre-existing asthma.[158] However, increased respiratory symptoms and mildly abnormal lung function have been reported in a group of histopathology laboratory workers in another case-control study.[159] Nonoccupational exposure occurs in buildings that contain urea formaldehyde foam insulation.[160–162] Symptoms have been produced in atopic subjects exposed to 2 ppm of formaldehyde for 40 minutes in an environmental chamber.[163]

Although formaldehyde has been considered to be a potential allergen that could cause skin and lung sensitization,[154] careful studies have failed to demonstrate any humoral immunologic response.[164] However, it is now generally accepted that exposure can cause eye irritation, rhinitis, skin rash, and upper respiratory symptoms.[160, 161, 165] One researcher has referred to the occasional case of acute pulmonary edema.[153] Few investigators have found evidence of long-term pathologic abnormalities from the inhalation of formaldehyde fumes;[155] however, tracheobronchial epithelial degeneration and metaplasia have been documented in monkeys exposed to 6 ppm for 6 weeks.[166] Despite these observations, most investigators have found no evidence of either acute or chronic impairment of pulmonary function.[153, 154, 157, 160–163, 167, 168] In one case study, there was an excess of nonspecific symptoms in occupants of homes insulated with urea formaldehyde foam insulation; although the symptoms decreased after attempts to remove the foam, the decrease in symptoms was not associated with a decrease in the detectable levels of formaldehyde vapor.[169]

METALS

Fumes or gaseous forms of several metals, including mercury, zinc (zinc chloride), manganese, cadmium, nickel (nickel carbonyl), and vanadium, can cause acute tracheobronchitis, diffuse lung injury associated with pulmonary edema (ARDS),[170, 171] interstitial pneumonitis and edema, or a syndrome called *fume fever*. The last named is a poorly understood systemic reaction characterized clinically by the sudden onset of thirst, a metallic taste in the mouth, substernal tightness, headache, fever, chills, muscle aches, an increased level of tumor necrosis factor in BAL,[172] and a neutrophil alveolitis.[171, 173, 174] It appears to be related to inhalation of the finely dispersed particles (<1 μm in diameter) that develop when zinc, copper, magnesium, iron, cadmium, nickel, and various other metals are heated to 93° C or higher. Symptoms usually appear within 12 hours of exposure and subside within 24 hours without complications or sequelae. Repeated exposure can result in increased tolerance, although re-exposure on Mondays after off-duty weekends is usually associated with a more severe episode. Moist crackles and rhonchi may be heard on auscultation, and there is leukocytosis (20,000/mm³ or more) with neutrophilia. The chest radiograph either is normal or shows increased prominence of bronchovascular markings. The illness has been reproduced in volunteers and in a patient who had the clinical history of recurring zinc fume fever who underwent experimental welding exposure.[175] Zinc chloride can stimulate neutrophils to produce oxygen radicals, which may in turn damage the lung.[176] Some patients who develop fume fever subsequently develop RADS.[177]

Mercury

Exposure to vaporized mercury usually occurs in a confined space such as a tank or boiler;[104] it has also been reported in a worker making fishing weights (sinkers) in a nonventilated space.[178] Accidental exposure can occur in the home when metallic mercury is allowed to burn on a stove.[179–181] Poisoning from metallic mercury usually occurs

by aspiration (*see* page 2513) or accidental or suicidal injection (*see* page 1863).

Symptoms and signs tend to develop 3 to 4 hours after exposure and include gingivostomatitis, crampy abdominal pain, and diarrhea; severe tracheitis, bronchitis, bronchiolitis, and pneumonitis can develop.[179–183] The condition is particularly serious in infants, in whom the bronchiolitis may be fatal; it is sometimes complicated by pneumothorax. Central nervous system symptoms are common and can develop in the absence of pulmonary disease.[183] Other manifestations include paronychia, erosion of the nails, and a metallic taste in the mouth.[182, 183] Pulmonary function tests performed 2 days after exposure have shown a combination of obstructive and restrictive disease and a lowered diffusing capacity.[181]

Zinc Chloride

The fumes of zinc chloride, a substance used in smoke bombs,[184] are extremely caustic and can cause severe damage to both the tracheobronchial mucosa and lung parenchyma.[185] Acute tracheobronchitis can cause death within hours;[186] in other cases, fatal ARDS ensues several days after exposure.[187] In one catastrophe, 70 people who were exposed to burning smoke generators in a tunnel developed symptoms, and 10 died.[186]

Manganese

Manganese oxide (pyrolusite) is employed in the smelting of manganese, in the dry-cell battery industry, and in the manufacture of coloring for glass bleaching. Exposed individuals have been said to be particularly susceptible to pneumonia.[188] The results of experimental studies in mice[188, 189] and the development of upper respiratory irritation and tracheobronchitis in exposed humans suggest a chemical origin of the pneumonia. However, the results of some animal studies suggest that inhalation of the metal increases the susceptibility to pulmonary infection with streptococci.[189a] Symptoms include dry cough and fever.

Cadmium

Cadmium is a toxic metal that is present in many foods and in tobacco. After ingestion or inhalation, it accumulates in the liver and kidneys.[190, 191] Acute exposure to a high concentration, usually of cadmium oxide which is evolved during the heating of cadmium-coated metal with an oxyacetylene torch, may result in metal fume fever, diffuse pneumonitis and ARDS, or delayed acute pulmonary edema.[192, 193]

There is conflicting evidence that chronic cadmium exposure contributes to the development of COPD and emphysema (*see* page 2175).[194–199] The lungs of patients who have emphysema contain a significantly higher content of cadmium than the lungs of those who do not;[200] however, because patients who have emphysema are usually heavy smokers and cigarette smoke contains cadmium, a cause-and-effect relationship has been controversial. In addition, not all investigators have found evidence of emphysema; in two studies of heavily exposed cadmium workers, a restrictive rather than an obstructive pulmonary function pattern was reported, and there was evidence of pulmonary fibrosis radiographically.[201, 202] Another survey of coppersmiths in Scotland who had been exposed to cadmium fumes revealed an incidence of restrictive disease greater than that observed in a control group (although there was no evidence of fibrosis radiographically).[203] Despite these observations, experiments in which animals have been exposed to aerosols of cadmium alone have established beyond doubt that the metal is toxic[204, 205] and that it can produce both emphysema and bronchiolitis.[206–208]

Pulmonary damage is not inevitable, even after substantial exposure to cadmium. One group measured pulmonary function in cadmium workers exposed to a relatively high concentration (sufficient to cause kidney toxicity in 42%) and found no evidence of pulmonary dysfunction in comparison with a control group.[209]

EPOXIDES, TRIMELLITIC ANHYDRIDE, AND POLYMERS

The first description of respiratory tract disease caused by epoxy resins was published in 1975.[210] It involved 210 rubber tire workers who developed conjunctivitis and bronchopulmonary disease that characteristically resolved while the affected individuals were on sick leave but recurred when they returned to work. In about 25% of the patients, the chest radiograph revealed patchy pneumonitis; in some, increased vascular markings, chiefly in the lower lobes, were also evident. Over one third of the workers who were tested showed abnormal expiratory flow rates and diffusing capacity. Subsequent investigators have described a syndrome consisting of hemoptysis, anemia,[211–213] and radiographic evidence of patchy air-space opacities resembling diffuse pulmonary edema. In one study, diffusing capacity was increased, perhaps reflecting uptake of carbon monoxide by erythrocytes sequestered in alveoli.[212]

It has been demonstrated that the agent responsible for these abnormalities is trimellitic anhydride (TMA), a low-molecular-weight chemical widely used in the manufacture of plastics, epoxy resin coatings, and paints.[213–218] Four syndromes have been associated with its inhalation: (1) an immediate-type airway response (asthma-rhinitis) that is mediated by immunoglobulin E (IgE) antibody directed against trimellityl-conjugated human respiratory tract proteins (*see* page 2117); (2) a syndrome characterized by cough, wheezing, dyspnea, myalgia, and arthralgia that develops 4 to 12 hours after exposure—in this variant, TMA reacts covalently with protein to form a hapten-protein complex that results in the induction of antibody, mostly IgG; (3) a hemoptysis-anemia syndrome that develops after high-dose exposure to fumes when materials containing TMA are sprayed on heated metal surfaces—high levels of antibodies to trimellityl-conjugated human proteins and erythrocytes have been found in affected patients, and biopsy specimens have shown alveolar hemorrhage and nonspecific alveolar epithelial damage;[212, 215] and (4) an occupational bronchitis resulting from direct irritant properties of TMA.[213–216] Rarely, TMA has been reported to produce a picture consistent with extrinsic allergic alveolitis.[219]

The first three syndromes have a latent period between initial exposure and the onset of symptoms, and there is good evidence, including the results of some experimental studies in animals, that they are immunologically mediated. It has been postulated that a TMA antigen-antibody response within the lung activates complement, attracting polymorphonuclear leukocytes and macrophages that, in turn, induce pulmonary damage through the production of superoxide radicals.[217] Removal from exposure usually results in rapid disappearance of symptoms and a decrease in the levels of serum antibodies.[212, 216] Hypoxemia, which may be severe, and the restrictive functional defect revert to normal in patients who have the hemoptysis-anemia syndrome.[212]

Polymer fume fever (polytetrafluoroethylene poisoning) is caused by inhalation of fumes that evolve as degradation products when polytetrafluoroethylene (Fluon, Teflon) is heated to high temperatures (above 250° C); the pyrolytic products of this plastic material have not been identified. Symptoms are similar to those of metal fume fever and include tightness in the chest, headache, shivering, fever, aching, weakness and, occasionally, shortness of breath.[220] Some patients have developed pulmonary edema.[221, 222] In most reported cases, fume inhalation has been associated with cigarette smoking,[220, 223] the high temperatures generated by the burning (879° C) of the tobacco being sufficient to produce pyrolysis products. In an influenza-like outbreak in a Massachusetts textile mill, 7 of 13 employees exposed to fluorocarbon polymer developed symptoms;[220] all were cigarette smokers. A case has been reported of a worker who had 40 episodes of fume fever before the cause was recognized.[223] In this instance and in the cases originating in the textile mill, the disease disappeared after workers washed their hands thoroughly before they smoked cigarettes.

BRONCHOPULMONARY DISEASE ASSOCIATED WITH BURNS

Burns caused by fire are a major cause of morbidity and mortality. Although the most significant pathophysiologic abnormalities that result are related to skin damage, secondary shock, and infection, pulmonary disease is also a common and important factor. In addition to infection and shock and the consequences of therapy, including overhydration,[224, 225] tracheobronchial and pulmonary damage can be caused by smoke and the materials it contains and by heat; assessment of the relative contribution of each of these mechanisms can be extremely difficult in an individual patient.[226]

The inhalation of smoke and the various toxic chemicals it contains is a particularly important mechanism of tracheobronchial injury, especially when exposure has occurred within a confined space. Smoke consists of gases and a suspension of small particles in hot air. The particles are composed of carbon that is coated with combustible products, such as organic acids and aldehydes. The gaseous fraction has a highly variable composition depending on the material that is burning; although most are unidentified, carbon monoxide and carbon dioxide are the main constituents and are always present. A list of toxic combustion products of common materials has been published,[227] but only two are discussed here. Cyanide is a product of fires involving material such as nylon, asphalt, wool, silk, and polyurethane;[228] high carboxyhemoglobin levels correlate with high cyanide levels in the blood of fire survivors. Polyvinyl chloride (PVC), a plastic solid widely used as a rubber substitute for covering electric and telephone wire and cable and in many manufactured products,[229] has been implicated as a major cause of bronchopulmonary damage because of the release of hydrogen chloride gas when it burns. PVC degrades and releases hydrochloric acid at temperatures higher than 225° C. The effect of the acid in the gas phase is largely restricted to irritability and chiefly involves the upper respiratory tract; however, hydrochloric acid can condense on soot aerosol and thereby gain access to the lower airway mucosa and lung parenchyma.

Direct trauma as a result of heat can cause severe tissue damage, particularly to the mucous membranes of the upper respiratory tract. Although the most frequent situation in which this occurs is fire, damage can also occur in other settings. For example, in an autopsy study of 27 individuals who died after the explosion of a steam tube in a ship's boiler room, airway abnormalities were found to extend from the trachea to the transitional airways and consisted of vacuolar swelling of epithelial cells and "coagulative" changes of the subepithelial connective tissue.[230] The lung parenchyma showed capillary congestion and air-space hemorrhage and edema.

The histologic changes observed in the lungs of patients who have died within 48 hours of a fire include congestion, edema, intravascular fibrin thrombi, and intra-alveolar hemorrhage.[231, 232] Ultrastructural studies have shown intracellular edema with focal bleb and vesicle formation in type I cells.[232] In both experimental animals and humans, smoke inhalation may be associated with necrosis of tracheal and proximal bronchial epithelium;[233] although this abnormality is probably diffuse in most cases, the injury occasionally results in the formation of localized endobronchial polyps composed of granulation tissue.[234] Carbon particles may be seen on the airway surface and provide a marker of inhalation. Atypical squamous cells, representing the result of reparative changes in the healing phase, can be identified in the sputum of many individuals.[235]

Pulmonary complications occur in 20% to 30% of burn victims admitted to a hospital.[236–238] The incidence correlates with the severity of the burn and with a history of being in an enclosed space.[236, 238, 239] During the first 24 hours, complications result from upper airway edema caused by direct heat injury or toxic products, usually in patients who have head and neck burns.[240] After a latent period of 12 to 48 hours, symptoms and radiographic evidence of lower respiratory tract involvement may be evident.[241, 242] Pulmonary complications that become evident 2 to 5 days after the burn consist of atelectasis, edema, and pneumonia. The first of these may be caused by mucous plugging of large bronchi;[243] the last occurs much more frequently in the presence

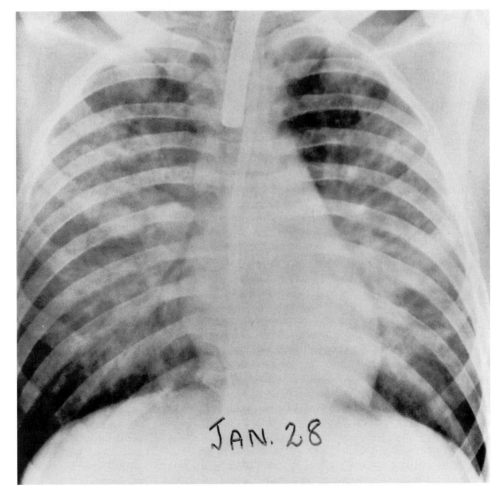

Figure 62–5. Acute Smoke Inhalation. This 30-year-old man was involved in a fire and inhaled large quantities of smoke before being rescued. He was brought to the emergency room in severe respiratory distress, and a tracheostomy was required. An anteroposterior radiograph reveals massive consolidation of both lungs in a pattern characteristic of acute pulmonary edema. The patient had an uneventful recovery.

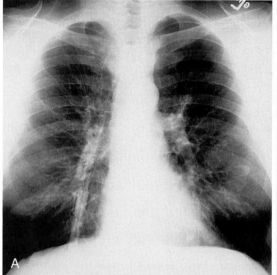

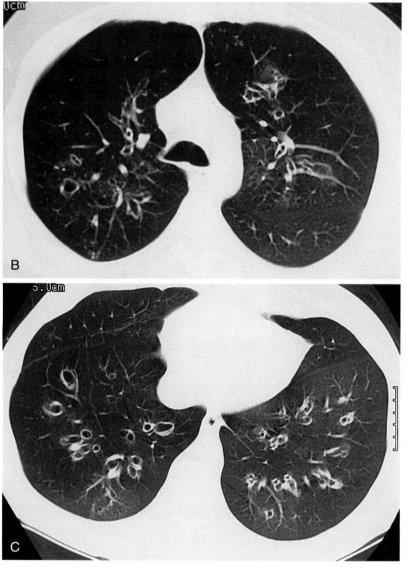

Figure 62–6. Bronchiectasis and Obliterative Bronchiolitis after Smoke Inhalation. A posteroanterior chest radiograph *(A)* in a 33-year-old man demonstrates increased lung volume, bronchiectasis, and decreased peripheral vascular markings. HRCT scan images *(B and C)* demonstrate extensive bronchiectasis and areas of decreased attenuation and vascularity as a result of obliterative bronchiolitis. The patient had experienced severe smoke inhalation several years earlier. (Courtesy of Dr. Christopher Griffin, Department of Radiology, Veterans Affairs Hospital, Portland, Oregon.)

of inhalation injury. In one review of the records of 1,058 burn patients treated at a single institution during a 5-year period, 373 (35%) suffered inhalation injury diagnosed by bronchoscopy, ventilation-perfusion scintigraphy, or both;[244] 141 of these patients (38%) subsequently developed pneumonia. Among the 685 patients who did not have inhalation injury, pneumonia occurred in only 60 (9%). Complications that arise after 5 days include pulmonary thromboembolism[245] and ARDS.[246] The acute effects of smoke exposure among firefighters have been reported to be greater in current cigarette smokers than among nonsmokers similarly exposed to smoke.[247] Acute smoke exposure can also cause transient bronchial hyper-responsiveness[248] or hypoxemia[249] and occasionally is complicated by the late development of bronchiectasis and obliterative bronchiolitis.[250]

The radiographic findings of acute smoke inhalation unassociated with skin burns were described in one study of 21 patients;[251] in 6, radiographs obtained 4 to 24 hours after the incident revealed focal opacities that were interpreted as atelectasis and that usually cleared within 3 days. In another study of 62 patients who required admission to a hospital

after smoke inhalation, 35 (63%) developed radiographic evidence of pulmonary edema, in most cases within 24 hours after the injury (Fig. 62–5).[242] In a third study of 29 patients who required ventilatory support after acute smoke inhalation and burns, 13 had radiologic findings consistent with inhalation injury, including interstitial or air-space edema or linear atelectasis.[252] Based on these studies, it can be concluded that the chest radiograph is a relatively insensitive indicator of airway and parenchymal injury after acute smoke inhalation. However, several groups of investigators have shown that patients who have an abnormal radiograph within 48 hours after inhalational injuries are more likely to require ventilatory support and have a worse prognosis than those who have normal radiographs.[242, 253, 254]

The pattern of deposition and the rate of clearance of aerosolized technetium-99m–DTPA has been used as a measure of the degree of acute inhalation injury in patients exposed to smoke; a pattern of inhomogeneous distribution and rapid uptake has been found to correlate with radiographic evidence, pulmonary function, and clinical markers of the severity of lung injury.[255]

Radiographic manifestations of large airway burns include subglottic edema and indistinctness of the trachea.[253, 256] Late manifestations include tracheal stenosis,[257] bronchiectasis,[258, 259] and evidence of obliterative bronchiolitis (increased lung volumes and decreased vascularity in the peripheral lung regions, Fig. 62–6).[259] Corresponding high-resolution computed tomography findings include bronchiectasis and areas of decreased attenuation and perfusion (*see* Fig. 62–6).

It might be expected that firefighters who are repeatedly exposed to smoke will show cumulative lung damage. Studies of more than 1,000 Boston firefighters demonstrated both clinical and physiologic evidence of impaired airway conductance (in addition to the effects ascribed to cigarette smoking).[260–262] However, follow-up of this cohort of firefighters 3 years later failed to confirm the original impression:[263] the annual decline in lung function was less than that observed over 1 year and could not be related to the number of fires fought or to other indices of acute fire exposure. In another study of lung function in retired firefighters, no evidence of severe impairment of respiratory function was identified over a 5-year follow-up period;[264] however, the average values were significantly lower than predicted. In addition, it was evident that subjects who had respiratory complaints and impaired ventilatory capacity tended to be selectively removed from active firefighting duty before retirement.

A number of other controlled studies in which pulmonary function has been assessed in firefighters have failed to show short-term deterioration in function;[265–269] however, they support the conclusion that a long-term risk of obstructive pulmonary disease exists in this occupation over and above that caused by cigarette smoking. An analysis of causes of death among 2,470 Boston firefighters employed during the period of 1915 to 1975 failed to reveal an association between occupation and cause-specific mortality.[270] By contrast, a determination of mortality by cause among 1,113 stationary engineers and firefighters revealed an excess of deaths from cancer of the buccal cavity, pharynx, rectum, and lung; in the same study, no evidence of an increase in the frequency of deaths from nonmalignant respiratory disease was detected.[271]

THESAUROSIS

In its broad connotation, thesaurosis designates storage in the body of unusual amounts of normal or foreign material. However, in the late 1950s and early 1960s, granulomatous pneumonitis resembling sarcoidosis was described in association with exposure to hair spray, and the term was used to describe this condition.[272, 273] In fact, there has been considerable controversy concerning the existence of hair spray–induced thesaurosis, and there have been few reports of the association since 1985.[274] It seems possible that the association represents no more than the chance coexistence of the use of hair spray and sarcoidosis.[275, 276] Although fairly rapid radiographic clearing and symptomatic improvement after cessation of exposure has been reported in some patients,[277] the available evidence casts doubts on the existence of this entity.

REFERENCES

1. Kleinfeld M: Acute pulmonary edema of chemical origin. Arch Environ Health 10:942, 1965.
2. Conner E, Dubois A, Comroe J: Acute chemical injury of the airway and lungs. Anesthesiology 23:538, 1962.
3. Baar HS, Galindo J: Bronchiolitis fibrosa obliterans. Thorax 21:209, 1966.
4. Thurston GD, Ito K, Hayes CG, et al: Respiratory hospital admissions and summertime haze air pollution in Toronto, Ontario: Consideration of the role of acid aerosols. Environ Res 65:271, 1994.
5. Currie WD, Pratt PC, Sanders AP: Hyperoxia and lung metabolism. Chest 66:19S, 1974.
6. Deneke SM, Fanburg BL: Normobaric oxygen toxicity of the lung. N Engl J Med 303:76, 1980.
7. Doelman CJ, Bast A: Oxygen radicals in lung pathology. Free Radical Biol Med 9:381, 1990.
8. Davreux CJ, Soric I, Nathens AB, et al: N-acetyl cysteine attenuates acute lung injury in the rat. Shock 8:432, 1997.
9. Cross CE, DeLucia AJ, Reddy AK, et al: Ozone interactions with lung tissue: Biochemical approaches. Am J Med 60:929, 1976.
10. Roehm JN, Hadley JH, Menzel DB: Antioxidants vs. lung disease. Arch Intern Med 128:88, 1971.
11. Putman E, van Golde LM, Haagsman HP: Toxic oxidant species and their impact on the pulmonary surfactant system. Lung 175:75, 1997.
12. Harada RN, Bowman CM, Fox RB, et al: Alveolar macrophage secretions: Initiators of inflammation in pulmonary oxygen toxicity. Chest 81(Suppl):S52, 1982.
13. Fox RB, Hoidal JR, Brown DM, et al: Pulmonary inflammation due to oxygen toxicity: Involvement of chemotactic factors and polymorphonuclear leukocytes. Am Rev Respir Dis 123:521, 1981.
14. Boatman ES, Sato S, Frank R: Acute effects of ozone on cat lungs. II. Structural. Am Rev Respir Dis 110:157, 1974.
15. Weibel ER: Oxygen effect on lung cells. Arch Intern Med 128:54, 1971.
16. Clark JM, Lambertsen CJ: Pulmonary oxygen toxicity: A review. Pharmacol Rev 23:37, 1971.
17. Fisher AB, Diamond S, Mallen S, et al: Effect of 48- and 72-hour oxygen exposure on the rabbit alveolar macrophage. Chest 66(Suppl):4S, 1974.
18. Simons JR, Theodore J, Robin ED: Common oxidant lesion of mitochondrial redox state produced by nitrogen dioxide, ozone and high oxygen in alveolar macrophages. Chest 66(Suppl):9S, 1974.
19. Huber GL, Mason RJ, LaForce M, et al: Alterations in the lung following the administration of ozone. Arch Intern Med 128:81, 1971.
20. Sackner MA, Hirsch JA, Epstein S, et al: Effect of oxygen in graded concentrations upon tracheal mucous velocity: A study in anesthetized dogs. Chest 69:164, 1976.
21. Frank L, Massaro D: Oxygen toxicity. Am J Med 69:117, 1980.
22. van Klaveren RJ, Demedts M, Nemery B: Cellular glutathione turnover in vitro with emphasis on type II pneumocyttes. Eur Respir J 10:1392, 1997.
23. Mohsenin V: Lipid peroxidation and antielastase activity in the lung under oxidant stress: Role of antioxidant defenses. J Appl Physiol 70:1456, 1991.
24. Tsan MF: Superoxide dismutase and pulmonary oxygen toxicity. Proc Soc Exp Biol Med 214:107, 1997.
25. Gilks CB, Price K, Wright JL, et al: Antioxidant gene expression in rat lung after exposure to cigarette smoke. Am J Pathol 152:269, 1998.
26. Folz RJ, Guan J, Seldin MF, et al: Mouse extracellular superoxide dismutase: Primary structure, tissue-specific gene expression, chromosomal localization, and lung in situ hybridization. Am J Respir Cell Mol Biol 17:393, 1997.
27. Su WY, Folz R, Chen JS, et al: Extracellular superoxide dismutase mRNA expressions in the human lung by in situ hybridization. Am J Respir Cell Mol Biol 16:162, 1997.
28. Crapo JD, Barry BE, Foscue HA, et al: Structural and biochemical changes in rat lungs occurring during exposure to lethal and adaptive doses of oxygen. Am Rev Respir Dis 122:123, 1980.
29. Wiester MJ, Tepper JS, Winsett DW, et al: Adaptation to ozone in rats and its association with ascorbic acid in the lung. Fund Appl Toxicol 31:56, 1996.
30. Crapo JD: Superoxide dismutase and tolerance to pulmonary oxygen toxicity. Chest 67(Suppl):39S, 1975.
31. Winter PM, Smith G, Wheelis RF: The effect of prior pulmonary injury on the rate of development of fatal oxygen toxicity. Chest 66(Suppl):1S, 1974.
32. Nash G, Blennerhassett JB, Pontoppidan H: Pulmonary lesions associated with oxygen therapy and artificial ventilation. N Engl J Med 276:368, 1967.
33. Northway WH Jr, Rosan RC, Porter DY: Pulmonary disease following respirator therapy of hyaline-membrane disease: Bronchopulmonary dysplasia. N Engl J Med 276:357, 1967.
34. Balentine JD: Pathologic effects of exposure to high oxygen tensions: A review. N Engl J Med 275:1038, 1966.
35. Kapanci Y, Tosco R, Eggerman J, et al: Oxygen pneumonitis in man: Light- and electron-microscopic morphometric studies. Chest 62:162, 1972.
36. Gillbe CE, Salt JC, Branthwaite MA: Pulmonary function after prolonged mechanical ventilation with high concentrations of oxygen. Thorax 35:907, 1980.
37. Pratt PC: Pulmonary capillary proliferation induced by oxygen inhalation. Am J Pathol 34:1033, 1958.
38. Paegle RD, Spain D, Davis S: Pulmonary morphology of chronic phase of oxygen toxicity in adult rats. Chest 66(Suppl):7S, 1974.
39. Pratt PC, Sanders AP, Currie WD: Oxygen toxicity and gas mixtures: Morphology. Chest 66(Suppl):8S, 1974.
40. Van DeWater JM, Kagey KS, Miller IT, et al: Oxygen response of the lung to six to twelve hours of 100 per cent inhalation in normal man. N Engl J Med 283:621, 1970.
41. Burger EJ Jr, Mead J: Static properties of lungs after oxygen exposure. J Appl Physiol 27:191, 1969.
42. Caldwell PR, Lee WL Jr, Schildkraut HS, et al: Changes in lung volume, diffusing capacity, and blood gases in men breathing oxygen. J Appl Physiol 21:1477, 1966.
43. Jackson RM: Pulmonary oxygen toxicity. Chest 88:900, 1985.
44. Pelled B, Shechter Y, Alroy G, et al: Deleterious effects of oxygen at ambient and hyperbaric pressure in the treatment of nitrogen dioxide-poisoned mice. Am Rev Respir Dis 108:1152, 1973.
45. Editorial: Ozone in smog. Lancet 2:1077, 1975.
46. Castleman WL, Dungworth DL, Schwartz LW, et al: Acute respiratory bronchiolitis: An ultrastructural and autoradiographic study of epithelial cell injury and renewal in rhesus monkeys exposed to ozone. Am J Pathol 98:811, 1980.
47. Wilson DW, Plopper CG, Dungworth DL: The response of the Macaque tracheobronchial epithelium to acute ozone injury. Am J Pathol 116:193, 1984.
48. Mellick PW, Dungworth DL, Schwartz LW, et al: Short-term morphologic effects of high ambient levels of ozone on lungs of Rhesus monkeys. Lab Invest 36:82, 1977.
49. Plopper CG, Dungworth DL, Tyler WS: Pulmonary lesions in rats exposed to ozone: A correlated light and electron microscopic study. Am J Pathol 71:375, 1973.
50. Harkema JR, Plopper CG, Hyde DM, et al: Response of macaque bronchiolar epithelium to ambient concentrations of ozone. Am J Pathol 143:857, 1993.
51. Watanabe S, Frank R, Yokoyama E: Acute effects of ozone on lungs of cats. I. Functional. Am Rev Respir Dis 108:1141, 1973.
52. Pinkerton KE, Dodge DE, Cederdahl-Demmler J, et al: Differentiated bronchiolar epithelium in alveolar ducts of rats exposed to ozone for 20 months. Am J Pathol 142:947, 1993.
53. Sato S, Kawakami N, Maeda S, et al: Scanning electron microscopy of the lungs of vitamin E-deficient rats exposed to a low concentration of ozone. Am Rev Respir Dis 113:809, 1976.
54. Hesterberg TW, Last JA: Ozone-induced acute pulmonary fibrosis in rats: Prevention of increased rates of collagen synthesis by methylprednisolone. Am Rev Respir Dis 123:47, 1981.
55. Boorman GA, Schwartz LW, Dungworth DL: Pulmonary effects of prolonged ozone insult in rats: Morphometric evaluation of the central acinus. Lab Invest 43:108, 1980.
56. Eustis SL, Schwartz LW, Kosch PC, et al: Chronic bronchiolitis in nonhuman primates after prolonged ozone exposure. Am J Pathol 105:121, 1981.
57. Gross KB, White HJ: Functional and pathologic consequences of a 52-week exposure to 0.5 ppm ozone followed by a clean air recovery period. Lung 165:283, 1987.
58. Hackney JD, Linn WS, Mohler JG, et al: Experimental studies on human health effects of air pollutants. II. Four-hour exposure to ozone alone and in combinations with other pollutant gases. Arch Environ Health 30:379, 1975.
59. Bates DV, Ball GM, Burnham CD, et al: Short-term effects of ozone on the lung. J Appl Physiol 32:176, 1972.
60. Kagawa J, Toyama T: Effects of ozone and brief exercise on specific airway conductance in man. Arch Environ Health 30:36, 1975.
61. Kagawa J: Respiratory effects of two-hour exposure with intermittent exercise to ozone, sulfur dioxide and nitrogen dioxide alone and in combination in normal subjects. Am Ind Hyg Assoc J 44:14, 1983.
62. Kagawa J: Exposure-effect relationship of selected pulmonary function measurements in subjects exposed to ozone. Int Arch Occup Environ Health 53:345, 1984.
63. Frampton MW, Morrow PE, Torres A, et al: Effects of ozone on normal and potentially sensitive human subjects. II. Airway inflammation and responsiveness to ozone in nonsmokers and smokers. Research Report—Health Effects Institute 78:39, 1997.
64. Hackney JD, Linn WS, Buckley RD, et al: Scientific communications: Experimental studies on human health effects of air pollutants. I. Design considerations. Arch Environ Health 30:373, 1975.
65. Kerr HD, Kulle TJ, McIlhany ML, et al: Effects of ozone on pulmonary function in normal subjects: An environmental-chamber study. Am Rev Respir Dis 111:763, 1975.
66. Hazucha M, Silverman F, Parent C, et al: Pulmonary function in a man after short-term exposure to ozone. Arch Environ Health 27:183, 1973.
67. Hazucha MJ, Madden M, Pape G, et al: Effects of cyclo-oxygenase inhibition on ozone-induced respiratory inflammation and lung function changes. Eur J Appl Physiol 73:17, 1996.
68. Hazucha MJ, Bates DV, Bromberg PA: Mechanism of action of ozone on the human lung. J Appl Physiol 67:1535, 1989.
69. Linn WS, Medway DA, Anzar UT, et al: Persistence of adaptation to ozone in volunteers exposed repeatedly for 6 weeks. Am Rev Respir Dis 125:491, 1982.
70. Bromberg PA, Hazucha MJ: Is "adaptation" to ozone protective? Am Rev Respir Dis 125:489, 1982.

71. Horvath SM, Gliner JA, Folinsbee LJ: Adaptation to ozone: Duration of effect. Am Rev Respir Dis 123:496, 1981.
72. Kulle TJ, Milman JH, Sauder LR, et al: Pulmonary function adaptation to ozone in subjects with chronic bronchitis. Environ Res 34:55, 1984.
73. Dejournette RL: Rocket propellant inhalation in the Apollo-Soyuz astronauts. Radiology 125:21, 1977.
74. Dowell AR, Kilburn KH, Pratt PC: Short-term exposure to nitrogen dioxide: Effects on pulmonary ultrastructure, compliance, and the surfactant system. Arch Intern Med 128:74, 1971.
75. Williams RA, Rhoades RA, Adams WS: The response of lung tissue and surfactant to nitrogen dioxide exposure. Arch Intern Med 128:101, 1971.
76. Evans MJ, Stephens RJ, Freeman G: Effects of nitrogen dioxide on cell renewal in the rat lung. Arch Intern Med 128:57, 1971.
77. Evans MJ, Cabral LC, Stephens RJ, et al: Acute kinetic response and renewal of the alveolar epithelium following injury by nitrogen dioxide. Chest 65(Suppl):62S, 1974.
78. Stephens RJ, Freeman G, Evans MJ: Ultrastructural changes in connective tissue in lungs of rats exposed to NO2. Arch Intern Med 127:873, 1971.
79. Ranga V, Kleinerman J: Lung injury and repair in the blotchy mouse: Effects of nitrogen dioxide inhalation. Am Rev Respir Dis 123:90, 1981.
80. Kleinerman J, Ip MPC, Sorensen J: Nitrogen dioxide exposure and alveolar macrophage elastase in hamsters. Am Rev Respir Dis 125:203, 1982.
81. Mohsenin V: Human exposure to oxides of nitrogen at ambient and supra-ambient concentrations. Toxicology 89:301, 1994.
82. Folinsbee LJ, Horvath SM, Bedi JF, et al: Effect of 0.62 ppm NO2 on cardiopulmonary function in young male nonsmokers. Environ Res 15:199, 1978.
82a. Linn WS, Shamoo DA, Spier CE, et al: Controlled exposure of volunteers with chronic obstructive pulmonary disease to nitrogen dioxide. Arch Environ Health 40:313, 1985.
83. Chaney S, Blomquist D, DeWitt P, et al: Biochemical changes in humans upon exposure to nitrogen dioxide while at rest. Arch Environ Health 36:53, 1981.
84. Gailitis J, Burns LE, Nally JB: Silo-filler's disease: Report of a case. N Engl J Med 258:543, 1958.
85. Becklake MR, Goldman HI, Bosman AR, et al: The long-term effects of exposure to nitrous fumes. Am Rev Tuberc 76:398, 1957.
86. Pfitzer EA, Yevich PP, Greene EA, et al: Acute toxicity of red fuming nitric acid-hydrofluoric acid vapor mixture. AMA Arch Ind Health 18:218, 1958.
87. Lafleche LR, Boivin C, Leonard C: Nitrogen dioxide: A respiratory irritant. Can Med Assoc J 84:1438, 1961.
88. Müller B: Nitrogen dioxide intoxication after a mining accident. Respiration 26:249, 1969.
89. Morgan WK. "Zamboni disease:" Pulmonary edema in an ice hockey player. Arch Intern Med 155:2479, 1995.
90. Horvath EP, doPico GA, Barbee RA, et al: Nitrogen dioxide-induced pulmonary disease: Five new cases and a review of the literature. J Occup Med 20:103, 1978.
91. Fleetham JA, Munt PW, Tunnicliffe BW: Silo-filler's disease. Can Med Assoc J 119:482, 1978.
92. Douglas WW, Hepper NG, Colby TV: Silo-filler's disease. Mayo Clin Proc 64:291, 1989.
93. Scott EG, Hunt WB Jr: Silo-filler's disease. Chest 63:701, 1973.
94. Ramirez RJ, Dowell AR: Silo-filler's disease: Nitrogen dioxide-induced lung injury. Long-term follow-up and review of the literature. Ann Intern Med 74:569, 1971.
95. Zwemer FL Jr, Pratt DS, May JJ: Silo filler's disease in New York State. Am Rev Respir Dis 146:650, 1992.
96. Ramirez FJ: The first death from nitrogen dioxide fumes: The story of a man and his dog. JAMA 229:1181, 1974.
97. Tse RL, Bockman AA: Nitrogen dioxide toxicity: Report of four cases in firemen. JAMA 212:1341, 1970.
98. Jones GR, Proudfoot AT, Hall JI: Pulmonary effects of acute exposure to nitrous fumes. Thorax 28:61, 1973.
99. Lowry T, Schuman LM: "Silo-filler's disease:" A syndrome caused by nitrogen dioxide. JAMA 162:153, 1956.
100. Cornelius EA, Betlach EH: Silo-filler's disease. Radiology 74:232, 1960.
101. Fleming GM, Chester EH, Montenegro HD: Dysfunction of small airways following pulmonary injury due to nitrogen dioxide. Chest 75:720, 1979.
102. Conrad E, Lo W, deBoisblanc BP, et al: Reactive airways dysfunction syndrome after exposure to dinitrogen tetroxide. South Med J 91:338, 1998.
103. Larson TV, Frank R, Covert DS, et al: Measurements of respiratory ammonia and the chemical neutralization of inhaled sulfuric acid aerosol in anesthetized dogs. Am Rev Respir Dis 125:502, 1982.
104. Morgan WKC, Seaton A: Occupational Lung Disease. Philadelphia, WB Saunders, 1975, p 241.
105. Kipen HM, Lerman Y: Respiratory abnormalities among photographic developers: A report of three cases. Am J Ind Med 9:341, 1986.
106. Hodgson MJ, Parkinson DK: Respiratory disease in a photographer. Am J Ind Med 9:349, 1986.
107. Koizumi A, Aoki T, Tsukada M, et al: Mercury, not sulphur dioxide, poisoning as cause of smelter disease in industrial plants producing sulphuric acid. Lancet 343(8910):1411, 1994.
108. Woodford DM, Coutu RE, Gaensler EA: Obstructive lung disease from acute sulfur dioxide exposure. Respiration 38:238, 1979.
109. Hamilton A, Hardy HL: Industrial Toxicology. 3rd ed. Acton MA, Publishing Sciences Group, 1974, p 210.
110. Charan NB, Myers CG, Lakshminarayan S, et al: Pulmonary injuries associated with acute sulfur dioxide inhalation. Am Rev Respir Dis 119:555, 1979.
111. Harkonen H, Nordman H, Korhonen O, et al: Long-term effects of exposure to sulfur dioxide: Lung function four years after a pyrite dust explosion. Am Rev Respir Dis 128:890, 1983.
112. Osbern LN, Crapo RO: Dung lung: A report of toxic exposure to liquid manure. Ann Intern Med 95:312, 1981.
113. Reiffenstein RJ, Hulbert WC, Roth SH: Toxicology of hydrogen sulfide. Ann Rev Pharmacol Toxicol 32:109, 1992.
114. Burnett WW, King EG, Grace M, et al: Hydrogen sulfide poisoning: Review of 5 years experience. Can Med Assoc J 117:1277, 1977.
115. Glass RI, Ford R, Allegra DT, et al: Deaths from asphyxia among fishermen. JAMA 244:2193, 1980.
116. Kilburn KH: Case report: Profound neurobehavioral deficits in an oil field worker overcome by hydrogen sulfide. Am J Med Sci 306:301, 1993.
117. Snyder JW, Safir EF, Summerville GP, et al: Occupational fatality and persistent neurological sequelae after mass exposure to hydrogen sulfide. Am J Emerg Med 13:199, 1995.
118. Price SK, Hughes JE, Morrison SC, et al: Fatal ammonia inhalation: A case report with autopsy findings. S Afr Med J 64:952, 1983.
119. Sobonya R: Fatal anhydrous ammonia inhalation. Hum Pathol 8:293, 1977.
120. Arwood R, Hammond J, Ward GG: Ammonia inhalation. J Trauma 25:444, 1985.
121. Hatton DV, Leach CS, Beaudet AL, et al: Collagen breakdown and ammonia inhalation. Arch Environ Health 34:83, 1979.
122. Caplin M: Ammonia gas-poisoning: Forty-seven cases in a London shelter. Lancet 241:95, 1941.
123. Klein J, Olson KR, McKinney HE: Caustic injury from household ammonia. Am J Emerg Med 3:320, 1985.
124. Hoeffler HB, Schweppe HI, Greenberg SD: Bronchiectasis following pulmonary ammonia burn. Arch Pathol Lab Med 106:686, 1982.
125. Kass I, Zamel N, Dobry CA, et al: Bronchiectasis following ammonia burns of the respiratory tract: A review of two cases. Chest 62:282, 1972.
126. Montague TJ, MacNeil AR: Mass ammonia inhalation. Chest 77:496, 1980.
127. Slot CMJ: Ammonia gas burns: An account of six cases. Lancet 235:1356, 1938.
128. Flury KE, Dines DE, Rodarte JR, et al: Airway obstruction due to inhalation of ammonia. Mayo Clin Proc 58:389, 1983.
129. Das R, Blanc PD: Chlorine gas exposure and the lung: A review. Toxicol Indust Health 9:439, 1993.
130. Shroff CP, Khade MV, Srinivasan M: Respiratory cytopathology in chlorine gas toxicity: A study in 28 subjects. Diagn Cytopathol 4:28, 1988.
131. Bherer L, Cushman R, Courteau JP, et al: Survey of construction workers repeatedly exposed to chlorine over a three to six month period in a pulpmill. II. Follow up of affected workers by questionnaire, spirometry, and assessment of bronchial responsiveness 18 to 24 months after exposure ended. Occup Environ Med 51:225, 1994.
132. Martinez TT, Long C: Explosion risk from swimming pool chlorinators and review of chlorine toxicity. J Toxicol Clin Toxicol 33:349, 1995.
133. Anonymous: Chlorine gas toxicity from mixture of bleach with other cleaning products—California. MMWR 40:619, 627, 1991.
134. Minami M, Katsumata M, Miyake K, et al: Dangerous mixture of household detergents in an old-style toilet: A case report with simulation experiments of the working environment and warning of potential hazard relevant to the general environment. Hum Exp Toxicol 11:27, 1992.
135. Demnati R, Fraser R, Ghezzo H, et al: Time-course of functional and pathological changes after a single high acute inhalation of chlorine in rats. Eur Respir J 11:922, 1998.
136. Weill H, George R, Schwarz M, et al: Late evaluation of pulmonary function after acute exposure to chlorine gas. Am Rev Respir Dis 99:374, 1969.
137. Chester EH, Gillespie DG, Krause FD: The prevalence of chronic obstructive pulmonary disease in chlorine gas workers. Am Rev Respir Dis 99:365, 1969.
138. Jones RN, Hughes JM, Glindmeyer H, et al: Lung function after acute chlorine exposure. Am Rev Respir Dis 134:1190, 1986.
139. Courteau J, Cushman R, Bouchard F, et al: Survey of construction workers repeatedly exposed to chlorine over a three to six month period in a pulpmill. I. Exposure and symptomatology. Occup Environ Med 51:219, 1994.
140. Adelson L, Kaufman J: Fatal chlorine poisoning: Report of two cases with clinicopathologic correlation. Am J Clin Pathol 56:430, 1971.
141. Rosenthal T, Baum GL, Frand U, et al: Poisoning caused by inhalation of hydrogen chloride, phosphorus oxychloride, phosphorus pentachloride, oxalyl chloride, and oxalic acid. Chest 73:623, 1978.
142. Hasan FM, Gehshan A, Fuleihan FJ: Resolution of pulmonary dysfunction following acute chlorine exposure. Arch Environ Health 38:76, 1983.
143. Rafferty P: Voluntary chlorine inhalation: A new form of self-abuse? BMJ 281:1178, 1980.
144. Lim SC, Yang JY, Jang AS, et al: Acute lung injury after phosgene inhalation. Korean J Intern Med 11:87, 1996.
145. Seidelin R: The inhalation of phosgene in a fire extinguisher accident. Thorax 16:91, 1961.
146. Everett ED, Overholt EL: Phosgene poisoning. JAMA 205:243, 1968.
147. Wyatt JP, Allister CA: Occupational phosgene poisoning: A case report and review. J Accid Emerg Med 12:212, 1995.
148. Polednak AP: Mortality among men occupationally exposed to phosgene in 1943–1945. Environ Res 22:357, 1980.
149. Gerritsen WB, Buschmann CH: Phosgene poisoning caused by the use of chemical paint removers containing methylene chloride in ill-ventilated rooms heated by kerosene stoves. Br J Ind Med 17:187, 1960.

150. English JM: A case of probable phosgene poisoning. BMJ 1:38, 1964.
151. Snyder RW, Mishel HS, Christensen GC 3d. Pulmonary toxicity following exposure to methylene chloride and its combustion product, phosgene. Chest 101:860, 1992.
152. Sjogren B, Plato N, Alexandersson R, et al: Pulmonary reactions caused by welding-induced decomposed trichloroethylene. Chest 99:237, 1991.
153. Yodaiken RE: The uncertain consequences of formaldehyde toxicity. JAMA 246:1677, 1981.
154. Bernstein RS, Stayner LT, Elliot LJ, et al: Inhalation exposure to formaldehyde: An overview of its toxicology, epidemiology, monitoring, and control. Am Ind Hyg Assoc J 45:778, 1984.
155. Alexandersson R, Kolmodin-Hedman B, Hedenstierna G: Exposure to formaldehyde: Effects on pulmonary function. Arch Environ Health 37:279, 1982.
156. Kwong F, Kraske G, Nelson AM, et al: Acute symptoms secondary to formaldehyde exposure in a pathology resident. Ann Allergy 50:326, 1983.
157. Levine RJ, DalCorso RD, Blunden PD, et al: The effects of occupational exposure on the respiratory health of West Virginia morticians. J Occup Med 26:91, 1984.
158. Uba G, Pachorek D, Bernstein J, et al: Prospective study of respiratory effects of formaldehyde among healthy and asthmatic medical students. Am J Ind Med 15:91, 1989.
159. Khamgaonkar MB, Fulare MB: Pulmonary effects of formaldehyde exposure: An environmental-epidemiological study. Indian J Chest Dis Allied Sci 33:9, 1991.
160. Harris JC, Rumack BH, Aldrich FD: Toxicology of urea formaldehyde and polyurethane foam insulation. JAMA 245:243, 1981.
161. Day JH, Lees REM, Clark RH, et al: Respiratory response to formaldehyde and off-gas of urea formaldehyde foam insulation. Can Med Assoc J 131:1061, 1984.
162. Norman GR, Pengelly LD, Kerigan AT, et al: Respiratory function of children in homes insulated with urea formaldehyde foam insulation. Can Med Assoc J 134:1135, 1986.
163. Witek TJ Jr, Schachter EN, Tosun T, et al: An evaluation of respiratory effects following exposure to 2.0 ppm formaldehyde in asthmatics: Lung function, symptoms, and airway reactivity. Arch Environ Health 42:230, 1987.
164. Grammer LC, Harris KE, Shaughnessy MA et al. Clinical and immunologic evaluation of 37 workers exposed to gaseous formaldehyde. J Allergy Clin Immunol 86:177, 1990.
165. Dally KA, Hanrahan LP, Woodbury MA, et al: Formaldehyde exposure in nonoccupational environments. Arch Environ Health 36:277, 1981.
166. Monticello TM, Morgan KT, Everitt JI, et al: Effects of formaldehyde gas on the respiratory tract of rhesus monkeys. Am J Pathol 134:515, 1989.
167. Marsh GM: Proportional mortality patterns among chemical plant workers exposed to formaldehyde. Br J Ind Med 39:313, 1982.
168. Nunn AJ, Craigen AA, Darbyshire JH, et al: Six year follow up of lung function in men occupationally exposed to formaldehyde. Br J Indust Med 47:747, 1990.
169. Broder I, Corey P, Brasher P, et al: Formaldehyde exposure and health status in households. Environ Health Perspect 95:101, 1991.
170. Graeme KA, Pollack CV Jr: Heavy metal toxicity. II. Lead and metal fume fever. J Emerg Med 16:171, 1998.
171. Nemery B: Metal toxicity and the respiratory tract. Eur Respir J 3:202, 1990.
172. Kuschner WG, D'Alessandro A, Wong H, et al: Early pulmonary cytokine responses to zinc oxide fume inhalation. Environ Res 75:7, 1997.
173. Gordon T, Fine JM: Metal fume fever. Occup Med 8:504, 1993.
174. Kuschner WG, D'Alessandro A, Wintermeyer S, et al: Pulmonary responses to purified zinc oxide fume. J Invest Med 43:371, 1995.
175. Vogelmeier C, Konig G, Bencze K, et al: Pulmonary involvement in zinc fume fever. Chest 92:946, 1987.
176. Lindahl M, Leanderson P, Tagesson C: Novel aspect of metal fume fever: Zinc stimulates oxygen radical formation in human neutrophils. Hum Exp Toxicol 17:105, 1998.
177. Langley RL: Fume fever and reactive airways dysfunction syndrome in a welder. South Med J 84:1034, 1991.
178. Gore I Jr, Harding SM: Sinker lung: Acute metallic mercury poisoning associated with the making of fish weights. Ala J Med Sci 24:267, 1987.
179. Hallee TJ: Diffuse lung disease caused by inhalation of mercury vapor. Am Rev Respir Dis 99:430, 1969.
180. Natelson EA, Blumenthal BJ, Fred HL: Acute mercury vapor poisoning in the home. Chest 59:677, 1971.
181. Lien DC, Todoruk DN, Rajani HR, et al: Accidental inhalation of mercury vapour: Respiratory and toxicologic consequences. Can Med Assoc J 129:591, 1983.
182. Haddad JK, Stenberg E Jr: Bronchitis due to acute mercury inhalation: Report of two cases. Am Rev Respir Dis 88:543, 1963.
183. Tamir M, Bronstein B, Behar M, et al: Mercury poisoning from an unsuspected source. Br J Ind Med 21:299, 1964.
184. Milliken JA, Waugh D, Kadish ME: Acute interstitial pulmonary fibrosis caused by a smoke bomb. Can Med Assoc J 88:36, 1963.
185. Hjortso E, Qvist J, Bud MI, et al: ARDS after accidental inhalation of zinc chloride smoke. Intens Care Med 14(1):17, 1988.
186. Evans EH: Casualties following exposure to zinc chloride smoke. Lancet 2:368, 1945.
187. Homma S, Jones R, Qvist J, et al: Pulmonary vascular lesions in the ARDS caused by inhalation of zinc chloride smoke: A morphometric study. Hum Pathol 23:45, 1992.
188. Davies TAL: Manganese pneumonitis. Br J Ind Med 3:111, 1946.
189. Davies TAL, Harding HK: Manganese pneumonitis: Further clinical and experimental observations. Br J Ind Med 6:82, 1949.

189a. Adkins B Jr, Luginbuhl GH, Miller FJ, et al: Increased pulmonary susceptibility to streptococcal infection following inhalation of manganese oxide. Environ Res 23:110, 1980.
190. Lewis GP, Coughlin LL, Jusko WJ, et al: Contribution of cigarette smoking to cadmium accumulation in man. Lancet 1:291, 1972.
191. Cadmium and the lung (editorial). Lancet 2:1134, 1973.
192. Seidal K, Jorgensen N, Elinder CG, et al: Fatal cadmium-induced pneumonitis. Scand J Work Environ Health 19:429, 1993.
193. Fuortes L, Leo A, Ellerbeck PG, et al: Acute respiratory fatality associated with exposure to sheet metal and cadmium fumes. J Toxicol Clin Toxicol 29:279, 1991.
194. Beton DC, Andrews GS, Davies HJ, et al: Acute cadmium fume poisoning: Five cases with one death from renal necrosis. Br J Ind Med 23:292, 1966.
195. Bonnell JA, Kazantzis G, King E: A follow-up study of men exposed to cadmium oxide fume. Br J Ind Med 16:135, 1959.
196. Kazantzis G, Flynn FV, Spowage JS, et al: Renal tubular malfunction and pulmonary emphysema in cadmium pigment workers. Q J Med 32:165, 1963.
197. Desilva PE, Donnan MB: Chronic cadmium poisoning in a pigment manufacturing plant. Br J Ind Med 38:76, 1981.
198. Lauwerys RR, Roels HA, Buchet J-P, et al: Investigations on the lung and kidney function in workers exposed to cadmium. Environ Health Perspect 28:137, 1979.
199. Davison AG, Fayers PM, Newman-Taylor AJ, et al: Cadmium fume inhalation and emphysema. Lancet 1:663, 1988.
200. Hirst RN, Perry HM, Cruz MG, et al: Elevated cadmium concentration in emphysematous lungs. Am Rev Respir Dis 108:30, 1973.
201. Smith TJ, Petty TL, Reading JC, et al: Pulmonary effects of chronic exposure to airborne cadmium. Am Rev Respir Dis 114:161, 1976.
202. Anthony JS, Zamel N, Aberman A: Abnormalities in pulmonary function after brief exposure to toxic metal fumes. Can Med Assoc J 119:586, 1978.
203. Scott R, Paterson PJ, McKirdy A, et al: Clinical and biochemical abnormalities in coppersmiths. Lancet 2:396, 1976.
204. Palmer KC, Snider GL, Hayes JA: Cellular proliferation induced in the lung by cadmium aerosol. Am Rev Respir Dis 112:173, 1975.
205. Snider GL, Hayes JA, Korthy AL, et al: Centrilobular emphysema experimentally induced by cadmium chloride aerosol. Am Rev Respir Dis 108:40, 1973.
206. Thurlbeck WM, Foley FD: Experimental pulmonary emphysema: The effect of intratracheal injection of cadmium chloride solution in the guinea pig. Am J Pathol 42:431, 1963.
207. Snider GL, Hayer JA, Korthy AL, et al: Centrilobular emphysema experimentally induced by cadmium chloride aerosol. Am Rev Respir Dis 108:40, 1973.
208. Janoff A: Elastases and emphysema: Current assessment of the protease-antiprotease hypothesis. Am Rev Respir Dis 132:417, 1985.
209. Edling C, Elinder CG, Randma E: Lung function in workers using cadmium containing solders. Br J Ind Med 43:657, 1986.
210. Dopico GA, Rankin J, Chosy LW, et al: Respiratory tract disease from thermosetting resins: Study of an outbreak in rubber tire workers. Ann Intern Med 83:177, 1975.
211. Herbert FA, Orford R: Pulmonary hemorrhage and edema due to inhalation of resins containing trimellitic anhydride. Chest 75:546, 1979.
212. Rice DL, Jenkins DE, Gray JM, et al: Chemical pneumonitis secondary to inhalation of epoxy pipe coating. Arch Environ Health 32:173, 1977.
213. Ahmad D, Morgan WK, Patterson R, et al: Pulmonary haemorrhage and haemolytic anaemia due to trimellitic anhydride. Lancet 2:328, 1979.
214. Patterson R, Addington W, Banner AS, et al: Antihapten antibodies in workers exposed to trimellitic anhydride fumes: A potential immunopathogenetic mechanism for the trimellitic anhydride pulmonary disease-anemia syndrome. Am Rev Respir Dis 120:1259, 1979.
215. Rivera M, Nicotra B, Byron GE, et al: Trimellitic anhydride toxicity: A cause of acute multisystem failure. Arch Intern Med 141:1071, 1981.
216. Zeiss CR, Wolkonsky P, Chacon R, et al: Syndromes in workers exposed to trimellitic anhydride: A longitudinal clinical and immunologic study. Ann Intern Med 98:8, 1983.
217. Leach CL, Hatoum NS, Ratajczak HV, et al: Evidence of immunologic control of lung injury induced by trimellitic anhydride. Am Rev Respir Dis 137:186, 1988.
218. Zeiss CR, Leach CL, Smith LJ, et al: A serial immunologic and histopathologic study of lung injury induced by trimellitic anhydride. Am Rev Respir Dis 137:191, 1988.
219. Piirila P, Keskinen H, Anttila S, et al. Allergic alveolitis following exposure to epoxy polyester powder paint containing low amounts (<1%) of acid anhydrides. Eur Respir J 10:948, 1997.
220. Wegman DH, Peters JM: Polymer fume fever and cigarette smoking. Ann Intern Med 81:55, 1974.
221. Robbins JJ, Ware RL: Pulmonary edema from Teflon fumes. N Engl J Med 271:360, 1964.
222. Evans EA: Pulmonary edema after inhalation of fumes from polytetrafluoroethylene (PTFE). J Occup Med 15:599, 1973.
223. Williams N, Smith K: Polymer fume fever, an elusive diagnosis. JAMA 219:1587, 1972.
224. The lung in burns (editorial). Lancet 2:673, 1981.
225. Moylan JA, Chan C-K: Inhalation injury: An increasing problem. Ann Surg 188:34, 1978.
226. Demling RH: Smoke inhalation injury. New Horizons 1:422, 1993
227. Done AK: The toxic emergency: Where there's smoke, there may be more than fire. Emerg Med 13:111, 1981.
228. Clark CJ, Campbell D, Reid WH: Blood carboxyhaemoglobin and cyanide levels in fire survivors. Lancet 1:1332, 1981.

229. Dyer RF, Esch VH: Polyvinyl chloride toxicity in fires, hydrogen chloride toxicity in fire fighters. JAMA 235:393, 1976.
230. Brinkmann B, Püschel K: Heat injuries to the respiratory system. Virchows Arch A Pathol Anat Histol 379:299, 1978.
231. Hasleton PS, McWilliam L, Haboubi NY: The lung parenchyma in burns. Histopathology 7:333, 1983.
232. Burns TR, Greenberg SD, Cartwright J, et al: Smoke inhalation: An ultrastructural study of reaction to injury in the human alveolar wall. Environ Res 41:447, 1986.
233. Thorning DR, Howard ML, Hudson LD, et al: Morphologic changes in rabbits exposed to pine wood smoke. Hum Pathol 13:355, 1982.
234. Williams DO, Vanecko RM, Glassroth J: Endobronchial polyposis following smoke inhalation. Chest 84:774, 1983.
235. Cooney W, Dzuira B, Harper R, et al: The cytology of sputum from thermally injured patients. Acta Cytol 16:433, 1972.
236. Achauer BM, Allyn PA, Furnas DW, et al: Pulmonary complications of burns: The major threat to the burn patient. Ann Surg 177:311, 1973.
237. Whitener DR, Whitener LM, Robertson KJ, et al: Pulmonary function measurements in patients with thermal injury and smoke inhalation. Am Rev Respir Dis 122:731, 1980.
238. Teixidor HS, Novick G, Rubin E: Pulmonary complications in burn patients. J Can Assoc Radiol 34:264, 1983.
239. Peters WJ: Inhalation injury caused by the products of combustion. Can Med Assoc J 125:249, 1981.
240. Raman TK, Dobbins JR, Berte JB: Respiratory burns during oxygen therapy. Chest 57:485, 1970.
241. Crapo RO: Smoke-inhalation injuries. JAMA 246:1694, 1981.
242. Teixidor HS, Rubin E, Novick GS, et al: Smoke inhalation: Radiologic manifestations. Radiology 149:383, 1983.
243. Pietak SP, Delahaye DJ: Airway obstruction following smoke inhalation. Can Med Assoc J 115:329, 1976.
244. Shirani KZ, Pruitt BA Jr, Mason AD Jr: The influence of inhalation injury and pneumonia on burn mortality. Ann Surg 205:82, 1987.
245. Achauer BM, Allyn PA, Furnas DW, et al: Pulmonary complications of burns: The major threat to the burn patient. Ann Surg 177:311, 1973.
246. Beachley MC, Ghahremani GG: The radiographic spectrum of pulmonary complications in burn victims. Am J Roentgenol 128:441, 1977.
247. Gu TL, Liou SH, Hsu CH, et al: Acute health hazards of firefighters after fighting a department store fire. Indust Health 34:13, 1996.
248. Kinsella J, Carter R, Reid WH, et al: Increased airways reactivity after smoke inhalation. Lancet 337(8741):595, 1991.
249. Tashkin DP, Genovesi MG, Chopra S, et al: Respiratory status of Los Angeles firemen: One-month follow-up after inhalation of dense smoke. Chest 71:445, 1977.
250. Tasaka S, Kanazawa M, Mori M, et al: Long-term course of bronchiectasis and bronchiolitis obliterans as late complication of smoke inhalation. Respiration 62:40, 1995.
251. Putman CE, Loke J, Matthay RA, et al: Radiographic manifestations of acute smoke inhalation. Am J Roentgenol 129:865, 1977.
252. Wittram C, Kenny JB: The admission chest radiograph after acute inhalation injury and burns. Br J Radiol 67:51, 1994.
253. Lee MJ, O'Connell DJ: The plain chest radiograph after acute smoke inhalations. Clin Radiol 39:3, 1988.
254. Darling GE, Keresteci MA, Ibanez D, et al: Pulmonary complications in inhalation injuries with associated cutaneous burn. J Trauma 40:83, 1996.
255. Lin WY, Kao CH, Wang SJ: Detection of acute inhalation injury in fire victims by means of technetium-99m DTPA radioaerosol inhalation lung scintigraphy. Eur J Nucl Med 24:125, 1997.
256. Griglak MJ: Thermal injuries. Emerg Med Clin North Am 10:369, 1992.
257. Gaissert HA, Lofgren RH, Grillo HC, et al: Upper airway compromise after inhalation injury: Complex strictures of the larynx and trachea and their management. Ann Surg 218:672, 1993.
258. Slutzker AD, Kinn R, Said SI: Bronchiectasis and progressive respiratory failure following smoke inhalation. Chest 95:1349, 1989.
259. Tasaka S, Kanazawa M, Mori M, et al: Long-term course of bronchiectasis and bronchiolitis obliterans as late complication of smoke inhalation. Respiration 62:40, 1995.
260. Sidor R, Peters JM: Prevalence rates of chronic non-specific respiratory disease in fire fighters. Am Rev Respir Dis 109:255, 1974.
261. Peters JM, Theriault GP, Fine LJ, et al: Chronic effect of fire fighting on pulmonary function. N Engl J Med 291:1320, 1974.
262. Sidor R, Peters JM: Fire fighting and pulmonary function: An epidemiologic study. Am Rev Respir Dis 109:249, 1974.
263. Musk AW, Peters JM, Wegman DH: Lung function in fire fighters. I. A three year follow-up of active subjects. Am J Public Health 67:626, 1977.
264. Musk AW, Peters JM, Wegman DH: Lung function in fire fighters. II. A five year follow-up of retirees. Am J Public Health 67:630, 1977.
265. Unger KM, Snow RM, Mestas JM, et al: Smoke inhalation in firemen. Thorax 35:838, 1980.
266. Loke J, Farmer W, Matthay RA, et al: Acute and chronic effects of fire fighting on pulmonary function. Chest 77:369, 1980.
267. Genovesi MG: Effects of smoke inhalation. Chest 77:335, 1980.
268. Young I, Jackson J, West S: Chronic respiratory disease and respiratory function in a group of fire fighters. Med J Aust 1:654, 1980.
269. Sparrow D, Bosse R, Rosner B, et al: The effect of occupational exposure on pulmonary function: A longitudinal evaluation of fire fighters and nonfire fighters. Am Rev Respir Dis 125:319, 1982.
270. Musk AW, Monson RR, Peters JM, et al: Mortality among Boston firefighters, 1915–1975. Br J Ind Med 35:104, 1978.
271. Decoufle P, Lloyd JW, Salvin LG: Mortality by cause among stationary engineers and stationary firemen. J Occup Med 19:679, 1977.
272. Bergmann M, Flance IJ, Blumenthal HT: Thesaurosis following inhalation of hair spray: A clinical and experimental study. N Engl J Med 258:471, 1958.
273. Bergmann M, Flance IJ, Cruz PT, et al: Thesaurosis due to inhalation of hair spray: Report of twelve new cases, including three autopsies. N Engl J Med 266:750, 1962.
274. Nagata N, Kawajiri T, Hayashi T, et al: Interstitial pneumonitis and fibrosis associated with the inhalation of hair spray. Respiration 64:310, 1997.
275. Herrero EU, Feigelson HH, Becker A: Sarcoidosis in a beautician. Am Rev Respir Dis 92:280, 1965.
276. Brunner MJ, Giovacchini RP, Wyatt JP, et al: Pulmonary disease and hair-spray polymers: A disputed relationship. JAMA 184:851, 1963.
277. Schraufnagel DE, Paré JAP, Wang NS: Micronodular pulmonary pattern: Association with inhaled aerosol. Am J Roentgenol 137:57, 1981.

Drugs

Knowledge of adverse drug reactions is important for the pulmonary physician for several reasons:

1. They are a significant cause of morbidity and mortality. It has been estimated that as many as 5% of all hospitalizations are the result of untoward effects of drug therapy, and about 0.3% of deaths that occur in the hospital are believed to be drug related.[1]

2. They are surprisingly common; for example, it has been estimated that about 5% of patients receiving amiodarone develop lung toxicity and that as many as 15% of patients taking angiotensin-converting enzyme (ACE) inhibitors develop an irritating cough.[1] Overall, up to 15% of patients have an adverse reaction to a drug given while in the hospital. If drugs causing lupus-like reactions and eosinophilic lung disease are included, more than 150 agents have been recognized to cause an adverse pulmonary reaction of one kind or another[1] (Table 63–1).

3. Their early recognition is important; unrecognized, the process can be progressive and fatal, whereas cessation of the drug may be followed by prompt reversibility of toxicity.[2]

Drug reactions can imitate virtually any pulmonary syndrome, and the *possibility* that an adverse drug response may explain a patient's illness must always be considered. Nevertheless, most drug reactions affecting the lungs can be categorized into one of six well-defined types (although it is important to remember that some drugs are capable of producing more than one response in different patients or simultaneously in the same patient):[1] (1) bronchospasm (*see* page 2112); (2) systemic lupus erythematosus-like syndrome (*see*

Table 63–1. DRUG-INDUCED DISEASE OF THE THORAX

DRUG	COMMENTS	SELECTED REFERENCES
Cytotoxic Antibiotics		
Bleomycin	Subacute to chronic interstitial pneumonitis with fibrosis is most common manifestation	5, 10
Mitomycin	Subacute to chronic interstitial pneumonitis with fibrosis is most common manifestation	84
Peplomycin		97
Zinostatin	Veno-occlusive disease	98
Alkylating Agents		
Busufan	Insidious onset of pulmonary fibrosis after long-term use	3
Cyclophosphamide	Disease uncommon when used as single agent	125, 126
Ifosfamide		130
Chlorambucil	Disease uncommon but frequently fatal	144
Melphalan		152
Nitrosureas (BCNU, CCNU)	Especially toxic when used in high-dose combined chemotherapy regimens	160
Vinca alkaloids	Diffuse alveolar damage (ARDS) and pulmonary fibrosis when used in combination with mitomycin	79
Antimetabolites		
Methotrexate	Acute to subacute disease is most common presentation; pulmonary injury can occur in patients receiving low-dose therapy	213, 215, 216
Cytosine arabinoside	Noncardiogenic pulmonary edema	270, 273
Azathioprine and 6-mercaptopurine		78, 274
Fludarabine		281
L-Asparaginase	Pulmonary thromboembolic disease	283
5-fluorouracil	Focal necrotizing pneumonia after accidental infusion by misplaced catheter	284
Miscellaneous Agents		
Cyclosporin A	Possible cause of ARDS	206
Procarbazine		210
Etoposide		211, 212
Hormonal Agents		
Tamoxifen	Possible association with pulmonary thromboembolic disease	200
Nilutamide	Interstitial pneumonitis and fibrosis	201, 204
Bicalutamide	Eosinophilic pneumonia	205
Biologic Response Modifiers		
Interleukin-2	Pulmonary edema	286
Tumor necrosis factor	Pulmonary edema or hemorrhage	296, 297
Granulocyte-macrophage colony-stimulating factor	Variable manifestations	6, 298
Interferon	Interstitial pneumonitis is the most common presentation	301, 302
Antimicrobial Agents		
Nitrofurantoin	Acute and chronic presentations are both seen	310, 312
Sulfasalazine	Usually associated with peripheral eosinophilia	340, 345
Tetracycline and minocycline	Simple pulmonary eosinophilia	352, 356
Sulfonamides	Simple pulmonary eosinophilia	365, 366
Penicillin	Simple pulmonary eosinophilia	367
Para-aminosalicylic acid	Simple pulmonary eosinophilia	368
Ethambutol	Simple pulmonary eosinophilia	369
Ampicillin	ARDS	370
Maloprim		371
Cephalosporins	Interstitial pneumonitis	372
Pyrimethamine	Noncardiogenic edema	373
Trimethoprim-sulfamethoxazole	Noncardiogenic edema	374
Amphotericin B (liposomal)	Pulmonary edema	375
Antiarrhythmic Drugs		
Amiodarone	Occurs in about 5% of users; usually, insidious onset of interstitial pneumonitis; about one third of affected patients have acute onset of symptoms	396
Lidocaine	Noncardiogenic edema	447
Tocainide	Interstitial pneumonitis and fibrosis	448, 449
Verapamil	Noncardiogenic edema with overdose	451
Procainamide	Myasthenia-like syndrome with chest wall weakness	452, 453
Sotalol	Bronchiolitis obliterans organizing pneumonia	455

Table 63–1. DRUG-INDUCED DISEASE OF THE THORAX *Continued*

DRUG	COMMENTS	SELECTED REFERENCES
Anticonvulsant Drugs		
Diphenylhydantoin	Interstitial pneumonitis with peripheral eosinophilia; lymph node enlargement sometimes seen in the absence of parenchymal lung changes	456, 461, 463
Carbamazepine	Interstitial pneumonitis with peripheral eosinophilia	480
Analgesic Drugs		
Acetylsalicylic acid	Pulmonary edema	486, 487
Mesalamine	Interstitial pneumonitis	495
Nonsteroidal Anti-Inflammatory Drugs		
Naproxen	Acute-onset air-space disease with peripheral eosinophilia	498
Sulindac	Acute-onset air-space disease with peripheral eosinophilia	501
Piroxicam	Acute-onset air-space disease with peripheral eosinophilia	502
Tolfenamic acid	Acute-onset air-space disease with peripheral eosinophilia	503
Diflunisal	Acute-onset air-space disease with peripheral eosinophilia	504
Diclofenac	Acute-onset air-space disease with peripheral eosinophilia	505
Antirheumatic Drugs		
Penicillamine	Varied presentation including lupus-like and myasthenia-like disease, diffuse alveolar hemorrhage, and obliterative bronchiolitis	510, 512, 522
Gold	Acute or subacute interstitial pneumonitis, often with skin rash; sometimes obstructive bronchiolitis	551
Sympathomimetic Drugs		
Tocolytics	Noncardiogenic edema	557, 560
Illicit Drugs, Narcotics, and Sedative Drugs		
Heroin	Noncardiogenic edema	569
Methadone	Noncardiogenic edema	568, 572
Buprenorphine	Noncardiogenic edema	573, 574
Propoxyphene	Noncardiogenic edema	575
Chlordiazepoxide	Noncardiogenic edema	576
Ethchlorvynol	Noncardiogenic edema	577
Paraldehyde	Noncardiogenic edema	578
Codeine	Noncardiogenic edema	579
Bromocarbamide	Noncardiogenic edema	580
Febarbamate	Noncardiogenic edema	581
Naloxone	Noncardiogenic edema	582, 583
Cocaine	Wide variety of manifestations, including edema, hemorrhage, and bronchiolitis obliterans organizing pneumonia	567, 608, 742
Antidepressant and Antipsychotic Drugs		
Amitriptyline	Bronchiolitis and interstitial pneumonitis	652
Clomipramine	Bronchiolitis obliterans organizing pneumonia	653
Fluoxetine	Pneumonia with eosinophilia; one case with lung nodules	654, 656
Contrast Media		
Lymphangiography	Noncardiogenic edema	659
Water-soluble contrast media—both low and high molecular weight	Noncardiogenic edema	674, 675, 669, 671
Angiotensin-Converting Enzyme Inhibitors		
Persistent cough, asthma (rare)		680, 685, 699
Miscellaneous Drugs		
Hydrochlorothiazide	Noncardiogenic edema	711
Inhaled beclomethasone	Eosinophilic pneumonia	716
Injected silicone	Acute interstitial pneumonitis	717, 718
Beta-adrenergic blockers	Varied manifestations, including lupus-like picture, acute interstitial pneumonitis, cardiogenic edema, and bronchospasm	721, 723, 724, 725
Ergotamine	Interstitial fibrosis	732
INH (isonicotinic acid hydrazide)	Interstitial pneumonitis	743
Desferrioxamine	Noncardiogenic edema	744
Diltiazem	Noncardiogenic edema with overdose	735

ARDS, adult respiratory distress syndrome.

page 1432); (3) responses due to illicit drug abuse; (4) eosinophilic lung reactions (*see* page 1751); (5) interstitial or air-space pneumonitis, which may be acute, subacute, or chronic and associated with a variable amount of fibrosis; and (6) increased permeability pulmonary edema. In this chapter, we discuss the last four categories. Other drug-induced thoracic disorders involving the pleura, the mediastinum, and the neuromuscular control of breathing are considered in the appropriate sections of the text.

Adverse drug reactions constitute one of the major diagnostic challenges in pulmonary medicine. This is especially so in the setting of the immunocompromised host, in which situation drug-induced lung disease is estimated to account for 5% to 30% of pulmonary complications.[1] Such reactions must be distinguished from the opportunistic infections and disease recurrence they mimic both clinically and radiologically.[3] In this setting and in others, the identification of a drug-related etiology for a patient's disease may be difficult because of a lack of specific clinical, functional, or radiologic findings. This difficulty is compounded in some cases because of the use of concomitant radiation or oxygen therapy, each of which has its own toxicity.

In most instances, the diagnosis is suspected because of the insidious onset of dyspnea and cough in a patient receiving a drug (or drugs) recognized as potentially damaging to the lungs. Onset with fever is common, and diffuse crackles are often audible. Drugs that initiate capillary leakage or bronchospasm tend to be associated with a more abrupt clinical presentation, and physical examination usually reveals profuse crackles or wheezes, respectively. Some patients may not have symptoms, and the presence of a drug reaction is suggested by the appearance of a diffuse reticulo-nodular pattern on the chest radiograph or by a significant reduction in diffusing capacity. Because the disease process can extend from the interstitium into the air spaces, the radiographic pattern may be mixed, or, in the case of drugs that cause noncardiogenic pulmonary edema, predominantly air space. Pulmonary dysfunction may be barely detectable or may be severe and require mechanical ventilation to maintain life; although generally restrictive in type with a low carbon monoxide diffusing capacity of the lungs (DLCO), the pattern may be mixed or even predominantly obstructive.

As with clinical and radiologic findings, histologic changes of drug-induced pulmonary disease tend to be relatively nonspecific and take four general forms: (1) alveolar interstitial inflammation, usually caused by lymphocytes, with a variable degree of fibrosis (usual interstitial pneumonia); (2) alveolar interstitial and/or air-space inflammation characterized by a large number of eosinophils and little or no fibrosis (eosinophilic pneumonia); (3) alveolar interstitial and air-space edema associated with a proteinaceous exudate, hyaline membranes, and relatively few inflammatory cells (diffuse alveolar damage); and (4) obliterative bronchiolitis with or without organizing pneumonia. Other reactions, such as granulomatous inflammation, pulmonary alveolar proteinosis, and the vascular abnormalities of veno-occlusive disease, occur rarely. None of these histologic patterns is specific; however, when one is found in association with a drug known to cause that particular reaction, the diagnosis of drug toxicity is clearly supported.

Mechanisms of drug-induced lung damage appear to be either immunologic (usually associated with a favorable

outcome) or cytotoxic (in many cases accompanied by irreparable damage and fibrosis); the latter may be by direct mechanisms, intracellular phospholipid deposition, or oxidant-related injury.[1] The toxicities of specific drugs vary; some are dose related and others not. It is likely that individual susceptibility also plays a role in the severity of a drug reaction, even with those agents known to cause cumulative, dose-related pulmonary damage.[4] In some cases, the simultaneous use of multiple drugs can make it difficult to be certain of identification of the specific agent responsible for the pulmonary disease.

CHEMOTHERAPEUTIC AND IMMUNOSUPPRESSIVE DRUGS

Bleomycin

Bleomycin is an antibiotic isolated from *Streptomyces verticillus* that has significant activity against a variety of cancers, including squamous cell carcinoma of the head and neck, cervix, and esophagus as well as germ cell tumors and Hodgkin's and non-Hodgkin's lymphomas.[5, 6] As an anticancer agent, it has the advantage of not inducing myelosuppression; unfortunately, its severe and relatively common pulmonary toxicity has limited its use.

The reported incidence of bleomycin-related lung toxicity varies from 2%[7] to more than 40%.[5, 6] This wide spectrum is related partly to variations in the prevalence of associated risk factors in the populations studied (*see* farther on) and partly to the sensitivity of the tests used for diagnosis. For example, in one study of 59 men who had testicular carcinoma and were treated with a bleomycin-containing regimen, 9 (15%) developed pulmonary symptoms considered to be the result of bleomycin toxicity, whereas 23 (39%) had significant changes on the chest radiograph.[8] In another report, bleomycin-related changes were seen on the chest radiograph in 15% of 100 patients, whereas computed tomography (CT) demonstrated changes in 38%.[9]

The spectrum of bleomycin toxicity is broad, varying from mild (asymptomatic) disease to severe interstitial pneumonitis with a mortality rate as high as 60%;[10] however, most patients develop subacute to chronic interstitial pneumonitis with fibrosis.[5] In a minority of patients, acute toxicity appears to be primarily immunologic in origin and to consist of reversible eosinophilic pneumonia;[11, 12] rarely, the drug causes pulmonary veno-occlusive disease.[13]

Pathogenesis

The observation that bleomycin produces reproducible and dose-related pulmonary fibrosis in a variety of animal species has led to the use of this agent in studies of the pathogenesis of lung fibrosis. As a result, there is considerable experimental information concerning the pathogenesis of bleomycin toxicity that may be relevant to an understanding of human disease.[9, 14–21] Animal models have demonstrated that bleomycin is concentrated predominantly in lung and skin, organs that are relatively deficient in the enzyme that inactivates the drug.[22] Once within its target cells, the drug has the ability to cleave DNA, possibly by generating oxygen radicals.[23] Theoretically, an imbalance between the production of such oxidants and the concentration of antioxidants within the alveolus could lead to epithelial damage and interstitial fibrosis.[24] In support of this hypothesis is the observation that augmentation of bleomycin toxicity is associated with oxygen administration and radiation therapy,[7, 25–29] both of which are also thought to cause toxicity by oxygen radical production. By contrast, hypoxia protects against bleomycin toxicity.[30]

A complex interaction among macrophages, lymphocytes, and fibroblasts appears to be responsible for both the initiation and the maintenance of chronic inflammation and for the fibrosis in bleomycin-induced pulmonary injury.[31] Inhibition of any part of this interaction may have an effect on the severity of the disease.[31, 32] In animal models, alveolar macrophages are affected early in the course of disease. This is manifested by the release of chemotactic, proinflammatory, and profibrotic cytokines[17, 31, 33–35a] and enhanced oxygen radical production, processes that lead to recruitment of other inflammatory cells, tissue injury, and, eventually, fibrosis.[14, 36] Factors that appear to be particularly important are the expression by alveolar macrophages and epithelial cells of monocyte chemoattractant protein-1 and macrophage inflammatory protein-1,[31] the actions of the profibrotic cytokine transforming growth factor-β,[9, 37] the loss of the capacity of regenerating epithelial cells to inhibit fibroblast proliferation,[38] the balance of pro- and anti-inflammatory prostaglandins produced in response to oxidant damage,[36] and the enhancement of collagen production by interstitial fibroblasts.[21]

The development of bleomycin-induced pulmonary disease is dose related, the overall incidence of 3% to 5% rising to 13% to 17% when the cumulative dose is more than 450 units.[5] However, disease has been reported after administration of as little as 49 units.[39] Risk is increased in older people,[40] in smokers,[22] and in patients receiving combined cytotoxic drug therapy (particularly with cyclophosphamide),[7, 41] a high concentration of inspired oxygen, or radiation therapy;[42, 43] impaired renal function may also be important.[5, 44, 45] Evidence for the enhancement of bleomycin toxicity by coadministration of granulocyte-macrophage colony-stimulating factor (GM-CSF) has been contradictory.[46, 47] The results of some studies suggest that continuous intravenous infusion of the drug is less likely to be toxic than biweekly administration;[27, 48] however, the results of other investigations make this conclusion suspect.[5]

Pathologic Characteristics

The characteristic pathologic findings in the lungs of patients and experimental animals[49] administered bleomycin consist of diffuse alveolar damage. The earliest changes appear to be related to endothelial cell damage and consist of interstitial and alveolar air-space edema, hemorrhage, and fibrin deposition.[7, 49] These histologic abnormalities may be reflected in physiologic evidence of a substantial decrease in the pulmonary capillary blood volume component (Vc) of the $DLCO_{38}$[50] and in biochemical evidence of a reduction in serum ACE.[51] The endothelial cell damage is followed by necrosis of type I pneumocytes,[7] hyperplasia of type II pneumocytes, and metaplasia (often squamous[52]) of airway and alveolar epithelium;[4, 49] in more advanced disease, collagen production within alveolar walls and air spaces results

in interstitial thickening.[49] Cytologically atypical pneumocytes that are sometimes apparent after the administration of alkylating agents (*see* page 2545) are not a common feature of the reaction.[25]

Uncommon histologic manifestations associated with bleomycin administration include bronchiolitis obliterans organizing pneumonia (BOOP), particularly with the nodular pattern of disease seen radiologically;[53, 54] eosinophilic pneumonia and pleuritis;[55] and veno-occlusive disease.[56, 57]

Radiologic Manifestations

Radiographic abnormalities usually consist of bilateral bibasilar reticular, reticulonodular, or fine nodular opacities, often showing a striking peripheral distribution.[58, 59] In one study of 20 patients with pulmonary complications associated with combination chemotherapy regimens containing bleomycin, the region of the costophrenic angles was involved in 90% of cases; in 33%, the opacities were confined to this region.[59] With more severe disease, the abnormalities may extend into the middle and upper lung zones[59] or progress to patchy or massive air-space consolidation[60] (Fig. 63–1). The radiographic abnormalities appear 6 weeks to 3 months after start of therapy[61] and may be seen before, synchronous with, or after the appearance of clinical symptoms.[28] An unusual manifestation is the development of multiple pulmonary nodules, occasionally cavitary,[62] simulating metastases; unlike the latter, they tend to disappear on drug withdrawal.[63–65]

Several groups have assessed the conventional and high-resolution computed tomography (HRCT) findings of bleomycin-induced lung disease.[66–68] In one series of 100 patients, parenchymal abnormalities were detected on conventional CT in 38% of patients and on the chest radiograph in 15%.[66] The CT findings consisted of bilateral irregular lines of attenuation or focal areas of consolidation. In patients who had mild disease, the abnormalities were pleural based and most marked in the posterior aspect of the lower lung zones; with more severe disease, the abnormalities became more diffuse throughout the lower lung zones and also involved the middle and upper lung zones[66] (Fig. 63–2). The findings on HRCT usually consist of bilateral irregular lines of attenuation, ground-glass attenuation, or focal areas of consolidation in a predominantly basal subpleural distribution.[68] Rarely, the abnormalities affect predominantly or exclusively the upper lobes or are unilateral.[66, 68] Follow-up CT scans may show complete resolution of the parenchymal abnormalities within 9 months or less after cessation of therapy. In one study, 40% of patients with mild to moderate parenchymal disease showed complete resolution on follow-up, and 60% showed no interval change;[66] persistent abnormalities were present in all patients who had severe disease, although some improvement was present in 50% of these patients.

Clinical Manifestations

Symptoms occur in both the acute hypersensitivity reaction and the more insidiously progressive diffuse interstitial disease and include fever, cough, and dyspnea on exertion;[5, 7, 25] substernal and pleuritic chest pain have also been reported.[5] In one series of 286 patients treated with continuous-

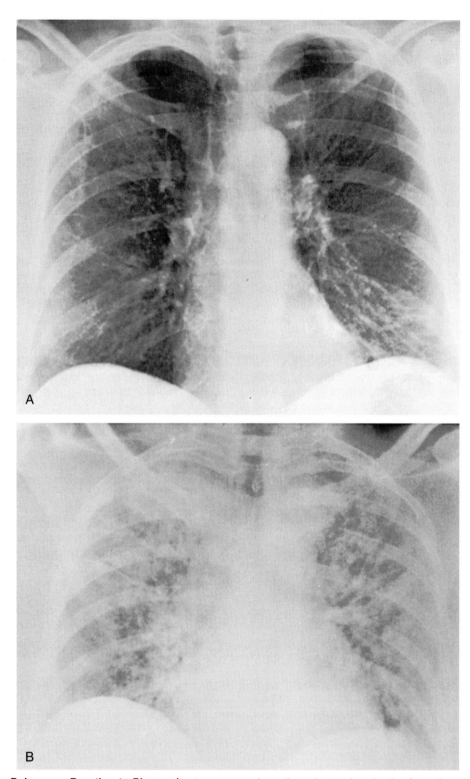

Figure 63–1. Acute Pulmonary Reaction to Bleomycin. A posteroanterior radiograph *(A)* taken shortly after a 6-week course of chemotherapy that included bleomycin, vincristine, and prednisone shows an almost normal appearance of the lungs apart from prominence of vascular markings. Five days later *(B)*, extensive disease had developed throughout both lungs, the pattern of which suggests diffuse interstitial and air-space involvement. An open-lung biopsy was performed that day from the lingula and left lower lobe. Pathologic examination showed interstitial pneumonitis. Shortly thereafter, the patient developed acute respiratory failure, from which recovery was prolonged.

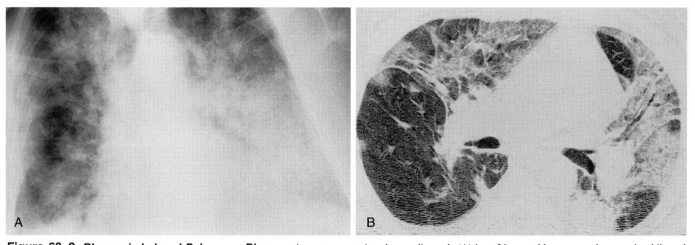

Figure 63–2. Bleomycin-Induced Pulmonary Disease. An anteroposterior chest radiograph *(A)* in a 36-year-old man reveals extensive bilateral air-space consolidation with relative sparing of the right lower lobe. HRCT *(B)* demonstrates bilateral areas of ground-glass attenuation, focal areas of consolidation, and a few linear areas of attenuation. Histologic assessment of a lung biopsy specimen demonstrated diffuse alveolar damage, focal areas of bronchiolitis obliterans organizing pneumonia–like reaction, and mild veno-occlusive disease consistent with a drug reaction.

infusion bleomycin, 8 (3%) experienced acute chest pain severe enough to lead to investigation for myocardial infarction or pulmonary embolism;[69] because there was no evidence of either of these and because several patients had clinical findings suggestive of pleuritis or pericarditis, one of the latter was considered to be the cause. Symptoms usually develop 4 to 10 weeks after treatment has finished,[5] although toxicity can occur while the drug is being given or shortly after completion of therapy.[10] Occasionally, patients are symptom free in the face of clear-cut findings of disease on radiographic, physical, or pathologic examination.[70]

Crackles may be detected, particularly at the lung bases, but may be absent even in the presence of radiologically evident disease;[70] rhonchi and wheezes have been noted occasionally. Cyanosis is a marker of serious disease.[5] The tendency for deposition of the drug in the skin can cause hyperpigmentation and swelling of the fingers, palms, and soles of the feet.

Pulmonary Function Tests

The most important clinical question with respect to bleomycin-related pulmonary function abnormalities is whether monitoring of lung function can reveal changes that predict the development of clinically important pulmonary damage. Vital capacity and diffusing capacity in particular have been used to monitor patients receiving the drug, and their measurement has been reported by some investigators to detect lung involvement at an early stage when the chest radiograph is still normal.[71, 72] A decrease in total lung capacity has also been found to predict the development of clinically evident lung toxicity.[8]

Because patients receiving bleomycin are often weakened or anemic as a result of underlying malignancy, and because progressive reduction in Vc and DLCO may be caused by these conditions alone, the results of these tests must be interpreted with caution.[73] In fact, some investigators have concluded that the DLCO is not a useful predictor of which patients will develop radiographic interstitial fibrosis.[73, 74] Vc is reduced in anemic patients, and it is necessary

to apply a correction factor before estimating diffusing capacity. After doing this, decreased Vc has been reported to reflect pulmonary endothelial damage[50] and in one study, was correlated with bleomycin toxicity.[75] Other investigators have found that maintenance of Vc in the face of a decrease in lung volumes predicts an increased risk of clinically evident toxicity.[45]

Prognosis and Natural History

In one study of 287 patients receiving bleomycin, severe lung toxicity was documented in 10 (3%);[10] 6 of these patients died, 3 early on and the others 12 to 15 months after diagnosis as a result of pulmonary fibrosis. Complete radiographic and clinical recovery can be associated with a persistent reduction in DLCO and the presence of fibrosis pathologically.[76] However, in one long-term follow-up of eight patients, previously documented pulmonary dysfunction eventually reverted to normal.[70] Some investigators have suggested that elevation of the erythrocyte sedimentation rate precedes the clinical manifestations and radiographic changes of bleomycin toxicity and that the monitoring of the erythrocyte sedimentation rate might prove useful in patient management.[77]

Mitomycin

Mitomycin is an alkylating antibiotic derived from *Streptomyces caespitosus* that is used mainly in the treatment of patients with gastrointestinal, breast, and cervical malignancies[7, 27] as well as in the therapy of non–small cell carcinoma of the lung.[78–80] It is frequently combined with vincristine or vindesine and 5-fluorouracil, drugs not generally regarded as toxic to the lungs when used as single agents.[7, 81]

More than 100 patients with mitomycin-related pulmonary toxicity have been reported.[78–80, 82–85] In four series, clinically evident toxicity was identified in 3% to 6.5% of treated patients.[79, 80, 86, 87] Although disease has been described with mitomycin alone,[88] most patients have been treated with other agents, usually the vinca alkaloids.[78, 79] Toxicity is more likely to occur at cumulative doses greater than 20 mg/m[2],[84, 89] although it has been reported after a single course of therapy.[78]

The mechanism by which mitomycin induces pulmonary damage has not been elucidated; however, because it possesses alkylating properties, its mode of action may be similar to that of cyclophosphamide and other alkylating agents. The ability of its metabolites to cross-link DNA may account, in part, for its cytotoxicity.[90] There is some evidence that oxygen (O_2) administration and radiation therapy enhance the risk of disease.[7]

Pathologic characteristics are similar to those associated with other cytotoxic drugs and include evidence of endothelial damage, necrosis of type I pneumocytes, proliferation of type II cells, and interstitial fibrosis (diffuse alveolar damage).[87] One group of investigators has described a syndrome consisting of noncardiogenic pulmonary edema, microangiopathic hemolytic anemia, and renal failure, accompanied by immunofluorescent evidence of vascular damage and fibrinogen-fibrin deposits.[92] Other reported vascular abnormalities include veno-occlusive disease[93] and capillary angiomatoid malformations.[94] BOOP has been described occasionally.[95]

The radiologic manifestations of mitomycin-induced pulmonary damage have been described in a small number of patients.[87, 88, 96] In one prospective study of 133 patients, 7 (5%) developed severe pulmonary toxicity.[96] The radiographic findings consist of bilateral reticular interstitial infiltrates that may be diffuse but tend to have a lower lung zone predominance.[87, 88, 96] Rarely, the radiographic and HRCT findings are those of adult respiratory distress syndrome (ARDS), with extensive bilateral areas of consolidation involving mainly the posterior aspects of the lungs[68, 96] (Fig. 63–3). Pleural effusion has been described in a number of patients and appears to be a more common feature of mitomycin toxicity than of other cytotoxic drug reactions.[88, 96]

Most affected patients have a clinical picture consistent with interstitial pneumonitis and fibrosis identical to that of

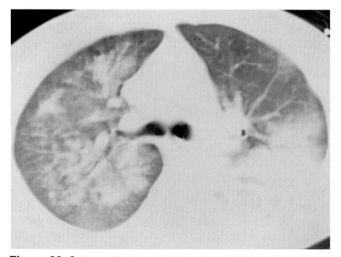

Figure 63–3. Acute Pulmonary Reaction to Mitomycin. A conventional CT scan in a 46-year-old woman demonstrates bilateral areas of consolidation involving mainly the posterior lung regions. The patient developed the disease after mitomycin treatment. The diagnosis of adult respiratory distress syndrome was confirmed at autopsy.

other cytotoxic agents.[78] The complication is usually suspected when the patient develops a dry cough and progressive dyspnea, symptoms that may subside with cessation of therapy.[87] Most patients remain afebrile.[7, 87] Physical examination may reveal bibasilar crackles.[78] Two additional rare but important effects have been described: (1) acute, severe asthma following the administration of a vinca alkaloid;[83] and (2) noncardiogenic pulmonary edema in the context of hemolytic-uremic syndrome induced by mitomycin. The latter complication may occur as long as 6 to 12 months after the initiation of therapy and may be precipitated by concomitant blood transfusion or therapy with 5-fluorouracil,[3] in which case the onset of dyspnea is abrupt. Diffuse alveolar hemorrhage has also been described in two patients who had mitomycin-induced hemolytic-uremic syndrome.[82]

Pulmonary function tests have been reported to show a restrictive defect and decreased DLCO.[7] In one prospective study of 40 patients receiving the drug, a greater than 20% decrease in DLCO was noted in 11 (28%);[80] although severe toxicity developed in 7 patients, this did not correlate with deterioration in the diffusing capacity.

The mortality rate exceeds 90% when mitomycin toxicity is associated with hemolytic-uremic syndrome and pulmonary edema; when edema is not present, about half of affected patients die.[3] Although initial improvement is the rule in patients who have interstitial pneumonitis and fibrosis and who are treated with systemic corticosteroids, about 40% develop progressive lung impairment despite continuation of therapy.[85]

Other Cytotoxic Antibiotics

In one report of 113 patients receiving *peplomycin*, a derivative of bleomycin, definite pulmonary toxicity was documented in 7 (6%);[97] 6 of the 7 died of pulmonary fibrosis despite prednisone therapy. Clinical, radiographic, and pathologic manifestations were identical to those of bleomycin toxicity. Two patients have been reported who developed histologic changes suggestive of veno-occlusive disease after receiving *neocarzinostatin*.[98, 99] Interstitial fibrosis and thrombocytopenia with pulmonary hemorrhage have also been reported in association with this agent.[6]

Busulfan

The chemotherapeutic agent busulfan was the first drug to be incriminated as a cause of diffuse interstitial fibrosis.[101, 102] It is used in the treatment of myeloproliferative disorders, particularly chronic myelogenous leukemia, and in preparation for autologous or allogenic bone marrow transplantation in patients with both hematologic and nonhematologic malignancies.[102–106] Although clinically recognized pulmonary toxicity occurs in only about 5% of patients,[3] some pathologic studies have found evidence of drug-induced damage in almost 50% of cases.[107] Patients who are treated with a conditioning regime of busulfan and cyclophosphamide before bone marrow transplantation have been found to have a 10% decline in pulmonary function, largely unassociated with clinical manifestations;[106] the abnormalities are generally reversible with time. The mechanism of damage is unknown, but the primary target appears to be epithelial cells.[7]

Clinically apparent pulmonary toxicity tends to occur only with long-term use, ranging from 8 months to 10 years in several studies (average, 3 to 4 years).[100, 101, 108, 109] Prior use of other cytotoxic drugs or radiation therapy increases the risk.[110] Although toxicity does not appear to be directly dose dependent, no patient receiving a total dose of less than 500 mg has developed pulmonary disease in the absence of other potentially toxic influences, such as radiation therapy or administration of other chemotherapeutic agents.[7, 108]

Patients receiving busulfan as part of a conditioning program before bone marrow transplantation may develop particularly serious and sometimes fatal lung disease, including pneumonitis, fibrosis, or hemorrhage.[102, 104, 105] However, the precise contribution of busulfan to toxicity in these patients is difficult to determine because it could just as easily be due to other chemotherapeutic drugs, such as etoposide or cyclophosphamide, to synergistic effects of all the agents used, or to associated radiation therapy.

The pathologic finding most characteristic of busulfan-induced pulmonary disease is the presence of large, cytologically atypical mononuclear cells[107, 111, 112] (Fig. 63–4) that have been identified on electron microscopy as altered type II pneumocytes.[113] Although similar atypical pneumocytes are also found in pulmonary disease induced by other drugs, the extent and severity of atypia are particularly common with busulfan. The finding of cytologic atypia in tissues other than the lung (such as the pancreas)[114] suggests that the abnormality is not the result of a reparative or inflammatory process but is rather a direct effect of the drug.

Other pathologic manifestations include an increase in fibroblasts associated with collagen deposition in both interstitium and air spaces, an infiltration of mononuclear cells, and (in the early stage) edema and hyaline membrane formation[107, 114] (*see* Fig. 63–4). Interstitial calcification is occasionally seen in association with pulmonary fibrosis;[100, 112] dendriform pulmonary ossification has been reported in one case.[115] Some patients with chronic myelogenous leukemia undergoing treatment with busulfan have developed pulmonary alveolar proteinosis,[1, 116, 117] an association more likely due to the relationship between the two diseases than to the drug (*see* page 2701).

The chest radiograph usually shows a bilateral reticular or reticulonodular pattern, which may be diffuse or have a lower lung zone predominance[7] (Fig. 63–5). Less common radiographic and HRCT findings include patchy or widespread bilateral air-space consolidation[7, 68] (Fig. 63–6). Pleural effusion has been reported occasionally.[118]

The onset of disease is usually insidious, and the major complaints are dry cough, fever, weakness, weight loss, and dyspnea.[100, 119] Many patients eventually become severely disabled by shortness of breath.[120] By removing an inhibitor of tyrosinase, busulfan accelerates the formation of melanin from tyrosine and thus results in hyperpigmentation of the skin; as a result, some patients have an appearance that resembles that of Addison's disease.[119] Once disease has become evident, lung volumes and diffusing capacity are usually reduced.[109, 111, 112, 121] There are no convincing data supporting the prospective use of pulmonary function tests in following patients on long-term busulfan therapy.[78]

The diagnosis of busulfan-induced pulmonary disease may be suggested by the finding of the atypical pneumocytes in expectorated or lavaged material;[26] however, as with other drugs, lung biopsy may be required to exclude other causes of the radiographic or clinical abnormalities. The prognosis is poor:[4, 25] the mean survival time after diagnosis of pulmonary fibrosis is 5 months,[108, 120, 122] and the mortality rate is estimated at greater than 80%.[123] The prognosis may be improved by early detection of disease and cessation of drug therapy.[78]

Cyclophosphamide

The alkylating drug cyclophosphamide is used widely in the treatment of malignancies and autoimmune connective tissue disease. Because it is often combined with other chemotherapeutic agents, it may not be apparent which agent is responsible for pulmonary disease or whether the toxicity is the result of a synergistic effect.[25, 124] Nevertheless, there are well-documented cases of pulmonary fibrosis following the use of cyclophosphamide as a single agent.[7, 125, 126] In addition, the results of both animal and *in vitro* experiments indicate that the drug is toxic by itself.[78, 127–129] A single case of interstitial pneumonitis has been reported following therapy with *ifosfamide*, a structural isomer of cyclophosphamide.[130]

The incidence of cyclophosphamide pulmonary toxicity is generally considered very low, probably less than 1%;[7] however, some authorities consider it likely that both the incidence and the severity of toxicity have been underestimated.[1, 3] The development of interstitial fibrosis has been reported after administration of as little as 150 mg of the drug,[108] although the risk of serious toxicity appears to be greater with higher doses.[7, 25] Unlike bleomycin, there appears to be no association between risk of toxicity and age.[3] Studies in humans[7] and animals[131] suggest that the risk of pulmonary damage is increased when cyclophosphamide is combined with oxygen; in addition, high-dose cyclophosphamide appears to sensitize the lung to radiation damage.[132]

Pathologic findings are usually similar to those of busulfan toxicity and consist of diffuse alveolar damage associated with the presence of cytologically atypical alveolar epithelial cells.[25, 133] Chronic interstitial pneumonitis and fibrosis[134, 135] and BOOP[136] have been reported in occasional cases.

The chest radiograph usually demonstrates a bilateral basilar reticular pattern, occasionally associated with focal areas of consolidation[7] (Fig. 63–7). In one review of five patients, pleural thickening accompanied the interstitial changes in all.[126] We have seen one patient who had ground-glass opacities on the radiograph and HRCT scan; a lung biopsy showed histologic features of extrinsic allergic alveolitis[68] (Fig. 63–8). In another patient who developed the abrupt onset of dyspnea, the radiograph revealed extensive bilateral air-space pulmonary edema.[137]

The onset of pulmonary disease is acute or subacute more often than chronic. The time interval between initiation of therapy and development of symptoms varies markedly:[25, 138] in some patients, symptoms develop within months,[138] whereas in others, they become apparent after years.[139] In one patient who had been receiving 50 to 100 mg of the drug daily, biopsy-proved interstitial fibrosis was

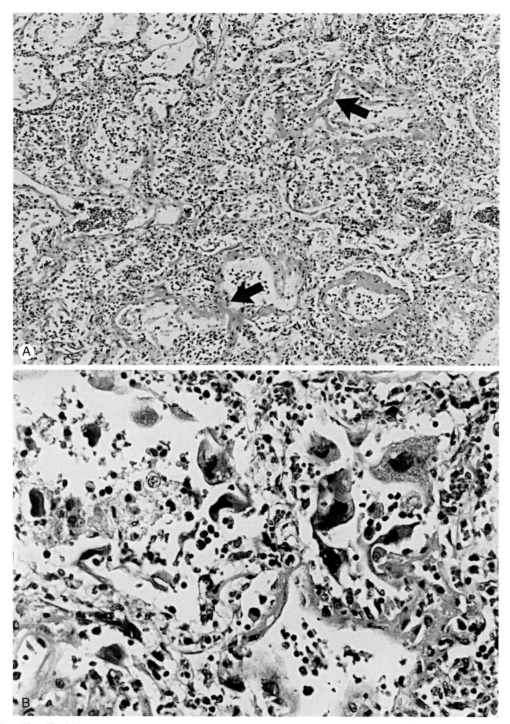

Figure 63–4. Busulfan Toxicity. A section of lung parenchyma *(A)* obtained at autopsy shows a moderate degree of interstitial thickening by lymphocytes, extensive air-space filling by macrophages and other mononuclear inflamatory cells, and multifocal hyaline membranes *(arrows)*. A magnified view of three alveoli *(B)* shows type II pneumocytes to be greatly increased in size and to contain hyperchromatic, cytologically atypical nuclei. The patient had been taking busulfan for therapy of acute myelogenous leukemia. *(A* ×80; *B* ×275.)

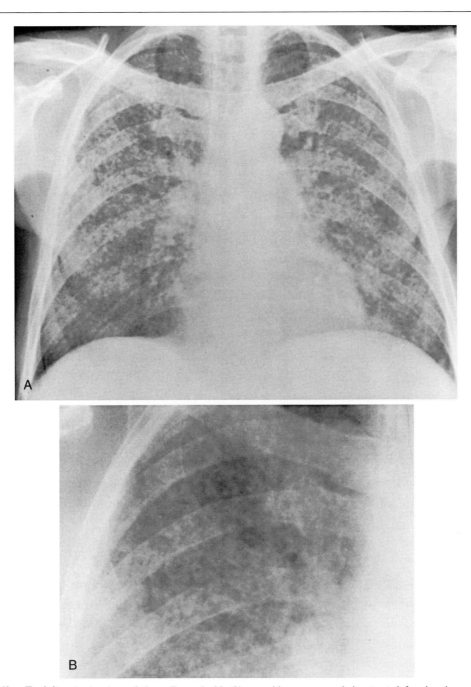

Figure 63–5. Busulfan Toxicity. At the time of the radiograph this 61-year-old woman was being treated for chronic myeloid leukemia and was complaining of severe exertional dyspnea. The posteroanterior radiograph *(A)* and magnified view of the right upper zone *(B)* reveal a widespread, coarse reticulonodular pattern throughout both lungs without anatomic predominance. The patient died about 1 year later; at autopsy, there was generalized alveolar interstitial fibrosis with preservation of lung architecture.

detected after 13 years.[140] Cough and dyspnea are the major complaints; fever occurs in more than 50% of patients.[25, 133, 141] Pulmonary function tests show a restrictive ventilatory defect and a reduced diffusing capacity.[25, 141]

The prognosis depends on how early toxicity is recognized and (perhaps) on whether corticosteroid therapy has been instituted; about 60% of patients recover.[25] There is evidence that patients who receive prednisone along with cyclophosphamide are protected from developing toxicity.[25] Cessation of cyclophosphamide therapy can be followed by resolution of the pulmonary disease,[141] especially when it is of early onset.[126]

Chlorambucil

The alkylating agent chlorambucil is used chiefly in the treatment of hematologic malignancies. It is a rare cause of pulmonary toxicity; less than 20 cases had been reported by 1996.[7, 142–145] Most patients have received more than 2.5 mg[146, 147] before toxicity is apparent.[6] There appears to be no synergistic effect with other oxidants.

Pathologic findings have been reported rarely but appear to consist of interstitial pneumonitis and fibrosis.[147, 148] The chest radiograph reveals a bilateral, predominantly bibasilar, reticular pattern,[7] on occasion said to be coarse.[147]

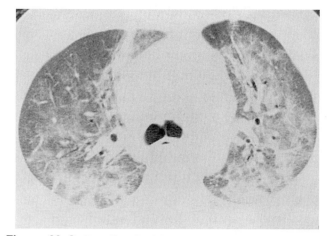

Figure 63–6. Busulfan Toxicity. HRCT in a 42-year-old man who had shortness of breath demonstrates extensive bilateral areas of ground-glass attenuation, focal areas of consolidation, and a few linear opacities. The diagnosis of busulfan pulmonary toxicity was based on the clinical and radiologic features. The clinical and radiographic findings improved rapidly after discontinuation of the drug.

In one patient, the interstitial disease was confined to the upper lobes.[149]

Onset of clinical symptoms generally ranges from 6 months to 3 years after the beginning of therapy[7] and may occur months to years after its cessation.[40] Symptoms tend to be subacute and include anorexia, weight loss, fatigue, fever, cough, and dyspnea.[147] One patient has been reported in whom recurrent attacks of respiratory distress developed 9 to 12 days after each treatment despite a normal chest radiograph.[150] Finger clubbing[149] and crackles[147] have been found on physical examination. Pulmonary function tests show a restrictive pattern and a decrease in DLco.[147, 148]

Chlorambucil pulmonary toxicity appears to be a serious complication; 5 of the 10 patients reported by 1986 died.[7] However, cessation of drug therapy and administration of steroids can result in resolution of disease.[147]

Melphalan

Melphalan is a phenylalanine derivative of nitrogen mustard used chiefly in the treatment of multiple myeloma. The incidence of clinically evident pulmonary toxicity is low, only eight cases having been reported by 1993.[7, 151, 152] Despite this, histologic abnormalities were identified in 5 of 10 patients exposed to the drug in one retrospective autopsy study.[153]

The pathologic appearance varies in reported cases, some showing interstitial pneumonitis and fibrosis associated with alveolar epithelial atypia[154, 155] and others demonstrating organizing diffuse alveolar damage.[156] The chest radiograph has been reported to show reticular[7] or predominantly nodular patterns.[157] Pleural effusion has been identified occasionally.[151]

Symptoms and signs tend to appear within 1 to 4 months of the initiation of therapy[7] and are identical to those associated with chlorambucil toxicity.[154] Pleuritic chest pain and pleural effusions have been reported in some cases.[6] Pulmonary function tests show a restrictive pattern and a

decrease in DLco.[154] Five of the eight reported patients died of respiratory failure;[7, 152] one of the other patients showed clearing of the radiographic abnormalities but persistence of symptoms and reduced diffusing capacity.[154]

Nitrosoureas

Nitrosoureas are used chiefly in the treatment of intracranial neoplasms, melanoma, breast and gastrointestinal carcinoma, and lymphoma.[7, 27, 158, 159] Following their increased use in the late 1960s and early 1970s, the number of reported cases of pulmonary damage increased. In a 1992 review from France, the number of reported cases was estimated to be about 70;[160] other patients have been described since then.[161–164] Most of these cases have been caused by BCNU (*carmustine* [1,3-bis (2-chloroethyl)-1-nitrosourea]); other nitrosoureas, such as *lomustine* (CCNU)[78, 165, 166] and *semustine* (methyl CCNU),[167] have been implicated rarely.

The pharmacologic action of the nitrosoureas is similar to that of other alkylating agents and consists of interference with DNA synthesis and impedance of DNA repair.[168] The propensity of the drug to reduce glutathione synthesis, an important antioxidant defense, may lead to oxidant-induced lung injury, particularly when combined with other agents that impair oxidant defense, such as cyclophosphamide.[169] Analysis of bronchiolar lavage (BAL) fluid in one patient with acute severe interstitial pneumonitis revealed a lymphocytosis, suggesting that immunologic reactions may also be important in some patients.[161]

Although many of the reported cases of pulmonary toxicity caused by BCNU have occurred in patients receiving this drug alone, some have developed in combination with other cytotoxic agents, particularly cyclophosphamide and cisplatinum.[158, 169, 170, 185] In this circumstance, the incidence of toxicity can be substantial; for example, in one series of 39 patients treated with cyclophosphamide and BCNU as part of an aggressive breast cancer treatment protocol before autologous bone marrow transplantation, 23 (39%) developed evidence of lung toxicity.[169] Because the dose of BCNU in these cases was lower than that generally recognized as producing interstitial fibrosis, a synergistic effect has been suggested.[4, 171] This synergism may depend in part on the pharmacokinetics of the administration of the BCNU;[170] studies in a rat model suggest that the prior administration of cyclophosphamide and cisplatinum prolongs the elimination of the drug.[158] The rate of drug administration also may be important: in one study of toxicity in a cyclophosphamide, cisplatinum, and BCNU regimen, more rapid infusion of the BCNU was associated with a syndrome of acute lung injury in 12 of 14 (86%) patients.[170]

The incidence of pulmonary toxicity following BCNU therapy as a single agent ranges from 1% to 20% in different series;[4, 171–174] by contrast, the incidence is as high as 40% to 60% of patients treated with high-dose combination chemotherapy protocols before autologous bone marrow transplantation.[158, 185] This large range reflects the total dose administered and the length of survival from the primary disease—the larger the dose and the longer the survival, the greater chance of a patient's developing pulmonary damage. An increased risk associated with a total dose of 1 gm or more has been well documented;[4, 175] for example, in a series

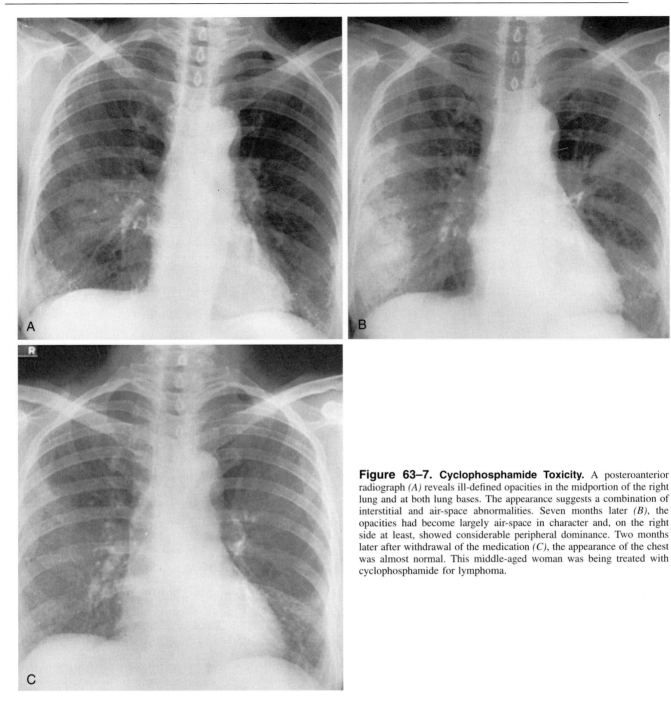

Figure 63–7. Cyclophosphamide Toxicity. A posteroanterior radiograph *(A)* reveals ill-defined opacities in the midportion of the right lung and at both lung bases. The appearance suggests a combination of interstitial and air-space abnormalities. Seven months later *(B)*, the opacities had become largely air-space in character and, on the right side at least, showed considerable peripheral dominance. Two months later after withdrawal of the medication *(C)*, the appearance of the chest was almost normal. This middle-aged woman was being treated with cyclophosphamide for lymphoma.

of 93 patients being treated for glioma, 50% of those who received 1.5 gm or more developed interstitial fibrosis.[174] In another study in which BCNU was the only chemotherapeutic agent employed in the treatment of 318 patients with glioma,[176] no clinical evidence of pulmonary damage was identified in patients who received a total dose of less than 900 mg/m²; by contrast, 10 of 107 patients who received more than this dose developed detectable pulmonary toxicity.

Several other factors may also increase the risk of BCNU pulmonary toxicity. For example, there is evidence that treatment at a young age favors the development of severe fibrosis at a later date; in one review, all five patients treated before the age of 5 years with BCNU had died of lung fibrosis, whereas nine long-term survivors received

treatment at a median age of 10 years.[163] Radiation may also be a factor; in one series, four patients who developed pulmonary toxicity from BCNU therapy had received prior mediastinal irradiation.[171] Another report of one patient documented "recall pneumonitis" in the radiation port when BCNU was administered after radiation therapy.[177] Finally, some investigators have suggested that underlying lung disease associated with abnormal lung function also serves as a risk factor for BCNU toxicity.[174]

Pathologic findings are similar to those of other forms of cytotoxic pulmonary damage:[7] interstitial pneumonitis and fibrosis with atypia of alveolar type II cells,[178] and exudative or organizing diffuse alveolar damage.[179] Pulmonary veno-occlusive disease has also been described in two patients

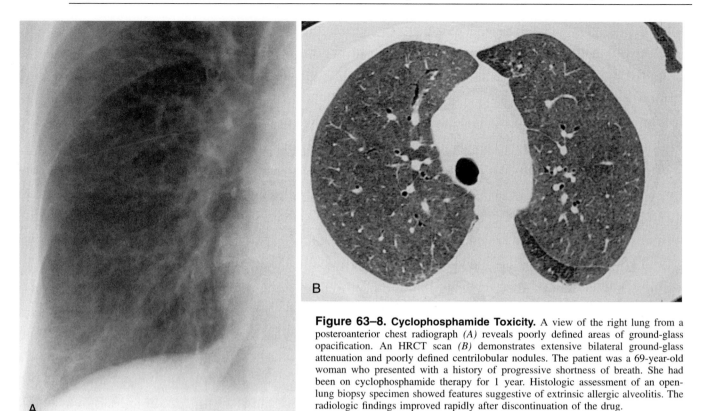

Figure 63–8. Cyclophosphamide Toxicity. A view of the right lung from a posteroanterior chest radiograph *(A)* reveals poorly defined areas of ground-glass opacification. An HRCT scan *(B)* demonstrates extensive bilateral ground-glass attenuation and poorly defined centrilobular nodules. The patient was a 69-year-old woman who presented with a history of progressive shortness of breath. She had been on cyclophosphamide therapy for 1 year. Histologic assessment of an open-lung biopsy specimen showed features suggestive of extrinsic allergic alveolitis. The radiologic findings improved rapidly after discontinuation of the drug.

who received the drug as a single agent for the treatment of glioma[180] and in three patients who received it with bleomycin as part of combination chemotherapy for other malignancies.[13, 181] Autopsy examination of one patient with late-onset disease showed alveolar air-space fibrosis and accentuated alveolar septal elastic tissue, particularly in the lung apices.[182]

The chest radiograph becomes abnormal late in the course of pulmonary toxicity, typically after the onset of symptoms.[183] Radiographic manifestations consist most commonly of a bibasilar reticular pattern.[183] Less common findings include focal or patchy bilateral areas of consolidation, upper lobe reticular opacities, or pneumothorax.[183, 184] The radiograph may be normal even in the presence of histologically proven pulmonary fibrosis,[172, 186] a feature that appears to be more common with nitrosoureas than with other cytotoxic agents.[7]

The findings on HRCT have been described in a small number of cases and consist of bilateral areas of ground-glass attenuation involving the lower lung zones[68, 187] (Fig. 63–9). Although the early radiographic and CT abnormalities tend to involve mainly the lower lung zones, in six patients with long-term follow-up (mean, 14 years), there was predominantly upper lobe fibrosis.[188, 189] The radiographic and CT findings consisted of irregular linear opacities involving mainly the subpleural lung regions and associated with elevation of the hila.[189] Gallium scans in these patients were normal.[188]

Clinical evidence of pulmonary damage usually appears from 1 month to 1 year after the institution of therapy;[4] however, fibrosis has been first identified as long as 17 years

after childhood therapy of brain tumors.[163, 188] Symptoms include dry cough, fatigue, and dyspnea.[168, 175, 179] The D_{LCO}, Pa_{O_2}, and V_C are reduced.[4, 7, 27, 163] The course of the disease is usually insidious over a period of months,[7] although it can be rapidly progressive and fatal.[191, 192] In one study of 17 patients who had pulmonary fibrosis that developed late after childhood therapy with BCNU, 8 had died;[163] the survivors continued to show deteriorating lung function. In a second investigation of 26 patients who had received BCNU for the treatment of relapsing Hodgkin's disease and who developed an "idiopathic pneumonia syndrome" within 1 year of administration of therapy, 14 had a complete recovery, 3 had persisting symptoms after 6 months of observation, and 9 died.[159] All patients who died had the first symptoms within 6 months of therapy, and all had received more than 475 mg/m^2 of BCNU; the risk was greater in women than in men.

Vinca Alkaloids

The vinca alkaloids *vinblastine* and *vindesine* are almost invariably used with other drugs, particularly mitomycin, a combination that has been reported to cause interstitial fibrosis[79, 193] and diffuse alveolar damage.[194] Whether the toxicity is caused by the vinca alkaloid, the mitomycin, or the combination of the two is difficult to determine. However, in a series of 387 patients treated with this regimen,[79] 25 developed acute dyspnea while being administered the vinca alkaloid; 22 of the 25 (88%) had new focal or diffuse interstitial infiltrates and impairment in gas exchange. Al-

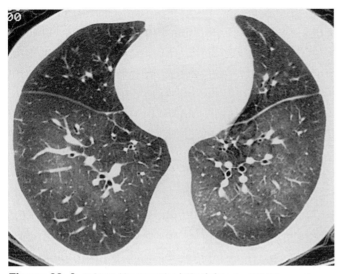

Figure 63–9. BCNU (Carmustine) Toxicity. An HRCT scan demonstrates bilateral areas of ground-glass attenuation in the lower lobes. The patient was a 28-year-old woman who had received BCNU as part of combination chemotherapy before bone marrow transplantation.

though substantial improvement occurred over 24 hours, 15 patients were left with chronic respiratory impairment.

Two patients were reported to have developed fatal pulmonary edema while receiving vinblastine and mitomycin;[193] however, it is likely that the toxicity was caused by the latter drug. A case has also been reported of a patient with acute basophilic leukemia treated with vincristine who developed an anaphylactoid reaction associated with disseminated intravascular coagulopathy and diffuse alveolar hemorrhage.[195] Vindesine and vinblastine appear to be capable of inducing bronchospasm;[6, 196] in one patient, this was associated with objective evidence of obstruction on pulmonary function testing.[196] Vindesine also may play a role in the development of progressive interstitial fibrosis when combined with radiation therapy.[197, 198] Interstitial lung disease has also developed rarely in patients treated with *vinorelbine*.[199]

Hormonal Agents

The administration of *tamoxifen*, an antiestrogen used in the treatment of breast cancer, has been associated with the development of thrombotic events in 1%[6] to 4.3%[200] of treated patients. However, most of these patients had other risk factors for the development of venous thrombosis and pulmonary thromboembolism,[200] and it is not clear whether tamoxifen conferred an additional risk of these complications.

Nilutamide, a specific synthetic antiandrogen used in the therapy of metastatic prostatic carcinoma,[201] has been associated with the development of interstitial pneumonitis[201–203] and fibrosis[204] in some patients. Recovery has been associated with drug withdrawal or dose reduction and with corticosteroid therapy.[201] In one patient, a hypersensitivity reaction was likely because BAL fluid analysis revealed a lymphocytic alveolitis, and rechallenge with the drug after initial recovery led to recurrence of disease.[202] *Bicalutamide*,

another antiandrogen agent used in the treatment of prostate cancer, was associated with an eosinophilic lung reaction in one patient.[205]

Miscellaneous Chemotherapeutic and Immunosuppressive Drugs

In one series of 29 patients receiving *cyclosporin A* to prevent graft-versus-host disease after bone marrow transplantation for leukemia and aplastic anemia, 5 patients developed ARDS 8 to 18 days after the initiation of therapy;[206] however, whether this was truly an effect of the drug or was simply a complication of transplantation is unclear. A prospective study of 21 patients treated with cyclosporine after renal transplantation failed to show any effect of therapy on lung function in the year after transplantation.[207]

The use of *procarbazine* has been associated with an acute allergic reaction characterized by eosinophilia, urticaria, abnormal liver function, and arthralgia.[208–210] In one series of eight patients with this syndrome, five developed pulmonary manifestations (three, interstitial pneumonitis and two, cough).[210]

Etoposide, a podophyllin derivative, is a cytotoxic agent that has activity against small cell cancer of the lung. Two patients have been described with drug-induced pneumonitis characterized by fever and diffuse interstitial disease;[211, 212] one died.

ANTIMETABOLIC DRUGS

Methotrexate

Methotrexate is employed in the treatment of malignancy and, in lower doses, in a variety of nonmalignant diseases, including psoriasis, pemphigus, asthma, primary biliary cirrhosis, and rheumatoid arthritis.[213–218] Use of the drug has been associated with pulmonary toxicity following oral, intravenous, or intrathecal administration. In contrast to other cytotoxic agents, methotrexate usually causes pulmonary disease that is reversible, apparently as a result of a hypersensitivity reaction (*see* farther on);[213, 219, 220] however, chronic interstitial fibrosis develops in some patients.[221] The latter complication can be difficult to diagnose in cases in which the condition being treated is itself associated with interstitial fibrosis (e.g., rheumatoid disease). Bronchitis has also been attributed to methotrexate therapy in some patients.[222]

According to published reports, methotrexate pneumonitis is uncommon: in 1994, it was estimated that only 60 to 65 cases had been reported since the condition was first described 25 years previously.[213, 223, 224] In a retrospective cohort and literature review in 1997, only 37 cases were considered to satisfy criteria for definite methotrexate-induced lung injury.[91] Despite these figures, it has been estimated that the incidence of disease in patients receiving low-dose methotrexate for rheumatoid arthritis is about 2% to 5%;[213, 225, 226] given the widespread use of such therapy, this constitutes a potentially serious health concern. In addition, there is evidence that when lung toxicity is defined by clinical events, the incidence of methotrexate lung injury may be substantial; in one study, 20% of patients treated with methotrexate for trophoblastic tumors developed transient symptoms.[227]

Pathogenesis

The pathogenesis of methotrexate lung toxicity is not clear. The drug is a folic acid analogue that inhibits cellular reproduction by causing an acute intracellular deficiency of folate coenzymes.[7] However, it is unlikely that this action is related to lung damage because leucovorin rescue does not appear to protect against toxicity.[213] Instead, there is evidence suggesting that a hypersensitivity reaction is the underlying pathogenetic mechanism. This evidence includes the finding of peripheral eosinophilia and granulomatous inflammation or eosinophil infiltration of lung tissue in some cases; the observation that pneumonitis is associated with a lymphocytic alveolitis in BAL fluid, with helper lymphocytes being predominant;[219, 228] the onset of disease shortly after initiation of therapy; clinical features of accompanying chills and fever;[3] and *in vitro* experiments in which peripheral lymphocytes from patients with methotrexate pneumonitis have been shown to elaborate leukocyte inhibitory factor.[229] Despite this evidence, the failure of some patients to experience recurrent pneumonitis after rechallenge with the drug argues against a hypersensitivity reaction.[1, 78]

The frequency of dosage and duration of therapy appear to be important risk factors.[4, 7] There is also some evidence that pre-existing lung disease increases the risk of a toxic reaction;[214, 230] in one investigation, 5 of 24 patients (20%) who had abnormal pretreatment chest radiographs developed interstitial pneumonitis during the course of therapy, compared with only 4 of 77 (5%) who did not have evidence of pre-existing lung pathology.[230] Risk factors for the development of pulmonary injury in patients receiving low-dose methotrexate for rheumatoid arthritis were evaluated in a case-control study that included 29 patients who had the complication.[231] Previous use of disease-modifying antirheumatic drugs and hypoalbuminemia were associated with very large attributable risks; older age, diabetes, and rheumatoid pleuropulmonary disease before the institution of methotrexate were also predictive of the complication.[231]

Pathologic Characteristics

Because interstitial pneumonitis is rapidly reversible in many patients receiving low-dose methotrexate therapy, histologic examination of affected tissue is uncommon. Interstitial pneumonitis and fibrosis, sometimes associated with granuloma formation resembling extrinsic allergic alveolitis, are the most frequent abnormalities.[232–234] Diffuse alveolar damage has been seen occasionally,[235] sometimes in patients who have received methotrexate intrathecally.[236] BOOP has been documented rarely.[237] Acute pleuritis with pleural effusion or basilar atelectasis has also been described in some patients treated with high doses.[6, 78]

Radiologic Manifestations

The radiographic changes are fairly characteristic and should suggest consideration of the diagnosis in the proper clinical setting. Initially, the chest radiograph reveals a basal or diffuse reticular or ground-glass pattern[223, 238] (Fig. 63–10). This progresses rapidly to patchy air-space consolidation (Fig. 63–11) that in time, reverts once again to an interstitial pattern followed by complete resolution.[223, 232, 239] Multiple nodules[233] and, in at least two patients, hilar lymph node enlargement have also been reported.[233, 240] Radiographically demonstrable disease may be present for periods ranging from a few days[241] to 1 year or longer.[223] The HRCT findings described in one patient consisted of bilateral areas of ground-glass attenuation.[68]

Clinical Manifestations

The duration of maintenance methotrexate therapy before symptoms and signs of toxicity become clinically apparent generally ranges from days to several years after initiation of therapy;[3, 25, 242] sometimes—as in one patient taking the medication for 18 years[243]—it is much longer. Onset after completion of therapy is unusual; however, toxicity has occasionally developed several weeks after drug cessation.[244]

In most cases, the onset is acute to subacute and is characterized by fever, cough, dyspnea, and headache;[91, 245, 246] pleuritic pain is unusual[213, 247] but well described.[227] A single case of asthma has been reported.[248] Tachypnea, crackles, and cyanosis are common findings on physical examination.[213] Digital clubbing has also been described,[243] and skin eruptions have been noted in about 15% of cases.[233] Liver disease, including cirrhosis, is a well-recognized complication of prolonged therapy.[240, 249–252] A moderate blood eosinophilia is common,[233, 242, 253] having been estimated to occur in about 40%[7] to 65%[26] of cases.

Pulmonary function tests show a restrictive pattern.[7] A very low PaO_2 may be apparent.[254] In one investigation of a cohort of patients with rheumatoid arthritis who were treated with weekly methotrexate and followed prospectively with serial measurements of lung function, the total dose of methotrexate was correlated over time with an increase in residual volume.[255] This finding was valid after controlling for age, sex, height, number of years of follow-up, prednisone use, and smoking history. No other evidence of lung toxicity was apparent in these patients, and the clinical significance of the functional abnormality is obscure. Monitoring lung function has not been found to permit early detection of lung injury before the onset of clinical symptoms.[256]

Despite hopes to the contrary, it has become apparent that low-dose methotrexate therapy is immunosuppressive and predisposes to a variety of opportunistic infections.[213] For example, patients with rheumatoid arthritis treated with methotrexate have developed *Pneumocystis carinii* pneumonia,[257–260] invasive pulmonary aspergillosis,[261] and pulmonary cryptococcosis.[262] A single case of lymphoma, which remitted after cessation of methotrexate, has also been reported.[260] Because there are no pathognomonic clinical, radiologic, or laboratory features that allow such infections to be distinguished from methotrexate pneumonitis, a thorough search for potential organisms must be made when drug toxicity is suspected, in some cases including biopsy, BAL, or both.

As indicated previously, the prognosis of methotrexate pneumonitis is usually favorable; most patients recover, although there is an overall estimated mortality rate of 1% to 10%.[78, 108, 233] Most patients on low-dose maintenance therapy experience rapid clearing of symptoms and radiographic

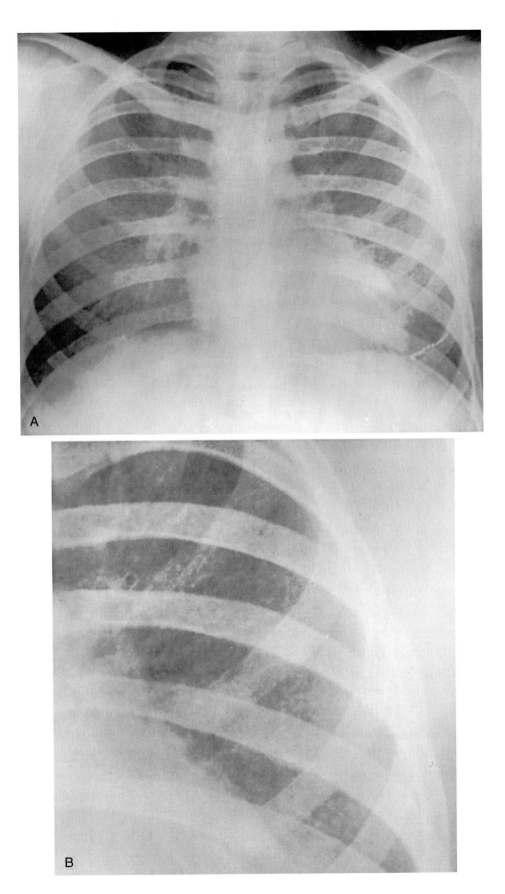

Figure 63–10. Methotrexate Toxicity.
A posteroanterior radiograph *(A)* and a magnified view of the left upper zone *(B)* reveal a diffuse ground-glass pattern. Lung volume is reduced. This middle-aged man complained of mild dyspnea on effort. He was receiving methotrexate therapy for psoriasis.

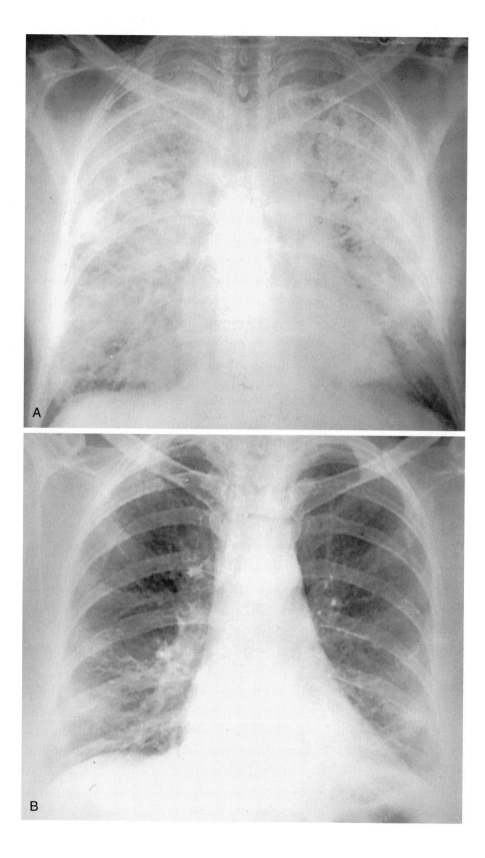

Figure 63–11. Methotrexate Toxicity. A posteroanterior radiograph *(A)* reveals massive bilateral air-space consolidation containing a well-defined air bronchogram. The heart size is within normal limits. This appearance is highly suggestive of permeability pulmonary edema. Almost 2 weeks later, after cessation of methotrexate therapy for rheumatoid arthritis *(B)*, the consolidation had cleared almost completely.

abnormality after withdrawal of the medication.[1, 225, 254, 263–265] Cases have also been reported in which clearing has occurred despite continuation or reinstitution of therapy.[108, 233]

Cytosine Arabinoside

Cytosine arabinoside is an antimetabolite that inhibits DNA synthesis. High-dose intravenous therapy is associated with a significant risk of pulmonary toxicity, having been reported in 15% to 30% of patients in several series involving hundreds of patients.[123, 266–270] Older age also appears to be a risk factor.[190] Most affected patients have been treated for acute leukemia.

Although diffuse alveolar damage is seen in some cases, an acellular proteinaceous alveolar exudate unassociated with a cellular inflammatory reaction or hyaline membranes resembling cardiogenic pulmonary edema have also been described.[267, 271] It is possible that the latter reaction is mediated by cytokine release induced by infusion of the drug[269] or by proteolytic enzymes released by tumor lysis.[2] BOOP has been reported to develop in children treated with a combination of cytosine arabinoside and anthracyclines.[271a]

The radiographic manifestations consist of bilateral irregular linear opacities, air-space consolidation, or, more commonly, both interstitial and air-space patterns.[272] In one review of 15 patients, the radiographic results at the time of clinical presentation were abnormal in 13 patients and normal in 2;[272] in 11 patients, the abnormalities were diffuse, and in 2 they were limited to the lower or upper lobes. Two patients had pleural effusion.

Clinical findings are those of noncardiogenic pulmonary edema and fever developing 1 to 38 days after therapy.[268, 270] The prognosis cited in published reports varies widely; for example, in one series of 13 patients, 9 died,[267] whereas in another study, fatality ensued in only 3 of 31 patients.[273]

Gemcitabine

Gemcitabine is a cytidine analogue that has activity against several neoplasms, including non–small cell pulmonary carcinoma.[273a] It is similar in structure and metabolism to cytosine arabinoside;[273b] like the latter, it has been associated with the development of noncardiogenic pulmonary edema.[273b, c]

Azathioprine and 6-Mercaptopurine

Azathioprine (Imuran) is the nitroimidazole derivative of 6-mercaptopurine; it interferes with purine base synthesis and therefore RNA and DNA synthesis.[274] It is commonly used to suppress rejection in patients who have received organ transplants and as an immunosuppressive agent in a variety of disorders. In view of its widespread use and the relatively few reports of associated complications, azathioprine must be considered an uncommon cause of pulmonary toxicity. Despite this, it has been implicated as a cause of interstitial pneumonitis and fibrosis,[275, 276] diffuse alveolar damage,[277] and diffuse alveolar hemorrhage.[278, 279] A study of renal allograft recipients on whom open-lung biopsy was

performed has suggested a dose-related effect.[275] Although some patients with interstitial fibrosis die of respiratory insufficiency,[275] others recover, possibly reflecting relatively low drug dose, treatment with corticosteroids, or early recognition of toxicity.[40, 275, 280] We are aware of only one case of restrictive lung disease reported in a patient receiving 6-mercaptopurine.[78]

Fludarabine

Fludarabine is a nucleotide analogue used in the treatment of refractory chronic lymphocytic leukemia. Several cases of interstitial pneumonitis or diffuse alveolar damage associated with its use have been reported.[281, 281a] The clinical course was characterized by cough, dyspnea, and fever occurring 1 week to several weeks after therapy. Exclusion of opportunistic infection is paramount because *P. carinii* and other pathogens are much more frequent causes of this clinical picture (73 of 2,269 patients [3%] in one study).[282]

Miscellaneous Antimetabolic Drugs

Thrombotic complications following the use of L-asparaginase developed in 10 of 238 patients treated for acute lymphoblastic leukemia in one study.[283] Of these, one patient had pulmonary thromboembolism and one deep venous thrombosis.

Focal necrotizing pneumonitis has been reported in a patient whose lung parenchyma was accidentally infused with *5-fluorouracil* by a misplaced Hickman catheter.[284]

BIOLOGIC RESPONSE MODIFIERS

Interleukin-2

Interleukin-2 (IL-2), with and without autologous lymphokine-activated killer (LAK) cell infusion, has been used in the treatment of a variety of malignancies, including melanoma and renal cell carcinoma.[285] Toxicity associated with these agents is prominent and includes a syndrome of cardiorespiratory failure with hypotension, weight gain, and peripheral and pulmonary edema.[6, 286] The chest radiographic manifestations range from mild interstitial to extensive air-space edema;[183] in one series of eight patients, two developed the former and three the latter.[287] In another retrospective review of 54 patients, 39 (72%) developed radiographic abnormalities, consisting of pleural effusions in 28 (52%), diffuse pulmonary edema in 22 (41%), and focal "infiltrates" in 12 (22%).[285] Although pulmonary edema developed at the time of LAK cell infusion in two of the patients, similar findings were seen in patients treated with IL-2 alone.

The mechanism of pulmonary edema in IL-2 toxicity is generally considered increased capillary permeability; however, careful monitoring of seven patients showed that small increases in pulmonary capillary wedge pressure and a decrease in blood oncotic pressure are also important.[288] Animal[289] and *in vitro*[290] experiments have implicated locally produced tumor necrosis factor-α (TNF-α) and leukotriene

B$_4$[291] in the pathogenesis. Methotrexate attenuates the vascular leak induced by IL-2 in a murine model of disease, perhaps owing to its inhibition of leukocyte adherence to IL-2–activated endothelium.[292]

Pulmonary toxicity is more likely to develop when IL-2 is administered as a bolus;[285] significant toxicity is rare when it is administered by continuous infusion.[293] A significant correlation has been described between the cumulative IL-2 dose and a decline in lung diffusing capacity during the first course of therapy.[294]

Tumor Necrosis Factor

TNF is a cytokine that has been used in a number of experimental protocols for the treatment of malignancy. It causes an isolated reduction in diffusing capacity that is unexplained by anemia or by progression of malignancy in the lung.[295, 296] It is possible that this is related to the development of subclinical noncardiogenic edema.[295] Exceptionally, air-space disease after TNF infusion has been the result of diffuse alveolar hemorrhage.[297]

Granulocyte-Macrophage Colony-Stimulating Factor

The use of the hematopoietic growth factor GM-CSF has been associated with a variety of pulmonary complications, including acute eosinophilic pneumonia,[298] dyspnea (caused by accumulation of aggregated neutrophils in the pulmonary vasculature), a capillary leak syndrome with pleural and pericardial effusions, and thromboembolism (possibly related to the development of thrombosis at the catheter tip as a result of local accumulation of granulocytes that damage the vascular endothelium).[6]

Interferon

Recombinant human interferon-α is used in the treatment of viral hepatitis.[299] A clinical and radiographic picture of interstitial pneumonitis has been reported in a number of patients.[299–302, 319] In most cases, biopsy material has not been obtained; however, BOOP has been documented in one patient.[299]

In an investigation of the rate of induction of autoantibodies in 30 patients with disseminated melanoma receiving various forms of immunotherapy, the development of antiphospholipid antibody was observed in 5 of 12 who had been treated with interferon-α and in none of 18 treated with IL-2 alone.[303] Four of these five patients developed deep venous thrombosis, which was followed by pulmonary embolism in one patient.

ANTIMICROBIAL DRUGS

Nitrofurantoin

Although almost 1,000 cases of pulmonary toxicity caused by nitrofurantoin (Furadantin) have been reported,[304–312] including 447 cases among 921 adverse reactions to the drug identified in Sweden during a 10-year period,[310] overall, adverse pulmonary reactions are rare. In a review of records of 16,101 patients treated with nitrofurantoin in the Group Health Cooperative of Puget Sound between 1976 and 1986, pulmonary disease requiring hospitalization and possibly related to drug toxicity occurred only three times;[312] of 742 patients receiving long-term therapy, only 1 developed fatal lung fibrosis. Despite a decrease in use of the drug during the 1980s, the incidence of toxic manifestations increased, a paradox interpreted by the authors of the Swedish study as an indication of sensitization of the Swedish population.[310] The incidence of adverse reactions in the United Kingdom is considerably lower than that in Sweden,[313] an observation that has been attributed either to differences in reporting or to dosages prescribed in the two countries. The higher incidence in women and the elderly is probably a reflection of the patient population receiving the medication.[308, 310]

There are two distinct presentations of nitrofurantoin-induced lung disease: (1) acute, developing hours to days after the onset of treatment; and (2) chronic and insidious, becoming manifest after weeks to years of continuous therapy. The former is the more common; in the Swedish series cited previously, 87% of cases were of this type.[310] This form of toxicity almost certainly constitutes a hypersensitivity reaction, a conclusion based on several observations, including the abrupt onset of disease and its reversibility with cessation of therapy, the presence of blood eosinophilia, and the results of *in vitro* and *in vivo* studies of lymphocytes from affected patients and experimental animals.[304]

The chronic form of disease probably represents direct tissue damage from oxidants.[314] This conclusion is based on experimental studies in animals that have shown hyperoxic enhancement and antioxidant suppression of pulmonary damage[304] as well as a deficiency in ability of the lung to detoxify reactive oxygen species after administration of the drug.[314] Histologic examination of the lungs shows interstitial pneumonitis and fibrosis indistinguishable from idiopathic pulmonary fibrosis in most patients;[309, 315, 316] rare cases showing diffuse alveolar damage[317] or resembling desquamative interstitial pneumonitis,[317] giant cell pneumonitis,[320] and extrinsic allergic alveolitis[320] have also been reported.

The radiographic manifestations of the acute form of nitrofurantoin-induced lung disease consist of a diffuse reticular pattern with some basilar predominance;[307, 321, 322] septal lines may be present[68] (Fig. 63–12). The pattern resembles interstitial pulmonary edema, and, in fact, the rapid clearing that occurs when the drug is withdrawn suggests that edema plays a considerable role in the production of the radiographic opacities.[323] Pleural effusions are relatively common and may be an isolated finding.[305, 308, 324] One patient has been reported in whom all the clinical and radiographic features of ARDS developed after 2 weeks of therapy.[325]

The radiographic manifestations of the chronic form of nitrofurantoin lung toxicity consist of a bilateral reticular pattern usually involving mainly the lower lung zones.[183] HRCT may demonstrate a predominantly subpleural or peribronchovascular distribution of consolidation and fibrosis[68] (Fig. 63–13). Pleural effusions are uncommon.[183] As with other drugs, clinical and physiologic evidence of pulmonary toxicity occasionally become evident in the absence of radiographic abnormality.[307, 310, 326]

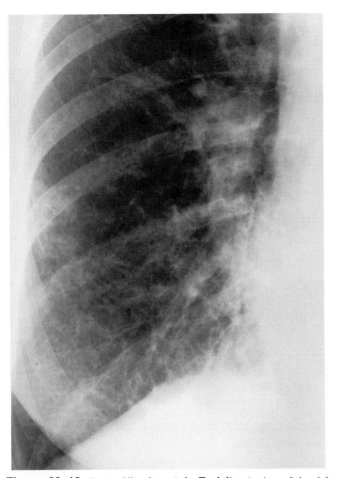

Figure 63–12. Acute Nitrofurantoin Toxicity. A view of the right lung from a posteroanterior chest radiograph demonstrates a reticular pattern involving predominantly the lower lung zones. A few septal lines and a small right pleural effusion are also evident. The patient was a 58-year-old woman who presented with progressive shortness of breath. The findings resolved within a few days after discontinuation of nitrofurantoin therapy.

Clinical manifestations in the acute form of the disease include fever, dyspnea, and a nonproductive cough developing within a few days of continuous medication; about 25% of patients complain of chest pain. A skin rash and arthralgia occur in 10% to 20%.[307, 308, 321, 327] Symptoms tend to develop more rapidly in patients who have received the drug previously. The chronic form of disease has a more insidious onset, with dry cough and gradually increasing shortness of breath on exertion developing after months to years of therapy.[308, 309, 315, 316, 328, 329] Crackles may be heard at the lung bases; pleural effusion[307, 328] and clubbing[316] develop in a minority of patients.

In the Swedish series, peripheral blood eosinophilia of 5% or more was present in almost 85% of patients with acute disease and in 40% of those with chronic disease;[310] pleural fluid eosinophilia has also been reported.[305] Profound lymphopenia caused by depletion of T cells was described in one series of five patients with an acute reaction.[305] In both the acute and chronic varieties, a restrictive pattern is found on physiologic assessment.[308, 310] The diffusing capacity and the PaO$_2$ may be very low, particularly in the acute form.[305, 316, 330]

The prognosis is excellent in the acute variety, with all evidence of disease usually disappearing within 4 to 8 weeks.[330] However, death can occur as a result of respiratory failure,[311, 312] as in 2 of 398 cases in the Swedish series.[310] In the latter study, 10% of patients with chronic disease died, although complete clearing has been reported following cessation of therapy.[309, 331] A fatal case of massive pulmonary hemorrhage occurring 24 hours after re-exposure to nitrofurantoin has been documented in an alcoholic who had cirrhosis and esophageal varices.[311] Diffuse alveolar hemorrhage has also been reported shortly after initiation of prophylactic nitrofurantoin therapy following cadaveric renal transplantation.[332] Improvement in function can occur after drug withdrawal despite persistence of radiographic abnormalities;[315, 328] by contrast, complete radiographic resolution can occur in the presence of residual impairment in the diffusing capacity.[316]

Sulfasalazine

When used in the treatment of inflammatory bowel disease, sulfasalazine (salazosulfapyridine, salicylazosulfapyridine, Salazopyrin, Azulfidine) is broken down into sulfapyridine and 5-aminosalicylate. Pulmonary toxicity has been reported in more than 24 patients.[304, 333–345] The complication probably represents a hypersensitivity reaction; in most patients, the presentation consists of acute, transitory radiographic opacities accompanied by peripheral blood eosinophilia. In addition, drug challenge after cessation of therapy has elicited a positive reaction in some patients.[333, 335, 340]

Most biopsy specimens have revealed interstitial pneumonitis and fibrosis or BOOP;[304, 334, 335, 339, 344] a histologic appearance resembling eosinophilic pneumonia or extrinsic allergic alveolitis has been documented occasionally.[344, 346] Analysis of BAL fluid showed a significant number of eosinophils in one patient[347] and evidence of a lymphocytic alveolitis without eosinophilia in another.[341]

The radiographic manifestations typically consist of poorly defined bilateral areas of consolidation that are commonly peripheral in distribution.[348] The areas of consolidation involve predominantly the upper lobes, although lower lobe or diffuse infiltrates occur in a small number of cases.[349] In one patient we have seen, blood eosinophilia and radiographic resolution after withdrawal of therapy simulated Löffler's syndrome. Another case has been reported in which the clinical and radiologic features mimicked those of Wegener's granulomatosis;[350] the chest radiograph revealed bilateral nodular infiltrates, and CT demonstrated bilateral peripheral wedge-shaped opacities and nodules, one of which had central cavitation. The opacities resolved after discontinuation of sulfasalazine therapy.

The clinical presentation varies little among patients and consists of dry cough, progressive dyspnea, and fever, often associated with a skin rash and blood eosinophilia;[333–337] these findings become manifest 1 to 6 months after initiation of treatment. Both restrictive[304, 339–341] and obstructive[304, 334] patterns have been found on pulmonary function testing. Follow-up studies usually reveal complete resolution of pulmonary disease; however, residual obliterative bronchiolitis and interstitial fibrosis have been reported rarely.[304, 334, 339, 340]

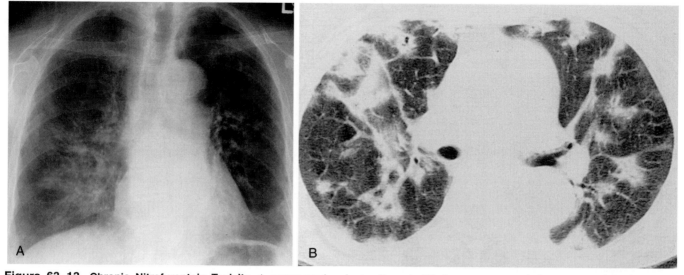

Figure 63–13. Chronic Nitrofurantoin Toxicity. A posteroanterior chest radiograph *(A)* shows a coarse reticular pattern and patchy areas of consolidation involving predominantly the middle and lower lung zones. An HRCT scan *(B)* demonstrates peribronchial distribution of the areas of consolidation and a few irregular linear opacities. The patient was an 81-year-old woman who presented with progressive shortness of breath. She had been on nitrofurantoin therapy for 2 years. Transbronchial biopsy demonstrated a bronchiolitis obliterans organizing pneumonia–like reaction. The radiologic findings improved within a few days after discontinuation of nitrofurantoin therapy; however, mild peribronchial reticulation was still present at 6-month follow-up.

Tetracycline and Minocycline

Both tetracycline[351] and minocycline,[352–357] a semisynthetic, long-acting tetracycline, have been reported to cause lung disease resembling simple pulmonary eosinophilia. A single case has also been reported of an association between minocycline and BOOP.[358]

Rechallenge with minocycline in several patients with eosinophilic lung disease has implicated a hypersensitivity reaction in the pathogenesis of disease.[355, 357, 359–361] A CD8-predominant lymphocytosis[356, 357] with an associated expansion of CD4 lymphocytes[357] has also been found in BAL fluid, suggesting a role for cell-mediated immunity in the pathogenesis.[357]

There have been few reports of the underlying histologic abnormalities. Transbronchial biopsy specimens have shown interstitial pneumonitis, in some cases with a large number of eosinophils.[356] A distinctive brownish coloration of alveolar macrophages has been noted by some investigators.[356] BOOP has been documented rarely.[358]

The radiographic findings resemble those of simple pulmonary eosinophilia and usually consist of bilateral, biapical, and predominantly subpleural areas of consolidation.[352] Less common findings include unilateral consolidation or a fine bilateral reticular pattern.[352, 363]

Patients present with a clinical picture of dyspnea, fever, and dry cough;[356] chest pain, fatigue, skin rash, and hemoptysis[356] have been noted in a minority of cases. Crackles can be appreciated on auscultation of the chest.[356] Hepatitis,[354] pleural effusion,[355, 364] and lymphadenopathy[354] are occasionally present. Typically, the peripheral[356] and BAL eosinophil[356, 357, 359, 361] counts are elevated. Hypoxemia is usual[356] and may be severe.[351] Lung function studies have revealed both obstructive and restrictive patterns.[356]

Pulmonary opacities resolve with discontinuation of the offending drug; corticosteroids appear to accelerate improvement when the process is severe.[355, 356]

Miscellaneous Antimicrobial Drugs

A number of other antibiotics have been associated with an eosinophilic lung reaction similar to that seen with sulfasalazine and tetracyclines, including *sulfonamides* (administered either orally or as vaginal creams),[26, 365, 366] *penicillin*,[367] *para-aminosalicylic acid*,[368] *ethambutol*,[369] *ampicilin*,[370] *maloprim*,[371] Fansidar (a *sulfadoxine-pyrimethamine* combination),[362] and *cephalosporins*.[372] A single case has been reported of a patient with polycythemia rubra vera treated with *pyrimethamine* who developed noncardiac pulmonary edema that resolved after discontinuation of the drug.[373] Recurrent noncardiac pulmonary edema has also been documented in one patient given a *trimethoprim-sulfamethoxazole* combination.[374]

Recurrent pulmonary edema of cardiac origin[375] and acute dyspnea in the absence of other findings[376] have been described occasionally in patients undergoing infusion of liposomal *amphotericin B*. Of potentially greater significance is a report of lethal pulmonary hemorrhage in 14 of 22 patients (64%) who were administered amphotericin B in conjunction with granulocyte infusion.[377] However, this finding was not reproduced in another series,[378] and it appears likely that most of the reactions seen with the combined infusion of amphotericin B and white blood cells are related to concurrent infection or granulocyte alloimmunization.[379]

Radiologically evident interstitial disease and BAL lymphocytosis similar to extrinsic allergic alveolitis have been described in patients treated with *piperacillin*,[380] *cephradine*,[381] and *penicillin*, the last-named following both occupational exposure[382] and oral therapy;[383] hilar and mediastinal adenopathy, in addition to the pulmonary disease, has been seen in some cases.[383]

ANTIARRHYTHMIC DRUGS

Amiodarone

Amiodarone hydrochloride is an iodinated benzofuran derivative used in the treatment of cardiac arrhythmias. It was originally believed that the drug lacked deleterious side effects, possibly because of the relatively low dosage employed in Europe, where it was first released. However, subsequent studies have revealed an important risk of pulmonary toxicity that has significantly limited its use.[384] Higher maintenance doses employed in the United States may be responsible for the observed increase in incidence of the complication.[304, 385–387] In the English language literature, a conservative estimate of the number of clinically and radiographically diagnosed cases is more than 200.[388–395] Given the vagaries of clinical presentation, different diagnostic criteria, and difficulties in distinguishing toxicity from congestive heart failure, thromboembolism, or infection, the precise incidence of pulmonary toxicity is uncertain; however, it has been suggested that with current patterns of use, 5% to 7% of treated patients develop the complication, of whom 5% to 10% die as a consequence.[396]

Pathogenesis

The pathogenesis of amiodarone lung toxicity is uncertain; however, it seems likely that both direct and indirect mechanisms are involved.[397] Although immune and inflammatory mechanisms could theoretically explain acute toxicity and direct tissue damage the findings in chronic fibrotic disease, no such distinction can be clearly drawn from published reports.

Amiodarone causes inhibition of phospholipid degradation within lysosomes of target cells, resulting in an increase in their phospholipid content and a foamy appearance pathologically.[385, 388, 398, 399] There is a strong correlation between the tissue concentration of amiodarone and its metabolite, desethylamidarone, and the degree of phospholipid accumulation.[400] This observation and the well-established relationship between the risk of toxicity and dose[386, 387] suggest that the increased intracellular phospholipids or tissue levels of the drug or its metabolites are directly responsible for cell changes. In fact, *in vitro* studies have shown that clinically achievable toxic tissue levels of amiodarone can induce cell injury and death.[401] Despite these observations, the presence of foamy macrophages in BAL fluid can be detected in patients without histologic evidence of pulmonary damage, and it appears more likely that the lipid accumulation represents a marker of amiodarone administration than an essential step in the pathogenesis of disease.[397, 402]

As a result of this uncertainty, other mechanisms have been hypothesized to account for cytotoxicity. *In vitro* and experimental animal studies have demonstrated that the metabolism of amiodarone produces a reactive aryl radical.[403] Although simultaneous treatment with an antioxidant revealed a reduction in lung cell lysosome formation in the latter study, no other marker of lung toxicity was altered; thus, the role of oxidant-induced lung damage remains to be established.

There is also evidence that an inflammatory or immune response is responsible for tissue damage, at least in some patients.[391, 393, 397, 401, 405] Examination of cells retrieved by BAL has revealed the presence of an increased number of neutrophils and lymphocytes in patients who have amiodarone toxicity.[391, 393, 406, 407] In some, analysis of the BAL lymphocyte profile has shown an increase of CD8 (suppressor and cytotoxic) lymphocytes, with reversal of the usual CD4-to-CD8 ratio.[393] Other patients with normal lavage lymphocyte numbers still have a low ratio of CD4 to CD8 cells.[393] This lavage pattern is similar to that seen in other forms of hypersensitivity lung disease, such as extrinsic allergic alveolitis.

A variety of other observations also implicate immunologic factors in disease pathogenesis. For example, rat models of amiodarone lung toxicity have been associated with the activation of lung, but not peripheral, natural killer cells[408] and with the release of TNF-α from drug-activated macrophages.[409] Peripheral immune cells also demonstrate increased reactivity to amiodarone.[397] In one investigation, leukocyte migration inhibition factor was produced by lymphocytes of patients who had pneumonitis but not by those of symptom-free patients receiving the drug.[410] A case has also been reported in which amiodarone-related lung fibrosis was associated with the presence of a circulating antibody to a lung antigen-amiodarone complex.[411]

Most patients reported in the literature have received 400 mg/d or more of amiodarone before the appearance of pulmonary disease.[384, 385, 387, 412, 413] The relationship of dose and toxicity is also supported by animal models.[414] However, interstitial pulmonary disease occurring with maintenance doses of less than 400 mg/d has been seen in some patients.[389, 404, 415–417] Some investigators have shown that the risk of developing an adverse reaction is related to the concentration of amiodarone in the serum,[416, 417] although this has not been a consistent finding.[396] As with other drugs, attempts have been made to evaluate whether pre-existing lung function abnormalities are a risk factor for the development of amiodarone toxicity;[417–419] however, no consistent relation has been found.

Lung damage has its onset months after the initiation of amiodarone therapy.[304, 384, 420] The drug is deposited in various organs and tissues throughout the body but particularly in the lungs, where the concentration has been found to be four to seven times higher than in other organs.[421] The drug is eliminated slowly—the half-life is estimated to be about 30 days[304]—which may explain the interval of 1 month or longer after the cessation of therapy before complete radiographic and clinical resolution occurs.

Pathologic Characteristics

Light microscopic examination of the lung in amiodarone toxicity typically reveals chronic inflammation and fibrosis of the alveolar septa, hyperplasia of type II pneumocytes, and accumulation of intra-alveolar macrophages[390, 422, 423] (Fig. 63–14). These macrophages and, to a lesser extent, the type II pneumocytes have coarsely vacuolated cytoplasm that can be seen ultrastructurally to contain nu-

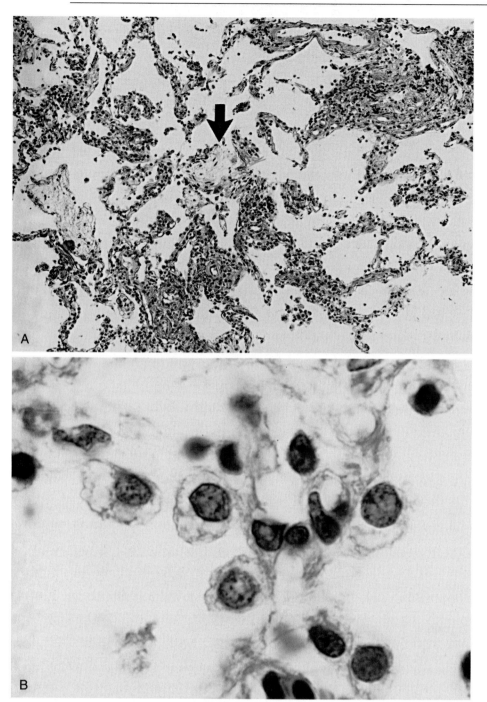

Figure 63–14. Amiodarone Toxicity: Interstitial Pneumonitis. A section of lung parenchyma from a transbronchial biopsy specimen *(A)* shows a moderate degree of interstitial fibrosis and lymphocytic infiltration; focal fibroblastic tissue is also present *(arrow)*. A magnified view of one alveolar wall *(B)* shows several type II pneumocytes with coarsely vacuolated cytoplasm.

merous, often enlarged lysosomal inclusions that have a characteristic appearance (*see* Fig. 63–14): one or more clusters of thin osmiophilic lamellae are surrounded by a layer of amorphous electron-dense material. The inclusions are also seen in pulmonary endothelial and interstitial cells as well as various extrapulmonary cells and have been shown by dispersive x-ray analysis to contain iodine, a constituent of the amiodarone molecule.[390] The inclusion-bearing macrophages can be identified in BAL specimens, supporting a diagnosis of amiodarone toxicity.[424] As indicated previously, however, such macrophages can also be seen in patients without evidence of disease,[423] and their presence is not diagnostic of drug-related tissue damage.

In addition to the typical histologic appearance described previously, there have also been reports of diffuse alveolar damage,[388, 423] necrotizing pneumonia (in a patient who also had hyperglycemia),[425] BOOP,[423, 427, 428] and necrotizing bronchiolitis associated with an infiltrate of eosinophils.[399] Complement has been demonstrated in alveolar septa in some cases,[413] although this finding has not been consistent.[401]

Radiologic Manifestations

Chest radiographs usually reveal a diffuse bilateral reticular pattern or bilateral areas of consolidation[183, 412, 429]

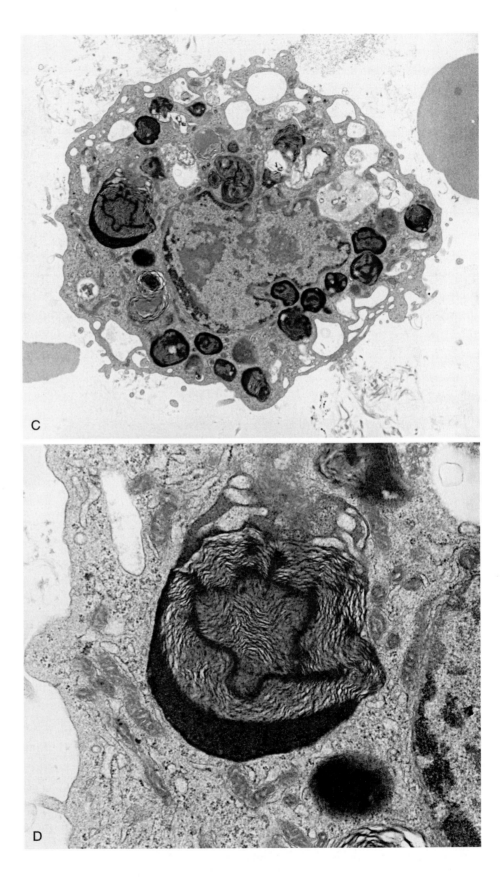

Figure 63–14 *Continued.* Ultrastructural examination of an alveolar macrophage within an alveolar space *(C)* shows the cytoplasm to contain numerous phagosomes, some of which are enlarged, and many of which contain densely osmiophilic material. A magnified view of one phagosome *(D)* shows a laminated inclusion organized in geographic segments with a crescent-shaped zone of amorphous electron-dense material at the periphery. The patient was a 63-year-old man who had been taking amiodarone daily for several months. (*A* ×110, *B* ×1500, *C* ×7720 and *D* ×28,370.)

(Fig. 63–15). The areas of consolidation may be peripheral in distribution and may involve predominantly the upper lobes, resembling chronic eosinophilic pneumonia.[384, 412] Less common manifestations include focal consolidation and nodular opacities.[183, 348] In one patient, cavitation occurred within one of the nodular infiltrates.[430] Pleural thickening has been described,[384] and one patient presented with bilateral exudative pleural effusions associated with toxic involvement of other organs.[431]

Because amiodarone contains about 37% iodine by weight, it has a high attenuation value on CT; as a result,

this procedure allows confident recognition of drug deposition within pulmonary and other tissues[432] (Fig. 63–16). In one review of the CT findings in 11 patients with symptoms of amiodarone pulmonary toxicity, high attenuation (82 to 175 HU), pulmonary lesions were present in 8 (73%), increased liver or spleen attenuation in 10 (91%), and increased myocardial attenuation in 2 (18%).[432] Similar findings have been reported by others.[68, 433] The pattern of the parenchymal abnormalities is variable and may consist of bilateral areas of consolidation (frequently wedge shaped and pleural based), a reticular pattern, linear atelectasis, or

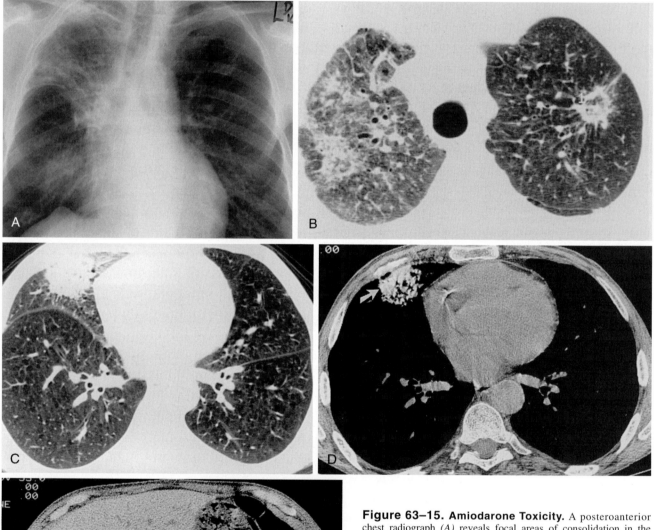

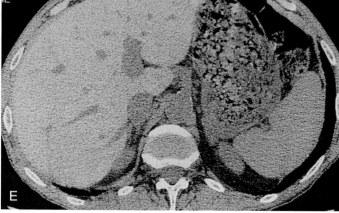

Figure 63–15. Amiodarone Toxicity. A posteroanterior chest radiograph *(A)* reveals focal areas of consolidation in the right upper and middle lobes and irregular linear opacities in the right upper and, to a lesser extent, left upper lobe. An HRCT scan *(B)* shows extensive ground-glass attenuation in the right upper lobe, a focal area of ground-glass attenuation in the left upper lobe, and bilateral irregular linear opacities. A scan at the level of the inferior pulmonary veins *(C)* reveals a focal area of consolidation in the right middle lobe. A scan at the same level as that in *C* and photographed using soft tissue windows *(D)* demonstrates that the consolidation in the right middle lobe *(arrow)* has an attenuation greater than that of chest wall and cardiac muscle. An HRCT scan through the upper abdomen *(E)* reveals high attenuation of the liver. The patient was a 61-year-old man who had clinical findings consistent with amiodarone pulmonary toxicity.

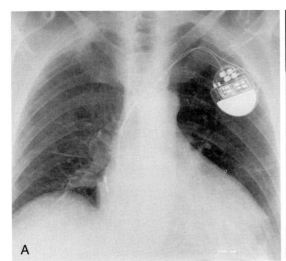

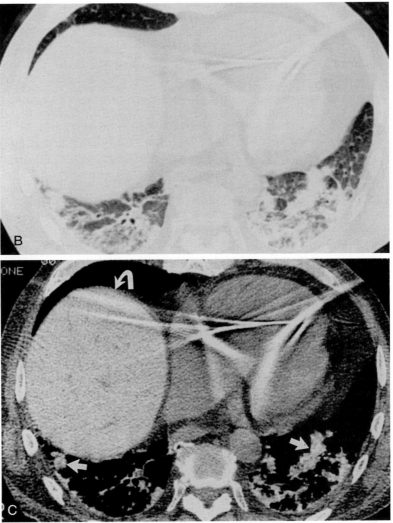

Figure 63–16. Amiodarone Toxicity. A posteroanterior chest radiograph *(A)* reveals a few linear opacities and small areas of consolidation in the lower lobes. Also noted are scarring in the right upper lobe as a result of previous tuberculosis, cardiomegaly, and a permanent pacemaker with sequential atrioventricular leads in place. An HRCT scan through the lung bases *(B)* reveals areas of ground-glass attenuation, focal areas of consolidation, and linear opacities. A scan photographed at soft tissue windows *(C)* demonstrates the high attenuation of the parenchymal infiltrates *(straight arrows)* and of the liver *(curved arrow)* related to amiodarone deposition. (Artifacts are due to pacemaker wires.) The patient was a 68-year-old man who had clinical findings consistent with amiodarone-induced lung disease.

(less commonly) focal round areas of consolidation.[68, 432, 433] Pleural effusions are seen on CT in about 50% of cases.[432] Visceral pleural thickening may also be seen.[434]

Distinction of amiodarone pneumonitis from congestive heart failure may also be made by the documentation of increased uptake on gallium 67 radionuclide lung scans.[435, 436]

Clinical Manifestations

Two distinct clinical patterns of pulmonary disease occur in amiodarone toxicity.[1, 395, 396] The most common corresponds to the interstitial pattern of abnormality described radiographically and is characterized by the insidious onset of dyspnea on exertion, dry cough, weight loss, weakness, and (occasionally) fever.[384, 385, 389, 396, 422] Hemoptysis has been described rarely.[436a] About one third of patients have a more acute onset of disease, which may be confused clinically with infection, pulmonary edema, or thromboembolism.[388, 396] Radiographs of such patients may show diffuse air-space disease in a patchy and somewhat peripheral distribution.[396] Physical findings in both forms of disease are inconsistent and nonspecific and include tachypnea, diffuse or focal crackles on chest auscultation, and occasionally, a pleural rub.[395] Clinically significant pleural effusion is rare.[437]

Manifestations of extrapulmonary toxicity are not uncommon and include blue-gray skin discoloration, skin rashes (such as photodermatitis), thyroid dysfunction (both hypothyroidism and hyperthyroidism), corneal microdeposits, gastrointestinal symptoms, neurotoxicity (manifested by muscle weakness, peripheral neuropathy, or extrapyramidal symptoms), hepatic dysfunction, and bradycardia.[304, 384, 420]

Laboratory Findings

Pulmonary function tests show restrictive impairment[384, 389, 424] and reduction in gas transfer.[389, 438] Prospective analyses of lung function have shown the ability to identify patients with lung toxicity, and a correlation has been found between dose or cumulative dose and the detection of decreased lung volumes, diffusing capacity, or both.[387, 390, 415, 417, 424] However, although an isolated reduction in diffusing capacity may be a sensitive finding in the diagnosis of amiodarone lung toxicity, it lacks specificity. This was illustrated in one cohort of 91 patients studied prospectively, of whom 15 developed asymptomatic reductions in diffusing capacity;[418] all remained well with continuation of the drug during the subsequent 11 months. The absence of lung function abnormalities, however, provides reasonable assurance of the absence of amiodarone lung toxicity.[418] Findings on BAL fluid analysis are not sufficiently specific to allow drug toxicity to be distinguished from confounding concurrent disease.[391, 406] The diagnosis remains one of exclusion and requires careful correlation of the results of the history, physical examination, functional and radiologic investigations, and, in some cases, BAL and biopsy. The finding of high attenuation of the parenchymal abnormalities on HRCT may be particularly useful in this regard.[68, 432]

Prognosis and Natural History

The response to withdrawal of medication and the initiation of corticosteroid therapy appears excellent, and few cases of irreversible damage have been reported. However, the long half-life of the drug creates considerable difficulty in assessing the value of corticosteroid therapy in the absence of a controlled clinical trial comparing this with drug withdrawal.[385, 387, 415, 439–441] Despite this, relapse of disease after steroid withdrawal has been reported in patients who had improvement following the institution of corticosteroid therapy.[442, 443] The prognosis might depend more on the underlying cardiovascular disease than on the effects of drug toxicity; continued use of the drug might be warranted when alternative therapy is not available and arrhythmia in the absence of amiodarone is life-threatening.[395] The development of ARDS in patients with previous amiodarone pulmonary toxicity or use who undergo cardiothoracic surgical procedures has been described.[444–446]

Miscellaneous Antiarrhythmic Drugs

Lidocaine used as a local anesthetic has been reported to cause noncardiogenic pulmonary edema on two separate occasions in the same patient.[447] *Tocainide*, an antiarrhythmic drug that possesses chemical and pharmacologic properties similar to those of *lidocaine*, has been reported to cause interstitial pneumonitis and fibrosis in six patients.[304, 448–450] Clinical and radiographic evidence of toxicity became apparent months after the onset of therapy and resolved after withdrawal of the drug;[448] however, two of the patients had residual impairment of diffusing capacity.[304] Noncardiogenic pulmonary edema has been attributed to *verapamil* in one patient who had a massive overdose.[451] A myasthenia-like syndrome resulting in ventilatory failure from chest wall weakness has been attributed to *procainamide* in two patients.[452, 453] The same agent can also cause lupus erythematosus and can therefore be associated with pleural effusion.[454] In one case, *sotalol* pulmonary toxicity was characterized histologically by features of both BOOP and eosinophilic pneumonia.[455]

ANTICONVULSANT DRUGS

Diphenylhydantoin

Diphenylhydantoin (phenytoin, Dilantin) is used principally to control seizures and is believed to act through stabilization of neuronal membranes.[304] It was originally thought that pulmonary toxicity could be manifested by both

an acute hypersensitivity reaction[456, 457] and a more chronic and insidious form of interstitial pneumonitis;[458] however, the existence of the latter syndrome has not been substantiated by prospective studies.[459, 460] Manifestations of the acute form of disease include blood eosinophilia and a diffuse reticulonodular pattern on chest radiograph, both of which resolve within 2 weeks after drug withdrawal.[456, 461] Analysis of BAL fluid in affected patients has suggested a predominantly lymphocytic type of alveolitis.[457, 462] Mediastinal lymph node enlargement simulating lymphoma has also been reported.[463, 464]

Pathologic reports are scarce; transbronchial biopsy specimens in some patients have revealed an infiltrate of lymphocytes within alveolar septa resembling lymphocytic interstitial pneumonia.[457, 461, 462] Necrotizing granulomatous vasculitis has been described in several patients who manifested fever, dermatitis, and peripheral eosinophilia;[465, 466] interstitial fibrosis was identified in the lower lobes of one patient.[465] A single case of BOOP was demonstrated on open-lung biopsy in a patient who had an acute hypersensitivity reaction characterized clinically by rhinorrhea, myalgia, fever, rash, dry cough, and dyspnea.[467]

Chest radiographs show a diffuse reticulonodular pattern, in some cases with hilar and mediastinal lymph node enlargement;[461, 463, 464, 468] occasionally, hilar and mediastinal adenopathy is seen without associated parenchymal abnormalities.[468] Rarely, patchy air-space consolidation similar to that associated with Loeffler's syndrome or miliary nodules may be present.[468–470] Although the lymphadenopathy is usually a reflection of hypersensitivity reaction, it must be remembered that there is a 4- to 10-fold increase in incidence of lymphoma in patients receiving the drug.[468, 471]

Acute pulmonary toxicity can result in severe impairment of gas exchange.[461] In one long-term study of pulmonary function in 50 patients who had taken phenytoin for 2 years or longer, abnormalities of gas exchange consisting of impaired diffusing capacity, low PaO_2 levels, and increased $P(A-a)O_2$ were found in 45%.[472] Unfortunately, there is no reference in this study to chest radiographs or to any change in function after cessation of therapy.

Carbamazepine

Carbamazepine (Tegretol) is used in the control of neuralgia and as an anticonvulsant. At least 12 patients with drug-induced pulmonary disease have been described.[473–480] However, one group documented a significant reduction in diffusing capacity in patients with normal chest radiographs who were suffering from systemic adverse reactions to carbamazepine,[481] suggesting that lung toxicity may be more common than the few case reports would suggest.

As with diphenylhydantoin, the onset of toxicity is acute, and symptoms consist of pneumonia, eosinophilia, and skin rash. A transbronchial biopsy specimen in one patient showed changes consistent with eosinophilic pneumonia.[482] Lung biopsy in another patient who had carbamazepine-induced lupus erythematosus revealed BOOP.[483] The radiographic findings have been described in a small number of cases and include reticular or reticulonodular patterns or focal areas of consolidation;[484, 485] hilar prominence consistent with lymph node enlargement may be evident.[484] In two patients, a lymphocyte-stimulation test with carbamazepine was strongly positive;[473, 480] in one of these studies, there was no reaction in healthy controls or in patients receiving carbamazepine therapy without adverse effects.[473] Analysis of BAL fluid in one patient revealed an inversion of the usual CD4-to-CD8 lymphocyte ratio, a finding in keeping with that described with other lung drug toxicities.[478] Lung function studies in another patient revealed a severe restrictive process with a low diffusing capacity.[477]

ANALGESIC DRUGS

Acetylsalicylic Acid

Acetylsalicylic acid (aspirin) is a well-known cause of acute pulmonary edema, particularly in middle-aged and elderly people who become habituated as a result of ingesting large doses to alleviate pain. Interestingly, younger patients admitted to the hospital because of intentional overdose rarely manifest overt pulmonary edema, even in the presence of coma.[486–488] Despite this, fatal salicylate-induced, pulmonary edema can occur even in children and has been correlated with high serum salicylate levels and anion gap.[489] Serum salicylate levels are usually 30 mg/mm^3 or more; however, there is not a clear dose relationship because many patients with similar blood levels do not develop edema.[486, 488–491] Cigarette smoking has been identified as a risk factor in some studies.[486, 488]

Studies of sheep in which pulmonary edema has been induced by salicylate ingestion have confirmed the clinical impression that the edema results from increased capillary permeability.[492] Pulmonary artery wedge pressure has been found to be normal in several studies,[486, 490, 493] and the constituents of airway fluid have been shown to be identical to those in plasma.[304, 491] Two mechanisms have been postulated for the increased permeability:[304, 486] (1) increased intracranial pressure, causing neurogenic edema as a result of deposition of the drug in brain tissue and (2) inhibition of prostaglandin production, resulting in vasodilation and increased permeability. Because patients tend to be dehydrated, it is possible that treatment of hypovolemia with crystalloid sometimes contributes to the development of edema.[491] In some cases, hypoproteinemia may also play a role.[491]

Chest radiographs reveal the typical diffuse air-space pattern of pulmonary edema.[486, 488, 490] Patients are dyspneic, lethargic, and confused; they tend to have proteinuria, perhaps reflecting increased capillary permeability in the systemic circulation. A history of long-term acetylsalicylic acid ingestion, usually in large quantities, is typical.[490, 491, 494] Because the pulmonary edema responds well to measures that decrease serum salicylate levels, the prognosis is good.[486]

Mesalamine, a 5-acetylsalicylic acid compound used in the treatment of inflammatory bowel disease, has been associated with the development of interstitial pneumonitis in some patients.[495, 496, 496a]

Nonsteroidal Anti-inflammatory Drugs

Pulmonary reactions to nonsteroidal anti-inflammatory agents are rare. In one population-based study of 100,000 users of *diclofenac*, *naproxen*, and *piroxicam*, no definite lung disease could be identified.[497] However, at least seven patients have been described who developed acute pulmonary air-space opacities while taking naproxen.[498–500] In all cases, the onset of symptoms was acute and consisted of weakness, fatigue, cough, low-grade fever, and blood eosinophilia. All abnormalities resolved within days to weeks after withdrawal of the drug. One patient was subsequently rechallenged and showed a similar reaction.[499] Air-space opacification of a similar nature has also been described in patients who have taken *sulindac*,[501] *piroxicam*,[502] *tolfenamic acid*,[503] *diflunisal*,[504] and *diclofenac*.[505] Pathologic examination in some cases has revealed poorly defined granulomas with admixed eosinophils.[498]

ANTIRHEUMATIC DRUGS

Penicillamine

Penicillamine is a derivative of penicillin that can chelate a variety of metals, including lead, copper, zinc, and mercury. It is used to treat lead poisoning, Wilson's disease, cystinuria, and connective tissue diseases, particularly rheumatoid disease.

The variety of pulmonary complications caused by this drug is probably greater than that of any other and includes lupus-like[506] and myasthenia-like[511, 512] disease as well as alveolitis,[513–516] obliterative bronchiolitis[517–524] and diffuse alveolar hemorrhage.[507–510] With the exception of bronchiolitis, the association of penicillamine with all these disorders appears to be causative. However, because rheumatoid disease is a well-recognized cause of bronchiolitis and because most published cases of penicillamine-associated bronchiolitis have occurred in patients who have had rheumatoid arthritis, it is possible that some, if not all, reported cases of obliterative bronchiolitis have been a manifestation of the underlying disease rather than the drug. However, BOOP has been documented in a patient who was being given penicillamine for scleroderma confined to the lower legs (morphea), an abnormality not normally complicated by pulmonary disease.[525] It is also reasonable to conclude that patients being treated with penicillamine for rheumatoid arthritis who develop reticulonodular disease that does not respond to withdrawal of the medication probably have an abnormality related to rheumatoid disease rather than penicillamine.

Judging by the number of reported cases and the frequency of penicillamine use, the incidence of penicillamine-induced pulmonary toxicity must be extremely low. The risk of toxicity is not dose related.[304] The mechanism of acute reversible pulmonary disease, usually accompanied by eosinophilia,[514, 516, 521] is likely a type I immunologic reaction, whereas limited pathologic findings suggest that the pulmonary-renal syndrome is type III.

Pathologic abnormalities vary with the type of disease. To the best of our knowledge, no patients with the acute eosinophilic syndrome have undergone biopsy. Biopsy specimens of some patients have shown interstitial pneumonitis and fibrosis.[304, 521] Histologic findings in patients with the pulmonary-renal syndrome have been those of diffuse alveolar hemorrhage without evidence of vasculitis;[507] in two patients, immunofluorescent studies showed an interrupted reaction pattern with immunoglobulin G and complement rather than the linear reaction typical of antiglomerular basement membrane antibody in Goodpasture's syndrome.[507, 526] The appearance of bronchiolitis is identical to that seen in rheumatoid disease.

Radiographic manifestations are of three types: (1) a reticular or reticulonodular pattern, with or without limited air-space opacities, indicating the presence of interstitial disease;[514] (2) overinflation unaccompanied by parenchymal abnormality, associated with advanced obliterative bronchiolitis; and (3) diffuse air-space consolidation, typically seen in patients with diffuse alveolar hemorrhage.[304, 527] In patients with obliterative bronchiolitis, the HRCT findings consist of areas of decreased attenuation and perfusion (mosaic attenuation) and bronchial dilation.[528]

Patients usually present with cough and dyspnea that develop insidiously over a period of weeks; however, the onset of dyspnea is typically abrupt in patients with pulmonary hemorrhage.[304] Crackles and, in some cases, rhonchi may be heard at the lung bases.[304, 514] Other manifestations include stomatitis, dermatitis,[304] and (rarely) cholestatic hepatitis.[515] In patients with bronchiolitis, pulmonary function tests can reveal evidence of severe obstruction, even when the chest radiograph is normal.[304]

The prognosis for patients with the acute hypersensitivity syndrome is excellent, the clinical and radiographic abnormalities characteristically resolving rapidly after withdrawal of medication and initiation of steroid therapy.[513, 514] By contrast, death is common in patients who have the pulmonary-renal syndrome or obliterative bronchiolitis.[304, 507]

Gold

Although chrysotherapy employing sodium aurothiomalate is effective in arthritis, side effects—usually involving the skin or mucous membranes—are common. Pulmonary toxicity is uncommon, having been estimated to occur in less than 1% of patients. In one investigation of 110 patients with rheumatoid arthritis receiving the agent, pulmonary function testing failed to find adverse effects in anyone.[304, 529] Despite these observations, more than 110 cases of gold-related pulmonary toxicity have been reported.[304, 530–551] The risk of toxicity does not appear to be dose related. However, a strong association between toxicity and the presence of certain major histocompatibility antigens has been reported.[544]

The mechanism of pulmonary damage is thought to be a hypersensitivity reaction; about one third of patients have peripheral eosinophilia.[533, 541] There is also evidence of a cell-mediated immune reaction: exposure of lymphocytes from affected patients to gold *in vitro* has been found to result in the elaboration of lymphokines (migration-inhibiting factor and macrophage chemotactic factor);[304, 531, 549, 550] normal controls and patients receiving gold therapy without pulmonary toxicity do not manifest this effect. Analysis of BAL fluid has revealed lymphocytic alveolitis in two patients.[549, 550]

Histologic examination reveals interstitial pneumonitis accompanied by varying degrees of fibrosis.[530, 531, 535] Gold can be identified within lysosomes of macrophages and pul-

monary capillary endothelial cells;[552] however, as with amiodarone, it has not been established whether this represents simply a marker of drug administration or is related to the pathogenesis of disease. Occasional patients have BOOP[553, 554] or pure obliterative bronchiolitis.[555] As with penicillamine, it is possible that the latter complication is the result of underlying rheumatoid disease rather than gold; however, we have seen one case of typical obliterative bronchiolitis in a patient treated for psoriatic arthritis, suggesting a true pathogenic effect in at least some cases.[555]

The chest radiograph has been described as showing diffuse interstitial and patchy air-space opacities;[532, 533, 556] in one report, the diffuse patchy (presumably air-space) opacities observed initially were subsequently replaced by a reticulonodular pattern.[535]

Clinical manifestations usually develop acutely or subacutely, thereby aiding in the differentiation from interstitial fibrosis associated with rheumatoid disease, the onset of which is insidious.[541, 556] Patients are often febrile and complain of progressive shortness of breath on exertion and a dry cough;[532, 535, 541] almost half have associated dermatitis.[304] Physical examination may reveal crackles.[532, 535] A restrictive pattern and hypoxemia are found on physiologic assessment.[531, 535, 541, 546] Rechallenge with the drug has been associated with recurrence of symptoms in some patients.[530, 531, 533]

The response to cessation of therapy is usually good; we are aware of only four reported deaths from pulmonary disease,[533, 547] although we have seen another in our own practice. Steroids are usually administered and may hasten recovery.[1] Residual restriction on pulmonary function testing or reticulonodularity on chest radiographs may be observed.[533, 537, 541, 542, 556]

SYMPATHOMIMETIC DRUGS

The tocolytic β-mimetics *terbutaline, ritodrine,* and *isoxsuprine,* used in the treatment of preterm labor, have been implicated in the development of permeability pulmonary edema.[304, 557–560] The complication has a low incidence: only 7 of 2,557 patients in one study[557] and 7 of 1,407[558] in another were affected. Because of underlying pregnancy, the certainty of diagnosis may be somewhat obscured by the possible presence of thromboemboli, amniotic fluid embolism, fluid overload, anemia and the necessity for transfusion, and the administration of other drugs, particularly corticosteroids,[557, 561] one or more of which could conceivably contribute to the development of the edema. Hemodynamic data suggest that the mechanism of edema formation is noncardiogenic.[557]

The chest radiograph reveals classic signs of air-space edema.[304] Symptoms and clinical findings develop within 2 to 3 days of the initiation of therapy and can be associated with extreme hypoxemia. The prognosis is excellent after discontinuation of the drug and the initiation of supportive measures.[304, 558]

The association of *fenfluramine, phentermine,* and related agents with the development of a primary pulmonary hypertension-like picture is discussed in detail in Chapter 50 (*see* page 1902). These agents have also been a cause of valvular heart disease, similar to that seen in association with carcinoid tumor.[562]

ILLICIT DRUGS

Although illicit drugs such as heroin and cocaine can induce a variety of specific pulmonary effects, it should always be remembered that their use may be associated with a number of nonspecific complications, the most important of which is infection.[563–566] For example, opportunistic infection associated with human immunodeficiency virus, including pneumonia due to *P. carinii, Mycobacterium tuberculosis*, and other bacteria,[563, 567] is now more common than septic pulmonary embolism and lung abscess among inner-city intravenous drug addicts. Aspiration pneumonia and atelectasis resulting from depressed levels of consciousness can also occur in those using sedating drugs.

This section is concerned with complications of narcotic drugs, cocaine, and marijuana. The consequences of inhalation of volatile hydrocarbons and injection of talc intravenously are discussed in Chapters 64 (*see* page 2588) and 49 (*see* page 1857), respectively.

Narcotic and Sedative Drugs

Opiates and related drugs are well-known causes of pulmonary edema. The incidence of the complication following heroin overdose ranges from 50% to 75%.[568, 569] Pulmonary edema has also been reported as a result of an overdose of *methadone,*[570–572] *buprenorphine,*[573, 574] *propoxyphene* (Darvon),[575] *chlordiazepoxide* (Librium),[576] *ethchlorvynol* (Placidyl),[577] *paraldehyde,*[578] *codeine,*[579] *bromocarbamide,*[580] *febarbamate,*[581] and *naloxone.*[582, 583]

A high protein content of the edema fluid has been well documented in affected patients,[584] indicating that the development of edema is related to increased capillary permeability. However, the mechanism by which capillary leakage occurs has not been elucidated. It is probable that the hypoxemia and acidosis that accompany severe respiratory center depression cause endothelial damage. Based on findings of reduced levels in the serum and deposition in the lungs of immunoglobulin M and complement components, some investigators have proposed an immunologic mechanism.[585, 586] Theoretically, the edema could also have a neurogenic origin. Opiate receptors can be identified near the medullary respiratory center,[587] and the application of drugs in this area has produced edema in dogs.[304] Such a mechanism could explain the paradoxical development of edema following the administration of the opiate antagonist naloxone.[582, 583]

The pathologic[588, 589] and radiographic[569, 590, 591] manifestations of pulmonary edema resulting from narcotic overdose are indistinguishable from those of other etiologies (Fig. 63–17). The findings usually consist of bilateral and symmetric air-space consolidation, often with a predominantly perihilar distribution.[591] Less commonly, the edema is focal, is unilateral, or has an upper lobe distribution.[591, 592] The heart size is normal. The appearance of pulmonary edema may be delayed after admission to the hospital, sometimes for as long as 6 to 10 hours;[593, 594] resolution characteristically occurs in as brief a time as 24 to 48 hours.[593, 595, 596] Pulmonary edema caused by methadone overdose is similar radiographically to that caused by heroin and other toxic drugs, except that it is somewhat slower to resolve (2 to 4 days).[570]

[571, 597] Prolonged absorption of methadone from the gastrointestinal tract has been suggested as the likeliest explanation for this delay.

Signs and symptoms usually develop within hours of narcotic use, although the onset may be delayed for as long as 24 hours and may first appear after assessment of the patient in the hospital.[566] The typical patient is stuporous or comatose and has frothy, pink fluid oozing from the nostrils and mouth. Constricted pupils and respiratory depression are usually evident; however, a depressed level of consciousness is not always present.[566] The peripheral blood may show leukocytosis in the absence of accompanying infection or (occasionally) leukopenia.[566, 593, 598]

Hypoxemia is severe and is accompanied by a mixed acidosis.[571, 593, 599, 600] By the time the first arterial blood gas is drawn, hypoxemia is probably the result of a combination of alveolar hypoventilation from depression of the respiratory center and shunt and ventilation-perfusion inequality related to air-space edema. Patients who manifest hypocapnia have presumably recovered from central nervous system depression; persisting hypoxemia and acidosis then reflect severe pulmonary edema and hypoperfusion of tissues. Lung function studies performed shortly after recovery from the edema show a severe restrictive ventilatory defect with reduced vital capacity and total lung capacity; the impairment disappears over a period of a few days.[601, 602]

Bronchiectasis has also been identified in some heroin addicts with a history of drug-induced pulmonary edema; it is likely explained by recurrent infection and aspiration.[566, 603] The observation in some retrospective studies that the onset of asthma occurs in close proximity to the initiation of heroin abuse has also suggested a relationship between the two;[566] however, the incidence of asthma in addicts is similar to that in the general population.[566]

Drug addicts with sclerosed peripheral veins seek alternate injection sites; one of the preferred routes is the veins in the neck ("the pocket shot"). (The latter term refers to the supraclavicular fossa, where the addict tries to gain access to the jugular, brachiocephalic, or subclavian veins.[604]) Complications are not infrequent; the most common are unilateral or bilateral pneumothorax.[604, 605] Hemothorax, hemopneumothorax, and pyopneumothorax have also been reported.[604, 606] Focal areas of increased opacity may be seen radiographically in the supraclavicular region secondary to cellulitis, abscess, soft tissue inflammation adjacent to osteomyelitis of the clavicle, or hematoma surrounding an arterial pseudoaneurysm.[604]

Cocaine

When smoked, the crystalline precipitate of free-base cocaine ("crack") reaches the cerebral circulation within 6 to 8 seconds, causing virtually instantaneous euphoria. This property, along with its ease of administration and wide availability, has made crack cocaine the most frequently abused controlled substance in the United States; for example, it has been estimated that 6% of high school seniors in the United States have used cocaine, most commonly as crack.[567] The use of this agent has been associated with an impressive variety of manifestations of lung toxicity.[566, 567, 607–610, 742] The presence of this variety in combination with the

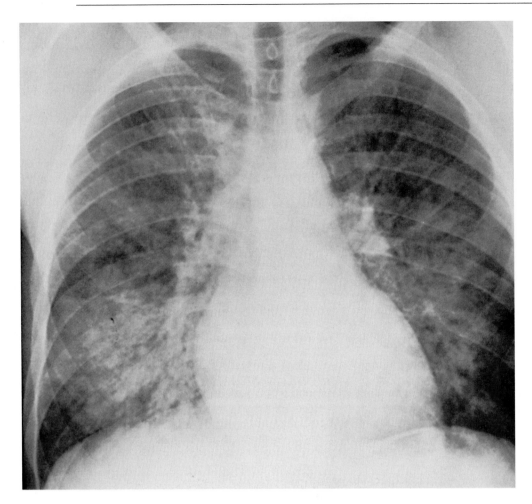

Figure 63–17. Acute Pulmonary Edema Caused by Drug Abuse. A posteroanterior chest radiograph reveals air-space consolidation typical of acute pulmonary edema of any etiology. Several hours previously, this 19-year-old man had injected a high dose of Demerol and methadone intravenously. He had an uneventful recovery.

drug's widespread abuse demands that inquiry concerning cocaine use be a routine part of history taking in pulmonary medicine.

Symptoms are common within minutes to hours of inhaling crack cocaine: more than 40% of users report intercurrent cough, production of black sputum, pleuritic or nonpleuritic chest pain, shortness of breath, exacerbation of asthma, or hemoptysis.[566, 567] Although the cause of chest pain is usually unclear following investigation, myocardial ischemia or infarction, pneumothorax, and pneumomediastinum must be excluded.[567] Despite the high prevalence of acute respiratory symptoms, cocaine inhalers do not appear to have more chronic respiratory symptoms than noninhalers with similar tobacco and marijuana use.[610]

Pulmonary edema has been reported as a complication of both cocaine[611] and crack[612] smoking. The pathogenesis of edema formation in this situation is not clear. Some observations suggest it is secondary to alveolar endothelial and epithelial damage. This is supported by the finding that long-term users of crack, even those who have normal pulmonary function, demonstrate increased lung epithelial permeability, as assessed by radioisotope testing.[613] In addition, analysis of BAL fluid in one patient showed a high protein content of the edema fluid.[567] It has also been shown that both intravenously injected and inhaled cocaine can cause activation of circulating neutrophils,[614] a process that

could contribute to lung injury. By contrast, the results of several animal experiments have implicated cardiac dysfunction as the cause of edema formation. Coronary artery vasoconstriction is induced by cocaine smoking, an effect enhanced by tobacco.[615] Significant myocardial depression may also occur when cocaine is combined with alcohol.[616] In a porcine model of cocaine toxicity, cardiogenic shock followed drug-induced reduction in coronary flow and (possibly) direct damage to cardiac muscle.[617]

Pulmonary hemorrhage is also an important complication of cocaine use. It is one histologic manifestation of "crack lung," a syndrome that is characterized by acute respiratory failure and diffuse parenchymal consolidation on chest radiographs.[608, 609] In one study of 20 patients who died of cocaine intoxication, 7 (35%) were found to have occult lung hemorrhage at autopsy.[617a] Hemoptysis with a normal chest radiograph is also a common complaint in crack cocaine users;[567] bronchoscopy reveals diffuse blood staining of the airways, but there appears to be no serious sequelae.

Inhalation of crack can lead to severe airway thermal injury[618] sometimes complicated by tracheal stenosis or the reactive airways dysfunction syndrome. Life-threatening asthma apparently precipitated by cocaine use has occurred in patients who smoked the drug[567] or inhaled it by nasal insufflation.[619] In one patient who had been inhaling freebase cocaine, an open-lung biopsy revealed BOOP;[620] after a stormy clinical course requiring positive end-expiratory pressure, the patient was found to have residual obstructive disease and air trapping. A second fatal case of BOOP following cocaine use has also been reported.[567] Surprisingly, airway hyper-reactivity has not been found to be a feature of habitual cocaine use.[621]

Pneumothorax, pneumomediastinum, and pneumopericardium have all been reported in users of crack cocaine.[567] In one study of 71 crack smokers who presented to the emergency department with chest pain,[612] two had a pneumomediastinum, one had a pneumothorax, and one a pneumohemothorax. Persistent reduction in diffusing capacity with otherwise normal pulmonary function has been described in long-term cocaine users,[610, 622, 623] although the precise pathogenesis of this finding is not known.

Pathologic correlates of the diffuse interstitial or alveolar infiltrates seen radiologically include a variety of abnormalities,[624] such as diffuse alveolar damage,[609] interstitial pneumonitis with[608] and without[609, 625] peripheral eosinophilia, frank eosinophilic pneumonia,[626] deposition of carbonaceous material in alveolar air spaces,[627] diffuse alveolar hemorrhage,[566] BOOP,[628] and pulmonary edema.[629] Granulomas have also been identified in the lungs of cocaine sniffers who denied intravenous injection of talc-based drugs;[630, 631] some have been considered to be related to the cellulose content of the cocaine mixture.[630] Specimens of BAL fluid submitted for cytologic analysis may be black and show abundant carbonaceous material in alveolar macrophages;[632] it has been speculated that this may be the result of addicts inhaling the tarry residue left on the inside of pipes or other instruments used for smoking.[632]

The radiographic manifestations of cocaine-induced pulmonary edema consist of bilateral, symmetric, and predominantly perihilar interstitial or air-space infiltrates.[633, 634] These abnormalities usually resolve within 24 to 72 hours, regardless of treatment.[633, 634] Pulmonary hemorrhage may result in transient focal or diffuse bilateral air-space consolidation.[529, 635] Less commonly, fleeting areas of consolidation may result from a Loeffler-like syndrome,[636] or diffuse consolidation from BOOP.[637, 638] As discussed previously, barotrauma related to cocaine abuse may result in pneumomediastinum,[634, 639] pneumothorax,[634, 640] or (rarely) hemopneumothorax[634] or pneumopericardium.[641, 642] Radiographic abnormalities have been reported in 13%[634] to 55%[604] of patients with cardiopulmonary symptoms following crack cocaine inhalation. The most common are focal air-space consolidation and atelectasis, the pathogenesis of which is uncertain.[604]

Marijuana

Habitual marijuana use is associated with the development of acute and chronic bronchitis similar to that seen in tobacco smokers.[643] Chronic, heavy use has no consistent effect on nonspecific airway reactivity;[621] the drug's bronchodilator effects become blunted with repeated use.[566] The common contamination of marijuana with *Aspergillus* species has been implicated in the development of both allergic bronchopulmonary aspergillosis in marijuana users who are asthmatic and opportunistic *Aspergillus* species infection in those who are immunocompromised.[566] A reduction in diffusing capacity has also been attributed to long-term marijuana use.[644]

ANTIDEPRESSANT AND ANTIPSYCHOTIC DRUGS

Antidepressant and antipsychotic agents have been associated with a variety of pulmonary abnormalities, the most common of which is ARDS.[645] In one investigation of 82 patients admitted to an intensive care unit with tricyclic antidepressant overdose, 32 (39%) had radiographic abnormalities, of which 9 were consistent with ARDS.[646] Although aspiration was documented by the finding of charcoal used in nasogastric lavage before intubation in the tracheal aspirate of 18 of 72 patients, there was no correlation between this observation and the radiographic findings of edema.

Imipramine,[647, 648] *trimipramine,*[649] and *chlorpromazine*[650] have all been associated with an acute, transient febrile disease associated with eosinophilia. Two patients have been described who developed severe bronchiolitis and interstitial pneumonitis while receiving *amitriptyline.*[651, 652] Evidence of CD8+ lymphocytic alveolitis on BAL and CT findings consistent with BOOP have also been reported with the use of *clomipramine.*[653] *Fluoxetine hydrochloride* (Prozac) has been reported to cause hypersensitivity pneumonitis,[654] interstitial lung disease,[655] and pulmonary nodules[656] in single case reports. In a retrospective review in which the lifetime drug use of patients who had developed idiopathic pulmonary fibrosis (IPF) was compared with that of a control group, the odds ratio for the development of IPF associated with a history of imipramine was 4.8;[656a] other antidepressants also demonstrated this relationship, albeit in a weaker fashion.

Another rare manifestation of tricyclic antidepressant toxicity is the malignant neuroleptic syndrome,[657] an acute febrile disease characterized by severe muscle rigidity, neurologic abnormalities, autonomic dysfunction, and pulmonary edema.[304] ARDS has also been reported in three patients suffering from an overdose of phenothiazines without other findings of the malignant neuroleptic syndrome.[658]

CONTRAST MEDIA

Embolization of *ethiodized oil* used for lymphangiography can result in a "subacute" form of ARDS that possesses clinical features resembling fat embolism and that may have a similar pathogenesis (*see* page 1861). A significant decrease in diffusing capacity has been recorded following lymphangiography that is maximal in 48 hours and returns to normal in 1 month.[659–663] These observations are comparable to those of animal studies in which complete restoration of normal pulmonary function and morphology has been shown to occur in 6 weeks.[664] Rarely, lymphography has been a cause of diffuse alveolar hemorrhage.[665]

Water-soluble contrast media occasionally have been reported to cause pulmonary edema. The pathogenesis of this complication has been debated.[666–671] Some investigators have suggested that it is a consequence of the high osmolarity of the solutions employed, particularly *sodium iothalamate* and *diatrizoate meglumine* (Gastrografin), the osmolarity of which is 5 to 10 times that of plasma.[669] In fact, in some patients with underlying heart disease, hyperosmolality created by the contrast media causes an overloading of the circulation, which undoubtedly plays a role in the development of disease.[669, 672] However, some affected patients are otherwise healthy, and the presence of a normal wedge pressure and a high protein content of the edema fluid indicates a permeability abnormality.[670, 671] Other observations supporting this mechanism are derived from experiments in rats, in which no difference in severity of edema between animals given low- or high-osmolality compounds has been identified,[673] and from occasional reports of noncardiogenic pulmonary edema in patients given nonionic, low-osmolality contrast media intravenously.[674, 675]

In one investigation of 336 patients undergoing transcatheter oily chemoembolization of hepatocellular carcinoma, 6 developed a clinical picture consistent with ARDS;[676] all were part of a group of 14 patients who had received excessive amounts of the oil.

Acute reactions to *ionic contrast medium* injected intravenously occur in 5% to 15% of cases.[677] These are usually mild; life-threatening reactions occur in only 0.05% to 0.1% of injections, with a mortality rate of about 1 in 75,000.[677, 678] Manifestations of minor reactions include nausea, vomiting, urticaria, and diaphoresis; more severe disease is associated with faintness, severe vomiting, laryngeal edema, and bronchospasm. Severe reactions are characterized by pulmonary edema, hypotensive shock, convulsions, respiratory arrest, and cardiac arrest.[677]

Reactions to intravascular contrast media are classified into anaphylactoid (idiosyncratic) and chemotoxic.[677] The former are independent of dose, occur unpredictably, and account for most cases. Chemotoxic reactions are due to specific physical and chemical effects of the contrast agent and are related to the concentration of the contrast medium.[677] The risk of anaphylactoid reaction is increased in patients who have allergies, asthma, or previous reactions to the contrast medium. Chemotoxic effects are more likely to cause clinically significant complications in patients who are debilitated or who have renal dysfunction or severe cardiovascular disease.[677]

In a nationwide study of Japanese patients (about 170,000 receiving ionic contrast media and 170,000 nonionic contrast media), the prevalence of adverse reactions was 12% for the former and 3% for the latter; the prevalence of severe reactions was 0.2% and 0.04%, respectively.[679] However, a meta-analysis of studies published before 1991 in which ionic and non-ionic contrast media were used showed no difference in the fatality rate.[679a] Furthermore, a review of the number and types of adverse drug reactions reported to the U.S. Food and Drug Administration between 1978 and 1994 showed no decrease in the number of nonfatal[679b] and fatal[679c] reactions to iodinated contrast media since the introduction of low-osmolality forms in 1986. The estimated 170 million contrast medium–enhanced studies performed in the United States between 1978 and 1994 produced 22,785 reports of mild or moderate adverse drug reactions, 2,639 reports of serious but nonfatal reactions, and 920 reports of death.[679b] Excluding 22 myelography-related deaths, 42% more deaths were reported each year between 1987 and 1994 than between 1978 and 1986; most of this increase was associated with non-ionic contrast media. In the period 1987 to 1994, 220 deaths were associated

with the use of high-osmolality ionic contrast media alone, 32 with ionic low-osmolality contrast media alone, 214 with non-ionic low-osmolality contrast media alone, and 8 with combinations of contrast media.[679c] It should be noted that the analysis of the data did not take into account the relative number of examinations performed using ionic versus non-ionic agents during the study period, the increase in the number of examinations using contrast media since 1986, or trends in reporting adverse drug reactions. In summary, although serious nonfatal and fatal reactions to contrast media are uncommon, they can occur with both ionic and nonionic agents.

ANGIOTENSIN-CONVERTING ENZYME INHIBITORS

Persistent nonproductive cough is a common side effect of ACE inhibitor therapy,[680–686] having been reported in up to 44% of users;[680] a reasonable estimate of its occurrence overall is probably about 10%.[685] Variation in cough prevalence in different studies may be related to the method by which the symptom is detected (self-reporting,[686] questionnaire,[685, 687] or interview[680, 684, 688]) and by the specific ACE inhibitor studied.[686, 689] Most[683, 686, 688, 690, 691] (albeit not all[680, 692]) investigators have reported a higher prevalence in women than in men.

The pathogenesis of ACE inhibitor–induced cough is unclear. It does not appear to be the result of inhibition of the renin-angiotensin system because treatment with angiotensin receptor blockers[681, 687, 693] and renin inhibitors has not caused the symptom.[694] More likely, it is related to stimulation of vagal afferents of the cough reflex in the airway by bradykinin or tachykinins, the accumulation of which is favored by ACE inhibition.[694]

Cough usually begins several months after starting the drug but may begin as early as the first dose or as late as 1 year after initiation of therapy. It is often very troublesome to the patient; in fact, cough is the most important cause of withdrawal of ACE inhibitor therapy, about half of affected patients stopping the drug because of the severity of the symptom.[684–686, 695–697] Despite adequate documentation of the drug-cough association, there is often lengthy delay in recognition of the cause of the symptom in office practice,[695] and unnecessary investigation and unwarranted therapies are often applied. Cough diminishes significantly within 3 days and disappears entirely within 10 days of drug cessation.[686, 698]

ACE inhibitors may also be a cause of asthma. In one investigation in Sweden, adverse reactions were reported in 424 patients, of whom 36 had symptoms suggesting asthma;[699] 33 of these patients had hypertension without heart failure, so that it is unlikely that asthma was confused with congestive heart failure. In another investigation, patients taking ACE inhibitors were compared retrospectively to those taking lipid-lowering drugs.[682] Although there was no difference between the two groups with respect to previous history of bronchospasm, the prevalence of bronchospasm was 5.5% in those taking ACE inhibitors, compared with 2.3% in those taking the lipid-lowering agents. ACE inhibitors have also been shown in some (albeit not all[700, 701]) studies to increase airway reactivity in patients with asthma[702] or with ACE inhibitor–related cough.[703] Despite this, administration of these agents to patients with established asthma has not been associated with deterioration in lung function or change in clinical status.[702, 704–706]

Other rare complications of ACE inhibitors include angioedema, occasionally associated with upper airway obstruction,[707] and peripheral eosinophilia.[708, 709]

MISCELLANEOUS DRUGS

Hydrochlorothiazide has been implicated rarely as a cause of permeability pulmonary edema[304, 710–714] (Fig. 63–18). Some patients have developed the complication after their first contact with the drug; others have received it previously.[304] The pathogenesis of edema formation is unknown; however, the acuteness of the reaction, the association with other clinical manifestations such as dermatitis and hepatitis,[304] the development of a similar reaction after re-exposure to the drug,[710, 715] and the rapid clinical and radiographic resolution on its withdrawal all point to a hypersensitivity reaction. Clinical symptoms and signs of edema develop 20 to 60 minutes after ingestion of the drug. Complete recovery typically occurs after cessation of therapy.[304]

Four reports have been published of patients who developed eosinophilia and air-space "pneumonia" after switching from oral corticosteroids to an aerosol of *beclomethasone diproprionate*.[716] The reaction may have represented an acute hypersensitivity reaction to the oleic acid used as a dispersing agent or to the hydrocarbon propellant. After reinstitution of the drug, one patient developed ARDS. A diagnosis of allergic bronchopulmonary aspergillosis was considered in all cases, but neither *Aspergillus* species nor mucous plugs were found. Clearing was prompt when the patients were restarted on oral corticosteroids.

Pulmonary disease has been reported in four transsexual men after subcutaneous injections of *silicone*.[717, 718] Three developed fever, chest pain, dyspnea, and radiographic evidence of acute interstitial and patchy air-space disease 24 hours after injection; silicone was identified in BAL fluid.

The fourth patient developed ARDS and died;[718] at autopsy, silicone was found in various organs of the body, particularly the lungs.

Beta-adrenergic blocking agents (β-blockers) can produce a systemic lupus erythematosus–like syndrome and can also precipitate acute bronchospasm. *Propranolol* has also been reported to cause cardiogenic edema in patients with pheochromocytoma,[719, 720] presumably by inducing β_1 and β_2 blockade, in turn resulting in unopposed alpha effects and sudden elevation of cardiac afterload. Propranolol[721, 722] and other β-blockers[723] have also been implicated as the cause of a hypersensitivity pneumonitis characterized by a lymphocytic alveolitis on BAL. Acute pulmonary edema[724] and bronchospasm[725] have been reported to accompany the use of β-blocker eye drops in the treatment of glaucoma.

ARDS has been reported in three patients in whom *talc* was instilled intrapleurally in the treatment of a malignant effusion.[726] Fever, increasing dyspnea, and finally ARDS developed over a 72-hour period following the injection; one patient died. All patients had normal pulmonary artery wedge pressures. A similar reaction has been documented in a single patient after intrapleural instillation of *streptokinase* followed 24 hours later by the intrapleural administration of urokinase.[727]

Multiple foci of ectatic pulmonary vessels ("pulmonary peliosis"), similar to those encountered in the liver in peliosis of that organ, have been described in one patient taking *anabolic steroids*.[728]

The use of *perfluorochemicals* as artificial blood has been reported to be associated with the presence of foamy macrophages throughout the reticuloendothelial system and the lungs in both humans[729] and experimental animals.[730] Clinical and functional consequences are not evident.

Although most strongly associated with pleural disease, *ergotamine* and its derivatives *bromocriptine* and *mesulergine* have been reported to cause pulmonary fibrosis.[731–733] Clinical and radiographic improvement after drug withdrawal suggests that this relationship was causal.[734]

Several agents have been associated with a variety of pulmonary complications in single case reports. The determi-

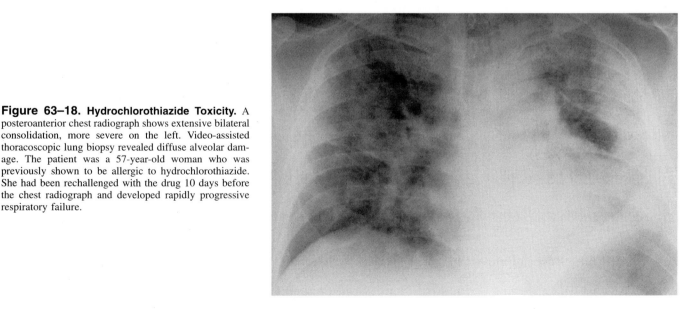

Figure 63–18. Hydrochlorothiazide Toxicity. A posteroanterior chest radiograph shows extensive bilateral consolidation, more severe on the left. Video-assisted thoracoscopic lung biopsy revealed diffuse alveolar damage. The patient was a 57-year-old woman who was previously shown to be allergic to hydrochlorothiazide. She had been rechallenged with the drug 10 days before the chest radiograph and developed rapidly progressive respiratory failure.

nation of causality is difficult because rechallenge has usually not been performed and the complications, if related, must be rare. Noncardiogenic pulmonary edema developed in a patient following massive *diltiazem* overdose.[735] Fever, pleural effusion, and perihilar lung infiltrates developed in a patient receiving intravenous *acyclovir*.[736] Lung fibrosis was noted in a patient receiving *bumetanide;*[737] antinuclear antibody had developed in this patient without other findings of lupus. Eosinophilic pleuritis occurred in a patient receiving *propylthiouracil*; all findings resolved with discontinuation of the drug.[738] Erythema, pruritus, and pulmonary edema followed the use of *bupivacaine* used for epidural anesthesia during labor;[739] the infant also developed lung edema subsequently. Pleural effusion with pleural and peripheral eosinophilia occurred in a patient given long-term *dantrolene* therapy for chronic spasticity.[740] Black pigmentation of rib cartilage has been reported after therapy with *levodopa* and *methyldopa*.[741]

REFERENCES

1. Rosenow EC III: Drug-induced pulmonary disease. Dis Mon 40:258, 1994.
2. Aronchick JM, Gefter WB: Drug-induced pulmonary disorders. Semin Roentgenol 30:18, 1995.
3. Rosenow EC III, Limper AH: Drug-induced pulmonary disease. Semin Respir Infect 10:86, 1995.
4. Demeter SL, Ahmad M, Tomashefski JF: Drug-induced pulmonary disease. Part I. Patterns of response. Part II. Categories of drugs. Part III. Agents used to treat neoplasms or alter the immune system including a brief review of radiation therapy. Clev Clin Q 46:89, 1979.
5. Jules-Elysee K, White DA: Bleomycin-induced pulmonary toxicity. Clin Chest Med 11(1):1, 1990.
6. Kreisman H, Wolkove N: Pulmonary toxicity of antineoplastic therapy. Semin Oncol 19:508, 1992.
7. Cooper JAD Jr, White DA, Matthay RA: Drug-induced pulmonary disease. Part 1. Cytotoxic drugs. Am Rev Respir Dis 133:321, 1986.
8. Wolkowicz J, Sturgeon J, Rawji M, et al: Bleomycin-induced pulmonary function abnormalities. Chest 101:97, 1992.
9. Santana A, Saxena B, Nobile NA, et al: Increased expression of transforming growth factor β isoforms (β_1, β_2, β_3) in bleomycin-induced pulmonary fibrosis. Am J Respir Cell Mol Biol 13:34, 1995.
10. White DA, Stover DE: Severe bleomycin-induced pneumonitis: Clinical features and response to corticosteroids. Chest 86:723, 1984.
11. Holoye PY, Luna MA, MacKay B, et al: Bleomycin hypersensitivity pneumonitis. Ann Intern Med 88:47, 1978.
12. Yousem SA, Lifson JD, Colby TV: Chemotherapy-induced eosinophilic pneumonia: Relation to bleomycin. Chest 88:103, 1985.
13. Rose AG: Pulmonary veno-occlusive disease due to bleomycin therapy for lymphoma. S Afr Med J 64:636, 1983.
14. Slosman DO, Sotabella PM, Roth M, et al: Bleomycin primes monocytes-macrophages for superoxide production. Eur Respir J 3:772, 1990.
15. Hernnäs, Nettelbladt O, Bjermer L, et al: Alveolar accumulation of fibronectin and hyaluronan precedes Bleomycin-induced pulmonary fibrosis in the rat. Eur Respir J 5:404, 1992.
16. Breuer R, Lossos IS, Or R, et al: Abatement of bleomycin-induced pulmonary injury by cell-impermeable inhibitor of phospholipase A2. Life Sci 57:237, 1995.
17. Sakanashi Y, Takeya M, Yoshimura T, et al: Kinetics of macrophage subpopulations and expression of monocyte chemoattractant protein-a (MCP-1) in bleomycin-induced lung injury of rats studied by a novel monoclonal antibody against rat MCP-1. J Leukoc Biol 56:741, 1994.
18. Nettelbladt O, Bergh J, Schenholm M, et al: Accumulation of hyaluronic acid in the alveolar interstitial tissue in bleomycin-induced alveolitis. Am Rev Respir Dis 139:759, 1989.
19. Piguet PF, Vesin C: Treatment by human recombinant soluble TNF receptor of pulmonary fibrosis induced by bleomycin or silica in mice. Eur Respir J 7:515, 1994.
20. Chandler DB, Barton JC, Briggs DD, et al: Effect of iron deficiency on bleomycin-induced lung fibrosis in the hamster. Am Rev Respir Dis 137:85, 1988.
21. Shahzeidi S, Mulier B, de Crombrugghe B, et al: Enhanced type III collagen gene expression during bleomycin induced lung fibrosis. Thorax 48:622, 1993.
22. Waid-Jones MI, Coursin DB: Perioperative considerations for patients treated with bleomycin. Chest 99:993, 1991.
23. Phan SH, Fantone JC: Inhibition of bleomycin-induced pulmonary fibrosis by lipopolysaccharide. Lab Invest 50:587, 1984.
24. Cantin AM, Hubbard RC, Crystal RC: Glutathione deficiency in the epithelial lining fluid of the lower respiratory tract in idiopathic pulmonary fibrosis. Am Rev Respir Dis 139:370, 1989.
25. Batist G, Andrews JL Jr: Pulmonary toxicity of antineoplastic drugs. JAMA 246:1449, 1981.
26. Lippman M: Pulmonary reactions to drugs. Med Clin North Am 61:1353, 1977.
27. Weiss RB, Muggia FM: Cytotoxic drug-induced pulmonary disease: Update 1980. Am J Med 68:259, 1980.
28. Samuels ML, Johnson DE, Holoye PY, et al: Large-dose bleomycin therapy and pulmonary toxicity: A possible role of prior radiotherapy. JAMA 235:1117, 1976.
29. Ingrassia TS, Ryu JH, Trastek VF, et al: Oxygen-exacerbated bleomycin pulmonary toxicity. Mayo Clin Proc 66:173, 1991.
30. Berend N: Protective effect of hypoxia on bleomycin lung toxicity in the rat. Am Rev Respir Dis 130:307, 1984.
31. Smith RE, Strieter RM, Phan SH, et al: C-C chemokines: Novel mediators of the profibrotic inflammatory response to bleomycin challenge. Am J Respir Cell Mol Biol 15:693, 1996.
32. Sharma SK, MacLean JA, Pinto C, et al: The effect of an anti-CD3 monoclonal antibody on bleomycin-induced lymphokine production and lung injury. Am J Respir Crit Care Med 154:193, 1996.
33. Smith RE, Strieter RM, Zhang K, et al: A role for C-C chemokines in fibrotic lung disease. J Leukoc Biol 57:782, 1995.
34. Phan SH, Kunkel SL: Lung cytokine production in bleomycin-induced pulmonary fibrosis. Exp Lung Res 18:29, 1992.
35. Everson MP, Chandler DB: Changes in distribution, morphology, and tumor necrosis factor-alpha secretion of alveolar macrophage subpopulations during the development of bleomycin-induced pulmonary fibrosis. Am J Pathol 140:503, 1992.

35a. Sleijfer S, Vujaskovic Z, Limburg PC, et al: Induction of tumor necrosis factor-alpha as a cause of bleomycin-related toxicity. Cancer 82:970, 1998.
36. Chandler DB: Possible mechanisms of bleomycin-induced fibrosis. Clin Chest Med 11(1):21, 1990.
37. Zhang HY, Gharaee-Kermani M, Zhang K, et al: Lung fibroblast alpha-smooth muscle actin expression and contractile phenotype in bleomycin-induced pulmonary fibrosis. Am J Pathol 148:527, 1996.
38. Young L, Adamson IY: Epithelial-fibroblast interactions in bleomycin-induced lung injury and repair. Environ Health Perspect 101:56, 1993.
39. Blum RH, Carter SK, Agre K: A clinical review of bleomycin: A new antineoplastic agent. Cancer 31:903, 1973.
40. Snyder LS, Hertz MI: Cytoxic drug-induced lung injury. Semin Respir Infect 3:217, 1988.
41. Ngan HY, Liang RH, Lam WK, et al: Pulmonary toxicity in patients with non-Hodgkin's lymphoma treated with bleomycin-containing combination chemotherapy. Cancer Chemother Pharmacol 32:407, 1993.
42. Lund MB, Kongerud J, Nome O, et al: Lung function impairment in long-term survivors of Hodgkin's disease. Ann Oncol 6:495, 1995.
43. Hirsch A, Vander Els N, Straus DJ, et al: Effect of ABVD chemotherapy with and without mantle or mediastinal irradiation on pulmonary function and symptoms in early-stage Hodgkin's disease. J Clin Oncol 14:1297, 1996.
44. McLeod BF, Lawrence HJ, Smith DW, et al: Fatal bleomycin toxicity from a low cumulative dose in a patient with renal insufficiency. Cancer 60:2617, 1987.
45. Van Barneveld PWC, van der Mark TW, Sleijfer DT, et al: Predictive factors for bleomycin-induced pneumonitis. Am Rev Respir Dis 130:1078, 1984.
46. Lei KI, Leung WT, Johnson PJ: Serious pulmonary complications in patients receiving recombinant granulocyte colony-stimulating factor during BACOP chemotherapy for aggressive non-Hodgkin's lymphoma. Br J Cancer 70:1009, 1994.
47. Saxman SB, Nichols CR, Einhorn LH: Pulmonary toxicity in patients with advanced-stage germ cell tumors receiving bleomycin with and without granulocyte colony stimulating factor. Chest 111:657, 1997.
48. Gerson R, Tellez BE, Lazaro LM, et al: Low toxicity with continuous infusion of high-dose bleomycin in progressive testicular cancer. Am J Clin Oncol 16:323, 1993.
49. Jones AW: Bleomycin lung damage: The pathology and nature of the lesion. Br J Dis Chest 72:321, 1978.
50. Luursema PB, Star-Kroesen MA, van der Mark TW, et al: Bleomycin-induced changes in the carbon monoxide transfer factor of the lungs and its components. Am Rev Respir Dis 128:880, 1983.
51. Sorensen PG, Romer FK, Cortes D: Angiotensin-converting enzyme: An indicator of bleomycin-induced pulmonary toxicity in humans. Eur J Cancer Clin Oncol 20:1405, 1984.
52. Adamson IYR, Bowden DH: Bleomycin-induced injury and metaplasia of alveolar type 2 cells: Relationship of cellular responses to drug presence in the lung. Am J Pathol 96:531, 1979.
53. Cohen MB, Austin JHM, Smith-Vaniz A, et al: Nodular bleomycin toxicity. Am J Clin Pathol 92:101, 1989.
54. Santrach PJ, Askin FB, Wells RJ, et al: Nodular form of bleomycin-related pulmonary injury in patients with osteogenic sarcoma. Cancer 64:806, 1989.
55. Yousem S, Lifson J, Colby T: Chemotherapy-induced eosinophilic pneumonia: Relation to bleomycin. Chest 88:103, 1985.
56. Joselson R, Warnock M: Pulmonary veno-occlusive disease after chemotherapy. Hum Pathol 13:88, 1983.
57. Lombard C, Churg A, Winokur S: Pulmonary veno-occlusive disease following therapy for malignant neoplasms. Chest 92:871, 1987.
58. Horowitz AL, Friedman M, Smith J, et al: The pulmonary changes of bleomycin toxicity. Radiology 106:65, 1973.
59. Balikian JP, Jochelson MS, Bauer KA, et al: Pulmonary complications of chemotherapy regimens containing bleomycin. Am J Roentgenol 139:455, 1982.
60. Iacovino JR, Leitner J, Abbas AK, et al: Fatal pulmonary reaction from low doses of bleomycin: An idiosyncratic tissue response. JAMA 235:1253, 1976.
61. Mills P, Husband J: Computed tomography of pulmonary bleomycin toxicity. Semin Ultrasound CT MR 11:417, 1990.
62. Talcott JA, Garnick MB, Stomper PC, et al: Cavitary lung nodules associated with combination chemotherapy containing bleomycin. J Urol 138:619, 1987.
63. Glasier CM, Siegel MJ: Multiple pulmonary nodules: Unusual manifestation of bleomycin toxicity. Am J Roentgenol 137:155, 1981.
64. McCrea ES, Diaconis JN, Wade JC, et al: Bleomycin toxicity simulating metastatic nodules to the lungs. Cancer 48:1096, 1981.
65. Dineen MK, Englander LS, Huben RP: Bleomycin-induced nodular pulmonary fibrosis masquerading as metastatic testicular cancer. J Urol 136:473, 1986.
66. Bellamy EA, Husband JE, Blaquiere RM, et al: Bleomycin-related lung damage: CT evidence. Radiology 156:155, 1985.
67. Rimmer MJ, Dixon AK, Flower CDR, et al: Bleomycin lung: Computed tomographic observations. Br J Radiol 58:1041, 1985.
68. Padley SPG, Adler B, Hansell DM, Müller NL: High-resolution computed tomography of drug-induced lung disease. Clin Radiol 46:232, 1992.
69. White DA, Schwartzberg LS, Kris MG, et al: Acute chest pain syndrome during bleomycin infusions. Cancer 59:1582, 1987.
70. Van Barneveld PWC, Sleijfer DT, van der Mark TW, et al: Natural course of bleomycin-induced pneumonitis: A follow-up study. Am Rev Respir Dis 135:48, 1987.

71. Pascual RS, Mosher MB, Sikand RS, et al: Effects of bleomycin on pulmonary function in man. Am Rev Respir Dis 108:211, 1973.

72. Perez-Guerra F, Harkleroad LE, Walsh RE, et al: Acute bleomycin lung. Am Rev Respir Dis 106:909, 1972.

73. Lewis BM, Izbicki R: Routine pulmonary function tests during bleomycin therapy: Tests may be ineffective and potentially misleading. JAMA 243:347, 1980.

74. Bell MR, Meredith DJ, Gill PG: Role of carbon monoxide diffusing capacity in the early detection of major bleomycin-induced pulmonary toxicity. Aust N Z J Med 15:235, 1985.

75. Sleijfer S, van der Mark TW, Schraffordt Koops H, et al: Decrease in pulmonary function during bleomycin-containing combination chemotherapy for testicular cancer: Not only a bleomycin effect. Br J Cancer 71:120, 1995.

76. Brown WG, Hasan FM, Barbee RA: Reversibility of severe bleomycin-induced pneumonitis. JAMA 239:2012, 1978.

77. Higa GM, AlKhouri N, Auber ML: Elevation of the erythrocyte sedimentation rate precedes exacerbation of bleomycin-induced pulmonary toxicity: Report of two cases and review of the literature. Pharmacotherapy 17:1315, 1997.

78. Twohig KJ, Matthay RA: Pulmonary effects of cytotoxic agents other than bleomycin. Clin Chest Med 11(1):31, 1990.

79. Rivera MP, Kris MG, Gralla RJ, et al: Syndrome of acute dyspnea related to combined mitomycin plus vinca alkaloid chemotherapy. Am J Clin Oncol 18:245, 1995.

80. Castro M, Veeder MH, Mailliard JA, et al: A prospective study of pulmonary function in patients receiving mitomycin. Chest 109:939, 1996.

81. Fielding JWL, Stockley RA, Brookes VS: Interstitial lung disease in a patient treated with 5-fluorouracil and mitomycin C. BMJ 2:602, 1978.

82. Torra R, Poch E, Torras A, et al: Pulmonary hemorrhage as a clinical manifestation of hemolytic-uremic syndrome associated with mitomycin C therapy. Chemotherapy 39:453, 1993.

83. Thomas P, Pradal M, Le Caer H, et al: Acute bronchospasm due to periwinkle alkaloid and mitomycin association. Rev Mal Respir 10:268, 1993.

84. Linette DC, McGee KH, McFarland JA. Mitomycin-induced pulmonary toxicity: Case report and review of the literature. Ann Pharmacother 26:481, 1992.

85. Okhuno SH, Frytak S: Mitomycin lung toxicity: Acute and chronic phases. Am J Clin Oncol 20:282, 1997.

86. Gunstream SR, Seidenfeld JJ, Sobonya RE, et al: Mitomycin-associated lung disease. Cancer Treat Rep 67:301, 1983.

87. Budzar AU, Legha SS, Luna MA, et al: Pulmonary toxicity of mitomycin. Cancer 45:236, 1980.

88. Orwoll ES, Kiessling PJ, Patterson JR: Interstitial pneumonia from mitomycin. Ann Intern Med 89:352, 1978.

89. Verweij J, van Zanten T, Souren T, et al: Prospective study on the dose relationship of mitomycin C-induced interstitial pneumonitis. Cancer 60:756, 1987.

90. Hoorn CM, Wagner JG, Petry TW, et al: Toxicity of mitomycin C toward cultured pulmonary artery endothelium. Toxicol Appl Pharmacol 130:87, 1995.

91. Kremer JM, Alarcon GS, Weinblatt ME, et al: Clinical, laboratory, radiographic, and histopathologic features of methotrexate-associated lung injury in patients with rheumatoid arthritis: A multicenter study with literature review. Arthritis Rheum 40:1829, 1997.

92. Jolivet J, Giroux L, Laurin S, et al: Microangiopathic hemolytic anemia, renal failure, and noncardiogenic pulmonary edema: A chemotherapy-induced syndrome. Cancer Treat Rep 67:429, 1983.

93. Waldhorn R, Tsou E, Smith F, et al: Pulmonary veno-occlusive disease associated with microangiopathic hemolytic anemia and chemotherapy of gastric adenocarcinoma. Med Pediatr Oncol 12:394, 1984.

94. Chang-Poon V, Hwang W, Wong A, et al: Pulmonary angiomatoid vascular changes in mitomycin C-associated hemolytic-uremic syndrome. Arch Pathol Lab Med 109:877, 1985.

95. Gunstream S, Seidenfeld J, Sobonya R, et al: Mitomycin-associated lung disease. Cancer Treat Rep 67:301, 1983.

96. Castro M, Veeder MH, Mailliard JA, et al: A prospective study of pulmonary function in patients receiving mitomycin. Chest 109:939, 1996.

97. Shinkai T, Saijo N, Tominaga K, et al: Pulmonary toxicity induced by pepleomycin 3-(S)-1-phenylethylaminol propylamino-bleomycin. Jpn J Clin Oncol 13:395, 1983.

98. Calvo D, Legha S, McKelvey E, et al: Zinostatin-related pulmonary toxicity. Cancer Treat Rep 65:165, 1981.

99. Selzer SE, Griffin T, D'Orsi C, et al: Pulmonary reaction associated with neocarzinostatin therapy. Cancer Treat Rep 62:1271, 1978.

100. Oliner H, Schwartz R, Rubio F, et al: Interstitial pulmonary fibrosis following busulfan therapy. Am J Med 31:134, 1961.

101. Leake E, Smith WG, Woodliff HJ: Diffuse interstitial pulmonary fibrosis after busulphan therapy. Lancet 2:432, 1963.

102. Crilley P, Topolsky D, Styler MJ, et al: Extramedullary toxicity of a conditioning regimen containing busulphan, cyclophosphamide and etoposide in 84 patients undergoing autologous and allogenic bone marrow transplantation. Bone Marrow Transplant 15:361, 1995.

103. Rosenthal MA, Grigg AP, Sheridan WP: High dose busulphan/cyclophosphamide for autologous bone marrow transplantation is associated with minimal non-hemapoietic toxicity. Leuk Lymphoma 14:279, 1994.

104. Ghalie R, Reynolds J, Valentino LA, et al: Busulfan-containing pre-transplant regimens for the treatment of solid tumors. Bone Marrow Transplant 14:437, 1994.

105. Przepiorka D, Dimopoulos M, Smith T, et al: Thiotepa, busulfan, and cyclophosphamide as a preparative regimen for marrow transplantation: Risk factors for early regimen-related toxicity. Ann Hematol 68:183, 1994.

106. Lund MB, Kongerud J, Brinch L, et al: Decreased lung function in one year survivors of allogenic bone marrow transplantation conditioned with high-dose busulfan and cyclophosphamide. Eur Respir J 8:1269, 1995.

107. Heard BE, Cooke RA: Busulphan lung. Thorax 23:187, 1968.

108. Ginsberg SJ, Comis RL: The pulmonary toxicity of antineoplastic agents. Semin Oncol 9:34, 1982.

109. Bates DV, Macklem PT, Christie RV: Respiratory Function in Disease: An Introduction to the Integrated Study of the Lung. 2nd ed. Philadelphia, WB Saunders, 1971.

110. Soble AR, Perry H: Fatal radiation pneumonia following subclinical busulfan injury. Am J Roentgenol 128:15, 1977.

111. Burns WA, McFarland W, Matthews MJ: Busulphan-induced pulmonary disease: Report of a case and review of the literature. Am Rev Respir Dis 101:408, 1970.

112. Koss LG, Melamed MR, Mayer K: The effect of busulfan on human epithelia. Am J Clin Pathol 44:385, 1965.

113. Littler WA, Kay JM, Hastleton PS, et al: Busulphan lung. Thorax 24:639, 1969.

114. Kirschner RH, Esterly JR: Pulmonary lesions associated with busulfan therapy of chronic myelogenous leukemia. Cancer 27:1074, 1971.

115. Kuplic JB, Higley CS, Niewoehner DE: Pulmonary ossification associated with long-term busulfan therapy in chronic myeloid leukemia: Case report. Am Rev Respir Dis 106:759, 1972.

116. Miyashita T, Ojima A, Tuji T, et al: Varied pulmonary lesions with intra-alveolar large lamellar bodies in an autopsy case with busulfan therapy. Acta Pathol Jpn 27:239, 1977.

117. Aymard J-P, Gyger M, Lavallee R, et al: A case of pulmonary alveolar proteinosis complicating chronic myelogenous leukemia: A peculiar pathologic aspect of busulfan lung? Cancer 53:954, 1984.

118. Smalley RV, Wall RL: Two cases of busulfan toxicity. Ann Intern Med 64:154, 1966.

119. Harrold BP: Syndrome resembling Addison's disease following prolonged treatment with busulphan. BMJ 1:463, 1966.

120. Podoll LN, Winkler SS: Busulfan lung: Report of two cases and review of the literature. Am J Roentgenol 120:151, 1974.

121. Littler WA, Ogilvie C: Lung function in patients receiving busulphan. BMJ 4:530, 1970.

122. Collis CH: Lung damage from cytotoxic drugs. Cancer Chemother Pharmacol 4:17, 1980.

123. Rosenow EC, Myers J, Swensen SJ, et al: Drug-induced pulmonary disease. Chest 102:239, 1992.

124. Wilczynski SW, Erasmus JJ, Petros WP, et al: Delayed pulmonary toxicity syndrome following high-dose chemotherapy and bone marrow transplantation for breast cancer. Am J Respir Crit Care Med 157:565, 1998.

125. Usui Y, Aida H, Kimula Y, et al: A case of cyclophosphamide-induced interstitial pneumonitis diagnosed by bronchoalveolar lavage. Respiration 59:125, 1992.

126. Malik SW, Myers JL, DeRemee RA, et al: Lung toxicity associated with cyclophosphamide use: Two distinct patterns. Am J Respir Crit Care Med 154:1851, 1996.

127. Gould VE, Miller J: Sclerosing alveolitis induced by cyclophosphamide: Ultrastructural observations on alveolar injury and repair. Am J Pathol 81:513, 1975.

128. Venkatesan N, Chandrakasan G: Cyclophosphamide induced early biochemical changes in lung lavage fluid and alterations in lavage cell function. Lung 172:147, 1994.

129. Kachel DL, Martin WJ II: Cyclophosphamide-induced lung toxicity: Mechanism of endothelial cell injury. J Pharmacol Exp Ther 268:42, 1994.

130. Baker WJ, Fistel SJ, Jones RV, et al: Interstitial pneumonitis associated with ifosfamide therapy. Cancer 65:2217, 1990.

131. Hakkinen PJ, Whiteley JW, Witschi HR: Hyperoxia, but not thoracic x-irradiation, potentiates bleomycin and cyclophosphamide-induced lung damage in mice. Am Rev Respir Dis 126:281, 1982.

132. Trask CW, Joannides T, Harper PG, et al: Radiation-induced lung fibrosis after treatment of small cell carcinoma of the lung with very high-dose cyclophosphamide. Cancer 55:47, 1985.

133. Burke DA, Stoddart JC, Ward MK, et al: Fatal pulmonary fibrosis occurring during treatment with cyclophosphamide. BMJ 285:696, 1982.

134. Karim F, Ayash R, Allam C, et al: Pulmonary fibrosis after prolonged treatment with low-dose cyclophosphamide. Oncology 40:174, 1983.

135. Mark G, Lehimgar-Zadeh A, Ragsdale B: Cyclophosphamide pneumonitis. Thorax 33:89, 1978.

136. Patel A, Shah P, Rhee H, et al: Cyclophosphamide therapy and interstitial pulmonary fibrosis. Cancer 38:1542, 1976.

137. Maxwell I: Reversible pulmonary edema following cyclophosphamide treatment. JAMA 229:137, 1974.

138. Spector JI, Zimbler H, Ross JS: Early-onset cyclophosphamide-induced interstitial pneumonitis. JAMA 242:2852, 1979.

139. Alvarado CS, Boat TF, Newman AJ: Late-onset pulmonary fibrosis and chest deformity in two children treated with cyclophosphamide. J Pediatr 92:443, 1978.

140. Abdel Karim FW, Ayash RE, Allam C, et al: Pulmonary fibrosis after prolonged treatment with low-dose cyclophosphamide: A case report. Oncology 40:174, 1983.

141. Mark GJ, Lehimgar-Zadeh A, Ragsdale BD: Cyclophosphamide pneumonitis. Thorax 33:89, 1978.

142. Giles FJ, Smith MP, Goldstone AH: Chlorambucil lung toxicity. Acta Haematol 83:156, 1990.

143. Carr ME Jr: Chlorambucil induced pulmonary fibrosis: Report of a case and review. Va Med 113:677, 1986.

144. Crestani B, Jaccard A, Israel-Biet D, et al: Chlorambucil-associated pneumonitis. Chest 105:634, 1994.

145. Mohr M, Kingreen D, Ruhl H, et al: Interstitial lung disease: An underdiagnosed side effect of chlorambucil? Ann Hematol 67:305, 1993.

146. Refvem O: Fatal intra-alveolar and interstitial lung fibrosis in chlorambucil-treated chronic lymphocytic leukemia. Mt Sinai J Med 44:847, 1977.

147. Cole SR, Myers TJ, Klatsky AU: Pulmonary disease with chlorambucil therapy. Cancer 41:455, 1978.

148. Godard P, Marty JP, Michel FB: Interstitial pneumonia and chlorambucil. Chest 76:471, 1979.

149. Clinicopathological conference. Two cases of drug-induced disease. Demonstration at the Royal College of Physicians of London. BMJ 2:1405, 1978.

150. Lane SD, Besa EC, Justh G, et al: Fatal interstitial pneumonitis following high-dose intermittent chlorambucil therapy for chronic lymphocytic leukemia. Cancer 47:32, 1981.

151. Major PP, Laurin S, Bettez P: Pulmonary fibrosis following therapy with melphalan: Report of two cases. Can Med Assoc J 123:197, 1980.

152. Morla J, Perez-Encinas M, Antela C, et al: Histiocytic lymphoma and pulmonary fibrosis in a female patient with essential thrombocythemia. Med Clin 100:104, 1993.

153. Taetle R, Dickman PS, Feldman PS, et al: Pulmonary histopathologic changes associated with melphalan therapy. Cancer 42:1239, 1978.

154. Goucher G, Rowland V, Hawkins J: Melphalan-induced pulmonary interstitial fibrosis. Chest 77:805, 1980.

155. Westerfield B, Michalski J, McCombs C, et al: Reversible melphalan-induced lung damage. Am J Med 68:767, 1980.

156. Codling BW, Chakera TM: Pulmonary fibrosis following therapy with melphalan for multiple myeloma. J Clin Pathol 25:668, 1972.

157. Westerfield BT, Michalski JP, McCombs C, et al: Reversible melphalan-induced lung damage. Am J Med 68:767, 1980.

158. Cherniack RM, Abrams J, Kalica AR: Pulmonary disease associated with breast cancer therapy. Am J Respir Crit Care Med 150:1169, 1994.

159. Rubio C, Hill ME, Milan S, et al: Idiopathic pneumonia syndrome after high-dose chemotherapy for relapsed Hodgkin's disease. Br J Cancer 75:1044, 1997.

160. Massin F, Coudert B, Foucher P, et al: Nitrosourea-induced lung diseases. Rev Mal Respir 9:575, 1992.

161. Lena H, Desrues B, Le Coz A, et al: Severe diffuse interstitial pneumonitis induced by carmustine (BCNU). Chest 105:1602, 1994.

162. Kalaycioglu M, Kavuru M, Tuason L, et al: Empiric prednisone therapy for pulmonary toxic reaction after high-dose chemotherapy containing carmustine (BCNU). Chest 107:482, 1995.

163. O'Driscoll BR, Kalra S, Gattamaneni HR, et al: Late carmustine lung fibrosis: Age at treatment may influence severity and survival. Chest 107:1355, 1995.

164. Patterson DL, Wiemann MC, Lee TH, et al: Carmustine toxicity presenting as a lobar infiltrate. Chest 104:315, 1993.

165. Cordonnier C, Vernant J-P, Mital P, et al: Pulmonary fibrosis subsequent to high doses of CCNU for chronic myeloid leukemia. Cancer 51:1814, 1983.

166. Dent RG: Fatal pulmonary toxic effects of lomustine. Thorax 37:627, 1982.

167. Lee W, Moore RP, Wampler GL: Interstitial pulmonary fibrosis as a complication of prolonged methyl-CCNU therapy. Cancer Treat Rep 62:1355, 1978.

168. Ryan BR, Walters TR: Pulmonary fibrosis: A complication of 1,3-bis(2-chloroethyl)-1-nitrosourea (BCNU) therapy. Cancer 48:909, 1981.

169. Todd NW, Peters WP, Ost AH, et al: Pulmonary drug toxicity in patients with primary breast cancer treated with high-dose combination chemotherapy and autologous bone marrow transplantation. Am Rev Respir Dis 147:1264, 1993.

170. Jones RB, Matthes S, Shpall EJ, et al: Acute lung injury following treatment with high-dose cyclophosphamide, cisplatin, and carmustine: Pharmacodynamic evaluation of carmustine. J Natl Cancer Inst 85:640, 1993.

171. Durant JR, Norgard, MJ, Murad TM, et al: Pulmonary toxicity associated with bischloroethylnitrosourea (BCNU). Ann Intern Med 90:191, 1979.

172. Selker RG, Jacobs SA, Moore PB: BCNU (1,3-bis(2-chloroethyl)-1-nitrosourea) induced pulmonary fibrosis. Neurosurgery 7:560, 1980.

173. Wolff SN, Phillips GL, Herzig GP: High-dose carmustine with autologous bone marrow transplantation for the adjuvant treatment of high-grade gliomas of the central nervous system. Cancer Treat Rep 71:183, 1987.

174. Aronin PA, Mahalev MS Jr, Rudnick SA, et al: Prediction of BCNU pulmonary toxicity in patients with malignant gliomas: An assessment of risk factors. N Engl J Med 303:83, 1980.

175. Melato M, Tuveri G: Pulmonary fibrosis following low-dose 1,3-bis(2-chloroethyl)-1-nitrosourea (BCNU) therapy. Cancer 45:1311, 1980.

176. Weinstein AS, Diener-West M, Nelson DF, et al: Pulmonary toxicity of carmustine in patients treated for malignant glioma. Cancer Treat Rep 70:943, 1986.

177. Thomas PS, Agrawal S, Gore M, et al: Recall lung pneumonitis due to carmustine after radiotherapy. Thorax 50:1116, 1995.

178. Holoye P, Jenkins D, Greenberg S: Pulmonary toxicity in long-term administration of BCNU. Cancer Treat Rep 60:1691, 1976.

179. Bellot PA, Valdiserri RO: Multiple pulmonary lesions in a patient treated with BCNU (1,3-bis(2-chloroethyl)-1-nitrosourea) for glioblastoma multiforme. Cancer 43:46, 1979.

180. Lombard CM, Churg A, Winokur S: Pulmonary veno-occlusive disease following therapy for malignant neoplasms. Chest 92:871, 1987.

181. Joselson R, Warnock M: Pulmonary veno-occlusive disease after chemotherapy. Hum Pathol 14:88, 1983.

182. Hasleton P, O'Driscoll B, Lynch P, et al: Late BCNU lung: A light and ultrastructural study on the delayed effect of BCNU on the lung parenchyma. J Pathol 164:31, 1991.

183. Aronchick JM, Gefter WB: Drug-induced pulmonary disorders. Semin Roentgenol 30:18, 1995.

184. Holoye P, Jenkins DE, Greenberg SD, et al: Pulmonary toxicity in long-term administration of BCNU. Cancer Treat Rep 60:1691, 1976.

185. Chap L, Shpiner R, Levine M, et al: Pulmonary toxicity of high-dose chemotherapy for breast cancer: A non-invasive approach to diagnosis and treatment. Bone Marrow Transplant 20:1063, 1997.

186. Weiss RB, Muggia FM: Pulmonary effects of carmustine. Ann Intern Med 91:131, 1979.

187. Brown MJ, Miller RR, Müller NL: Acute lung disease in the immunocompromised host: CT and pathologic examination findings. Radiology 190:247, 1994.

188. O'Driscoll BR, Hasleton PS, Taylor PM, et al: Active lung fibrosis up to 17 years after chemotherapy with carmustine (BCNU) in childhood. N Engl J Med 323:378, 1990.

189. Taylor PM, O'Driscoll BR, Gattamaneni HR, et al: Chronic lung fibrosis following carmustine (BCNU) chemotherapy: Radiological features. Clin Radiol 44:299, 1991.

190. Kumar M, Saleh A, Rao PV, et al: Toxicity associated with high-dose cytosine arabinoside and total body irradiation as conditioning for allogeneic bone marrow transplantation. Bone Marrow Transplant 19:1061, 1997.

191. Patten GA, Billi JE, Rotman HH: Rapidly progressive fatal pulmonary fibrosis induced by carmustine. JAMA 244:687, 1980.

192. Mitsudo SM, Greenwald ES, Banerji B, et al: BCNU (1,3-bis-(2-chloroethyl)-1-nitrosourea) lung: Drug-induced pulmonary changes. Cancer 54:751, 1984.

193. Rao SX, Ramaswamy G, Levin M, et al: Fatal acute respiratory failure after vinblastine-mitomycin therapy in lung carcinoma. Arch Intern Med 145:1905, 1985.

194. Konits P, Aisner J, Sutherland J, et al: Possible pulmonary toxicity secondary to vinblastine. Cancer 50:2771, 1982.

195. Bernini JC, Timmons CF, Sandler ES: Acute basophilic leukemia in a child: Anaphylactoid reaction and coagulopathy secondary to vincristine-mediated degranulation. Cancer 75:110, 1995.

196. Luedke D, McLaughlin TT, Daughaday C, et al: Mitomycin C and vindesine associated pulmonary toxicity with variable clinical expression. Cancer 55:542, 1985.

197. Figueredo AT, Jones G, Kay MJ, et al: Kaposi's sarcoma of the lung: Remission followed by fatal pneumonitis after vinblastine and thoracic irradiation. Acta Oncol 34:532, 1995.

198. Bott SJ, Stewart FM, Prince-Fiocco MA: Interstitial lung disease associated with vindesine and radiation therapy for carcinoma of the lung. South Med J 79:894, 1986.

199. Kouroukis C, Hings I: Respiratory failure following vinorelbine tartrate infusion in a patient with non-small cell lung cancer. Chest 112:846, 1997.

200. Cutuli B, Petit JC, Fricker JP, et al: Thromboembolic accidents in postmenopausal patients with adjuvant treatment by tamoxifen: Frequency, risk factors and prevention possibilities. Bull Cancer 82:51, 1995.

201. Pfitzenmeyer P, Foucher P, Piard F, et al: Nilutamide pneumonitis: A report on eight patients. Thorax 47:622, 1992.

202. Akoun GM, Liote HA, Liote F, et al: Provocation test coupled with bronchoalveolar lavage in diagnosis of drug (nilutamide)-induced hypersensitivity pneumonitis. Chest 97:495, 1990.

203. Gomez JL, Dupont A, Cusan L, et al: Simultaneous liver and lung toxicity related to the nonsteroidal antiandrogen Nilutamide (Anandron): A case report. Am J Med 92:563, 1992.

204. Seigneur J, Trechot PF, Hubert J, et al: Pulmonary complications of hormone treatment in prostate carcinoma. Chest 93:1106, 1988.

205. Wong PW, Macris N, DiFabrizio L, et al: Eosinophilic lung disease induced by bicalutamide: A case report and review of the medical literature. Chest 113:548, 1998.

206. Bacigalupo A, Frassoni F, van Lint MT, et al: Cyclosporin A in marrow transplantation for leukemia and aplastic anemia. Exp Hematol 13:244, 1985.

207. Morales P, Cremades MJ, Pallardo L, et al: Effect of cyclosporin on lung diffusing capacity in renal transplant patients. Transpl Int 8:481, 1995.

208. Cersosimo RJ, Licciardello JT, Matthews SJ, et al: Acute pneumonitis associated with MOPP chemotherapy of Hodgkin's disease. Drug Intell Clin Pharm 18:609, 1984.

209. Ecker MD, Jay B, Keohane MF: Procarbazine lung. Am J Roentgenol 131:527, 1978.

210. Coyle T, Bushunow P, Winfield J, et al: Hypersensitivity reactions to procarbazine with mechlorethamine, vincristine and procarbazine chemotherapy in the treatment of glioma. Cancer 69:2532, 1992.

211. Araki N, Matsumot K, Ikuta N, et al: A case of drug induced pneumonitis caused by oral etoposide. Nippon Kyobu Shikkan Gakkai Zasshi 31:903, 1993.

212. Dajczman E, Srolovitz H, Kreisman H, et al: Fatal pulmonary toxicity oral etoposide therapy. Lung Cancer 12:81, 1995.

213. Barrera P, Laan RF, van Riel PL, et al: Methotrexate-related pulmonary complications in rheumatoid arthritis. Ann Rheum Dis 53:434, 1994.

214. Carroll GC, Thomas R, Phatouros CC, et al: Incidence, prevalence and possible risk factors for pneumonitis in patients with rheumatoid arthritis receiving methotrexate. J Rheumatol 21:51, 1994.

215. Hargreaves MR, Mowat AG, Benson MK: Acute pneumonitis associated with low dose methotrexate treatment for rheumatoid arthritis: Report of five cases and review of published reports. Thorax 47:628, 1992.

216. Goodman TA, Polusson RP: Methotrexate: Adverse reactions and major toxicities. Rheum Dis Clin North Am 20:513, 1994.

217. Tsai JJ, Shin JF, Chen CH, et al: Methotrexate pneumonitis in bronchial asthma. Int Arch Allergy Immunol 100:287, 1993.
218. Sharma A, Provenzale D, McKusick A, et al: Interstitial pneumonitis after low-dose methotrexate therapy in primary biliary cirrhosis. Gastroenterology 107:266, 1994.
219. White DA, Rankin JA, Stover DE, et al: Methotrexate pneumonitis: Bronchoalveolar lavage findings suggest an immunologic disorder. Am Rev Respir Dis 139:18, 1989.
220. Leduc D, De Vuyst P, Lheureux P, et al: Pneumonitis complicating low-dose methotrexate therapy for rheumatoid arthritis: Discrepancies between lung biopsy and bronchoalveolar lavage findings. Chest 104:1620, 1993.
221. Bedrossian CWM, Miller WC, Luna MA: Methotrexate-induced diffuse interstitial pulmonary fibrosis. South Med J 72:313, 1979.
222. Hilliquin P, Renoux M, Perrot S, et al: Occurrence of pulmonary complications during methotrexate therapy in rheumatoid arthritis. Br J Rheumatol 35:441, 1996.
223. Clarysse AM, Cathey WJ, Cartwright GE, et al: Pulmonary disease complicating intermittent therapy with methotrexate. JAMA 209:1861, 1969.
224. Cooperative study. Acute lymphocytic leukemia in children: Maintenance therapy with methotrexate administered intermittently. Acute leukemia group B. JAMA 207:923, 1969.
225. Carson CW, Cannon GW, Egger MJ, et al: Pulmonary disease during the treatment of rheumatoid arthritis with low-dose pulse methotrexate. Semin Arthritis Rheum 16:186, 1987.
226. Salaffi F, Manganelli P, Carotti M, et al: Methotrexate-induced pneumonitis in patients with rheumatoid arthritis and psoriatic arthritis: Report of five cases and review of the literature. Clin Rheumatol 16:296, 1997.
227. Gillespie AM, Lorigan PC, Radstone CR, et al: Pulmonary function in patients with trophoblastic disease treated with low-dose methotrexate. Br J Cancer 76:1382, 1997.
228. Schnabel A, Richter C, Bauerfeind S, et al: Bronchoalveolar lavage cell profile in methotrexate induced pneumonitis. Thorax 52:377, 1997.
229. Akoun GM, Gauthier-Rahman S, Mayaud CM, et al: Leukocyte migration inhibition in methotrexate induced pneumonitis: Evidence for an immunologic cell-mediated mechanism. Chest 91:96, 1987.
230. Golden MR, Katz RS, Balk RA, et al: The relationship of preexisting lung disease to the development of methotrexate pneumonitis in patients with rheumatoid arthritis. J Rheumatol 22:1043, 1995.
231. Alarcon GS, Kremer JM, Macaluso M, et al: Risk factors for methotrexate-induced lung injury in patients with rheumatoid arthritis. Ann Intern Med 127:356, 1997.
232. Everts CS, Westcott JL, Bragg DG: Methotrexate therapy and pulmonary disease. Radiology 107:539, 1973.
233. Sostman HD, Matthay RA, Putman CE, et al: Methotrexate-induced pneumonitis. Medicine 55:371, 1976.
234. Leduc D, De Vuyst P, Lheureux P, et al: Pneumonitis complicating low-dose methotrexate therapy for rheumatoid arthritis: Discrepancies between lung biopsy and bronchoalveolar lavage findings. Chest 104:1620, 1993.
235. St. Clair E, Rice J, Snyderman R: Pneumonitis complicating low-dose methotrexate therapy in rheumatoid arthritis. Arch Intern Med 145:2035, 1985.
236. Bernstein M, Sobel D, Wimmer R: Noncardiogenic pulmonary edema following injection of methotrexate into the cerebrospinal fluid. Cancer 50:866, 1982.
237. Cannon G, Ward J, Clegg D, et al: Acute lung disease associated with low-dose pulse methotrexate therapy in patients with rheumatoid arthritis. Arthritis Rheum 26:1269, 1983.
238. Case Records of the Massachusetts General Hospital. N Engl J Med 323:737, 1990.
239. Lisbona A, Schwartz J, Lachance C, et al: Methotrexate-induced pulmonary disease. J Can Assoc Radiol 24:215, 1973.
240. Filip DJ, Logue GL, Harle TS, et al: Pulmonary and hepatic complications of methotrexate therapy of psoriasis. JAMA 216:881, 1971.
241. Schwartz IR, Kajani MK: Methotrexate therapy and pulmonary disease. JAMA 210:1924, 1969.
242. Whitcomb ME, Schwarz MI, Tormey DC: Methotrexate pneumonitis: Case report and review of the literature. Thorax 27:636, 1972.
243. Kaplan RL, Waite DH: Progressive interstitial lung disease from prolonged methotrexate therapy. Arch Dermatol 114:1800, 1978.
244. Elsasser S, Dalquen P, Soler M, et al: Methotrexate-induced pneumonitis: Appearance four weeks after discontinuation of treatment. Am Rev Respir Dis 140:1089, 1989.
245. Kremer JM, Alarcon GS, Weinblatt ME, et al: Clinical, laboratory, radiographic, and histopathologic features of methotrexate-associated lung injury in patients with rheumatoid arthritis: A multicenter study with literature review. Arthritis Rheum 40:1829, 1997.
246. Schnabel A, Dalhoff K, Bauerfeind S, et al: Sustained cough in methotrexate therapy for rheumatoid arthritis. Clin Rheumatol 15:277, 1996.
247. Cooper JAD Jr, White DA, Matthay RA: Drug-induced pulmonary disease. Part 1. Cytotoxic drugs. Am Rev Respir Dis 133:321, 1986.
248. Jones G, Mierins E, Karsh J: Methotrexate-induced asthma. Am Rev Respir Dis 143:179, 1991.
249. Colsky J, Greenspan EM, Warren TN: Hepatic fibrosis in children with acute leukemia after therapy with folic acid antagonists. Arch Pathol 59:198, 1955.
250. Muller SA, Farrow GM, Martalock DL: Clinical studies: Cirrhosis caused by methotrexate in the treatment of psoriasis. Arch Dermatol 100:523, 1969.
251. Epstein EH Jr, Croft JD Jr: Cirrhosis following methotrexate administration for psoriasis. Arch Dermatol 100:531, 1969.
252. Coe RO, Bull FE: Cirrhosis associated with methotrexate treatment of psoriasis. JAMA 206:1515, 1968.
253. Robertson HH: Medical memoranda: Pneumonia and methotrexate. BMJ 2:156, 1970.
254. Clair EW, Rice JR, Snyderman R: Pneumonitis complicating low-dose methotrexate therapy in rheumatoid arthritis. Arch Intern Med 145:2035, 1985.
255. Dayton CS, Schwartz DA, Sprince NL, et al: Low-dose methotrexate may cause air trapping in patients with rheumatoid arthritis. Am J Respir Crit Care Med 151:1189, 1995.
256. Cottin V, Tebib J, Massonet B, et al: Pulmonary function in patients receiving long-term low-dose methotrexate. Chest 109:933, 1996.
257. Kuitert LM, Harrison AC: *Pneumocystis carinii* pneumonia as a complication of methotrexate treatment of asthma. Thorax 46:936, 1991.
258. Kane GC, Troshinsky MB, Peters SP, et al: *Pneumocystis carinii* pneumonia associated with weekly methotrexate: Cumulative dose of methotrexate and low CD4 cell count may predict this complication. Respir Med 87:153, 1993.
259. Okuda Y, Oyama T, Oyama H, et al: *Pneumocystis carinii* pneumonia associated with low dose methotrexate treatment for malignant rheumatoid arthritis. Ryumachi 35:699, 1995.
260. Shiroky JB, Frost A, Skelton JD, et al: Complications of immunosuppression associated with weekly low dose methotrexate. J Rheumatol 18:1172, 1991.
261. O'Reilly S, Hartley P, Jeffers M, et al: Invasive pulmonary aspergillosis associated with low dose methotrexate therapy for rheumatoid arthritis: A case report of treatment with itraconazole. Tuber Lung Dis 72:153, 1994.
262. Law KF, Aranda CP, Smith RL, et al: Pulmonary cryptococcosis mimicking methotrexate pneumonitis. J Rheumatol 20:872, 1993.
263. Cannon GW, Ward JR, Clegg DO, et al: Acute lung disease associated with low-dose pulse methotrexate therapy in patients with rheumatoid arthritis. Arthritis Rheum 26:1269, 1983.
264. Engelbrecht JA, Calhoon SL, Scherrer JJ: Methotrexate pneumonitis after low-dose therapy for rheumatoid arthritis. Arthritis Rheum 26:1275, 1983.
265. Manni JJ, Van den Broek P: Pulmonary complications of methotrexate therapy. Clin Otolaryngol 2:131, 1977.
266. Andersson BS, Cogan BM, Keating MJ, et al: Subacute pulmonary failure complicating therapy with high-dose ara-C in acute leukemia. Cancer 56:2181, 1985.
267. Hui KK, Keating MJ, McCredie KB: Fatal pulmonary failure complicating high-dose cytosine arabinoside therapy in acute leukemia. Cancer 65:1079, 1990.
268. Shearer P, Katz J, Bozeman P, et al: Pulmonary insufficiency complicating therapy with high dose cytosine arabinoside in five pediatric patients with relapsed acute myelogenous leukemia. Cancer 74:1953, 1994.
269. Chiche D, Pico JL, Bernaudin JF, et al: Pulmonary edema and shock after high-dose aracytosine-C for lymphoma: Possible role of TNF-alpha and PAF. Eur Cytokine Netw 4:147, 1993.
270. Reed CR, Glauser FL: Drug-induced noncardiogenic pulmonary edema. Chest 100:1120, 1991.
271. Haupt H, Hutchins G, Moore G: Ara-C lung: Noncardiogenic pulmonary edema complicating cytosine arabinoside therapy of leukemia. Am J Med 70:256, 1981.
271a. Battistini E, Dini G, Savioli C, et al: Bronchiolitis obliterans organizing pneumonia in three children with acute leukaemias treated with cytosine arabinoside and anthracyclines. Eur Respir J 10:1187, 1997.
272. Tjon A, Tham RTO, Peters WG, de Bruine FT, et al: Pulmonary complications of cytosine-arabinoside therapy: Radiographic findings. Am J Roentgenol 149:23, 1987.
273. Tham RT, Peters WG, de Bruine FT, et al: Pulmonary complications of cytosine-arabinoside therapy: Radiographic findings. Am J Roentgenol 149:23, 1987.
273a. Hui YF, Reitz J: Gemcitabine: A cytidine analogue active against solid tumors. Am J Health-Syst Pharm 54:162, 1997.
273b. Pavlakis N, Bell DR, Millward MJ, et al: Fatal pulmonary toxicity resulting from treatment with gemcitabine. Cancer 80:286, 1997.
273c. Marruchella A, Fiorenzano G, Merizzi A, et al: Diffuse alveolar damage in a patient treated with gemcitabine. Eur Respir J 11:504, 1998.
274. Saway PA, Heck LW, Bonner JR, et al: Azathioprine hypersensitivity: Case report and review of the literature. Am J Med 84:960, 1988.
275. Bedrossian CWM, Sussman J, Conklin RH, et al: Azathioprine-associated interstitial pneumonitis. Am J Clin Pathol 82:148, 1984.
276. Krowka M, Breuer R, Kehoe T: Azathioprine-associated pulmonary dysfunction. Chest 83:696, 1983.
277. Weisenburger D: Interstitial pneumonitis associated with azathioprine therapy. Am J Clin Pathol 69:181, 1978.
278. Stetter M, Schmidl M, Krapf R, et al: Azathioprine hypersensitivity mimicking Goodpasture's syndrome. Am J Kidney Dis 23:874, 1994.
279. Refabert L, Sinnassamy P, Leroy B, et al: Azathioprine-induced pulmonary haemorrhage in a child after renal transplantation. Pediatr Nephrol 9:470, 1995.
280. Weisenburger DD: Interstitial pneumonitis associated with azathioprine therapy. J Clin Pathol 69:181, 1978.
281. Kane GC, McMichael AJ, Patrick H, et al: Pulmonary toxicity and acute respiratory failure associated with fludarabine monophosphate. Respir Med 86:261, 1992.
281a. Cutler C, Samman Y, Fraser R, et al: Recurrent acute pulmonary toxicity and respiratory failure associated with fludarabine monophosphate. Can Respir J 4:331, 1997.
282. Byrd JC, Hargis JB, Kester KE, et al: Opportunistic pulmonary infections with fludarabine in previously treated patients with low-grade lymphoid malignancies: A role for pneumocystis carinii pneumonia prophylaxis. Am J Hematol 49:135, 1995.

283. Gugliotta L, Mazzucconi MG, Leone G, et al: Incidence of thrombotic complications in adult patients with acute lymphoblastic leukaemia receiving L-asparaginase during induction therapy: A retrospective study. The GIMEMA group. Eur J Haematol 49:63, 1992.

284. Manheimer F, Aranda CP, Smith RL: Necrotizing pneumonitis caused by 5-fluorouracil infusion: A complication of a Hickman catheter. Cancer 70:554, 1992.

285. Vogelzang PJ, Bloom SM, Mier JW, et al: Chest roentgenographic abnormalities in IL-2 recipients. Chest 101:746, 1992.

286. Baluna R, Vitetta ES: Vascular leak syndrome: A side effect of immunotherapy. Immunopharmacology 37:117, 1997.

287. Conant EF, Fox KR, Miller WT: Pulmonary edema as a complication of interleukin-2 therapy. Am J Roentgenol 152:749, 1989.

288. Berthiaume Y, Boiteau P, Fick G, et al: Pulmonary edema during IL-2 therapy: Combined effect of increased permeability and hydrostatic pressure. Am J Respir Crit Care Med 152:329, 1995.

289. Rabinovici R, Feuerstein G, Abdullah F, et al: Locally produced tumor necrosis factor-alpha mediates interleukin-2-induced lung injury. Circ Res 78:329, 1996.

290. Dubinett SM, Huang M, Lichtenstein A, et al: Tumor necrosis factor-alpha plays a central role in interleukin-2-induced pulmonary vascular leak and lymphocyte accumulation. Cell Immunol 157:170, 1994.

291. Klausner JM, Goldman G, Skornick Y, et al: Interleukin-2-induced lung permeability is mediated by leukotriene B4. Cancer 1:2357, 1990.

292. DeJoy SQ, Jeyaseelan R Sr, Torley LW, et al: Attenuation of interleukin 2-induced pulmonary vascular leak syndrome by low doses of oral methotrexate. Cancer Res 55:4929, 1995.

293. Ardizzoni A, Bonavia M, Viale M, et al: Biologic and clinical effects of continuous infusion interleukin-2 in patients with non-small cell lung cancer. Cancer 73:1353, 1994.

294. Villani F, Galimberti M, Rizzi M, et al: Pulmonary toxicity of recombinant interleukin-2 plus lymphokine-activated killer cell therapy. Eur Respir J 6:828, 1993.

295. Kuei JH, Tashkin DP, Figlin RA: Pulmonary toxicity of recombinant human tumour necrosis factor. Chest 96:334, 1989.

296. Villani F, Galimberti M, Mazzola G, et al: Pulmonary toxicity of alpha tumor necrosis factor in patients treated by isolation perfusion. J Chemother 7:452, 1995.

297. Schilling PJ, Murray JL, Markowitz AB: Novel tumor necrosis factor toxic effects: Pulmonary hemorrhage and severe hepatic dysfunction. Cancer 69:256, 1992.

298. Seebach J, Speich R, Fehr J, et al: GM-CSF-induced eosinophilic pneumonia. Br J Haematol 90:963, 1995.

299. Ogata K, Koga T, Yagawa K: Interferon-related bronchiolitis obliterans organizing pneumonia. Chest 106:612, 1994.

300. Harris J, Bines S, Das Gupta T: Therapy of disseminated malignant melanoma with recombinant alpha 2b-interferon and piroxicam: Clinical results with a report of an unusual response-associated feature (vitiligo) and unusual toxicity (diffuse pulmonary interstitial fibrosis). Med Pediatr Oncol 22:103, 1994.

301. Chin K, Tabata C, Satake N, et al: Pneumonitis associated with natural and recombinant interferon alpha therapy for chronic hepatitis C. Chest 105:939, 1994.

302. Moriya K, Yasuda K, Koike K, et al: Induction of interstitial pneumonitis during interferon treatment for chronic hepatitis C. J Gastroenterol 29:514, 1994.

303. Becker JC, Winkler B, Klingert S, et al: Antiphospholipid syndrome associated with immunotherapy for patients with melanoma. Cancer 73:1621, 1994.

304. Cooper JAD Jr, White DA, Matthay RA: Drug-induced pulmonary disease. Part 2. Noncytotoxic drugs. Am Rev Respir Dis 133:488, 1986.

305. Geller M, Flaherty DK, Dickie HA, et al: Lymphopenia in acute nitrofurantoin pleuropulmonary reactions. J Allergy Clin Immunol 59:445, 1977.

306. Koch-Weser J, Sidel VW, Dexter M, et al: Adverse reactions to sulfisoxazole, sulfamethoxazole and nitrofurantoin, manifestations and specific reaction rates during 2,118 courses of therapy. Arch Intern Med 128:399, 1971.

307. Murray MJ, Kronenberg R: Pulmonary reactions simulating cardiac pulmonary edema caused by nitrofurantoin. N Engl J Med 273:1185, 1965.

308. Hailey FJ, Glascock HW Jr, Hewitt WF: Pleuropneumonic reactions to nitrofurantoin. N Engl J Med 281:1087, 1969.

309. Simonian SJ, Kroeker EJ, Boyd DP: Chronic interstitial pneumonitis with fibrosis after long-term therapy with nitrofurantoin. Ann Thorac Surg 24:284, 1977.

310. Holmberg L, Boman G, Bottiger LE, et al: Adverse reactions to nitrofurantoin: Analysis of 921 reports. Am J Med 69:733, 1980.

311. Averbuch SD, Yungbluth P: Fatal pulmonary hemorrhage due to nitrofurantoin. Arch Intern Med 140:271, 1980.

312. Jick SS, Jick H, Walker AM, et al: Hospitalizations for pulmonary reactions following nitrofurantoin use. Chest 96:512, 1989.

313. Penn RG, Griffin JP: Adverse reactions to nitrofurantoin in the United Kingdom, Sweden, and Holland. BMJ 284:1440, 1982.

314. Suntres ZE, Shek PN: Nitrofurantoin-induced pulmonary toxicity: *In vivo* evidence of oxidative stress-mediated mechanisms. Biochem Pharmacol 43:1127, 1992.

315. Rosenow EC III, DeRemee RA, Dines DE: Chronic nitrofurantoin pulmonary reaction: Report of five cases. N Engl J Med 279:1258, 1968.

316. Willcox PA, Maze SS, Sandler M, et al: Pulmonary fibrosis following long-term nitrofurantoin therapy. S Afr Med J 61:714, 1982.

317. Bone RC, Wolfe J, Sobonya RE, et al: Desquamative interstitial pneumonia following long term nitrofurantoin therapy. Am J Med 60:697 1976.

318. Geller M, Dickie H, Kass D, et al: The histopathology of acute nitrofurantoin-associated pneumonitis. Ann Allergy 37:275, 1976.

319. Nakamura F, Andoh A, Minamiguchi H, et al: A case of interstitial pneumonitis associated with natural alpha-interferon threapy for myelofibrosis. Acta Haematol 97:222, 1997.

320. Magee F, Wright J, Chan N, et al: Two unusual pathological reactions to nitrofurantoin: Case reports. Histopathology 10:701, 1986.

321. Muir DCF, Stanton JA: Allergic pulmonary infiltration due to nitrofurantoin. BMJ 1:1072, 1963.

322. Nicklaus TM, Snyder AB: Nitrofurantoin pulmonary reaction. A unique syndrome. Arch Intern Med 121:151, 1968.

323. Ngan H, Millard RJ, Lant AF, et al: Nitrofurantoin lung. Br J Radiol 44:21, 1971.

324. Holmberg L, Boman G: Pulmonary reactions to nitrofurantoin: 447 cases reported to the Swedish Adverse Drug Reaction Committee 1966-1976. Eur J Respir Dis 62:180, 1981.

325. Israel RH, Gross RA, Bomba PA: Adult respiratory distress syndrome associated with acute nitrofurantoin toxicity: Successful treatment with continuous positive airway pressure. Respiration 39:318, 1980.

326. Strauss WG, Griffin LM: Nitrofurantoin pneumonia. JAMA 199:765, 1967.

327. Lee NK, Slavin JD Jr, Spencer RP: Ventilation-perfusion lung imaging in nitrofurantoin-related pulmonary reaction. Clin Nucl Med 17:94, 1992.

328. Bone RC, Wolfe J, Sobonyar RE, et al: Desquamative interstitial pneumonia following chronic nitrofurantoin therapy. Chest 69(Suppl):296, 1976.

329. Sollaccio PA, Ribaudo CA, Grace WJ: Subacute pulmonary infiltration due to nitrofurantoin. Ann Intern Med 65:1284, 1966.

330. Taskinen E, Tukiainen P, Sovijarvi AR: Nitrofurantoin-induced alterations in pulmonary tissue: A report on five patients with acute or subacute reactions. Acta Pathol Microbiol Scand (A) 85:713, 1977.

331. Robinson BW: Nitrofurantoin-induced interstitial pulmonary fibrosis: Presentation and outcome. Med J Aust 22:72, 1983.

332. Meyer MM, Meyer RJ: Nitrofurantoin-induced pulmonary hemorrhage in a renal transplant recipient receiving immunosuppressive therapy: Case report and review of the literature. J Urol 152:938, 1994.

333. Berliner S, Neeman A, Shoenfeld Y, et al: Salazopyrin-induced eosinophilic pneumonia. Respiration 39:119, 1980.

334. Williams T, Eidus L, Thomas P: Fibrosing alveolitis, bronchiolitis obliterans, and sulfasalazine therapy. Chest 81:766, 1982.

335. Sigvaldason A, Sorenson S: Interstitial pneumonia due to sulfasalazine. Eur J Respir Dis 64:229, 1983.

336. Averbuch M, Halpern Z, Hallak A, et al: Sulfasalazine pneumonitis. Am J Gastroenterol 80:343, 1985.

337. Yaffe BH, Korelitz BI: Sulfasalazine pneumonitis. Am J Gastroenterol 78:493, 1983.

338. Cazzadori A, Braggio P, Bontempini L: Salazopyrin-induced eosinophilic pneumonia. Respiration 47:158, 1985.

339. Teague WG, Sutphen JL, Fechner RE: Desquamative interstitial pneumonitis complicating inflammatory bowel disease of childhood. J Pediatr Gastroenterol Nutr 4:663, 1985.

340. Abdulgany M, Atkinson J, Smith LJ: Sulfasalazine-induced pulmonary disease. Chest 101:1033, 1992.

341. Moss SF, Ind PW: Time course of recovery of lung function in sulphasalazine-induced alveolitis. Respir Med 85:73, 1991.

342. Kolbe J, Caughey D, Rainer S: Sulphasalazine-induced sub-acute hyper-sensitivity pneumonitis. Respir Med 88:149, 1994.

343. Timmer R, Duurkens VA, van Hees PA: Sulphasalazine-induced eosinophilic pneumonia. Neth J Med 41:153, 1992.

344. Gabazza EC, Taguchi O, Yamakami T, et al: Pulmonary infiltrates and skin pigmentation associated with sulfasalazine. Am J Gastroenterol 87:1654, 1992.

345. Yamakado S, Yoshida Y, Yamada T, et al: Pulmonary infiltration and eosinophilia associated with sulfasalazine therapy for ulcerative colitis: A case report and review of literature. Intern Med 31:108, 1992.

346. Kolbe J, Caughey D, Rainer S: Sulphasalazine-induced sub-acute hyper-sensitivity pneumonitis. Respir Med 88:149, 1994.

347. Valcke Y, Pauwels R, Van der Straeten M: Bronchoalveolar lavage in acute hypersensitivity pneumonitis caused by sulfasalazine. Chest 92:572, 1987.

348. Cooper JAD Jr, Matthay RA: Drug-induced pulmonary disease. *In* Bone RC (ed): Disease-a-Month. Vol 33. Chicago, Year Book Medical Publishers, 1987, pp 61.

349. Camus P, Piard F, Ashcroft T, et al: The lung in inflammatory bowel disease. Medicine 72:151, 1993.

350. Salerno SM, Ormseth EJ, Roth BJ, et al: Sulfasalazine pulmonary toxicity in ulcerative colitis mimicking clinical features of Wegener's granulomatosis. Chest 110:556, 1996.

351. Ho D, Tashkin DP, Bein ME, et al: Pulmonary infiltrates with eosinophilia associated with tetracycline. Chest 76:33, 1979.

352. Dykhuizen RS, Zaidi AM, Godden DJ, et al: Minocycline and pulmonary eosinophilia. BMJ 310:1520, 1995.

353. Dykhuizen RS, Legge JS: Minocycline induced pulmonary eosinophilia. Respir Med 89:61, 1995.

354. Kaufmann D, Pichler W, Beer JH: Severe episode of high fever with rash, lymphadenopathy, neutropenia, and eosinophilia after minocycline therapy for acne. Arch Intern Med 154:1983, 1994.

355. Bando T, Fujimura M, Noda Y, et al: Minocycline-induced pneumonitis with bilateral hilar lymphadenopathy and pleural effusion. Intern Med 33:177, 1994.

356. Sitbon O, Bidel N, Dussopt C, et al: Minocycline pneumonitis and eosinophilia: A report on eight patients. Arch Intern Med 154:1633, 1994.

357. Guillon JM, Joly P, Autran B, et al: Minocycline-induced cell-mediated hypersensitivity pneumonitis. Ann Intern Med 117:476, 1992.
358. Piperno D, Donne C, Loire R, et al: Bronchiolitis obliterans organizing pneumonia associated with minocycline therapy: A possible cause. Eur Respir J 8:1018, 1995.
359. Dussopt C, Mornez JF, Cordier JF, et al: Acute eosinophilic lung after a course of minocycline. Rev Mal Respir 11:67, 1994.
360. Horikx PE, Gooszen HC: Minocycline as a cause of acute eosinophilic pneumonia. Ned Tijdschr Geneeskd 136:530, 1992.
361. Haruna T, Mochizuki Y, Nakahara Y, et al: A case of minocycline-induced pneumonitis with bronchial asthma. Nippon Kyobu Shikkan Gakkai Zasshi 32:671, 1994.
362. Daniel PT, Holzschuh J, Berg PA: Sulfadoxine specific lymphocyte transformation in a patient with eosinophilic pneumonia induced by sulfadoxine-pyrimethamine (Fansidar). Thorax 44:307, 1989.
363. Otero M, Goodpasture HC: Pulmonary infiltrates and eosinophilia from minocycline. JAMA 250:2602, 1983.
364. Osanai S, Fukuzawa J, Akiba Y, et al: Minocycline-induced pneumonia and pleurisy: A case report. Nippon Kyobu Shikkan Gakkai Zasshi 30:322, 1992.
365. Fiegenberg DS, Weiss H, Kirshman H: Migratory pneumonia with eosinophilia associated with sulfonamide administration. Arch Intern Med 120:85, 1967.
366. Donlan CJ, Scutero JV: Transient eosinophilic pneumonia secondary to use of a vaginal cream. Chest 67:232, 1975.
367. Reichlin S, Loveless MH, Kane EG: Loeffler's syndrome following penicillin therapy. Ann Intern Med 38:113, 1953.
368. Wold DE, Zahn DW: Allergic (Löffler's) pneumonitis occurring during antituberculous chemotherapy: Report of three cases. Am Rev Tuberc 74:445, 1956.
369. Wong PC, Yew WW, Wong CF, et al: Ethambutol-induced pulmonary infiltrates with eosinophilia and skin involvement. Eur Respir J 8:866, 1995.
370. Poe R, Condemi J, Weinstein S, et al: Adult respiratory distress syndrome related to ampicillin sensitivity. Chest 77:449, 1980.
371. Begbie S, Burgess KR: Maloprim-induced pulmonary eosinophilia. Chest 103:305, 1993.
372. Dreis DF, Winterbauer RH, Van Norman GA, et al: Cephalosporin-induced interstitial pneumonitis. Chest 86:138, 1984.
373. Pang JA: Non-cardiogenic pulmonary oedema associated with pyrimethamine. Respir Med 83:247, 1989.
374. Cass RM: Adult respiratory distress syndrome and trimethoprim sulfamethoxazole (letter). Ann Intern Med 106:331, 1987.
375. Levine SJ, Walsh TJ, Martinez A, et al: Cardiopulmonary toxicity after liposomal amphotericin B infusion. Ann Intern Med 114:664, 1991.
376. Arning M, Heer-Sonderhoff AH, Wehmeier A, et al: Pulmonary toxicity during infusion of liposomal amphotericin B in two patients with acute leukemia. Eur J Clin Microbiol Infect Dis 14:41, 1995.
377. Wright DG, Robichaud KJ, Pizzo PA, et al: Lethal pulmonary reactions associated with the combined use of amphotericin B and leukocyte transfusions. N Engl J Med 304:1185, 1981.
378. Dana BW, Durie BGM, White RF, et al: Concomitant administration of granulocyte transfusions and amphotericin B in neutropenic patients: Absence of significant pulmonary toxicity. Blood 57:90, 1981.
379. Dutcher JP, Kendall J, Norris D, et al: Granulocyte transfusion therapy and amphotericin B: Adverse reactions? Am J Hematol 31:102, 1989.
380. Inoue M, Tanigawa S, Masutani M, et al: A case of piperacillin-induced pneumonitis. Nippon Kyobu Shikkan Gakkai Zasshi 31:530, 1993.
381. Dreis DF, Winterbauer RH, Van Norman GA, et al: Cephalosporin-induced interstitial pneumonitis. Chest 86:138, 1984.
382. de Hoyos A, Holness DL, Tarlo SM: Hypersensitivity pneumonitis and airways hyperreactivity induced by occupational exposure to penicillin. Chest 103:303, 1993.
383. Yonemaru M, Mizuguchi Y, Kasuga I, et al: Hilar and mediastinal lymphadenopathy with hypersensitivity pneumonitis induced by penicillin. Chest 102:1907, 1992.
384. Marchlinski FE, Gansler TS, Waxman HL, et al: Amiodarone pulmonary toxicity. Ann Intern Med 97:839, 1982.
385. Rakita L, Sobol SM, Mostow N, et al: Amiodarone pulmonary toxicity. Am Heart J 106(4 Pt 2):906, 1983.
386. Kowey PR, Friehling TD, Marinchak RA, et al: Safety and efficacy of amiodarone: The low-dose perspective. Chest 93:54, 1988.
387. Adams GD, Kehoe R, Lesch M, et al: Amiodarone-induced pneumonitis: Assessment of risk factors and possible risk reduction. Chest 93:253, 1988.
388. Dean PJ, Groshart KD, Porterfield JG, et al: Amiodarone-associated pulmonary toxicity: A clinical and pathologic study of eleven cases. J Clin Pathol 87:7, 1987.
389. Cazzadori A, Braggio P, Barbieri E, et al: Amiodarone-induced pulmonary toxicity. Respiration 49:157, 1986.
390. Adams PC, Gibson GJ, Morley AR, et al: Amiodarone pulmonary toxicity: Clinical and subclinical features. Q J Med 59:449, 1986.
391. Coudert B, Bailly F, Lombard JN, et al: Amiodarone pneumonitis: Bronchoalveolar lavage findings in 15 patients and review of the literature. Chest 102:1005, 1992.
392. Heras JR, Rodriguez-Roisin R, Magrina J, et al: Pulmonary complications after long term amiodarone treatment. Thorax 47:372, 1992.
393. Akoun GM, Cadranel JL, Blanchette G, et al: Bronchoalveolar lavage cell data in amiodarone-associated pneumonitis. Chest 99:1177, 1991.
394. Zhu YY, Botvinick E, Dae M, et al: Gallium lung scintigraphy in amiodarone pulmonary toxicity. Chest 93:1124, 1988.

395. Kennedy JI: Clinical aspects of amiodarone pulmonary toxicity. Clin Chest Med 11:119, 1990.
396. Martin WJ II, Rosenow EC III: Amiodarone pulmonary toxicity: Recognition and pathogenesis (Part 1). Chest 93:1067, 1988.
397. Martin WJ: Mechanisms of amiodarone pulmonary toxicity. Clin Chest Med 11:131, 1990.
398. Dake MD, Madison JM, Montgomery CK, et al: Electron microscopic demonstration of lysosomal inclusion bodies in lung, liver, lymph nodes, and blood leukocytes of patients with amiodarone pulmonary toxicity. Am J Med 78:506, 1985.
399. Costa-Jussa FR, Corrin B, Jacobs JM: Amiodarone lung toxicity: A human and experimental study. J Pathol 144:73, 1984.
400. Martin WJ, Standing JE: Amiodarone pulmonary toxicity: Biochemical evidence for a cellular phospholipidosis in the bronchoalveolar lavage of human subjects. J Pharmacol Exp Ther 244:774, 1988.
401. Martin WJ II, Rosenow EC III: Amiodarone pulmonary toxicity: Recognition and pathogenesis (Part 2). Chest 93:1242, 1988.
402. Nicolet-Chatelain G, Prevost MC, Escamilla R, et al: Amiodarone-induced pulmonary toxicity: Immunoallergologic tests and bronchoalveolar lavage phospholipid content. Chest 99:363, 1991.
403. Vereckei A, Blazovicx A, Gyorgy I, et al: The role of free radicals in the pathogenesis of amiodarone toxicity. J Cardiovasc Electrophysiol 4:161, 1993.
404. Vorperian VR, Havighurst TC, Miller S: Adverse effects of low dose amiodarone: A meta-analysis. J Am Coll Cardiol 30:791, 1997.
405. Akoun GM, Gauthier-Rahman S, Milleron BJ, et al: Amiodarone-induced hypersensitivity pneumonitis: Evidence of an immunological cell-mediated mechanism. Chest 85:133, 1984.
406. Ohar JA, Jackson F, Dettenmeier PA, et al: Bronchoalveolar lavage cell count and differential are not reliable indicators of amiodarone-induced pneumonitis. Chest 102:999, 1992.
407. Akoun GM, Milleron BJ, Badaro DM, et al: Pleural T-lymphocyte subsets in amiodarone-associated pleuropneumonitis. Chest 95:596, 1989.
408. Karpel JP, Mitsudo S, Norin AJ: Natural killer cell activity in a rat model of amiodarone-induced interstitial lung disease. Chest 99:230, 1991.
409. Reinhart PG, Gairola CG: Amiodarone-induced pulmonary toxicity in Fischer rats: Release of tumor necrosis factor alpha and transforming growth factor beta by pulmonary alveolar macrophages. J Toxicol Environ Health 52:353, 1997.
410. Akoun GM, Gauthier-Rahman S, Liote H, et al: Leukocyte migration inhibition in amiodarone-associated pneumonitis. Chest 94:1050, 1988.
411. Fan K, Bell R, Eudy S, et al: Amiodarone-associated pulmonary fibrosis: Evidence of an immunologically mediated mechanism. Chest 92:625, 1987.
412. Gefter WB, Epstein DM, Pietra GG, et al: Lung disease caused by amiodarone, a new antiarrhythmia agent. Radiology 147:339, 1983.
413. Suarez LD, Poderoso JJ, Elsner B, et al: Subacute pneumopathy during amiodarone therapy. Chest 83:566, 1983.
414. Wilson BD, Clarkson CE, Lippmann ML: Amiodarone-induced pulmonary inflammation: Correlation with drug dose and lung levels of drug, metabolite and phospholipid. Am Rev Respir Dis 143:1110, 1991.
415. Kudenchuk PJ, Pierson DJ, Greene HL, et al: Prospective evaluation of amiodarone pulmonary toxicity. Chest 86:541, 1984.
416. Rotmensch HH, Belhassen B, Swanson BN, et al: Steady-state serum amiodarone concentrations: Relationships with antiarrhythmic efficacy and toxicity. Ann Intern Med 101:462, 1984.
417. Ulrik CS, Backer V, Aldershvile J, et al: Serial pulmonary function tests in patients treated with low-dose amiodarone. Am Heart J 123:1550, 1992.
418. Gleadhill IC, Wise RA, Schonfeld SA, et al: Serial lung function testing in patients treated with amiodarone: A prospective study. Am J Med 86:4, 1989.
419. Graille V, Lapeyre-Mestre M, Montastruc JL: Amiodarone-induced pleuropneumopathies: Experience 1983–1993 in a drug vigilance regional center. Therapie 49:421, 1994.
420. Raeder EA, Podrid PJ, Lown B: Side effects and complications of amiodarone therapy. Am Heart J 109(5 Pt 1):975, 1985.
421. Darmanata JI, van Zandwijk N, Düren DR, et al: Amiodarone pneumonitis: Three further cases with a review of published reports. Thorax 39:57, 1984.
422. Kennedy JI, Myers JL, Plumb VJ, et al: Amiodarone pulmonary toxicity: Clinical, radiologic, and pathologic correlations. Arch Intern Med 147:50, 1987.
423. Myers JL, Kennedy JI, Plumb VJ: Amiodarone lung: Pathologic findings in clinically toxic patients. Hum Pathol 18:349, 1987.
424. Liu FL, Cohen RD, Downar E, et al: Amiodarone pulmonary toxicity: Functional and ultrastructural evaluation. Thorax 41:100, 1986.
425. Pollak PT, Sami M: Acute necrotizing pneumonitis and hyperglycemia after amiodarone therapy: Case report and review of amiodarone-associated pulmonary disease. Am J Med 76:935, 1984.
426. Lahita RG, Chiorazzi N, Gibofsky A, et al: Familial systemic lupus erythematosus in males. Arthritis Rheum 26:39, 1983.
427. Conte SC, Pagan V, Murer B: Bronchiolitis obliterans organizing pneumonia secondary to amiodarone: Clinical, radiological and histological pattern. Monaldi Arch Chest Dis 52:24, 1997.
428. Jessurun GA, Hoogenberg K, Crijns HJ: Bronchiolitis obliterans organizing pneumonia during low-dose amiodarone. Clin Cardiol 20:300, 1997.
429. Olson LK, Forrest JV, Friedman PJ, et al: Pneumonitis after amiodarone therapy. Radiology 150:327, 1984.
430. Pollak PT, Sami M: Acute necrotizing pneumonitis and hyperglycemia after amiodarone therapy. Am J Med 76:935, 1994.
431. Gonzalez-Rothi RJ, Hannan SE, Hood CI, et al: Amiodarone pulmonary toxicity presenting as bilateral exudative pleural effusions. Chest 92:179, 1987.

432. Kuhlman JE, Teigen C, Ren H, et al: Amiodarone pulmonary toxicity: CT findings in symptomatic patients. Radiology 177:121, 1990.

433. Nicholson AA, Hayward C: The value of computed tomography in the diagnosis of amiodarone-induced pulmonary toxicity. Clin Radiol 40:564, 1989.

434. Ren H, Kuhlman JE, Hruban RH, et al: CT-pathology correlation of amiodarone lung. J Comput Assist Tomogr 14:760, 1990.

435. Van Rooiji WJ, Vandermeer SC, Van Royen EA, et al: Pulmonary gallium-67 uptake in amiodarone pneumonitis. J Nucl Med 25:211, 1984.

436. Zhu YY, Botvinick E, Dae M, et al: Gallium lung scintigraphy in amiodarone pulmonary toxicity. Chest 93:1126, 1988.

436a. Vizioli LD, Cho S: Amiodarone-associated hemoptysis. Chest 105:305, 1994.

437. McNeil KD, Firouz-Abadi A, Oliver W, et al: Amiodarone pulmonary toxicity: Three unusual manifestations. Aust N Z J Med 22:14, 1992.

438. Riley SA, Williams SE, Cooke NJ: Alveolitis after treatment with amiodarone. BMJ 284:161, 1982.

439. Pozzi E, Sada E, Luisetti M, et al: Interstitial pneumopathy and low-dosage amiodarone. Eur J Respir Dis 65:620, 1984.

440. Quyyumi AA, Ormerod LP, Clarke SW, et al: Pulmonary fibrosis: A serious side-effect of amiodarone therapy. Eur Heart J 4:521, 1983.

441. Koslin DB, Chapman P, Youker JE, et al: Amiodarone-induced pulmonary toxicity. J Can Assoc Radiol 35:195, 1984.

442. Parra O, Ruiz J, Ojanguren I, et al: Amiodarone toxicity: Recurrence of interstitial pneumonitis after withdrawal of the drug. Eur Respir J 2:905, 1989.

443. Chendrasekhar A, Barke RA, Druck P: Recurrent amiodarone pulmonary toxicity. South Med J 89:85, 1996.

444. Nalos PC, Kass RM, Gang ES, et al: Life-threatening postoperative pulmonary complications in patients with previous amiodarone pulmonary toxicity undergoing cardiothoracic operations. J Thorac Cardiovasc Surg 93:904, 1987.

445. Van Mieghem W, Coolen L, Malysse I, et al: Amiodarone and the development of ARDS after lung surgery. Chest 105:1642, 1994.

446. Kupferschmid JP, Rosengart TK, McIntosh CL, et al: Amiodarone-induced complications after cardiac operation for obstructive hypertrophic cardiomyopathy. Ann Thorac Surg 48:359, 1989.

447. Howard JJ, Mohsenifar Z, Simons SM: Adult respiratory distress syndrome following administration of lidocaine. Chest 81:644, 1982.

448. Perlow GM, Jain BP, Pauker SG, et al: Tocainide-associated interstitial pneumonitis. Ann Intern Med 94:489, 1981.

449. Feinberg L, Travis WD, Ferrans V, et al: Pulmonary fibrosis associated with tocainide: Report of a case with literature review. Am Rev Respir Dis 141:505, 1990.

450. Stein MG, DeMarco T, Gamsu G, et al: Computed tomography: Pathologic correlation in lung disease due to tocainide. Am Rev Respir Dis 137:458, 1988.

451. Leesar MA, Martyn R, Talley JD, et al: Noncardiogenic pulmonary edema complicating massive verapamil overdose. Chest 105:606, 1994.

452. Putnam JB, Bolling SF, Kirsh MM: Procainamide-induced respiratory insufficiency after cardiopulmonary bypass. Ann Thorac Surg 51:482, 1991.

453. Miller B, Skupin A, Rubenfire M, et al: Respiratory failure produced by severe procainamide intoxication in a patient with preexisting peripheral neuropathy caused by amiodarone. Chest 94:663, 1988.

454. Smith PR, Nacht RI: Drug-induced lupus pleuritis mimicking pleural space infection. Chest 101:268, 1992.

455. Faller M, Quoix E, Popin E, et al: Migratory infiltrates in a patient treated with sotalol. Eur Respir J 10:2159, 1997.

456. Fruchter L, Laptook A: Diphenylhydantoin hypersensitivity reaction associated with interstitial pulmonary infiltrates and hypereosinophilia. Ann Allergy 47:453, 1981.

457. Chamberlain DW, Hyland RH, Ross DJ: Diphenylhydantoin-induced lymphocytic interstitial pneumonia. Chest 90:458, 1986.

458. Moore MT: Pulmonary changes in hydantoin therapy. JAMA 171:1328, 1959.

459. Low NL, Yahr MD: The lack of pulmonary fibrosis in patients receiving diphenylhydantoin. JAMA 174:1201, 1960.

460. Livingston S, Whitehouse D, Pauli LL: Study of the effects of diphenylhydantoin sodium on the lungs. N Engl J Med 264:648, 1961.

461. Michael JR, Rudin ML: Acute pulmonary disease caused by phenytoin. Ann Intern Med 95:452, 1981.

462. Munn NJ, Baughman RP, Ploysongsang Y, et al: Bronchoalveolar lavage in acute drug-hypersensitivity pneumonitis probably caused by phenytoin. South Med J 77:1594, 1984.

463. Saltzstein SL, Ackerman LV: Lymphadenopathy induced by anticonvulsant drugs and mimicking clinically and pathologically malignant lymphomas. Cancer 12:164, 1959.

464. Heitzman ER: Lymphadenopathy related to anticonvulsant therapy: Roentgen findings simulating lymphoma. Radiology 89:311, 1967.

465. Yermakov VM, Hitti IF, Sutton AL: Necrotizing vasculitis associated with diphenylhydantoin: Two fatal cases. Hum Pathol 14:182, 1983.

466. Gaffey CM, Chun B, Harvey JC, et al: Phenytoin-induced systemic granulomatous vasculitis. Arch Pathol Lab Med 110:131, 1986.

467. Angle P, Thomas P, Chiu B, et al: Bronchiolitis obliterans organizing pneumonia and cold agglutinin disease associated with phenytoin hypersensitivity syndrome. Chest 112:1697, 1997.

468. Miller WT: Pleural and mediastinal disorders related to drug use. Semin Roentgenol 30:35, 1995.

469. Fruchter L, Laptook A: Diphenylhydantoin hypersensitivity reaction associated with interstitial pulmonary infiltrates and hypereosinophilia. Ann Allergy 47:453, 1981.

470. Bayer AS, Targan SR, Pitchon HE, et al: Dilantin toxicity: Miliary pulmonary infiltrates and hypoxemia. Ann Intern Med 85:475, 1976.

471. Li FP, Willard DR, Goodman R, et al: Malignant lymphoma after diphenylhydantoin (Dilantin) therapy. Cancer 36:1359, 1975.

472. Hazlett DR, Ward GW, Madison DS: Pulmonary function loss in diphenylhydantoin therapy. Chest 66:660, 1974.

473. De Swert LF, Ceuppens JL, Teuwen D, et al: Acute interstitial pneumonitis and carbamazepine therapy. Acta Paediatr Scand 73:285, 1984.

474. Cullinan SA, Bower GC: Acute pulmonary hypersensitivity to carbamazepine. Chest 68:580, 1975.

475. Stephan WC, Parks RD, Tempest B: Acute hypersensitivity pneumonitis associated with carbamazepine therapy. Chest 74:463, 1978.

476. Lee T, Cochrane GM, Amlot P: Pulmonary eosinophilia and asthma associated with carbamazepine. BMJ 282:440, 1981.

477. Barreiro B, Manresa F, Valldeperas J: Carbamazepine and the lung. Eur Respir J 3:930, 1990.

478. Fernandez Alvarez R, Gullom Blanco JA, Riesgo Alonso C, et al: Acute pulmonary toxicity caused by carbamazepine: Apropos of a case. Arch Broncopneumol 30:471, 1994.

479. King GG, Barnes DJ, Hayes MJ: Carbamazepine-induced pneumonitis. Med J Aust 160:126, 1994.

480. Takahashi N, Aizawa H, Takata S, et al: Acute interstitial pneumonitis induced by carbamazepine. Eur Respir J 6:1409, 1993.

481. Tijhuis GJ, Strijbos JH, van Ermen A, et al: Generalized side effects with the use of carbamazepine. Ned Tijdschr Geneeskd 139:2265, 1995.

482. Stephan WC, Parks RD, Tempest B: Acute hypersensitivity pneumonitis associated with carbamazepine therapy. Chest 74:463, 1978.

483. Milesi-Lecat AM, Schmidt J, Aumaitre O, et al: Lupus and pulmonary nodules consistent with bronchiolitis obliterans organizing pneumonia induced by carbamazepine. Mayo Clin Proc 72:1145, 1997.

484. Lee T, Cochrane GM, Amlot P: Pulmonary eosinophilia and asthma associated with carbamazepine. BMJ 282:440, 1981.

485. De Vriese ASP, Philippe J, Van Renterghem DM: Carbamazepine hypersensitivity syndrome: Report of 4 cases and review of the literature. Medicine (Baltimore) 74:144, 1995.

486. Heffner JE, Sahn SA: Salicylate-induced pulmonary edema: Clinical features and prognosis. Ann Intern Med 95:405, 1981.

487. Leatherman JW, Drage CW: Adult respiratory distress syndrome due to salicylate intoxication. Minn Med 65:677, 1982.

488. Walters JS, Woodring JH, Stelling CB, et al: Salicylate-induced pulmonary edema. Radiology 146:289, 1983.

489. Fisher CJ Jr, Albertson TE, Foulke GE: Salicylate-induced pulmonary edema: Clinical characteristics in children. Am J Emerg Med 3:33, 1985.

490. Liebman RM, Katz HM: Pulmonary edema in a 52-year-old woman ingesting large amounts of aspirin. JAMA 246:2227, 1981.

491. Hormaechea E, Carlson RW, Rogove H, et al: Hypovolemia, pulmonary edema and protein changes in severe salicylate poisoning. Am J Med 66:1046, 1979.

492. Bowers RE, Brigham KL, Owen PJ: Salicylate pulmonary edema: The mechanism in sheep and review of the clinical literature. Am Rev Respir Dis 115:261, 1977.

493. Heffner J, Starkey T, Anthony P: Salicylate-induced noncardiogenic pulmonary edema. West J Med 130:263, 1979.

494. Andersen R, Refstad S: Adult respiratory distress syndrome precipitated by massive salicylate poisoning. Intensive Care Med 4:211, 1978.

495. Reinoso MA, Schroeder KW, Pisani RJ: Lung disease associated with orally administered mesalazine for ulcerative colitis. Chest 101:1469, 1992.

496. Lagler U, Schultess HK, Kuhn M: Acute alveolitis due to mesalazine. Schweiz Med Wochenschr 122:1332, 1992.

496a. Sviri S, Gafanovich I, Kramer MR, et al: Mesalamine-induced hypersensitivity pneumonitis. A case report and review of the literature. J Clin Gastroenterol 24:34, 1997.

497. Jick H, Derby LE, Garcia Rodriguez LA, et al: Nonsteroidal antiinflammatory drugs and certain rare, serious adverse events: A cohort study. Pharmacotherapy 13:212, 1993.

498. Goodwin SD, Glenny RW: Nonsteroidal anti-inflammatory drug-associated pulmonary infiltrates with eosinophilia: Review of the literature and Food and Drug Administration Adverse Drug Reaction reports. Arch Intern Med 152:1521, 1992.

499. Nader DA, Schillaci RF: Pulmonary infiltrates with eosinophilia due to naproxen. Chest 83:280, 1983.

500. Buscaglia AJ, Cowden FE, Brill H: Pulmonary infiltrates associated with naproxen. JAMA 251:65, 1984.

501. Takimoto CH, Lynch D, Stulbarg MS: Pulmonary infiltrates associated with sulindac therapy. Chest 97:230, 1990.

502. Pfitzenmeyer P, Meier M, Zuck P, et al: Piroxicam induced pulmonary infiltrates and eosinophilia. J Rheumatol 21:1573, 1994.

503. Nakatsumi Y, Nomura M, Yasui M, et al: A case of eosinophilic pneumonia due to tolfenamic acid. Nippon Kyobu Shikkan Gakkai Zasshi 31:1322, 1993.

504. Rich MW, Thomas RA: A case of eosinophilic pneumonia and vasculitis induced by diflunisal. Chest 111:1767, 1997.

505. Khalil H, Molinary E, Stoller JK: Diclofenac (Voltaren)-induced eosinophilic pneumonitis: Case report and review of the literature. Arch Intern Med 153:16491, 1993.

506. Gould DM, Daves ML: A review of roentgen findings in systemic lupus erythematosus (SLE). Am J Med Sci 235:596, 1958.

507. Fuleihan FJD, Abboud RT, Hubaytar R: Idiopathic pulmonary hemosiderosis:

Case report with pulmonary function tests and review of the literature. Am Rev Respir Dis 98:93, 1968.

508. Ewan PW, Jones HA, Rhodes CG, et al: Detection of intrapulmonary hemorrhage with carbon monoxide uptake: Application in Goodpasture's syndrome. N Engl J Med 295:1391, 1976.

509. Robboy SJ, Minna JD, Coleman RW, et al: Pulmonary hemorrhage syndrome as a manifestation of disseminated intravascular coagulation: Analysis of ten cases. Chest 63:718, 1973.

510. Macarron P, Garcia Diaz JE, Azofra JA, et al: D-penicillamine therapy associated with rapidly progressive glomerulonephritis. Nephrol Dial Transplant 7:161, 1992.

511. Bocanegra T, Espinoza LR, Vasey FB, et al: Myasthenia gravis and penicillamine therapy of rheumatoid arthritis. JAMA 244:1822, 1980.

512. Adelman HM, Winters PR, Mahan CS, et al: D-penicillamine-induced myasthenia gravis: Diagnosis obscured by coexisting chronic obstructive pulmonary disease. Am J Med Sci 309:191, 1995.

513. Eastmond CJ: Diffuse alveolitis as complication of penicillamine treatment for rheumatoid arthritis. BMJ 1:1506, 1976.

514. Davies D, Jones JKL: Pulmonary eosinophilia caused by penicillamine. Thorax 35:957, 1980.

515. Kumar A, Bhat A, Gupta DK, et al: D-penicillamine-induced acute hypersensitivity pneumonitis and cholestatic hepatitis in a patient with rheumatoid arthritis. Clin Exp Rheumatol 3:337, 1985.

516. Petersen J, Moller I: Miliary pulmonary infiltrates and penicillamine. Br J Radiol 51:915, 1978.

517. Estes D, Christian CL: The natural history of systemic lupus erythematosus by prospective analysis. Medicine 50:85, 1971.

518. Fessel WJ: Systemic lupus erythematosus in the community. Arch Intern Med 134:1027, 1974.

519. Wallace SL, Diamond H, Kaplan D: Recent advances in rheumatoid diseases: The connective tissue diseases other than rheumatoid arthritis—1970 and 1971. Ann Intern Med 77:455, 1972.

520. Cohen AS, Reynolds WE, Franklin EC, et al: Preliminary criteria for the classification of systemic lupus erythematosus. Bull Rheum Dis 21:643, 1971.

521. Camus P, Degat OR, Justrabo E, et al: D-penicillamine-induced severe pneumonitis. Chest 81:376, 1982.

522. Honda T, Hachiya T, Hayasaka M, et al: A case of rheumatoid arthritis with obstructive bronchiolitis appearing after D-penicillamine therapy. Nippon Kyobu Shikkan Gakkai Zasshi 31:1195, 1993.

523. Yam LY, Wong R: Bronchiolitis obliterans and rheumatoid arthritis: Report of a case in a Chinese patient on D-penicillamine and review of the literature. Ann Acad Med Singapore 22:365, 1993.

524. Padley SP, Adler BD, Hansell DM, et al: Bronchiolitis obliterans: High resolution CT findings and correlation with pulmonary function tests. Clin Radiol 47:236, 1993.

525. Boehler A, Vogt P, Speich R, et al: Bronchiolitis obliterans in a patient with localized scleroderma treated with D-penicillamine. Eur Respir J 9:1317, 1996.

526. Clinical Pathologic Conference: Pulmonary hemorrhage and renal failure. Am J Med 60:397, 1976.

527. Zitnik RJ, Cooper JAD: Pulmonary disease due to antirheumatic agents. Clin Chest Med 11:139, 1990.

528. Padley SPG, Adler BD, Hansell DM, Müller NL: Bronchiolitis obliterans: High resolution CT findings and correlations with pulmonary function tests. Clin Radiol 47:236, 1993.

529. Cooke NT, Bamji AN: Gold and pulmonary function in rheumatoid arthritis. Br J Rheumatol 22:18, 1983.

530. Winterbauer RH, Wilske KR, Wheelis RF: Diffuse pulmonary injury associated with gold treatment. N Engl J Med 294:919, 1976.

531. Geddes DM, Brostoff J: Pulmonary fibrosis associated with hypersensitivity to gold salts. BMJ 1:1444, 1976.

532. Scharf J, Nahir M, Kleinhaus U, et al: Diffuse pulmonary injury associated with gold therapy. JAMA 237:2412, 1977.

533. Gould PW, McCormack PL, Palmer DG: Pulmonary damage associated with sodium aurothiomalate therapy. J Rheumatol 4:252, 1977.

534. Sepuya SM, Grzybowski S, Burton JD, et al: Diffuse lung changes associated with gold therapy. Can Med Assoc J 118:816, 1978.

535. James DW, Whimeter WF, Hamilton EBD: Gold lung. BMJ 1:1523, 1978.

536. Weaver LT, Law JS: Lung changes after gold salts. Br J Dis Chest 72:247, 1978.

537. Tala E, Jalava S, Nurmela T, et al: Pulmonary infiltrates associated with gold therapy: Report of a case. Scand J Rheumatol 8:97, 1979.

538. Terho EO, Torkko M, Vaita R: Pulmonary damage associated with gold therapy: A report of two cases. Scand J Respir Dis 60:345, 1979.

539. McCormick J, Cole S, Lahirir B, et al: Pneumonitis caused by gold salt therapy: Evidence for the role of cell-mediated immunity in its pathogenesis. Am Rev Respir Dis 122:145, 1980.

540. Ettensohn DB, Roberts NJ Jr, Condemi JJ: Bronchoalveolar lavage in gold lung. Chest 85:569, 1984.

541. Morley TF, Komansky HJ, Adelizzi RA, et al: Pulmonary gold toxicity. Eur J Respir Dis 65:627, 1984.

542. Schapira D, Nahir M, Scharf Y: Pulmonary injury induced by gold salts treatment. Med Interna 23:259, 1985.

543. Gortenuti G, Parrinello A, Vicentini D: Diffuse pulmonary changes caused by gold salt therapy: Report of a case. Diagn Imag Clin Med 54:298, 1985.

544. Partanen J, van Assendelft AH, Koskimies S, et al: Patients with rheumatoid arthritis and gold-induced pneumonitis express two high-risk major histocompatibility complex patterns. Chest 92:277, 1987.

545. Vernhet H, Bousquet C, Cover S, et al: The use of high resolution x-ray computed tomography in the diagnosis of hypersensitivity pneumopathy to gold salts: Apropos of a case. Rev Mal Respir 12:317, 1995.

546. Blackwell TS, Gossage JR: Gold pulmonary toxicity in a patient with normal chest radiograph. South Med J 88:644, 1995.

547. Mack U, Schmidt K, Heine M: Fatal diffuse alveolar damage after gold medication. Pneumologie 48:405, 1994.

548. Breton JL, Westeel V, Garnier G, et al: Gold salt-induced pneumonia and CD4 alveolitis. Rev Pneumol Clin 49:27, 1993.

549. Bando M, Takishita Y, Bando H, et al: A case of gold-induced pneumonitis showing a positive reaction in the drug lymphocyte stimulation test (DLST) for gold. Nippon Kyobu Shikkan Gakkai Zasshi 30:128, 1992.

550. Matsumura Y, Miyake A, Ishida T: A case of gold lung with positive lymphocyte stimulation test to gold, using bronchoalveolar lymphocytes. Nippon Kyobu Shikkan Gakkai Zasshi 30:472, 1992.

551. Tomioka H, King TE: Gold-induced pulmonary disease: Clinical features, outcome, and differentiation from rheumatoid lung disease. Am J Respir Crit Care Med 155:1011, 1997.

552. Nickels J, van Assendelft AHW, Tukiainen P: Diffuse pulmonary injury associated with gold treatment. Acta Pathol Microbiol Immunol Scand (A) 91:265, 1983.

553. Fort J, Scovern H, Abruzzo J: Intravenous cyclophosphamide and methylprednisolone for the treatment of bronchiolitis obliterans and interstitial fibrosis associated with crysotherapy. J Rheumatol 15:850, 1988.

554. Morley T, Komansky H, Adelizzi R, et al: Pulmonary gold toxicity. Eur J Respir Dis 65:627, 1984.

555. Schwartzman KJ, Bowie DM, Yeadon C, et al: Constrictive bronchiolitis obliterans following gold therapy for psoriatic arthritis. Eur Respir J 8:2191, 1995.

556. Evans RB, Ettensohn DB, Fawaz-Estrup F, et al: Gold lung: Recent developments in pathogenesis, diagnosis, and therapy. Semin Arthritis Rheum 16:196, 1987.

557. Mabie WC, Pernoll ML, Witty JB, et al: Pulmonary edema induced by betamimetic drugs. South Med J 76:1354, 1983.

558. Nimrod C, Rambihar V, Fallen E, et al: Pulmonary edema associated with isoxsuprine therapy. Am J Obstet Gynecol 148:625, 1984.

559. Pisani RJ, Rosenow EC III: Pulmonary edema associated with tocolytic therapy. Ann Intern Med 110:714, 1989.

560. Gupta RC, Foster S, Romano PM, et al: Acute pulmonary edema associated with the use of oral ritodrine for premature labor. Chest 95:479, 1989.

561. Evron S, Samueloff A, Mor-Yosef S, et al: Pulmonary edema occurring after isoxsuprine and dexamethasone treatment for preterm labor: Case report. J Perinat Med 11:272, 1983.

562. Connolly HM, Crary JL, McGoon MD, et al: Valvular heart disease associated with fenfluramine-phentermine. N Engl J Med 337:581, 1997.

563. O'Donnell AE, Selig J, Aravamuthan M, et al: Pulmonary complications associated with illicit drug use. Chest 108:460, 1995.

564. Glassroth J, Adams GD, Schnoll S: The impact of substance abuse on the respiratory system. Chest 91:596, 1987.

565. O'Donnell AE, Pappas LS: Pulmonary complications of intravenous drug abuse. Chest 94:251, 1988.

566. Heffner JE, Harley RA, Schabel SI: Pulmonary reactions from illicit substance abuse. Clin Chest Med 11:151, 1990.

567. Haim DY, Lippmann ML, Goldberg SK, et al: The pulmonary complications of crack cocaine. Chest 107:233, 1995.

568. Wilen SB, Ulreich S, Rabinowitz JG: Roentgenographic manifestations of methadone-induced pulmonary edema. Radiology 114:51, 1975.

569. Duberstein JL, Kaufman DM: A clinical study of an epidemic of heroin intoxication and heroin-induced pulmonary edema. Am J Med 51:704, 1971.

570. Frand UI, Shim CS, Williams MH Jr: Methadone-induced pulmonary edema. Ann Intern Med 76:975, 1972.

571. Schaaf JT, Spivack ML, Rath GS, et al: Pulmonary edema and adult respiratory distress syndrome following methadone abuse. Am Rev Respir Dis 107:1047, 1973.

572. Hunt G, Bruera E: Respiratory depression in a patient receiving oral methadone for cancer pain. J Pain Symptom Manage 10:401, 1995.

573. Gould DB: Buprenorphine causes pulmonary edema just like all other mu-opioid narcotics (letter). Chest 107:1478, 1995.

574. Thammakumpee G, Sumpatanukule P: Noncardiogenic pulmonary edema induced by sublingual buprenorphine. Chest 106:306, 1994.

575. Bogartz LJ, Miller WC: Pulmonary edema associated with propoxyphene intoxication. JAMA 215:259, 1971.

576. Richman S, Harris RD: Acute pulmonary edema associated with Librium abuse: A case report. Radiology 103:57, 1972.

577. Glauser FL, Smith WR, Caldwell A, et al: Ethchlorvynol (Placidyl)-induced pulmonary edema. Ann Intern Med 84:46, 1976.

578. Mountain R, Ferguson S, Fowler A, et al: Noncardiac pulmonary edema following administration of parenteral paraldehyde. Chest 82:371, 1982.

579. Sklar J, Timms RM: Codeine-induced pulmonary edema. Chest 72:230, 1977.

580. Sugihara H, Hagedorn M, Böttcher D, et al: Interstitial pulmonary edema following bromocarbamide intoxication. Am J Pathol 75:457, 1974.

581. Gali JM, Vilanova JL, Mayos M, et al: Febarbamate-induced pulmonary eosinophilia: A case report. Respiration 49:231, 1986.

582. Flacke JW, Flacke WE, Williams GD: Acute pulmonary edema following naloxone reversal of high-dose morphine anesthesia. Anesthesiology 47:376, 1977.

583. Taff RH: Pulmonary edema following naloxone administration in a patient without heart disease. Anesthesiology 59:576, 1983.

584. Katz S, Aberman A, Frand UI, et al: Heroin pulmonary edema: Evidence for increased pulmonary capillary permeability. Am Rev Respir Dis 106:472, 1972.

585. Smith WR, Wells ID, Glauser FL, et al: Immunologic abnormalities in heroin lung. Chest 68:651, 1975.

586. Smith WR, Glauser FL, Dearden LC, et al: Deposits of immunoglobulin and complement in the pulmonary tissue of patients with "heroin lung." Chest 73:471, 1978.

587. Snyder SH: Opiate receptors in the brain. N Engl J Med 296:266, 1977.

588. Helpern M, Rho Y-M: Deaths from narcotism in New York City: Incidence, circumstances, and postmortem findings. N Y J Med 66:2391, 1966.

589. Siegel H: Human pulmonary pathology associated with narcotic and other addictive drugs. Hum Pathol 3:55, 1972.

590. Morrison WJ, Wetherill S, Zyroff J: The acute pulmonary edema of heroin intoxication. Radiology 97:347, 1970.

591. Stern WZ, Subbarao K: Pulmonary complications of drug addiction. Semin Roentgenol 18:183, 1983.

592. Heffner JE, Harley RA, Schabel SI: Pulmonary reactions from illicit substance abuse. Clin Chest Med 11:151, 1990.

593. Steinberg AD, Karliner JS: The clinical spectrum of heroin pulmonary edema. Arch Intern Med 122:122, 1968.

594. Saba GP II, James AE Jr, Johnson BA, et al: Pulmonary complications of narcotic abuse. Am J Roentgenol 122:733, 1974.

595. Light RW, Dunham TR: Severe slowly resolving heroin-induced pulmonary edema. Chest 67:61, 1975.

596. Master K: Heroin pulmonary edema. Chest 64:147, 1973.

597. Zyroff J, Slovis TL, Nagler J: Pulmonary edema induced by oral methadone. Radiology 112:567, 1974.

598. Alexander M: Surveillance of heroin-induced deaths in Atlanta 1971 to 1973. JAMA 229:677, 1974.

599. Kjeldgaard JM, Hahn GW, Heckenlively JR, et al: Methadone-induced pulmonary edema. JAMA 218:882, 1971.

600. Fraser DW: Methadone overdose: Illicit use of pharmaceutically prepared parenteral narcotics. JAMA 217:1387, 1971.

601. Karliner JS, Steinberg AD, Williams MH Jr: Lung function after pulmonary edema associated with heroin overdoses. Arch Intern Med 124:350, 1969.

602. Frand UI, Shim CS, Williams MH Jr: Heroin-induced pulmonary edema: Sequential studies of pulmonary function. Ann Intern Med 77:29, 1972.

603. Banner A, Rodriquez J, Sunderrajan E, et al: Bronchiectasis: A cause of pulmonary symptoms in heroin addicts. Respiration 37:232, 1979.

604. McCarroll KA, Roszler MH: Lung disorders due to drug abuse. J Thorac Imaging 6:30, 1991.

605. Douglass RE, Levison MA: Pneumothorax in drug abusers: An urban epidemic? Am Surg 52:377, 1986.

606. Kurtzman RS: Complications of narcotic addiction. Radiology 96:23, 1970.

607. Ettinger NE: A review of the respiratory effects of smoking cocaine. Am J Med 87:664, 1989.

608. Kissner DG, Lawrence WD, Selis JE, et al: Crack lung: Pulmonary disease caused by cocaine abuse. Am Rev Respir Dis 136:1250, 1987.

609. Forrester JM, Steele AW, Waldron JA, et al: Crack lung: An acute pulmonary syndrome with a spectrum of clinical and histopathologic findings. Am Rev Respir Dis 142:462, 1990.

610. Tashkin DP, Khalsa ME, Gorelick D, et al: Pulmonary status of habitual cocaine smokers. Am Rev Respir Dis 145:92, 1992.

611. Hoffman CK, Goodman PC: Pulmonary edema in cocaine smokers. Radiology 172:463, 1989.

612. Eurman DW, Potash HI, Eyler WR, et al: Chest pain and dyspnea related to "crack" cocaine smoking: Value of chest radiography. Radiology 172:459, 1989.

613. Susskind H, Weber, Volkow ND, et al: Increased lung permeability following long-term use of free-base cocaine (crack). Chest 100:903, 1991.

614. Baldwin GC, Buckley DM, Roth MD, et al: Acute activation of circulating polymorphonuclear neutrophils following *in vivo* administration of cocaine: A potential etiology for pulmonary injury. Chest 111:698, 1997.

615. Moliterno DJ, Willard JE, Lange RA, et al: Coronary artery vasoconstriction induced by cocaine, cigarette smoking or both. N Engl J Med 330:454, 1994.

616. Henning RJ, Wilson LD, Glauser JM: Cocaine plus ethanol is more cardiotoxic than cocaine or ethanol alone. Crit Care Med 22:1896, 1994.

617. Nunez BD, Miao L, Kuntz RE, et al: Cardiogenic shock induced by cocaine in swine with normal coronary arteries. Cardiovasc Res 28:105, 1994.

617a. Murray RJ, Smialek JE, Golle M, et al: Pulmonary artery medial hypertrophy in cocaine users without foreign particle microembolization. Chest 96:1050, 1989.

618. Taylor RF, Bernard GR: Airway complications from free-basing cocaine. Chest 95:476, 1989.

619. Averbach M, Casey KK, Frank E: Near fatal status asthmaticus induced by nasal insufflation of cocaine. South Med J 89:340, 1996.

620. Patel RC, Dutta D, Schonfeld SA: Free-base cocaine use associated with bronchiolitis obliterans organizing pneumonia. Ann Intern Med 107:186, 1987.

621. Tashkin DP, Simmons MS, Chang P, et al: Effects of smoked substance abuse on nonspecific airway hyperresponsiveness. Am Rev Respir Dis 147:97, 1993.

622. Weiss RD, Goldenheim PD, Mirin SM, et al: Pulmonary dysfunction in cocaine smokers. Am J Psychiatry 138:1110, 1981.

623. Itkonen J, Schnoll S, Glassroth J: Pulmonary dysfunction in "free base" cocaine users. Arch Intern Med 144:2195, 1984.

624. Bailey ME, Fraire AE, Greenberg SD, et al: Pulmonary histopathology in cocaine abusers. Hum Pathol 25:203, 1994.

625. O'Donnell AE, Mappin G, Sebo TJ, et al: Interstitial pneumonitis associated with "crack" cocaine abuse. Chest 100:1155, 1991.

626. Anonymous: Clinical Pathologic Conference. Respiratory failure and eosinophilia in a young man. Am J Med 94:533, 1993.

627. Klinger JR, Bensadoun E, Corrao WM: Pulmonary complications from alveolar accumulation of carbonaceous material in a cocaine smoker. Chest 101:1171, 1992.

628. Patel RC, Dutta D, Schonfeld SA: Free-base cocaine use associated with bronchiolitis obliterans organizing pneumonia. Ann Intern Med 107:186, 1987.

629. Kline JN, Hirasuna JD: Pulmonary edema after freebase cocaine smoking: Not due to an adulterant. Chest 97:1009, 1990.

630. Cooper CB, Bai TR, Heyderman E, et al: Cellulose granuloma in the lungs of a cocaine sniffer. BMJ 286:2021, 1983.

631. Oubeid M, Bickel JT, Ingram EA, et al: Pulmonary talc granulomatosis in a cocaine sniffer. Chest 98:237, 1990.

632. Greenebaum E, Copeland A, Grewal R: Blackened bronchoalveolar lavage fluid in crack smokers: A preliminary study. Am J Clin Pathol 100:481, 1993.

633. Hoffman CK, Goodman PC: Pulmonary edema in cocaine smokers. Radiology 172:463, 1989.

634. Eurman DW, Potash HI, Eyler WR: Chest pain and dyspnea related to "crack" cocaine smoking: Value of chest radiography. Radiology 172:459, 1989.

635. Murray RJ, Albin RJ, Mergner W, et al: Diffuse alveolar hemorrhage temporally related to cocaine smoking. Chest 93:427, 1988.

636. Kissner DG, Lawrence DW, Selis JE, et al: Crack lung: Pulmonary disease caused by cocaine abuse. Am Rev Respir Dis 136:1250, 1987.

637. Patel RC, Dutta D, Schonfeld SA: Free-base cocaine use associated with bronchiolitis obliterans pneumonia. Ann Intern Med 107:186, 1987.

638. Haim DY, Lippmann ML, Goldberg SK, et al: The pulmonary complications of crack cocaine: a comprehensive review. Chest 107:233, 1995.

639. Goldberg REA, Lipuma JP, Cohen AM: Pneumomediastinum associated with cocaine abuse: Case report and review of the literature. J Thorac Imaging 2:88, 1987.

640. Cregler L, Mark H: Medical complications of cocaine abuse. N Engl J Med 315:1495, 1986.

641. Mundinger MO: Pneumopericardium from cocaine inhalation. N Engl J Med 313:46, 1985.

642. Leitman BS, Greengart A, Wasser HJ: Pneumomediastinum and pneumopericardium after cocaine abuse. Am J Roentgenol 151:614, 1988.

643. Gong H Jr, Fligiel S, Tashkin DP, et al: Tracheobronchial changes in habitual heavy smokers of marijuana with and without tobacco. Am Rev Respir Dis 136:142, 1987.

644. Tilles DS, Goldenheim PD, Johnson DC, et al: Marijuana smoking as a cause of reduction in single-breath carbon monoxide diffusing capacity. Am J Med 80:601, 1986.

645. Varnell RM, Godwin JD, Richardson ML, et al: Adult respiratory distress syndrome from overdose of tricyclic antidepressants. Radiology 170:667, 1989.

646. Roy TM, Ossorio MA, Cipolla LM, et al: Pulmonary complications after tricyclic antidepressant overdose. Chest 96:852, 1989.

647. Wilson IC, Gambill JM, Sandifer MG: Loeffler's syndrome occurring during imipramine therapy. Am J Psychiatry 119:892, 1963.

648. Joynt RJ, Clancy J: Extreme eosinophilia during imipramine therapy. Am J Psychiatry 118:170, 1961.

649. Paré JAP: Unpublished data, 1975.

650. Shear MK: Chlorpromazine-induced PIE syndrome. Am J Psychiatry 135:492, 1978.

651. Marshall A, Moore K: Pulmonary disease after amitriptyline overdosage. BMJ 1:716, 1973.

652. Sunshine P, Yaffe SJ: Amitriptyline poisoning: Clinical and pathological findings in a fatal case. Am J Dis Child 106:501, 1963.

653. Kummer F, Salzmann H, Wieckowski A: Progressive interstitial lung disease in a 75 year old woman. Monaldi Arch Chest Dis 50:118, 1995.

654. Gonzales-Rothi RJ, Zander DS, Ros PR: Fluoxetine hydrochloride (Prozac)-induced pulmonary disease. Chest 107:1763, 1995.

655. Vandezande LM, Lamblin C, Wallaert B: Interstitial lung disease linked to fluoxetine. Rev Mal Respir 14:327, 1997.

656. de Kerviler E, Tredaniel J, Revlon G, et al: Fluoxetine-induced pulmonary granulomatosis. Eur Respir J 9:615, 1996.

656a. Hubbard R, Venn A, Smith C, et al: Exposure to commonly prescribed drugs and the etiology of cryptogenic fibrosing alveolitis: A case-control study. Am J Respir Crit Care Med 157:743, 1998.

657. Smego RA, Durack DT: The neuroleptic malignant syndrome. Arch Intern Med 142:1183, 1982.

658. Li C, Gefter WB: Acute pulmonary edema induced by overdosage and phenothiazines. Chest 101:102, 1992.

659. Fraimow W, Wallace S, Lewis P, et al: Changes in pulmonary function due to lymphangiography. Radiology 85:231, 1965.

660. Fallat RJ, Powell MR, Youker JE, et al: Pulmonary deposition and clearance of ^{131}I-labeled oil after lymphography in man: Correlation with lung function. Radiology 97:511, 1970.

661. Weg JG, Harklerload LE: Aberrations in pulmonary function due to lymphangiography. Dis Chest 53:534, 1968.

662. Gold WM, Youker J, Anderson S, et al: Pulmonary-function abnormalities after lymphangiography. N Engl J Med 273:519, 1965.

663. White RJ, Webb JAW, Tucker AK, et al: Pulmonary function after lymphography. BMJ 4:775, 1973.

664. Silvestri RC, Huseby JS, Rughani I, et al: Respiratory distress syndrome from lymphangiography contrast medium. Am Rev Respir Dis 122:543, 1980.

665. Tapper DP, Taylor JR: Diffuse pulmonary infiltrates following lymphography. Chest 96:915, 1989.

666. Ansell G: A national survey of radiological complications: Interim report. Clin Radiol 19:175, 1968.

667. Reich SB: Production of pulmonary edema by aspiration of water-soluble nonabsorbable contrast media. Radiology 92:367, 1969.

668. Chiu CL, Gambach RR: Hypaque pulmonary edema: A case report. Radiology 111:91, 1974.

669. Malins AF: Pulmonary oedema after radiological investigation of peripheral occlusive vascular disease: Adverse reaction to contrast media. Lancet 1:413, 1978.

670. Greganti MA, Flowers WM Jr: Acute pulmonary edema after the intravenous administration of contrast media. Radiology 132:583, 1979.

671. Chamberlin WH, Stockman GD, Wray NP: Shock and noncardiogenic pulmonary edema following meglumine diatrizoate for intravenous pyelography. Am J Med 67:684, 1979.

672. Cameron JD: Pulmonary edema following drip-infusion urography. Radiology 111:89, 1974.

673. Hayashi H, Kumazaki T, Asano G: Pulmonary edema induced by intravenous administration of contrast media: Experimental study in rats. Radiat Med 12:47, 1994.

674. Goldsmith SR, Steinberg P: Noncardiogenic pulmonary edema induced by nonionic low-osmolality radiographic contrast media. J Allergy Clin Immunol 96:698, 1995.

675. Hudson ER, Smith TP, McDermott VG, et al: Pulmonary angiography performed with iopamidol: Complications in 1,434 patients. Radiology 198:61, 1996.

676. Chung JW, Park JH, Im JG, et al: Pulmonary oil embolism after transcatheter oily chemoembolization of hepatocellular carcinoma. Radiology 187:689, 1993.

677. Bush WH, Swanson DP: Acute reactions to intravascular contrast media: Types, risk factors, recognition, and specific treatment. Am J Roentgenol 157:1153, 1991.

678. Hartman GW, Hattery RR, Witten DM, et al: Mortality during excretion urography: Mayo Clinic experience. Am J Roentgenol 139:919, 1982.

679. Katayama H, Yamaguchi K, Kozuka T, et al: Adverse reactions to ionic and nonionic contrast media: A report from the Japanese Committee on the Safety of Contrast Media. Radiology 175:621, 1990.

679a. Caro JJ, Trindade E, McGregor M: The risks of death and of severe nonfatal reactions with high- versus low-osmolality contrast media: A meta-analysis. Am J Roentgenol 156:825, 1991.

679b. Spring DB, Bettmann MA, Barkan HE: Nonfatal adverse reactions to iodinated contrast media: Spontaneous reporting to the U.S. Food and Drug Administration, 1978–1994. Radiology 204:325, 1997.

679c. Spring DB, Bettmann MA, Barkan HE: Deaths related to iodinated contrast media reported spontaneously to the U.S. Food and Drug Administration, 1978–1994: Effect of the availability of low-osmolality contrast media. Radiology 204:333, 1997.

680. Woo KS, Nicholls MG: High prevalence of persistent cough with angiotensin converting enzyme inhibitors in Chinese. Br J Clin Pharmacol 40:141, 1995.

681. Lacourcière Y, Lefebvre J: Modulation of the renin-angiotensin-aldosterone system and cough. Can J Cardiol 11:33, 1995.

682. Wood R: Bronchospasm and cough as adverse reactions to the ACE inhibitors captopril, enalapril and lisinopril: A controlled retrospective cohort study. Br J Clin Pharmacol 39:265, 1995.

683. Visser LE, Stricker BH, Van der Velden J, et al: Angiotensin converting enzyme inhibitor associated cough: A population-based case-control study. J Clin Epidemiol 48:851, 1995.

684. Ravid D, Lishner M, Lang R, et al: Angiotensin-converting enzyme inhibitors and cough: A prospective evaluation in hypertension and in congestive heart failure. J Clin Pharmacol 34:1116, 1994.

685. Fletcher AE, Palmer AJ, Bulpitt CJ: Cough with angiotensin converting enzyme inhibitors: How much of a problem? J Hypertens Suppl 12:43, 1994.

686. Yesil S, Yesil M, Bayata S, et al: ACE inhibitors and cough. Angiology 45:805, 1994.

687. Goldberg AI, Dunlay MC, Sweet CS: Safety and tolerability of losartan potassium, an angiotensin II receptor antagonist, compared with hydrochlorothiazide, atenolol, felodipine, ER and angiotensin-converting enzyme inhibitors for the treatment of systemic hypertension. Am J Cardiol 75:793, 1995.

688. Os I, Bratland B, Dahlof B, et al: Female preponderance for lisinopril-induced cough in hypertension. Am J Hypertens 7:1012, 1994.

689. Punzi HA: Safety update: Focus on cough. Am J Cardiol 72:45, 1993.

690. Israili ZH, Hall WD: Cough and angioneurotic edema associated with angiotensin-converting enzyme inhibitor therapy: A review of the literature and pathophysiology. Ann Intern Med 117:234, 1992.

691. Gibson GR: Enalapril-induced cough. Arch Intern Med 149:2701, 1989.

692. Lefebvre J, Poirier L, Lacourcière Y: Prospective trial on captopril-related cough. Ann Pharmacother 26:161, 1992.

693. Lacourcière Y, Brunner H, Irwin R, et al: Effects of modulators of the renin-angiotensin-aldosterone system on cough. Losartan Cough Study Group. J Hypertens 12:1387, 1994.

694. Semple PF: Putative mechanisms of cough after treatment with angiotensin converting enzyme inhibitors. J Hypertens 13:17, 1995.

695. Olsen CG: Delay of diagnosis and empiric treatment of angiotensin-converting enzyme inhibitor-induced cough in office practice. Arch Fam Med 4:525, 1995.

696. Berkin KE: Respiratory effects of angiotensin converting enzyme inhibition. Eur Respir J 2:198, 1989.

697. Meeker DP, Wiedemann HP: Drug-induced bronchospasm. Clin Chest Med 11:163, 1990.

698. Reisin L, Schneeweiss A: Complete spontaneous remission of cough induced by ACE inhibitors during chronic therapy in hypertensive patients. J Hum Hypertens 6:333, 1992.

699. Lunde H, Hedner T, Samuelsson O, et al: Dyspnea, asthma and bronchospasm in relation to treatment with angiotensin converting enzyme inhibitors. BMJ 308:18, 1994.

700. Boulet LP, Milot J, Lampron N, et al: Pulmonary function and airway responsiveness during long term therapy with captopril. JAMA 261:413, 1989.

701. Mue S, Tamura G, Yamauchi K, et al: Bronchial responses to enalapril in asthmatic, hypertensive patients. Clin Ther 12:335, 1990.

702. Talwar D, Jindal SK: Effects of enalapril in ACE-inhibitor, on bronchial responsiveness in asthmatics. Indian J Physiol Pharmacol 37:217, 1993.

703. Bucknall CE, Neilly JB, Carter R, et al: Bronchial hyperreactivity in patients who cough after receiving angiotensin converting enzyme inhibitors. BMJ (Clin Res Ed.) 296:86, 1988.

704. Riska H, Sovijarvi AR, Ahonen A, et al: Effects of captopril on blood pressure and respiratory function compared to verapamil in patients with hypertension and asthma. J Cardiovasc Pharmacol 15:57, 1990.

705. Overlack A, Muller B, Schmidt L, et al: Airway responsiveness and cough induced by angiotensin converting enzyme inhibition. J Hum Hypertens 6:387, 1992.

706. Kaufman J, Schmitt S, Barnsard J, et al: Angiotensin-converting enzyme inhibitors in patients with bronchial responsiveness and asthma. Chest 101:922, 1992.

707. Jain M, Armstrong L, Hall J: Predisposition to and late onset of upper airway obstruction following angiotensin-converting enzyme inhibitor therapy. Chest 102:871, 1992.

708. Schatz PL, Mesologites D, Hyun J, et al: Captopril-induced hypersensitivity lung disease. Chest 95:685, 1989.

709. Watanabe K, Nishimura K, Shiode M, et al: Captopril, an angiotensin-converting enzyme inhibitor, induced pulmonary infiltration with eosinophilia. Intern Med 35:142, 1996.

710. Dorn MR, Walker BK: Noncardiogenic pulmonary edema associated with hydrochlorothiazide therapy. Chest 79:482, 1981.

711. Bell RT, Lippmann M: Hydrochlorothiazide-induced pulmonary edema: Report of a case and review of the literature. Arch Intern Med 139:817, 1979.

712. Anderson TJ, Berthiaume Y, Matheson D, et al: Hydrochlorothiazide-associated pulmonary edema. Chest 96:695, 1989.

713. Leser C, Bolliger CT, Winnwisser J, et al: Pulmonary edema and hypotension induced by hydrochlorothiazide. Monaldi Arch Chest Dis 49:308, 1994.

714. Fine SR, Lodha A, Zoneraich S, et al: Hydrochlorothiazide-induced acute pulmonary edema. Ann Pharmacother 29:701, 1995.

715. Shieh CM, Chen CH, Tao CW, et al: Hydrochlorothiazide-induced pulmonary edema: A case report and literature review. Chung Hua I Hsueh Tsa Chih (Taipei) 50:495, 1992.

716. Mollura JL, Bernstein R, Fine SR, et al: Pulmonary eosinophilia in a patient receiving beclomethasone diproprionate aerosol. Ann Allergy 42:326, 1979.

717. Chastre J, Basset F, Viau F, et al: Acute pneumonitis after subcutaneous injections of silicone in transsexual men. N Engl J Med 308:764, 1983.

718. Coulaud JM, Labrousse J, Carli P, et al: Adult respiratory distress syndrome and silicone injection. Toxicol Eur Res 5:171, 1983.

719. Wark JD, Larkins RG: Pulmonary oedema after propranolol therapy in two cases of phaeochromocytoma. BMJ 1:1395, 1978.

720. Sloand EM, Thompson BT: Propranolol-induced pulmonary edema and shock in a patient with pheochromocytoma. Arch Intern Med 144:173, 1984.

721. Akoun GM, Milleron BJ, Mayaud CM, et al: Provocation test coupled with bronchoalveolar lavage in diagnosis of propanolol-induced hypersensitivity pneumonia. Am Rev Respir Dis 139:247, 1989.

722. Gauthier-Rahman S, Akoun GM, Milleron BJ, et al: Leukocyte migration inhibition in propranolol-induced pneumonitis. Chest 97:238, 1990.

723. Lombard JN, Bonnotte B, Maynadie M, et al: Celiprolol pneumonitis. Eur Respir J 6:588, 1993.

724. Johns MD, Ponte CD: Acute pulmonary edema associated with ocular metopranol use. Ann Pharmacother 29:370, 1995.

725. Diggory P, Heyworth P, Chau G, et al: Unsuspected bronchospasm in association with topical timolol: A common problem in elderly people. Can we easily identify those affected and do cardioselective agents lead to improvement? Age Aging 23:17, 1994.

726. Rinaldo JE, Owens GR, Rogers RM: Adult respiratory distress syndrome following intrapleural instillation of talc. J Thorac Cardiovasc Surg 85:523, 1983.

727. Frye MD, Jarratt M, Sahn SA: Acute hypoxemic respiratory failure following intrapleural thrombolytic therapy for hemothorax. Chest 105:1596, 1994.

728. Lie JT: Pulmonary peliosis. Arch Pathol Lab Med 109:878, 1985.

729. Ohnishi Y, Kitazawa M: Application of perfluorochemicals in human beings: A morphological report of a human autopsy case with some experimental studies using rabbit. Acta Pathol Jpn 30(3):489, 1980.

730. Kitazawa M, Ohnishi Y: Long-term experiment of perfluorochemicals using rabbits. Virchows Arch Pathol Anat 398:1, 1982.

731. Wiggins J, Skinner C: Bromocriptine-induced pleuropulmonary fibrosis. Thorax 41:328, 1986.

732. Taal BG, Spierings ELH, Hilvering C: Pleuropulmonary fibrosis associated with chronic and excessive intake of ergotamine. Thorax 38:396, 1983.

733. McElvaney NG, Wilcox PG, Churg A, et al: Pleuropulmonary disease during bromocriptine treatment of Parkinson's disease. Arch Intern Med 14:2231, 1988.

734. Melmed S, Braunstein GD: Bromocriptine and pleuropulmonary disease. Arch Intern Med 149:258, 1989.

735. Humbert VH Jr, Munn NJ, Hawkins RF: Noncardiogenic pulmonary edema complicating massive diltiazem overdose. Chest 99:258, 1991.

736. Pusateri DW, Muder RR: Fever, pulmonary infiltrates and pleural effusion following acyclovir therapy for herpes zoster opthalmicus. Chest 98:754, 1990.

737. Barnett R, Israel HL, Scott R, et al: Pulmonary fibrosis in a patient treated with bumetanide: Clinical improvement associated with transition from a granulocytic to lymphocytic alveolitis. Respir Med 84:71, 1990.

738. Middleton KL, Santella R, Couser JI Jr: Eosinophilic pleuritis due to propylthiouracil. Chest 103:955, 1993.

739. Thomas AD, Caunt JA: Anaphylactoid reaction following local anaesthesia for epidural block. Anaesthesia 48:50, 1993.

740. Mahoney JM, Bachtel MD: Pleural effusion associated with chronic dantrolene administration. Ann Pharmacother 28:587, 1994.

741. Rausing A, Rosen U: Black cartilage after therapy with levodopa and methyldopa. Arch Pathol Lab Med 118:531, 1994.

742. Brody SL, Slovis CM, Wrenn KD: Cocaine related medical problems: Consecutive series of 233 patients. Am J Med 88:325, 1990.

743. Miyai M, Tsubota T, Asano K: Isoniazid-induced interstitial pneumonia. Respir Med 83:517, 1989.

744. Tenenbein M, Kowalski S, Sienko A, et al: Pulmonary toxic effects of continuous desferrioxamine administration in acute iron poisoning. Lancet 339:1601, 1992.

Poisons

In contrast to drug-induced pulmonary disease, which in most cases represents a side effect of medication used as treatment for a symptom or clinical disorder, poison-induced pulmonary toxicity often occurs as a result of accidental exposure or suicidal intent. Most of the involved toxic substances are inhaled as gases or aerosols (see page 2519); a minority, including insecticides, herbicides, various aromatic hydrocarbons, and the toxin responsible for the Spanish toxic-allergic syndrome, usually reach the lungs by absorption through the skin or after ingestion or intravenous injection. Although most of the poisons that cause pulmonary disease are well known, unusual agents can also be seen. For example, in one report of eight young people who inhaled strychnine by mistake, believing it was cocaine, most suffered convulsions and required mechanical ventilation; one died.[1]

INSECTICIDES AND HERBICIDES

There is substantial evidence that a variety of pesticides are toxic and that every effort should be made to avoid inhalation of these chemicals when they are used as sprays.[2] In one study of fruit growers and farmers questioned during the spraying season, 41% of the 181 respondents stated that they had developed symptoms during the period of exposure.[3] Subsequent examination showed a decrease in peak flow rates in 19% of individuals studied and abnormal chest radiograph results in 24%. The radiographic pattern was predominantly interstitial, although cases of air-space consolidation were also observed, sometimes associated with cavitation.

Difficulty in identifying the specific chemicals responsible for the pulmonary toxicity in these cases is at least partly related to the great variety of available insecticides and the multiple ingredients that they contain. About 600 active pesticide ingredients are currently in use; toxicologic information is available for only 100.[2] The organophosphates—particularly parathion and malathion—constitute one group that has been definitely incriminated. These chemicals can be absorbed through the skin or from the respiratory tract, gastrointestinal tract, or conjunctiva; they can also cause pulmonary injury when injected intravenously. In addition to the acute toxic effects caused by these and other insecticides, there is evidence that some (particularly those containing arsenic) have a pathogenetic role in the development of pulmonary carcinoma (see page 1076).

Organophosphates

Poisoning with organophosphates occurs most commonly in agricultural workers during or shortly after the spraying of crops and less often in industrial workers during manufacture and transport; it can also happen accidentally in children and intentionally in suicide attempts.[4, 5] Parathion is the major cause of fatal poisoning; more than 50 deaths were reported during one 6-month period in Florida.[6]

Parathion and malathion are converted to paraxon and malaxon in the liver, the toxicity of the latter being greater than that of the parent forms. They exert their effects by inhibiting acetylcholinesterase at nerve endings.[7] Symptoms and signs are thus attributable mainly to the accumulation of acetylcholine at cholinergic synapses, resulting in an initial stimulation and later inhibition of synaptic transmission. Miosis, diaphoresis, increased salivation, bronchorrhea, bronchoconstriction, bradycardia, and hyperperistalsis develop. At automatic ganglia and neuromuscular junctions, nicotinic action is manifested by muscular fasciculations, particularly of the diaphragm,[8] followed by fatigue and eventual paralysis. Stimulation of cholinergic receptors in the central nervous system is followed by depression and results in coma. Depending on the route and the amount of poison taken, the time interval between exposure and the onset of symptoms ranges from 5 minutes (after a massive dose) to 24 hours.

In one review of 13 cases, the radiographic findings consisted of acute bilateral interstitial or air-space pulmonary edema, usually associated with cardiomegaly (Fig. 64–1).[9] All patients presented with coma or depressed levels of consciousness; excessive lacrimation and salivation were seen 30 minutes to 9 hours after ingestion. In patients who survived, the radiographic findings cleared within 2 to 4 days.

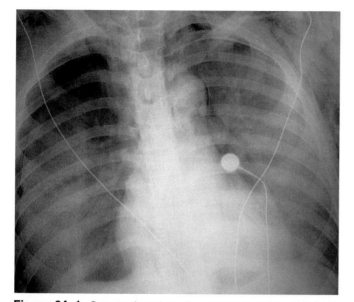

Figure 64–1. Organophosphate Poisoning. A chest radiograph in a 32-year-old man 4 days after ingestion of organophosphate pesticide demonstrates extensive bilateral consolidation with associated bilateral pneumothoraces and subcutaneous emphysema. The findings are essentially those of increased permeability pulmonary edema. (Courtesy of Dr. Kyung-Soo Lee, Department of Radiology, Samsung Medical Center, Seoul, Korea.)

The condition is serious; for example, in one group of 157 patients treated for organophosphate insecticide poisoning in South Africa, 41 were admitted to an intensive care unit, and 12 died.[10] In another series of 107 patients from China, respiratory failure, multifactorial in origin, developed in 43 (40%);[11] 22 of these patients died. Death can result from central nervous system depression or from diaphragmatic paralysis; the effects of the latter are compounded by bronchoconstriction, hypersecretion of airway mucus,[4] and pulmonary edema.[9, 13]

Paraquat

Paraquat is a bipyridylium herbicide that has been available in the United Kingdom since 1962 as a 20% concentrate (Gramoxone) and as a 5% solid form (Weedol). It was introduced in North America in 1964 in the form of three solutions of variable concentration (Orthoparaquat, Orthodualparaquat, and Ortho-spot).

Usually, poisoning results from ingestion of the drug, sometimes by mistake but, more often, for suicidal purposes; homicidal poisoning has also been described.[14] In addition, there are well-documented cases of respiratory failure and death resulting from absorption of the poison through the skin.[15-19] Such cases have been reported in fruit growers and farmers (in whom cutaneous lesions often develop)[15-17, 19] and in individuals from Papua New Guinea who applied the agent to their skin in an attempt to treat scabies and body lice.[17] In one remarkable case, a patient received a lung transplant for paraquat-induced pulmonary damage some weeks after ingestion of the poison and subsequently developed paraquat toxicity in the transplanted lung as a result of poison released from tissue stores.[20] However, transplanta-

tion was performed successfully in another patient 44 days after poisoning.[21] Poisoning has also occurred occasionally in the apparent absence of ingestion or skin exposure,[19] leading to speculation that inhalation may be the mechanism by which the poison gains access to the lungs. A patient has been described in whom chest tightness and dyspnea developed after the spraying of a field with paraquat;[22] the patient's garden (which was adjacent to the field) was subsequently defoliated, revealing a number of dead mice and moles, suggesting that inhaled paraquat was responsible for the symptoms.

As might be suspected, the likelihood of developing disease and the rapidity of its onset are dependent on the amount of paraquat ingested. When 200 ml or more is taken in an attempt to commit suicide, death usually ensues in 24 hours or less, whereas accidental poisoning, which usually occurs from imbibing a mouthful of concentrated solution (15 or 20 ml, commonly from an unlabeled container),[23] tends to cause irreversible respiratory failure in 5 to 10 days. The form of poisoning that occurs in individuals who absorb paraquat through the skin is less acute and less severe than that which follows ingestion, presumably reflecting a smaller dosage; however, even this is often fatal.[15, 17]

There is also both experimental and pathologic evidence that pulmonary damage may occur as a result of prolonged absorption of low concentrations of paraquat.[16, 24] In one investigation of 10 vineyard sprayers (one of whom developed paraquat-related skin lesions and a subacute course of respiratory failure), the diffusing capacity was reduced in 6;[16] lung biopsy performed in 2 patients showed medial hypertrophy and fresh and organized thrombi in pulmonary arteries. Application of low concentrations of paraquat to the skin of rats produced similar vascular changes. These morphologic findings are consistent with the results of experiments in which mice injected intraperitoneally with paraquat showed a linear dose-response increase in serum levels of angiotensin-converting enzyme, a substance present in large quantity in pulmonary endothelial cells.[25]

Pathogenesis

It is believed that paraquat acts in the same fashion as other oxidants (such as oxygen, ozone, and some cytotoxic drugs),[26] a concept that has been supported by studies in which poisoned rats administered oxygen died much more rapidly than those that breathed ambient air.[27] In addition, the results of experiments in which low doses of ozone and paraquat have been administered to rats have shown similar histologic and biochemical manifestations.[28]

The mechanisms by which oxidant damage occurs are likely complex. Biochemical reactions may result in peroxidation of cell lipid membranes,[29] a metabolic process that is reflected in an increase in the serum malondialdehyde level.[30] The results of experiments with cultured epithelial cells suggest that toxicity of this agent is isolated to DNA injury.[12] In isolated guinea pig lungs, nitric oxide synthesis is markedly stimulated by the acute oxidant injury induced by paraquat;[31] protection against or attenuation of toxic effects is provided by inhibition of nitric oxide synthase. Oxygen radical–mediated inhibition of phospholipase A_2, an enzyme that catalyzes the reduction of lipid hydroperoxides, has been shown to favor the accumulation of these cytotoxic oxidative compounds in rats.[32] However, the role that this enzyme plays is uncertain.[32a] In the rat model, neutrophils that migrate into the lung after intoxication have been found to be a major source of oxidants. In this respect, increased expression of the neutrophil chemotactic cytokine interleukin-8 (IL-8) has been found in human lung epithelial cell lines treated with paraquat.[33] Undoubtedly, other cytokines will be found to be important in the pathogenesis of paraquat injury, as suggested by the excess production of IL-1 and tumor necrosis factor by peripheral blood monocytes stimulated by endotoxin and exposed to paraquat.[34] *In vitro* studies have shown that paraquat also damages mitochondria[35, 36] and can cause irreversible disruption of the cellular actin cytoskeleton.[37]

Pathologic Characteristics

Large doses of paraquat cause severe pulmonary edema and hemorrhage, resulting in rapid death. Ultrastructural studies of the lungs of rats administered the poison intravenously have shown type I alveolar epithelial cell damage, with little evidence of endothelial cell injury.[38] In individuals who survive for several days, hyaline membranes and an intra-alveolar fibrinous exudate are often present (histologically identical to the exudative phase of diffuse alveolar damage seen after other forms of pulmonary injury).[39–41] Fibrous tissue begins to appear in relation to alveolar septa as early as the sixth day after poisoning[40] and increases in amount thereafter,[42] often with significant parenchymal remodeling. It has been hypothesized that fibrosis is progressive once a threshold tissue concentration of the poison has been reached.[40] Medial hypertrophy of pulmonary arteries

can be seen by the eighth day and progresses in concert with the interstitial fibrosis.[43]

Radiologic Manifestations

The radiographic findings include extensive bilateral areas of consolidation (in about 60% of patients), pneumomediastinum with or without pneumothorax (in 40%), and cardiomegaly associated with widening of the superior mediastinum (in 20%).[44] Consolidation may be seen at presentation or may develop over several days in patients whose radiographs were previously normal or had a ground-glass opacity (Fig. 64–2).[44, 45] In patients who survive, the consolidation may resolve completely or evolve into a chronic interstitial pattern consisting of irregular linear opacities or cystic spaces measuring 2 to 9 mm in diameter.[44]

The HRCT findings were reviewed in one study of 16 patients.[45a] The most common pattern, seen up to 14 days after ingestion, consisted of diffuse bilateral areas of ground-glass attenuation. Associated areas of parenchymal consolidation involving mainly the lower lung zones were present in 40% of cases (Fig. 64–3). In some patients, the areas of ground-glass attenuation progressed to consolidation over several days. CT scans performed more than 14 days after ingestion in two patients demonstrated consolidation in one and irregular lines consistent with fibrosis in the other.

Clinical Manifestations

In most cases, the diagnosis is suggested from a history of accidental ingestion or a suicide attempt. The patient

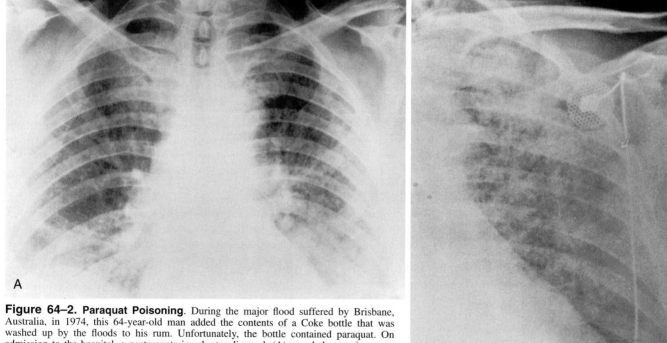

Figure 64–2. Paraquat Poisoning. During the major flood suffered by Brisbane, Australia, in 1974, this 64-year-old man added the contents of a Coke bottle that was washed up by the floods to his rum. Unfortunately, the bottle contained paraquat. On admission to the hospital, a posteroanterior chest radiograph *(A)* revealed extensive areas of ground-glass opacity throughout both lungs and focal areas of consolidation in the lung bases. Three days later *(B)*, there was more extensive parenchymal involvement with consolidation present in the upper lobes. The patient died a few days later. (Courtesy of Dr. Peter Goy and Dr. Sid Moro, Royal Brisbane Hospital, Brisbane, Australia.)

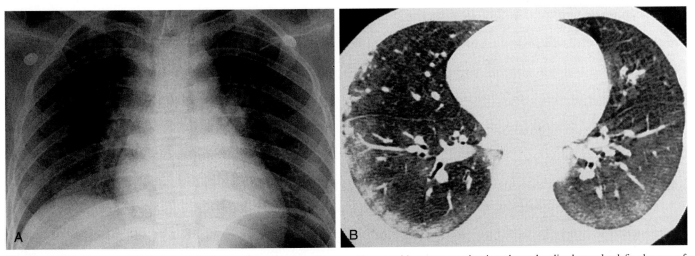

Figure 64–3. Paraquat Poisoning. A chest radiograph in an 18-year-old man with paraquat poisoning shows localized, poorly defined areas of increased opacity in the lower lung zones *(A)*. An HRCT scan *(B)* demonstrates extensive bilateral areas of ground-glass attenuation. Focal areas of consolidation are present, particularly in the subpleural lung regions in the right lower lobe, right middle lobe, and posterior basal segment of the left lower lobe. The patient recovered with complete resolution of the radiologic abnormalities. (Courtesy of Dr. Kyung-Soo Lee, Department of Radiology, Samsung Medical Center, Seoul, Korea.)

presents with vomiting, abdominal pain, and burning of the mouth and throat. An oropharyngeal membrane has been described that closely resembles that of diphtheria, except that it is situated predominantly on the tongue rather than the pharynx.[46] Death may occur within hours to a few days from pulmonary edema and renal and hepatic failure.[47] However, some patients show a brief period of apparent recovery before developing respiratory failure 5 to 10 days after admission.[48] Eighteen percent methemoglobinemia has been reported in one alcoholic patient who imbibed paraquat and survived following methylene blue therapy.[49]

Measurement of blood and urine levels of paraquat may be useful, not only in diagnosis but also in establishing prognosis.[47] In one patient, however, the herbicide was absent in multiple urine and blood specimens and yet was detected in high concentration in all major organs at autopsy.[50]

Prognosis

Although relatively uncommon, paraquat poisoning is a serious disorder: during the 13-year period since the initial fatal cases were recognized, more than 560 deaths were reported to the manufacturers.[51] Overall, about 30% to 55% of affected individuals die,[47, 48] and serious suicide attempts are almost always successful.[48a] Once there is clinical or radiographic evidence of pulmonary involvement, death is common;[47] for example, in one investigation of 42 patients who developed radiographic abnormalities, the mortality rate was 96% (26 of 27 cases) for patients who had a history of suicidal ingestion and 40% (6 of 15 cases) for patients with accidental ingestion.[44] Patients who survive may manifest residual pulmonary dysfunction,[47, 52] although this may improve with time.[53, 54] Prompt treatment may be of benefit; if at all possible, oxygen therapy should be avoided.[23, 29]

Miscellaneous Insecticides and Herbicides

The possibility that *carbamate insecticides* might be a cause of asthma was suggested by a report from Saskatche-

wan in which the prevalence of the disease in farmers exposed to these agents was greater than that of farmers not so exposed, regardless of age, smoking history, or history of allergic rhinitis.[55]

Propoxur (Baygon), a member of the carbamylester family, has an acetylcholinesterase-binding capacity similar to that of the organophosphates. Pulmonary edema, coma, bronchorrhea, and miosis have been described in patients who have used it in suicide attempts.[56]

Toxaphene, a chlorinated camphene, is a solid, waxy material containing about 68% chlorine. Its inhalation has been found to result in extensive bilateral "allergic bronchopneumonia."[57] The radiographic pattern has been reported to vary with the severity of exposure, from "simple bronchopneumonia" of middle and lower lung zones to extensive "miliary" disease.[57] Hilar lymph nodes may be enlarged. In the few reported cases, resolution has usually taken about 3 weeks. Pulmonary function tests reveal an obstructive pattern. Blood eosinophilia and elevation of serum globulin levels can be seen.

Thallium, a drug formerly utilized as a rodenticide and insecticide, is now used industrially in the production of optic lenses, low-temperature thermometers, semiconductors, pigments, and scintillation counters. Although it is more commonly associated with central nervous system and gastrointestinal toxicity, it has been responsible for the adult respiratory distress syndrome in four patients, two of whom died.[58]

The inhalation of an *amitrole-containing herbicide*, which is commonly used for spraying grass, was associated with severe alveolar damage in a single case report.[59] In another study from Taiwan, ingestion of large amounts of the herbicide *Roundup* was associated with noncardiac pulmonary edema in a minority of patients.[60]

SPANISH TOXIC OIL SYNDROME

In the summer of 1981, a previously unrecognized pneumonic-paralytic-eosinophilic syndrome occurred in

Spain in epidemic form.[61–63] Epidemiologic studies strongly indicated that the agent responsible for this disease was rapeseed oil that was denatured by the addition of 2% aniline and illegally marketed as a cooking oil. More than 20,000 people have been officially recognized by the Spanish government as suffering from the resulting toxic oil syndrome;[64] of these, about 12,000 were hospitalized and more than 300 died in the first year of the epidemic,[65] restrictive lung disease being an important cause of death.[66] The incidence of the syndrome decreased dramatically when the Spanish government removed all suspected oil from the market; however, a few late cases have been described in patients who ingested stored oil.[67]

The agent responsible for the disorder has not been identified with certainty. Although aniline was a potential candidate, it is now considered to be no more than a marker for the contaminated oil that caused the syndrome because aniline poisoning does not cause the same type of disease in humans, and the disease cannot be reproduced in animals.[66] Instead, there is evidence that the responsible agent may have been one of two esters of PAP (3-*N*-[phenylamino]-1,2-propanediol), which have been found in high concentrations in denatured rapeseed oil responsible for the syndrome but not in other aniline-denatured oils that did not result in disease.[68] This hypothesis is strengthened by the observation that PAP is structurally similar to PAA (3-[phenylamino]alanine), a contaminant of L-tryptophan, which may be responsible for a clinically related disorder, the eosinophilia-myalgia syndrome.[69]

Pathologic changes in the early stages of the syndrome were those of pulmonary edema accompanied by a scanty, largely mononuclear inflammatory infiltrate. Ultrastructural studies at this time showed degenerative changes in both type I and type II pneumocytes.[70] Some individuals who survived the acute event showed pulmonary vascular changes consistent with hypertension; in some of these, a lymphocytic vasculitis was also present.[71] In one study of individuals who died of pulmonary hypertension, pathologic abnormalities included plexiform lesions, thrombosis, and severe intimal fibrosis of veins.[72]

Clinically, the initial phase of the syndrome consisted of an acute respiratory illness characterized by cough, fever, dyspnea, and hypoxemia. Radiography showed lung opacities described as "atypical pneumonia" and pleural effusions. Half of the patients recovered from this acute illness without apparent sequelae. The remaining patients developed chronic disease consisting of severe myalgia, eosinophilia, abnormal liver function, peripheral nerve dysfunction, scleroderma-like skin lesions, sicca syndrome, alopecia, and joint contractures.[65]

Most patients improve,[66, 73, 74] the excess mortality rate seen in the early phases of disease returning to that of a comparable control population.[64] In one study of patients evaluated in 1993, 58% had persistent symptoms consisting of muscle cramping (60%), fatigue (55%), arthralgia (43%), subjective cognitive impairment (44%), psychiatric disease (27%), and soft tissue tenderness (23%).[73] Severe neuromuscular sequelae, sclerodermatous skin changes, and pulmonary hypertension were not identified. In another cohort followed for 8 years after the initial illness, chronic lung disease was noted, although only 16% of patients had evidence of extrapulmonary disease, and only 7% had any

functional impairment, as assessed clinically.[66] One group of 436 patients had a more detailed evaluation 4 years after the onset of illness, consisting of clinical examination, chest radiograph, lung function studies, and electrocardiogram.[74] Dyspnea and cough were still noted in most patients; reduced vital capacity and reduced diffusing capacity were present in 35% and 22%, respectively. Six patients (1.4%) had pulmonary hypertension, a complication seen more often in the early phase of disease and that, although potentially fatal,[72] tended to resolve with time.

HYDROCARBONS

It has been estimated that 5% of all poisonings in children result from the ingestion of petroleum products,[75] the most common of which is kerosene.[76–79] Other potentially harmful agents include gasoline,[80] furniture polish,[81] lighter fluid, automatic transmission fluid,[82] cleaning fluid, insecticides, other household cleaners (such as Dettol),[83, 84] and citronella.[85] Rarely, intravenous injection of small quantities of hydrocarbons has also been reported to result in fever, pleural and abdominal pain, and hemoptysis;[86, 87] chest radiographs showed bilateral patchy air-space opacities that cleared completely in 3 days and in 1 week. Cases of pulmonary disease have also been reported following the accidental aspiration of petroleum in performers demonstrating the art of fire-eating;[88] other reports suggest that this complication is a common occupational hazard in these individuals.[89–91]

Although poisoning by these routes is important in terms of the number of individuals affected, the resulting disease is fortunately of relatively mild severity. For example, in one survey of 950 children younger than 5 years of age who were suspected of having ingested products containing hydrocarbons, 800 were symptom free at the time of initial evaluation and remained so during a 6- to 8-hour period of observation; they were managed as outpatients.[75] The remaining 150 were admitted to the hospital; although 71 were symptom free, all had abnormal chest radiograph results. Complications occurred only in the 79 children who had both symptoms and abnormal radiographs; of these, 2 died and 5 developed progressive pulmonary disease. Despite these observations, the number of children who develop radiographic changes varies considerably among studies, with some groups reporting radiographic changes in 70% to 90% of such patients.[76] Such variation may be related to the inclusion in some investigations of children who either did not actually swallow the poison or ingested such small amounts that they would have been excluded from other series.[75]

There is some controversy concerning the pathogenesis of this form of poison-induced pulmonary disease, one hypothesis supporting absorption from the intestinal tract with subsequent transport to the pulmonary capillaries, and another invoking emesis and aspiration of vomitus with direct alveolocapillary damage. Experimental studies in animals have produced conflicting results. There is no doubt that intratracheal injection of aromatic hydrocarbons into animals can produce hemorrhagic edema, necrosis, and acute inflammation.[76, 92–95] However, although the instillation of hydrocarbons into the peritoneal cavity or stomach of animals (unaccompanied by esophageal regurgitation) has resulted in the development of pulmonary disease in some studies,[96] in others, there has been no significant reaction.[92, 97] These contradictory results may be related to the varying toxicity and dosage of the hydrocarbon used; for example, in one study, it was estimated that the dose instilled into a dog's stomach had to be 140 times that instilled into the trachea to produce a chemical pneumonitis.[86]

The chest radiograph is usually abnormal within an hour of the ingestion of kerosene;[76, 77] however, changes have been found to appear somewhat later after furniture polish ingestion.[81] The severity of the pulmonary abnormality varies with the amount ingested.[76] The typical radiographic pattern is one of patchy bilateral air-space consolidation involving predominantly the basal portions of the lung.[76, 77, 81, 98] The hila are sometimes indistinct and hazy as a result of contiguous pulmonary disease, a finding that can occur alone but is more often associated with basal changes. Radiographic resolution tends to be slow (up to 2 weeks) and usually lags well behind clinical improvement.[76, 77] Pneumatoceles may develop;[99–101] for example, in one investigation of 338 children, 134 (40%) developed acute pneumonia, of whom 14 demonstrated pneumatocele formation during resolution;[101] the pneumatoceles were often large, septate, and irregular and sometimes contained fluid levels.

In the absence of witnesses to the incident, the diagnosis may be suspected from the odor of the offending agent on the patient's breath. Vomiting follows shortly after ingestion and in many cases is probably associated with aspiration. Symptoms are usually mild; however, the greater the amount of hydrocarbon ingested, the greater the severity of clinical findings and the extent of radiographic abnormalities.[76]

REFERENCES

1. O'Callaghan WG, Joyce N, Counihan HE, et al: Unusual strychnine poisoning and its treatment: Report of eight cases. Br Med J 285:478, 1982.
2. Weisenburger DD: Human health effects of agrichemical use. Hum Pathol 24:571, 1993.
3. Lings S: Pesticide lung: A pilot investigation of fruit-growers and farmers during the spraying season. Br J Ind Med 39:370, 1982.
4. Namba T, Nolte CT, Jackrel J, et al: Poisoning due to organophosphate insecticides: Acute and chronic manifestations. Am J Med 50:475, 1971.
5. Bardin PG, van Eeden SF, Joubert JR: Intensive care management of acute organophosphate poisoning: A 7-year experience in the Western Cape. S Afr Med J 72:593, 1987.
6. Bledsoe FH, Seymour EQ: Acute pulmonary edema associated with parathion poisoning. Radiology 103:53, 1972.
7. Neal EA: Enzymic mechanism of metabolism of the phosphorothionate insecticides. Arch Intern Med 128:118, 1971.
8. Hunter D: Devices for the protection of the worker against injury and disease. Part II. Br Med J 1:506, 1950.
9. Li C, Miller WT, Jiang J: Pulmonary edema due to ingestion of organophosphate insecticide. Am J Roentgenol 152:265,1989.
10. Du Toit PW, Muller FO, Van Tonder WM, et al: Experience with the intensive care management of organophosphate insecticide poisoning. S Afr Med J 60:227, 1981.
11. Tsao TCY, Juang YC, Lan RS, et al: Respiratory failure of acute organophosphate and carbamate poisoning. Chest 98:631, 1990.
12. Dusinska M, Kovacikova Z, Vallova B, et al: Responses of alveolar macrophages and epithelial type II cells to oxidative DNA damage caused by paraquat. Carcinogenesis 19:809, 1998.
13. Betrosian A, Balla M, Kafiri G, et al: Multiple systems organ failure from organophosphate poisoning. J Toxicol Clin Toxicol 33:257, 1995.
14. Stephens BG, Moormeister SK: Homicidal poisoning by paraquat. Am J Forensic Med Pathol 18:33, 1997.
15. Newhouse M, McEvoy D, Rosenthal D: Percutaneous paraquat absorption: An association with cutaneous lesions and respiratory failure. Arch Dermatol 114:1516, 1978.
16. Levin PJ, Klaff LJ, Rose AG, et al: Pulmonary effects of contact exposure to paraquat: A clinical and experimental study. Thorax 34:150, 1979.
17. Wohlfahrt DJ: Fatal paraquat poisonings after skin absorption. Med J Aust 1:512, 1982.
18. Papiris SA, Maniati MA, Kyriakidis V, et al: Pulmonary damage due to paraquat poisoning through skin absorption. Respiration 62:101, 1995.
19. Wesseling C, Hogstedt C, Picado A, et al: Unintentional fatal paraquat poisonings among agricultural workers in Costa Rica: Report of 15 cases. Am J Ind Med 32:433, 1997.
20. The Toronto Lung Transplant Group: Sequential bilateral lung transplantation for paraquat poisoning: A case report. J Thorac Cardiovasc Surg 89:734, 1985.
21. Walder B, Brundler MA, Spiliopoulos A, et al: Successful single-lung transplantation after paraquat intoxication. Transplantation 64:789, 1997.
22. George M, Hedworth-Whitty RB: Non-fatal lung disease due to inhalation of nebulised paraquat. Br Med J 280:902, 1980.
23. Fairshter RD, Wilson AF: Paraquat poisoning: Manifestations and therapy. Am J Med 59:751, 1975.
24. Shinozaki S, Kobayashi T, Kubo K, et al: Pulmonary hemodynamics and lung function during chronic paraquat poisoning in sheep: Possible role of reactive oxygen species. Am Rev Respir Dis 146:775, 1992.
25. Hollinger MA, Patwell SW, Zuckerman JE, et al: Effect of paraquat on serum angiotensin-converting enzyme. Am Rev Respir Dis 121:795, 1980.
26. Van der Wal NA, Smith LL, van Oirschot JF, et al: Effect of iron chelators on paraquat toxicity in rats and alveolar type II cells. Am Rev Respir Dis 145:180, 1992.
27. Fisher HK, Clements JA, Wright RR: Enhancement of oxygen toxicity by the herbicide paraquat. Am Rev Respir Dis 107:246, 1973.
28. Montgomery MR, Casey PJ, Valls AA, et al: Biochemical and morphological correlation of oxidant-induced pulmonary injury: Low dose exposure to paraquat, oxygen, and ozone. Arch Environ Health 34:396, 1979.
29. Fairshter RD: Paraquat toxicity and lipid peroxidation. Arch Intern Med 141:1121, 1981.
30. Yasaka T, Ohya I, Matsumoto J, et al: Acceleration of lipid peroxidation in human paraquat poisoning. Arch Intern Med 141:1169, 1981.
31. Berisha HI, Pakbaz H, Absood A, et al: Nitric oxide as a mediator of oxidant lung injury due to paraquat. Proc Natl Acad Sci U S A 91:7445, 1994.
32. Giulivi C, Lavagno CC, Lucesoli F, et al: Lung damage in paraquat poisoning and hyperbaric oxygen exposure: Superoxide-mediated inhibition of phospholipase A2. Free Radical Biol Med 18:203, 1995.
32a. Fabisiak JP, Kagan VE, Tyurina YY, et al: Paraquat-induced phosphatidylserine oxidation and apoptosis are independent of activation of PLA2. Am J Physiol 274:L793, 1998.
33. Bianchi M, Fantuzzi G, Bertini R, et al: The pneumotoxicant paraquat induces IL-8 mRNA in human mononuclear cells and pulmonary epithelial cells. Cytokine 5:525, 1993.
34. Erroi A, Bianchi M, Ghezzi P: The pneumotoxicant paraquat potentiates IL-1 and TNF production by human mononuclear cells. Agents Actions 36:66, 1992.
35. Costantini P, Petronilli V, Colonna R, et al: On the effects of paraquat on isolated mitochondria: Evidence that paraquat causes opening of the cyclosporin A-sensitive permeability transition pore synergistically with nitric oxide. Toxicology 99:77, 1995.
36. Fukushima T, Yamada K, Hojo N, et al: Mechanism of cytotoxicity of paraquat. III. The effects of acute paraquat exposure on the electron transport system in rat mitochondria. Exp Toxicol Pathol 46:437, 1994.
37. Cappelletti G, Incani C, Maci R: Paraquat induces irreversible actin cytoskeleton disruption in cultured human lung cells. Cell Biol Toxicol 10:255, 1994.
38. Thurlbeck WM, Thurlbeck SM: Pulmonary effects of paraquat poisoning. Chest 69(Suppl):276, 1976.
39. Rebello G, Mason JK: Pulmonary histological appearances in fatal paraquat poisoning. Histopathology 2:53, 1978.
40. Takahashi T, Takahashi Y, Nio M: Remodeling of the alveolar structure in the paraquat lung of humans: A morphometric study. Hum Pathol 25:702, 1994.
41. Soontornniyomkij V, Bunyaratvej S: Fatal paraquat poisoning: A light microscopic study in eight autopsy cases. J Med Assoc Thai 75(Suppl 1):98, 1992.
42. Yamaguchi M, Takahashi T, Togashi H, et al: The corrected collagen content in paraquat lungs. Chest 90:251, 1986.
43. Sawai T, Fujiyama J, Takahashi M, et al: The site of elevated vascular resistance in early paraquat lungs: A morphometric study of pulmonary arteries. Tohoku J Exp Med 174:129, 1994.
44. Im JG, Lee KS, Han MC, et al: Paraquat poisoning: Findings on chest radiography and CT in 42 patients. Am J Roentgenol 157:697, 1991.
45. Davidson JK, MacPherson P: Pulmonary changes in paraquat poisoning. Clin Radiol 23:18, 1972.
45a. Lee SH, Lee KS, Ahn JM, et al: Paraquat poisoning of the lung: thin-section CT findings. Radiology 195:271, 1995.
46. Stephens DS, Walker DH, Schaffner W, et al: Pseudodiphtheria: Prominent pharyngeal membrane associated with fatal paraquat ingestion. Ann Intern Med 94:202, 1981.
47. Higenbottam T, Crome P, Parkinson C, et al: Further clinical observations on the pulmonary effects of paraquat ingestion. Thorax 34:161, 1979.
48. Editorial: Paraquat poisoning. Lancet 2:1018, 1971.
48a. Hudson M, Patel SB, Ewen SWB, et al: Paraquat induced pulmonary fibrosis in three survivors. Thorax 46:201, 1991.
49. Ng LL, Naik RB, Polak A: Paraquat ingestion with methaemoglobinaemia treated with methylene blue. Br Med J 284:1445, 1982.
50. Conradi SE, Olanoff LS, Dawson WT Jr: Fatality due to paraquat intoxication: Confirmation by postmortem tissue analysis. J Clin Pathol 80:771, 1983.
51. Harley JB, Grinspan S, Root RK: Paraquat suicide in a young woman: Results of therapy directed against the superoxide radical. Yale J Biol Med 50:481, 1977.
52. Anderson CG: Paraquat and the lung. Australas Radiol 14:409, 1970.
53. Bismuth C, Hall AH, Baud FJ, et al: Pulmonary dysfunction in survivors of acute paraquat poisoning. Vet Hum Toxicol 38:220, 1996.
54. Lin JL, Liu L, Leu ML: Recovery of respiratory function in survivors with paraquat intoxication. Arch Environ Health 50:432, 1995.
55. Senthilselvan A, McDuffie HH, Dosman JA: Association of asthma with use of pesticides: Results of a cross-sectional survey of farmers. Am Rev Respir Dis 146:884, 1992.
56. Salisburg BD, Tate CF, Davies JE: Baygon-induced pulmonary edema. Chest 65:455, 1974.
57. Warraki S: Respiratory hazards of chlorinated camphene. Arch Environ Health 7:253, 1963.
58. Roby DS, Fein AM, Bennett RH, et al: Cardiopulmonary effects of acute thallium poisoning. Chest 85:236, 1984.
59. Balkisson R, Murray D, Hoffstein V: Alveolar damage due to inhalation of amitrole-containing herbicide. Chest 101:1174, 1992.
60. Talbot AR, Shiaw MH, Huang JS, et al: Acute poisoning with a glyphosate-surfactant herbicide. Hum Exp Toxicol 10:1, 1991.
61. Tabuenca JM: Toxic-allergic syndrome caused by ingestion of rapeseed oil denatured with aniline. Lancet 2:567, 1981.
62. Rigau-Pérez JG, Pérez-Alvarez L, Duñas-Castro S, et al: Epidemiologic investigation of an oil-associated pneumonic paralytic eosinophilic syndrome in Spain. Am J Epidemiol 119:250, 1984.
63. De la Cruz JL, Oteo LA, López C, et al: Toxic-oil syndrome: Gallium-67 scanning and bronchoalveolar lavage studies in patients with abnormal lung function. Chest 88:398, 1985.
64. Abaitua Borda I, Kilbourne EM, Posada de la Paz M, et al: Mortality among people affected by toxic oil syndrome. Int J Epidemiol 22:1077, 1993.
65. Kilbourne EM, Posada de la Paz M, Abaitua Borda I, et al: Toxic oil syndrome: A current clinical and epidemiologic summary, including comparisons with the eosinophilia-myalgia syndrome. J Am Coll Cardiol 18:711, 1991.
66. Alonso-Ruiz A, Calabozo M, Perez-Ruiz F, et al: Toxic oil syndrome. Medicine 72:285, 1993.
67. Posada de la Paz M, Abaitua Borda I, Kilbourne EM, et al: Late cases of toxic oil syndrome: Evidence that the aetiologic agent persisted in oil stored for up to one year. Food Chem Toxicol 27:517, 1989.
68. Hill RH Jr, Schurz HH, Posada de la Paz M, et al: Possible etiologic agents for toxic oil syndrome: Fatty acid esters of 3-(N-phenylamino)-1,2-propanediol. Arch Environ Contam Toxicol 28:259, 1995.

69. Mayeno AN, Belongia EA, Lin F, et al: 3-(Phenylamino) alanine, a novel aniline-derived amino acid associated with the eosinophilia-myalgia syndrome: A link to the toxic oil syndrome? Mayo Clin Proc 67:1134, 1992.

70. Martinez-Tello FJ, Navas-Palacios JJ, Ricoy JR, et al: Pathology of a new toxic syndrome caused by ingestion of adulterated oil in Spain. Virchows Arch (Pathol Anat) 397:261, 1982.

71. Fernández-Segoviano P, Esteban A, Martínez-Cabruja R: Pulmonary vascular lesions in the toxic oil syndrome in Spain. Thorax 38:724, 1983.

72. Gómez-Sánchez MA, Mestre de Juan MJ, Gómez-Pajuelo C, et al: Pulmonary hypertension due to toxic oil syndrome: A clinicopathologic study. Chest 95:325, 1989.

73. Kaufman LD, Izquierdo Martinez M, Serrano JM, et al: 12-Year follow up study of epidemic Spanish toxic oil syndrome. J Rheumatol 22:282, 1995.

74. Martin Escribano P, Diaz de Atauri MJ, Gómez Sánchez MA: Persistence of respiratory abnormalities four years after the onset of toxic oil syndrome. Chest 100:336, 1991.

75. Anas N, Namasonthi V, Ginsburg CM: Criteria for hospitalizing children who have ingested products containing hydrocarbons. JAMA 246:840, 1981.

76. Reynolds J, Bonte FJ: Kerosene pneumonitis. Tex Med 56:34, 1960.

77. Brünner S, Rovsing H, Wulf H: Roentgenographic changes in the lungs of children with kerosene poisoning. Am Rev Respir Dis 89:250, 1964.

78. Fagbule DO, Joiner KT: Kerosene poisoning in childhood: A 6-year prospective study at the University of Ilorin Teaching Hospital. West Afr J Med 11:116, 1992.

79. Singh H, Chugh JC, Shembesh AH, et al: Management of accidental kerosene ingestion. Ann Trop Paediatr 12:105, 1992.

80. Nome O, Ditlefsen EML: Acute gasoline poisoning: Four cases. Nord Med 61:140, 1959.

81. Jimenez JP, Lester RG: Pulmonary complications following furniture polish ingestion: A report of 21 cases. Am J Roentgenol 98:323, 1966.

82. Perrot LJ, Palmer H: Fatal hydrocarbon lipoid pneumonia and pneumonitis secondary to automatic transmission fluid ingestion. J Forensic Sci 37:1422, 1992.

83. Chan TY, Critchley JA, Lau JT: The risk of aspiration in Dettol poisoning: A retrospective cohort study. Hum Exp Toxicol 14:190, 1995.

84. Chan TY, Lau MS, Critchley JA: Serious complications associated with Dettol poisoning. Q J Med 86:735, 1993.

85. Temple WA, Smith NA, Beasley M: Management of oil of citronella poisoning. J Toxicol Clin Toxicol 29:257, 1991.

86. Neeld EM, Limacher MC: Chemical pneumonitis after the intravenous injection of hydrocarbon. Radiology 129:36, 1978.

87. Vaziri ND, Jeeminson-Smith P, Wilson AF: Hemorrhagic pneumonitis after intravenous injection of charcoal lighter fluid. Ann Intern Med 90:794, 1979.

88. Brander PE, Taskinen E, Stenius-Aarniala B: Fire-eater's lung. Eur Respir J 5:112, 1992.

89. Borer H, Koelz AM: Fire eater's lung (hydrocarbon pneumonitis). J Suisse de Medecine 124:362, 1994.

90. Ewert R, Lindemann I, Romberg B, et al: The accidental aspiration and ingestion of petroleum in a "fire eater." Deutsche Medizinische Wochenschrift 117:1594, 1992.

91. Iversen E, Christensen BE: Pulmonary complications in flame swallowers. Ugeskr Laeger 146:26, 1984.

92. Wolfe BM, Brodeur AE, Shields JB: The role of gastrointestinal absorption of kerosene in producing pneumonitis in dogs. J Pediatr 76:867, 1970.

93. Gross P, McNerney JM, Babyak MA: Kerosene pneumonitis: An experimental study with small doses. Am Rev Respir Dis 88:656, 1963.

94. Steele RW, Conklin RH, Mark HM: Corticosteroids and antibiotics for the treatment of fulminant hydrocarbon aspiration. JAMA 219:1434, 1972.

95. Scharf SM, Heimer D, Goldstein J: Pathologic and physiologic effects of aspiration of hydrocarbons in the rat. Am Rev Respir Dis 124:625, 1981.

96. Thurlbeck WM: Conference summary. Chest 66(Suppl):40, 1974.

97. Heinisch HM, Levejohann R: The pathogenesis of radiological changes in the lungs after ingestion of petroleum distillates: An experimental study in rabbits and extrapolation of the results to children. Ann Radiol 16:263, 1973.

98. Bonte FJ, Reynolds J: Hydrocarbon pneumonitis. Radiology 71:391, 1958.

99. Baghdassarian OM, Weiner S: Pneumatocele formation complicating hydrocarbon pneumonitis. Am J Roentgenol 95:104, 1965.

100. Campbell JB: Pneumatocele formation following hydrocarbon ingestion. Am Rev Respir Dis 101:414, 1970.

101. Harris VJ, Brown R: Pneumatoceles as a complication of chemical pneumonia after hydrocarbon ingestion. Am J Roentgenol 125:531, 1975.

Irradiation

Within the therapeutic range of doses usually administered, the pulmonary parenchyma can be assumed to react to ionizing radiation in virtually all patients. Many variables, however, affect this reaction and its clinical and radiologic manifestations, including the volume of lung tissue irradiated, the radiation dose administered, the time over which it is given, and the nature of the radiation.[1, 2] In addition, the lung can be affected by radiation in the absence of a demonstrable abnormality on conventional radiographs.[3, 4] There is semantic confusion in the literature, however; the term *radiation pneumonitis* is used by some to denote a radiographic abnormality and by others to describe a clinical syndrome. For all these reasons, the incidence of pulmonary damage after radiotherapy varies considerably from series to series.

Pulmonary tissue is usually damaged by radiation aimed directly at the lungs; however, it also can be injured when the beam is directed elsewhere in the thorax, such as at the mediastinum or chest wall. In a review of 18 studies involving 5,534 patients reported before 1992, 7% of patients (range 1% to 34%) developed symptomatic pneumonitis after radiation treatment for carcinoma of the lung, breast, or mesothelioma or for Hodgkin's disease;[5] 43% of patients (range, 13% to 100%) developed radiologic changes. In a more recent report, the incidence of radiation pneumonitis following combined modality therapy for lung cancer that was reported in 24 separate series and included 1,911 patients.[6] The total radiation dose used in these studies ranged from 25 to 63 Gy, with a median dose of 50 Gy (1 Gray = 100 rad). Symptomatic radiation pneumonitis occurred in 7.8% of patients. The risk was greater with total radiation dose, daily radiation fractions greater than 2.67 Gy, and use of once-daily as opposed to twice-daily irradiation. Symptomatic radiation pneumonitis occurred in 6% of patients receiving a total radiation dose lower than 45 Gy, in 9% of patients receiving doses between 45 and 54 Gy, and in 12% of patients with total radiation doses of 55 Gy or greater.

Focal radiation injury to the airways can occur after brachytherapy, a procedure that is used with increasing frequency for palliation of obstructing pulmonary carcinoma.[7–9] The technique consists of intraluminal endobronchial irradiation with a radioactive substance, usually iridium 192. Radiation injury to the lungs can also follow inhalation of β-emitting radionuclides.[10–12] Rarely, it follows internal selective radiotherapy of the liver when radioactive microspheres injected into the hepatic artery enter the pulmonary circulation through arterioportal shunts.[13] Pulmonary fibrosis associated with remote Thorotrast administration has also been reported.[14]

PATHOGENESIS

Radiologic and Clinical Factors

Volume of Lung Irradiated. The likelihood of clinical symptoms and radiologic evidence of pulmonary injury is proportional to the volume of lung irradiated.[2] In fact, this variable is considered by some investigators to be the most important factor associated with lung damage.[15, 16] For example, it has been estimated that a total dose of 30 Gy delivered in fractions to 25% of total lung volume may not produce any symptoms, whereas an identical dose delivered in the same manner to the entire volume of both lungs would probably prove fatal.[15]

Recognition of the importance of the volume of irradiated lung has led to the development of tangential ports to deliver radiotherapy, thereby limiting radiation dose to normal structures. The prevalence of symptomatic radiation pneumonitis after treatment of breast carcinoma decreased from about 60% to 7% with the use of tangential ports rather than direct irradiation.[17, 18] Refinements in the tangential ports have led to further reduction in the incidence of symptomatic radiation pneumonitis. For example, in one study of 1,624 patients treated for carcinoma of the breast with tangential field irradiation, only 17 (1%) developed symptomatic pneumonitis.[19] All 17 had radiographic changes that corresponded to the treatment portals; in 12, the radiographs became normal within 1 to 12 months after radiotherapy. Only 5 patients had persistent radiation fibrosis, and none had late or persistent pulmonary symptoms. In another study, the incidence of symptomatic radiation pneumonitis after therapy for Hodgkin's disease was compared in patients receiving only mantle irradiation for mediastinal lymph nodes and those receiving additional low-dose lung irradiation.[20] The mantle-field radiation dose ranged from 36 to 44 Gy, and the total-lung radiation dose was 15 Gy. Twelve of

395 patients (3%) receiving mantle irradiation alone developed radiation pneumonitis, as compared with 7 of 47 (15%) who received mantle-field plus total-lung irradiation.

Dose. Radiation pneumonitis seldom occurs with doses below 30 Gy,[2, 21, 22] is variably present with doses between 30 and 40 Gy, and is almost always present with doses greater than 40 Gy.[2, 5, 22] There is, however, considerable individual variability in the pulmonary response, and it is therefore impossible to predict which patients will develop radiologic changes or symptomatic radiation pneumonitis.[2, 18] For example, radiation pneumonitis has been reported in some patients who received less than 0.5 Gy,[23] whereas others who have received more than 40 Gy have developed no complication.[2] Furthermore, despite the fact that the average dose to patients in whom radiographically demonstrable changes develop is significantly higher than the average dose to those whose lungs remain normal, statistically significant differences between the doses that result in minimal, moderate, or severe pulmonary changes have not been found.[24]

Time and Dose Factor. The effect of radiation on the lung is related less to the total dose than to the rate at which it is delivered because fractionation permits time for repair of sublethal damage between fractions.[10] This variable biologic effect of equivalent doses of radiation is related to the total dose absorbed, the number of fractions, and the time elapsed between first and last treatments.[25–27] The severity of radiation effect increases with increased dose per fraction or when the same dose is given over a shorter period of time.[2]

Previous or Concurrent Therapy. The susceptibility to radiation pneumonitis is increased in patients who have had previous pulmonary irradiation[5, 18, 23] or previous or concurrent chemotherapy[2, 18] and in whom corticosteroid has been withdrawn.[28–30] Drugs known to enhance the effects of radiation include actinomycin D, doxorubicin, bleomycin, busulfan, cyclophosphamide, mitomycin C, methotrexate, and vincristine.[18, 31–35] In one study of 328 patients with breast cancer who received radiotherapy and chemotherapy, 11 (3%) developed symptomatic radiation pneumonitis, as compared with only 6 of 1296 (0.5%) of those who received radiotherapy alone.[36] The risk of radiation pneumonitis is increased when irradiation and chemotherapy are administered simultaneously.[5, 36] For example, in one investigation of 92 patients with breast cancer treated concurrently with chemotherapy and radiotherapy, 8 (9%) developed symptomatic radiation pneumonitis, as compared with only 3 of 326 (1.3%) who were treated sequentially.[36] Radiation recall—the development of pneumonitis in a previously irradiated site following the administration of chemotherapeutic agents—can occur within hours to days of drug administration and can be seen a few days up to 15 years after radiotherapy.[36a–c]

Cellular and Molecular Factors

The molecular basis of radiation-induced pulmonary disease is complex and not completely understood.[37] It is believed that x-rays or gamma rays exert their effects by colliding with and exciting electrons, which, in turn, generate ion pairs and a variety of free radicals. The latter cause breakage of covalent bonds in both small and large molecules; such damage can be repaired in some instances but may be irreversible, particularly in the presence of oxygen.

The resulting molecular changes can lead to significant biochemical, structural, and functional abnormalities. These abnormalities are caused by two classes of molecules: (1) those such as DNA that are concerned with genetic effects and (2) a variety of non-DNA macromolecules contained in the cell cytoplasm, organelles, and membranes. Damage to the latter group can result in several immediate effects, such as "leaky" cell membranes or impaired transport of intracellular material; if sufficiently severe, these can lead directly to cell death. Such injury may be the mechanism of capillary endothelial and type I epithelial cell damage in early radiation pneumonitis.[37] Damage to both types of cell at this stage results in an increase in capillary permeability and the accumulation of intra-alveolar fluid.[37] Increased transudation of fluid and serum proteins into the alveoli also occurs secondary to the increased alveolar surface tension as a consequence of injury to type II pneumocyte and surfactant loss.

Less obvious in its effect, at least in the early stages of radiation pneumonitis, is injury to DNA. This may take several forms, including breaks that are incorrectly repaired, abnormal cross-links, and chromosomal rearrangements. Cells containing such DNA can remain viable and apparently unharmed until they divide, at which time the progeny may die or show functional disturbances. These effects are most evident in cells with a rapid turnover rate and least obvious in highly differentiated cells. In the lungs, the cells most sensitive to radiation-induced chromosomal abnormalities are capillary endothelial, bronchial epithelial, and alveolar type II cells. The cytologic atypia of type II pneumocytes in radiation pneumonitis presumably reflects this genetic damage.

The precise pathogenesis of delayed pulmonary fibrosis that occurs after radiation is unclear. Although it may be caused by a direct effect of radiation on parenchymal interstitial cells, there is experimental evidence that it is the result of endothelial damage that causes an alteration of the normal endothelial-fibroblast interaction.[38] Endothelial cells synthesize plasminogen activator, an enzyme that cleaves plasminogen in the fibrinolysis cascade. Decreased activity of plasminogen activator has been demonstrated in rats 1 month after irradiation and has been shown to correlate with decreased fibrinolysis in irradiated lungs compared with that in control lungs.[39] Murine strains prone to radiation-induced pulmonary fibrosis have also been shown to have lower plasminogen activator activity than strains not prone to radiation fibrosis.[40]

It has also been suggested that one of the main mechanisms for the development of radiation pneumonitis and fibrosis is radiation-induced cytokine production and release by pulmonary macrophages.[5, 41, 42] One of the most important stimulator of collagen synthesis is believed to be transforming growth factor-β (TGF-β).[41] Experiments in rabbits have shown increased release of TGF, including TGF-β, within days to weeks after irradiation;[42–44] this increase persists until the development of fibrosis. Irradiation can also lead to release of fibroblast growth factors from endothelial cells.[41]

It has been suggested that the involvement of lung tissue outside the radiation field may be the result of a delayed hypersensitivity reaction in response to a radiation-damaged antigen.[45] A variety of observations support this hypothesis, including the discordance between the severity of clinical findings and volume of irradiated lung, the latent period for the reaction, the beneficial response to corticosteroid therapy, the lymphocytosis that can be observed in bronchoalveolar lavage fluid, and the increased gallium uptake that occurs in the contralateral lung when irradiation is confined to one hemithorax.[41, 42, 45, 46]

PATHOLOGIC CHARACTERISTICS

Knowledge of the pathologic features of the earliest stage of radiation pneumonitis derives primarily from animal experiments. Although such knowledge is useful, there are significant interspecies differences in the pattern of the reaction.[47, 48] In addition, some investigators have employed very large doses (up to 70 Gy[49]) or have exposed a whole lung rather than part of a lung to the irradiation; thus, extrapolation of experimental findings to humans must be made with caution.

One of the earliest and most consistent abnormalities in experimental animals is endothelial damage, manifested initially as swelling and vacuolization of the cytoplasm, followed by necrosis and detachment from the basement membrane.[50, 51] Platelet thrombi develop and are organized by either recanalization or fibrosis; this in turn can cause significant vascular narrowing and obstruction, decreased lung perfusion,[52] and pulmonary arterial hypertension.[53] Soon after irradiation, type I cells become necrotic,[50] although there is evidence that this occurs later than the damage to capillary endothelial cells.[47]

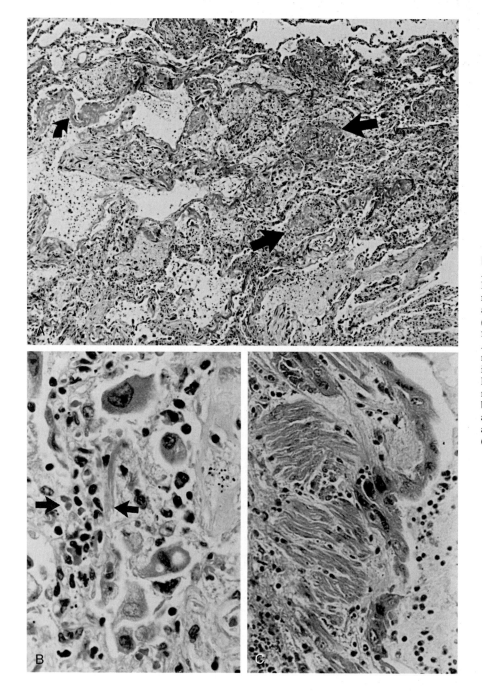

Figure 65–1. Acute Radiation Pneumonitis. A section of lung parenchyma *(A)* from the upper lobe of a patient treated 3 months before death with radiotherapy for breast carcinoma reveals extensive air-space filling by a proteinaceous exudate *(straight arrows)*, mild interstitial thickening, and focal hyaline membrane formation *(curved arrow)*. A magnified view of a single alveolus *(B)* shows a mononuclear inflammatory infiltrate in the septal interstitium *(between arrows)* and several irregularly shaped type II pneumocytes with hyperchromatic and cytologically atypical nuclei. A section of bronchial wall *(C)*, also within the field of radiation, again shows a mononuclear inflammatory infiltrate as well as markedly abnormal epithelial lining cells. *(A,* ×60; *B,* ×400; *C,* ×200.)

In humans, two stages of radiation damage can be recognized, an early or acute reaction (radiation pneumonitis) and a late or fibrotic stage. Many reports of pathologic changes in the early stage have been derived from autopsies of patients who died 4 to 12 weeks after completion of radiotherapy at a time when secondary changes from superimposed infection or heart failure may have obscured or been difficult to separate from the effects of irradiation. However, enough information is available from apparently uncomplicated cases and from lung biopsies to permit a reasonable description.[21, 47, 54]

Typically, the reaction in the acute stage is characterized by a pattern of diffuse alveolar damage (Fig. 65–1), consisting of an exudate of proteinaceous material in the alveolar air spaces associated with hyaline membranes, especially in alveolar ducts and distal respiratory bronchioles. The parenchymal interstitium is thickened by congested capillaries, edema, and, with time, fibroblasts and loose connective tissue; an inflammatory cellular infiltrate is usually minimal. Type II cells are hyperplastic and often have large nuclei, which are sometimes bizarre in shape (*see* Fig. 65–1). Although this latter feature can be seen in diseases of other etiologies, provided the changes are sufficiently extensive and the effect of cytotoxic drugs can be excluded, it is suggestive of radiation damage. Evidence of epithelial injury also can be present in membranous bronchioles and bronchi, typically in the form of a loss of the normal respiratory epithelium and its replacement by a cuboidal or flattened epithelium; these epithelial cells can also show nuclear atypia (*see* Fig. 65–1).

The late or fibrotic stage of radiation damage is characterized by fibrosis of both parenchymal air spaces and interstitium that may be so severe that underlying architecture is difficult to identify; an increased number and fragmentation of elastic fibers are common (Fig. 65–2). Although somewhat distorted by the adjacent fibrosis, airways can appear remarkably unaffected. However, bronchiolitis obliterans and (occasionally) endobronchial fibrosis are present. Vessels—particularly veins but also arteries[55]—often show intimal thickening as a result of myofibroblast proliferation and connective tissue deposition; focal medial hyalinization and intimal foam cells also may be seen.

RADIOLOGIC MANIFESTATIONS

Radiographic evidence of acute radiation pneumonitis usually becomes evident about 8 weeks after completion of radiotherapy with doses of 40 Gy and about 1 week earlier for every additional 10 Gy increment.[2, 22] Abnormalities are usually most marked 3 to 4 months after completion of radiotherapy;[2, 56] they are seen rarely immediately after completion of therapy[57] and occasionally within 1 to 4 weeks (Fig. 65–3).[3, 23, 57]

The radiographic manifestations may be subtle, consisting of hazy ground-glass opacities with slight indis-

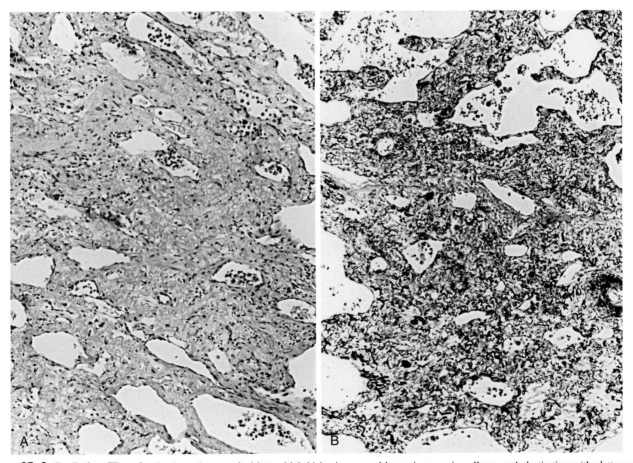

Figure 65–2. Radiation Fibrosis. Sections show marked interstitial thickening caused by an increase in collagen and elastic tissue (the latter seen as *curly black lines* in *B*). The patient had received radiation 6 months before death for metastatic breast carcinoma.

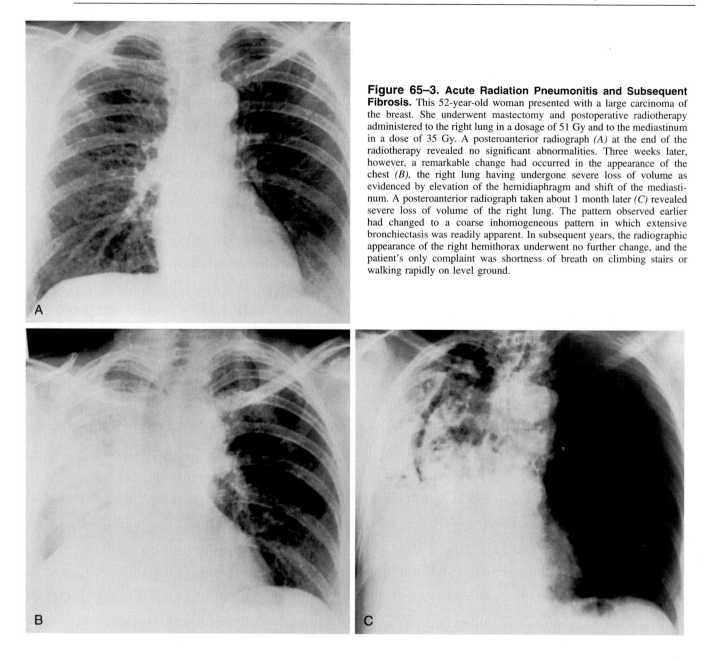

Figure 65–3. Acute Radiation Pneumonitis and Subsequent Fibrosis. This 52-year-old woman presented with a large carcinoma of the breast. She underwent mastectomy and postoperative radiotherapy administered to the right lung in a dosage of 51 Gy and to the mediastinum in a dose of 35 Gy. A posteroanterior radiograph *(A)* at the end of the radiotherapy revealed no significant abnormalities. Three weeks later, however, a remarkable change had occurred in the appearance of the chest *(B)*, the right lung having undergone severe loss of volume as evidenced by elevation of the hemidiaphragm and shift of the mediastinum. A posteroanterior radiograph taken about 1 month later *(C)* revealed severe loss of volume of the right lung. The pattern observed earlier had changed to a coarse inhomogeneous pattern in which extensive bronchiectasis was readily apparent. In subsequent years, the radiographic appearance of the right hemithorax underwent no further change, and the patient's only complaint was shortness of breath on climbing stairs or walking rapidly on level ground.

tinctness of the pulmonary vessels, or more marked, consisting of patchy or homogeneous air-space consolidation (Fig. 65–4).[2, 18, 58, 58a] Air bronchograms are commonly present.[2, 58] The abnormalities usually have sharp boundaries corresponding to the radiation portals and therefore cross normal anatomic structures without segmental or lobar distribution (Fig. 65–5).[2, 59] Occasionally, mild abnormalities are seen beyond the radiation ports (Fig. 65–6).[3, 58a] Rarely, pneumonitis progresses to diffuse consolidation involving the entire lung[58, 60] or both lungs (adult respiratory distress syndrome).[61, 62] Another rare manifestation of radiation pneumonitis is hyperlucent lung (Fig. 65–7);[63–65] we have seen one patient whose left lung became replaced by a multitude of large bullae after irradiation of the mediastinum for Hodgkin's disease.

Radiation pneumonitis is usually associated with considerable loss of volume (Fig. 65–8), presumably as a result of a surfactant deficit and adhesive atelectasis.[58, 66] Atelecta-

sis may also occur secondary to obstruction shortly after radiotherapy for an endobronchial lesion;[67] this is caused by radiation-induced edema of the bronchial wall that is already severely narrowed by the endobronchial lesion. A lung scan pattern suggesting pulmonary thromboembolism may result from vascular obliteration.[68] An uncommon but highly suggestive sign of previous mediastinal radiation consists of bilateral superomedial hilar displacement in the absence of radiographic evidence of parenchymal irradiation fibrosis.[69]

Evidence of acute radiation pneumonitis is seen more commonly and earlier on CT scan than on the chest radiograph (Fig. 65–9)[3, 4, 70] and is better seen on high-resolution than on conventional scans.[3, 71] In one review of 83 CT scans performed at relatively short intervals in 17 patients who had received 24 to 60 Gy, radiation-induced abnormalities were detected on CT in 15 of 17 patients (88%) and on chest radiographs in 12 (71%).[3] In 13 patients, the earliest changes were evident on CT 1 to 4 weeks after completion

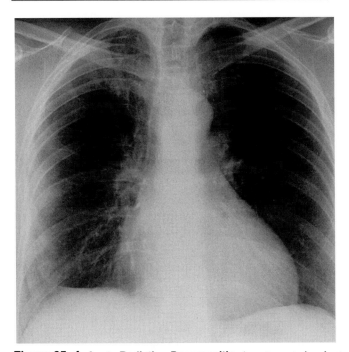

Figure 65–4. Acute Radiation Pneumonitis. A posteroanterior chest radiograph shows areas of consolidation with poorly defined margins in the axillary portion of the right lung. The patient was a 54-year-old woman who had undergone radiotherapy for carcinoma of the right breast 6 weeks previously. (Courtesy of Dr. Jackie Morgan-Parkes, British Columbia Cancer Agency, Vancouver.)

of therapy; in the remaining 2, the abnormalities became evident after 8 weeks and 13 weeks. In 3 of the 12 patients who developed radiographic abnormalities, these became evident 1 to 8 weeks after they had been first detected on CT; in the remaining 9 patients, the abnormalities were identified at the same time that they were first seen on CT.

A second group of investigators assessed the CT and radiographic findings in 18 patients who received 40 Gy of radiotherapy for Hodgkin's disease.[57] Parenchymal abnormalities were evident immediately after completion of radiotherapy on CT in 7 (39%) patients and on radiography in 2 (11%).[57] One month after completion of radiotherapy, radiation pneumonitis was visualized on CT in 78% of cases and on the radiograph in 55%. Four months after irradiation, 17 of 18 patients (94%) had evidence of radiation pneumonitis on both chest CT and radiography.

The CT manifestations of acute radiation pneumonitis consist of homogeneous areas of ground-glass attenuation or patchy or diffuse consolidation involving the radiated portions of the lungs; well-defined borders conforming to the shape of the radiation portals are usually present (Fig. 65–10).[3, 71, 72] In a small number of cases, areas of consolidation within the radiated lung are patchy in distribution and do not conform to the shape of the radiation portal;[72] occasionally, they extend beyond the radiation portals.[3, 73] Other characteristic findings include the presence of air bronchograms, loss of volume, and extension across normal anatomic boundaries.[58a, 71–74]

The late or chronic stage of radiation damage is characterized by evidence of fibrosis (Fig. 65–11). Typically, this starts after 3 to 4 months, develops gradually, and becomes stable 9 to 12 months after completion of radiotherapy.[2, 56]

The affected lung shows severe loss of volume, with obliteration of all normal architectural markings (Fig. 65–12), and the peripheral parenchyma is characteristically airless and opaque as a result of replacement by fibrous tissue. Dense fibrotic strands frequently extend from the hilum to the periphery. Radiation fibrosis develops in most patients who receive therapeutic doses of radiation, and may be seen even in patients with no radiographic evidence of acute radiation pneumonitis.[2] The radiographic findings may occasionally be subtle and consist only of mild elevation of one or both hila, mild retraction of pulmonary vessels, or mild pleural thickening.[2] The CT findings consist of dense consolidation or linear strands conforming to the radiation portals and associated with volume loss, architectural distortion, and bronchial dilation (traction bronchiectasis) (Figs. 65–13 and 65–14).[2, 70, 72]

Pleural effusions are seldom seen on the chest radiograph during acute radiation pneumonitis,[24, 75, 76] although small effusions are not uncommonly detected on CT.[2] By contrast, pericardial effusion following radiotherapy to the mediastinum is not uncommon; for example, in one group of 31 patients with a variety of malignancies who developed pericarditis, 3 (10%) developed radiation-induced pericarditis 2, 11, and 20 months after completion of radiotherapy;[77] 2 had pericardial effusion at echocardiography. Although this complication usually develops within a few months after initiation of therapy, it can be delayed for a considerable time, sometimes years.[78, 79] Other pleural complications of radiotherapy include spontaneous pneumothorax (in patients with pulmonary carcinoma who develop thin-walled cavities)[79a] and bronchopleural fistula (related to necrosis of a postlobectomy or pneumonectomy stump).[58a, 79b] Some degree of pleural thickening, occasionally extensive, develops in most patients in association with radiation-induced pulmonary fibrosis (*see* Fig. 65–12); it is also more readily assessed on CT than on the radiograph.[4, 58]

Additional late complications within the radiation field include myocardial fibrosis, premature atherosclerosis (associated with an increased incidence of coronary artery disease and myocardial infarction) (Fig. 65–15),[80–82] calcification of the aorta,[83] stenosis of the subclavian and carotid arteries, tracheal or bronchial stricture,[58a] and pericardial calcification (Fig. 65–16).[82] Bone changes within the radiation field include demineralization, small lytic areas, aseptic necrosis, and spontaneous fractures.[81, 84, 85] Fractures of the ribs or clavicle may be associated with nonunion or with atypical callus formation with irregular calcification mimicking radiation-induced osteosarcoma.[81] CT is superior to radiography in demonstrating subtle fractures, changes in bone architecture, and dystrophic soft tissue calcification.[85a] Osteonecrosis of the spine results in high signal intensity on T1-weighted MR images and intermediate intensity on T2-weighted images as a result of replacement of hematopoietic elements by fat.[85a]

CT can be helpful in the detection of recurrent tumor within the irradiated field.[2] Findings suggestive of this include the presence of a mass lesion or development of a focal opacity not containing air bronchograms.[2, 86] Distinction of tumor recurrence from radiation fibrosis may also be made using magnetic resonance imaging.[87] Radiation fibrosis has a low signal intensity on T2-weighted images, the signal

Text continued on page 2604

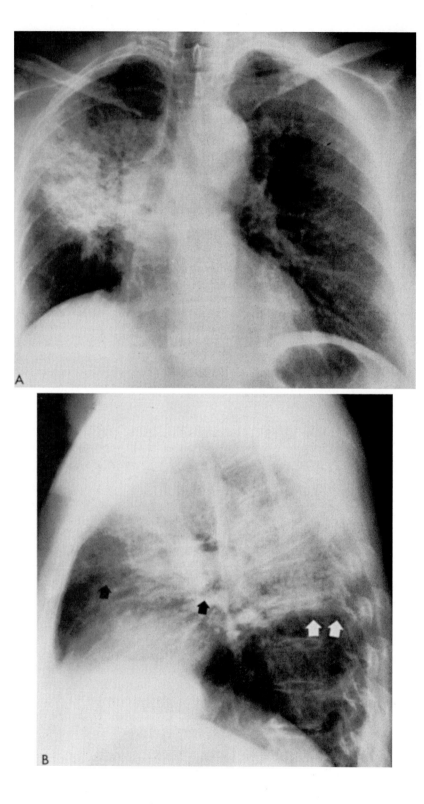

Figure 65–5. Acute Radiation Pneumonitis Illustrating "Through-and-Through" Effect. Posteroanterior *(A)* and lateral *(B)* radiographs reveal inhomogeneous consolidation of the upper half of the right lung associated with a prominent air bronchogram. In the lateral projection *(B)*, the lower border of the consolidation is almost a straight line *(arrows),* conforming precisely to the lower margin of the collimated beam of radiation. These films were of a 48-year-old woman about 3 months after an intensive course of cobalt therapy for pulmonary carcinoma.

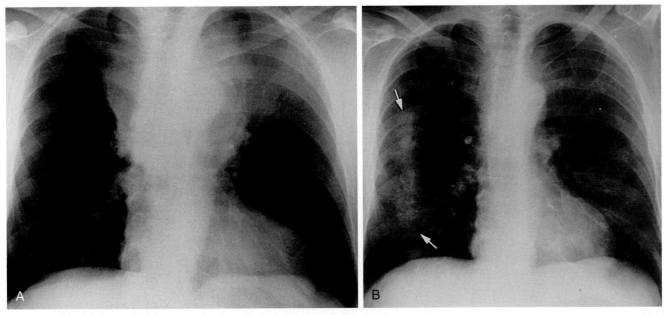

Figure 65–6. Acute Radiation Pneumonitis. A posteroanterior chest radiograph *(A)* before radiotherapy for Hodgkin's disease demonstrates widening of the mediastinum. A chest radiograph 5 weeks later *(B)* shows consolidation in the right lung *(arrows)*. The consolidation resolved slowly over the following months. The diagnosis of radiation pneumonitis outside the radiation ports was made clinically. (Courtesy of Dr. Jackie Morgan-Parkes, British Columbia Cancer Agency, Vancouver.)

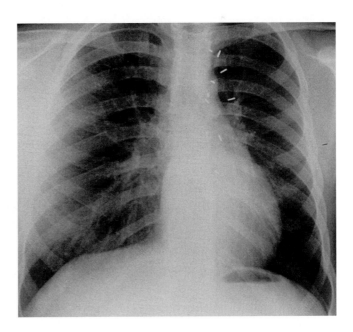

Figure 65–7. Hyperlucent Lung Following Radiotherapy. A posteroanterior chest radiograph demonstrates decreased size of the left lung and diffuse oligemia. The patient had undergone left thoracotomy and received radiotherapy to the left hemithorax during infancy for a neurogenic tumor. (Courtesy of Dr. Jackie Morgan-Parkes, British Columbia Cancer Agency, Vancouver.)

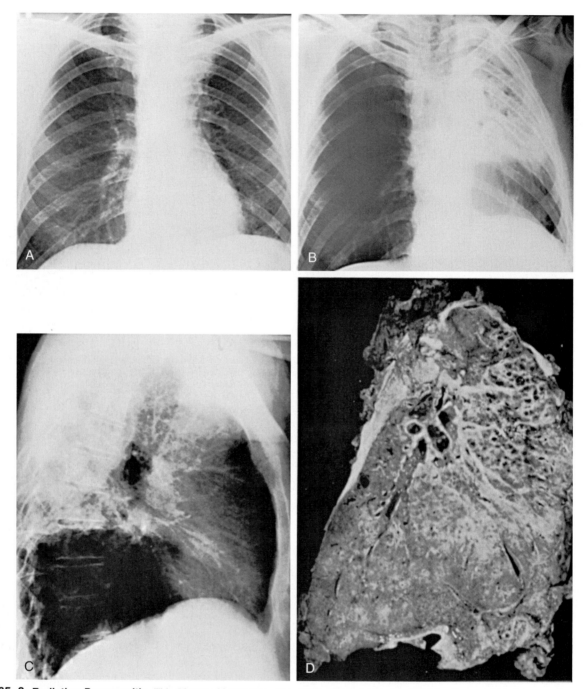

Figure 65–8. Radiation Pneumonitis. This 56-year-old man presented with metastases to cervical and lumbar vertebrae from an adenocarcinoma of the left upper lobe. A radiograph at that time *(A)* demonstrated moderate loss of volume of the left upper lobe as a result of endobronchial tumor. He received radiotherapy to the left upper lung and mediastinum through opposing fields. Two courses were administered, each delivering 30 Gy to the left upper lung. Six weeks after the end of the second course of treatment, radiographs of the chest in posteroanterior *(B)* and lateral *(C)* projections revealed a severe loss of volume of the left lung, with marked mediastinal displacement and elevation of the hemidiaphragm. The posterior portion of the left upper lobe and the superior portion of the left lower lobe were the sites of extensive inhomogeneous consolidation and atelectasis. The patient expired 2 weeks later. At autopsy, the left upper lobe and upper third of the lower lobe showed fibrosis, bronchiectasis, and atelectasis *(D)*. Note the sharp line of definition of affected lung parenchyma corresponding to the radiographic appearance in *C*.

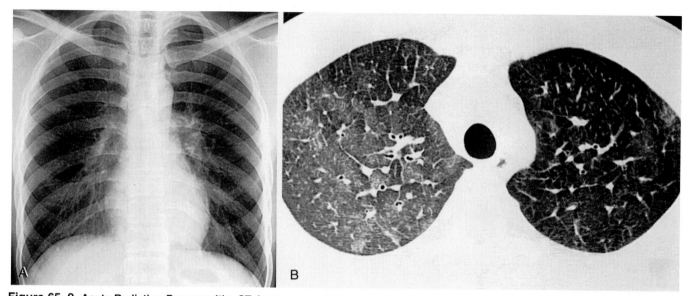

Figure 65–9. Acute Radiation Pneumonitis: CT Appearance. A posteroanterior chest radiograph *(A)* in a patient with acute radiation pneumonitis shows no definite abnormality. A high-resolution CT scan *(B)* performed the same day as the chest radiograph demonstrates extensive bilateral areas of ground-glass attenuation. (Courtesy of Dr. Kyung Soo Lee, Samsung Medical Center, Seoul.)

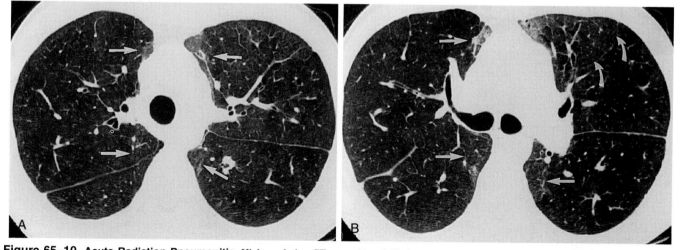

Figure 65–10. Acute Radiation Pneumonitis. High-resolution CT scans *(A* and *B)* demonstrate areas of ground-glass attenuation *(straight arrows)* in the paramediastinal regions of both lungs. Mild focal extension of radiation pneumonitis outside of the radiation portal *(curved arrows)* in *(B)* is present in the anterior aspect of the left upper lobe. The patient was a 37-year-old man who had completed a course of radiotherapy for Hodgkin's disease 2 months previously.

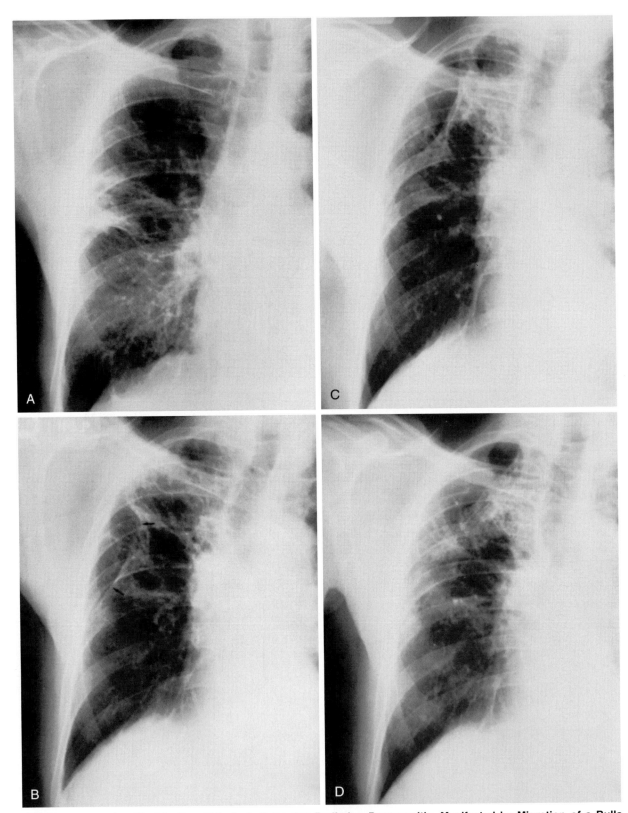

Figure 65–11. Progressive Cicatrization Atelectasis Following Radiation Pneumonitis, Manifested by Migration of a Bulla. Several months after completion of a course of radiotherapy to the right hemithorax for inoperable pulmonary carcinoma, a radiograph *(A)* of this 66-year-old man reveals some loss of volume of the right lung and a few patchy opacities in the axillary portion of the right upper lobe. Almost 1.5 years later *(B)*, the loss of volume was more severe, and a well-circumscribed cystic space had developed in the axillary portion of the right lung *(arrows)*, representing a bulla. Three months later *(C)*, the bulla had enlarged somewhat and had migrated superiorly in response to progressive fibrosis of the right upper lobe. A further 3 months later *(D)*, the bulla occupied the apical zone of the right hemithorax.

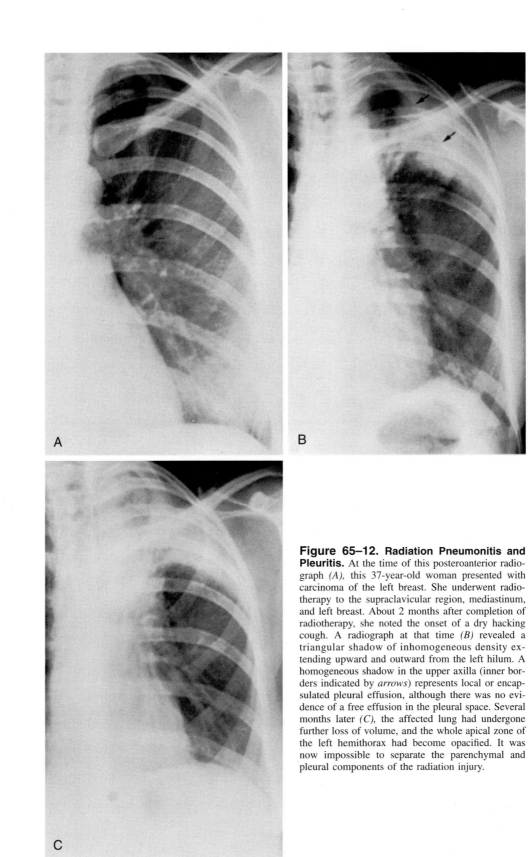

Figure 65–12. Radiation Pneumonitis and Pleuritis. At the time of this posteroanterior radiograph *(A)*, this 37-year-old woman presented with carcinoma of the left breast. She underwent radiotherapy to the supraclavicular region, mediastinum, and left breast. About 2 months after completion of radiotherapy, she noted the onset of a dry hacking cough. A radiograph at that time *(B)* revealed a triangular shadow of inhomogeneous density extending upward and outward from the left hilum. A homogeneous shadow in the upper axilla (inner borders indicated by *arrows*) represents local or encapsulated pleural effusion, although there was no evidence of a free effusion in the pleural space. Several months later *(C)*, the affected lung had undergone further loss of volume, and the whole apical zone of the left hemithorax had become opacified. It was now impossible to separate the parenchymal and pleural components of the radiation injury.

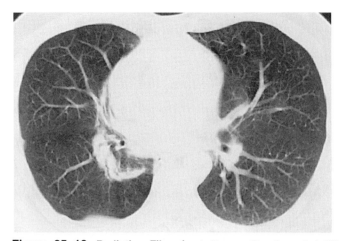

Figure 65–13. Radiation Fibrosis. A 7-mm collimation spiral CT scan demonstrates a sharply marginated focal area of ground-glass attenuation with associated linear opacities and air bronchograms. Focal pleural thickening is also evident. This 47-year-old man had undergone thymectomy and radiotherapy for invasive thymoma 4 years previously.

being similar to or lower than that of muscle, whereas a neoplasm has greater signal intensity than muscle.[87] Persistence of an inflammatory process, infection, or hemorrhage, however, may also lead to increased signal intensity on T2-weighted images.[87, 88] Persistent inflammation may also result in enhancement in the affected area following intravenous administration of gadolinium-DTPA.[88]

Ventilation-perfusion nuclear medicine scan results are frequently abnormal after radiotherapy;[89–91] perfusion abnormalities in the irradiated lung have been reported in 50% to 95% of patients and ventilation abnormalities in 35% to 45%.[91] The most common abnormality is ventilation of poorly perfused areas of lung,[91, 92] in some cases mimicking thromboembolism.[93] Single photon emission computed tomography ventilation-perfusion scans are more sensitive than conventional planar ventilation-perfusion scans and chest radiographs in the detection of regional lung injury after radiotherapy.[4, 91, 94] There is also evidence that gallium-67

scintigraphy may be superior to chest radiography in the demonstration of the spatial extent of radiation pneumonitis. In one study of 12 patients who developed radiation pneumonitis after radiotherapy for pulmonary carcinoma, gallium-67 uptake was confined to the radiated lung in 7 patients and was diffuse in 5;[95] histopathologic assessment of the lung outside the radiated field in 4 of the 5 patients with diffuse uptake revealed findings consistent with radiation pneumonitis. Evidence of radiation pneumonitis outside of the irradiated field was not apparent on chest radiographs.

Thymic cysts, sometimes with a thin rim of calcification, may develop after radiotherapy for Hodgkin's disease, progressively enlarge, and simulate recurrent tumor.[96, 97] Other abnormalities that may be seen after radiotherapy for Hodgkin's disease include calcification of mediastinal lymph nodes[98, 99] and presternal soft tissue.[100] Calcification of mediastinal lymph nodes may also occur after radiotherapy for lymphoma.[101]

Complications of brachytherapy include mucosal fibrosis with bronchostenosis, localized radiation pneumonitis, bronchoesophageal fistula, and hemoptysis.[7–9] In one study of 46 patients receiving endobronchial brachytherapy, 4 (9%) developed self-limited radiation pneumonitis and 3 (7%) suffered fatal hemoptysis.[8] (The authors of this study, however, concluded that the former abnormality was probably the result of the external-beam irradiation that these patients had received because previous or concurrent external-beam irradiation did not correlate with an increased risk of fatal hemoptysis.)

In a study of 342 patients receiving brachytherapy (three fractions of 7.5 to 10 Gy at a calculated depth of 5 to 10 mm), 41 (12%) developed radiation bronchitis and stenosis.[9] At bronchoscopy, predominantly inflammatory changes were seen at a mean of about 16 weeks from the date of first brachytherapy, and predominantly fibrotic changes were seen at 40 weeks. Twenty-five patients (9%) developed fatal hemoptysis. Variables associated with an increased risk of complications included large cell carcinoma, prior laser photoresection, and concurrent external-beam irradiation.

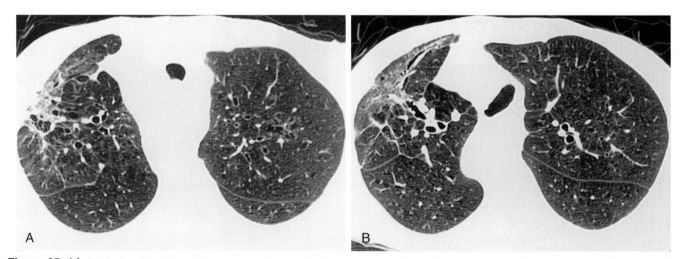

Figure 65–14. Radiation Fibrosis. High-resolution CT scans (*A* and *B*) reveal areas of ground-glass attenuation, irregular linear opacities, and traction bronchiectasis in the axillary portion of the right upper lobe. Note the associated loss of volume with anterior displacement of the right major fissure. This 83-year-old woman had undergone radiotherapy for breast carcinoma several years previously. Incidental note is made of a right aortic arch.

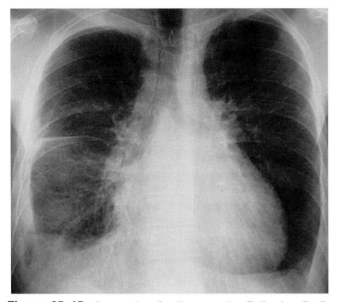

Figure 65–15. Congestive Cardiomyopathy Following Radiotherapy. An anteroposterior chest radiograph in a 31-year-old man demonstrates cardiomegaly, interstitial pulmonary edema, and small bilateral pleural effusions. The patient had experienced two myocardial infarcts and developed cardiomyopathy several years after radiotherapy for Hodgkin's disease. (Courtesy of Dr. Jackie Morgan-Parkes, British Columbia Cancer Agency, Vancouver.)

CLINICAL MANIFESTATIONS

Many patients with radiographic evidence of radiation damage remain symptom free.[24] When symptoms do develop, they usually appear between 2 and 3 months, and occasionally as late as 6 months, after the completion of therapy; rarely, they arise during the first month. As indicated previously, discontinuation of corticosteroids in patients receiving combined steroid and radiotherapy can precipitate severe symptomatic pneumonitis.[28, 29]

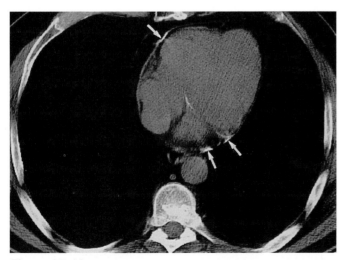

Figure 65–16. Pericardial Calcification Following Radiotherapy. A CT scan in a 51-year-old man demonstrates focal areas of pericardial calcification *(arrows)*. The patient had undergone radiotherapy for Hodgkin's disease 21 years previously. The calcification was limited to the irradiation field. (Courtesy of Dr. Jackie Morgan-Parkes, British Columbia Cancer Agency, Vancouver.)

Symptoms generally have an insidious onset and consist of nonproductive cough, weakness, and shortness of breath on exertion. Cough may be troublesome and occur in spasms. The patient may have a sensation of inability to inspire to total-lung capacity and, when encouraged to do so, coughs. Chest pain develops occasionally;[102] hemoptysis is rare.[24, 103] Dyspnea is generally mild; however, extreme respiratory distress may occur. Fever also may be a prominent finding; it is usually low grade but is sometimes high and spiking.[10] Tachycardia out of proportion to the fever may be observed. Inspiratory crackles at end inspiration are common, and there may be signs of lung consolidation in patients with severe pneumonitis. Rarely, a pleural friction rub can be heard.

Acute radiation pneumonitis may persist for up to 1 month and can either resolve completely or progress to pulmonary fibrosis. With the onset of fibrosis, symptoms of the acute pneumonitis gradually abate. In a minority of patients, fibrosis develops insidiously without an acute phase being recognized. Death may be caused by respiratory insufficiency.

As previously mentioned, the institution of radiotherapy for an endobronchial neoplasm can induce edema and narrowing of the airway lumen. In our experience and that of others,[104] this effect can have disastrous consequences if the tumor is in the trachea.

PULMONARY FUNCTION STUDIES

In most patients, the impairment in lung function following radiotherapy is mild and transient.[5] Measurable changes usually occur 2 to 3 months after irradiation, are maximal after 4 to 6 months, and return to normal after 8 to 24 months.[5, 105–107] The main impairment in function is restrictive in nature, with a greater decrease in the vital capacity than in the forced expiratory volume in 1 second (FEV_1). Diffusing capacity is decreased when a large volume of lung is involved; it may return to normal as the acute process subsides but more commonly remains decreased as fibrosis ensues.[91, 105, 108] In a prospective study of 34 patients who underwent radiotherapy for breast carcinoma, the D_{LCO} decreased a mean of 22% from baseline 1 to 4 months after radiotherapy but returned to normal within 24 months;[105] similar results have been found by other investigators.[109] As might be expected, the greater the amount of lung affected, the more severe the diffusion defect.[110]

In a study of the effect of unilateral thoracic irradiation on lung function in dogs, differential lung function tests were performed for 6 months after stopping the irradiation.[111] Measurement of the diffusing capacity by the steady-state method in the damaged lung showed reduction after 6 to 10 weeks, with simultaneous ipsilateral reduction in blood flow and ventilation; it was concluded that hypoxemia resulted from ventilation-perfusion imbalance. In another experimental study in rats, changes in expandability of the lungs and thorax were measured after single-fraction irradiation of the lungs following exposures up to 30 Gy.[112] Six weeks after irradiation, compliance (as measured by the slope of the pressure-volume curve) was found to be markedly reduced in all lungs receiving more than 15 Gy.

In a physiologic-radiographic correlative study in humans, repeated regional measurements of pulmonary blood flow and ventilation were performed on 25 patients who underwent radiotherapy for breast cancer.[113] Patients were studied before and at varying times after (16 to 407 days) the start of radiotherapy. Measured blood flow showed the earliest and greatest decrease. In another prospective study of patients with Hodgkin's disease in whom there was no evidence of intrathoracic involvement but who received pro-phylactic mantle-field radiotherapy to the chest, a 10% reduction in both forced vital capacity and diffusing capacity were noted at an interval of 6 weeks to 6 months after the initiation of therapy.[114]

Pulmonary function may improve initially in some patients receiving radiotherapy for endobronchial tumors, presumably as a result of the therapeutic effect on neoplastic tissue.[115, 116]

REFERENCES

1. Chacko DC: Considerations in the diagnosis of radiation injury. JAMA 245:1255, 1981.
2. Libshitz HI: Radiation changes in the lung. Semin Roentgenol 28:303, 1993.
3. Ikezoe J, Takashima S, Morimoto S, et al: CT appearance of acute radiation-induced injury in the lung. Am J Roentgenol 150:765, 1988.
4. Bell D, McGivern J, Bullimore J, et al: Diagnostic imaging of post-irradiation changes in the chest. Clin Radiol 39:109, 1988.
5. Movas B, Raffin TA, Epstein AH, et al: Pulmonary radiation injury. Chest 111:1061, 1997.
6. Roach M III, Gandara DR, Yuo HS, et al: Radiation pneumonitis following combined modality therapy for lung cancer: Analysis of prognostic factors. J Clin Oncol 13:2606, 1995.
7. Khanavkar B, Stern P, Alberti W, et al: Complications associated with brachytherapy alone or with laser in lung cancer. Chest 99:1062, 1991.
8. Gustafson G, Vicini F, Freedman L, et al: High dose rate endobronchial brachytherapy in the management of primary and recurrent bronchogenic malignancies. Cancer 75:2345, 1995.
9. Speiser BL, Spratling L: Radiation bronchitis and stenosis secondary to high dose rate endobronchial irradiation. Int J Radiat Oncol Biol Phys 25:589, 1993.
10. Gross NJ: Pulmonary effects of radiation therapy. Ann Intern Med 86:81, 1977.
11. Pickrell JA, Harris DV, Mauderly JL, et al: Altered collagen metabolism in radiation-induced interstitial pulmonary fibrosis. Chest 69:311, 1976.
12. Case of acute radiation injury. BMJ 2:574, 1974.
13. Lin M: Radiation pneumonitis caused by yttrium-90 microspheres: Radiologic findings. Am J Roentgenol 162:1300, 1994.
14. de Vuyst P, Dumortier P, Ketelbant P, et al: Lung fibrosis induced by Thorotrast. Thorax 45:899, 1990.
15. Rubin P, Casarett GW: Clinical Radiation Pathology. Vol I. Philadelphia, WB Saunders, 1968.
16. Bloomer WD, Hellman S: Normal tissue responses to radiation therapy. N Engl J Med 293:80, 1975.
17. Chu FCH, Phillips R, Nickson JJ, McPhee JG: Pneumonitis following radiation therapy of cancer of the breast by tangential technique. Radiology 64:642, 1955.
18. Davis SD, Yankelevitz DF, Henschke CI: Radiation effects on the lung: Clinical features, pathology, and imaging findings. Am J Roentgenol 159:1157, 1992.
19. Lingos TI, Recht A, Vicini F, et al: Radiation pneumonitis in breast cancer patients treated with conservative surgery and radiation therapy. Int J Radiat Oncol Biol Phys 21:355, 1991.
20. Tarbell NJ, Thompson L, Mauch P: Thoracic irradiation in Hodgkin's disease: Disease control and long-term complications. Int J Radiat Oncol Biol Phys 18:275, 1990.
21. Jennings FL, Arden A: Development of radiation pneumonitis: Time and dose factors. Arch Pathol 74:351, 1962.
22. Libshitz HI, Brosof AB, Southard ME: Radiographic appearance of the chest following extended field radiation therapy for Hodgkin's disease: A consideration of time-dose relationships. Cancer 32:206, 1973.
23. Roswit B, White DC: Severe radiation injuries of the lung. Am J Roentgenol 129:127, 1977.
24. Lougheed MN, Maguire GH: Irradiation pneumonitis in the treatment of carcinoma of the breast. J Can Assoc Radiol 11:1, 1960.
25. Ellis F: Dose, time and fractionation: A clinical hypothesis. Clin Radiol 20:1, 1969.
26. Wara WM, Phillips TL, Margolis LW, et al: Radiation pneumonitis: A new approach to the derivation of time-dose factors. Cancer 32:547, 1973.
27. Gish JR, Coates EO, DuSault LA, et al: Pulmonary radiation reaction: A vital-capacity and time-dose study. Radiology 73:679, 1959.
28. Parris TM, Knight JG, Hess CE, et al: Severe radiation pneumonitis precipitated by withdrawal of corticosteroids: A diagnostic and therapeutic dilemma. Am J Roentgenol 132:284, 1979.
29. Pezner RD, Bertrand M, Cecchi GR, et al: Steroid-withdrawal radiation pneumonitis in cancer patients. Chest 85:816, 1984.
30. Gez E, Sulkes A, Isacson R, et al: Radiation pneumonitis: A complication resulting from combined radiation and chemotherapy for early breast cancer. J Surg Oncol 30:116, 1985.
31. Sostman HD, Putnam CE, Gamsu G: Diagnosis of chemotherapy lung. Am J Roentgenol 136:33, 1981.
32. Phillips TL: Effects of chemotherapy and irradiation on normal tissues. Front Radiat Ther Oncol 26:45, 1992.
33. Catane R, Schwade JG, Turrisi AT, et al: Pulmonary toxicity after radiation and bleomycin: A review. Int J Radiat Oncol Biol Phys 5:1513, 1979.
34. Mah K, Keane TJ, Van Dyk J, et al: Quantitative effect of combined chemotherapy and fractionated radiotherapy on the incidence of radiation-induced lung damage: A prospective clinical study. Int J Radiat Oncol Biol Phys 28:563, 1994.
35. Ma LD, Taylor GA, Wharam MD, et al: "Recall" pneumonitis: Adriamycin potentiation of radiation pneumonitis in two children. Radiology 187:465, 1993.
36. Lingos TI, Recht A, Vicini F, et al: Radiation pneumonitis in breast cancer patients treated with conservative surgery and radiation therapy. Int J Radiat Oncol Biol Phys 21:355, 1991.
36a. Burdon J, Bell R, Sullivan J, Henderson M: Adriamycin-induced recall phenomenon 15 years after radiotherapy. J Am Med Assoc 239:931, 1978.
36b. McInerney DP: Reactivation of radiation pneumonitis by adriamycin. Br J Radiol 50:224, 1977.
36c. Soh LT, Koo WH, Ang PT: Case report: Delayed radiation pneumonitis induced by chemotherapy. Clin Radiol 52:720, 1997.
37. Gross NJ: The pathogenesis of radiation-induced lung damage. Lung 159:115, 1981.
38. Adamson IYR, Bowden DH: Endothelial injury and repair in radiation-induced pulmonary fibrosis. Am J Pathol 112:224, 1983.
39. Ward WF, Shih-Hoellworth A, Tuttle RD: Collagen accumulation in irradiated rat lung: Modification by D-penicillamine. Radiology 146:533, 1983.
40. Ward WF, Sharplin J, Franko AJ, et al: Radiation-induced pulmonary endothelial dysfunction and hydroxyproline accumulation in four strains of mice. Radiat Res 120:113, 1989.
41. Morgan GW, Breit SN: Radiation and the lung: A reevaluation of the mechanisms mediating pulmonary injury. Int J Radiat Oncol Biol Phys 31:361, 1995.
42. Rubin P, Finkelstein J, Shapiro D: Molecular biology mechanisms in the radiation induction of pulmonary injury syndromes: Interrelationship between the alveolar macrophage and the septal fibroblast. Int J Radiat Oncol Biol Phys 24:93, 1992.
43. Finkelstein JN, Johnston CJ, Baggs R, et al: Early alterations in extracellular matrix and transforming growth factor beta gene expression in mouse lung indicative of late radiation fibrosis. Int J Radiat Oncol Biol Phys 28:621, 1994.
44. Rubin P, Johnston CJ, Williams JP, et al: A perpetual cascade of cytokines postirradiation leads to pulmonary fibrosis. Int J Radiat Oncol Biol Phys 33:99, 1995.
45. Roswit B, White DC: Severe radiation injuries of the lung. Am J Roentgenol 129:127, 1977.
46. Gibson PG, Bryant DH, Morgan GW, et al: Radiation-induced lung injury: A hypersensitivity pneumonitis? Ann Intern Med 109:288, 1988.
47. Fajardo LF, Berthrong M: Radiation injury in surgical pathology. Am J Surg Pathol 2:159, 1978.
48. Heppleston AG, Young AE: Population and ultrastructural changes in murine alveolar cells following 239PuO2 inhalation. J Pathol 146:155, 1985.
49. Slauson DO, Hahn FF, Chiffelle TL: The pulmonary vascular pathology of experimental radiation pneumonitis. Am J Pathol 88:635, 1977.
50. Adamson IYR, Bowden DH, Wyatt JP: A pathway to pulmonary fibrosis: An ultrastructural study of mouse and rat following radiation to the whole body and hemithorax. Am J Pathol 58:481, 1970.
51. Phillips TL: An ultrastructural study of the development of radiation injury in the lung. Radiology 87:49, 1966.
52. Teates CD: The effects of unilateral thoracic irradiation on pulmonary blood flow. Am J Roentgenol 102:875, 1968.
53. Schreiner BF Jr, Michaelson SM, Yuile CL: The effects of thoracic irradiation upon cardiopulmonary function in the dog. Am Rev Respir Dis 99:205, 1969.
54. Bennett DE, Million RR, Ackerman LV: Bilateral radiation pneumonitis: A complication of the radiotherapy of bronchogenic carcinoma. (Report and analysis of seven cases with autopsy.) Cancer 23:1001, 1969.
55. Wilkinson MJ, MacLennan KA: Vascular changes in irradiated lungs: A morphometric study. J Pathol 158:229, 1989.
56. Slanina J, Maschitzki R, Wannenmacher M: Die pulmonale strahlenreaktion im Röntgenbild des thorax nach megavolttherapie bei mammakarzinom. Radiologe 27:182, 1987.
57. Frija J, Fermé C, Baud L, et al: Radiation-induced lung injuries: A survey by computed tomography and pulmonary function tests in 18 cases of Hodgkin's disease. Eur J Radiol 8:18, 1988.
58. Fennessy JJ: Irradiation damage to the lung. J Thorac Imag 1:68, 1987.
58a. Logan PM: Thoracic manifestations of external beam radiotherapy. Am J Roentgenol 171:569, 1998.
59. Polansky SM, Ravin CE, Prosnitz LR: Pulmonary changes after primary irradiation for early breast carcinoma. Am J Roentgenol 134:101, 1980.
60. DoPico GA, Wiley AL, Rao P, et al: Pulmonary reaction to upper mantle radiation therapy for Hodgkin's disease. Chest 75:688, 1979.
61. Fulkerson WJ, McLendon RE, Prosnitz LR: Adult respiratory distress syndrome after limited thoracic radiotherapy. Cancer 57:1941, 1986.
62. Byhardt RW, Abrams R, Almagro U: The association of adult respiratory distress syndrome (ARDS) with thoracic irradiation (RT). Int J Radiat Oncol Biol Phys 15:1441, 1988.
63. Fleming JAC, Filbee JF, Wiernik G: Sequelae to radical irradiation in carcinoma of the breast. An inquiry into the incidence of certain radiation injuries. Br J Radiol 34:713, 1961.
64. Farmer W, Ravin C, Schachter EN: Hyperlucent lung after radiation therapy. Am Rev Respir Dis 112:255, 1975.
65. Berdon WE, Baker DH, Boyer J: Unusual benign and malignant sequelae to childhood radiation therapy including "unilateral hyperlucent lung." Am J Roentgenol 93:545, 1965.
66. Gross NJ: The pathogenesis of radiation-induced lung damage. Lung 159:115, 1981.
67. Goldman AL, Enquist R: Hyperacute radiation pneumonitis. Chest 67:613, 1975.
68. Bateman NT, Croft DN: False-positive lung scans and radiotherapy. BMJ 1:807, 1976.
69. Harnsberger HR, Armstrong JD II: Bilateral superomedial hilar displacement: A unique sign of previous mediastinal radiation. Radiology 147:35, 1983.
70. Schratter-Sehn AU, Schurawitzki H, Zach M: High-resolution computed tomography of the lungs in irradiated breast cancer patients. Radiother Oncol 27:198, 1993.

71. Ikezoe J, Morimoto S, Takashima S, et al: Acute radiation-induced pulmonary injury: Computed tomography evaluation. Semin Ultrasound CT MRI 11:409, 1990.

72. Libshitz HI, Shuman LS: Radiation-induced pulmonary change: CT findings. J Comput Assist Tomogr 8:15, 1984.

73. Mah K, Poon PY, Van Dyk J, Keane T, et al: Assessment of acute radiation-induced pulmonary changes using computed tomography. J Comput Assist Tomogr 10:736, 1986.

74. Nabawi P, Mantravadi R, Breyer D, et al: Computed tomography of radiation-induced lung injuries. J Comput Assist Tomogr 5:568, 1981.

75. Bachman AL, Macken K: Pleural effusions following supervoltage radiation for breast carcinoma. Radiology 72:699, 1959.

76. Whitcomb ME, Schwarz MI: Pleural effusion complicating intensive mediastinal radiation therapy. Am Rev Respir Dis 103:100, 1971.

77. Posner MR, Cohen GI, Skarin AT: Pericardial disease in patients with cancer: The differentiation of malignant from idiopathic and radiation-induced pericarditis. Am J Med 71:407, 1981.

78. Gomm SA, Stretton TB: Chronic pericardial effusion after mediastinal radiotherapy. Thorax 36:149, 1981.

79. Applefield MM, Cole JF, Pollock SH, et al: The late appearance of chronic pericardial disease in patients treated by radiotherapy for Hodgkin's disease. Ann Intern Med 94:338, 1981.

79a. Okada M, Ebe K, Matsumoto T, et al: Case report: Ipsilateral spontaneous pneumothorax after rapid development of large thin-walled cavities in two patients who had undergone radiation therapy for lung cancer. Am J Roentgenol 170:932, 1998.

79b. Deslauriers J, Ferraro P: Non-small cell lung cancer: Late complications. *In* Pearson FG, Deslauriers J, Ginsberg RJ, et al (eds.): Thoracic Surgery. New York, Churchill Livingstone, 1995, pp 763–782.

80. Wallgren A: Late effects of radiotherapy in the treatment of breast cancer. Acta Oncol 31:237, 1992.

81. Iyer RB, Libshitz HI: Late sequelae after radiation therapy for breast cancer: Imaging findings. Am J Roentgenol 168:1335, 1997.

82. Schultz-Hector S, Kallfab, Sund M: Strahlenfolgen an groben Arterien: Übersicht über klinische und experimentelle Daten. Strahlenther Onkol 171:427, 1995.

83. Coblentz C, Martin L, Tuttle R: Calcified ascending aorta after radiation therapy. Am J Roentgenol 147:477, 1986.

84. Libshitz HI: Radiation changes in bone. Semin Roentgenol 29:15, 1994.

85. Pierce SM, Recht A, Lingos TI, et al: Long-term radiation complications following conservative surgery (CS) and radiation therapy (RT) in patients with early stage breast cancer. Int J Radiat Oncol Biol Phys 23:915, 1992.

85a. Mitchell MJ, Logan PM: Radiation-induced changes in bone. Radiographics 18:1125, 1998.

86. Bourgouin P, Cousineau G, Lemire P, et al: Differentiation of radiation-induced fibrosis from recurrent pulmonary neoplasm by CT. Can Assoc Radiol J 38:23, 1987.

87. Glazer HS, Lee JKT, Levitt RG, et al: Radiation fibrosis: Differentiation from recurrent tumor by MR imaging. Radiology 156:721, 1985.

88. Werthmuller WC, Schiebler ML, Whaley RA, et al: Gadolinium-DTPA enhancement of lung radiation fibrosis. J Comput Assist Tomogr 13:946, 1989.

89. Prato FS, Kurdyak R, Saibil EA, et al: Regional and total lung function in patients following pulmonary irradiation. Invest Radiol 12:224, 1977.

90. Prata FS, Kurdyak R, Saibil EA, et al: Physiological and radiographic assessment during the development of pulmonary radiation fibrosis. Radiology 122:389, 1977.

91. McDonald S, Rubin P, Phillips TL, et al: Injury to the lung from cancer therapy: Clinical syndromes, measurable endpoints, and potential scoring systems. Int J Radiat Oncol Biol Phys 31:1187, 1995.

92. Pezzulli F, Posner D, Mask K: Reverse V/P mismatch in radiation pneumonitis. Australas Radiol 38:135, 1994.

93. Slavin Jr JD, Friedman NC, Spencer RP: Radiation effects on pulmonary ventilation and perfusion. Clin Nucl Med 18:81, 1993.

94. Marks LB, Spencer DP, Bentel GC, et al: The utility of SPECT lung perfusion scans in minimizing and assessing the physiological consequences of thoracic irradiation. Int J Radiat Oncol Biol Phys 26:659, 1993.

95. Kataoka M, Kawamura M, Ueda N, et al: Diffuse gallium-67 uptake in radiation pneumonitis. Clin Nucl Med 15:707, 1990.

96. Baron RL, Sagel SS, Baglan RJ: Thymic cysts following radiation therapy for Hodgkin disease. Radiology 141:593, 1981.

97. Lindfors KK, Neyer JE, Dedrick CG, et al: Thymic cysts in mediastinal Hodgkin disease. Radiology 156:37, 1985.

98. Brereton HD, Johnson RE: Calcification in mediastinal lymph nodes after radiation therapy of Hodgkin's disease. Radiology 112:705, 1974.

99. Strickland B: Intrathoracic Hodgkin's disease. II. Peripheral manifestations of Hodgkin's disease in the chest. Br J Radiol 40:930, 1967.

100. Vainright JR, Diaconis JN, Haney PJ: Presternal soft tissue calcifications following mediastinal radiotherapy for Hodgkin's disease. Chest 91:136, 1987.

101. Fishman EK, Kuhlman JE, Jones RJ: CT of lymphoma: Spectrum of disease. Radiographics 11:647, 1991.

102. Lichtenstein H: X-ray diagnosis of radiation injuries of the lung. Dis Chest 38:294, 1960.

103. Smith JC: Radiation pneumonitis: A review. Am Rev Respir Dis 87:647, 1963.

104. Cameron SJ, Grant IWB, Lutz W, et al: The early effect of irradiation on ventilatory function in bronchial carcinoma. Clin Radiol 20:12, 1969.

105. Kimsey FC, Price Mendenhall N, Ewald LM, et al: Is radiation treatment volume a predictor for acute or late effect on pulmonary function? Cancer 73:2549, 1994.

106. Host H, Vale JR: Lung function after mantle field irradiation in Hodgkin's disease. Cancer 32:328, 1973.

107. Evans RF, Sagerman RH, Ringrose TL, et al: Pulmonary function following mantle-field irradiation for Hodgkin's disease. Radiology 111:729, 1974.

108. Groth S, Johansen H, Sørensen PG, et al: The effect of thoracic irradiation for cancer of the breast on ventilation, perfusion and pulmonary permeability. Acta Oncol 28:671, 1989.

109. Cudkowicz L, Cunningham M, Haldane EV: Effects of mediastinal irradiation upon respiratory function following mastectomy for carcinoma of breast. Thorax 24:359, 1969.

110. Brady LW, Germon PA, Cander L: The effects of radiation therapy on pulmonary function in carcinoma of the lung. Radiology 85:130, 1965.

111. Teates CD: Effect of unilateral-thoracic irradiation on lung function. J Appl Physiol 20:628, 1965.

112. Shrivastava PN, Hans L, Concannon JP: Changes in pulmonary compliance and production of fibrosis in x-irradiated lungs of rats. Radiology 112:439, 1974.

113. Prato FS, Kurdyak R, Saibil EA, et al: Physiological and radiographic assessment during the development of pulmonary radiation fibrosis. Radiology 122:389, 1977.

114. Jones PW, Al-Hillawi A, Wakefield JM, et al: Differences in the effect of mediastinal radiotherapy on lung function and the ventilatory response to exercise. Clin Sci 67:389,1984.

115. Hoffbrand BI, Gillam PMS, Heaf PJD: Effect of chronic bronchitis on changes in pulmonary function caused by irradiation of the lungs. Thorax 20:303, 1965.

116. Deeley TJ: The effects of radiation on the lungs in the treatment of carcinoma of the bronchus. Clin Radiol 11:33, 1960.

PART XIII

TRAUMATIC CHEST DISEASE

CHAPTER 66

Penetrating and Nonpenetrating Chest Trauma

Trauma to the thorax can result in a wide variety of effects on the chest wall, diaphragm, mediastinum, trachea, and lungs.[1] The results may be direct (e.g., fractures of the ribs, spine, or shoulder girdles; diaphragmatic hernia; esophageal rupture; and pulmonary contusion or laceration) or indirect (e.g., air embolism resulting from the escape of air into pulmonary veins subsequent to parenchymal laceration). Because the manifestations of such trauma are dissimilar in different sites, each is considered separately. As might be anticipated, however, a great deal of overlap occurs. Also, the effects of penetrating and nonpenetrating trauma may differ markedly and thus require separate consideration. The consequences of iatrogenic "trauma" are considered in Chapter 67. The adult respiratory distress syndrome (ARDS), one of the most ominous consequences of prolonged shock in the immediate post-traumatic period, is discussed in Chapter 51 (*see* page 1976).

Although diagnosis of most traumatic abnormalities of the thorax can be established with reasonable confidence by conventional radiographic methods, in some cases, significant abnormalities may be apparent only on CT.[2-4] Furthermore, certain conditions, such as laceration of the aorta, often require special diagnostic procedures, including aortography, to confirm the injury and establish its extent.

EFFECTS ON THE LUNGS OF NONPENETRATING TRAUMA

Pulmonary Contusion

Pulmonary contusion consists of traumatic extravasation of blood into the parenchyma of the lung unaccompanied by substantial tissue disruption.[5] It is considered to be the most common pulmonary complication of chest trauma.[5] In a review of the findings in 515 patients with blunt chest trauma, it was identified radiographically in 133 (26%);[6] 35 (26%) had no evidence of bony thoracic injury. The severity of the injury necessary to produce contusion varies from a trivial glancing blow to major trauma resulting from motor vehicle or aircraft accidents.[7] Nonmilitary blast injuries account for a small percentage of cases.[8, 9] The complication has also been reported following extracorporeal shock-wave lithotripsy.[10]

Histologic assessment of pulmonary contusion resulting from motor vehicle accidents or falls has shown that the hemorrhage results from torn vessels and that the extravasated blood fills the adjacent air spaces and bronchi.[2] In some cases, such as those resulting from blast injuries, interstitial edema and interstitial and air-space hemorrhage appear to result from disruption of small parenchymal vessels.[2, 11]

Radiographically, the pattern varies from irregular, patchy areas of air-space consolidation to diffuse and extensive homogeneous consolidation (Fig. 66–1). As might be expected, the distribution of the contused areas does not conform to lobes or segments.[12–14] Although the major change is usually in the lung directly deep to the traumatized areas, damage may occur also, or even predominantly, on the opposite side as a result of a contrecoup effect.[15, 16] In blast injuries, the contusion is typically bilateral,[15] although again the major change occurs in the area that faced the blast. Increase in the size and loss of definition of the vascular markings extending out from the hila indicates the presence of hemorrhage and edema in the peribronchovascular interstitial tissue.[6, 14] Extensive bilateral contusion may lead to respiratory failure and ARDS.[5, 17]

The time between the trauma and the detection of radiographic abnormality is important, particularly in the differentiation of pulmonary contusion from traumatic fat embolism. In contusion, changes are apparent radiographically soon after trauma (almost invariably within 6 hours),[7, 14] whereas in fat embolism, they usually become manifest only 1 to 2 days or more after injury. Resolution of lung contusion typically occurs rapidly, with improvement noted within 24 to 48 hours[18, 19] and clearing complete within 3 to 10 days (Fig. 66–2).[12, 18, 20]

The CT findings consist of areas of consolidation that may be patchy or homogeneous. They involve mainly the lung directly deep to the area of trauma;[5, 21, 22] however, 1 to 2 mm of subpleural lung parenchyma adjacent to the injured chest wall is often spared.[23] Air bronchograms are commonly present.[5] Occasionally, CT demonstrates a contusion not apparent on the radiograph.[21, 22] In an experimental study in dogs, 100% of pulmonary contusions were visible on CT immediately after trauma, compared with only 37% on chest radiography.[24] After 30 minutes, 75% of lesions were seen on the radiograph.[24] Although contusion is by definition unassociated with radiographic evidence of pulmonary laceration, small lacerations—seen as small round or ovoid air collections with or without an air-fluid level—are commonly evident on CT;[25] in one study, they were detected in 95% of patients with a radiographic diagnosis of contusion.[2]

Clinical findings are seldom striking; in fact, symptoms may be entirely absent[14, 26] or may be masked by other injuries.[27] Pain is not a prominent feature, except in relation to other injuries. Hemoptysis is said to occur in 50% of cases, and there may be mild fever; shortness of breath may develop in the presence of severe contusion.[7, 14] Rarely, the contused region is the site of secondary infection.[28] Lacerations detected by CT but not by radiography are of limited clinical significance.[22]

The mortality rate in patients with pulmonary contusion

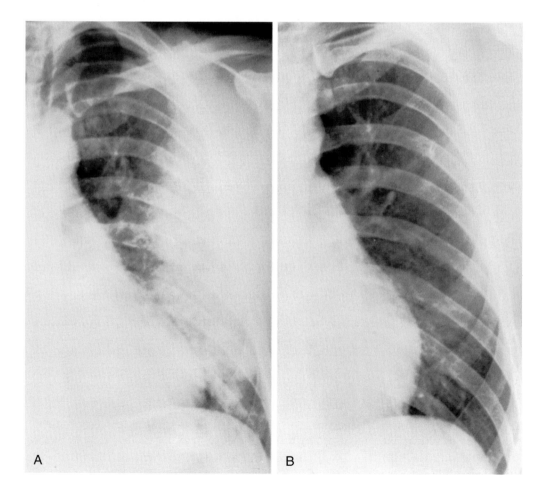

A   B

Figure 66–1. Pulmonary Contusion. Six hours before the radiographic examination illustrated in *(A)*, this 33-year-old man was involved in a car accident in which he suffered severe trauma to the posterior portion of his left chest. A view of the left hemithorax from an anteroposterior radiograph reveals homogeneous consolidation of the posterolateral portion of the left lung in nonsegmental distribution. The margins of the consolidation are indistinctly defined, and there is no air bronchogram. No ribs were fractured. The right lung was clear. Six days later *(B)*, complete clearing had occurred.

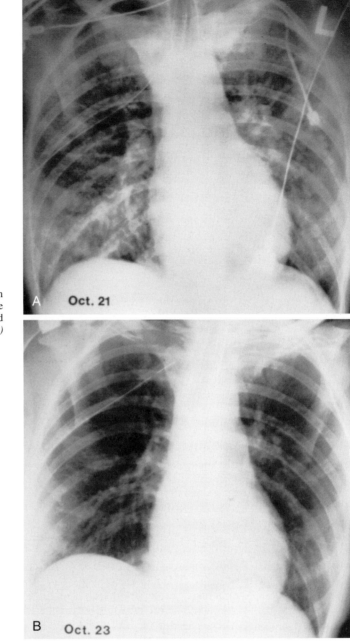

Figure 66–2. Pulmonary Contusion with Rapid Resolution. An anteroposterior chest radiograph *(A)* performed shortly after arrival in the emergency room following an automobile accident shows poorly defined bilateral areas of consolidation. A radiograph performed 48 hours later *(B)* shows complete resolution.

ranges from 10% to 40% and varies with the severity and extent of contusion and with the presence of other thoracic and nonthoracic injuries.[5, 17]

Pulmonary Laceration, Traumatic Pneumatocele, and Hematoma

Rather uncommonly, closed chest trauma results in the development of radiographically detectable cystic spaces within the lung that can remain air filled or that can fill partly or completely with blood. The trauma usually is blunt and often severe, as in automobile accidents. Children and young adults appear to be particularly prone, probably because of the greater flexibility of their thoracic walls; in fact,

in young patients, the trauma can be relatively minor and still result in rather large parenchymal lacerations.[29]

The pathologic features of traumatic pneumatoceles have been described infrequently; the occasional excised specimen has shown the wall to be composed of fibrous or granulation tissue.[30] A parenchymal hematoma consists of a collection of blood of variable size that compresses adjacent lung tissue (Fig. 66–3); an acute inflammatory reaction is occasionally present at the periphery.

Radiographically, traumatic pneumatoceles (Fig. 66–4) and hematomas (Fig. 66–5) are not usually seen until a few hours or even several days after trauma, often being initially masked by the surrounding contusion.[32] They may be single or multiple,[16, 33] unilocular or multilocular,[32] oval or spherical, and from 2 to 14 cm in diameter (Fig. 66–6).[34] They are

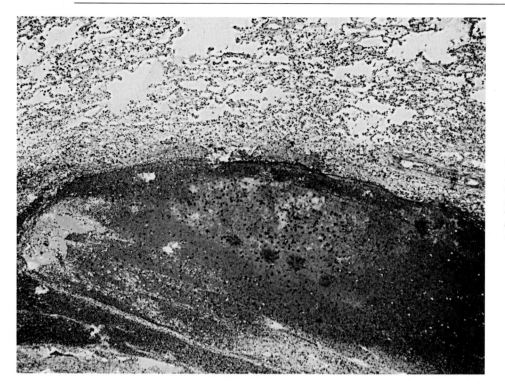

Figure 66–3. Pulmonary Hematoma. A section of lung taken from the lower lobe of a person involved in a motor vehicle accident 24 hours before death shows a well-defined focus of hemorrhage somewhat compressing adjacent lung parenchyma. (×40.)

typically located in the subpleural parenchyma.[7, 32] In most cases, they develop under the point of maximal injury; occasionally, they occur in a remote location as a result of a contrecoup effect.

Their appearance depends in large measure on whether hemorrhage has occurred into them. About half the lesions present as thin-walled, air-filled spaces with or without fluid levels (Fig. 66–7);[35] the remainder appear as homogeneous, well-circumscribed masses of soft tissue density—pulmonary hematomas (Fig. 66–8). Traumatic pneumatoceles may enlarge rapidly in patients receiving high-pressure mechanical ventilation.[5] Occasionally, they have a markedly irregular contour and resemble multiple cavities (*see* Fig. 66–4). The development of a pneumatocele at the base of the left lung after trauma has been confused with a ruptured diaphragm;[36] however, identification of the diaphragmatic contour should make such a misdiagnosis unlikely.

A characteristic of these lesions is their tendency to persist for a long time, frequently up to 4 months[20, 37, 38] and occasionally as long as 1 year[25, 39] (*see* Fig. 66–8). Rarely, a traumatic hematoma increases in size, in which case it has been termed *chronic expanding hematoma*.[25] More commonly, they decrease in size progressively; if this is not apparent within 6 weeks, the possibility must be considered that trauma may have been purely coincidental with a solitary nodule of other etiology.[7, 40]

The CT findings of pulmonary laceration consist of one or more round, oval, or multiloculated air collections with or without air-fluid levels (Fig. 66–9).[2, 22, 31, 41] CT can be particularly useful in the demonstration of paramediastinal pneumatoceles.[33] Hemorrhage related to a pulmonary laceration may result in an air-fluid level, an air crescent sign, or, when the lacerated region is completely filled by blood, a round or oval soft tissue density.[39, 42] The appearance may be indistinguishable from pulmonary masses of other etiology.[39]

Hematomas persisting for several months may have a central attenuation slightly greater than that of water and a rim enhancement.[39] Magnetic resonance (MR) imaging in one patient with a persistent hematoma 6 months after a motor vehicle accident demonstrated hyperintensity on both T1- and T2-weighted images and an even greater rim intensity on T1-weighted images;[39] follow-up 6 months later showed substantial decrease in size of the lesion.

Based on the CT findings, mechanism of injury, location of associated rib fracture, or surgical findings, pulmonary laceration may be classified into four types.[2] Type 1 lacerations are the most common and result from sudden compression of a pliable chest wall leading to rupture of the underlying lung; the CT appearance is usually that of a focal air collection with or without a fluid level and often located deep within the lung parenchyma. Type 2 lacerations result from sudden compression of a pliable lower chest wall causing the lower lobe to shift suddenly across the vertebral body and producing a shear injury; the appearance is similar to type 1 laceration, but the location is in the paravertebral regions of the lower lobes.[2] Type 3 lacerations result from a fractured rib that punctures the lung; it is considered to be present when a focal air collection or linear lucency in the subpleural region lies close to a fractured rib and is usually associated with a pneumothorax. Type 4 lacerations occur when pre-existing pleural adhesions cause the lung to tear when the chest wall is suddenly moved inward; they can be confidently diagnosed only at surgery or autopsy.

Most patients do not have symptoms related to the pulmonary lesion itself. Hemoptysis occurs rarely and is probably attributable to the emptying of a hematoma.[35] Rare pneumatoceles appear to have been secondarily infected.[43] Pulmonary hematomas indistinguishable from those caused by closed chest trauma sometimes develop after segmental or wedge resection of the lung.[16, 44] In addition, bleeding into

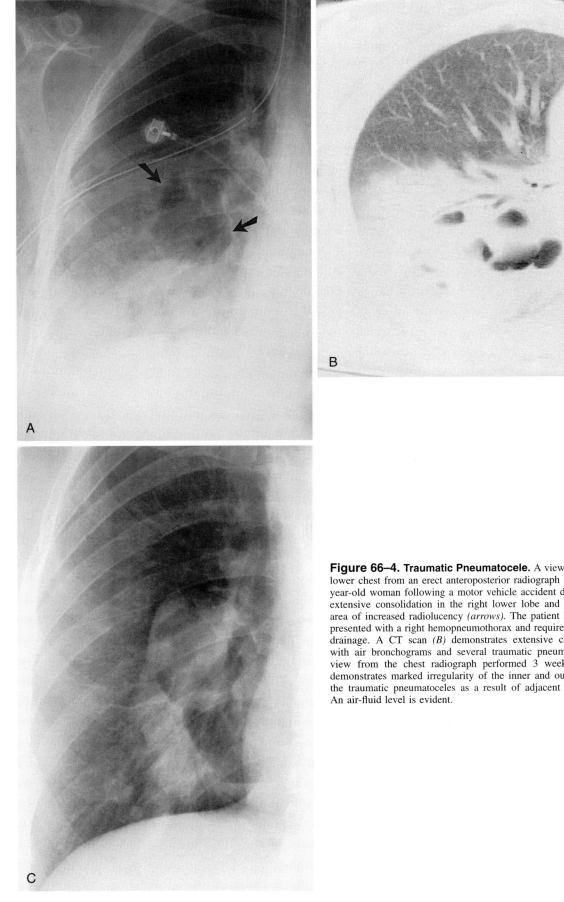

Figure 66–4. Traumatic Pneumatocele. A view of the right lower chest from an erect anteroposterior radiograph *(A)* in a 29-year-old woman following a motor vehicle accident demonstrates extensive consolidation in the right lower lobe and an irregular area of increased radiolucency *(arrows)*. The patient had initially presented with a right hemopneumothorax and required chest tube drainage. A CT scan *(B)* demonstrates extensive consolidation with air bronchograms and several traumatic pneumatoceles. A view from the chest radiograph performed 3 weeks later *(C)* demonstrates marked irregularity of the inner and outer walls of the traumatic pneumatoceles as a result of adjacent hematomas. An air-fluid level is evident.

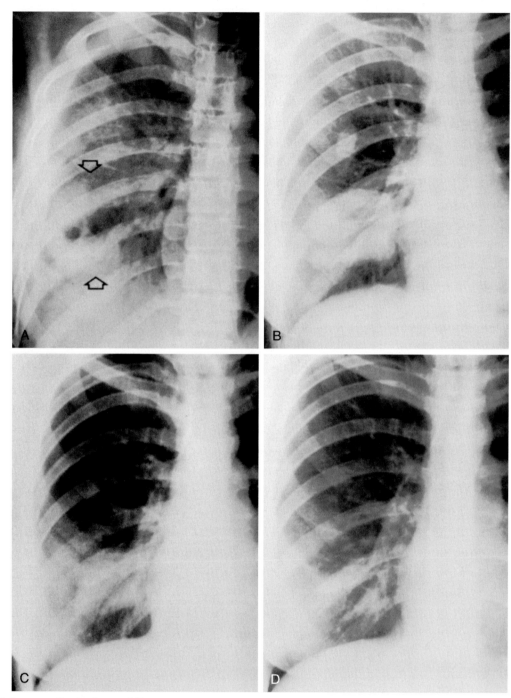

Figure 66–5. Pulmonary Contusion and Hematoma. This 15-year-old girl suffered a severe blow to the right side of her chest in a car accident. Three hours after the accident, an anteroposterior radiograph *(A)* demonstrates extensive consolidation of the parenchyma of the right lung due to pulmonary contusion (the left lung was clear). In addition to the diffuse opacity, an indistinctly defined shadow of greater density is present in the right base *(arrows)*, containing a central radiolucency; there is a large hemothorax. Three weeks later *(B)*, the general opacity caused by contusion has completely cleared, as has the hemothorax. However, there remains a large, sharply circumscribed, lobulated shadow that represents the hematoma vaguely visible in *(A)*. A much smaller hematoma can be identified in the lung directly above the major lesion. About 1 month later *(C)*, the mass has undergone considerable decrease in size and is not as sharply defined. One month later *(D)*, the hematoma is still present in the form of an elliptical shadow. Complete clearing did not occur until 6 months later. (Courtesy of Dr. J. G. Monks, Rosetown Union Hospital, Rosetown, Saskatchewan.)

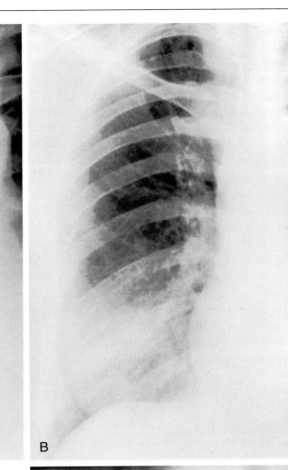

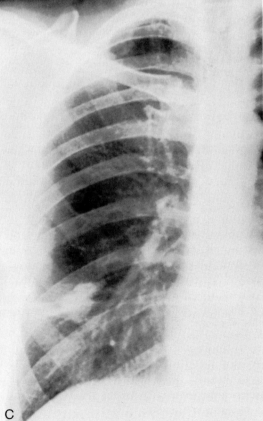

Figure 66–6. Traumatic Pulmonary Contusion, Hematoma, and Pneumothorax. This 38-year-old man suffered a severe blow to the right side of the chest in a car accident. Two hours later, a posteroanterior radiograph *(A)* revealed a hemopneumothorax with about 50% collapse of the right lung (the left lung was normal); ribs 6 and 7 were fractured in the posterior axillary line. A poorly defined shadow of inhomogeneous density is present in the lower portion of the right lower lobe. Three days later *(B)*, the pneumothorax has disappeared following closed-tube drainage, and the shadow in the right lower lobe is still poorly defined because of surrounding contusion. Three weeks later *(C)*, the shadow has undergone considerable decrease in size; it did not disappear completely until 2 months later.

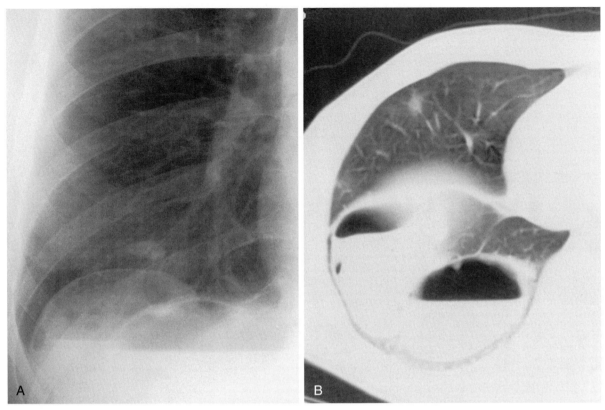

Figure 66–7. Traumatic Pneumatocele. A view of the right lower chest from a posteroanterior radiograph *(A)* in a 26-year-old man 2 weeks after a motor vehicle accident reveals thin-walled cystic lesions with air-fluid levels. A CT scan *(B)* essentially confirms the radiographic findings. The appearance is characteristic of traumatic pneumatoceles.

bullae during mechanical ventilation of patients with severe chronic obstructive pulmonary disease (COPD) has been reported, the resulting shadows simulating traumatic pneumatoceles.[45]

Fractures of the Trachea and Bronchi

Fractures (rupture, transection) of the tracheobronchial tree as a result of nonpenetrating trauma usually result from blunt trauma to the anterior chest in vehicular accidents;[45a] occasionally, they occur as a result of overdistention of the cuff of an endotracheal tube.[46] Although tracheobronchial fractures may occur in the absence of thoracic skeletal injury,[6] this is often present. The incidence of rib fractures varies considerably in different series; for example, such fractures were observed in 53% of patients in one series,[47] in an astonishing 91% in another,[48] and only 2% in a third.[49] In another review of nine patients, four had fractures involving the clavicles, scapula, or sternum, but only two had rib fractures.[50]

Most tracheobronchial fractures associated with blunt trauma follow rapid anteroposterior compression of the chest.[51, 52] This may result in a sudden increase in airway pressure, causing "burst" tracheobronchial injury; alternatively, the sudden lateral widening of the thorax may pull the lung apart, avulsing a bronchus.[51–53]

Fractures of the bronchi are more common than those of the trachea and constitute about 80% of all tracheobronchial injuries.[20, 52] They are usually parallel to the cartilage rings and involve the main bronchi 1 to 2 cm distal to the carina.[20, 52, 54] The right side is affected more often than the left; pulmonary vessels are rarely damaged.[55] Fractures of the intrathoracic trachea are horizontal and usually occur just above the carina.[20, 54, 56] Occasionally, the proximal trachea ruptures as a result of blunt trauma to the throat, in which case, other cervical structures are usually involved;[56] the tracheal tear tends to be vertical in the membranous portion and can be associated with vascular damage.[20, 57]

As might be expected, the most common radiographic findings are pneumomediastinum and pneumothorax.[50, 58] In one review of nine patients with tears or transection of the trachea or main bronchi after blunt trauma, seven had pneumomediastinum and subcutaneous emphysema, and six had pneumothorax;[50] in five, the pneumothorax was present on the initial radiograph, and in one, it was not evident until the 13th day after admission. Tension pneumothorax occurred in four of the six patients. Four patients had upper thoracic fractures involving the clavicles, scapula, or sternum; only two had rib fractures. Certain combinations of findings related to pneumomediastinum and pneumothorax are highly suggestive of tracheobronchial fracture in a patient who has undergone trauma: (1) a large pneumothorax that does not respond to chest tube drainage (because of the free communication between the fractured airway and the pleural space);[54, 59, 60] (2) pneumothorax and pneumomediastinum in the absence of pleural effusion;[61] and (3) mediastinal and deep cervical emphysema in a patient who is not receiving positive-pressure ventilation.[62]

Other radiologic findings are less common. After bron-

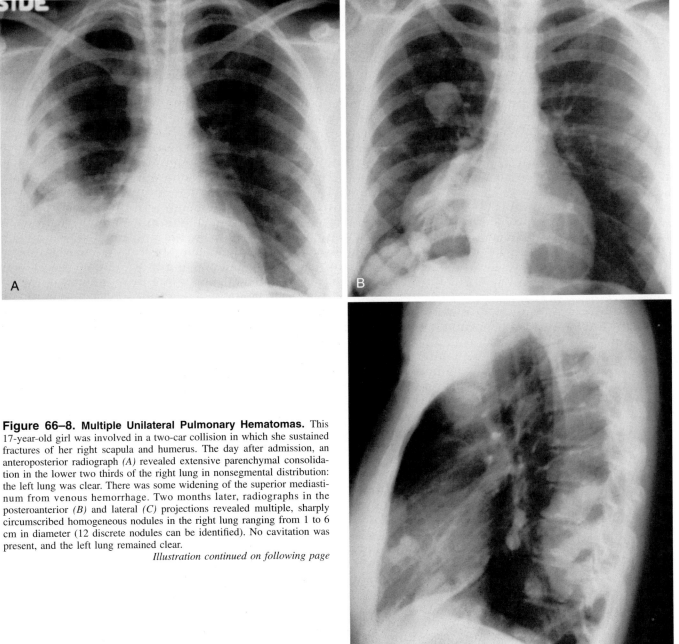

Figure 66–8. Multiple Unilateral Pulmonary Hematomas. This 17-year-old girl was involved in a two-car collision in which she sustained fractures of her right scapula and humerus. The day after admission, an anteroposterior radiograph *(A)* revealed extensive parenchymal consolidation in the lower two thirds of the right lung in nonsegmental distribution: the left lung was clear. There was some widening of the superior mediastinum from venous hemorrhage. Two months later, radiographs in the posteroanterior *(B)* and lateral *(C)* projections revealed multiple, sharply circumscribed homogeneous nodules in the right lung ranging from 1 to 6 cm in diameter (12 discrete nodules can be identified). No cavitation was present, and the left lung remained clear.

Illustration continued on following page

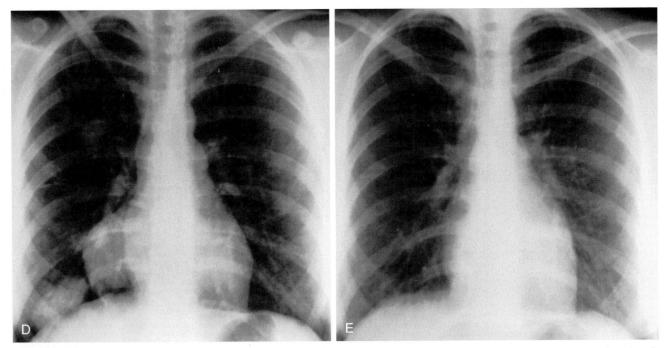

Figure 66–8 *Continued.* About 1 month later *(D),* the nodules had diminished considerably in size, and several had disappeared altogether. Seven months after the injury, all signs of disease had disappeared, and the chest radiograph *(E)* was normal. (Courtesy of Dr. John D. Armstrong, Jr., University of Utah College of Medicine, Salt Lake City.)

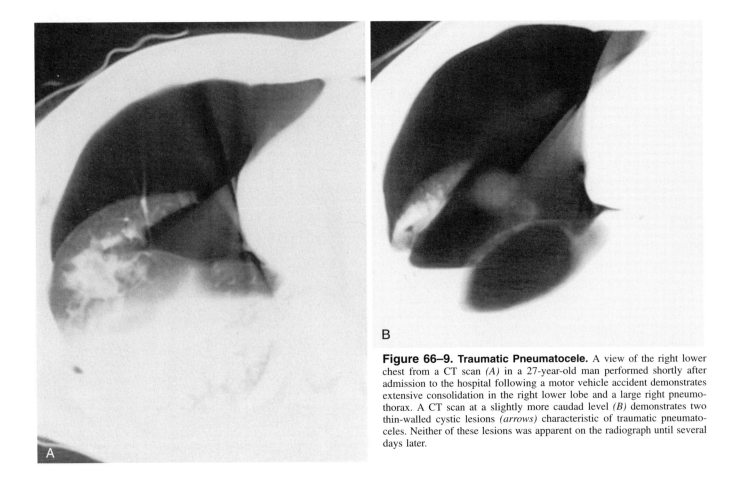

Figure 66–9. Traumatic Pneumatocele. A view of the right lower chest from a CT scan *(A)* in a 27-year-old man performed shortly after admission to the hospital following a motor vehicle accident demonstrates extensive consolidation in the right lower lobe and a large right pneumothorax. A CT scan at a slightly more caudad level *(B)* demonstrates two thin-walled cystic lesions *(arrows)* characteristic of traumatic pneumatoceles. Neither of these lesions was apparent on the radiograph until several days later.

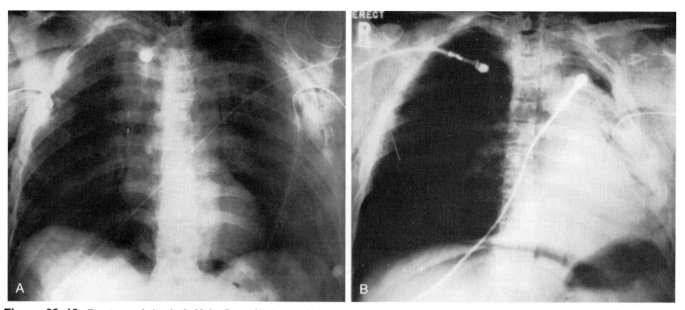

Figure 66–10. Fracture of the Left Main Bronchus. On admission to the hospital following a crush injury to his chest, this 33-year-old man showed radiographic evidence *(A)* of severe subcutaneous and mediastinal emphysema and fractures of multiple left ribs, including the first, second, and third (not visible on the illustration). Bilateral pneumothorax had been treated in the emergency room by chest tube insertion. At this time, both lungs were well expanded. Six days later *(B)*, there had occurred almost total collapse of the left lung. Bronchoscopy revealed an obstruction in the midportion of the left main bronchus. The obstructing material resembled a blood clot, although in some areas, the bronchoscopist thought he was looking at the edge of a cartilaginous ring. At thoracotomy, the left main bronchus was found to be completely disrupted just proximal to its bifurcation. (Courtesy of Dr. Harold Stolberg, Hamilton Civic Hospitals, Hamilton, Ontario.)

chial rupture, a small amount of air can escape from the airway and remain localized to the surrounding connective tissues, where it can be demonstrated radiologically.[18] However, this is an uncommon finding (having been seen, for example, in only one of nine patients in one study).[50] Displacement of fracture ends can cause bronchial obstruction and atelectasis of an entire lung (Fig. 66–10);[13, 18, 58] it is important to recognize that atelectasis may be a late development, and the discovery of such a change some time after an accident should strongly suggest the diagnosis. A diagnostic but uncommon sign of complete bronchial transsection is the "fallen lung sign," in which the collapsed lung falls away from the hilum toward the lateral and posterior chest wall or diaphragm (Fig. 66–11).[63–65] This may be more readily apparent on CT than on the radiograph.[50] In one patient with unsuspected rupture of the left main bronchus, a prospective diagnosis was made on the basis of discontinuity of the left bronchus and deviation of the trachea and right main bronchus to the right on CT.[66] In another case, CT demonstrated focal narrowing of the left main bronchus (Fig. 66–12). Occasionally, overdistention of the endotracheal balloon cuff may be the only sign of a tracheal rupture, the overdistention resulting from herniation of the balloon through the tracheal tear into the mediastinum.[67]

In about 10% of patients, tracheobronchial fracture is unassociated with any radiographically demonstrable abnormality or with much in the way of symptoms or signs.[20] In such cases, it is likely that the peribronchial connective tissue is preserved, preventing passage of air into the mediastinum or pleura. Thus, the consequence of the trauma may not become evident until the patient presents with atelectasis of a lobe or lung as a result of bronchial stenosis.[68] A review of 90 such cases showed that the condition was not diagnosed until 1 month to 19 years after the traumatic episode in one third of the patients.[69]

Traumatic tracheobronchial fracture is uncommon; it has been estimated that about 2% to 3% of patients who die

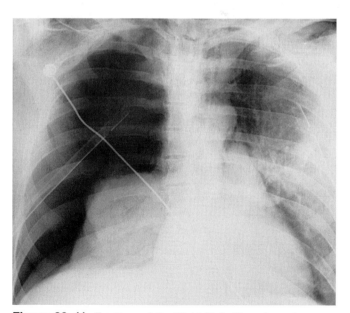

Figure 66–11. Fracture of the Right Main Bronchus. An anteroposterior chest radiograph in a 24-year-old man following a motor vehicle accident demonstrates large right and small left pneumothoraces, extensive pneumomediastinum, and multiple rib fractures. Despite the presence of a chest tube, the right lung is collapsed and displaced inferior to the right hilum ("fallen-lung sign"). A few air bronchograms are still visible within the collapsed lung. Complete transection of the right main bronchus was identified at surgery.

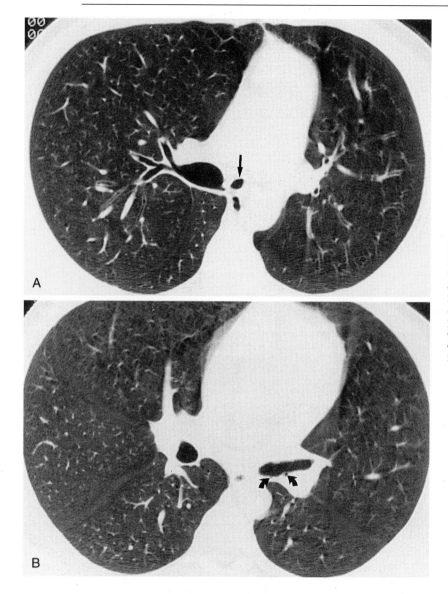

Figure 66–12. Fracture of the Left Main Bronchus. An HRCT scan *(A)* in a 26-year-old man demonstrates focal narrowing of the left main bronchus *(straight arrow)*. A scan at a more caudad level *(B)* demonstrates focal collections of air within the wall of the left main and left upper lobe bronchi *(curved arrows)*. The patient presented with a history of cough and progressive shortness of breath 1 month following a motor vehicle accident. The diagnosis of fracture of the left main bronchus was confirmed bronchoscopically.

as a result of trauma have the complication.[45a] Its rarity probably contributes to the infrequency with which it is recognized early. In one series, 68% of cases were not diagnosed until obstructive pneumonitis had developed in the lung distal to the fracture.[48] Symptoms and signs include cyanosis, hemoptysis, shock, and cough; rarely, there is pain caused by hemorrhage into the pleural space.[69] Air is often identifiable in the subcutaneous tissues, initially involving the neck and upper thorax and later becoming generalized.[54] Air may also escape directly from a wound in the neck in cases of tracheal fracture.[45a]

The overall mortality of patients who suffer tracheobronchial fracture resulting from blunt trauma is about 20% to 30%; more than half of these patients die within 1 hour of injury.[47, 52] Early diagnosis is extremely important because primary surgical repair can result in anatomic and functional restoration.[53, 70, 71] If the presence of tracheobronchial fracture goes unrecognized, the eventual development of stenosis and stricture can result in destruction of distal parenchyma. In such circumstances, resectional rather than reparative surgery is usually indicated,[56] although successful late repair has been reported.[72]

Traumatic bronchial rupture can cause severe $\dot{V}/\dot{Q}$ inequality as a result of persistent perfusion of unventilated lung.[73] However, in a follow-up study of seven patients in whom a transected main bronchus had been repaired 2 to 14 (average, 7.5) years previously, all showed normal $\dot{V}/\dot{Q}$ scans and normal flow-volume curves while breathing air and an air-helium mixture.[74]

Pulmonary Torsion

Torsion of a lobe or lung occurs most commonly as a complication of blunt chest trauma or of thoracic surgery (usually lobectomy or lingulectomy).[75–78] It has also been described after lung transplantation,[79] after fine-needle aspiration biopsy,[80–82] and in patients with spontaneous pneumothorax.[83, 84] Occasionally, it develops spontaneously, usually in association with an underlying pulmonary abnormality, such as pneumonia,[78, 85, 86] carcinoma,[78, 85] or carcinoid tumor.[78]

As a complication of trauma, torsion of a whole lung occurs most commonly in children, presumably because of the easy compressibility of a child's thoracic cage. Typically, the trauma is severe, such as when a child is run over by a vehicle; torsion occurs most often when the major force is applied to the relatively more compressible lower thorax. The lung is twisted through 180 degrees so that its base comes to lie at the apex of the hemithorax and its apex at the base. If the torsion is not relieved, the vascular supply can be compromised and the lung can become radiographically opaque as a result of exudation of edema fluid and blood into the air spaces.[85]

In an analysis of nine cases of pulmonary torsion associated with a variety of intrathoracic abnormalities (not necessarily trauma), the following manifestations were found:[85] (1) a collapsed or consolidated lobe that was situated in an unusual location on the radiograph, CT, or angiogram; (2) hilar displacement in a direction inappropriate for that lobe; (3) alteration in the normal position and sweep of the pulmonary vasculature; (4) rapid opacification of an ipsilateral lobe after trauma or thoracic surgery; (5) marked change in position of an opacified lobe on sequential radiographs; and (6) a bronchial cut-off, with no evidence of a mass (Fig. 66–13). In some cases, posteroanterior and lateral chest radiographs with the patient upright may show findings characteristic of lobar consolidation, with the torsion evident only on the radiograph or CT scan performed with the patient supine.[85] CT may demonstrate not only the abnormal position of the lobe but also the abnormal orientation of the vessels and the site of bronchial obstruction.[79, 85] Angiography may show abnormally oriented vessels as well as fusiform tapering at the site of the torsion.[85, 86a, b]

Post-traumatic Atelectasis

Post-traumatic atelectasis of a lobe—or of a whole lung—is not common but, when present, constitutes a cause of significant intrapulmonary shunting and hypoxemia at a time when a patient's clinical status may be critical. The cause of the atelectasis is not always clear, although it is probable that most cases result from bronchial obstruction from blood clots or mucous plugs.[6] In such circumstances, bronchoscopy readily reveals the cause and permits prompt relief of the obstruction. Occasionally, total collapse of a lobe or even a lung occurs without apparent reason, and bronchoscopy reveals no evidence of bronchial fracture or occlusion.[87] Whether the atelectasis in such cases is related to surfactant deficit is not certain. The affected parenchyma usually re-expands spontaneously without radiographic or functional residua.[87]

There is also evidence that mechanical percussion or hand clapping of the chest wall during physiotherapy can result in focal atelectasis. Studies of gas exchange in patients undergoing these procedures have shown variable results; some investigators have found a decrease in arterial PaO_2,[88, 89] and others an increase.[90] Experiments on dogs have shown small foci of subpleural atelectasis adjacent to the region of clapping or percussion.[91] Although the pathogenesis of this process is unclear, it has been suggested that differences in the amount of atelectasis may underlie the variation in the results of gas-exchange studies noted clinically.[91]

EFFECTS ON THE PLEURA OF NONPENETRATING TRAUMA

Hemothorax and pneumothorax are common manifestations of nonpenetrating trauma, and each may develop from a variety of causes. Blood can enter the pleural space from injury to vessels of the chest wall, diaphragm, lung, or mediastinum. Although pneumothorax most commonly develops as a consequence of pulmonary interstitial emphysema (*see* farther on), it may also result from tracheobronchial fracture and esophageal rupture, both of which are associated with potentially grave consequences. Those conditions in which hydrothorax has resulted from trauma to mediastinal structures (rupture of the aorta, the thoracic duct, or the esophagus) are considered in the section on mediastinal trauma. Similarly, pneumothorax caused by tracheobronchial fracture has been dealt with in the previous section, and that caused by esophageal rupture is discussed in the section on the mediastinum that follows. We are concerned here with hemothorax and pneumothorax developing as a consequence of damage to the pleura.

Hemothorax

Although hemorrhage may result from laceration of the parietal or visceral pleura by fractured ribs, hemothorax or pneumothorax (or both) may also occur in closed chest trauma without evidence of fracture. When blood enters the pleural space, it coagulates rapidly; however, presumably as a result of physical agitation produced by movement of the heart and lungs, the clot may be defibrinated and leave fluid indistinguishable radiographically from effusion from any other cause. On CT, acute hemorrhage into the pleural space may be recognized by the increased attenuation of the pleural fluid or by the presence of a fluid-fluid level.[92, 93] As in empyema, loculation tends to occur early in hemothorax. The site of hemorrhage influences the quantity of hemothorax:[18] when bleeding is from a vessel in the chest wall, diaphragm, or mediastinum, the hemothorax tends to increase despite the quantity of blood present; by contrast, when the blood originates in the pulmonary vasculature, the expanding hemothorax compresses the lung, with resultant pulmonary vascular tamponade that may produce hemostasis.

The radiographic demonstration of small quantities of blood requires examination of the patient in the lateral decubitus position.[20] Although an accumulation of pleural fluid after trauma is usually the result of hemorrhage, occasionally it results from other causes, such as traumatic subarachnoid pleural fistula[94] or rupture of the esophagus (*see* farther on). Similarly, widening of the pleural line, particularly over the apex, may be produced by faulty placement of a central venous catheter, with resultant hemorrhage from a subclavian vein or the instillation of fluid through the catheter.[95] Traumatic hemothorax may be associated with pneumothorax, thereby producing hemopneumothorax. The blood in traumatic hemothorax may contain a large number of eosinophils,[96] a finding that is rarely accompanied by blood eosinophilia.[97, 98]

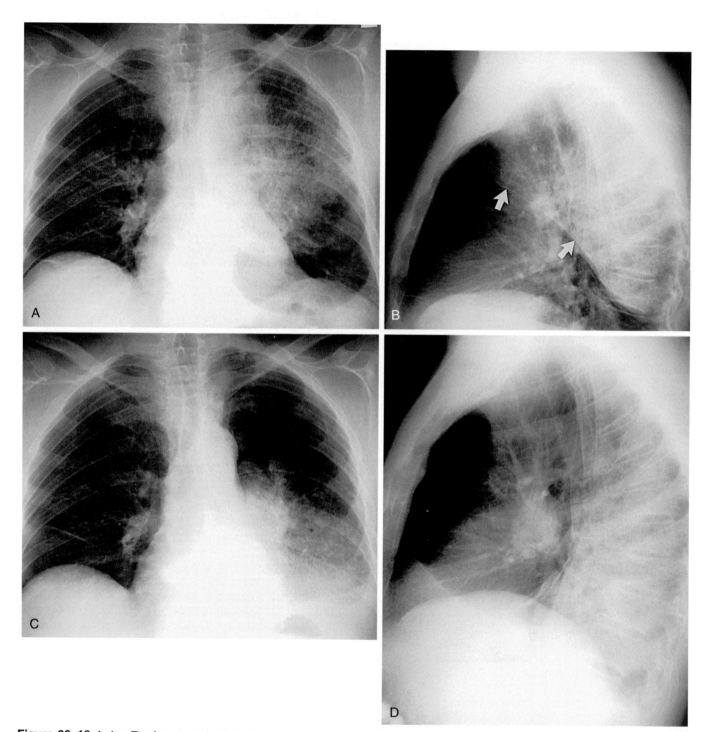

Figure 66–13. Lobar Torsion. A previously healthy adult man developed sudden-onset left chest pain. A posteroanterior radiograph at admission *(A)* demonstrates increased opacity of the left upper hemithorax. The lateral view *(B)* demonstrates inversion of the left major fissure *(arrows)*, a finding diagnostic of lobar torsion. The diagnosis was confirmed at bronchoscopy. The torsion resolved spontaneously. Posteroanterior *(C)* and lateral *(D)* radiographs 2 days later demonstrate mild loss of volume of the left lower lobe, which has returned to a normal position. Note the normal orientation of the interlobar fissures. The consolidation and left pleural effusion were presumably the result of ischemia-related pulmonary hemorrhage. (Courtesy of Dr. Peter Hicken, Lions Gate Hospital, Vancouver.)

Pneumothorax

Pneumothorax occurs in 15% to 40% of patients with blunt chest trauma.[99, 100] Pneumothorax complicating trauma may occur without radiographic evidence of rib fracture; for example, in one series of 15 survivors of attempted suicide who jumped into water from a considerable height (50 M), 10 patients developed a pneumothorax within 12 hours, and in only 4 of these was there an associated rib fracture.[101] When fracture is present, the likely mechanism is laceration of the visceral pleura by rib fragments; in such circumstances, hemothorax may be expected as a concomitant finding. When no fractures are visible, it is likely that pneumothorax is secondary to pulmonary laceration.

As indicated previously, small parenchymal lacerations are seen on CT in most patients with radiographically evident pulmonary contusion; pneumothorax is frequently present in these patients, even in the absence of rib fractures.[2] Pneumomediastinum and subcutaneous emphysema without rib fracture may also result from pulmonary interstitial emphysema, with subsequent tracking of air to the mediastinum and through the thoracic inlet into the neck and lateral chest wall (Fig. 66–14). In this regard, it is noteworthy that subcutaneous emphysema may result from closed chest trauma without associated pneumothorax (as in 13 of 166

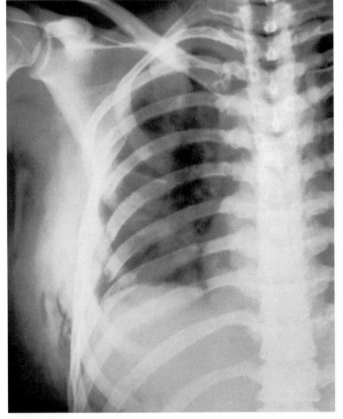

Figure 66–14. Subcutaneous Emphysema Associated with Multiple Fractured Ribs in the Absence of Pneumothorax. An anteroposterior radiograph in the supine position reveals multiple grossly displaced fractures of the right rib cage in the posterior axillary line. There is considerable subcutaneous emphysema in the adjacent soft tissues but no pneumothorax. (However, a small pneumothorax might not be visible on this radiograph, which is exposed with the patient supine.)

patients in one report[102]). Traumatic pneumothorax sometimes develops on the undamaged side, presumably as a result of a contrecoup effect.[103]

When a pneumothorax is small and the visceral pleural line is poorly visualized, radiography at full expiration may reveal the partially collapsed lung to better advantage. When a patient's condition does not warrant radiography in the erect position, examination in the lateral decubitus position permits identification of small quantities of air in the pleural space.[95]

Pneumothorax is more commonly detected on CT than on the radiograph.[2] For example, in one series of 85 patients with pulmonary contusion, pneumothorax was detected on the radiograph in 34 cases and on CT in 70 cases.[2] In another review of abdominal CT scans performed for evaluation of blunt trauma, 35 patients had pneumothorax, 10 (29%) of which had not been previously diagnosed on chest radiography;[104] of the 10 cases, 7 required chest tube drainage. Therefore, in all patients undergoing abdominal CT for blunt trauma, images should be obtained through the lung bases and viewed on lung settings to assess the presence of pneumothorax.[42, 99]

EFFECTS ON THE MEDIASTINUM OF NONPENETRATING TRAUMA

The abnormalities with which we are primarily concerned in nonpenetrating trauma to the mediastinum include pneumomediastinum, hemorrhage, rupture of the aorta and major vessels, perforation of the esophagus, and rupture of the thoracic duct. Traumatic abnormalities of the heart and pericardium are not within the scope of this book.

Pneumomediastinum

Traumatic pneumomediastinum may develop after closed chest trauma, in which case it is probably produced by the same mechanism as spontaneous pneumomediastinum—rupture of alveoli as a result of an abrupt increase in pressure or sheer stress followed by tracking of gas into the peribronchovascular interstitial tissue. The abnormality may also follow traumatic rupture of the esophagus or fracture of the tracheobronchial tree; in either case, the mediastinal emphysema may be associated with acute mediastinitis. Sometimes, perforation of the esophagus or the tracheobronchial tree occurs during or after diagnostic instrumentation, either directly due to the trauma or from the paroxysmal coughing engendered by these procedures.[105, 106] Air may also enter the mediastinum along deep fascial planes as a result of trauma or surgical procedures to the neck or in association with zygomaticomaxillary fractures.[107] The radiographic signs are identical to those of pneumomediastinum from any cause (*see* page 2865).

Mediastinal Hemorrhage

Most cases of mediastinal hemorrhage result from trauma, usually of a severe nature, such as that associated with a motor vehicle accident or a fall from a height.[108, 109]

The source of bleeding in these cases is often the aorta; other sources include veins and smaller arteries. Mediastinal blood also may originate in traumatized retropharyngeal soft tissue. In some cases, the trauma is iatrogenic (e.g., after faulty placement of a central venous line[110, 111] or perforation of the superior vena cava[112]).

Radiographically, extensive hemorrhage typically results in uniform, symmetric widening of the mediastinum (Fig. 66–15). Local accumulation of blood in the form of a

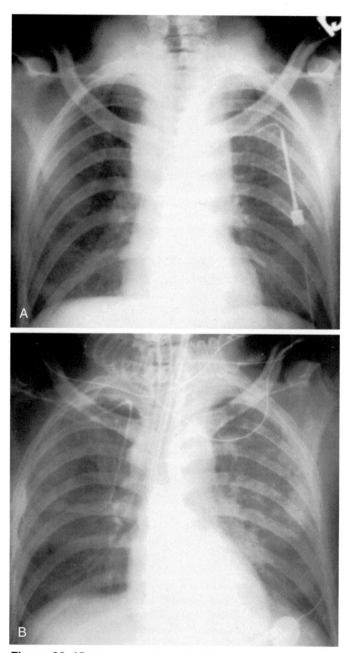

Figure 66–15. Traumatic Mediastinal Hemorrhage. A radiograph of the chest in anteroposterior projection, supine position *(A)* of this young man following severe closed chest trauma reveals moderate widening of the upper half of the mediastinum, roughly symmetric on both sides. The lungs are unremarkable. About 36 hours later *(B)*, the widening had diminished considerably. There is now evidence of a uniform opacity over both lungs, which in a supine view, is good evidence for bilateral pleural effusions, in this case hemothorax.

hematoma is manifested by a homogeneous focal opacity that may project to one or both sides of the mediastinum and may be situated in any compartment.[113, 114] The most important diagnostic consideration in these cases is traumatic aortic rupture. However, only 10% to 20% of patients with radiographic findings suggestive of mediastinal hemorrhage in this situation have an aortic injury.[4] Therefore, further diagnostic procedures, including contrast-enhanced CT, transesophageal ultrasound, or aortography, are required for definitive diagnosis (*see* farther on).[108, 109, 115]

Symptoms and signs of mediastinal hemorrhage are seldom striking. Suspicion of aortic rupture should be aroused when retrosternal pain that radiates into the back develops in a patient who suffered chest trauma recently. A hematoma of sufficient size and appropriate location may compress the superior vena cava.[116, 117]

Rupture of the Thoracic Aorta and Its Branches

Rupture of the aorta is a well-recognized sequela of closed chest injury. About 80% to 90% of cases follow severe motor vehicle accidents, and 5% to 10% automobile-pedestrian accidents; an additional 5% to 10% result from falls from a height, usually greater than 9 M (30 feet).[109, 118]

About 90% of thoracic aortic injuries diagnosed clinically and radiologically involve the region of the aortic isthmus immediately distal to the left subclavian artery;[4, 119] tears of the ascending aorta, the distal descending aorta, and abdominal aorta are much less common.[120–122] The most commonly accepted mechanism is a deceleration-related shearing stress on the relatively mobile anterior portion of the aortic arch between the more fixed posterior arch and descending aorta.[120, 123] It has also been suggested that laceration may be caused by sudden chest compression pinching the aorta between the anterior and posterior components of the bony thorax.[124, 125] According to this hypothesis, compressive forces depress the anterior thoracic osseous structures, causing them to rotate posteriorly and inferiorly around the posterior rib articulation, pinching and shearing the interposed vascular structures.

Laceration of the ascending aorta represents only about 5% of all thoracic aortic injuries identified clinically; however, the incidence of this injury at autopsy is higher, ranging from 8% to almost 25%.[121, 122, 126] This disparity is caused by the association of severe and often fatal cardiac injury in roughly 80% of cases (compared with 25% when the laceration is at the isthmus). Although these injuries are rarely recognized during life,[127] it is nevertheless important to opacify the entire aorta from the aortic valve to the diaphragm in any patient in whom the possibility of aortic laceration is entertained.

Occasionally, mediastinal hemorrhage following severe chest trauma results from damage to one of the great vessels arising from the aortic arch. In fact, avulsion of the innominate artery from the arch has been stated to be the second most common type of aortic injury in which the patient survives long enough for diagnostic evaluation.[128] The radiographic findings are similar to those of rupture of the aortic isthmus, with the possible exception that the outline of the descending aorta may be preserved.[128] Fractures of the upper thoracic spine may also cause radiographic findings similar to those of aortic rupture. In a retrospective analysis of the frontal chest radiographs of 54 patients with traumatic fractures of at least one vertebral body from C-6 to T-8, 37 patients (69%) were identified with signs generally considered to be consistent with aortic laceration;[129] the spinal fracture could be identified on the initial radiograph in about half of the 37 patients.

Radiographic Signs

A wide variety of radiographic signs have been described as being useful in the diagnosis of aortic rupture. Some—particularly mediastinal widening and poor definition of the aortic arch—have a relatively high sensitivity but a low specificity, whereas others, such as rightward deviation of the trachea, downward displacement of the left main bronchus, rightward displacement of a nasogastric tube, and thickening of the right paratracheal stripe, have greater specificity but lower sensitivity.[4] The greatest value of the chest radiograph is in excluding traumatic aortic injury; the negative predictive value of a normal erect frontal chest radiograph is about 98%.[4, 118] However, the positive predictive value of an abnormal chest radiograph is relatively low, only 10% to 20% of patients with abnormalities suggestive of mediastinal hemorrhage having aortic injury.[4, 31, 126]

Widening of the Upper Half of the Mediastinum

Plain radiographs of the chest frequently reveal widening of the superior mediastinum as a result of hemorrhage (Fig. 66–16), although the hemorrhage eventually may prove to be of venous origin because of either direct trauma or iatrogenic causes, such as malpositioning of a central venous line.[130] Hemorrhage resulting from aortic injury tends to widen the mediastinum predominantly to the left of the midline while, at the same time, causing disappearance of the shadow of the tracheal stripe and the azygos vein.[131] This combination of changes contrasts with the situation pertaining in the presence of an increase in systemic blood volume (or the supine position), in which the vascular pedicle widens predominantly to the right and the azygos vein dilates concomitantly.[131]

Assessment of mediastinal widening may be based solely on subjective criteria or on measurements.[115, 132] Most radiologists use either the former or measurement of mediastinal diameter at the level of the aortic arch (a figure greater than 8 cm indicating pathologic widening).[4, 119] Measurement of the mediastinal width-to-chest width ratio has also been used; in one study of 20 patients with proven traumatic aortic rupture, a ratio of 0.25 or greater was seen in 95% of those who had a ruptured aorta.[132] However, this ratio was found in a subsequent study to have insufficient sensitivity and specificity to be clinically useful in confirming or excluding rupture.[133] A retrospective review of chest radiographs from 205 patients with blunt chest trauma who also underwent aortography revealed that a widened mediastinum, defined by either subjective impression, width greater

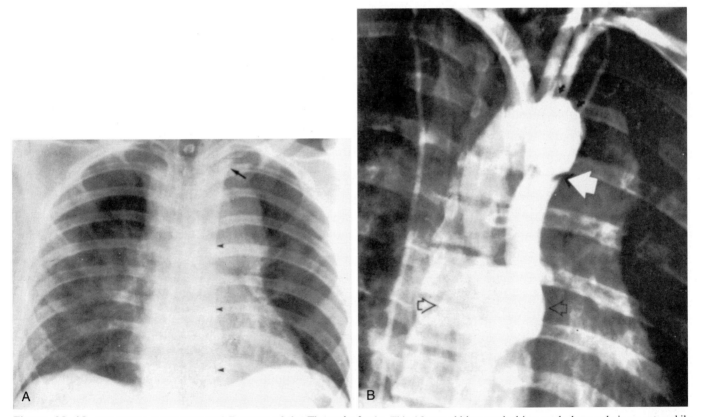

Figure 66–16. Traumatic Aneurysm and Rupture of the Thoracic Aorta. This 16-year-old boy crashed into a telephone pole in an automobile traveling at 85 mph. Shortly after his arrival in the emergency room, a chest radiograph in anteroposterior projection *(A)* revealed marked widening of the upper mediastinum and loss of visualization of the aortic arch. A wide paravertebral opacity *(arrowheads)* extends to the apex, creating an extrapleural apical cap *(arrow)*. The suspicion of aortic rupture was confirmed by aortography *(B)*. The site of primary aortic laceration is indicated by a thick arrow, the irregular bulge immediately above *(small arrows)* representing dissection proximally. Several centimeters distally is a large, well-circumscribed collection of contrast medium *(open arrows)*, which represents an extra-aortic hematoma from a second rupture. The patient exsanguinated following section of the mediastinal pleura at thoracotomy.

than 8 cm at the level of aortic arch, or a mediastinal width-to-chest width ratio of greater than 0.25, had a sensitivity of 36% and a specificity of 81% in the diagnosis of aortic rupture on erect anteroposterior chest radiographs and a sensitivity of 67% and specificity of 45% on radiographs performed with the patient supine.[118]

Compared with the appearance on the upright radiograph, the mediastinum is widened and magnified on the supine radiograph, decreasing the diagnostic usefulness of mediastinal widening. For example, in one study of 123 patients radiographed in the supine position, mediastinal widening greater than 8 cm was present in 87% of patients with traumatic aortic rupture but also in 69% of patients without rupture.[134]

Abnormal Contour of the Aortic Arch

Irregularity (Fig. 66–17) or obscuration of the contour of the aortic arch (Fig. 66–18) is probably the most reliable sign of aortic rupture. In a study of 205 patients with blunt chest trauma who underwent aortography, this sign had a sensitivity of 63% and a specificity of 62% on erect radiographs and a sensitivity of 81% and a specificity of 45% on radiographs performed with the patient supine.[118] Other related signs that have also been found to be helpful include obscuration of the aortopulmonary window[118, 134, 135] and obscuration of the proximal descending thoracic aorta.[118]

Deviation of the Trachea and Left Main Bronchus

As the hematoma enlarges, the left main bronchus may be deviated anteriorly, inferiorly, and to the right, and the trachea may be displaced to the right. Shift of the left tracheal wall to the right of the T-4 spinous process has a specificity of greater than 90% for the detection of traumatic aortic tears but has a low sensitivity, the finding being present on erect frontal views of the chest in only 15% of patients.[118] Depression of the left main bronchus greater than 40 degrees below the horizontal in the absence of left lower lobe atelectasis is also suggestive of the diagnosis but is seen in only a small number of patients.[118, 136]

Deviation of a Nasogastric Tube

Displacement of a nasogastric tube to the right of the T-4 spinous process also has a high specificity and a low sensitivity, being present in only about 10% of patients with aortic rupture in one study (*see* Fig. 66–18).[118]

Displacement of the Right Paraspinous Interface

Displacement or widening of the right paraspinous interface is highly suggestive of the diagnosis;[118, 137] however, it is again present in less than 10% of patients.[118]

Widening of the Right Paratracheal Stripe

Another sign that has been suggested as a possible indicator of aortic tear is widening of the right paratracheal stripe to a thickness greater than 5 mm[138] (*see* Fig. 66–16). In one investigation of 102 consecutive patients with blunt chest trauma, all those with a right paratracheal stripe less

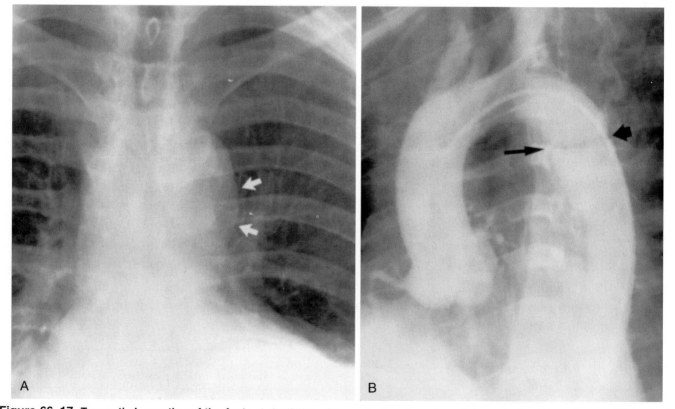

Figure 66–17. Traumatic Laceration of the Aorta. A detail view of the mediastinum in posteroanterior projection *(A)* reveals a small bulge on the descending arch of the aorta *(arrows);* there is also a left pleural effusion of moderate size. An aortogram in right posterior oblique projection *(B)* reveals a lucent defect in the descending arch *(arrows),* representing the tear in the aortic wall.

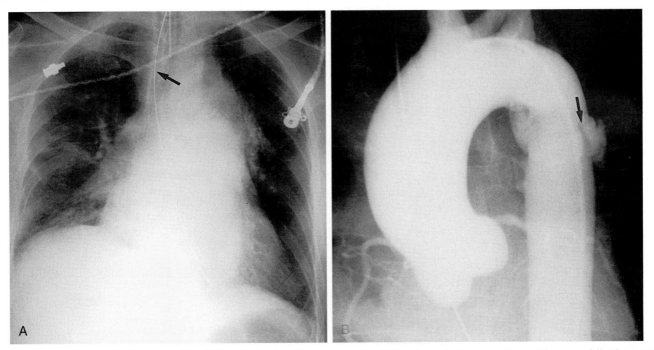

Figure 66–18. Traumatic Rupture of the Thoracic Aorta. An anteroposterior chest radiograph *(A)* in an 80-year-old woman following a motor vehicle accident reveals increased soft tissue opacity with obscuration of the aortic arch. Note the deviation of the nasogastric tube *(curved arrow)* to the right of the spinous process of T-4. An aortogram *(B)* demonstrates transection of the aorta *(arrow)*.

than 5 mm in width had a normal aortogram;[138] by contrast, aortography revealed major arterial injury in 23% of patients whose right tracheal stripe measured 5 mm or greater. In another study of 87 patients, 83% of those with an aortic tear had widening of the right paratracheal stripe, compared with only 29% without aortic injury.[134]

The Left Apical Cap

A potential space exists between the isthmus of the aorta and the parietal pleura of the left lung. Provided that the parietal pleura is intact, extravasated blood can track cephalad along the course of the left subclavian artery between the parietal pleura and the extrapleural soft tissues, resulting in a homogeneous opacity over the apex of the left hemithorax—the extrapleural apical cap.[139] A left apical cap by itself constitutes an unreliable sign of acute aortic rupture.[118, 140] For example, in one study in which angiograms were performed solely because of the presence of an apical cap, aortic ruptures were seen in only 2 of 12 patients;[140] in another series, the finding was present in only 10% of patients with aortic rupture.[118]

Left Hemothorax

Hemothorax complicating traumatic rupture of the aorta is common and is almost invariably left sided.[141] It should not be attributed erroneously to left-sided rib fractures.

Fracture of the First and Second Ribs

Formerly considered a potential indicator of aortic and brachiocephalic artery trauma, fractures of the first and second ribs are now thought to represent unreliable signs on the strength of several well-documented studies.[118, 142–144]

Summary

A number of papers have been published in which an attempt has been made to assess the relative value of the many radiographic signs described previously.[118, 136, 145, 146] The majority opinion, with which we agree, is that the most reliable features are mediastinal widening and an abnormal outline of the aortic arch. However, no single sign or combination of signs on conventional chest radiographs has sufficient sensitivity to avoid the performance of a large number of negative aortographic studies. As a result, the use of additional, noninvasive techniques—primarily CT and echocardiography—is indicated in most patients.

On the basis of the many studies that we have reviewed, we believe that in any patient who has suffered severe chest trauma in whom conventional chest radiographs reveal upper mediastinal widening or loss of normal contour of the aortic arch, further investigation by contrast-enhanced spiral CT, transesophageal echocardiography, or aortography is indicated to establish the diagnosis and reveal the anatomic extent of rupture. Patients with equivocal radiographic findings or in whom only supine radiographs can be obtained should undergo contrast-enhanced spiral CT[108, 147, 148] or transesophageal echocardiography.[149, 150] Unstable patients with obvious mediastinal abnormalities on the chest radiograph should proceed directly to aortography or surgery.

Computed Tomography

CT permits ready distinction of a mediastinal hematoma from mediastinal widening related to tortuous vessels, fat, or radiographic magnification. The findings include both indirect and direct signs.[151] Mediastinal hematoma (Fig. 66–19) is an indirect sign, whereas irregularity of the wall (Fig. 66–20), the presence of an aortic pseudoaneurysm, abrupt

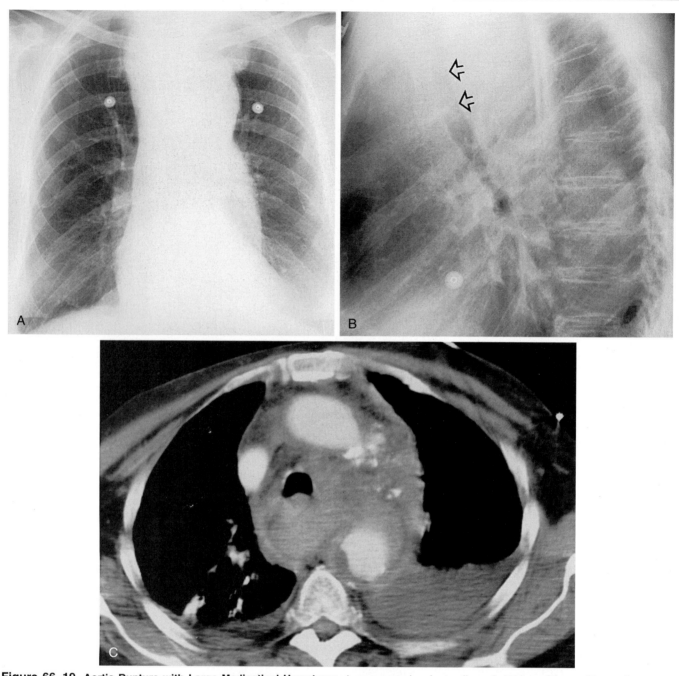

Figure 66–19. Aortic Rupture with Large Mediastinal Hematoma. A posteroanterior chest radiograph *(A)* in an 84-year-old man demonstrates widening of the mediastinum. The lateral view *(B)* shows marked anterior displacement of the trachea *(arrows)*. A contrast-enhanced CT scan *(C)* demonstrates abnormal contour of the descending aorta and an extensive mediastinal hematoma associated with displacement of the trachea anteriorly and to the right. Bilateral pleural effusions are also evident. The diagnosis of aortic rupture was confirmed at surgery.

caliber change of the aorta, or (less commonly) extravasation of contrast material from the aorta or the presence of an intraluminal radiolucent filling defect (intimal flap) (Fig. 66–21) constitutes a direct sign.[108, 148, 151]

Several groups have assessed the role of CT in the diagnosis of aortic injury.[108, 109, 147, 152, 153] In one study, 5-mm collimation contrast-enhanced CT scans were performed in 160 consecutive patients with radiographic findings considered to indicate low to moderate probability of aortic injury following blunt trauma;[152] aortography was performed in patients with evidence of mediastinal hemorrhage on CT.

The investigators found no evidence of mediastinal hemorrhage in any of the 132 patients with normal chest radiographs. CT excluded mediastinal hemorrhage in 22 of 28 (78%) patients with abnormal radiographs. Six patients had mediastinal hematoma at CT, one of whom had an aortic laceration at angiography. In another study, CT scans demonstrated mediastinal hemorrhage in 15 of 199 (8%) patients with normal radiographs, 2 of whom had an aortic tear at aortography;[109] scans showed mediastinal hematoma in 39 of 127 (31%) patients with abnormal radiographs, 8 of whom had aortic tear demonstrated at aortography. In a third inves-

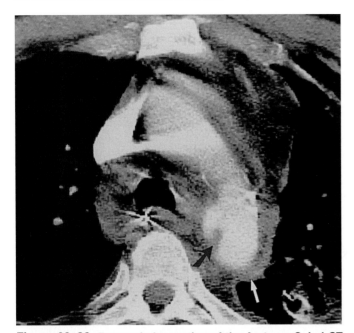

Figure 66–20. Traumatic Laceration of the Aorta on Spiral CT. A contrast-enhanced 7-mm collimation spiral CT scan performed in a 53-year-old man following an automobile accident reveals focal irregularity of the proximal descending thoracic aorta *(black arrow)*, diagnostic of an aortic laceration. A small amount of blood can be seen adjacent to the aorta *(white arrow)*.

tigation, contrast-enhanced CT was performed in 677 patients with equivocal or positive radiographic findings.[148] CT findings were negative in 570 cases, positive in 100, and equivocal in 7. Mediastinal hemorrhage was the only abnor-

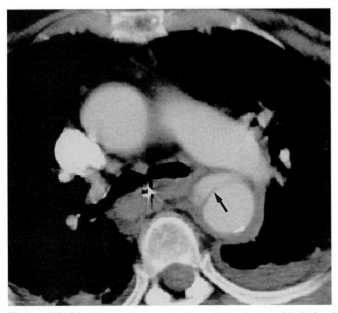

Figure 66–21. Traumatic Laceration of the Aorta with Intimal Flap. A contrast-enhanced spiral CT demonstrates irregularity of the lateral wall of the aorta and an intimal flap *(arrow)*. A small amount of blood is evident around the proximal descending thoracic aorta, and there are small bilateral pleural effusions. The patient was a 79-year-old woman being assessed following a motor vehicle accident. The diagnosis of aortic laceration was confirmed at surgery.

mality on CT in 79 cases; aortography was negative in 77 of these (97%). In the remaining 21 cases with positive CT findings, CT demonstrated direct evidence of aortic injury, including contour abnormality or pseudoaneurysm in 19 patients, intimal flap in 8, and pseudocoarctation in 3.

Although the studies described previously suggest that contrast-enhanced CT has a 100% sensitivity in the diagnosis of aortic laceration, some investigators have documented cases of false-negative CT scans.[153–155] For example, in one prospective investigation of 153 consecutive patients with suspected aortic injury, 49 underwent immediate angiography without chest CT;[153] 11 of these (22%) had major thoracic arterial injuries. Data from the remaining 104 cases showed that CT detected 5 of 11 cases of major thoracic arterial injuries (sensitivity 55%, specificity of 65%); aortic injury was missed on CT in 2 patients and major aortic branch injury in 3.

Meta-analysis of the data from a total of 3,334 cases published in the literature by 1996 showed that when the presence of either mediastinal hematoma or direct signs of aortic injury was considered as an indicator for a positive examination the sensitivity of CT was 99.3%, the specificity 87.1%, positive predictive value 19.9%, and negative predictive value 99.9%.[148] A cost-effectiveness analysis study published in 1995 compared six diagnostic strategies combining chest radiography, CT, and angiography in various sequences.[147] The authors concluded that selecting hemodynamically stable patients with suspected aortic injury after blunt chest trauma for angiography on the basis of CT findings is more effective than doing so based on chest radiographic findings.[147]

Most studies published before 1996 used conventional CT. The relatively long interval between each individual slice and the difference in inspiratory effort among slices often resulted in suboptimal contrast-enhancement and interslice artifacts. The shortened scanning time of spiral CT has resulted in greatly improved vascular contrast enhancement *(see* Figs. 66–20 and 66–21).[156] Rapid scanning of multiple levels during a single breath-hold eliminates interslice artifacts and permits CT angiography with excellent direct visualization of the aortic injury.[157]

The efficacy of spiral CT as a screening device to detect aortic injury was assessed in a prospective study of 1,518 consecutive patients with nontrivial blunt chest trauma.[157] The chest radiograph was not used in the triage process. In 92% of patients, the CT scans showed no evidence of mediastinal hematoma and no suggestion of aortic abnormality, and no further investigation was undertaken. One hundred and twenty-seven patients (about 8%) had abnormal or indeterminate CT scans and underwent aortography. In 89 (70%) of these, CT demonstrated mediastinal hematoma and a normal aorta; none had evidence of aortic injury (in 85 patients the aorta was normal at aortography; in 3, aortography was indeterminate or falsely positive because of the presence of prominent atherosclerotic plaques; and in 1, it was falsely positive because of a large ductus diverticulum proven at surgery). Thirty-eight of the 127 patients (21%) with abnormal CT scans had either direct evidence of thoracic injury (contour abnormality, localized area of narrowing, intimal flap, pseudoaneurysm, or contrast extravasation), indeterminate scans, or inadequate spiral CT scans; 17 of these patients had aortic injury demonstrated at aortography, all of whom had direct signs of aortic injury on CT. In 1 patient, angiography was falsely negative—the presence of an intimal flap missed at aortography was confirmed by transesophageal echocardiography. In this study, therefore, spiral CT was more sensitive than aortography (100% versus 94%, respectively) but less specific (82% versus 96%, respectively) in the detection of aortic injury. The main limitation of the study is its assumption that patients with normal CT scans do not have traumatic aortic injury. Furthermore, two branch vessel injuries were missed with direct CT visualization (although adjacent hematoma suggested their presence); this is an important consideration, because about 5% of aortic arch injuries involve major branch vessels.[158, 159] Furthermore, because of cardiac motion artifact, ascending aortic injuries may be missed on spiral CT.[157, 159]

In a subsequent study from the same institution, investigators evaluated the use of spiral CT aortography in the assessment of thoracic aortic rupture.[160] This procedure consisted of two-dimensional multiplanar reconstructions and three-dimensional analysis based on maximal-intensity projection or shaded-surface display reconstructions.[160] Thirty-eight injuries of the aorta and great vessels were detected in 36 of 3,229 patients with nontrivial blunt chest trauma. The extent of injury was identified in 100% of cases on standard transverse spiral CT images, compared with 82% of cases on two-dimensional reconstructions, 82% on three-dimensional maximal-intensity projection reconstructions, 71% on the three-dimensional surface shading reconstructions, and 88% on transcatheter thoracic aortograms.[160] All nondiagnostic images from transcatheter aortograms involved patients who had subtle intimal flaps. CT angiography accurately demonstrated the presence and extent of aortic injuries when these were greater than 15 mm long but was inferior to standard transverse CT images for small tears.

Some workers have suggested that a normal aorta on spiral CT effectively excludes the possibility of aortic injury and that aortography is not necessary in this situation, even when there is mediastinal hematoma.[160, 175] However, the majority of investigators consider that aortography is mandatory in patients who have hematoma.[42a, 160a–c] In one study of 21 patients who underwent spiral CT for the assessment of aortic injury, 8 of the 11 patients who had periaortic hematoma identified on CT had aortic injury proven at aortography;[160b] the other 3 had normal angiograms. All 10 patients who did not have a periaortic hematoma had normal findings at angiography. Thus, the presence of periaortic hematoma had a sensitivity of 100%, a specificity of 77%, a negative predictive value of 100%, and a positive predictive value of 73% in predicting traumatic aortic rupture.

Based on our review of the literature, we believe that the following recommendations are reasonable in a patient who has had blunt chest trauma:

1. A normal chest radiograph performed with the patient erect has a 98% negative predictive value for aortic injury, and a normal supine view has a 96% negative predictive value.[118] Because of these high values, further investigation is seldom warranted in patients with normal chest radiographs. However, because it may provide important diagnostic information, spiral CT of the chest is indicated in patients who are undergoing CT of the abdomen and pelvis after trauma regardless of the chest radiographic findings.[157]

2. Patients with abnormal chest radiographs who are unstable should proceed directly to aortography or surgery.

3. Patients who are stable and who have suboptimal or abnormal chest radiographs should undergo CT of the chest, preferably using spiral technique. Patients with normal spiral CT need no further evaluation, unless serial radiographs show progressive mediastinal widening.[152] Depending on the experience of the radiologist and surgeon, patients with direct signs of aortic injury on CT may undergo transcatheter aortography or proceed directly to surgery. Patients who have a periaortic hematoma evident on CT and patients with indeterminate or inadequate chest CT scans should undergo emergency aortography.

It cannot be overemphasized that assessment of traumatic aortic injury on spiral CT requires not only interpretive expertise, but also careful attention to technique.[160a, 160c] We currently use intravenous contrast material (300 mg I/ml) administered with a power injector at a rate of 2 to 3 ml per second for a total of 100 to 150 ml. Optimal scan delay can be determined by using a 20-ml test injection and obtaining images at a preselected level (such as the aortic arch), or by using a standard software package provided with the CT scanner. In the majority of patients, a 30-second delay provides adequate visualization of the aorta. CT scans are obtained during a single breath-hold from 2 cm above the aortic arch to 2 cm below the tracheal carina using 3-mm collimation and a pitch of 1.7; the images are reconstructed at 1-mm intervals. The remainder of the chest is scanned using 7-mm collimation.

Transesophageal Echocardiography

The results of several studies suggest that transesophageal echocardiography is a highly sensitive and specific method of detecting thoracic aortic injuries.[149, 150, 161, 162] In one study, the procedure was compared with aortography in 101 patients with suspected traumatic rupture of the aorta.[150] It was successfully performed in 93 patients but could not be completed in 8 because of lack of cooperation or extensive maxillofacial trauma. Comparison of the results of transesophageal echocardiography with those of aortography, surgery, or autopsy demonstrated that echocardiography had detected all 11 cases of aortic injury (sensitivity 100%) and demonstrated true negative results in 82 patients and one false-positive result (specificity, 98%; positive predictive value, 99%).[150]

Although results such as these are encouraging, transesophageal echocardiography has a number of disadvantages. The procedure is more operator dependent and invasive than CT, takes an average of 30 minutes to complete, and, in patients who are awake, requires intravenous sedation.[150] In one investigation of 34 patients who had blunt chest trauma, transesophageal echocardiography and aortography were performed prospectively.[162a] In 5 (15%) patients, echocardiography was unsuccessful; 2 of these 5 had aortic injury at aortography, and the unsuccessful echocardiography resulted in substantial delay in diagnosis. In the remaining patients, echocardiography had a 57% sensitivity and a 91% specificity for the diagnosis of aortic injury. Transesophageal echocardiography cannot be performed in patients who are uncooperative or who have maxillofacial trauma and should not be attempted in those with unstable neck and spine injuries.[150] The echocardiographic signs of aortic injury are complex and often limited to a short section of the vessel.[163] In addition, although the procedure yields detailed images of most of the thoracic aorta, a 3- to 5-cm portion of the ascending portion cannot be adequately assessed;[164] thus, injuries limited to this region, although rare, may be missed.[150] Finally, the procedure does not allow visualization of the great vessels coming off the aortic arch.

Aortography

Transfemoral aortography remains the definitive imaging modality to diagnose the presence, location, and extent of aortic injury.[119, 147, 152] At least two projections must be obtained, most commonly the left anterior oblique and anteroposterior views.[119] The examination must include the entire thoracic aorta and great branch vessels.[119] Angiographic findings diagnostic of aortic injury include tear of the intima, extravasation of contrast material, dissection with an intimal flap, pseudoaneurysm, and pseudocoarctation (*see* Fig. 66–16).[119]

Although aortography is the gold-standard imaging modality for the diagnosis of aortic injury, false-positive and false-negative interpretations may occur. The main reasons for the former are the presence of an atypical ductus diverticulum or an ulcerated atherosclerotic plaque.[165] In one study of 314 patients assessed for possible aortic trauma, the aortogram was falsely positive in 3 (1%) and equivocal in 9 (3%);[165] postoperative diagnoses in the false-positive cases were ductus diverticulum in 2 patients and ulcerating atherosclerotic plaque in 1. A ductus diverticulum—defined as a focal bulge or convexity at the level of the aortic isthmus—was seen in 51 patients (26%).[165] Distinction of a ductus diverticulum from an aortic injury can usually be made based on the absence of contrast-material retention or intimal flap;[165, 166] however, a diverticulum may fold back against the aorta, creating an appearance of intimal radiolucency indistinguishable from an aortic tear.[165]

Aortography has a sensitivity of about 95% in the detection of aortic injuries and a negative predictive value of 99%.[157] Missed findings include the presence of a small traumatic intimal flap and a small localized rupture through the intima and media.[150, 157] The procedure is relatively safe; however, complications occur, including entry of the catheter into a false channel due to atherosclerotic or traumatic dissection and (rarely) rupture at the site of injury with subsequent exsanguination and death.[119, 167]

Clinical Manifestations

Although evidence of penetrating thoracic trauma is usually present, significant internal injury may occur with blunt trauma in the absence of obvious external injury to the thorax; in this situation, certain features related to the trauma may suggest such injury.[168] Attention should be paid to features associated with the severity of deceleration injury (e.g., a high-speed automobile accident) and the magnitude of the trauma (e.g., associated fatalities); a history of lower extremity paresis or paralysis and evidence of hemodynamic instability during transport also suggest the possibility of serious internal injury. Clinical signs may also be important. For example, the patient may have respiratory distress as a result of hemothorax, an initial rush of blood after tube thoracostomy may indicate great vessel injury,[168] and signs of pericardial tamponade may be evident. Other signs of potential large vessel injury include[168] (1) external evidence of major chest trauma, such as steering wheel imprint on the chest, palpable fracture of the sternum, left flail chest, or palpable fracture of the thoracic vertebrae; (2) an expanding hematoma at the thoracic outlet; (3) an interscapular murmur; (4) upper extremity hypertension; (5) diminished or absent pulses in the upper extremity (from innominate or subclavian injury, which can accompany aortic injury) or lower extremity (related to pseudocoarctation syndrome); (6) elevated central venous pressure; and (7) hypotension.

Some aneurysms of traumatic origin are unrecognized at the time and may remain so for many years until a screening chest radiograph of an asymptomatic patient reveals the abnormality (Fig. 66–22).[169–173] Rarely, a patient presents with symptoms and signs of rupture of an aortic aneurysm that was caused by severe trauma many years previously but was not recognized (Fig. 66–23). In a review of 413 cases of chronic traumatic thoracic aorta aneurysms reported from 1950 to 1980, signs or symptoms of aneurysm expansion developed within 5 years of injury in 42% of the patients and within 20 years in 85%.[174] The most common symptom was pain, usually accompanied by radiographic evidence of progressive enlargement of the aortic shadow. A follow-up of the 60 patients who did not undergo surgery showed that 20 had died of their aortic lesions, most of them in the absence of symptoms. Of the 300 patients who had surgery, only about 5% died, most as a result of hemorrhage.

As might be expected, traumatic aortic rupture is a serious condition; only 10% to 20% of affected patients live longer than 1 hour, and many of these succumb shortly thereafter.[120, 122, 126] In a retrospective study of 90 motor vehicle fatalities related to aortic injury, death was immediate in 44% of cases, within 1 hour in 50%, between 1 and 24 hours in 5%, and after 24 hours in 1%.[122] In another series of 142 fatal cases, death occurred at the scene of the accident in 43%, on arrival at the hospital in 15%, less than 30 minutes after arrival in 4%, between 30 minutes and 4 hours after arrival in 30%, and more than 4 hours after arrival in 8%.[121] Several groups of investigators have shown that death from aortic hemorrhage or associated injuries occurs within the first few hours after admission to hospital in about 10% to 15% of patients who have traumatic aortic rupture.[175–178] Moreover, it has been estimated that without surgical repair, about 30% of initial survivors would die within 24 hours, and more than 50% would die within 1 week.[42]

Perforation of the Esophagus

Rupture of the esophagus from closed chest trauma is rare and results in changes localized to the mediastinum and pleura.[103, 179, 180] Manifestations include mediastinal widening related to acute mediastinitis, pneumomediastinum, left pleural effusion, pneumothorax, and hydropneumothorax.[42] In most cases, the site of rupture can be identified precisely—although sometimes with considerable difficulty—only by radiographic evidence of extravasation of ingested contrast material. CT may show pneumomediastinum not

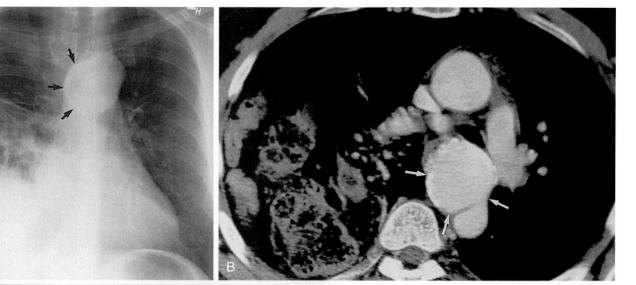

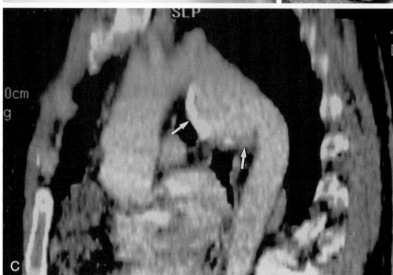

Figure 66–22. Chronic Traumatic Pseudoaneurysm of the Aorta. A 47-year-old man was referred for further assessment of chronic changes in the right lower lobe. A posteroanterior chest radiograph *(A)* reveals inhomogeneous areas of increased opacity and focal areas of lucency in the right lower hemithorax. A round area of increased opacity *(arrows)* can be seen projecting over the lower trachea and left main bronchus. A contrast-enhanced spiral CT scan *(B)* demonstrates a pseudoaneurysm *(arrows)* originating from the region of the aortic isthmus. Also note loops of large bowel in the right lower chest secondary to traumatic rupture of the right hemidiaphragm. The location of the traumatic aortic pseudoaneurysm *(arrows)* is easier to appreciate on the oblique sagittal reconstruction *(C)*. The patient had been involved in a motor vehicle accident 32 years previously.

apparent on the radiograph,[3] as well as leakage of ingested contrast material into the mediastinum or pleural space and mediastinitis or empyema secondary to delayed diagnosis (Fig. 66–24).[42]

Chills and high fever are common, and effects of obstruction of the superior vena cava may be apparent. Vomitus may contain blood.[179] Physical examination usually reveals subcutaneous emphysema in the soft tissues of the neck or Hamman's sign (a crunching or clicking sound during systole heard during auscultation over the apex of the heart). When the diagnosis is not suspected initially and treatment is not instituted promptly, abscess formation, sometimes complicated by extension into a bronchus or the pleural cavity, may ensue. The resultant esophagobronchial or esophagopleural fistulae usually can be identified by contrast radiographic examination or, with esophagopleural fistula, by the identification of foreign material in pleural fluid on microscopic examination.[180a] Analysis of pleural fluid may also show an amylase concentration higher than that of the blood as a result of contamination by saliva.

The morbidity and mortality increase considerably with delay in treatment;[180, 181] for example, in one series, mortality

increased three-fold when surgery was delayed beyond 24 hours.[182]

Rupture of the Thoracic Duct

In addition to nonpenetrating injury, rupture of the thoracic duct may develop from surgical procedures or penetrating wounds from a bullet or knife.[183–186] The most common cause is iatrogenic: chylothorax is reported as a complication in about 0.2% of patients undergoing thoracic surgery.[183] Thoracic duct injury from penetrating chest trauma is usually overshadowed by associated vascular or tracheoesophageal injuries;[185, 186] in a review of more than 13,000 patients treated for penetrating chest or neck trauma, only 8 patients with isolated thoracic duct injury were identified.[186] Thoracic duct injury from blunt trauma is rare: only 20 cases were reported by 1988.[187] It is thought to be secondary to hyperextension of the thoracic spine.[186]

The anatomic course of the thoracic duct and the site of damage establish on which side the chylothorax develops. As it enters the thorax, the duct lies slightly to the right of

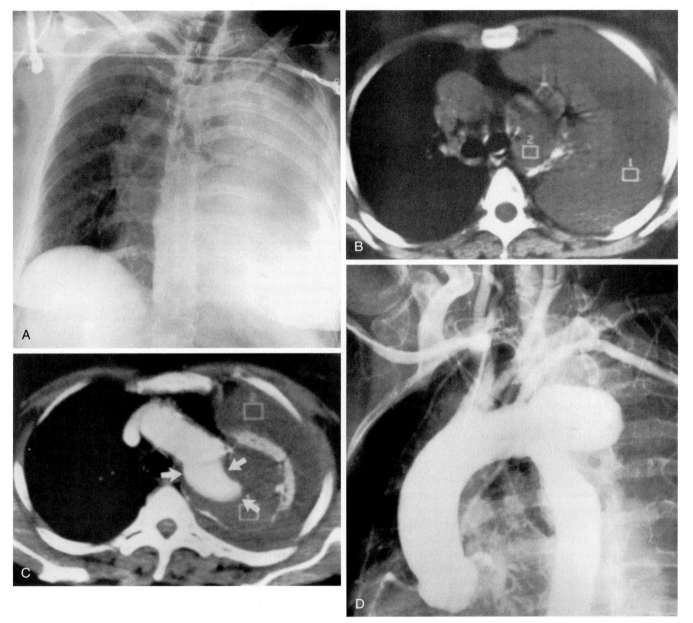

Figure 66–23. Traumatic Aneurysm of the Aorta: Delayed Rupture 20 Years after Trauma. This 53-year-old woman was admitted to the hospital about 24 hours after the abrupt onset of severe chest pain and worsening dyspnea. A radiograph of the chest in anteroposterior projection, supine position *(A)* discloses a massive left pleural effusion that, on thoracentesis, proved to be blood. A CT scan at the level of the tracheal bifurcation *(B)* shows the left pleural space to be filled with fluid, the density of which is identical to that of the blood in the descending thoracic aorta. Marked calcification of the wall of the aorta can be identified. A CT scan at the level of the aortic arch following a bolus injection of contrast medium *(C)* reveals a large saccular aneurysm extending off the left side of the arch *(arrows)*. An aortogram in left anterior oblique projection *(D)* shows the aneurysm arising from the aorta just distal to the takeoff of the left subclavian artery. The patient had been involved in an automobile accident about 20 years previously in which she suffered a severe injury to her thorax against a steering wheel. She had not been investigated for possible thoracic injury at that time.

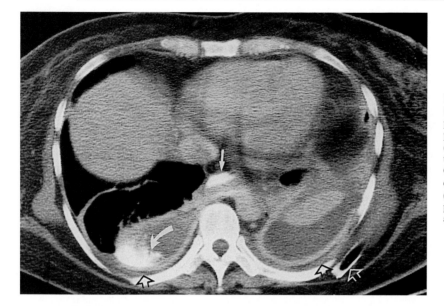

Figure 66–24. Bilateral Empyema Following Esophageal Rupture. A CT scan demonstrates bilateral pleural effusions with associated smooth thickening of the pleura and increased attenuation of the extrapleural fat *(open black arrows)* consistent with empyema. A left chest tube lies outside the pleural space *(open white arrow).* Orally administered contrast medium can be seen in the esophagus *(straight arrow)* and in the right pleural space *(curved arrow),* indicating the presence of an esophageal-pleural fistula. The patient was a 41-year-old man who had a delayed diagnosis of esophageal rupture.

the midline, so that rupture in its lower third—an unusual site in crushing injuries—leads to right-sided chylothorax. The duct crosses the midline to the left in the midthorax, so that its disruption above this point tends to produce left-sided chylothorax. Although usually unilateral, chylothorax may be bilateral.[188]

Several days to weeks may elapse between the time of chest trauma and the development of radiographically demonstrable pleural fluid,[18, 103, 189] a time lag that should strongly suggest this entity. It has been postulated that the delay occurs because the extravasated chyle is initially confined to the mediastinal space and ruptures into the pleural space only when the accumulation has acquired sufficient pressure.[18] Rarely, the lymph collection remains contained within the mediastinum, where it is manifested as a rounded mass (lymphocele) on the radiograph several weeks to months after injury.[190, 191]

The site of injury to the thoracic duct is best demonstrated by lymphangiography. In a study of 12 patients with chylous ascites or chylothorax after surgery, the site of injury was identified on lymphangiography in 7 patients. The authors did not consider CT to provide any additional information.[192] The CT appearance of chylous effusions is similar to that of other effusions. In one case, a traumatic mediastinal lymphocele was assessed by CT and MR imaging and the diagnosis confirmed by CT-guided needle aspiration;[191] CT demonstrated a homogeneous fluid collection that on MR had the characteristics of proteinaceous fluid with increased signal intensity on T1-weighted spin-echo images and homogeneous high-signal intensity on T2-weighted images. In another case, a traumatic lymphocele was demonstrated by lymphoscintigraphy with modified technetium-99m sulfur colloid.[193]

Apart from symptoms related to the inciting traumatic event, clinical findings of thoracic duct rupture are usually absent. Occasionally, spillage of large quantities of chyle from the mediastinum into the pleural space gives rise to the abrupt onset of respiratory difficulty. Thoracentesis yielding milky fluid of high triglyceride content confirms the diagnosis *(see* page 2768).

EFFECTS ON THE CHEST WALL AND DIAPHRAGM OF NONPENETRATING TRAUMA

Rupture of the Diaphragm

Diaphragmatic rupture is diagnosed in 1% to 4% of patients admitted to the hospital with blunt trauma[6, 194, 195] and in about 5% of patients undergoing laparotomy or thoracotomy for trauma.[194] Of the penetrating injuries to the lower chest, about 15% of stab wounds and 45% of gunshot wounds are associated with this complication.[194, 196] In a review of 1,000 diaphragmatic injuries in 980 patients reported in the literature by 1995, 75% of ruptures were the result of blunt trauma and 25% of penetrating injury.[194] Rarely, rupture is iatrogenic,[194] usually in association with hiatus hernia repair,[197] or follows a bout of severe vomiting.[198, 199]

Several mechanisms have been postulated for the development of diaphragmatic rupture during blunt trauma, including sudden increase in intrathoracic or intra-abdominal pressure against a fixed diaphragm, shearing stress on a stretched diaphragm, and avulsion of the diaphragm from its points of attachment;[194] the first of these is the most commonly accepted.[200, 201] The greater prevalence of left-sided ruptures has been ascribed to a variety of causes, including the buffer action of the liver, greater strength of the right hemidiaphragm (experimental studies in cadavers having shown a greater weakness of the left hemidiaphragm), and underdiagnosis of right-sided injuries.[194] Although ruptures may occur in any area, most develop through the weakest portion (posterolateral surface along the embryonic fusion lines).[6]

As might be expected, patients with diaphragmatic rupture frequently have other serious injuries.[194, 202] In one review of 25 patients with diaphragmatic rupture following blunt trauma, associated findings included rib fractures (52%), pelvic fractures (52%), splenic laceration or rupture (48%), closed head injury (32%), and liver laceration (16%).[202] In the same study, of 43 patients with penetrating diaphragmatic injuries, 44% had liver laceration, 30% had splenic laceration, and 30% had gastrointestinal injury.[202] These associated abnormalities often obscure the findings related to the diaphragmatic rupture. In one review of 1,000 diaphragmatic injuries, the diagnosis was made at the time of admission in 44% of cases and incidentally at thoracotomy, laparotomy, or autopsy in 41% of cases;[194] in the remaining 15%, the diagnosis was delayed 24 hours or more.

Following diaphragmatic rupture, intra-abdominal viscera may herniate into the chest. The hernial contents depend on the size and position of the rupture and can include the omentum, stomach, small and large intestines, spleen, kidney, and even pancreas. Such traumatic herniated material frequently strangulates, particularly if the diagnosis is delayed beyond 24 hours. Although traumatic hernias account for only about 5% of diaphragmatic hernias,[203] 90% of strangulated diaphragmatic hernias are traumatic in origin.[194, 204]

Radiologic Manifestations

The radiographic findings are influenced by mechanism of injury (blunt or penetrating), the site of injury (left or right), the presence of herniated viscera, and the presence of concomitant pleural or pulmonary injury (which may be associated with obscuration of the diaphragm as a result of pleural effusion or atelectasis).[194, 202] Depending on these factors, a preoperative diagnosis based on the radiographic findings in various studies has ranged from 4% to 63% of cases.[194, 205, 206] The likelihood of diagnosis is higher in patients with left-sided perforation and with blunt rather than perforating injury.[202, 207, 207a] In one study of 50 patients with diaphragmatic rupture following blunt trauma, radiographic findings diagnostic or highly suggestive of rupture were present in 20 of 44 patients (46%) with rupture on the left side and in only 1 of 6 (17%) with rupture on the right.[207] The radiographic findings of penetrating diaphragmatic injury are usually normal or nonspecific and include hemothorax, pneumothorax, or apparent elevation of the hemidiaphragm.[207a]

Diagnostic signs of diaphragmatic rupture include visualization of herniated stomach or bowel in the chest and cephalad extension of an intragastric tube above the level of the diaphragm (Fig. 66–25).[99, 194, 207] Suggestive findings include irregularity of the diaphragmatic contour, inability to visualize the diaphragm, a persistent basilar opacity that may mimic atelectasis or a supradiaphragmatic mass (Fig. 66–26), an elevated hemidiaphragm in the absence of atelectasis, and a contralateral shift of the mediastinum in the absence of a large pleural effusion or pneumothorax.[99, 194, 207]

When the rupture occurs in the left hemidiaphragm, the stomach and the colon are the viscera that most commonly herniate into the thorax (Fig. 66–27). The diagnosis can be confirmed by contrast-enhanced studies of these two organs, CT, or MR imaging.[99, 208, 209] A diagnostic finding is the presence of a focal constriction ("collar sign") in the stomach or afferent and efferent loop of bowel where they traverse the orifice of the diaphragmatic rupture (Fig. 66–28). This finding may be sometimes seen on plain chest radiographs but is more readily visualized on contrast-enhanced stomach or colon studies or CT scans.[204, 209] When strangulation occurs, unilateral pleural effusion may be present.[210, 211]

When rupture occurs in the right hemidiaphragm, a portion of the liver may herniate through the rent and create

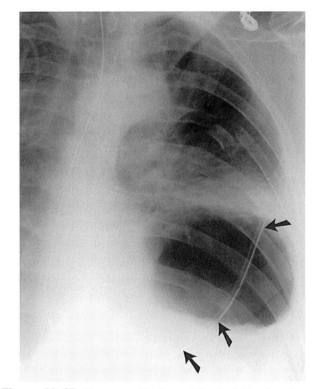

Figure 66–25. Traumatic Rupture of the Left Hemidiaphragm. A view of the left chest from an anteroposterior radiograph demonstrates an intrathoracic stomach with cephalad extension of the nasogastric tube *(arrows).* Also noted are left rib fractures, areas of atelectasis in the left lung, and mediastinal shift to the right. The patient was a 44-year-old man who had been involved in a motor vehicle accident.

a mushroom-like mass within the right hemithorax, with the herniated liver constricted by the tear. In such circumstances, herniation may be suspected by the high position of the lower border of the liver as indicated by the position of the hepatic flexure.[212, 213] The diagnosis of rupture of the right hemidiaphragm may be confirmed by CT (Fig. 66–29), MR imaging (Fig. 66–30), radionuclide liver scan, or ultrasound.[99, 209, 214–216]

Radionuclide liver scans may show nonspecific cephalad displacement of the liver or a diagnostic photopenic waist where the liver traverses the diaphragmatic orifice.[84, 207a, 214, 216] In one study, seven surgically proven cases of traumatic rupture of the right hemidiaphragm with a hepatic herniation were diagnosed preoperatively using technetium-99m sulfur colloid liver-spleen imaging;[216] in all cases, there was distortion of liver configuration with superior and posterior displacement of the right lobe and a focal area of narrowing at the site of perforation.

Ultrasonography permits direct visualization of the hemidiaphragm and may show focal disruption or interruption of diaphragmatic echoes at the site of rupture.[217, 218] However, although the procedure is helpful in the diagnosis of rupture of the right hemidiaphragm, it is of limited value in left rupture because the presence of gas within adjacent large bowel or stomach does not allow visualization of the hemidiaphragm.

Several groups have assessed the use of CT in the diagnosis of diaphragmatic rupture.[205, 209, 219, 220] Characteristic findings include sharp discontinuity of the diaphragm,

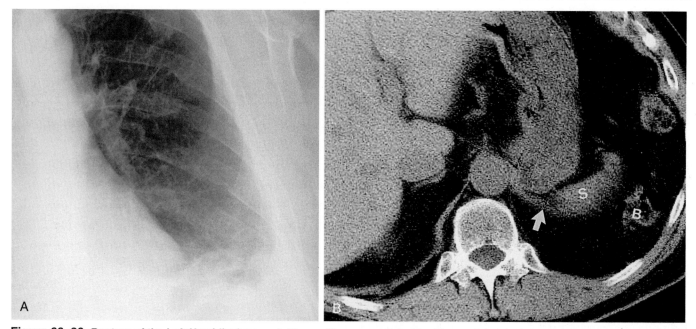

Figure 66–26. Rupture of the Left Hemidiaphragm. A 60-year-old man presented with a history of chronic changes in the left lower lobe following a motor vehicle accident. A view of the left chest from a posteroanterior radiograph *(A)* demonstrates poorly defined opacities and areas of lucency in the region of the left hemidiaphragm. Healing rib fractures are also evident. A CT scan *(B)* demonstrates the torn end of the left hemidiaphragm *(arrow)* with intrathoracic herniation of omental fat and bowel *(B)*. The torn portion of the hemidiaphragm abuts the spleen (S). The diagnosis was confirmed at surgery.

intrathoracic visceral herniation, lack of visualization of a hemidiaphragm (absent diaphragm sign), and constriction of bowel or stomach at the site of herniation (collar sign).[41, 160a, 209, 220]

Focal discontinuity of the diaphragm is seen on CT in 70% to 80% of patients with diaphragmatic rupture (Fig. 66–31).[209, 220] However, focal defects are occasionally seen in healthy people, particularly the elderly. For example, in one review of CT scans in 120 patients without a history of trauma, localized defects were seen in 13 patients (11%), all at least 40 years old;[221] the abnormality was seen in only 1 patient between 40 and 49 years, but in 7 of 20 (35%) who were 70 years or older. Most diaphragmatic ruptures occur in young adults,[205, 219] in whom discontinuity of the diaphragm is not normally seen. However, regardless of age, the diagnosis of diaphragmatic rupture based solely on the presence of diaphragmatic discontinuity may result in false-positive diagnosis and therefore should be made with caution.[209, 220]

The diagnosis of diaphragmatic rupture can be made more confidently on CT when there is associated herniation of omental fat[222] or abdominal viscera;[209, 220] the latter includes bowel, liver, kidney, and spleen and is seen in 50% to 60% of cases (Fig. 66–32).[209, 220] Herniation of viscera may not be seen while patients are on positive-pressure ventilation and may develop after discontinuation of ventilatory support.[205, 220] A waistlike narrowing of the stomach, bowel, or liver *(see* Fig. 66–29) at the site of herniation (collar sign) is seen on CT in 30% to 40% of cases;[209, 220] occasionally, it is the only CT abnormality.[209]

Most ruptures involve the posterolateral portion of the diaphragm at the junction of its central tendon and posterior leaves and are therefore well seen on CT.[41] Less commonly, the rupture involves the dome of the diaphragm, a region that is difficult to assess on conventional transverse CT

images because it is tangential to the plane of section.[209] It may therefore be difficult to distinguish a focal diaphragmatic injury in this region from an eventration or elevation of the diaphragm.[222] Optimal assessment of the diaphragmatic dome with detection of diaphragmatic ruptures that might otherwise be missed can be obtained using spiral CT with multiplanar coronal and sagittal reconstructions (Fig. 66–33).[160a, 207a, 222]

Initial studies suggested a poor sensitivity of CT in the detection of diaphragmatic injuries.[205, 219] However, refinements in technology and the use of dynamic scanning of several levels during a single breath-hold or spiral CT have resulted in marked improvement in the detection of diaphragmatic abnormalities. In a review of the findings in 11 patients with proven diaphragmatic rupture following blunt trauma, a preoperative diagnosis was made on CT in 6 of 8 patients (75%) with left-sided rupture and in all 3 patients with right-sided lesions.[209] In a second study, CT scans performed in 11 patients with diaphragmatic rupture and 21 patients with an intact diaphragm after blunt trauma were independently reviewed by three observers who were unaware of the surgical findings.[220] Ten of the 11 cases of diaphragmatic rupture were correctly identified on CT by at least one observer. The average sensitivity for the three observers in the detection of diaphragmatic rupture was 61% and the average specificity 87%. False-negative results were related to hemothorax or hemoperitoneum that obscured the diaphragm; false-positive diagnosis occurred when the diagnosis was based solely on the presence of a diaphragmatic defect.

Clinical Manifestations

Signs and symptoms of diaphragmatic injury can be immediate or delayed. Bleeding from the torn edge of the diaphragm is seldom of sufficient severity to cause hemody-

Text continued on page 2643

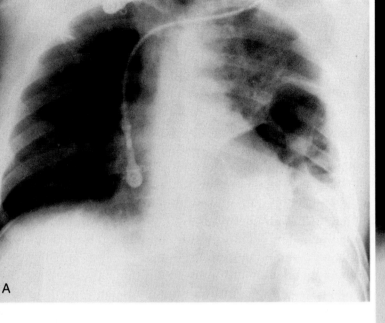

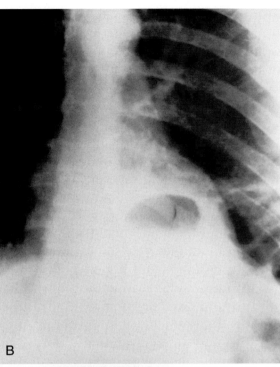

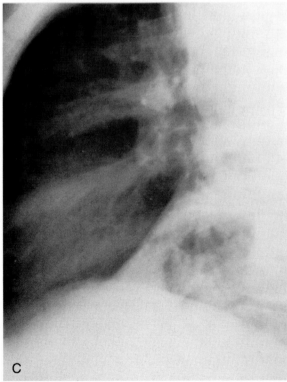

Figure 66–27. Acute Traumatic Rupture of the Left Hemidiaphragm.
This 22-year-old man was involved in a car accident in which he suffered severe
trauma to the left side of his chest and abdomen. On his arrival in the hospital
emergency department, an anteroposterior radiograph of his chest in the supine
position (A) revealed no evidence of a left hemidiaphragm. Multiple gas-containing
structures could be identified in the lower portion of the left hemithorax. Later the
same day, anteroposterior (B) and lateral (C) radiographs in the erect position
revealed a gas-containing structure in the medial portion of the left hemithorax
posteriorly, showing a prominent air-fluid level in the erect position; this is the
stomach. In addition, there is almost total airlessness of the left lower lobe as a
result of atelectasis. A large left diaphragmatic laceration was satisfactorily repaired.

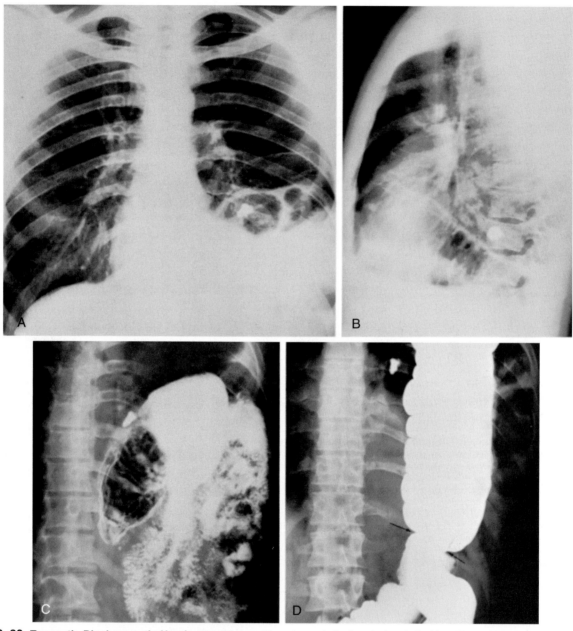

Figure 66–28. Traumatic Diaphragmatic Hernia. This 25-year-old man was admitted to the hospital with a 12-year history of discomfort in the left chest and upper abdomen, a symptom that had been present more or less continuously since he was wounded in 1944 by a piece of shrapnel that entered the left side of his chest between the eighth and ninth ribs. On admission, posteroanterior *(A)* and lateral *(B)* radiographs revealed numerous air-containing viscera within the lower portion of the left hemithorax. The left hemidiaphragm could not be identified clearly along any of its surface. The metallic foreign body was readily visualized. Barium examination of the upper gastrointestinal tract *(C)* showed much of the stomach and several loops of small bowel within the left hemithorax. Barium opacification of the colon *(D)* demonstrated a long segment of splenic flexure within the left hemithorax, the point at which the colon passed through the rent in the diaphragm being indicated by arrows. At thoracotomy, a defect measuring 3 inches in diameter was found in the left hemidiaphragm; most of the stomach, part of the large bowel, and a considerable amount of small bowel were situated within the left hemithorax.

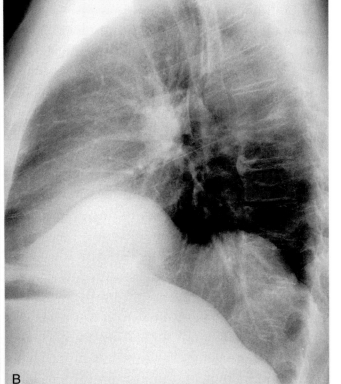

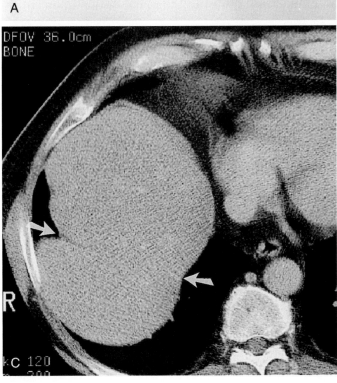

Figure 66–29. Traumatic Rupture of the Right Hemidiaphragm. A 53-year-old man was referred for further evaluation of an unusual diaphragmatic contour on the radiograph. Views of the right chest from posteroanterior *(A)* and lateral *(B)* radiographs demonstrate elevation of the right hemidiaphragm with a biconvex upper contour. A CT scan *(C)* demonstrates superior herniation of the liver and a focal constriction *(arrows)*, characteristic of traumatic tear. The diagnosis was confirmed at surgery.

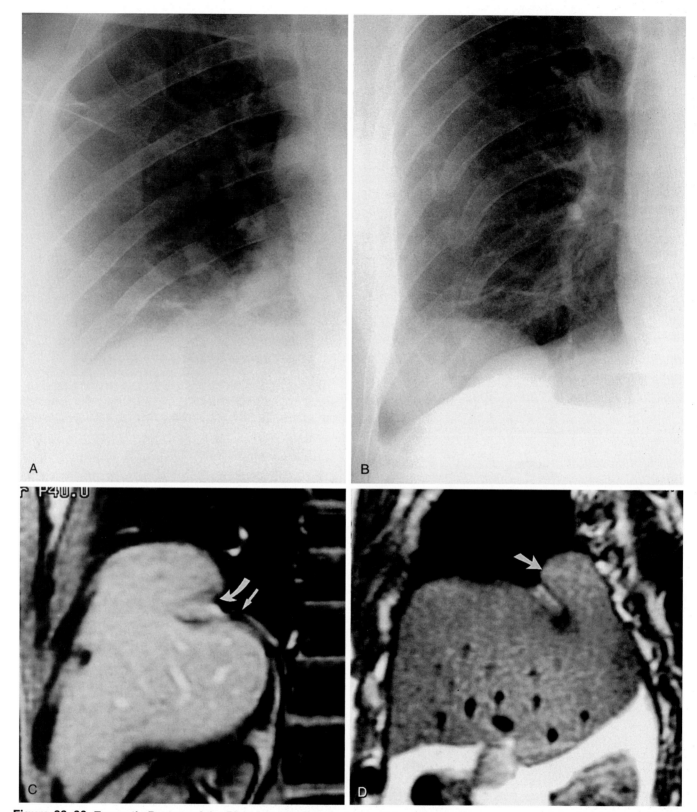

Figure 66–30. Traumatic Rupture of the Right Hemidiaphragm. A view of the right chest from an anteroposterior radiograph *(A)* performed in a 46-year-old man following a motor vehicle accident shows right rib fractures, a right pleural effusion, and apparent elevation of the right hemidiaphragm. The patient recovered and was discharged without further evaluation. Eleven months later, he presented with a 4-month history of right upper quadrant pain. A view of the right chest from a posteroanterior radiograph *(B)* demonstrates a mushroom-like mass in the right lower hemithorax. Several rib fractures and blunting of the right hemidiaphragm are also evident. A coronal spin-echo T1-weighted MR image *(C)* demonstrates discontinuity of the right hemidiaphragm *(straight arrow)* and waistlike constriction of the liver *(curved arrow)* where it traverses the diaphragmatic tear. A sagittal MR image *(D)* demonstrates the posterior location of the herniated liver *(arrow)*.

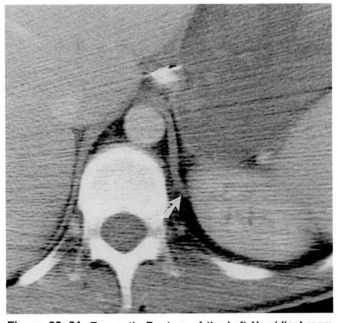

Figure 66–31. Traumatic Rupture of the Left Hemidiaphragm. A contrast-enhanced CT scan demonstrates abrupt discontinuity of the left hemidiaphragm *(arrow)* at the level of the medial arcuate ligament. The patient was a 24-year-old man being assessed for unresolving pulmonary contusions 10 days after a motor vehicle accident. The diagnosis of traumatic tear of the hemidiaphragm was confirmed at surgery.

namic compromise; however, the displacement of abdominal contents into the pericardial cavity rarely produces the hemodynamic equivalent of pericardial tamponade.[223] Respiratory distress can be caused by mechanical displacement of lung or by pneumothorax following intrathoracic rupture of an abdominal viscus. Strangulation of herniated abdominal viscera may cause nausea and vomiting. Failure to make the diagnosis has been associated with a mortality of 20% to 35%.[224, 225]

As indicated previously, associated injuries are common and may dominate the clinical picture;[223, 226] the most frequent are rupture of the spleen, perforation of a hollow abdominal viscus, and fractured ribs. Intestinal obstruction as a result of strangulation occurs most commonly in cases of long-standing hernia.[227] After blunt trauma, an extremely scaphoid anterior abdominal wall (Gibson's sign) should make one suspicious of the complication.[28]

Diaphragmatic rupture can be associated with several unusual complications, including concomitant involvement of the pericardial sac with passage of various organs into this space[228, 229] or of the pancreas with the development of a bronchopancreatic fistula (an abnormality that occurs more frequently after acute pancreatitis);[230, 231] the diagnosis can be confirmed in the latter instance by finding a high level of amylase in the sputum.[231] A thoracobiliary fistula can also develop. In one review of 16 cases, 7 patients had biloptysis, and two thirds developed bile empyema;[232] the chest radiograph usually revealed an elevated right hemidiaphragm and pleural effusion.

Herniation of abdominal contents through a rent in the diaphragm may be delayed for several years or longer.[223] In fact, the true incidence of diaphragmatic injury that heals without ever coming to medical attention is unknown. The longer the interval from the initial injury to current symptoms, the more astute must be the clinician to consider the diagnosis. In one series of 57 patients recognized as having blunt injury to the diaphragm, the diagnosis was delayed in 7 (12%).[233] Acute chest pain, epigastric distress, breathlessness, signs of small or large bowel obstruction, and sepsis may develop quickly; however, vague and nonlocalizing symptoms may occur intercurrently when strangulation is intermittent.[223]

Another unusual complication of thoracoabdominal trauma associated with diaphragmatic rupture is thoracic splenosis. Splenosis is defined as the autotransplantation of splenic tissue; it usually occurs after splenic rupture and affects the peritoneum, omentum, and mesentery. Thoracic involvement may occur after combined diaphragmatic and splenic injury from blunt trauma[234, 235] or gunshot wounds.[236] The complication is uncommon: only 20 cases had been reported in the English literature by 1994.[235] However, it is likely that the incidence has been underestimated; in one study of 17 patients who had rupture of the spleen and left

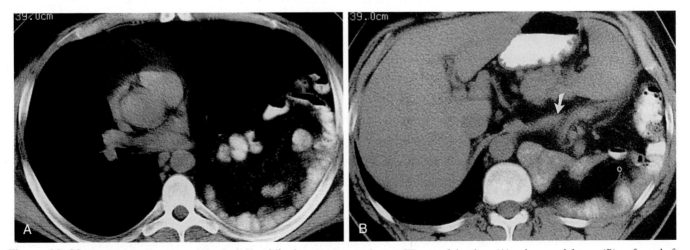

Figure 66–32. Traumatic Rupture of the Left Hemidiaphragm. Images from a CT scan of the chest *(A)* and upper abdomen *(B)* performed after oral administration of contrast demonstrate the torn end of the left hemidiaphragm *(arrow)* and intrathoracic herniation of bowel. There is marked contralateral shift of the mediastinum. The patient was a 28-year-old man who presented with a history of abdominal pain 1 year after trauma during wrestling.

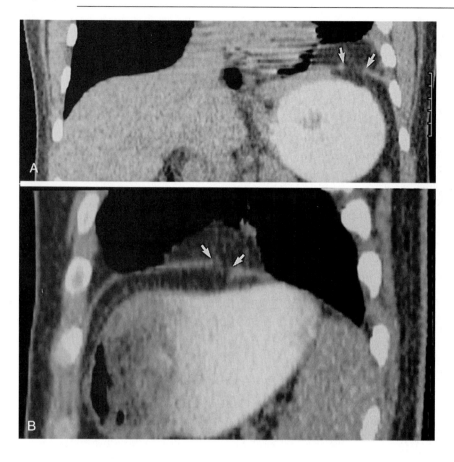

Figure 66–33. Spiral CT in the Diagnosis of Traumatic Rupture of the Left Hemidiaphragm. Coronal *(A)* and sagittal *(B)* reconstructions from a spiral CT obtained during a single breath-hold demonstrate a focal defect in the left hemidiaphragm (arrows) with intrathoracic herniation of omental fat. (Courtesy of Dr. Steven Primack, Oregon Health Sciences University.)

hemidiaphragm after a motor vehicle accident, 3 (18%) showed evidence of ectopic splenic activity in the left hemithorax on technetium-99m–tagged heated–red blood cell scintigraphy.[234]

In a review of 20 cases published by 1994, thoracic splenosis was identified 6 to 42 years after injury.[235] All lesions were pleural based and involved the left hemithorax. Nodules were solitary in 10 patients and multiple in 10. They measured from a few millimeters up to 7.5 cm in diameter.[235] The splenic implants may involve either the visceral or parietal pleura or the interlobar fissures.[234] They have not been described in the lung parenchyma. The nodules usually grow after implantation,[235] but occasionally regress.[237]

The radiographic and CT findings include single or multiple pleural-based or paraspinal soft tissue nodules.[234, 235, 238] Most are seen on the left side; rarely, disease is bilateral (Fig. 66–34). Findings such as healed fractures of a lower rib, diaphragmatic irregularity, or bullet fragments in the abdomen and left hemithorax provide helpful clues to the diagnosis.[238] The measured attenuation on CT may be similar to that of normal spleen (30 to 70 Hounsfield units) or slightly lower.[234] The signal intensity on both T1- and T2-weighted MR images is comparable to that of the signal intensity of normal spleen.[234, 239] Also similar to the spleen, the foci of splenosis are isointense with respect to the paraspinal muscles on T1-weighted images and isointense with respect to subcutaneous fat on T2-weighted images.[234, 239] Although these CT and MR imaging findings are characteristic of splenosis, confident radiologic diagnosis requires the use of technetium-99m–tagged heated-red blood cell scintig-

raphy.[234, 240] This technique permits identification of the splenic nature of nodules seen on radiographs and CT as well as visualization of nodules not visible on chest radiographs.[234]

In most cases, thoracic splenosis is unassociated with symptoms, and surgery is not indicated; in the literature review cited previously, one patient had recurrent episodes of hemoptysis, and the other 19 were symptom free.[235] It has been suggested that overwhelming sepsis develops less commonly in patients who have undergone post-traumatic splenectomy than in those who have had splenectomies performed for other reasons because of the presence of splenosis in the peritoneal cavity and chest.[241]

Fractures of the Ribs

Rib fractures occur in about half of all patients who have had major blunt chest trauma.[242, 243] Most commonly, they involve the fourth to tenth ribs. The fractures are often missed on the posteroanterior radiograph because the lateral portions of the ribs are frequently affected and the fracture line is not tangential to the x-ray beam.[244, 245] The presence of fractures is easier to detect on oblique rib views.[246] However, the presence or absence of rib fractures *per se* is of limited clinical significance,[246] the main value of the radiograph being the detection of associated pleural and pulmonary complications.[246] CT may demonstrate rib fractures not evident on the radiograph as well as unsuspected complications such as pneumothorax and hemothorax.[3, 242]

Fractures of certain ribs have specific clinical implications. For example, fractures of the ninth, tenth, or eleventh

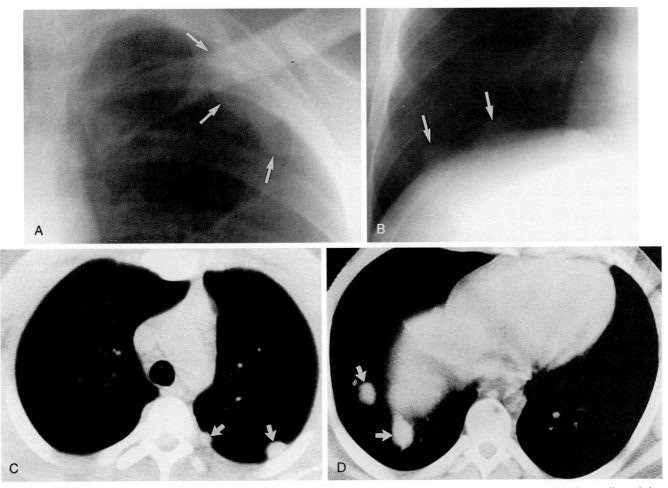

Figure 66–34. Thoracic Splenosis. Views of the left upper *(A)* and right lower hemithorax *(B)* from a posteroanterior chest radiograph in an asymptomatic 18-year-old man demonstrate several pleural-based nodules *(arrows)*. The radiographic findings are confirmed by CT scans at the level of the aortic arch *(C)* and right hemidiaphragm *(D)*. The diagnosis was confirmed by technetium-99m–tagged heated–red blood cell scintigraphy. This case constitutes a rare example of bilateral thoracic splenosis secondary to splenic injury and bilateral diaphragmatic tears that the patient sustained when he was hit by a bus at the age of 2 years. (Courtesy of Dr. Robert Pugatch, University of Maryland Medical Center, Baltimore.)

ribs are apt to be associated with splenic or hepatic injury and sometimes with serious intra-abdominal hemorrhage.[28, 242] Because they are relatively protected, fractures of the first, second, and third ribs usually imply severe trauma.[244] In one study of 75 patients with 90 first-rib fractures, the authors divided the patients into two groups. Group I consisted of 13 patients with a fracture of one or both first ribs only, and group II (62 patients) had multiple rib fractures that included the first rib.[247] In group I, intrathoracic injuries were mild and included none involving major vessels, whereas in group II, many of the patients sustained severe intrathoracic injury, 58% involving the aorta.

Cough fractures of the ribs occur more often in women than in men[248, 249] and almost invariably involve the sixth to ninth ribs, most often the seventh and usually in the posterior axillary line.[248, 249] Unless special care is taken to obtain radiographs of superior quality that detail the involved ribs, these fractures may go undetected until evidenced by callus formation some time later.

The diagnosis of fractured ribs may be suggested clinically by the abrupt onset of chest pain after blunt trauma or a severe bout of coughing. The pain is accentuated by breathing; in some cases, a sensation of "something snap-ping" is noted by the patient. Involvement of multiple ribs may result in focal chest wall instability, in which case paradoxical motion of the "flail" chest may lead rapidly to severe respiratory failure. This complication is usually apparent clinically as paradoxical movement of the chest wall; blood gas analysis is imperative to assess the presence and course of respiratory failure in these cases.

Severe sudden compression of the thorax, regardless of whether it is associated with rib fractures, can result in a dramatic clinical picture of ecchymosis and edema of the face known as *traumatic asphyxia*.[250] This complication is believed to be the result of reflux of blood from the right side of the heart into the great veins of the head and neck. Ninety percent of patients who present with this clinical picture as the sole manifestation of trauma and who survive the first few hours after injury recover; the survival rate is inversely proportional to the extent and severity of associated injuries.[250]

Dislocation of the Clavicle

Potential serious morbidity and even death have been associated with posterior dislocation of the clavicle at the sternoclavicular joint.[251] Although retrosternal dislocation of the clavicle is rare—only 3 examples were identified among 63 sternoclavicular dislocations recorded at the Mayo Clinic over a 50-year period[252]—the displaced clavicle may produce serious morbidity by impinging on the trachea, esophagus, or great vessels or major nerves in the superior mediastinum. Prompt diagnosis is important, not only because of the serious consequences of compression of major structures but also because closed reduction can usually be achieved if treatment is instituted within 24 to 48 hours of the injury. Open surgical reduction is required if diagnosis is delayed.[251] Sternoclavicular dislocation, as well as sternal fractures and associated retrosternal hematoma, are better depicted by CT than by plain radiography.[3, 42]

Fractures of the Spine

Fractures of the thoracic spine account for about 15% to 30% of all spine fractures.[253, 254] They may result in extraosseous hemorrhage and the development of unilateral or bilateral paraspinal masses (Fig. 66–35) or diffuse widening of the mediastinum.[255, 256] The findings on the chest radiograph may mimic those of aortic rupture.[255] About 70% to 90% of fractures are visible on plain radiographs.[4] CT

and MR imaging allow detection of otherwise occult fractures and assessment of the relationship between the fracture fragments and the spinal cord.[4, 253] When pleural effusion develops in association with signs of spinal cord injury at the thoracic level, the possibility of subarachnoid-pleural fistula should be considered; the complication can be confirmed by myelography.[94]

Early recognition of thoracic spinal fractures is important because of the frequency with which they lead to neurologic deficits.[4] About 60% of patients with fracture-dislocations of the thoracic spine have complete neurologic deficits, compared with 30% of patients with similar injuries to the cervical spine and 2% with injury of the lumbar spine.[4]

Post-traumatic Pulmonary Herniation

Protrusion of a portion of lung through an abnormal aperture of the thoracic cage may be congenital or acquired and may be cervical, thoracic, or (rarely) diaphragmatic in position.[257–259] The protrusion is covered by both parietal and visceral pleura. Congenital hernias occur most frequently in the supraclavicular fossa and less often at the costochondral junction. Traumatic hernias may follow chest trauma or surgery[257, 258] or chest tube drainage;[258] in one patient with

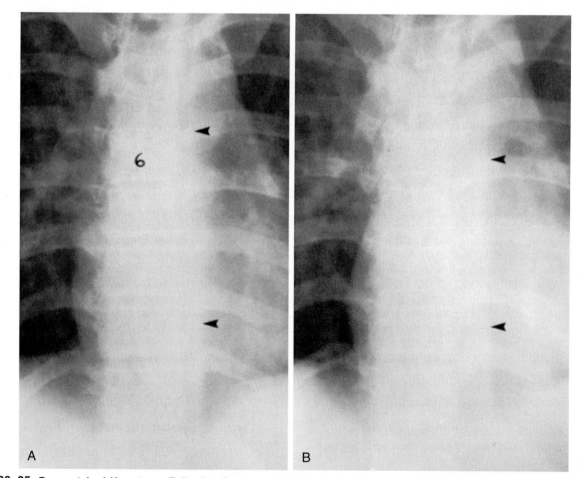

Figure 66–35. Paravertebral Hematoma Following Fracture of the Thoracic Spine. Shortly after this 20-year-old man fell from a moderate height, an anteroposterior view of the thoracic spine *(A)* revealed a slight reduction in the vertical diameter of the sixth thoracic vertebral body. The paraspinal soft tissues showed no abnormality *(arrowheads)*. Three days later *(B)*, there has occurred a moderate lateral displacement of the paraspinal line *(arrowheads)* as a result of hemorrhage.

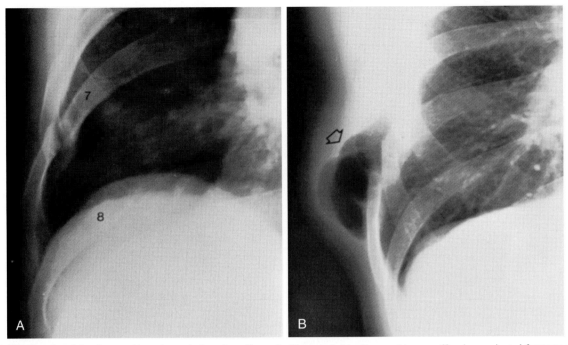

Figure 66–36. Hernia of the Lung. About 1 year before the radiographs illustrated, this 46-year-old man suffered comminuted fractures of the axillary portions of ribs 6, 7, and 8 on the right in a crush injury to his chest. Healing of the fractures had occurred such that there was considerable separation between ribs 7 and 8 *(A)*. The patient noted a soft, fluctuant bulge in the axillary region of his chest on coughing and straining. Radiography of the chest in full inspiration during a Valsalva maneuver *(B)* demonstrated herniation of a sizable portion of lung through the defect in the rib cage into the contiguous soft tissues *(arrow)*. The radiograph illustrated in *(A)* was exposed at full expiration and shows no evidence of lung herniation. The defect was successfully repaired surgically.

multiple rib fractures and a flail chest, positive end-expiratory pressure was considered to play a role in herniation.[260] In a small number of cases, the weakened area is the result of inflammatory or neoplastic damage to the chest wall.[261]

The most common location of posttraumatic herniation is the parasternal region just medial to the costochondral junction, where the intercostal musculature is thinnest. The patient usually complains of a bulge appearing during coughing and straining. In most cases, the diagnosis can be made by the observation of a soft crepitant mass that develops under these conditions and disappears during expiration or rest. Chest radiographs reveal pulmonary parenchymal tissue herniating through an obvious defect in the rib cage (Fig. 66–36) or through the supraclavicular fossa.[262] Optimal visualization requires peformance of a Valsalva maneuver, with or without tangential radiographic projection[258, 263] or CT.[258]

A rare consequence of blunt trauma has been described in a patient in whom a pocket of air collected in the chest wall at the site of the injury; it was postulated that air had replaced the blood in a hematoma.[264]

EFFECTS ON THE LUNGS OF NONTHORACIC TRAUMA

A number of pleuropulmonary abnormalities occur as a consequence of trauma in which the pathogenesis is unrelated to direct injury to the thorax (although chest injury may have occurred as well). Some of these effects are specific to trauma, including fat embolism, air embolism, and the hypoxemia associated with severe head trauma, whereas others are nonspecific, such as thromboembolism and ARDS. In a prospective study of 119 patients with multiple fractures or with fractures of long bones or hip, 42 patients (35%) were found to have PaO_2 values less than 79 mm Hg on the first day.[265] The lowest levels were observed in patients with multiple fractures. Only 11 patients had abnormal chest radiographs; in 1 patient with a PaO_2 of 47 mm Hg, the chest radiograph was considered to be normal. In most patients, the PaO_2 had returned to normal by the sixth day, and all patients survived. The hypoxemia that sometimes follows isolated severe head injury is also complex; in some patients it is the result of pulmonary edema, whereas in others it has been clearly shown to be caused by ventilation-perfusion mismatching in the absence of apparent edema.[266, 267]

If there is reason to believe that the chest was also injured, the only other condition that need be considered in the differential diagnosis of a radiographic pattern of diffuse opacification following trauma is severe pulmonary contusion. Sometimes, this distinction can be difficult, although contusion tends to be less diffuse and to clear more rapidly.

EFFECTS ON THE THORAX OF PENETRATING TRAUMA

The usual radiographic appearance of the path of a bullet through lung parenchyma is a rather poorly defined homogeneous shadow that, as might be expected, is more or less circular when viewed in the direction in which the bullet passed and longitudinal when viewed in perpendicular projection (Fig. 66–37). The indistinct definition is caused

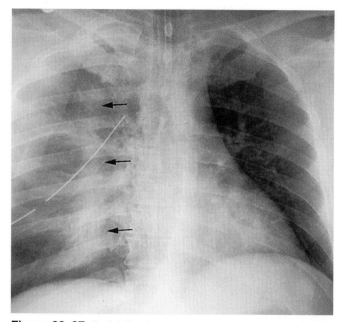

Figure 66–37. Bullet Track. A 40-year-old man was shot in the back of the neck, the bullet traversing the pleura, lung, diaphragm, and anterior aspect of the liver. An anteroposterior chest radiograph demonstrates the bullet track in the lung *(arrows)* as well as a right hemopneumothorax. A chest tube is in place.

by hemorrhage and edema in the parenchyma surrounding the bullet track; both usually resolve within 3 to 8 days, permitting clear visualization of the bullet track, which now contains blood and therefore is seen as a soft tissue density that is circular when seen *en face* and tubular when seen in profile.[268] The hematoma in the bullet track slowly decreases in size from its periphery.[268] In a small number of cases, a central radiolucency may be apparent along the bullet's course and reveal communication between the central core of blood and the bronchial tree (Fig. 66–38).[268, 269] In such circumstances, a history of hemoptysis can usually be elicited. In most cases, the bullet track resolves completely within a few months. Delay or failure in resolution should suggest the possibility of superimposed infection.[263, 268] In one remarkable case, the track persisted for many years, its dense fibromuscular wall lined by and presumably derived from bronchial epithelium.[270]

Usually, bullets follow straight paths through the chest. Occasionally, they ricochet off body structures, particularly vertebrae and ribs; rarely, they move along an artery, vein, or the tracheobronchial tree.[271] Determination of the bullet path and location of a missile within the chest require two views at 90 degrees (i.e., frontal and lateral radiographs) or CT.[271] The size and configuration of the bullet track are influenced by the mass and velocity of the bullet, the shape of the projectile, whether the bullet fragments are deformed on impact, and the characteristics of the tissue through which it passes.[268, 271] Because the lung has a relatively low specific gravity and a high elastin content, it is more resistant to gunshot wounds than tissues with higher specific gravity and lower elastin content, such as the brain and liver.[268] Several reviews of the radiology and ballistics of gunshot wounds have been published.[271, 272]

Penetrating wounds of the thorax from a knife or bullet

may induce pneumothorax or hemopneumothorax (*see* Fig. 66–37), although the searing effect of a bullet as it passes through the pleura may cauterize the tissues sufficiently to prevent escape of air into the pleural space. In one series of 250 consecutive patients who had gunshot wounds involving the thorax, 90% presented with hemothorax or hemopneumothorax and only 3% with pneumothorax alone.[273] Hemothorax sometimes results in calcific fibrothorax (Fig. 66–39).

For obvious reasons, penetrating injury to the lungs may be associated with damage to other intrathoracic structures with corresponding radiologic and clinical manifestations. For example, laceration of the esophagus results in pneumomediastinum, mediastinitis, and pleural effusion (Fig. 66–40). The diaphragm can be damaged without evidence of visceral injury and with negative radiographic findings;[274] patients usually complain of abdominal pain, and examination reveals tenderness and rigidity of the abdominal wall. When present, the radiographic abnormalities associated with penetrating diaphragmatic injury are nonspecific and consist of hemothorax, pneumothorax, or apparent elevation of the hemidiaphragm.[207a]

Stab wounds of the chest are often initially unassociated with respiratory symptoms. In a prospective study of 4,106 such cases, 87% were successfully treated as outpatients after negative findings on a repeat chest radiograph performed 6 hours after presentation;[275] 12% of patients required chest tube drainage for delayed pneumothoraces or hemothoraces, 0.2% required thoracotomy for delayed and continued bleeding or cardiac injuries, 1% with small pneumothoraces (less than 20%) were observed, and 68% remained symptom free. The negative predictive value of the initial chest radiograph in excluding delayed pneumothorax was only 87%; therefore, a patient with a stab wound of the chest and a normal chest radiograph should have a repeat radiograph 6 hours after injury.[275, 276] (Although the pulmonary injury from a knife wound is often difficult to detect on the initial radiograph, follow-up radiographs often demonstrate a pulmonary hematoma [Fig. 66–41].) More than 98% of delay pneumothoraces occur within 6 hours of injury; however, delayed pneumothorax can occur as late as 48 hours or, rarely, as late as 5 days after injury.[275, 277]

Occasionally, a foreign body enters the pleural cavity, where it may cause chronic empyema. The foreign body may have been left in the vicinity of the pleura at the time of surgery[278] or may be the direct result of a gunshot or shrapnel wound.[279] When it is metallic or otherwise opaque, it should be easily identifiable radiographically. The history and the scar on the skin of the chest wall provide suggestive evidence. Rarely, a knife or bullet traverses a pulmonary artery and vein lying in close proximity, leading to the formation of an arteriovenous fistula.[280, 281] The penetrating object may also traverse the aorta and lead to rapidly fatal hemothorax or, rarely, remain in close contact with the aorta; in these cases, CT can be helpful in demonstrating the relationship between the foreign body and the aorta and other intrathoracic structures (Fig. 66–42). We have seen one case of angiographically and surgically proven fistula between the aorta and superior vena cava following a self-inflicted stab wound to the lower neck and upper chest; CT scan demonstrated mediastinal hematoma and increased size of the superior vena cava (Fig. 66–43).

The bullet causing a gunshot wound to the chest can

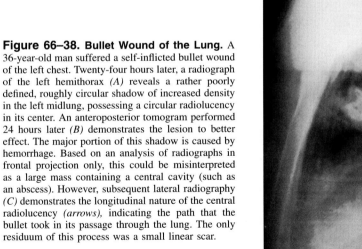

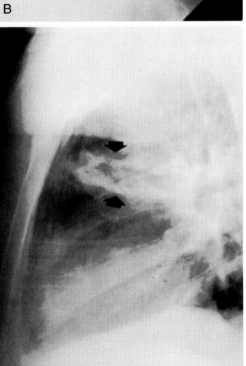

Figure 66–38. Bullet Wound of the Lung. A 36-year-old man suffered a self-inflicted bullet wound of the left chest. Twenty-four hours later, a radiograph of the left hemithorax *(A)* reveals a rather poorly defined, roughly circular shadow of increased density in the left midlung, possessing a circular radiolucency in its center. An anteroposterior tomogram performed 24 hours later *(B)* demonstrates the lesion to better effect. The major portion of this shadow is caused by hemorrhage. Based on an analysis of radiographs in frontal projection only, this could be misinterpreted as a large mass containing a central cavity (such as an abscess). However, subsequent lateral radiography *(C)* demonstrates the longitudinal nature of the central radiolucency *(arrows)*, indicating the path that the bullet took in its passage through the lung. The only residuum of this process was a small linear scar.

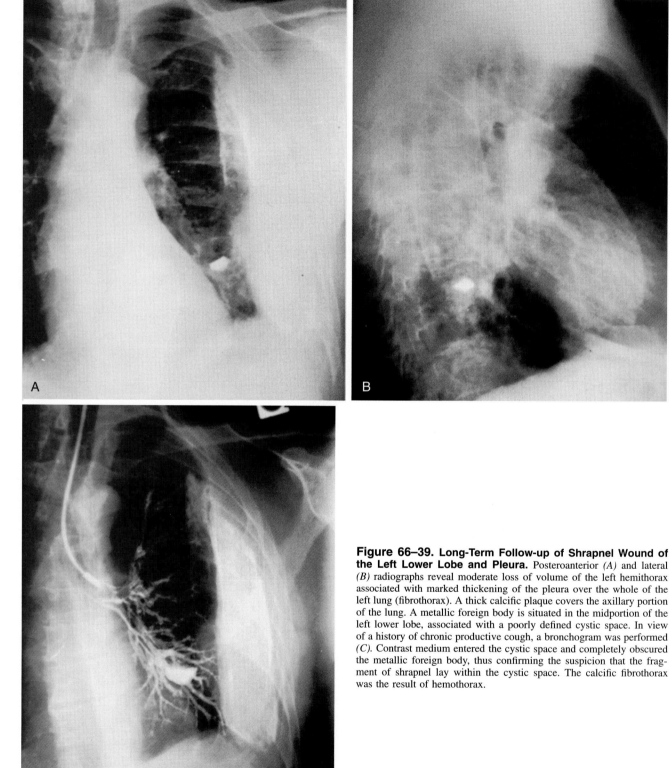

Figure 66–39. Long-Term Follow-up of Shrapnel Wound of the Left Lower Lobe and Pleura. Posteroanterior *(A)* and lateral *(B)* radiographs reveal moderate loss of volume of the left hemithorax associated with marked thickening of the pleura over the whole of the left lung (fibrothorax). A thick calcific plaque covers the axillary portion of the lung. A metallic foreign body is situated in the midportion of the left lower lobe, associated with a poorly defined cystic space. In view of a history of chronic productive cough, a bronchogram was performed *(C)*. Contrast medium entered the cystic space and completely obscured the metallic foreign body, thus confirming the suspicion that the fragment of shrapnel lay within the cystic space. The calcific fibrothorax was the result of hemothorax.

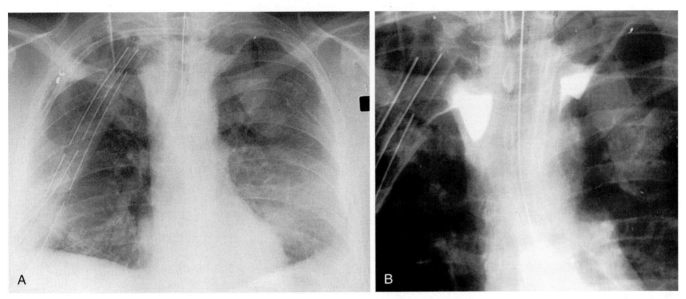

Figure 66–40. Gunshot Wound to the Esophagus. A 30-year-old man presented with a large right hemopneumothorax following a gunshot wound. The abnormality required three chest tubes for appropriate drainage. An anteroposterior chest radiograph *(A)* demonstrates widening of the superior mediastinum. Metallic fragments can be seen over the upper chest and left axilla. A view from a chest radiograph performed after oral administration of contrast *(B)* demonstrates extravasation into the mediastinum and communication with the pleural spaces. The esophageal perforation was successfully corrected surgically.

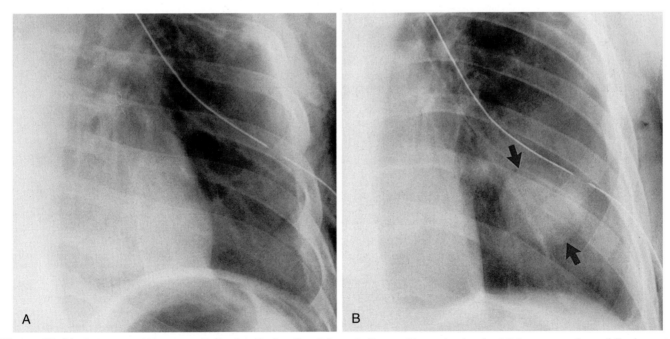

Figure 66–41. Pulmonary Hematoma Following Perforating Injury. A 40-year-old man developed a left hemopneumothorax following a stab wound to the lower chest. A view from an anteroposterior radiograph *(A)* following insertion of a chest tube shows a poorly defined focal lucency in the left lower lobe. A radiograph performed 3 days later *(B)* demonstrates a pulmonary hematoma *(arrows)*. The scarring in the left upper lobe was the result of previous tuberculosis.

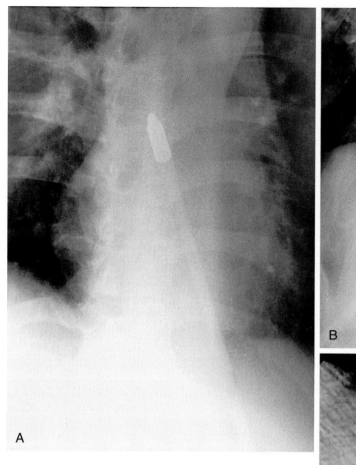

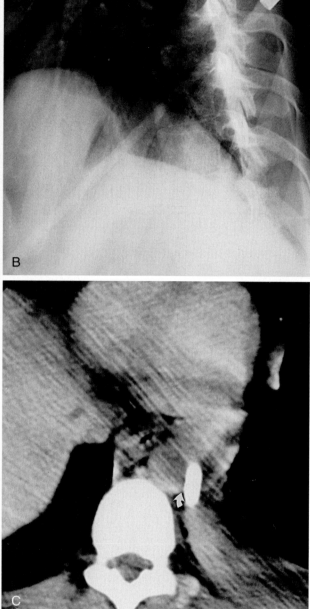

Figure 66–42. Penetrating Injury to the Aorta. Views of the lower chest and upper abdomen from an anteroposterior *(A)* and lateral chest radiographs *(B)* in a 33-year-old man demonstrate a bolt traversing the upper abdomen and lower chest. A CT scan *(C)* demonstrates the bolt traversing the aorta *(curved arrow).* Also noted is an associated left hemothorax. The injury was self-inflicted and apparently occurred accidentally while the patient was trying to load a cross-bow. The diaphragmatic perforation and the injury to the aorta were successfully corrected surgically.

also enter the aorta and be carried distally to a peripheral artery.[282] The younger patient appears to have a better chance of survival after bullet perforation of the aorta, possibly because greater elasticity permits the defect in the vessel to close without exsanguination and death. Whenever a patient with a gunshot wound of entry and no wound of exit shows no radiologic evidence of the projectile in the thorax, embolization should be suspected. Similarly, a bullet or its fragments may enter an extrathoracic vein and be carried to the lung, where its presence is readily apparent. Intrapulmonary migration of metallic foreign bodies used to stabilize the vertebrae or shoulder joint also has been reported;[283, 284] this occurs most often across the pleural space into lung

parenchyma but has also been reported to occur through the trachea, with the foreign body eventually residing in the bronchi.[283] This complication can develop during the postoperative period immediately after insertion of the pin[283] or many years later.[284] The radiologic appearance and clinical history should be diagnostic.

Bullets, shrapnel, and other metallic fragments that have penetrated lung parenchyma occasionally cause intrathoracic complications many years later. Hemoptysis is the most common complication;[285–287] others include bronchial obstruction with atelectasis,[285] abscess formation, and (as discussed previously) empyema.[279] The factors that govern the onset of disease, usually after many years of quiescence, are

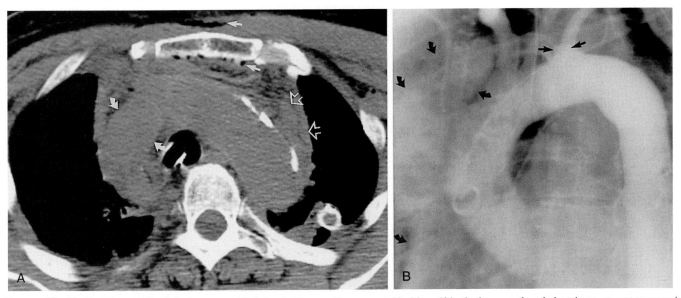

Figure 66–43. Post-traumatic Arteriovenous Fistula. A 61-year-old woman stabbed herself in the lower neck and chest in an attempt to commit suicide. A CT scan performed without intravenous contrast *(A)* demonstrates subcutaneous and mediastinal air *(straight arrows)*, mediastinal hemorrhage *(open arrows)*, and increased diameter of the superior vena cava *(curved arrows)*. A view from a digital aortogram *(B)* demonstrates the proximal site of the fistula *(straight arrows)* originating from the aorta and opacification of the superior vena cava and right atrium *(curved arrows)* immediately after contrast injection as a result of communication between the aorta and the left brachiocephalic vein. The injury was successfully treated surgically.

not precisely known but are presumably related to a slowly developing change in the position of the metallic fragments and their erosion through significant structures, such as bronchi, vessels, or pleura. These changes in position may be noted radiologically, providing a diagnostic clue.[279, 286] Another uncommon long-term complication is the development of carcinoma in relation to scarring associated with a metallic fragment.[270, 288–290] In this case, the carcinoma can arise either in relation to the metallic fragment itself or in the fibrous tract linking the fragment with the pleura.[290]

Despite the impressive list of complications described previously, penetrating injuries of the lung have a surprisingly good prognosis, and the incidence of such complica-

tions is low. For example, in one series of 373 patients seen during a period of 1 year, 282 were treated with intercostal thoracostomy tube only;[291] 91 patients required thoracotomy, and there were 29 deaths. Associated intra-abdominal injuries are common, however, in patients with penetrating thoracic trauma; for example, in one series of 250 consecutive cases of gunshot wounds of the thorax, 20% of the patients also had injuries involving the diaphragm or one or more abdominal viscera.[273] Injury involving the thoracic trachea is often associated with damage to the heart and great vessels or surrounding lung parenchyma and has a particularly poor prognosis;[181] more than 50% of gunshot wounds and 10% of stab wounds involving the trachea are rapidly fatal.[292]

REFERENCES

1. Boyd AD, Glassman LR: Trauma to the lung. Chest Surg Clin North Am 7:263, 1997.
2. Wagner RB, Crawford WO Jr, Schimpf PP: Classification of parenchymal injuries of the lung. Radiology 167:77, 1988.
3. Kerns SR, Gay SB: CT of blunt chest trauma. Am J Roentgenol 154:55, 1990.
4. Groskin SA: Selected topics in chest trauma. Semin Ultrasound CT MRI 17:119, 1996.
5. Greene R: Lung alterations in thoracic trauma. J Thorac Imag 2:1, 1987.
6. Shorr RM, Crittenden M, Indeck M, et al: Blunt thoracic trauma: Analysis of 515 patients. Ann Surg 206:200, 1987.
7. Errion AR, Houk VN, Kettering DL: Pulmonary hematoma due to blunt, nonpenetrating thoracic trauma. Am Rev Respir Dis 88:384, 1963.
8. Schneider M, Klein CP: Blast injury of the lungs: With report of a case occurring in peace time. Radiology 54:548, 1950.
9. Hirsch M, Bazini J: Blast injury of the chest. Clin Radiol 20:362, 1969.
10. Roth RA, Beckmann CF: Complications of extracorporeal shock-wave lithotripsy and percutaneous nephrolithotomy. Urol Clin North Am 15:155, 1988.
11. Huller T, Bazini Y: Blast injuries of the chest and abdomen. Arch Surg 100:24, 1970.
12. Williams JR, Bonte FJ: Pulmonary changes in nonpenetrating thoracic trauma. Tex Med 59:27, 1963.
13. Williams JR, Bonte FJ: Pulmonary damage in nonpenetrating chest injuries. Radiol Clin North Am 1:439, 1963.
14. Stevens E, Templeton AW: Traumatic nonpenetrating lung contusion. Radiology 85:247, 1965.
15. Williams JR, Stembridge VA: Pulmonary contusion secondary to nonpenetrating chest trauma. Am J Roentgenol 91:284, 1964.
16. Williams JR: The vanishing lung tumor: Pulmonary hematoma. Am J Roentgenol 81:296, 1959.
17. Kollmorgen DR, Murray KA, Sullivan JJ, et al: Predictors of mortality in pulmonary contusion. Am J Surg 168:659, 1994.
18. Reynolds J, Davis JT: Injuries of the chest wall, pleura, pericardium, lungs, bronchi and esophagus. Radiol Clin North Am 4:383, 1966.
19. Ting YM: Pulmonary parenchymal findings in blunt trauma to the chest. Am J Roentgenol 98:343, 1966.
20. Wiot JF: The radiologic manifestations of blunt chest trauma. JAMA 231:500, 1975.
21. Toombs BD, Sandler CM, Lester RG: Computed tomography of chest trauma. Radiology 140:733, 1981.
22. Smejkal R, O'Malley KF, David E, et al: Routine initial computed tomography of the chest in blunt torso trauma. Chest 100:667, 1991.
23. Donnelly LF, Klosterman LA: Subpleural sparing: A CT finding of lung contusion in children. Radiology 204:385, 1997.
24. Schild HH, Strunk H, Weber W, et al: Pulmonary contusion: CT vs plain radiograms. J Comput Assist Tomogr 13:417, 1989.
25. Reid JD, Kommareddi S, Lankerani M, et al: Chronic expanding hematomas: A clinicopathologic entity. JAMA 244:2441, 1980.
26. Schwartz A, Borman JB: Contusion of the lung in childhood. Arch Dis Child 36:557, 1961.
27. Hussey HH: Pulmonary contusion (editorial). JAMA 230:264, 1974.
28. Wilson RF, Murray C, Antonenko DR: Nonpenetrating thoracic injuries. Surg Clin North Am 57:17, 1977.
29. Cochlin DL, Shaw MRP: Traumatic lung cysts following minor blunt chest trauma. Clin Radiol 29:151, 1978.
30. Shirakusa T, Araki Y, Tsutsui M, et al: Traumatic lung pseudocyst. Thorax 42:516, 1987.
31. Kuhlman JE, Pozniak MA, Collins J, Knisely BL: Radiographic and CT findings of blunt chest trauma: Aortic injuries and looking beyond them. Radiographics 18:1085, 1998.
32. Greening R, Kynette A, Hodes PJ: Unusual pulmonary changes secondary to chest trauma. Am J Roentgenol 77:1059, 1957.
33. Shirakusa T, Araki Y, Tsutsui M, et al: Traumatic lung pseudocyst. Thorax 42:516, 1987.
34. Fagan CJ: Traumatic lung cyst. Am J Roentgenol 97:186, 1966.
35. Santos GH, Mahendra T: Traumatic pulmonary pseudocysts. Ann Thorac Surg 27:359, 1979.
36. Cochlin DL, Shaw MRP: Traumatic lung cysts following minor blunt chest trauma. Clin Radiol 29:151, 1978.
37. Sorsdahl OA, Powell JW: Cavitary pulmonary lesions following nonpenetrating chest trauma in children. Am J Roentgenol 95:118, 1965.
38. Chester EH: Chest injury resulting in bullae in the lung: Report of a case. N Engl J Med 268:1068, 1963.
39. Takahashi N, Murakami J, Murayama S, et al: MR evaluation of intrapulmonary hematoma. J Comput Assist Tomogr 19:125, 1995.
40. Joynt GHC, Jaffe F: Solitary pulmonary hematoma. J Thorac Cardiovasc Surg 43:291, 1962.
41. Kang EY, Müller NL: CT in blunt chest trauma: Pulmonary, tracheobronchial, and diaphragmatic injuries. Semin Ultrasound CT MRI 17:114, 1996.
42. Mirvis SE, Templeton P: Imaging in acute thoracic trauma. Semin Roentgenol 27:184, 1992.
43. Ganske JG, Dennis DL, Vanderveer JB Jr: Traumatic lung cyst: Case report and literature review. J Trauma 21:493, 1981.
44. Beumer HM, Mellema TL: Excavated hematomas after pulmonary segmental resection. Dis Chest 37:163, 1960.
45. Bonmarchand G, Lefebvre E, Lerebours-Pigeonniere G, et al: Intrapulmonary hematoma complicating mechanical ventilation in patients with chronic obstructive pulmonary disease. Intensive Care Med 14:246, 1988.
45a. Rossbach MM, Johnson SB, Gomez MA, et al: Management of major tracheobronchial injuries: A 28-year experience. Ann Thorac Surg 65:182, 1998.
46. Roxburgh JC: Rupture of the tracheobronchial tree. Thorax 42:681, 1987.
47. Chesterman JT, Satsangi PN: Rupture of the trachea and bronchi by closed injury. Thorax 21:21, 1966.
48. Burke JF: Early diagnosis of traumatic rupture of the bronchus. JAMA 181:682, 1962.
49. Woodring JH, Fried AM, Hatfield DR, et al: Fractures of first and second ribs: Predictive value for arterial and bronchial injury. Am J Roentgenol 138:211, 1982.
50. Unger JM, Schuchmann GG, Grossman JE, et al: Tears of the trachea and main bronchi caused by blunt trauma: Radiologic findings. Am J Roentgenol 153:1175, 1989.
51. Bertelsen S, Howitz P: Injuries of the trachea and bronchi. Thorax 27:188, 1972.
52. Barmada H, Gibbons JR: Tracheobronchial injury in blunt and penetrating chest trauma. Chest 106:74, 1994.
53. Eastridge CE, Hughes FA Jr, Pate JW, et al: Tracheobronchial injury caused by blunt trauma. Am Rev Respir Dis 101:230, 1970.
54. Larizadeh R: Rupture of the bronchus. Thorax 21:28, 1966.
55. Collins JP, Ketharanathan V, McConchie I: Rupture of major bronchi resulting from closed chest injuries. Thorax 28:371, 1973.
56. Bertelsen S, Howitz P: Injuries of the trachea and bronchi. Thorax 27:188, 1972.
57. Heceta WG, Torpoco J, Richardson RL: Extensive linear "blow-out" of the thoracic membranous trachea with innominate artery avulsion secondary to blunt chest trauma. Chest 67:247, 1975.
58. Silbiger ML, Kushner LN: Tracheobronchial perforation: Its diagnosis and treatment. Radiology 85:242, 1965.
59. Harvey-Smith W, Bush W, Northrop C: Traumatic bronchial rupture. Am J Roentgenol 134:1189, 1980.
60. Travis SP, Layer GT: Traumatic transection of the thoracic trachea. Ann R Coll Surg Engl 65:240, 1983.
61. Döpper TH: Zur Röntgendiagnostik stumpfer Thoraxtrauman. (Roentgen diagnosis of injuries of the thorax due to blunt trauma.) Fortschr Roentgenstr 92:524, 1960.
62. Lotz PR, Martel W, Rohwedder JJ, et al: Significance of pneumomediastinum in blunt trauma to the thorax. Am J Roentgenol 132:817, 1979.
63. Oh KS, Fleishner FG, Wyman SM: Characteristic pulmonary finding in traumatic complete transection of a mainstem bronchus. Radiology 92:371, 1969.
64. Kumpe DA, Oh KS, Wyman SM: A characteristic pulmonary finding in unilateral complete bronchial transection. Am J Roentgenol 110:704, 1970.
65. Peterson C, Deslauriers J, McClish A: A classic image of complete right main bronchus avulsion. Chest 96:1415, 1989.
66. Weir IH, Müller NL, Connell DG: CT diagnosis of bronchial rupture. J Comput Assist Tomogr 12:1035, 1988.
67. Rollins RJ, Tocino I: Early radiographic signs of tracheal rupture. Am J Roentgenol 148:695, 1987.
68. Vidinel I: Displacement of the mediastinum. Chest 62:215, 1972.
69. Hood RM, Sloan HE: Injuries to the trachea and major bronchi. J Thorac Cardiovasc Surg 38:458, 1959.
70. Streete BG, Stull FE Jr: Primary repair of fracture of the left main-stem bronchus. J Thorac Surg 36:76, 1958.
71. Weisel W, Watson RR, O'Connor TM: Long-term follow-up study of patients with bronchial anastomosis or tracheal replacement. Chest 61:141, 1972.
72. van der Schaar H, Wagenaar JPM, Swierenga J, et al: Successful late repair of a post-traumatic bronchial stricture. Thorax 27:769, 1972.
73. Lynne-Davis P, Ganguli PC, Sterns LP: Pulmonary function following traumatic rupture of the bronchus. Chest 61:400, 1972.
74. Deslauriers J, Beaulieu M, Archambault G, et al: Diagnosis and long-term follow-up of major bronchial disruptions due to non-penetrating trauma. Ann Thorac Surg 33:32, 1982.
75. Weisbrod GL: Left upper lobe torsion following left lingulectomy. J Can Assoc Radiol 38:296, 1987.
76. Kelly MV II, Kyger ER, Miller WC: Postoperative lobar torsion and gangrene. Thorax 32:501, 1977.
77. Larsson S, Lepore V, Dernevik L, et al: Torsion of a lung lobe: Diagnosis and treatment. J Thorac Cardiovasc Surg 36:281, 1988.
78. Groskin SA: Selected topics in chest trauma. Semin Ultrasound CT MRI 17:119, 1996.
79. Collins J, Love RB: Pulmonary torsion: Complication of lung transplantation. Clin Pulm Med 3:297, 1996.
80. Graham RJ, Heyd RL, Raval VA, et al: Lung torsion after percutaneous needle biopsy of lung. Am J Roentgenol 159:35, 1992.
81. Callol L, Navarro S, Galvez A, et al: Total pulmonary torsion without vascular compromise: A case report. Angiology 43:529, 1992.
82. Brath LK, Glauser FL, Zeilender S: The case of the disappearing mass. Chest 110:550, 1996.

83. Berkmen YM: Uncomplicated torsion of the right upper lobe secondary to spontaneous pneumothorax. Chest 87:695, 1985.
84. Berkmen YM, Yankelevitz D, Davis SD, et al: Torsion of the upper lobe in pneumothorax. Radiology 173:447, 1989.
85. Felson B: Lung torsion: Radiographic findings in nine cases. Radiology 162:631, 1987.
86. Shorr RM, Rodriguez A: Spontaneous pulmonary torsion. Chest 91:927, 1987.
86a. Munk PL, Vellet AD, Zwirewich C: Torsion of the upper lobe of the lung after surgery: Finding on pulmonary angiography. Am J Roentgenol 157:471, 1991.
86b. Spizarny DL, Shetty PC, Lewis JW Jr: Lung torsion: Preoperative diagnosis with angiography and computed tomography. J Thorac Imaging 13:42, 1998.
87. Crawford WO Jr: Pulmonary injury in thoracic and non-thoracic trauma. Radiol Clin North Am 11:527, 1973.
88. Connors AF, Hammon WE, Martin RJ, et al: Chest physical therapy: The immediate effect on oxygenation in acutely ill patients. Chest Physical Ther 78:559, 1980.
89. Huseby J, Hudson L, Stark K, et al: Oxygenation during chest physiotherapy. Chest 70:430, 1976.
90. Wynn-Williams N, Young RD: Cough fracture of the ribs: Including one complicated by pneumothorax. Tubercle 40:47, 1959.
91. Zidulka A, Chrome JF, Wight DW, et al: Clapping or percussion causes atelectasis in dogs and influences gas exchange. J Appl Physiol 66:2833, 1989.
92. Wolverson MK, Crepps LF, Sundaram M, et al: Hyperdensity of recurrent hemorrhage at body computed tomography: Incidence and morphologic variation. Radiology 148:779, 1983.
93. McLoud TC, Flower CDR: Imaging the pleura: Sonography, CT, and MR imaging. Am J Roentgenol 156:1145, 1991.
94. Higgins CB, Mulder DG: Traumatic subarachnoid-pleural fistula. Chest 61:189, 1972.
95. Paredes S, Hipona FA: The radiologic evaluation of patients with chest trauma. Med Clin North Am 59:37, 1975.
96. Campbell GD, Webb WR: Eosinophilic pleural effusion: A review with the presentation of seven new cases. Am Rev Respir Dis 90:194, 1964.
97. Kumar UN, Varkey B, Mathal G: Posttraumatic pleural-fluid and blood eosinophilia. JAMA 234:625, 1975.
98. Beekman JF, Bosniak S, Canter HG: Eosinophilia and elevated IgE concentration in a serous pleural effusion following trauma. Am Rev Respir Dis 110:484, 1974.
99. Groskin SA: Selected topics in chest trauma. Radiology 183:605, 1992.
100. Ashbaugh DG, Peters GN, Halgrimson CG, et al: Chest trauma: Analysis of 685 patients. Arch Surg 95:546, 1967.
101. Robertson HT, Lakshminarayan S, Hudson LD: Lung injury following a 50-metre fall into water. Thorax 33:175, 1978.
102. Craighead CC, Glass BA: Management of nonpenetrating injuries of the chest. JAMA 172:1138, 1960.
103. Williams JR, Bonte FJ: The Roentgenologic Aspect of Nonpenetrating Chest Injuries. Springfield, IL, Charles C Thomas, 1961.
104. Wall SD, Federle MP, Jeffrey RB, et al: CT diagnosis of unsuspected pneumothorax after blunt abdominal trauma. Am J Roentgenol 141:919, 1983.
105. Tsai SH, Cohen SS, Fenger EPK: Bronchial perforation as a complication of bronchoscopy. Am Rev Tuberc 78:106, 1958.
106. Armen RN, Morrow CS, Sewell S: Mediastinal emphysema: A complication of bronchoscopy. Ann Intern Med 48:1083, 1958.
107. Switzer P, Pitman RG, Fleming JP: Pneumomediastinum associated with zygomatico-maxillary fracture. J Can Assoc Radiol 25:316, 1974.
108. Raptopoulos V, Sheiman RG, Phillips DA, et al: Traumatic aortic tear: Screening with chest CT. Radiology 182:667, 1992.
109. Fisher RG, Chasen MH, Lamki N: Diagnosis of injuries of the aorta and brachiocephalic arteries caused by blunt chest trauma: CT vs aortography. Am J Roentgenol 162:1047, 1994.
110. Langston CS: The aberrant central venous catheter and its complications. Radiology 100:55, 1971.
111. Mitchell SE, Clark RA: Complications of central venous catheterization. Am J Roentgenol 133:467, 1979.
112. Tocino IM, Watanabe A: Impending catheter perforation of superior vena cava: Radiographic recognition. Am J Roentgenol 146:487, 1986.
113. Raphael MJ: Mediastinal haematoma: A description of some radiological appearances. Br J Radiol 36:921, 1963.
114. Leigh TF: Mass lesions of the mediastinum. Radiol Clin North Am 1:377, 1963.
115. Kearney PA, Smith W, Johnson SB, et al: Use of transesophageal echocardiography in the evaluation of traumatic aortic injury. J Trauma 34:696, 1993.
116. Laforet EG: Traumatic hemomediastinum. J Thorac Surg 29:597, 1955.
117. Strax TE, Ryvicker MJ, Elguezabal A: Superior vena caval syndrome due to a mediastinal hematoma secondary to a dissecting aortic aneurysm. Dis Chest 55:338, 1969.
118. Mirvis SE, Bidwell JK, Buddemeyer EU, et al: Value of chest radiography in excluding traumatic aortic rupture. Radiology 163:487, 1987.
119. Creasy JD, Chiles C, Routh WD, et al: Overview of traumatic injury of the thoracic aorta. Radiographics 17:27, 1997.
120. Sanborn JC, Heitzman R, Markarian B: Traumatic rupture of the thoracic aorta: Roentgen-pathological correlations. Radiology 95:293, 1970.
121. Feczko JD, Lynch L, Pless JE, et al: An autopsy case review of 142 nonpenetrating (blunt) injuries of the aorta. J Trauma 33:846, 1992.
122. Williams JS, Graff JA, Uku JM, et al: Aortic injury in vehicular trauma. Ann Thorac Surg 57:726, 1994.
123. Lundevall J: The mechanism of traumatic rupture of the aorta. Acta Pathol Microbiol Scand 62:34, 1964.
124. Crass JR, Cohen AM, Motta AO, et al: A proposed new mechanism of traumatic aortic rupture: The osseous pinch. Radiology 176:645, 1990.
125. Cohen AM, Crass JR, Thomas HA, et al: CT evidence for the "osseous pinch" mechanism of traumatic aortic injury. Am J Roentgenol 159:271, 1992.
126. Pretre R, Chilcott M: Blunt trauma to the heart and great vessels. N Engl J Med 336:626, 1997.
127. Lundell CJ, Quinn MF, Finck EJ: Traumatic laceration of the ascending aorta: Angiographic assessment. Am J Roentgenol 145:715, 1985.
128. Eller JL, Ziter FMH Jr: Avulsion of the innominate artery from the aortic arch: An evaluation of roentgenographic findings. Radiology 94:75, 1970.
129. Dennis LN, Rogers LF: Superior mediastinal widening from spine fractures mimicking aortic rupture on chest radiographs. Am J Roentgenol 152:27, 1989.
130. Hewes RC, Smith DC, Lavine MH: Iatrogenic hydromediastinum simulating aortic laceration. Am J Roentgenol 133:817, 1979.
131. Milne ENC, Imray TJ, Pistolesi M, et al: The vascular pedicle and the vena azygos. III. In trauma: The "vanishing" azygos. Radiology 153:25, 1984.
132. Seltzer SE, D'Orsi C, Kirshner R, et al: Traumatic aortic rupture: Plain radiographic findings. Am J Roentgenol 137:1011, 1981.
133. Marnocha KE, Maglinte DDT, Woods J, et al: Mediastinal-width/chest-width ratio in blunt chest trauma: A reappraisal. Am J Roentgenol 142:275, 1984.
134. Heystraten FM, Rosenbusch G, Kingma LM, et al: Chest radiography in acute traumatic rupture of the thoracic aorta. Acta Radiol 29:411, 1988.
135. Gundry SR, Williams S, Burney RE: Indications for aortography. Radiography after blunt chest trauma: A reassessment of the radiographic findings associated with traumatic rupture of the aorta. Invest Radiol 18:230, 1983.
136. Sefczek DM, Sefczek RJ, Deeb ZL: Radiographic signs of acute traumatic rupture of the thoracic aorta. Am J Roentgenol 141:1259, 1983.
137. Peters DR, Gamsu G: Displacement of the right paraspinous interface: A radiographic sign of acute traumatic rupture of the thoracic aorta. Radiology 134:599, 1980.
138. Woodring JH, Pulmano CM, Stevens RK: The right paratracheal stripe in blunt chest trauma. Radiology 143:605, 1982.
139. Simeone JF, Minagi H, Putman CE: Traumatic disruption of the thoracic aorta: Significance of the left apical extrapleural cap. Radiology 117:265, 1975.
140. Simeone JF, Deren MM, Cagle F: The value of the left apical cap in the diagnosis of aortic rupture: A prospective and retrospective study. Radiology 139:35, 1981.
141. Williams JR, Bonte FJ: The Roentgenological Aspect of Non-Penetrating Chest Injuries. Springfield, IL, Charles C Thomas, 1961.
142. Yee ES, Thomas AN, Goodman PC: Isolated first rib fracture: Clinical significance after blunt chest trauma. Ann Thorac Surg 32:278, 1981.
143. Fisher RG, Ward RE, Ben-Menachem Y, et al: Arteriography and the fractured first rib: Too much for too little? Am J Roentgenol 138:1059, 1982.
144. Woodring JH, Fried AM, Hatfield DR, et al: Fractures of first and second ribs: Predictive value for arterial and bronchial injury. Am J Roentgenol 138:211, 1982.
145. Marnocha KE, Maglinte DDT: Plain-film criteria for excluding aortic rupture in blunt chest trauma. Am J Roentgenol 144:19, 1985.
146. Mirvis SE, Bidwell JK, Buddemeyer EU, et al: Imaging diagnosis of traumatic aortic rupture: A review and experience at a major trauma center. Invest Radiol 22:187, 1987.
147. Hunink MGM, Bos JJ: Triage of patients to angiography for detection of aortic rupture after blunt chest trauma: Cost-effectiveness analysis of using CT. Am J Roentgenol 165:27, 1995.
148. Mirvis SE, Shanmuganathan K, Miller BH, et al: Traumatic aortic injury. Diagnosis with contrast-enhanced thoracic CT: Five-year experience at a major trauma center. Radiology 200:413, 1996.
149. Braithwaite CE, Cilley JM, O'Connor WH, et al: The pivotal role of transesophageal echocardiography in the management of traumatic thoracic aortic rupture with associated intra-abdominal hemorrhage. Chest 105:1899, 1994.
150. Smith MD, Cassidy JM, Souther S, et al: Transesophageal echocardiography in the diagnosis of traumatic rupture of the aorta. N Engl J Med 332:356, 1995.
151. Marotta R, Franchetto AA: The CT appearance of aortic transection. Am J Roentgenol 166:647, 1996.
152. Morgan PW, Goodman LR, Aprahamian C, et al: Evaluation of traumatic aortic injury: Does dynamic contrast-enhanced CT play a role? Radiology 182:661, 1992.
153. Miller FB, Richardson D, Thomas HA, et al: Role of CT in diagnosis of major arterial injury after blunt thoracic trauma. Surgery 106:596, 1989.
154. McLead TR, Olinger GN, Thorsten MK: Computed tomography in the evaluation of the aorta in patients sustaining blunt chest trauma. J Trauma 31:254, 1991.
155. Tomiak MM, Rosenblum JD, Messersmith RN, et al: Use of CT for diagnosis of traumatic rupture of the thoracic aorta. Ann Vasc Surg 7:130, 1993.
156. Rigauts H, Marchal G, Baert AL, et al: Initial experience with volume CT scanning. J Comput Assist Tomogr 14:675, 1990.
157. Gavant ML, Menke PG, Fabian T, et al: Blunt traumatic aortic rupture: Detection with helical CT of the chest. Radiology 197:125, 1995.
158. Sanders C: Current role of conventional and digital aortography in the diagnosis of aortic disease. J Thorac Imaging 5:48, 1990.
159. Trerotola SO: Can helical CT replace aortography in thoracic trauma? Radiology 197:13, 1995.
160. Gavant ML, Flick P, Menke P, et al: CT aortography of thoracic aortic rupture. Am J Roentgenol 166:955, 1996.
160a. Van Hise ML, Primack SL, Israel RS, Müller NL: CT in blunt chest trauma: Indications and limitations. Radiographics 18:1071, 1998.

160b. Wong Y-C, Wang L-J, Lim K-E, et al: Periaortic hematoma on helical CT of the chest: A criterion for predicting blunt traumatic aortic rupture. Am J Roentgenol 170:1523, 1998.

160c. Patel NH, Stephens KE Jr, Mirvis SE, et al: Imaging of acute thoracic aortic injury due to blunt trauma: A review. Radiology 209:335, 1998.

161. Shapiro MJ, Yanofsky SD, Trapp J, et al: Cardiovascular evaluation in blunt chest trauma using transesophageal echocardiography. J Trauma 31:835, 1991.

162. Brooks SW, Young JC, Cmolik B, et al: The use of transesophageal echocardiography in the evaluation of chest trauma. J Trauma 32:761, 1992.

162a. Minard G, Schurr MJ, Croce MA, et al: A prospective analysis of transesophageal echocardiography in the diagnosis of traumatic disruption of the aorta. J Trauma 40:225, 1996.

163. Goarin JP, Catoire P, Jacquens Y, et al: Use of transesophageal echocardiography for diagnosis of traumatic aortic injury. Chest 112:71, 1997.

164. Seward JB, Khandheria BK, Edwards WD, et al: Biplanar transesophageal echocardiography: Anatomic correlations, image orientation, and clinical applications. Mayo Clin Proc 65:1193, 1990.

165. Morse SS, Glickman MG, Greenwood LH, et al: Traumatic aortic rupture: False-positive aortographic diagnosis due to atypical ductus diverticulum. Am J Roentgenol 150:793, 1988.

166. Goodman PC, Jeffrey RB, Minagi H, et al: Angiographic evaluation of the ductus diverticulum. Cardiovasc Intervent Radiol 5:1, 1982.

167. LaBerge JM, Jeffrey RB: Aortic lacerations: Fatal complications of thoracic aortography. Radiology 165:367, 1987.

168. Mattox KL: Injury to the thoracic great vessels. *In* Moore EE, Mattox KL, Feliciano DV (eds): Trauma. 2nd ed. Norwalk, CT, Appleton & Lange, 1991.

169. Parmley LF, Mattingly TW, Manion WC, et al: Nonpenetrating traumatic injury of the aorta. Circulation 17:1086, 1958.

170. Langbein IE, Brandt PWT: Traumatic rupture of the aorta. Australas Radiol 12:102, 1968.

171. Verdant A: Chronic traumatic aneurysm of the descending thoracic aorta with compression of the tracheobronchial tree. Can J Surg 27:278, 1984.

172. Chew FS, Panicek DM, Heitzman ER: Late discovery of a posttraumatic right aortic arch aneurysm. Am J Roentgenol 145:1001, 1985.

173. Heystraten FM, Rosenbusch G, Kingma LM, et al: Chronic posttraumatic aneurysm of the thoracic aorta: Surgically correctable occult threat. Am J Roentgenol 146:303, 1986.

174. Finkelmeier BA, Mentzer RM Jr, Kaiser DL, et al: Chronic traumatic thoracic aneurysm: Influence of operative treatment on natural history. An analysis of reported cases, 1950–1980. J Thorac Cardiovasc Surg 84:257, 1982.

175. Zeiger MA, Clark DE, Morton JR: Reappraisal of surgical treatment of traumatic transection of the thoracic aorta. J Cardiovasc Surg 31:607, 1990.

176. Kipfer B, Leupi F, Schuepback P, et al: Acute traumatic rupture of the thoracic aorta: Immediate or delayed surgical repair? Eur J Cardiothorac Surg 8:30, 1994.

177. von Oppell UO, Dunne TT, De Groot MK, et al: Traumatic aortic rupture: Twenty-year metaanalysis of mortality and risk of paraplegia. Ann Thorac Surg 58:585, 1994.

178. Pate JW, Fabian TC, Walker W: Traumatic rupture of the aortic isthmus: An emergency? World J Surg 19:119, 1995.

179. Stanbridge RD: Tracheo-oesophageal fistula and bilateral recurrent laryngeal nerve palsies after blunt chest trauma. Thorax 37:548, 1982.

180. Parkin GJS: The radiology of perforated oesophagus. Clin Radiol 24:324, 1973.

180a. Eriksen KR: Oesophageal fistula diagnosed by microscopic examination of pleural fluid. Acta Chir Scand 128:771, 1964.

181. Burnett CM, Rosemurgy AS, Pfeiffer EA: Life-threatening acute posterior mediastinitis due to esophageal perforation. Ann Thorac Surg 49:979, 1990.

182. Wichern WA: Perforation of the esophagus. Am J Surg 119:534, 1970.

183. Cevese PG, Vecchioni R, D'Amico DF, et al: Postoperative chylothorax: Six cases in 2,500 operations, with a survey of the world literature. J Thorac Cardiovasc Surg 89:966, 1975.

184. Engevik L: Traumatic chylothorax. Scand J Cardiovasc Surg 10:77, 1976.

185. Grant PW, Brown SW: Traumatic chylothorax: A case report. Aust N Z J Surg 61:798, 1991.

186. Worthington MG, de Groot M, Gunning AJ, et al: Isolated thoracic duct injury after penetrating chest trauma. Ann Thorac Surg 60:272, 1995.

187. Dulchavsky SA, Ledgerwood AM, Lucas CE: Management of chylothorax after blunt chest trauma. J Trauma 28:1400, 1988.

188. Brook MP, Dupree DW: Bilateral traumatic chylothorax. Ann Emerg Med 17:69, 1988.

189. Rea D: Traumatic chylothorax in a closed chest injury: Report of a case. Br J Dis Chest 54:82, 1960.

190. Thorne PS: Traumatic chylothorax. Tubercle 39:29, 1958.

191. Hom M, Jolles H: Traumatic mediastinal lymphocele mimicking other thoracic injuries: case report. J Thorac Imaging 7:78, 1992.

192. Sachs PB, Zelch MG, Rice TW, et al: Diagnosis and localization of laceration of the thoracic duct: Usefulness of lymphangiography and CT. Am J Roentgenol 157:703, 1991.

193. Ellis MC, Gordon L, Gobien RP, et al: Traumatic lymphocele: Demonstration by lymphoscintigraphy with modified 99mTc sulfur colloid. Am J Roentgenol 140:973, 1983.

194. Shah R, Sabanathan S, Mearns AJ, et al: Traumatic rupture of diaphragm. Ann Thorac Surg 60:1444, 1995.

195. Ward RE, Flynn TC, Clark WP: Diaphragmatic disruption due to blunt abdominal trauma. J Trauma 21:35, 1981.

196. Broos PLO, Rommens PM, Carlier H, et al: Traumatic rupture of the diaphragm: Review of 62 successive cases. Int Surg 74:88, 1989.

197. Keshishian JA, Cox PA: Diagnosis and management of strangulated diaphragmatic hernias. Surg Gynecol Obstet 115:626, 1962.

198. Desforges G, Strieder JW, Lynch JP, et al: Traumatic rupture of the diaphragm: Clinical manifestations and surgical treatment. J Thorac Surg 34:779, 1957.

199. Efron G, Hyde I: Non-penetrating traumatic rupture of the diaphragm. Clin Radiol 18:394, 1967.

200. de la Rocha AG, Creel RJ, Mulligan GWN, et al: Diaphragmatic rupture due to blunt abdominal trauma. Surg Gynecol Obstet 154:175, 1982.

201. Leaman PL: Rupture of the right hemidiaphragm due to blunt trauma. Ann Emerg Med 12:351, 1983.

202. Meyers BF, McCabe CJ: Traumatic diaphragmatic hernia: Occult marker of serious injury. Ann Surg 218:783, 1993.

203. Marchand P: Traumatic hiatus hernia. BMJ 1:754, 1962.

204. Carter BN, Giuseffi J, Felson B: Traumatic diaphragmatic hernia. Am J Roentgenol 65:56, 1951.

205. Miller LW, Bennett EV, Root DH: Management of blunt and penetrating diaphragmatic injury. J Trauma 24:403, 1984.

206. Beauchamp G, Khalfallah A, Girard R, et al: Blunt diaphragmatic rupture. Am J Surg 148:292, 1984.

207. Gelman R, Mirvis SE, Gens D: Diaphragmatic rupture due to blunt trauma: Sensitivity of plain chest radiographs. Am J Roentgenol 156:51, 1991.

207a. Shackleton KL, Stewart ET, Taylor AJ: Traumatic diaphragmatic injuries: Spectrum of radiographic findings. Radiographics 18:49, 1998.

208. Shanmuganathan K, Mirvis SE, White CS, et al: MR imaging evaluation of hemidiaphragms in acute blunt trauma: experience with 16 patients. Am J Roentgenol 167:397, 1996.

209. Worthy SA, Kang EY, Hartman TE, et al: Diaphragmatic rupture: CT findings in 11 patients. Radiology 194:885, 1995.

210. Aronchick JM, Epstein DM, Gefter WB, et al: Chronic traumatic diaphragmatic hernia: The significance of pleural effusion. Radiology 168:675, 1988.

211. Radin DR, Ray MJ, Halls JM: Strangulated diaphragmatic hernia with pneumothorax due to colopleural fistula. Am J Roentgenol 146:321, 1986.

212. Laws HL, Waldschmidt ML: Rupture of diaphragm (letter). JAMA 243:32, 1980.

213. Salomon NW, Zukoski CF: Rupture of the right hemidiaphragm with eventration of the liver. JAMA 241:1929, 1979.

214. Estrera A, Landay M, McClelland R: Blunt traumatic rupture of the right hemidiaphragm: Experience in 12 patients. Ann Thorac Surg 39:525, 1985.

215. Carter EA, Cleverley JR, Delany DJ, et al: Case report: Cine MRI in the diagnosis of a ruptured right hemidiaphragm. Clin Radiol 51:137, 1996.

216. Kim EE, McConnell BJ, McConnell RW, et al: Radionuclide diagnosis of diaphragmatic rupture with hepatic herniation. Surgery 94:36, 1983.

217. Somers JM, Gleeson FV, Flower CD: Rupture of the right hemidiaphragm following blunt trauma: The use of ultrasound in diagnosis. Clin Radiol 42:97, 1990.

218. Ammann A, Brewer W, Maull K, et al: Traumatic rupture of the diaphragm: Real-time sonographic diagnosis. Am J Roentgenol 140:915, 1983.

219. Voeller GR, Reisser JR, Fabian TC, et al: Blunt diaphragm injuries. Am Surg 56:28, 1990.

220. Murray JG, Caoili E, Gruden JF, et al: Acute rupture of the diaphragm due to blunt trauma: Diagnostic sensitivity and specificity of CT. Am J Roentgenol 166:1035, 1996.

221. Caskey CI, Zerhouni EA, Fishman EK, et al: Aging of the diaphragm: A CT study. Radiology 171:385, 1989.

222. Israel RS, Mayberry JC, Primack SL: Diaphragmatic rupture: Use of helical CT scanning with multiplanar reformations. Am J Roentgenol 167:1201, 1996.

223. Root HD, Harmen PK: Injury to the diaphragm. *In* Moore EE, Mattox KL, Feliciano DV (eds): Trauma. 2nd ed. Norwalk, CT, Appleton & Lange, 1991.

224. Lindsey I, Woods SD, Nottle PD: Laparascopic management of blunt diaphragmatic injury. Aust N Z J Surg 67:619, 1997.

225. Mansour KA. Trauma to the diaphragm. Chest Surg Clin North Am 7:373, 1997.

226. Holm A, Bessey PQ, Aldrete JS: Diaphragmatic rupture due to blunt trauma: Morbidity and mortality in 42 cases. South Med J 81:956, 1988.

227. Ebert PA, Gaertner RA, Zuidema GD: Traumatic diaphragmatic hernia. Surg Gynecol Obstet 125:59, 1967.

228. Fagan CJ, Schreiber MH, Amparo EG, et al: Traumatic diaphragmatic hernia into the pericardium: Verification of diagnosis by computed tomography. Case report. J Comput Assist Tomog 3:405, 1979.

229. Glasser DL, Shanmuganathan K, Mirvis SE: General case of the day. Radiographics 18:799, 1998.

230. Bell JW: Pancreatic-bronchial fistula. Am Rev Respir Dis 106:97, 1972.

231. Cox CL Jr, Anderson JN, Guest JL Jr: Bronchopancreatic fistula following traumatic rupture of the diaphragm. JAMA 237:1461, 1977.

232. Oparah SS, Mandal AK: Traumatic thoracobiliary (pleurobiliary and bronchobiliary) fistulas: Clinical and review study. J Trauma 18:539, 1978.

233. Guth AA, Pachter HL, Kim U: Pitfalls in the diagnosis of blunt diaphragmatic injury. Am J Surg 170:5, 1995.

234. Normand JP, Rioux M, Dumont M, et al: Thoracic splenosis after blunt trauma: Frequency and imaging findings. Am J Roentgenol 161:739, 1993.

235. Madjar S, Weissberg D: Thoracic splenosis. Thorax 49:1020, 1994.

236. Dalton ML Jr, Strange WH, Downs EA: Intrathoracic splenosis: Case report and review of the literature. Am Rev Respir Dis 103:827, 1971.

237. Dalton ML Jr, Strange WH, Downs EA: Intrathoracic splenosis. Am Rev Respir Dis 103:827, 1971.

238. Bordlee RP, Eshaghi N, Oz O: Thoracic splenosis: MR demonstration. J Thorac Imaging 10:146, 1995.

239. Mirowitz SA, Brown JJ, Lee JKT, et al: Dynamic gadolinium-enhanced MR imaging of the spleen: Normal enhancement patterns and evaluation of splenic lesions. Radiology 179:681, 1991.
240. Bidet AC, Dreyfus-Schmidt G, Combe J, et al: Diagnosis of splenosis: The advantages of splenic scintiscanning with Tc99m heat damaged red blood cells. Eur J Nucl Med 12:357, 1986.
241. Pearson HA, Johnston D, Smith KA, et al: The born-again spleen: Return of splenic function after splenectomy for trauma. N Engl J Med 198:1389, 1978.
242. Tocino I, Miller MH: Computed tomography in blunt chest trauma. J Thorac Imaging 2:45, 1987.
243. Dougall AM, Paul ME, Finley RJ, et al: Chest trauma: Current morbidity and mortality. J Trauma 17:547, 1977.
244. Stark P: Radiology of thoracic trauma. Invest Radiol 25:1265, 1990.
245. Shulman HS, Samuels TH: The radiology of blunt chest trauma. J Can Assoc Radiol 34:204, 1983.
246. DeLuca SA, Rhea JT, O'Malley T: Radiographic evaluation of rib fractures. Am J Roentgenol 138:91, 1982.
247. Albers JE, Rath RK, Glaser RS, et al: Severity of intrathoracic injuries associated with 1st rib fractures. Ann Thorac Surg 33:614, 1982.
248. Wynn-Williams N, Young RD: Cough fracture of the ribs: Including one complicated by pneumothorax. Tubercle 40:47, 1959.
249. Pearson JEG: Cough fracture of the ribs. Br J Tuberc 51:251, 1957.
250. Moore JD, Mayer JH, Gago O: Traumatic asphyxia. Chest 62:634, 1972.
251. Lee FA, Gwinn JL: Retrosternal dislocation of the clavicle. Radiology 110:631, 1974.
252. Nettles JL, Linscheid RL: Sternoclavicular dislocations. J Trauma 8:158, 1968.
253. Meyer S: Thoracic spine trauma. Semin Roentgenol 27:254, 1992.
254. Pal J, Mulder D, Brown R, et al: Assessing multiple trauma: Is the cervical spine enough? J Trauma 28:1282, 1988.
255. Dennis L, Rogers L: Superior mediastinal widening from spine fractures mimicking aortic rupture on chest radiographs. Am J Roentgenol 152:27, 1989.
256. Bolesta MJ, Bohlman HH: Mediastinal widening associated with fractures of the upper thoracic spine. J Bone Joint Surg Am 73:447, 1991.
257. Sebba L, Baigelman W: Post-surgical lung hernia. Am J Med Sci 284:40, 1982.
258. Bhalla M, Leitman BS, Forcade C, et al: Lung hernia: Radiographic features. Am J Roentgenol 154:51, 1990.
259. George PY, Goodman P: Radiographic appearance of bullet tracks in the lung. Am J Roentgenol 159:967, 1992.
260. Kyosola K, Reinikainen M, Siitonen P, et al: Lung hernia after blunt thoracic trauma. Acta Chir Scand 150:425, 1984.
261. Bidstrup P, Nordentoft JM, Petersen B: Hernia of the lung: Brief survey and report of two cases. Acta Radiol [Diagn] (Stockh) 4:490, 1966.
262. Taylor DA, Jacobson HG: Posttraumatic herniation of the lung. Am J Roentgenol 87:896, 1962.
263. Spees EK, Strevey TE, Geiger JP, et al: Persistent traumatic lung cavities resulting from medium- and high-velocity missiles. Ann Thorac Surg 4:133, 1967.
264. Banerjee A, Khanna SK, Narayanan PS: Chest wall pneumonia: A hitherto unreported clinical entity. Thorax 37:388, 1982.
265. Cole WS: Respiratory sequels to non-thoracic injury. Lancet 1:555, 1972.
266. Schumacker PT, Rhodes GR, Newell JC, et al: Ventilation-perfusion imbalance after head trauma. Am Rev Respir Dis 119:33, 1979.
267. Popp AJ, Shah DM, Berman RA, et al: Delayed pulmonary dysfunction in head-injured patients. J Neurosurg 57:784, 1982.
268. George PY, Goodman P: Radiographic appearance of bullet tracks in the lung. Am J Roentgenol 159:967, 1992.
269. Larose JH: Cavitation of missile tracks in the lung. Radiology 90:995, 1968.
270. Dubeau L, Fraser RS: Long-term effects of pulmonary shrapnel injury: Report of a case with carcinoma and residual shrapnel tract. Arch Pathol Lab Med 108:407, 1984.
271. Hollerman JJ, Fackler ML: Gunshot wounds: Radiology and wound ballistics. Emerg Radiol 2:171, 1995.
272. Hollerman JJ, Fackler ML, Coldwell DM, et al: Gunshot wounds. 1. Bullets, ballistics, and mechanisms of injury. Am J Roentgenol 155:685, 1990.
273. Oparah SS, Mandal AK: Penetrating gunshot wounds of the chest in civilian practice: Experience with 250 consecutive cases. Br J Surg 65:45, 1978.
274. Sandrasagra FA: Penetrating thoracoabdominal injuries. Br J Surg 64:638, 1977.
275. Ordog GJ, Wasserberger J, Balasubramanium S, et al: Asymptomatic stab wounds of the chest. J Trauma 36:680, 1994.
276. Weigelt JA: Management of asymptomatic patients following stab wounds to the chest. J Trauma 22:41, 1982.
277. Muckart DJ: Delayed pneumothorax and hemothorax following observation for stab wounds of the chest. J Trauma 16:247, 1985.
278. Trombold JS, McCuistion AC, Harris HW: Slowly expanding intrapleural lesion due to a foreign body: Report of a case. N Engl J Med 264:172, 1961.
279. Wellington JL: The shrapnel awakes: Pyopneumothorax and chronic empyema resulting from a foreign body retained for 17 years. Can Med Assoc J 87:349, 1962.
280. Ekstrom D, Weiner M, Baier B: Pulmonary arteriovenous fistula as a complication of trauma. Am J Roentgenol 130:1178, 1978.
281. Gavant ML, Winer-Muram HT: Traumatic pulmonary artery pseudoaneurysm. J Can Assoc Radiol 37:108, 1986.
282. Klein CP: Gunshot wounds of the aorta with peripheral arterial bullet embolism: Report of 2 cases. Am J Roentgenol 119:547, 1973.
283. Richardson M, Gomes M, Tsou E: Transtracheal migration of an intravertebral Steinmann pin to the left bronchus. J Thorac Cardiovasc Surg 93:939, 1987.
284. Singh A, Singh B, Singh P: An interesting and unusual cause of hemoptysis. Chest 62:339, 1972.
285. Vogt-Moykopf I, Krumhaar D: Treatment of intrapulmonary shell fragments. Surg Gynecol Obstet 123:1233, 1966.
286. Kovnat DM, Anderson WM, Rath GS, et al: Hemoptysis secondary to retained transpulmonary foreign body. Am Rev Respir Dis 109:279, 1974.
287. Le Roux BT: Intrathoracic foreign bodies. Thorax 19:203, 1964.
288. Raeburn C, Spencer H: Lung scar cancers. Br J Tuberc 51:237, 1957.
289. Siddons AHM, MacArthur AM: Carcinomata developing at the site of foreign bodies in the lung. Br J Surg 39:542, 1952.
290. Strauss FH, Dordal E, Kappas A: The problem of pulmonary scar tumors. Arch Pathol 76:693, 1963.
291. Graham JM, Mattox KL, Beall AC Jr: Penetrating trauma of the lung. J Trauma 19:665, 1979.
292. Stark P: Imaging of tracheobronchial injuries. J Thorac Imaging 10:206, 1995.

CHAPTER 67

Complications of Therapeutic, Biopsy, and Monitoring Procedures

COMPLICATIONS OF THORACIC SURGERY

Most complications related to thoracic surgery occur in the immediate postoperative period (up to day 10), although certain manifestations may not become apparent for several weeks or even months postoperatively (e.g., after pneumonectomy). When considering these complications, we find it convenient to divide postoperative radiographs into three broad groups, depending on the abnormalities observed and the requirement for immediate clinical attention.

1. Radiographs that show changes that are ordinarily anticipated after thoracotomy, such as subcutaneous emphysema or the accumulation of a minimal amount of pleural fluid, unassociated with major pulmonary abnormality; in such cases, we employ the designation "satisfactory postoperative appearance" without going into any detail about the changes observed.

2. Radiographs that show abnormalities that may or may not be of importance in patient care, but whose nature requires that follow-up studies be performed; examples include a pneumothorax or hydrothorax greater in amount than ordinarily anticipated, a large hematoma following wedge resection, and mediastinal widening following mediastinotomy.

3. Radiographs that show findings that require immediate attention and require a telephone call to the attending physician or surgeon; for example, acute atelectasis, a large pneumothorax or hydrothorax, malposition of an endotracheal tube, or findings suggestive of thromboembolism.

Although radiographic changes observed in the soft tissues of the chest wall, thoracic cage, pleura, mediastinum, diaphragm, and lungs are in many ways interdependent and therefore should be considered together in interpretation, it is convenient to deal with them separately.

Soft Tissues of the Chest Wall

Although soft tissue swelling caused by hemorrhage and edema in the vicinity of the incision is common, it seldom leads to difficulty in radiologic interpretation and, in fact, is often not radiographically apparent. Subcutaneous emphysema, manifested by linear streaks of gas density in the lateral chest wall and frequently in the neck, is almost invariably apparent for 2 or 3 days postoperatively. It need cause concern only when it is present in exceptionally large quantities, in which case it may be the result of ongoing leak from the surgical anastomosis; such an event is rare.

Thoracic Cage

The absence of a rib, usually the fifth or sixth, is an occasional finding after thoracotomy. Nowadays, however, the ribs usually are spread rather than resected in both pulmonary and cardiac procedures, so that an intact rib cage is compatible with prior thoracotomy; ribs that have been spread may be fractured. The only evidence of previous sternotomy may be the presence of wire sutures.

The major abnormality detectable in the rib cage relates to the size of one hemithorax in comparison with the other—approximation of ribs and a smaller hemithorax in the presence of atelectasis and separation of ribs and a larger hemithorax in the presence of pneumothorax. As discussed farther on, enlargement of one hemithorax may be the only sign of pneumothorax in a patient whose radiograph was exposed in the supine position; in such circumstances, a pleural line may not be visible when the pneumothorax is small.

Median sternotomy has become the principal surgical approach to the heart and great vessels and to a variety of mediastinal abnormalities. Although the incidence of complications following the procedure is low (less than 5%), the overall mortality rate of three of the major events (sternal dehiscence, mediastinitis, and osteomyelitis) approaches 50%.[1, 2] Complications usually become manifest 1 to 2 weeks postoperatively and are associated with six clinical presentations: (1) serosanguineous discharge with a stable sternum; (2) unstable sternum with or without a serosanguineous discharge; (3) sternal dehiscence without mediastinitis; (4) superficial wound infection without mediastinitis; (5) subcutaneous infection with retrosternal extension and an unstable sternum; and (6) mediastinitis with or without sternal separation.[3] In one study, all patients in groups 1 and 2 survived with appropriate therapy;[3] by contrast, the mortality rate of patients in groups 3 and 4 was about 25%, and that of groups 5 and 6 was more than 70%. The clinical manifestations of mediastinitis are reviewed in Chapter 73 (*see* page 2851).

Conventional radiography plays a limited role in the assessment of these abnormalities, and CT is required for adequate evaluation, particularly when the presence of retrosternal collections or mediastinitis is suspected clinically. In one CT study of 32 patients in the immediate poststernotomy period, focal edema, focal hematomas, and minor sternal irregularities were common in the 20 patients who suffered no clinical problems.[1] Twelve patients had clinical problems such as sternal clicks, sternal pain, draining sinuses, and other signs of infection; 6 of these showed only minor abnormalities on CT that did not differ from those seen in the 20 control patients and that were successfully treated nonoperatively. The other 6 patients had evidence of presternal or mediastinal abscess formation on CT (confirmed surgically or at autopsy).

Normal postoperative findings that may persist on CT for 2 to 3 weeks after sternotomy include minimal presternal and retrosternal soft tissue infiltration with edema and blood, localized hematoma, postincisional bone defect, minor sternal irregularities such as slight misalignment, and minimal

pericardial thickening.[4] Small localized collections of air also may be present in the immediate postoperative period but usually resolve by 7 days after surgery.[1, 4] Presternal complications, including inflammation or infection, draining sinus tracts, or frank abscess formation, can be readily identified using CT. The presence and extent of mediastinal communication of draining sinus tracts can be documented with CT contrast sinography.[4] Although retrosternal complications, such as hematoma, abscess formation, mediastinitis, pericardial effusion, and empyema, can be diagnosed with CT (Fig. 67–1),[4] the procedure is of limited value in the

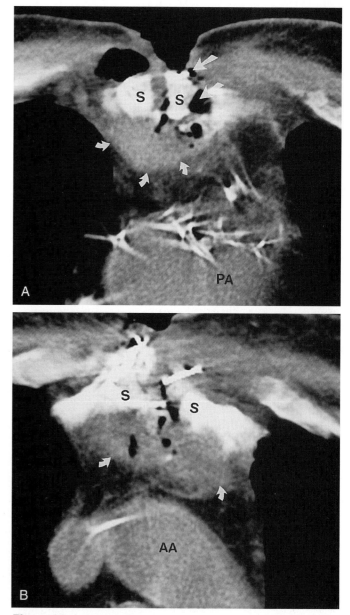

Figure 67–1. Retrosternal Abscess Following Sternotomy. A 64-year-old patient had persistent wound infection 5 weeks after coronary artery bypass surgery. A CT scan at the level of the main pulmonary artery (PA) *(A)* demonstrates a draining sinus *(straight arrows)* communicating with a retrosternal collection *(curved arrows)*. The collection extended cephalad to the level of the aortic arch (AA) *(B)*. Note sternal (S) dehiscence and broken sternal wires. The presence of a retrosternal abscess was confirmed at surgery. Cultures grew *Staphylococcus aureus.*

early detection of sternal osteomyelitis. When the latter is suspected clinically and the CT findings are equivocal, ^{99m}Tc-phosphate or gallium-67 scintigraphy can be helpful in establishing the diagnosis.[4]

A 2- to 4-mm gap at the sternotomy site (the "midsternal stripe") can be recognized in 30% to 60% of patients sometime during the postoperative period and is of no diagnostic or prognostic significance.[5] Of much greater importance in establishing sternal separation is migration or reorientation of the sternal wires.

Fracture of the first rib is occasionally seen after midline sternotomy; in a review of 50 randomly selected cases in one study, such fractures were visualized on the chest radiograph in 3 cases (6%).[6] On radionuclide bone scans, first-rib fractures are identified in about 50% of patients who have undergone sternal retraction.[7]

Pleura

After pneumonectomy, fluid gradually fills the empty hemithorax. The rate of accumulation is variable; in most cases, about one half to two thirds of the hemithorax fills with fluid within the first week; complete filling usually occurs within 2 to 4 months (*see* farther on),[8] although occasionally it takes up to 6 months.[9] Long-term follow-up studies of postpneumonectomy patients have shown partial or complete resorption of the pleural fluid. In one series of patients examined by CT, this outcome was established in about one third of patients.[10] In these patients, there was marked ipsilateral shift of the mediastinum, elevation of the hemidiaphragm, and overinflation of the contralateral lung. In the other two thirds, a variable amount of fluid was still evident several years after pneumonectomy; this was associated with less marked shift of the mediastinum.

On spin-echo magnetic resonance (MR) imaging, the postpneumonectomy space has a heterogeneous signal intensity irrespective of the interval between pneumonectomy and the MR examination.[11] The contents of the space have a low to medium signal intensity on T1-weighted images (the signal intensity is usually less than that of muscle) and medium to high signal intensity on T2-weighted images. MR imaging is comparable to CT in the assessment of tumor recurrence after pneumonectomy.[12] Usually, it can be identified by its inhomogeneous appearance and its mass effect;[12] tumor has a relatively low signal intensity on T1-weighted images and a high intensity on T2-weighted ones.

In patients who have not undergone pneumonectomy, little or no fluid is evident during the first 2 or 3 days after thoracotomy because the pleural space is effectively drained. After removal of the drainage tube, however, a small amount of fluid often appears, only to disappear quickly during convalescence. Minimal residual pleural thickening may remain, particularly over the lung base.

The accumulation of fluid in larger-than-expected amounts may result from a variety of causes, including poor positioning of the drainage tube, hemorrhage from an intercostal vessel (Fig. 67–2), or infection (empyema). In the presence of pleural adhesions, fluid may loculate in areas that are not in communication with the drainage tube, a finding that is particularly common after pleural decortication. In this circumstance, absorption of the fluid may be prolonged, sometimes requiring several weeks. Such local intrapleural collections may be simulated by an extrapleural hematoma secondary to the thoracotomy incision; however, in either event, the finding is not of major importance unless the accumulation is very large or infected. Extrapleural hematomas are particularly common after surgery over the lung apex and sometimes create a rather ominous-looking shadow (Fig. 67–3), which actually is of little or no clinical significance.

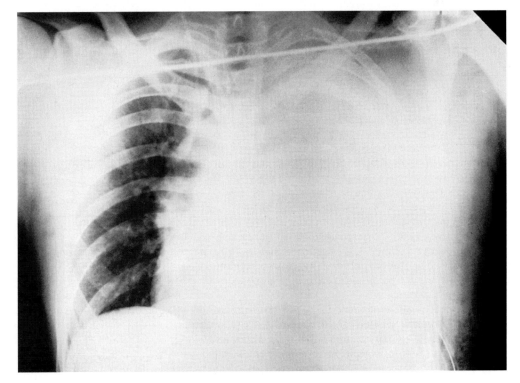

Figure 67–2. Massive Hemothorax Complicating Thoracotomy. Twenty-four hours before the radiograph, this 20-year-old man was subjected to left thoracotomy for repair of a coarctation of the aorta (minimal rib notching was apparent). The radiograph illustrates a massive effusion in the left pleural space with considerable shift of the mediastinum to the right. This represents a massive hemothorax caused by bleeding into the pleural space from an intercostal artery. The unusually severe hemorrhage was related to hypertrophy of the intercostal circulation secondary to coarctation.

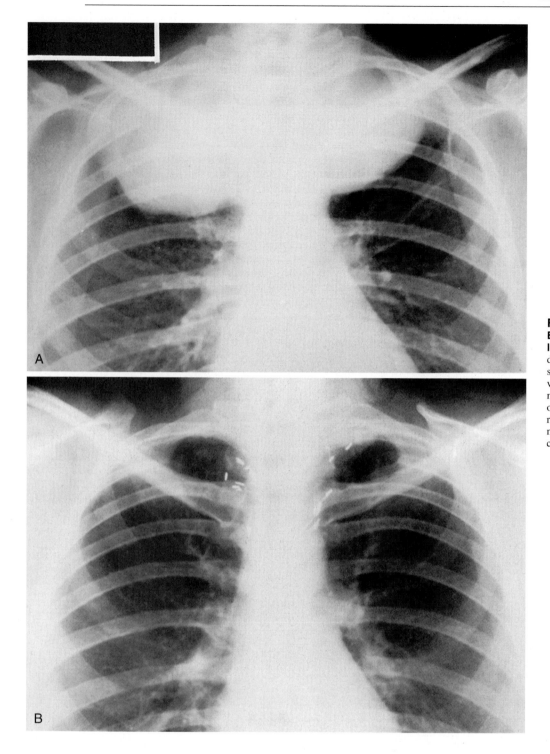

A

B

Figure 67–3. Bilateral Apical Extrapleural Hematomas Following Sympathectomy. Several days after bilateral upper thoracic sympathectomy, a radiograph *(A)* reveals sharply defined homogeneous masses occupying the apical portion of both hemithoraces (a preoperative radiograph was normal). Three months later *(B)*, the hematomas had completely resolved.

In contrast to the small amount of fluid that often accumulates, gas is seldom visible in the pleural space after removal of the drainage tube, even on radiographs exposed with the patient erect. A word of caution regarding the assessment of possible pneumothorax is required. In the immediate postoperative period, radiographs are often exposed with the patient supine; in this position, any intrapleural gas tends to be situated at the base of the hemithorax anteriorly, where it may not be in communication with the drainage tube. Even a small pneumothorax in this location is usually of sufficient size to permit identification of the visceral pleural line at the base of the lung. If the line is not visible, however, suspicion of pneumothorax still should be raised by the presence of enlargement of the ipsilateral hemithorax as a result of a loss of the inward retractile force of the elastic recoil of the lung. A pneumothorax of such small size usually does not cause symptoms; however, when there is clinical concern, radiography should be performed in the lateral decubitus or erect position to confirm or eliminate the presence of pneumothorax. Physicians should be particularly aware of the possibility of pneumothorax in circumstances in which it is unexpected, for example, after mediastinotomy for cardiac surgery, during which the mediastinal pleura may be accidentally nicked.

Postoperative pneumothorax has a variety of causes. Lack of communication with the drainage tube is probably the most common, particularly if the gas is loculated or the tube is incorrectly positioned (e.g., in the major fissure). Other causes include leakage into the pleural space from a "blown" bronchial stump (bronchopleural fistula) or from a bare area of lung after wedge or segmental resection of lung (Fig. 67–4). In the presence of pleural adhesions, a loculated collection of gas may remain for a considerable period of time because of lack of communication with the drainage tube; it may be associated with a collection of fluid in the form of hydropneumothorax.

The incidence of bronchopleural fistula as a complication of pulmonary resection is about 2%[13, 14] and the mortality rate ranges from 30% to 70%.[13–15] It occurs as a result of necrosis of bronchial stump tissue or dehiscence of sutures. It is most common after right pneumonectomy and occurs rarely after lower lobectomy on either side. In one investigation of 2,359 pulmonary resections, bronchopleural fistulas developed in 52 (2%);[14] multivariate analysis revealed an increased risk in association with more extensive surgery (e.g., pneumonectomy), residual carcinoma at the bronchial stump, preoperative radiation, and diabetes. Characteristically, the development of a fistula is heralded by the sudden onset of dyspnea and expectoration of bloody fluid during the first 10 days postoperatively; dehiscence is uncommon more than 90 days after resection.[15] The chest radiograph

may reveal an unexpected disappearance of fluid as a result of emptying of the pleural space by way of the tracheobronchial tree.[16] Radiologic evaluation of this complication can be facilitated by CT,[17] particularly with the use of thin sections (2-mm collimation) and spiral technique.[17a, b]

Esophageal-pleural fistulas may develop after esophagectomy, anterior fusion of the cervical spine, or esophageal dilation.[18] Radiographic findings include mediastinal widening, pleural effusion, pneumothorax, and hydropneumothorax.[18, 19] Mediastinal widening may be absent because of drainage of the esophageal contents into the pleural space.[18] The diagnosis is readily made by demonstration of orally administered contrast material in the pleural space by fluoroscopically guided esophagography or CT.[19, 20] The latter procedure is superior to esophagography because it requires little cooperation of the patient, allows evaluation of both the pleura and mediastinum, and may demonstrate a fistula even in patients who have a normal esophagogram.[18, 20]

Mediastinum

The two major radiologic abnormalities of the mediastinum that occur in the postoperative period are enlargement and displacement. The former results from the accumulation of either gas or fluid. Pneumomediastinum is a frequent finding after mediastinotomy and should not occasion alarm; however, its persistence in the absence of other potential causes (such as tracheostomy) should raise the suspicion of

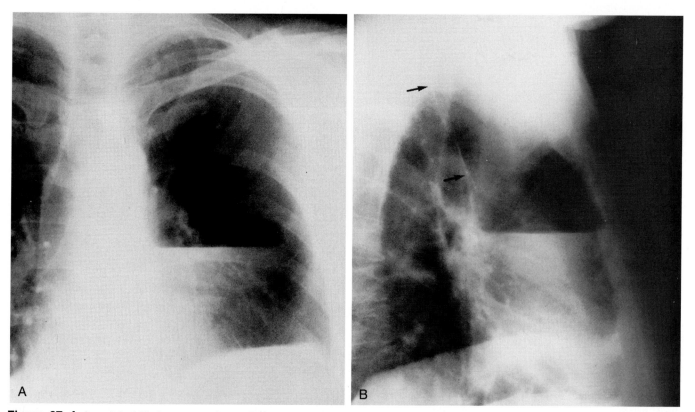

Figure 67–4. Loculated Hydropneumothorax Following Lobectomy. Posteroanterior *(A)* and lateral *(B)* radiographs reveal a large loculated collection of gas and fluid in the anterior portion of the left hemithorax (the upper half of the lower lobe major fissure is indicated by *arrows* in *B*). These films were made about 2 weeks after left upper lobectomy; the persistence of pneumothorax was caused by an air leak from lower lobe parenchyma. Several weeks were required for spontaneous absorption.

interstitial pulmonary emphysema associated with some form of pulmonary disease.[21] Venous hemorrhage and edema are also common after mediastinotomy and should not be considered serious unless widening is excessive or progressive. Severe bleeding should be suspected when there is an abrupt increase in the mediastinal width or change in contour after sternotomy.[22] Although the radiographic findings may be helpful in diagnosis, in most cases, it is made based on excessive bloody mediastinal tube drainage.[23] For example, in one series of 100 patients, 7 required re-exploration for mediastinal bleeding after cardiac surgery;[23] only 1 of the 7 had mediastinal widening. In this patient, the diagnosis was first suggested because of a rapid increase in mediastinal width in the early postoperative period; mediastinal tube drainage was deceptively normal as a result of partial blockage of the tube.

Other causes of mediastinal widening after cardiac surgery include aortic dissection and traumatic venous catheter insertion.[23] Rarely, focal mediastinal widening or an anterior mediastinal mass following coronary artery bypass surgery represents a saphenous vein graft aneurysm[24] or intrathoracic fat from an internal mammary artery pedicle.[25] Distinction of mediastinal hemorrhage from these two abnormalities can be readily made with contrast-enhanced CT.[24, 25] A sponge is rarely retained in the pericardial cavity following cardiac surgery;[26] it is usually located posteriorly, since this region is not visible to the surgeon. Detection is difficult on standard anteroposterior chest radiographs because of exposure factors but can readily be made on the lateral view or on CT.[26]

Alterations in contour of the mediastinum after thoracic surgery may be caused by transposed muscle or by omental or pericardial fat used to obliterate spaces, to promote repair

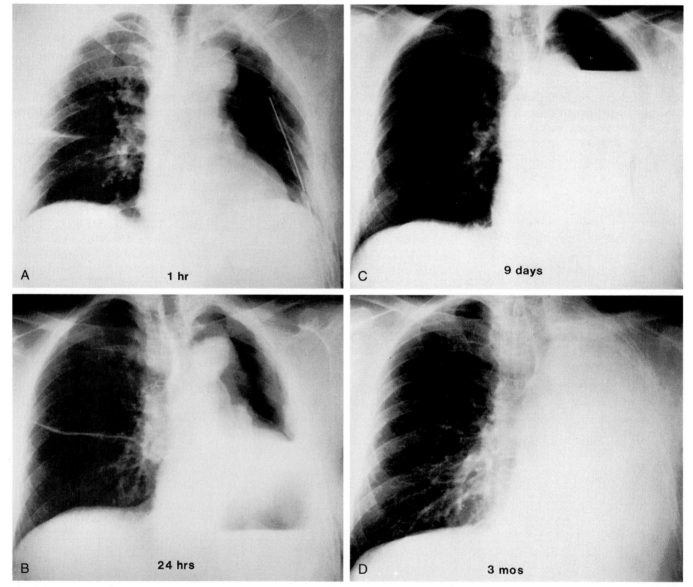

Figure 67–5. Postpneumonectomy Course: Normal. An anteroposterior radiograph obtained in the supine position at the bedside 1 hour after left pneumonectomy *(A)* reveals a slight reduction in the volume of the left hemithorax. The space is air filled, and the mediastinum is in the midline. After 24 hours, a radiograph in the erect position *(B)* shows moderate elevation of the left hemidiaphragm (as indicated by the gastric air bubble), a moderate shift of the mediastinum to the left, and a prominent air-fluid level in the plane of the third interspace anteriorly. By 9 days *(C)*, fluid has filled about two thirds of the cavity of the left hemithorax, but the mediastinum is still displaced to the left (note the curvature of the tracheal air column). By 3 months *(D)*, the left hemithorax has become completely airless. Note the persistent shift of the mediastinum to the left and the prominent curve of the air column of the trachea.

and healing, to cover a bronchial stump, or to reinforce airway and esophageal anastomosis.[27, 28] Blood supply to these transpositions, known as *surgical flaps*, is maintained by keeping their vascular pedicle intact. On CT, surgical flaps are visualized as vascularized structures that, depending on their nature, have soft tissue or adipose tissue attenuation.[27, 28]

Position of the mediastinum is one of the most important indicators of pulmonary abnormality during the postoperative period. Displacement may occur toward or away from the side of the thoracotomy. Ipsilateral displacement is an expected finding after lobectomy or pneumonectomy. In the former situation, it is temporary, and the normal midline position is regained as the remainder of the lung undergoes compensatory overinflation. Excessive displacement toward the operated side may be a sign of atelectasis in the ipsilateral lung. In the case of pneumonectomy, ipsilateral mediastinal displacement is progressive and permanent (*see* farther on). Mediastinal displacement away from the operated side may occur as a result of atelectasis in the contralateral lung or an accumulation of excessive fluid or gas in the ipsilateral pleural space.

The changes on the chest radiograph after pneumonectomy were assessed in one review of 110 cases.[8] Within 24 hours of the procedure, the ipsilateral pleural space is air containing, the mediastinum is shifted slightly to the ipsilateral side, and the hemidiaphragm is slightly elevated (Fig. 67–5). The postpneumonectomy space then begins to fill with serosanguineous fluid in a progressive and predictable manner at a rate of about two rib spaces per day. In most cases, there is 80% to 90% obliteration of the space at the end of 2 weeks and complete obliteration by 2 to 4 months. Such obliteration occurs as a result of fluid accumulation as well as by progressive ipsilateral displacement of the mediastinum and elevation of the hemidiaphragm. Mediastinal displacement is an almost invariable finding and constitutes the most reliable indicator of a normal postoperative course. It generally requires 6 to 8 months to reach its maximum. Failure of the mediastinum to shift in the postoperative period almost always indicates an abnormality in the postpneumonectomy space, regardless of the character or level of the air-fluid interface.

The postpneumonectomy space tends to fill more rapidly on the left than on the right and when the pneumonectomy is extrapleural (i.e., when it includes the parietal pleura).[8] In one study, the character of the fluid level was found to have little or no diagnostic or prognostic significance; the contour of the air-fluid interface was less important than the appearance of bubbles or a drop in the level of fluid by more than 2 cm. The hallmark of a normal course of events after pneumonectomy was progressive shift of the mediastinum to the operative side, associated with compensatory overinflation of the contralateral lung (*see* Fig. 67–5). The absence of such a shift in the immediate postoperative period indicated the presence of bronchopleural fistula, empyema (Fig. 67–6), hemorrhage, or (occasionally) chylothorax.

The most sensitive indicator of late complications was a return to the midline of a previously shifted mediastinum, particularly the tracheal air column.[8] This indicated the presence within the postpneumonectomy space of recurrent neoplasm (Fig. 67–7), bronchopleural fistula, hemorrhage, chy-

lothorax, or empyema (Fig. 67–8). In some patients with recurrent carcinoma after pneumonectomy, conventional radiographs of the thorax do not manifest signs of such an expanding process within the ipsilateral hemithorax. In these cases, CT can be of great value in documenting tumor recurrence, either as enlarged mediastinal lymph nodes or as a soft tissue mass projecting into the near-water-density postpneumonectomy space.[29]

CT is also helpful in the assessment of patients with suspected postpneumonectomy empyema. Although a shift of the trachea and mediastinal contents back to midline and a sudden appearance of an air-fluid level on the radiograph are helpful clues to the diagnosis, they are present in a minority of cases. For example, in one series of 9 patients with late-onset postpneumonectomy empyema, only 1 had shift of the trachea towards the remaining lung.[30] On CT, the mediastinal border of the postpneumonectomy space normally has a concave margin;[31] loss of this margin with development of convex expansion of the postpneumonectomy space has been described as a characteristic finding of empyema.[31] The clinical and additional radiologic manifestations of empyema are reviewed in Chapter 69 (*see* page 2739).

A rare but potentially catastrophic event is herniation of the heart through a pericardial defect after radical pneumonectomy in which partial pericardiectomy has been carried out or in which intrapericardial ligation of pulmonary vessels has been performed.[32, 33] Only 50 cases had been reported by 1997.[9] The herniation occurs at the end of the surgical procedure or in the immediate postoperative period.[9] It may occur on either side and is frequently associated with the abrupt onset of circulatory collapse or superior vena cava obstruction. Radiologically, the appearance varies with the side on which the pneumonectomy has been performed: if on the right, the heart is dextrorotated into the right hemithorax, producing an unmistakable appearance;[34, 35] when on the left, the heart may rotate posteriorly or laterally, and herniation is usually less evident, particularly if there is a sizable accumulation of pleural fluid. On the left side, an indentation or notch may become apparent between the great vessels and the heart, simulating the appearance of congenital absence of the left side of the pericardium. In one case, herniation resulted in displacement of a left chest tube, which constituted the initial evidence that something was amiss.[36] In the correct clinical setting, this grave complication should be readily recognizable radiologically, leading to life-saving thoracotomy.[37] The diagnosis can be confirmed by thoracoscopy.[38]

Another rare complication of pneumonectomy that tends to occur a considerable time after surgery (often less than 1 year but occasionally as long as 37 years[39]) is the so-called postpneumonectomy syndrome.[40] The condition typically follows right pneumonectomy and is usually seen in children and adolescents (although in one report, it was identified in a patient 50 years of age).[39] Radiographic manifestations following right pneumonectomy include marked rightward and posterior displacement of the mediastinum, clockwise rotation of the heart and great vessels, and displacement of the overinflated left lung into the anterior portion of the right hemithorax. As a result of the rotation of the heart and great vessels, the distal trachea and left main bronchus become compressed between the aorta and pulmonary artery, with resulting dyspnea and recurrent left-

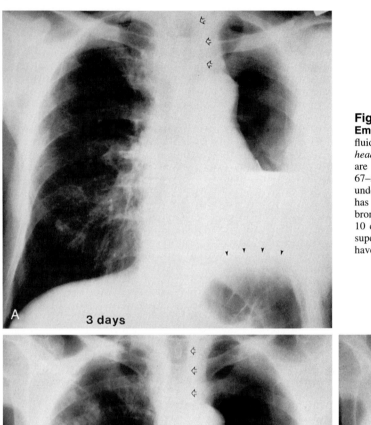

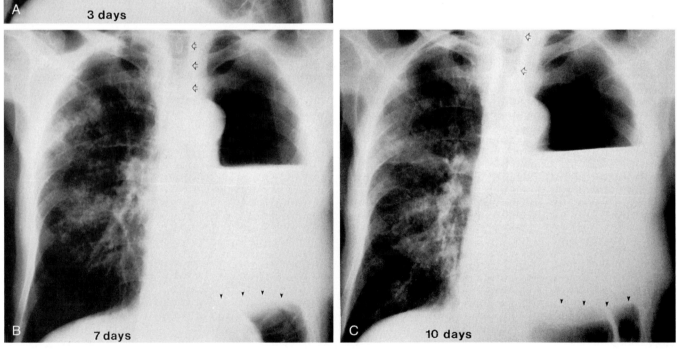

Figure 67–6. Postpneumonectomy Course Complicated by Empyema. Three days after left pneumonectomy *(A)*, the amount of fluid that has accumulated, the position of the left hemidiaphragm *(arrowheads)*, and the shift of the tracheal air column to the left *(open arrows)* are all consistent with a normal postoperative course (compare with Fig. 67–5). At 7 days *(B)*, however, the left hemidiaphragm *(arrowheads)* has undergone some depression, and the tracheal air column *(open arrows)* has returned to the midline. Such a change should suggest empyema, bronchopleural fistula, pleural hemorrhage, or (possibly) chylothorax. By 10 days *(C)*, the left hemidiaphragm *(arrowheads)* has become concave superiorly, and the mediastinum and tracheal air column *(open arrows)* have shifted farther to the right.

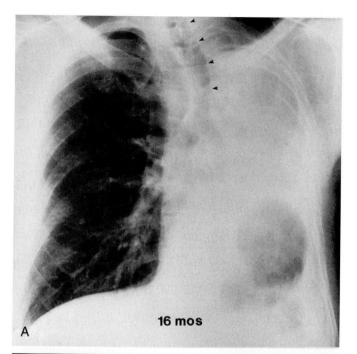

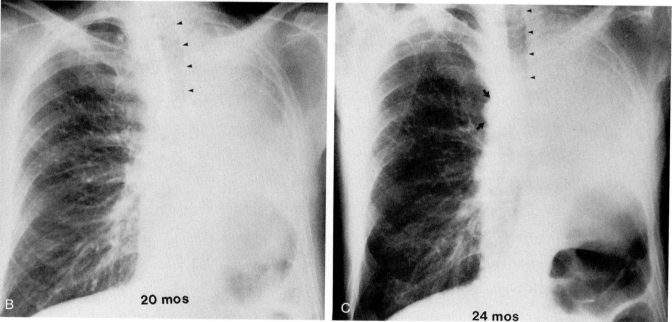

Figure 67–7. Postpneumonectomy Course: Recurrence of Neoplasm. Sixteen months after left pneumonectomy for pulmonary carcinoma, a posteroanterior radiograph *(A)* reveals a normal appearance (compare with Fig. 67–5). The left hemidiaphragm is markedly elevated, and the heart and tracheal air column *(arrowheads)* are shifted into the left hemithorax. By 20 months *(B)*, the left side of the tracheal air column has a flatter appearance *(arrowheads)*, suggesting the presence of an expanding process in the left hemithorax. By 24 months *(C)*, the trachea is in the midline *(arrowheads)* and a soft tissue mass has developed in the region of the right tracheobronchial angle *(arrows)*, suggesting a metastasis to the azygos lymph node. Recurrence of neoplasm in the pleural space and contralateral node metastasis were subsequently proved pathologically.

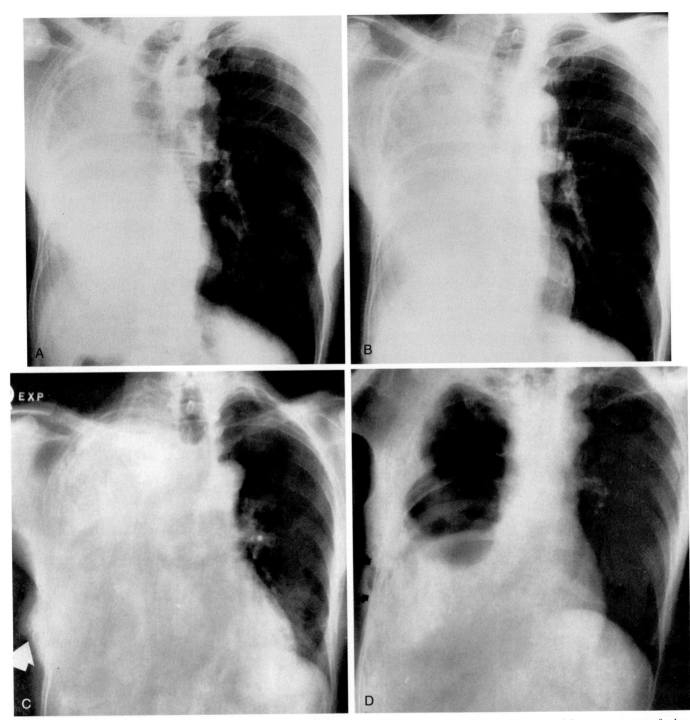

Figure 67–8. Empyema Necessitatis in a Postpneumonectomy Space. This 53-year-old man had undergone a right pneumonectomy for lung gangrene about 1 year before this radiograph *(A)*; at the time of this study, he was asymptomatic. Note the marked reduction in volume of the right hemithorax, as indicated by shift of the trachea and heart to the right. Ten months later *(B)*, he was admitted with fever and pain in the right side of his chest; note that both the tracheal air column and heart show less displacement to the right. Two weeks later *(C)*, both the tracheal air column and the heart have reached a midline position as a result of the presence of a large expanding process in the right postpneumonectomy space. In addition, a smooth soft tissue mass has developed in the right lateral chest wall *(arrow)*. After drainage of a large amount of pus from the right pleural space and replacement with air *(D)*, a gas shadow can be seen extending outside the rib cage *(arrows)* in the identical position of the soft tissue mass previously identified. This represents extension of pus through the parietal pleura and intercostal musculature into the subcutaneous tissues of the chest wall—empyema necessitatis.

sided pneumonia. Rarely, postpneumonectomy syndrome develops after left pneumonectomy.[40–42] Marked rotation of the mediastinal structures to the left and herniation of the right lung into the left hemithorax in these cases is associated with narrowing of the right upper lobe and right middle lobe bronchi or the bronchus intermedius as they are splayed anterior to the spine.[42] The bronchus intermedius may also be compressed between the right pulmonary artery anteriorly and the vertebral body posteriorly.[42] A case has also been reported in which recurrent episodes of dyspnea were associated with swallowing solid food, presumably as a result of bronchial compression by a distended esophagus.[43] CT can facilitate identification of the syndrome.[39, 42]

Diaphragm

The value of diaphragmatic position in the assessment of the postoperative chest radiograph depends largely on the position of the patient at the time of radiography. In the supine position, the normally higher position of the right hemidiaphragm is accentuated, presumably because of the mass of the liver, and this must not be mistaken for evidence of intrathoracic abnormality. With the patient erect, the usual rules regarding diaphragmatic position pertain.

After pneumonectomy or lobectomy, the ipsilateral hemidiaphragm is almost invariably elevated during the first few days. With pneumonectomy, this elevation persists along with ipsilateral mediastinal shift, despite accumulation of fluid in the pleural space; with lobectomy, elevation and mediastinal displacement disappear over a period of several days or weeks as the remainder of the ipsilateral lung undergoes compensatory overinflation.

Marked elevation of a hemidiaphragm can result from injury to the phrenic nerve sustained during surgery. Elevation can also be caused by a number of pathologic states within the lungs, including atelectasis, bronchopneumonia, and thromboembolism. Differentiation of these conditions may be difficult on the basis of radiographic signs alone, although the time interval following surgery may be of some assistance (*see* farther on).

Depression of one hemidiaphragm is an uncommon postoperative abnormality and is invariably caused by a massive pneumothorax or hydrothorax.

Lungs

The radiographic changes that can be anticipated after thoracotomy depend on the nature of the surgical procedure. For example, after lobectomy, there is a predictable pattern of reorientation of the remaining lobe or lobes that rotate and hyperinflate to occupy the residual space.[44] The rearrangement of fissures resulting from reorientation of lobes should not be misinterpreted as evidence of atelectasis. Similarly, the vascular markings become more widely spaced, and lung density is reduced as a result of compensatory overinflation, signs that must not be confused with those resulting from atelectasis or from reduced perfusion from thromboembolism. Hematoma formation is common after wedge or segmental resection and results from hemorrhage at the site of excision (Fig. 67–9). Provided that the radiolo-

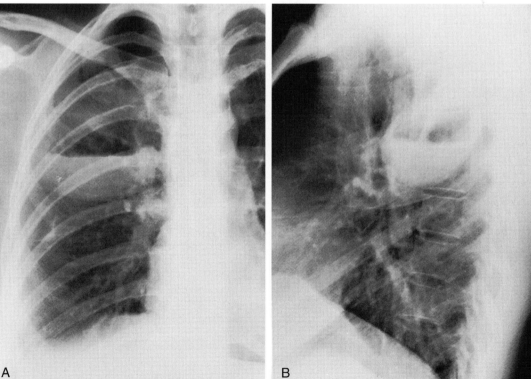

Figure 67–9. Postoperative Pulmonary Hematoma. Views of the right hemithorax from posteroanterior *(A)* and lateral *(B)* radiographs reveal a large, well-defined circular shadow in the upper portion of the right lung, possessing a prominent air-fluid level. It is very thin walled. These radiographs were made about 3 days after wedge resection of a bulla of the right upper lobe. The shadow represents an accumulation of blood and gas in the bare area after resection. Over a period of 4 weeks, it underwent slow but progressive resolution and left no significant residuum. The patient was a 39-year-old woman.

gist is aware of the type of surgical procedure carried out, these rather ominous-looking, yet clinically insignificant, opacities should present little difficulty in diagnosis.

To attribute an opacity in the lungs on a postoperative radiograph to residual atelectasis resulting from compression by a retractor or the surgeon's hand during the surgical procedure is tenuous; to the best of our knowledge, such effects have never been documented. Any local pulmonary opacity identified in the postoperative period must be regarded as one of the "big four"—atelectasis, pneumonia, infarction, or edema. The manifestations of these complications are no different from those that develop in a nonsurgical setting. As might be anticipated, diffuse pulmonary edema is much more common in patients who have undergone cardiac surgery. Additional rare complications of thoracic surgery include pulmonary herniation and torsion.

Atelectasis

Undoubtedly, the most common pulmonary complication of surgical procedures is atelectasis, whether the surgery is thoracic or abdominal.[45] The abnormality varies widely in extent, in some cases affecting an entire lobe and in others a number of lobular units whose airlessness causes insufficient density to be appreciated radiographically. In the latter circumstance, atelectasis may be evidenced only by alterations in lung function and gas exhange.[46] The mechanisms by which postoperative atelectasis develops also vary considerably. The most common cause is mucous plugging, which occurs chiefly as a result of diminished diaphragmatic excursion (caused, e.g., by phrenic nerve paralysis[47] or by splinting as a result of pain).[46] Disruption of mucociliary clearance and pooling of mucus associated with atelectasis after major surgery have also been documented.[48]

Atelectasis is the most common complication following lobectomy, and various degrees are present in up to 60% of cases.[49] In one review of the radiographic findings in 218 patients undergoing lobectomy or bilobectomy, 8% were found to have developed complete ipsilateral lobar or bilobar collapse with white-out of the involved lobe or lobes and mediastinal shift.[49] Patients who had severe atelectasis had significantly longer intensive care unit and hospital stays than patients who did not have complications. Right upper lobectomy, alone or in combination with the right middle lobe, was associated with a five-fold greater incidence of severe atelectasis than all other types of resection.

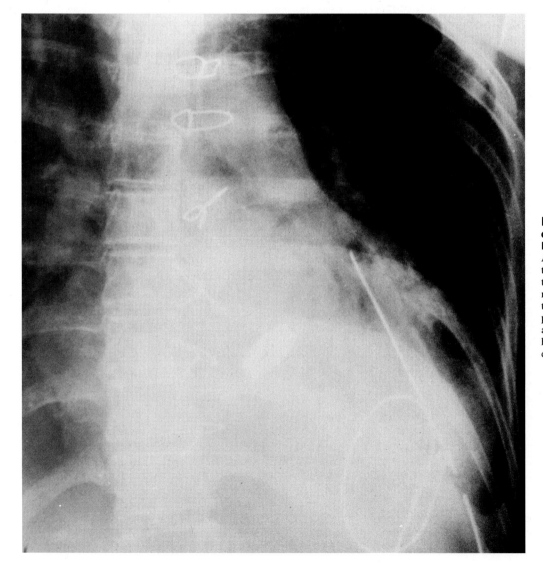

Figure 67–10. Adhesive Atelectasis of the Left Lower Lobe Following Open Heart Surgery. A view of the left lung from an anteroposterior radiograph exposed at the patient's bedside reveals airlessness and loss of volume of much of the left lower lobe associated with a prominent air bronchogram. Such an appearance is so common after open heart surgery that it represents an expected finding.

A common abnormality that occurs postoperatively in patients who have undergone cardiopulmonary bypass for open heart surgical procedures is left lower lobe atelectasis, usually seen as a homogenous opacity behind the heart and often associated with an air bronchogram (Fig. 67–10). Right lower lobe atelectasis may also occur but is less common and less severe. In one review of radiographs from 99 patients, atelectasis was identified in 84;[23] the abnormality involved the left lower lobe in 40 patients, both lower lobes in 43, and only the right lower lobe in 1 patient. In another series, review of the daily chest radiographs after coronary artery bypass surgery in 57 patients demonstrated evidence of left lower lobe atelectasis at some time between surgery and discharge in about 90% of cases and right lower lobe atelectasis in 60%.[50] The atelectasis increased progressively until the fourth postoperative day and then gradually improved; it was more severe in the left lower lobe than the right on all postoperative days.

Although the etiology remains obscure, it appears most logical to ascribe this complication to adhesive atelectasis resulting from surfactant loss.[51] However, it has also been suggested that intraoperative hypothermic injury may lead to paralysis or paresis of the left hemidiaphragm with subsequent left lower lobe atelectasis.[50, 52] In one study, retrospective and prospective analyses of chest radiographs of patients after coronary artery bypass surgery revealed a left lower lobe opacity in 13 of 40 patients (32%) who were operated on without topical cooling of the heart with ice and in 111 of 162 (70%) who underwent this procedure.[52] The investigators explained this difference, at least partly, on the effect of ice cooling on the phrenic nerve. In another study, the frequency of acute postoperative atelectasis was compared in 331 patients, half of whom underwent the normothermic (warm) technique and half the hypothermic (cold) technique; no difference was observed in the incidence of abnormal radiographs between the two groups.[53]

The importance of operative variables in the development of postoperative atelectasis was assessed in another investigation of 57 patients undergoing coronary artery bypass surgery.[50] Transcutaneous stimulation was used to evaluate phrenic nerve function preoperatively and postoperatively. Postoperative phrenic nerve paresis was present in only 5 patients. Discriminate analysis of intraoperative variables showed more severe atelectasis with a larger number of grafts, with a longer operative and bypass time, when the pleural space was entered, when a right atrial drain and a cardiac insulating pad were not used, and with a lower body temperature.[50] The researchers concluded that the atelectasis is probably multifactorial in etiology; although phrenic nerve paresis may occur after coronary bypass surgery, other factors must explain the atelectasis in most patients.

The left and right lower lobe atelectasis appear to cause little clinical disability and are such a frequent finding after bypass surgery that they can be regarded as an expected part of a satisfactory postoperative appearance. Small pleural effusions are also seen in most of these patients. Blood gas measurements have shown a 25% decrease in PaO_2 on the second preoperative day, with gradual improvement thereafter.[54]

During the postoperative period, there are some patients in whom blood gas measurements reveal evidence of pulmonary arteriovenous shunt despite the presence of a normal radiograph. In most cases, however, areas of atelectasis are evident on the radiograph. In one study of 23 patients whose arterial blood gases were measured while they breathed 100% oxygen before and after surgery, calculation revealed a mean true shunt of 12% during the postoperative period;[55] shunting averaged 7% in the 12 patients whose chest radiographs were normal, 13% in the 5 patients whose radiographs showed linear atelectasis, and 19% in the 6 patients whose radiographs revealed segmental collapse.

Postoperative PaO_2 levels appear to relate to the presence or absence of complications. In one investigation of 40 patients who had undergone elective cholecystectomy, a PaO_2 below 70 mm Hg was found in 30 patients;[56] this finding was associated with abnormal auscultatory or chest radiographic findings, whereas none of the 10 patients with normal chest examinations had a PaO_2 below 70. Similar findings have been reported after left thoracotomy for benign esophageal disease in 14 patients in whom no lung tissue was resected:[57] in all patients, a decrease in PaO_2 was observed postoperatively, with a mean reduction of 31%. The hypoxemia was at its worst during the first 2 days, after which time levels gradually returned to preoperative values.

Edema

Pulmonary edema, usually mild, is seen in most patients in the immediate postoperative period after cardiac surgery.[22] It may be caused by fluid overload, intrinsic left ventricular dysfunction, or increased capillary permeability related to cardiopulmonary bypass.[22] The edema usually resolves within 24 to 48 hours. Pulmonary edema may also occur after lung surgery as a result of fluid overload, congestive heart failure, thromboembolism, or adult respiratory distress syndrome (ARDS) secondary to aspiration, pneumonia, or sepsis.[58] Occasionally, no cause is apparent. The latter situation is known as *postpneumonectomy pulmonary edema* and has a high mortality rate. For example, in one retrospective study of 197 patients who underwent pneumonectomy, it was present in 54 (27%);[58] all 5 patients in whom no cause was identified died. This abnormality is discussed in greater detail on page 2001.

Miscellaneous Complications

An uncommon complication of thoracotomy or chest tube drainage is herniation of lung through the surgical defect.[59, 60] Such hernias may not be detectable on conventional chest radiographs performed at end inspiration but are usually readily demonstrated on radiographs performed at end expiration, during cough or a Valsalva maneuver, or on CT (Fig. 67–11). Lung hernias may also be congenital or result from direct trauma, lifting heavy weights, or playing wind instruments.[59]

Another rare complication of thoracotomy is torsion of a lobe or lung.[61, 62] Early recognition is essential because complete 180-degree torsion leads to infarction.[61] Lobar torsion occurs most commonly after lobectomy but may also be seen after wedge resection, severance of pleural adhesions, pleurectomy, or lung transplantation.[62-64] The radiologic findings consist of atelectasis due to airway obstruction, abnormal positioning and orientation of pulmonary vessels and bronchi within the atelectatic lobe, abnormal position of

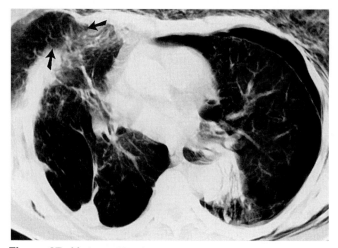

Figure 67–11. Lung Hernia. A CT scan in a 74-year-old man demonstrates herniation of a portion of the right lung *(arrows)* through a defect in the chest wall. The patient had undergone right thoracotomy and bullectomy several years previously and was being evaluated for recurrent left pneumothorax. Evidence of emphysema and scarring in both lungs, left lower lobe atelectasis, left pneumothorax, and subcutaneous emphysema are also evident.

the hilum in relation to the atelectatic lobe, and rapid expansion of an abnormally located consolidated lobe.[62–64] CT demonstrates twisting and narrowing or occlusion of the bronchus as well as abnormal orientation of the pulmonary vessels and delayed opacification following intravenous administration of contrast (Fig. 67–12).[64, 65] Fusiform tapering of the pulmonary artery is particularly well seen on angiography.[65]

Occasionally, a sponge is accidentally left in the chest after thoracotomy (Fig. 67–13). Rarely, it serves as a focus for the development of infection. In one case, the sponge was retained for 43 years, the patient presenting at age 73 with a history of long-standing hemoptysis.[66] Chest radiographs and CT demonstrated a retrocardiac mass. At surgery, the mass was shown to represent a 4-cm-diameter sponge that had eroded through the pleura into the lung parenchyma and was surrounded by chronic inflammation.

The pulmonary artery or bronchial stumps left after pneumonectomy can be the site of a process that leads to subsequent intrathoracic disease. Thrombosis of the artery stump is common and usually innocuous; rarely, however, it may embolize to the residual lung and lead to radiologic and clinical findings (Fig. 67–14). *Aspergillus* species can colonize the bronchial stump and grow into a fungus ball;[67, 68] extension of the organism across the wall into the adjacent pleural space has been followed by empyema.

COMPLICATIONS OF NONTHORACIC SURGERY

The major thoracic complications of abdominal surgery are atelectasis, pneumonia, thromboembolism, subphrenic abscess, cardiogenic pulmonary edema, and ARDS.[69–71] The reported incidence of such complications has varied from about 20% to 75%;[72] series associated with the higher figures have undoubtedly included patients who had radiographic abnormalities of little clinical significance.

A number of risk factors for pulmonary complications

of nonresectional thoracic surgery have been identified. One of the most important is chronic obstructive pulmonary disease (COPD). For example, in one investigation of 78 patients, serious pulmonary complications occurred in 6 (23%) of 26 patients who had severe COPD, of whom 5 died;[71] by contrast, only 2 of the 52 patients who did not have underlying lung disease had a serious pulmonary complication, of whom 1 died.[71] It seems likely that risk of surgery increases with the presence of an increasing number of risk factors and their increasing severity. The results of several studies have shown that both cigarette smoking and older age are also risk factors for postoperative pulmonary complications.[73–75] In a study of 3,156 cardiac operations, logistic regression was used to identify 11 variables that predicted postoperative complications, including those related to the lungs;[76] the results were used to construct an additive model to calculate the probability of serious morbidity. The model was then validated prospectively in another 394 patients. Identified risks for pulmonary complications included chronic pulmonary disease, emergency surgery, recent myocardial infarction, congestive heart failure, renal insufficiency, and advanced age.

Predictors of postoperative pulmonary complications after abdominal surgery specifically have also been evaluated.[77–79] In one study of 400 patients who underwent abdominal surgery, six independent risk factors were associated with an increased risk of postoperative atelectasis or pneumonia, including age 60 years or older, impaired preoperative cognitive function, smoking history within the previous 8 weeks, body mass index of 27 or higher, history of cancer, and incision in the upper or lower and upper abdomen.[77] Both the nature of the operation and its location also influence the risk of pulmonary complications.[79–81] For example, in an investigation of 95 patients, only 1 of 37 (2.7%) had postoperative pulmonary complications after laparoscopic cholecystectomy, compared with 10 of 58 (17%) who had open cholecystectomy.[81] Similarly, lower abdominal procedures (e.g., laparoscopic gynecologic surgery) result in less frequent pulmonary complications than do upper abdominal ones (e.g., laparoscopic cholecystectomy).[80] In another study of 361 consecutive adult patients admitted to the hospital for abdominal surgery, the risk of serious postoperative pulmonary complications was greater in those who had mucous hypersecretion, hyperinflation, reduced forced expiratory volume in 1 second, and reduced DCO on lung function testing.[78]

As discussed previously, atelectasis is undoubtedly the most common complication of surgery and in most patients is related to retention of secretions and airway mucous plugging. Such secretions can become infected;[72] with and without such infection, the separation of atelectasis from pneumonia in the postoperative setting can be difficult because symptoms of cough, sputum production, and fever do not permit an accurate distinction of one from the other.[72] The radiographic and clinical features of acute pneumonia and pulmonary thromboembolism are no different from those observed in other clinical settings. Subphrenic abscess, although uncommon, is almost always a complication of abdominal surgery; its clinical signs (pain in the hypochondrium, limitation of respiratory motion, and fever), timing (10 days after surgery), and radiographic manifestations

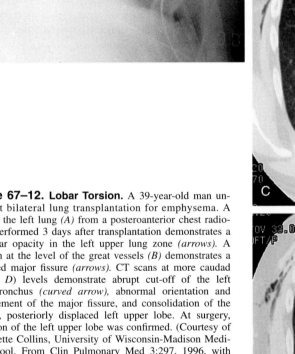

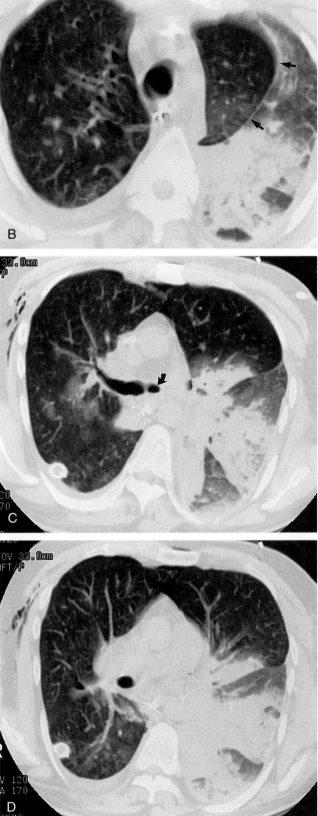

Figure 67–12. Lobar Torsion. A 39-year-old man underwent bilateral lung transplantation for emphysema. A view of the left lung *(A)* from a posteroanterior chest radiograph performed 3 days after transplantation demonstrates a triangular opacity in the left upper lung zone *(arrows)*. A CT scan at the level of the great vessels *(B)* demonstrates a displaced major fissure *(arrows)*. CT scans at more caudad *(C* and *D)* levels demonstrate abrupt cut-off of the left main bronchus *(curved arrow)*, abnormal orientation and displacement of the major fissure, and consolidation of the torqued, posteriorly displaced left upper lobe. At surgery, infarction of the left upper lobe was confirmed. (Courtesy of Dr. Janette Collins, University of Wisconsin-Madison Medical School. From Clin Pulmonary Med 3:297, 1996, with permission.)

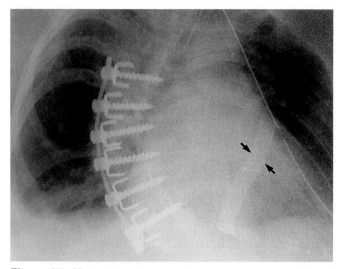

Figure 67–13. Retained Sponge. An anteroposterior chest radiograph in a 42-year-old woman who had fever 3 days after left thoracotomy and extensive thoracic spine surgery demonstrates a radiopaque sponge *(arrows)* in left pleural space. The patient recovered uneventfully after its removal.

(pleural effusion and diaphragmatic elevation) do not allow its easy distinction from thromboembolism.

A number of uncommon thoracic abnormalities have been seen in association with specific surgical interventions. Examples include gastrobronchial fistula (secondary to a benign ulcer located in mediastinal gastric mucosa following a gastric pull-up in the treatment of esophageal carcinoma),[82] aortobronchial fistula (subsequent to aortic valve replacement[83] or coarctation repair [sometimes many years after surgery][83a]), and hypercapnia and respiratory acidosis (as a result of absorption of CO_2 used in preparation for laparoscopic cholecystectomy).[84, 85] Pulmonary air embolism has also been described as a complication of the latter procedure.[85a]

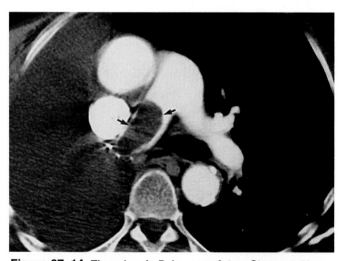

Figure 67–14. Thrombus in Pulmonary Artery Stump. A 79-year-old woman presented with a history of recurrent episodes of dyspnea after right pneumonectomy. Confirmation of the clinical diagnosis of recurrent pulmonary thromboembolism was made by ventilation-perfusion scintigraphy. A contrast-enhanced spiral CT scan demonstrates thrombus *(arrows)* within the right pulmonary artery stump, presumed to be the site of origin of the recurrent emboli. (Courtesy of Dr. J. Stephen Kwong, Richmond General Hospital, Richmond, British Columbia.)

COMPLICATIONS OF THERAPEUTIC PROCEDURES

Tracheostomy

Tracheal stenosis, tracheomalacia, and tracheal perforation are well-recognized complications of tracheostomy. The first of these is the most common and can occur at the level of the stoma or at the site at which an endotracheal tube impinged on the mucosa. The pathogenesis and radiologic and clinical manifestations are discussed in Chapter 52 (*see* page 2033). The efficacy of routine chest radiography was assessed in a retrospective chart review of 268 patients who had undergone tracheostomy;[85a] abnormalities were identified in only 9 patients (a small apical pneumothorax in 1 and foci of subsegmental atelectasis in 8). Detection of these abnormalities did not result in significant management changes.

Airway and Vascular Stents

Expandable metal or silicone stents have been used in the definitive or (more often) palliative therapy of a number of intrathoracic diseases.[86] The most common has been carcinoma, usually pulmonary[87–89] and occasionally esophageal.[90] Benign conditions causing airway stenosis, including airway compression secondary to congenital pulmonary artery aneurysm,[91] relapsing polychondritis,[92] tuberculosis,[93] postpneumonectomy syndrome,[94] and lung transplantation,[95, 96] have also been treated in this manner. Stenting of vascular stenoses as a result of congenital cardiovascular disease,[97–99] thromboemboli,[100] or lung transplantation[101] has also been used.

The incidence of complications associated with these stents is low. In one study of four patients who had wire stents inserted into the trachea or main bronchi for the control of tracheobronchial malacia, strut fracture and progressive airway widening were observed and suggested the possibility of airway perforation.[102] The formation of obstructing granulation tissue or mucous webs has been reported by some investigators.[103] Erosion of an esophageal stent into a bronchus has been associated with the development of recurrent pneumonia.[104] Recurrent vascular stenosis secondary to intimal fibrosis at the stent site has been reported in a small number of patients.[98] Focal pulmonary edema has also been documented during stent insertion into a stenotic pulmonary artery.[105]

Pulmonary hemorrhage following coronary artery stent placement has also been reported. In one study of 88 patients, the complication was diagnosed in 4 (5%);[106] the authors speculated it was related to anticoagulation therapy given to prevent stent thrombosis.

Brachytherapy

Complications of brachytherapy include mucosal fibrosis with bronchostenosis, localized radiation pneumonitis, bronchoesophageal fistula, and hemoptysis.[107–109] In one study of 46 patients who had received endobronchial brachytherapy, 4 (9%) developed self-limited radiation pneumonitis and 3 (7%) suffered fatal hemoptysis.[108] (The authors of this study, however, concluded that the former abnormality was probably the result of the external-beam irradiation that these patients had received because previous or concurrent external-beam irradiation did not correlate with an increased risk of fatal hemoptysis.) In a second study of 342 patients who had undergone brachytherapy (three fractions of 7.5 to 10 Gy at a calculated depth of 5 to 10 mm), 41 (12%) developed radiation bronchitis and stenosis.[109] At bronchoscopy, predominantly inflammatory changes were seen at a mean of about 16 weeks from the date of first brachytherapy, and predominantly fibrotic changes were seen after 40 weeks. Twenty-five patients (9%) developed fatal hemoptysis. Variables associated with an increased risk of complications included large cell carcinoma, prior laser photoresection, and concurrent external-beam irradiation.

Photodynamic Therapy

Photodynamic therapy is an experimental technique used primarily for abnormalities of the tracheobronchial mucosa, particularly malignancy such as early squamous cell carcinoma but also (in one case) hereditary hemorrhagic telangiectasia.[110–112] The procedure consists of systemic injection of a photosensitizer such as porfimer sodium, following which tumor is illuminated with light of a specific wavelength using a laser; the combination of the sensitizer and the light result in cell death. Skin photosensitivity is the most important factor limiting the use of the technique. Experimental studies of rat tracheas have shown mucosal necrosis with subsequent healing and no effect on cartilage, suggesting that airway perforation (at least with the doses used) is unlikely to occur.[113] This conclusion has been supported by an absence of serious complications in clinical series.[114] Despite these observations, a case of esophagopleural fistula has been reported as a complication of the treatment of mesothelioma.[115]

Laser Therapy

The use of lasers to ablate endobronchial or endotracheal tumor and re-establish airway patency has become a valuable means of palliation in selected patients who have pulmonary carcinoma and of primary therapy in some who have benign neoplasms or carcinoma *in situ*.[116] Several laser systems have been used, including carbon dioxide, argon, and neodymium:yttrium-aluminum-garnet (Nd-YAG); for various reasons, the last is the most useful. The mechanism of the Nd-YAG laser includes photocoagulation and thermal necrosis. Complications include hemorrhage from necrotic tumor or a vessel adjacent to the bronchial wall, perforation with bronchopleural fistula, and (in the healing stage) recurrent airway obstruction secondary to granulation tissue.[112] An endobronchial "fire" is an uncommon but dramatic event.[117]

Esophageal Procedures

Esophageal rupture occurs most commonly as a complication of esophagoscopy or gastroscopy[118] but also follows a variety of therapeutic procedures, such as dilation of a stricture or achalasia, esophageal resection and anastomosis (followed by disruption of the suture line), variceal sclerotherapy, or (rarely) passage of an esophageal obturator airway by paramedical personnel during cardiopulmonary resuscitation.[119] About 75% of esophageal ruptures are the result of such iatrogenic interventions; perforation occurs in 0.1% of all esophageal endoscopies, 5% of esophageal dilations, and 10% to 35% of Sengstaken-Blakemore tube placements.[120, 121] The most common sites of perforation are below the cricopharyngeal muscle, at the level of the left main bronchus, and immediately above the gastroesophageal junction.[120] Rupture can be associated with fistulas from the esophagus to the pleura, mediastinum, or bronchi, with corresponding consequences.

The usual result of esophageal rupture is acute mediastinitis, manifested radiographically by mediastinal widening that typically possesses a smooth, sharply defined margin. Other manifestations include pneumomediastinum, left pleural effusion, pneumothorax, hydropneumothorax, and chylothorax (Fig. 67–15).[122]

Clinical manifestations include chills, fever, subcutaneous emphysema in the soft tissues of the neck, or Hamman's sign on auscultation over the apex of the heart. Abscess formation, sometimes complicated by esophagobronchial or esophagopleural fistulas, may ensue, particularly if the diagnosis of rupture is delayed. In the latter situation, the pleural fluid contains a concentration of amylase that is higher than that of the blood because of contamination by saliva.

Pleural Plombage and Thoracoplasty

In the late nineteenth and early twentieth centuries, thoracoplasty was performed in many patients with pulmonary tuberculosis and in some with emphysema.[123] Although much less common today, it is still used occasionally for the former purpose;[124–126] as a somewhat less extensive operation, it is also used in the treatment of some patients with empyema.[127] The instillation of inert material, such as paraffin, adipose tissue, plastic, or Lucite spheres, in the pleural space (plombage) was used as a substitute for thoracoplasty in patients with tuberculosis to preserve lung function and engender less deformity. (Interestingly, the first recorded use of plombage may have been by Hippocrates more than 2,400 years ago when, for unknown reasons, he inserted a pig's bladder into a patient's chest and inflated it![128])

Both procedures have been associated with complications many years after the initial surgery. Thoracoplasty has been followed by *Aspergillus* infection of the residual pleural space, often in association with a bronchopleural fistula,[129, 130] and with primary pleural lymphoma.[131] A localized chest wall mass related to leakage of instilled material is the most common long-term complication of plombage;[132] some of these masses have become infected and have developed sinuses with the skin, mediastinum, and lung.[133] In one case, a Lucite ball passed through an esophageal fistula to the jejunum, where it caused intestinal obstruction.[128] Additional rare complications of plombage include bronchopleural fistula[134] and the development of carcinoma or sarcoma adjacent to the plombage space.[135, 136]

COMPLICATIONS OF INTUBATION AND MONITORING APPARATUS

The intubation and monitoring apparatus discussed in this section includes endotracheal tubes, transtracheal cathe-

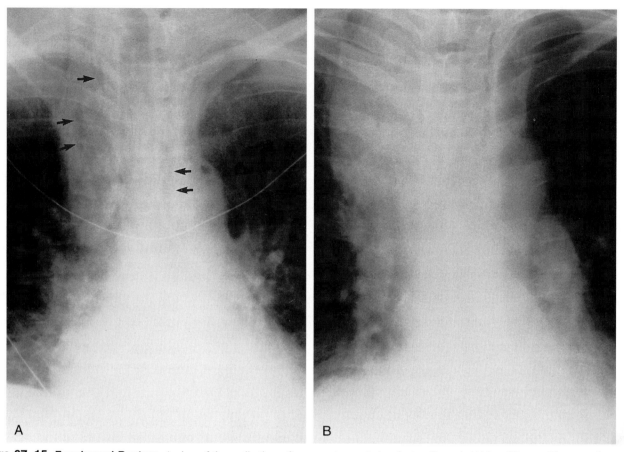

Figure 67–15. Esophageal Rupture. A view of the mediastinum from an anteroposterior chest radiograph *(A)* in a 39-year-old woman demonstrates pneumomediastinum *(arrows)* and mild mediastinal widening. A radiograph taken 5 days later *(B)* demonstrates increased mediastinal widening. Esophageal rupture at the level of the T1 vertebral body, which occurred during attempted endotracheal intubation, was confirmed by Gastrografin swallow.

ters, chest tubes for drainage of the pleural space, abdominal drainage tubes, nasogastric tubes, venous catheters for measurement of central venous pressure or for hyperalimentation, arterial catheters for measurement of pulmonary arterial and wedge pressures (Swan-Ganz), cardiac pacemaker leads, and the intra-aortic assist balloon.

Chest Drainage Tubes

Complications of chest drainage tubes are uncommon and are usually readily apparent clinically.[137, 138] They include laceration of an intercostal artery or vein; laceration of the diaphragm, liver, spleen, or stomach; malposition of the tube (such as in the chest wall, abdomen, or interlobar fissure); pulmonary perforation; infection (predominantly empyema); and formation of a systemic artery–pulmonary artery shunt.[137, 139–141]

Hemorrhage from a lacerated intercostal vessel can be avoided by insertion of the tube in the intercostal space as close as possible to the superior surface of a rib; however, intercostal vessels may be tortuous, especially in the elderly, and insertion elsewhere carries a risk.[139] Laceration of an intercostal vessel can also occur during insertion of a needle into the chest.

Malposition of the chest tube can occur within the pleural space, in which case the complication is only one of

inadequate drainage. Such malposition can occur in several ways. For example, a tube inserted anterolaterally and directed posteriorly will drain the posterior pleural space but, with the patient lying in a supine position, will not drain a pneumothorax situated anteriorly. Obviously, a drainage tube in any position will not drain a loculated accumulation of fluid or gas in an area not in communication with the tube's holes. The incidence of malposition of a chest tube within a major fissure probably is higher than generally believed.[142–144] Such malposition often cannot be convincingly recognized on a single anteroposterior radiograph; however, when drainage of a pneumothorax or hydrothorax is not occurring satisfactorily, the abnormal position can be confirmed, if necessary, by lateral radiography. In some cases, suboptimal tube positioning may be unrecognized even when frontal and lateral radiographs are obtained.[145, 146] CT may demonstrate such unexpected tube malplacement, including extrapleural location, intraparenchymal course, transdiaphragmatic course, trans-splenic course, and impingement on the trachea or posterior mediastinum.[145–147]

Although draining of intrafissural tubes may be suboptimal,[144] there is evidence that most chest tubes placed within interlobar fissures drain adequately. For example, in one prospective study of 58 consecutive patients who presented to the emergency department with chest trauma requiring tube thoracostomy, assessment of frontal and lateral radiographs showed 58% of tubes to be within an interlobar fissure;[148] no significant difference was found in the duration of thoracoscopy drainage, need for further tubes, or need for surgical intervention between patients whose tubes were located within a fissure and other patients. However, as the authors pointed out, although these observations would be applicable to patients with trauma or transudates, they would not be relevant for patients with empyema. In the latter situation, adhesions and loculation develop rapidly, and precise tube placement is important. Thus, although only frontal radiographs are required for assessment of chest tube location in most patients, both frontal and lateral radiographs are recommended after every tube insertion for empyema unless the tube was placed under CT or ultrasound guidance.[145, 148]

Pulmonary perforation is rarely recognized radiographically as a complication of tube insertion[137, 138] but can readily be detected on CT.[147] It is likely that the condition is underdi-

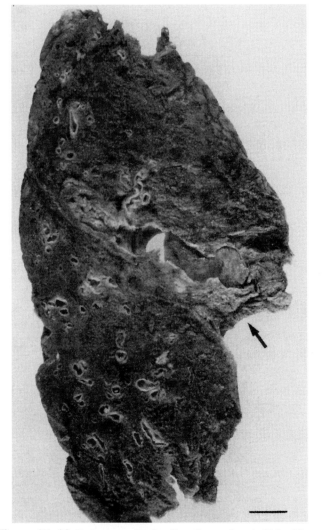

Figure 67–16. Pulmonary Perforation Secondary to Tube Thoracostomy. A section of right lung obtained at autopsy shows a linear track extending from the middle lobe *(arrow)* into the posterior aspect of the upper lobe. The patient was a 75-year-old man who had a thoracostomy tube inserted with aid of a trocar for spontaneous pneumothorax. He did not complain of chest pain, nor did he have hemoptysis. He died 7 weeks later. The origin of the track in the middle lobe corresponded to the chest wall scar where the tube had been inserted (bar = 1.5 cm). (From Fraser RS: Hum Pathol 19:512, 1988.)

agnosed. In one autopsy study in which three cases were identified, two were part of a series of 18 patients who had had chest tubes inserted and had subsequently died, because of underlying disease indicating an incidence of perforation of about 10%.[149] Such perforation is usually minimal in extent but is occasionally substantial (Fig. 67–16). It is often associated with the use of a trocar to aid tube insertion; underlying pulmonary parenchymal consolidation or fibrous interpleural adhesions appear to increase the risk, probably by decreasing or eliminating the possibility of the lung retracting when the pleural space is entered. Radiographic and clinical findings are absent in most cases; rarely, parenchymal hemorrhage can result in hemoptysis and the production of a linear opacity in the region of the chest tube.[149] In some cases, the complication only becomes apparent by the presence of a track after removal of the tube (Fig. 67–17). CT demonstrates the intraparenchymal location of the tube as well as the presence of associated laceration and hematoma[147] (Fig. 67–18). Care must be taken, however, in assessing the lung periphery, particularly near the lung apex and diaphragm, where partial volume averaging and indentation of the lung by a chest tube in the pleural space may mimic perforation.[147]

Infection of the pleural space related to the presence of a thoracostomy tube is uncommon; in one study of 1,249 trauma patients, it was documented in only 30 (2.4%).[137] A rare complication of closed-tube thoracostomy is systemic-to-pulmonary artery vascular shunt.[150–152] In one case, the fistula was fed by large, tortuous, intercostal artery collaterals originating from the lateral thoracic and thoracoacromial branches of the right axillary artery and anterior intercostal branches of the internal mammary artery;[152] the chest radiograph showed an ill-defined opacity projecting over the right-third anterior interspace. Aids to the diagnosis of this complication include the presence of a continuous murmur and radiographic evidence of unilateral rib notching.[153]

Other rare complications of chest tube insertion include Horner's syndrome,[154] necrotizing fasciitis of the chest wall in association with empyema,[155] and entrapment and "infarction" of pulmonary tissue within one of the side holes or the end hole of the tube.[156]

Abdominal Drainage Tubes

Potentially serious complications can follow transgression of the pleural space during placement of interventional drainage catheters into the liver and upper abdomen.[157, 158] Two groups of investigators have emphasized the importance of not puncturing the ninth intercostal space in the midaxillary line, because needles inserted through this interspace have traversed the pleura in virtually all cadaver studies.[157, 158] Complications of percutaneous catheter drainage of an abdominal abscess through the intercostal space include hemothorax, pneumothorax, and empyema.[158, 159]

Nasogastric Tubes

Because most nasogastric tubes are opaque, any malposition should be readily apparent radiographically. The two most common abnormalities are coiling within the esophagus

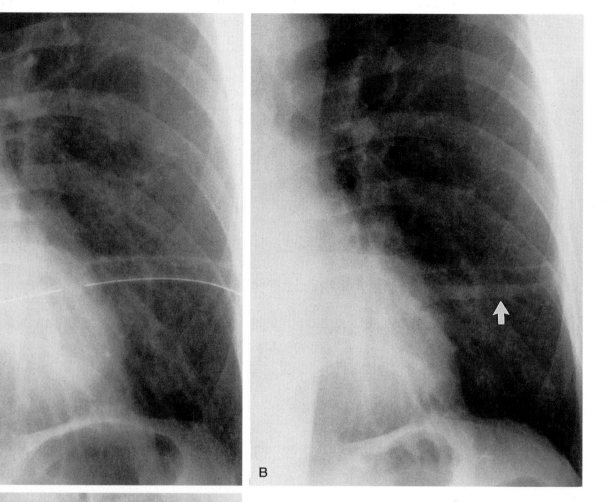

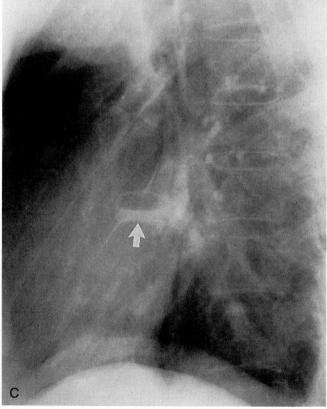

Figure 67–17. Chest Tube Track. A view of the left chest from an anteroposterior chest radiograph *(A)* in a 27-year-old man with spontaneous pneumothorax shows a left chest tube in an apparently adequate position. Posteroanterior *(B)* and lateral *(C)* radiographs taken after removal of the tube show a tube track *(arrows)* with a fluid level.

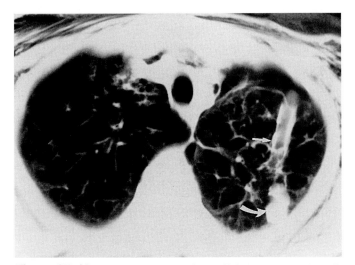

Figure 67–18. Intraparenchymal Chest Tube. A CT scan in a 69-year-old patient demonstrates a left chest tube *(straight arrow)* with its tip in the left upper lobe; a small hematoma *(curved arrow)* is present. Severe emphysema, a small left pneumothorax, pneumomediastinum, and subcutaneous emphysema are also evident.

into the esophagus, a complication that has been reported in about 0.2% to 0.3% of feeding tube placements[160–162] and that can lead to intrabronchial infusion of feedings, pneumonia, lung abscess, pneumothorax, hydropneumothorax, and empyema.[163–165] In these cases, the tip of the tube sometimes ends up in an unusual location, such as the mediastinum (Fig. 67–19) or abdomen (Fig. 67–20). Such malposition can be particularly hazardous if the tube is meant for hyperalimentation, because the injection of a large amount of fluid into the lungs or pleural cavity, rather than the stomach, can have disastrous consequences (Fig. 67–21).

Despite the presence of inflatable cuffs on endotracheal tubes, the low pressure within them does not prevent passage of the tube into the distal airways.[166] A patient receiving mechanical ventilation in whom a feeding tube has been inadvertently placed in the tracheobronchial tree close to the pleural surface is in danger of developing a large pneumothorax on removal of the tube.[167] In this situation, the attending physician or surgeon should be warned that the feeding tube may be acting as a "finger in the dike" and that insertion of a thoracostomy tube into the pleural space

and incomplete insertion; in each situation, the function of the nasogastric tube clearly is not being served. Of far greater clinical importance is the faulty insertion of the nasogastric tube into the tracheobronchial tree rather than

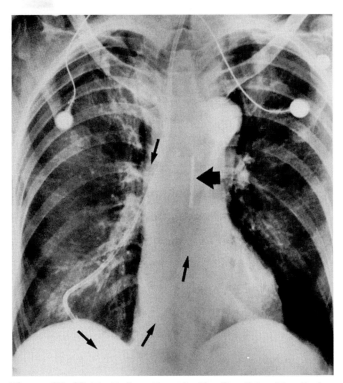

Figure 67–19. Faulty Insertion of a Feeding Tube. The circuitous course taken by this feeding tube can be established only partly from this anteroposterior radiograph. Obviously, it passed into the right lower lobe. As it turned to the left, it presumably penetrated the visceral pleura covering this lobe and then passed superiorly either within the mediastinum or in the pleural space adjacent to the azygoesophageal recess to a point where its tip overlies the region of the tracheal carina *(large arrow)*. Remarkably, the patient suffered no ill effects after removal of the tube.

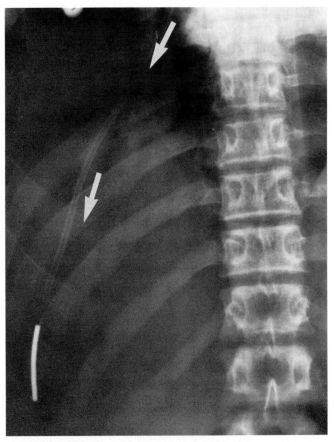

Figure 67–20. Faulty Insertion of a Feeding Tube. A view of the lower portion of the right hemithorax and upper abdomen in an anteroposterior projection reveals a feeding tube that has passed through the bronchi of the right lower lobe to a point projected over the lower portion of the liver and the posterolateral portion of the right tenth rib *(arrows indicate the course of the tube)*. Judging from this single projection, it is almost certain that the visceral pleura has been penetrated; however, whether the tip has penetrated the diaphragm was not established. After removal of the tube, the patient developed a right pneumothorax that required thoracostomy tube insertion; she subsequently developed a right-sided empyema that required thoracotomy for drainage.

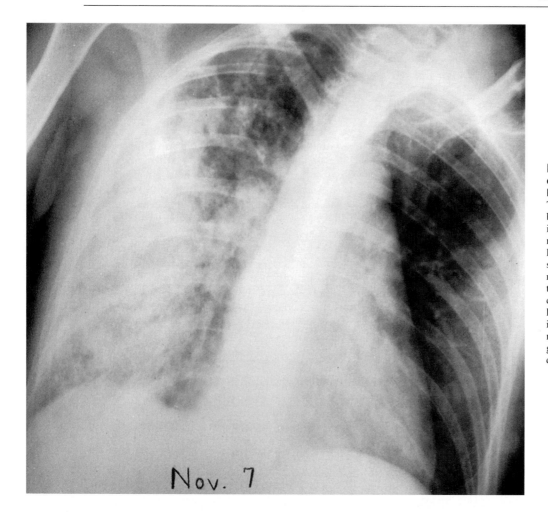

Nov. 7

Figure 67–21. Faulty Insertion of a Nasogastric Tube into the Right Tracheobronchial Tree. This middle-aged woman was brought to the emergency department in a coma after a drug overdose. A nasogastric tube was introduced to lavage the stomach, and 1,000 ml of saline was injected. An anteroposterior radiograph taken shortly thereafter reveals massive air-space consolidation throughout the right lung; the left lung is clear. The saline had been injected into the right lung through a malpositioned tube. Complete radiographic clearing had occurred 3 days later.

may be advisable before the feeding tube is withdrawn. Inadvertent placement of feeding tubes into the tracheobronchial tree, with subsequent insertion into the pleural space, appears to be a particular complication of the use of the narrow-bore nasogastric tube with stylet[168–170] and is most apt to occur in patients with impaired mental status or diminished gag, cough, or swallowing reflexes.[170, 171]

Endotracheal Tubes

During the first few days after insertion of an endotracheal tube, serious complications are infrequent; they occur more often in association with emergency resuscitation than with more routine interventions.[172] The chief complication is large airway obstruction resulting from malpositioning of the tube too low in the trachea or in the major bronchi. In most instances, the endotracheal tube enters the right main bronchus (in 27 of 28 cases in one series[172]), and the orifice of the left main bronchus is occluded by the balloon cuff of the endotracheal tube, resulting in complete obstruction and atelectasis of the left lung. If the tube is advanced sufficiently down into the right main bronchus, the right upper lobe bronchus may also be occluded, resulting in atelectasis of this lobe as well as the left lung or of the right upper lobe alone.[172] Occasionally, the tube enters the left rather than the right main bronchus, leading to atelectasis of the right lung.

The rate at which atelectasis occurs depends on the gas content of the lung at the moment of occlusion. Total collapse requires 18 to 24 hours if the parenchyma is air containing but may occur in a matter of minutes if the lung contains 100% oxygen (often the case in acute respiratory emergencies). Withdrawal of the tube typically results in rapid re-expansion of the collapsed lung or lobe.

With the head and neck in a neutral position, the ideal distance between the tip of the endotracheal tube and the carina is 5 ± 2 cm.[173] Flexion and extension of the neck cause a 2-cm descent and ascent, respectively, of the tip of the endotracheal tube; if the position of the neck can be established from the radiograph (through visualization of the mandible), the ideal distance between the tip of the endotracheal tube and the carina should be 3 ± 2 cm with the neck flexed and 7 ± 2 cm with the neck extended.[173] When the carina is not visualized, it is sufficient to establish the relationship of the tip of the endotracheal tube to the fifth, sixth, or seventh thoracic vertebral bodies; this relationship pertained in 92 of 100 patients whose bedside chest radiographs were reviewed in one study.[174]

The radiographic findings of airway obstruction by an endotracheal tube are typical and should present no difficulty in interpretation. Clinically, the examining physician should not be misled by hearing breath sounds transmitted from the normal or overinflated contralateral lung through the atelectatic lung.

Malpositioning of an endotracheal tube in the esophagus is uncommon and is usually evident clinically. Because the trachea and esophagus are superimposed on an anteroposterior radiograph, such malpositioning is seldom apparent radiographically; when present, findings include projection of the tip of the endotracheal tube lateral to the trachea, gaseous distention of the distal esophagus or stomach, and (rarely) deviation of the trachea by an overinflated balloon cuff[175] (Fig. 67–22).

Traumatic intubation may result in injury to the larynx or trachea. Most often, this is relatively localized and limited to the mucosa; occasionally, it is more extensive and associated with necrosis of the entire tracheal wall.[176] Perforation of the trachea usually involves the posterior (membranous) wall and results in subcutaneous emphysema, pneumomediastinum, and pneumothorax; additional complications include mediastinitis, cervical abscess, and mediastinal abscess.[177] Persistent angulation of the endotracheal tube can lead to tracheal ulceration and eventual perforation by the tip of the tube. Persistent anterolateral angulation can result in a tracheoinnominate or tracheocarotid fistula, whereas persistent posterior angulation can result in a tracheoesophageal fistula.[177] Additional rare complications of tracheal intubation include cardiac arrhythmia[178] and trachea and innominate artery fistulas.[176]

Complications that result from prolonged inflation of the cuff of an endotracheal tube, such as tracheal stenosis, are discussed in Chapter 52 in relation to large airway obstruction (*see* page 2033).

Transtracheal Catheters

The use of long-term indwelling transtracheal catheters to administer oxygen to patients with COPD was developed in the 1980s to cut the cost and increase the ease of home oxygen care.[179] The catheters may be inserted directly into the trachea through the skin of the neck (percutaneous catheters) or may be implanted through an incision in the suprasternal notch, stitched to the tracheal wall, and tunneled under the skin to exit in the upper abdomen (tunneled catheters).[179]

Complications of such transtracheal catheters include subcutaneous emphysema, localized skin infection or hemorrhage, abnormal tracheal mucus production, breakage of catheter parts into the trachea, and formation of partly occlusive mucous or mucopurulent plugs around the catheter tip.[180, 181] Increase in the size or dislodgment of such a plug may result in tracheal or bronchial obstruction that can significantly compromise air flow.[181, 182]

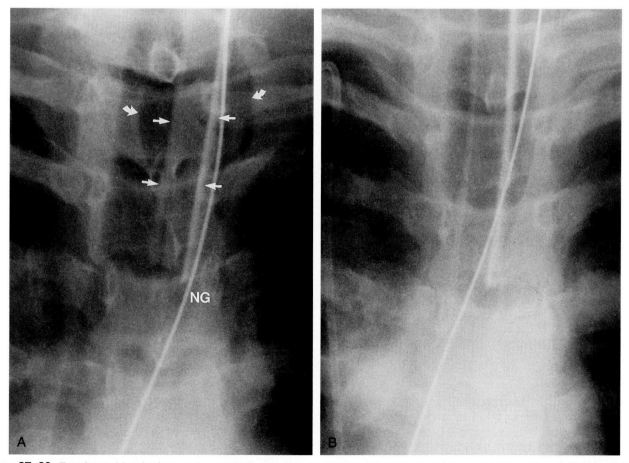

Figure 67–22. Esophageal Intubation. A view of the thoracic inlet from an anteroposterior chest radiograph *(A)* in a 22-year-old patient following a motor vehicle accident demonstrates an endotracheal tube *(straight arrows)* lying lateral to the trachea and in close proximity to the nasogastric tube (NG); the appearance is consistent with esophageal intubation. Note the inflated cuff of endotracheal tube *(curved arrows)*. A view after reintubation *(B)* shows a normal endotracheal position.

Percutaneous Central Venous Catheters

Several extensive reviews of the literature have been published on the complications of central venous catheterization,[182a, 183–186] and the reader cannot avoid being impressed by their great variety and potentially serious consequences. Some complications pertain to the catheterization procedure itself and relate to abnormalities within or around the catheterized vein; others—perhaps most—arise from incorrect positioning of the tip of the catheter.

Faulty Insertion

Central venous catheters can be inserted through an arm vein, a subclavian vein (by either an infraclavicular or supraclavicular route), or an external or internal jugular vein. Most faulty placements occur in arm and infraclavicular subclavian approaches. Only about 65% to 75% of catheters reach their proper location following arm vein insertion; the results through external jugular placement are even less satisfactory.[187] Supraclavicular, subclavian, and internal jugular approaches result in a relatively small percentage of improper placements. In one review, only 186 (62%) of 300 central venous lines were positioned in the subclavian or innominate veins or superior vena cava at the time of the initial chest radiograph obtained immediately after catheterization.[188] Of the remainder, 48 (16%) were in the internal jugular vein (Fig. 67–23), 39 (13%) in the right atrium or right ventricle, 2 in the azygous vein, 1 in a left-sided superior vena cava that drained into the coronary sinus, and 2 coiled in the subclavian vein; 22 were in extrathoracic sites other than the internal jugular vein. In none of these cases was the incorrect position recognized clinically. The problem with faulty placement is that pressure recorded in the jugular vein is not equivalent to central venous pressure. Because it is often within the normal range and may show only slightly diminished dynamics, however, it is unlikely that the malposition of the catheter can be recognized through pressure measurements alone.

Phlebothrombosis

Phlebothrombosis is probably the most common complication of venous catheterization and can be manifested in two ways: sleeve thrombosis and mural thrombosis.[182a] Autopsy studies have shown that circumferential fibrin sleeves develop around indwelling venous catheters as early as 24 hours after insertion in 80% to 100% of cases.[188a, b] Although this seldom gives rise to symptoms or signs, parts of the thrombus may embolize to the lungs, particularly as the catheter is removed.[182a, 188b, 189]

Mural thrombosis can lead to partial or complete venous obstruction.[188b] It has been estimated that venous catheters account for 30% to 40% of axillary and subclavian venous obstructions in the United States.[190, 191] In an autopsy series of 139 burn patients who had thoracic venous catheters, 37% had central venous thrombosis.[192] In one investigation of 204 patients in the intensive care unit who had internal jugular or subclavian catheters, color Doppler ultrasound examination performed just before or within 24 hours of catheter removal showed thrombosis at the catheter site in 33%.[252] The thrombus was limited (2 to 4 mm) in 8%, large ($\geq$ 4 mm) in 22%, and occlusive in 3%. The risk of

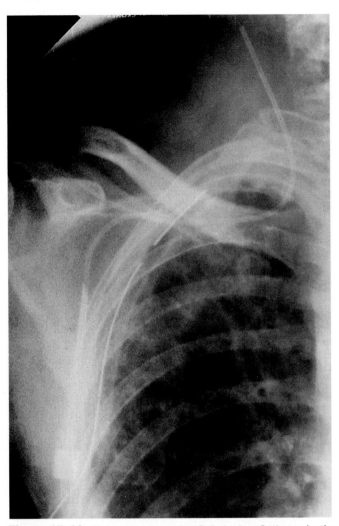

Figure 67–23. Malpositioning of a Subclavian Catheter in the Jugular Vein. The catheter occupies a correct position in the subclavian vein but then ascends the jugular vein. Central venous pressure cannot be properly recorded with a catheter in this position.

catheter-associated sepsis was 2.6-fold greater when thrombus was present. The prevalence of venous obstruction is related to the duration in which the catheter is left in place; as many as 75% of thoracic venous catheters cause mural thrombosis after 14 days.[189] Complications of the thrombosis include loss of central venous access, superior vena cava syndrome, septic thrombophlebitis, and pulmonary thromboembolism.[188b, 190, 191]

The radiographic findings are neither sensitive nor specific and include enlargement of the vena cava, pleural effusion, and dilated collateral vessels (including the arch of the azygous vein or left superior intercostal vein).[188b] The diagnosis can be confirmed by venography, color-flow Doppler ultrasonography, CT, or MR imaging.[188b, 193–196] All these modalities have limitations, and the technique of choice is influenced by the suspected localization of the thrombosis, cost, and local experience. Venography allows diagnosis of partial and complete obstruction, but does not permit confident distinction of intrinsic from extrinsic compression. This distinction can be readily made on CT or MR imaging; however, both procedures may fail to demonstrate small nonocclusive thrombi that are readily seen on phlebography.[182a] Color-flow Doppler has been shown to be an accurate noninvasive method;[182a, 194] its major limitation is inability to image the midportion of the subclavian veins and superior vena cava.[182a]

Although most venous thromboses are sterile, catheter-related septic thrombosis may also occur, particularly in patients who have long-term indwelling central venous catheters.[185] These catheters are inserted into a central vein and advanced so that the distal tip lies just above the level of the right atrium; the proximal portion is tunneled subcutaneously to a skin exit site (e.g., the Hickman catheter) or to a subcutaneous reservoir on the anterior chest wall (e.g., the Mediport or Broviac catheter).[185] It has been estimated that the incidence of infections associated with the long-term use of central venous catheters is between 15% and 20% in most institutions, or about 1.4 infections per 1,000 patient days of catheter use.[185] This incidence is considerably lower than that of other catheters, including peripheral lines and Swan-Ganz catheters.[185] One of the most important factors associated with infection is catheter thrombosis: in a review of 129 cases of Hickman catheter infections, 5 of 6 catheters with thrombosis were infected, as compared with only 10 of 123 catheters without evidence of thrombosis.[197] Other infectious complications include mediastinitis, osteomyelitis of the clavicle, and exit site or tunnel infections.[185]

Perforation of a Vein

A vein can be perforated either at the time of catheter insertion[198–200] or some time later;[201–203] late perforation is caused by gradual erosion of a relatively thin-walled intra-thoracic vessel by the catheter, partly as a result of cardiac and respiratory movements affecting the catheter tip.[204] Most perforations occur after introduction of catheters for pressure measurements and hyperalimentation; they occur less often with electrode insertion for cardiac pacing[205] and with catheter placement for providing vascular access for plasmapheresis and hemodialysis.[206]

Depending on the vein involved, perforation can result in pneumothorax, hemothorax, hydrothorax, mediastinal hemorrhage (Fig. 67–24), bronchopulmonary-venous fistula, or extrapleural hematoma[186, 200, 207–209] (Fig. 67–25). Unilateral pneumothorax is undoubtedly the most common of these. A particularly serious consequence is bilateral pneumothorax,[198] a complication that arises when an unsuspected perforation with consequent pneumothorax occurs in an unsuccessful attempt on one side followed by induction of a pneumothorax with a catheter insertion on the contralateral side. Rarely, pleural effusion also is bilateral and massive.[203, 210, 211] It is obvious that when venous perforation occurs into the pleura, lung, or mediastinum, patients receiving hyperalimentation are at greater risk of serious complications[184, 212] (Fig. 67–26). "Pneumonia" has been reported after the development of a venopulmonary fistula,[213] and lung abscess has occurred after passage of a catheter through the heart and pulmonary artery.[214]

Vascular erosion by central venous catheters usually affects the superior vena cava and is considerably more common with left-sided catheters: in one review of 61 patients with catheter-induced hydrothorax, the route of catheterization was left sided in 74% and right sided in 26%.[186] It

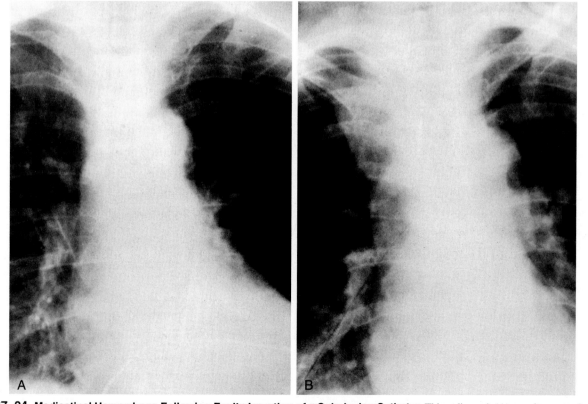

Figure 67–24. Mediastinal Hemorrhage Following Faulty Insertion of a Subclavian Catheter. This radiograph *(A)* reveals a normal appearance of the upper mediastinum. Three days later *(B)*, after attempted insertion of a right subclavian line, there has occurred moderate widening of the superior mediastinum as a result of venous hemorrhage secondary to perforation of a vein by the catheter.

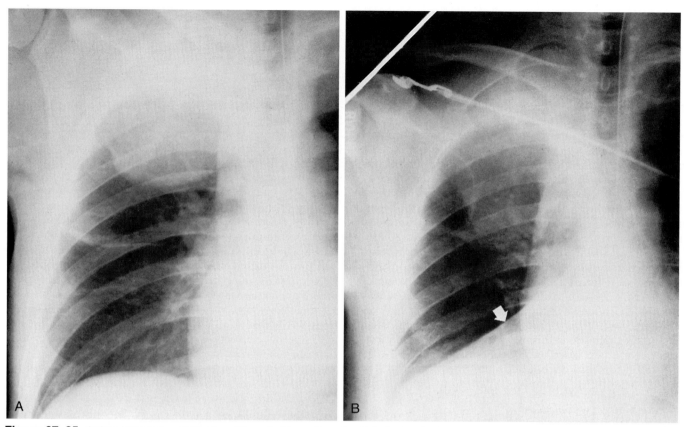

Figure 67–25. Apical Hematoma Following Attempted Insertion of a Subclavian Catheter. Several hours after attempted insertion of a right subclavian catheter, an anteroposterior radiograph *(A)* reveals a large homogeneous opacity in the upper third of the right hemithorax (a previous radiograph was normal). One week later *(B)*, the opacity is slightly larger and less well defined. Coincidentally, there had developed complete airlessness of the right lower lobe caused by atelectasis, presumably from an obstructing mucous plug *(arrow* points to downward displaced major fissure).

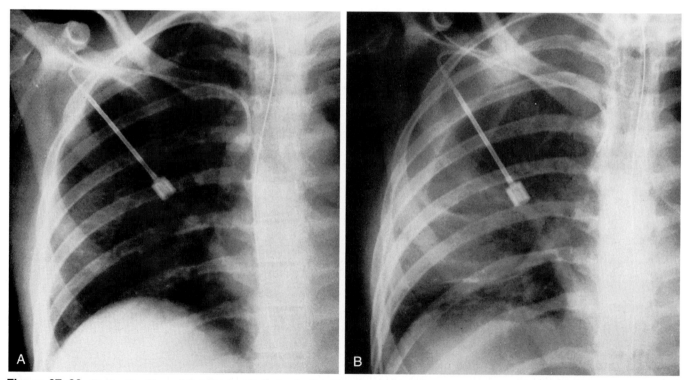

Figure 67–26. Faulty Position of Subclavian Catheter in the Pleural Space. Immediately after insertion of a right subclavian catheter, an anteroposterior radiograph *(A)* reveals the tip to lie in a position consistent with the superior vena cava, although it could be argued that it is more medial than usual. After injection of several hundred milliliters of fluid for hyperalimentation, a second radiograph exposed in the supine position *(B)* reveals a large accumulation of fluid in the right pleural space, indicating that the tip of the catheter had perforated the vein and mediastinal parietal pleura.

has been postulated that the predisposition of left-sided catheters to perforate derives from the horizontal orientation of the left brachiocephalic vein compared with the right. As a consequence, the tip of a left-sided catheter inserted an insufficient length tends to abut against the right lateral wall of the superior vena cava within 45 degrees of perpendicular.[186] An early sign of impending perforation of the superior vena cava is a gentle curvature of the distal portion of the catheter with the tip directed toward the right lateral vein wall.[204] Venous erosion may also occur with catheter tips located in the right and left brachiocephalic veins.[186]

Air embolism has also been reported as a complication of subclavian vein catheterization, during either insertion or withdrawal of the catheter.[215–217] In fact, asymptomatic air embolism is probably a common complication following central or peripheral vein injection of any kind[218] (Fig. 67–27). In one study of 100 patients who underwent contrast-enhanced CT (contrast was injected through a 19-gauge needle inserted into either a hand or forearm vein), venous air embolism was detected in 23% of patients.[218] In 20, the amount of air was minimal, consisting of small bubbles of air within the blood; however, the amount of air was sufficient to form air-fluid levels in the other 3 patients. The amount of air in all cases was considered to be only a few milliliters, and no patients had symptoms.

Perforation of the Myocardium

It is not uncommon for the tip of a central venous catheter to reside in one of the right heart chambers; for example, in one investigation of 300 patients, it was identified in the right atrium or right ventricle in 40 (13%).[188] This is obviously a potentially hazardous position, particularly if the catheter has a firm or sharp tip; perforation of the atrium

or ventricle may result in fatal pericardial tamponade (from either blood or infused fluid),[219] and irritation of the myocardium may cause arrhythmias.

Catheter Coiling, Knotting, and Breaking

Coiled catheters traumatize the vein and are much more likely to perforate, break, and embolize (Figs. 67–28 and 67–29). They also show a much greater tendency to twist into knots; although these can sometimes be manipulated free, this is not always possible, and thoracotomy is occasionally required for removal.[220]

Miscellaneous Complications

Other complications of percutaneous central venous catheter insertion include sepsis,[207, 221] embolization of catheter fragments to the lungs[207, 221, 222] (Fig. 67–30), thoracic duct laceration,[207] entanglement in an intravenous filter inserted to prevent pulmonary thromboemboli,[223] and damage to the brachial plexus, sympathetic chain, or phrenic, recurrent laryngeal, or ninth to twelfth cranial nerves.[207, 221, 224, 225]

Indwelling Balloon-Tipped Pulmonary Arterial Catheters

Flow-directed balloon-tipped (Swan-Ganz) catheters for monitoring circulatory hemodynamics in critically ill patients have been used with increasing frequency since their first description in 1970.[226] Complications associated with their use have been reviewed by several groups[227–230] and include atrial and ventricular arrhythmias, rupture of the balloon, knotting of the catheter, perforation of the pulmonary artery, perforation of the visceral pleura (resulting in

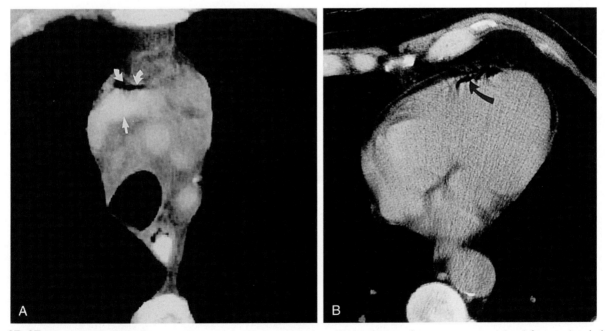

Figure 67–27. Venous Air Embolism. A CT scan in a 65-year-old patient *(A)* demonstrates intravenous contrast *(straight arrow)* and air *(curved arrows)* within the left brachiocephalic vein. Injection of air presumably occurred concomitantly with injection of contrast. A CT scan in another patient *(B)* demonstrates air *(curved arrow)* within the right ventricle. In this patient, the scan was performed after starting an intravenous infusion of saline. Neither patient developed symptoms.

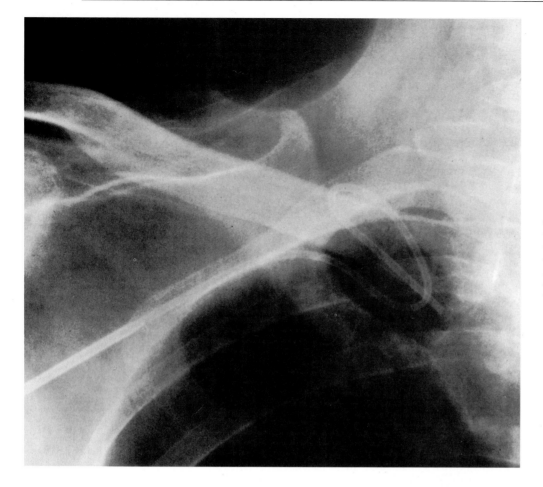

Figure 67–28. Malpositioning (Coiling) of a Subclavian Catheter. An anteroposterior radiograph of the apical portion of the right hemithorax reveals a subclavian catheter that has coiled through a 360-degree arc. It is almost certain that the tip of this catheter does not lie within the subclavian vein.

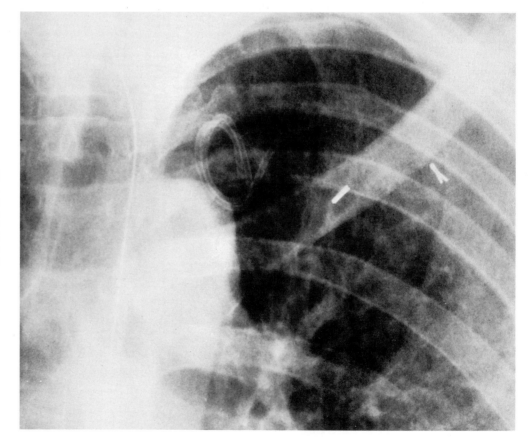

Figure 67–29. Broken Central Venous Pressure (CVP) Line. A tightly coiled CVP catheter can be identified overlying the upper portion of the left lung. The catheter had broken at its point of entry and had retracted inward to constitute a foreign body in the soft tissues of the anterior chest wall.

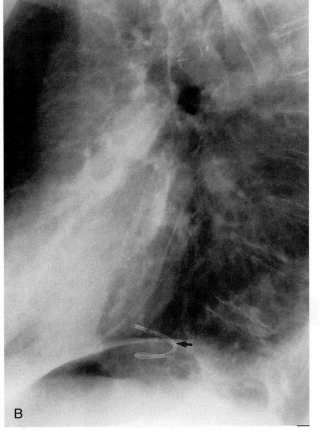

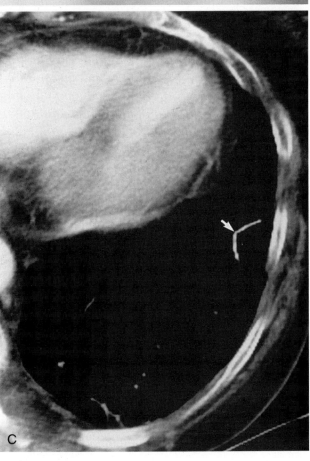

Figure 67–30. Embolization of Broken Central Venous Line. Views of the left lung from posteroanterior *(A)* and lateral *(B)* chest radiographs and a CT scan *(C)* demonstrate the broken distal portion of an intravenous catheter *(arrows)* in the left lower lobe. The tip presumably lies within a pulmonary artery. The patient did not have symptoms, and the catheter was left in place; no associated symptoms were observed over a 4-year follow-up.

pneumothorax or hemothorax[230, 231]), false aneurysms of the pulmonary artery,[232-234] tears of the pulmonary valve,[235] pulmonary artery occlusion with pulmonary infarction, and air embolism.[236] The catheters can also act as a nidus for bacterial colonization[237] and platelet consumption,[238] with the potential of causing sepsis or contributing to hemorrhage. As a group, these events are not rare; in one prospective study of 528 catheterizations, serious complications were considered to have occurred in 23 (4.4%).[239]

Pulmonary artery occlusion, with or without infarction, is probably the most common pulmonary complication. In one series of 125 patients undergoing catheterization, some sort of ischemic lesion was identified in 9 patients (7.2%);[228] in another review of 391 patients, evidence of thromboembolism was found in 16 (4%).[240] Pulmonary artery occlusion can result from one or more of four mechanisms: (1) irrita-

tion of the endothelium of the vena cava, right-sided heart chambers, or a major pulmonary artery by the catheter tip or inflated balloon, resulting in thrombus formation and subsequent embolization; (2) formation of thrombus around the distal end of the catheter itself, followed by embolization; (3) prolonged inflation of the balloon for recording of wedge pressure, resulting in peripheral ischemia and infarction; and (4) tightening of a large intracardiac loop of the catheter by hemodynamic action, followed by propulsion of the tip of the catheter to a point where it occludes a small peripheral artery with resultant infarction (Fig. 67–31). The last mechanism can be avoided if the technique described by Swan and associates is strictly adhered to—the balloon is inflated as soon as a large-caliber vein is encountered, and the catheter is permitted to float into the pulmonary artery.[241]

The incidence of pulmonary artery occlusion rises

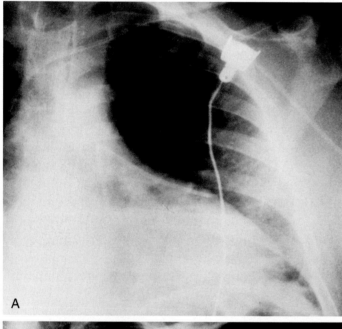

Figure 67–31. Pulmonary Infarction Associated with a Swan-Ganz Catheter. In the anteroposterior radiograph *(A)*, a Swan-Ganz catheter is in position in the left lower lobe, its tip in a position consistent with a subsegmental artery. Twenty-four hours later *(B)*, the intrapulmonary extent of the catheter had increased considerably, such that its tip now lies less than 2 cm from the visceral pleural surface. Several days later *(C)*, a wedge-shaped opacity had appeared in the left axillary lung zone, which was highly suggestive of a pulmonary infarct; its position corresponds precisely to what was undoubtedly an impacted Swan-Ganz catheter tip.

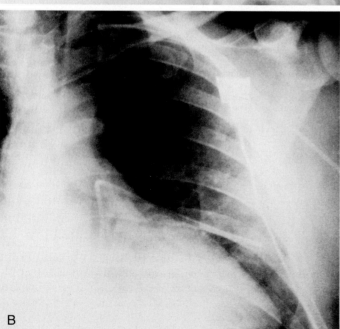

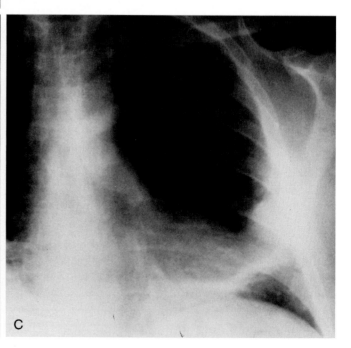

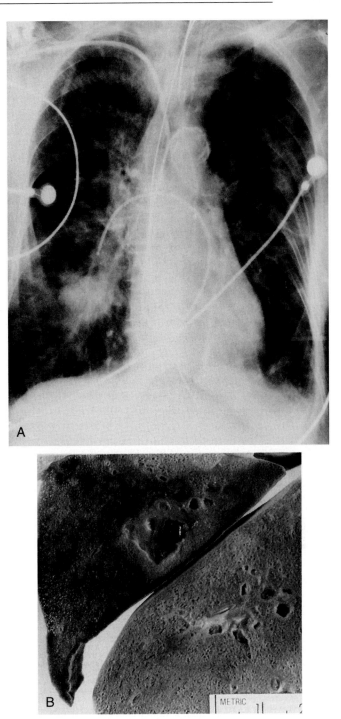

Figure 67–32. Pulmonary Artery Perforation by a Swan-Ganz Catheter. A posteroanterior radiograph *(A)* shows the tip of a Swan-Ganz catheter in the region of the right interlobar artery. Distal to it is a fairly well-defined opacity that could be situated in either the middle or lower lobe. Shortly thereafter, this 83-year-old woman coughed up a small amount of blood and died. At autopsy, the right middle lobe *(B)* showed extensive air-space hemorrhage and a defect in a subsegmental pulmonary artery associated with an irregularly shaped intraparenchymal hematoma. (From Fraser RS: Hum Pathol 18:1246, 1987.)

sharply as the length of time the catheter is left *in situ* increases. For example, in one series, all five patients in whom the catheter was maintained in position for more than 72 hours developed infarcts.[229] Two cases have been reported in which septic infarction occurred distal to the catheter tip, with resultant abscess formation and the development of large cavities after expulsion of liquefied material into the tracheobronchial tree.[242]

Although it has been estimated that the pulmonary artery is perforated in only about 0.001% to 0.5% of all cases of catheter insertion,[243] there is evidence that it may be a more common event. For example, in one autopsy review, 4 such cases were identified in a consecutive series of 270 cases (1.5%);[244] in only 1 was the perforation suspected clinically. The most common clinical situation associated with perforation is cardiac surgery, an observation attributed to one or more of three factors: (1) shrinkage of heart chambers as a result of evacuation of blood with distal migration of the catheter during surgery; (2) cooling of the perfusate and cardiovascular tissue leading to increased rigidity of the tubing and vessel walls; and (3) manipulation of the heart causing increased movement of the catheter.[245]

As might be expected, the usual result of pulmonary artery perforation is hemorrhage, generally into pulmonary parenchyma but on occasion predominantly into the bronchovascular interstitium or pleural space.[246] Only a few cases have been examined pathologically;[244] in many, the site of rupture has been undetected, whereas in others, a localized intraparenchymal hematoma or nodule of intraparenchymal thrombus (false aneurysm) reveals the location (Fig. 67–32).

Shortly after pulmonary artery perforation, the chest radiograph may show localized areas of consolidation with hazy margins.[234, 247] The consolidation is replaced within 1 to 3 weeks by a round, well-circumscribed nodule or mass ranging from 2 to 8 cm in diameter, corresponding to the development of a false aneurysm.[234, 247] Contrast-enhanced CT demonstrates the latter as an enhancing mass associated with a vessel and sometimes containing a partially thrombosed lumen.[234, 248, 249] The mass may be surrounded by a halo of ground-glass attenuation as a result of recent hemorrhage.[234, 250] The chest radiograph may be unremarkable or show nonspecific findings: in one review of seven false aneurysms in five patients, chest radiographs were unremarkable in two and revealed focal consolidation in one and a pulmonary mass consistent with false aneurysm in two.[234] The diagnosis can be readily confirmed with pulmonary angiography.[234]

Perforation should be suspected whenever a new airspace opacity develops in association with hemoptysis,[231, 251, 253] which can be massive.[254, 255] The mortality rate associated with clinically evident pulmonary artery perforation has been estimated to be 45% to 65%.[256] Patients who develop false aneurysms can also have recurrent life-threatening hemorrhage; the rate of this complication has been estimated to be about 30% to 40% and the mortality rate 40% to 70%.[234, 257]

The prime purpose of the Swan-Ganz catheter is the determination of pressure within the pulmonary artery and within the left atrium as measured through the wedged catheter. It has been shown in both experimental animals[258] and humans at the time of open heart surgery[259] that when the tip of the catheter is positioned at or above the level of the left atrium, the wedge pressure measured by the catheter is not an accurate estimate of left atrial pressure when positive end-expiratory pressure (PEEP) is being administered; in such positions, the catheter consistently recorded pressures higher than left atrial pressure. In all other situations in which catheters were located below the left atrium, they were accurate at every level of PEEP tested. The admonition is obvious: when PEEP is being used, the position of a Swan-Ganz catheter should be confirmed by a lateral chest radiograph; when the catheter is situated anterior to the level of the left atrium, it should be repositioned.

Intra-aortic Counterpulsation Balloons

The intra-aortic counterpulsation balloon catheter has been used in conditions characterized by low-output cardiac decompensation and cardiogenic shock. It provides augmentation of diastolic coronary artery perfusion as well as reduced impedance to ventricular ejection.[260, 261] Reported complications resulting from its use include aortic dissection, laceration, and subadventitial hematoma formation; red blood cell destruction; embolic phenomena, such as vascular insufficiency of the catheterized limb; and balloon rupture

with secondary gas embolism.[261, 262] The most common complication observed by radiologists is improper positioning.[165] The ideal position of the tip is just distal to the origin of the left subclavian artery. A more proximal position can occlude the left subclavian artery, and one more distal can result in decreased effectiveness of diastolic counterpulsation. Angulation of the catheter tip suggests incorrect positioning within the transverse portion of the aortic arch.[165]

Cardiac Pacemakers

The impact that radiology can make in determining the cause of pacemaker malfunction and in the evaluation of lead position and integrity can be considerable and has been reviewed.[263–265] Complications include electrode malposition, redundant or taut leads, infection of the subcutaneous pacemaker pouch or along the lead, myocardial perforation, pneumothorax, pleural effusion, and fracture of the lead.[264, 265] Wire fracture causes loss of pacing and the potential risk of embolism of the distal segment to the pulmonary artery.[165] Venous thrombosis may lead to partial or complete occlusion of the subclavian and brachiocephalic veins or superior vena cava[264, 265] (Fig. 67–33). The complications from automatic

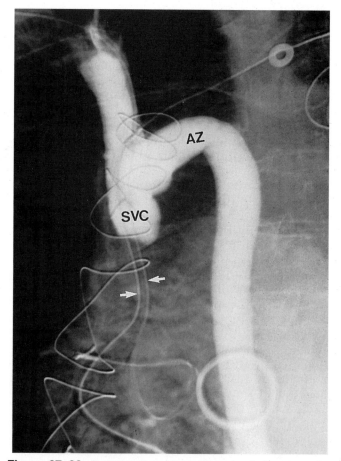

Figure 67–33. Superior Vena Cava Thrombosis Due to a Cardiac Pacemaker. A view of a digital venogram demonstrates complete obstruction of the superior vena cava (SVC) and collateral flow through the azygos vein (AZ). The patient had undergone insertion of sequential atrioventricular pacemaker leads *(arrows)* 11 years previously and had subsequently developed the SVC syndrome.

implantable cardioverter defibrillators have also been reviewed[266] and include hemoptysis as a result of erosion of the ventricular patch into a bronchus.[267, 268]

COMPLICATIONS OF DIAGNOSTIC BIOPSY PROCEDURES

Pleuropulmonary complications of diagnostic biopsy procedures, such as transbronchial biopsy, transthoracic needle aspiration, and closed-chest pleural biopsy, are well known. Because these procedures necessarily cause tissue disruption to obtain material for diagnosis, infiltration of air or blood into the pleural cavity, mediastinum, lung parenchyma, or bronchovascular interstitium is, to some extent, an inevitable consequence. In most instances, the extent of this infiltration is limited, so that related clinical problems are minimal or nonexistent. Details of the incidence and type of complications with the different procedures are discussed at greater length in Chapters 14 and 15.

REFERENCES

1. Goodman LR, Kay HR, Teplick SK, et al: Complications of median sternotomy: Computed tomographic evaluation. Am J Roentgenol 141:225, 1983.
2. Carrol CL, Jeffrey RB Jr, Federle MP, et al: CT evaluation of mediastinal infections. J Comput Assist Tomogr 11:449, 1987.
3. Serry C, Bleck PC, Javid H, et al: Sternal wound complications: Management and results. J Thorac Cardiovasc Surg 80:861, 1980.
4. Templeton PA, Fishman EK: CT evaluation of poststernotomy complications. Am J Roentgenol 159:45, 1992.
5. Goodman LR: Review: Postoperative chest radiograph. II. Alterations after major intrathoracic surgery. Am J Roentgenol 134:803, 1980.
6. Curtis JA, Libshitz HI, Dalinka MK: Fracture of the first rib as a complication of midline sternotomy. Radiology 115:63, 1975.
7. Greenwald LV, Baisden CE, Symbas PN. Rib fractures in coronary artery bypass patients: Radionuclide detection. Radiology 48:553, 1983.
8. Hanson RE, Kloiber R, Lesperance RR, et al: Unpublished data.
9. Tsukada G, Start P: Postpneumonectomy complications. Am J Roentgenol 169:1363, 1997.
10. Biondetti PR, Fiore D, Sartore F, et al: Evaluation of the postpneumonectomy space by computed tomography. Comput Assist Tomogr 6:238, 1982.
11. Laissy JP, Rebibo G, Iba-Zizen MT, et al: MR appearance of the normal chest after pneumonectomy. J Comput Assist Tomogr 13:248, 1989.
12. Heelan RT, Panicek DM, Burt ME, et al: Magnetic resonance imaging of the postpneumonectomy chest: Normal and abnormal findings. J Thorac Imaging 12:200, 1997.
13. Williams NS, Lewis CT: Bronchopleural fistula: A review of 86 cases. Br J Surg 63:520, 1976.
14. Asamura H, Naruke T, Tsuchiya R, et al: Bronchopleural fistulas associated with lung cancer operations. Univariate and multivariate analysis of risk factors, management, and outcome. J Thorac Cardiovasc Surg 104:1456, 1992.
15. Hollaus PH, Lax F, el-Nashef BB, et al: Natural history of bronchopleural fistula after pneumonectomy: A review of 96 cases. Ann Thorac Surg 63:1391, 1997.
16. Leading article: Bronchopleural fistula. BMJ 2:1093, 1976.
17. Heater K, Revzani L, Rubin JM: CT evaluation of empyema in the postpneumonectomy space. Am J Roentgenol 145:39, 1985.
17a. Westcott JL, Volpe JP: Peripheral bronchopleural fistula: CT evaluation in 20 patients with pneumonia, empyema, or postoperative air leak. Radiology 196:175, 1995.
17b. Stern EJ, Sun H, Haramati LB: Peripheral bronchopleural fistulas: CT imaging features. Am J Roentgenol 167:117, 1996.
18. Wechsler RJ: CT of esophageal-pleural fistulae. Am J Roentgenol 147:907, 1986.
19. Wechsler RJ, Steiner RM, Goodman LR, et al: Iatrogenic esophageal-pleural fistula: Subtlety of diagnosis in the absence of mediastinitis. Radiology 144:239, 1982.
20. Heiken JP, Balfe DM, Roper CL: CT evaluation after esophagogastrectomy. Am J Roentgenol 143:555, 1984.
21. Westcott JL, Cole SR: Interstitial pulmonary emphysema in children and adults: Roentgenographic features. Radiology 111:367, 1974.
22. Henry DA, Jolles H, Berberich JJ, et al: The post-cardiac surgery chest radiograph: A clinically integrated approach. J Thorac Imaging 4:20, 1989.
23. Carter AR, Sostman HD, Curtis AM, et al: Thoracic alterations after cardiac surgery. Am J Roentgenol 140:475, 1983.
24. Doyle MT, Spizarny DL, Baker DE: Saphenous vein graft aneurysm after coronary artery bypass surgery. Am J Roentgenol 168:747, 1997.
25. Benya EC, Joseph AE, Nemcek AA: Mediastinal mass after coronary artery bypass surgery with internal mammary artery grafts. J Thorac Imaging 6:40, 1991.
26. Scott WW, Beall DP, Wheeler PS: The retained intrapericardial sponge: Value of the lateral chest radiograph. Am J Roentgenol 171:595, 1998.
27. Bhalla M, Wain JC, Shepard JAO, et al: Surgical flaps in the chest: Anatomic considerations, applications, and radiologic appearance. Radiology 192:825, 1994.
28. Coppage L, Jolles H, Wornom IL III: Computed tomography findings in patients who have undergone muscle flap and omental transposition procedures in the treatment of poststernotomy mediastinitis. J Thorac Imaging 9:14, 1994.
29. Peters JC, Desai KK: CT demonstration of postpneumonectomy tumor recurrence. Am J Roentgenol 141:259, 1983.
30. Kerr WF: Late-onset post-pneumonectomy empyema. Thorax 32:149, 1977.
31. Heater K, Revzani L, Rubin JM: CT evaluation of empyema in the postpneumonectomy space. Am J Roentgenol 145:39, 1985.
32. Gates GF, Sette RS, Cope JA: Acute cardiac herniation with incarceration following pneumonectomy. Radiology 94:561, 1970.
33. Tschersich HU, Skopara V Jr, Fleming WH: Acute cardiac herniation following pneumonectomy. Radiology 120:546, 1976.
34. Brady MB, Brogdon BG: Cardiac herniation and volvulus: Radiographic findings. Radiology 161:657, 1986.
35. Castillo M, Oldham S: Cardiac volvulus: Plain film recognition of an often fatal condition. Am J Roentgenol 145:271, 1985.
36. Hidvegi RS, Abdulnour EM, Wilson JAS: Herniation of the heart following left pneumonectomy. J Can Assoc Radiol 32:185, 1981.
37. Arndt RD, Frank CG, Schmitz AL, Haveson SB: Cardiac herniation with volvulus after pneumonectomy. Am J Roentgenol 130:155, 1978.
38. Rodgers BM, Moulder PV, DeLaney A: Thoracoscopy: New method of early diagnosis of cardiac herniation. J Thorac Cardiovasc Surg 78:623, 1979.
39. Shepard JO, Grillo HC, McLoud TC, et al: Right-pneumonectomy syndrome: Radiologic findings and CT correlation. Radiology 161:661, 1986.
40. Grillo HC, Shepard JO, Mathisen DJ, et al: Postpneumonectomy syndrome: Diagnosis, management, and results. Ann Thorac Surg 54:638, 1992.
41. Quillin SP, Shackelford GD: Postpneumonectomy syndrome after left lung resection. Radiology 179:100, 1991.
42. Boiselle PM, Shepard JAO, McLoud TC, et al: Postpneumonectomy syndrome: Another twist. J Thorac Imaging 12:209, 1997.
43. Fong KM, McNeil KD, Kennedy KP, et al: Asphyxia while swallowing solid food caused by bronchial compression: A variant of the pneumonectomy syndrome. Thorax 49:382, 1994.
44. Holbert JM, Libshitz HI, Chasen MH, et al: The postlobectomy chest: Anatomic considerations. Radiographics 7:889, 1987.
45. Carter AR, Sostman HD, Curtis AM, et al: Thoracic alterations after cardiac surgery. Am J Roentgenol 140:475, 1983.
46. Hamilton W: Atelectasis, pneumothorax, and aspiration as postoperative complications. Anesthesiology 22:708, 1961.
47. Culiner MM, Reich SB, Abouav J: Nonobstructive consolidation atelectasis following thoracotomy. J Thorac Surg 37:371, 1959.
48. Gamsu G, Singer MM, Vincent HH, et al: Postoperative impairment of mucous transport in the lung. Am Rev Respir Dis 114:673, 1976.
49. Korst RJ, Humphrey CB: Complete lobar collapse following pulmonary lobectomy: Its incidence, predisposing factors, and clinical ramifications. Chest 111:1285, 1997.
50. Wilcox P, Baile EM, Hards J, et al: Phrenic nerve function and its relationship to atelectasis after coronary artery bypass surgery. Chest 93:693, 1988.
51. Templeton AW, Almond CH, Seaber A, et al: Postoperative pulmonary patterns following cardiopulmonary bypass. Am J Roentgenol 96:1007, 1966.
52. Benjamin JJ, Cascade PN, Rubenfire M, et al: Left lower lobe atelectasis and consolidation following cardiac surgery: The effect of topical cooling on the phrenic nerve. Radiology 142:11, 1982.
53. Thomas JA, Cusimano RJ, Hoffstein V: Is atelectasis following aortocoronary bypass related to temperature? Chest 111:1290, 1997.
54. Singh NP, Vargas FS, Cukier A, et al: Arterial blood gases after coronary artery bypass surgery. Chest 102:1337, 1992.
55. Diament ML, Palmer KNV: Venous/arterial pulmonary shunting as the principal cause of postoperative hypoxemia. Lancet 1:15, 1967.
56. Hansen G, Drablos PA, Steinert R: Pulmonary complications, ventilation and blood gases after upper abdominal surgery. Acta Anaesthesiol Scand 21:211, 1977.
57. Bainbridge ET, Matthews HR: Hypoxaemia after left thoracotomy for benign oesophageal disease. Thorax 35:264, 1980.
58. van der Werff YD, van der Houwen HK, Heijmans PJM, et al: Postpneumonectomy pulmonary edema: A retrospective analysis of incidence and possible risk factors. Chest 111:1278, 1997.
59. Bhalla M, Leitman BS, Forcade C, et al: Lung hernia: Radiographic features. Am J Roentgenol 154:51, 1990.
60. DiMarco AF, Oca O, Renston JP: Lung herniation: A cause of chronic chest pain following thoracotomy. Chest 107:877, 1995.
61. Kelly MV II, Kyger ER, Miller WC: Postoperative lobar torsion and gangrene. Thorax 32:501, 1977.
62. Moser ES Jr, Proto AV: Lung torsion: Case report and literature review. Radiology 162:639, 1987.
63. Felson B: Lung torsion: Radiographic findings in nine cases. Radiology 162:631, 1987.
64. Collins J, Love RB: Pulmonary torsion: Complication of lung transplantation. Clin Pulmonary Med 3:297, 1996.
65. Munk PL, Vellet AD, Zwirewich C: Torsion of the upper lobe of the lung after surgery: Findings on pulmonary angiography. Am J Roentgenol 157:471, 1991.
66. Taylor FH, Zollinger RW II, Edgerton TA, et al: Intrapulmonary foreign body: Sponge retained for 43 years. J Thorac Imaging 9:56, 1994.
67. Sawasaki H, Horie K, Yamada M, et al: Bronchial stump aspergillosis: Experimental and clinical study. J Thorac Cardiovasc Surg 58:198, 1969.
68. Parry MF, Coughlin FR, Zambetti FX: Aspergillus empyema. Chest 81:768, 1982.
69. Goodman LR: Review: Postoperative chest radiograph. I. Alterations after abdominal surgery. Am J Roentgenol 134:533, 1980.
70. Harman E, Lillington G: Pulmonary risk factors in surgery. Med Clin North Am 63:1289, 1979.
71. Kroenke K, Lawrence VA, Theroux JF, et al: Postoperative complications after thoracic and major abdominal surgery in patients with and without obstructive lung disease. Chest 104:1445, 1993.
72. Hall JC, Tarala RA, Hall JL, et al: A multivariate analysis of the risk of pulmonary complications after laparotomy. Chest 99:923, 1991.
73. Wiren JE, Janzon L: Respiratory complications following surgery: Improved prediction with preoperative spirometry. Acta Anaesthesiol Scand 27:476, 1983.
74. Martin LF, Asher EF, Casey JM, et al: Postoperative pneumonia: Determinants of mortality. Arch Surg 119:379, 1984.
75. Poe RH, Kallay MC, Dass T, et al: Can postoperative pulmonary complications after elective cholecystectomy be predicted? Am J Med Sci 295:29, 1988.

76. Tuman KJ, McCarthy RJ, McCarthy RJ, et al: Morbidity and duration of ICU stay after cardiac surgery: A model for preoperative risk assessment. Chest 102:36, 1992.

77. Brooks-Brunn JA: Predictors of postoperative pulmonary complications following abdominal surgery. Chest 111:564, 1997.

78. Barisione G, Rovida S, Gazzaniga GM, et al: Upper abdominal surgery: Does a lung function test exist to predict early severe postoperative respiratory complications? Eur Respir J 10:1301, 1997.

79. Lawrence VA, Dhanda R, Hilsenbeck SG, et al: Risk of pulmonary complications after elective abdominal surgery. Chest 110:744, 1996.

80. Joris J, Kaba A, Lamy M: Postoperative spirometry after laparoscopy for lower abdominal or upper abdominal surgical procedures. Br J Anaesth 79:422, 1997.

81. Hall JC, Tarala RA, Hall JL: A case-control study of postoperative pulmonary complications after laparoscopic and open cholecystectomy. J Laparoendosc Surg 6:87, 1996.

82. Stal JM, Hanly PJ, Darling GE: Gastrobronchial fistula: An unusual complication of esophagectomy. Ann Thorac Surg 58:886, 1994.

83. Ninan M, Hunter S, Parker DJ: Aortobronchial fistula following aortic valve surgery. J R Soc Med 87:558, 1994.

83a. Foster CL, Kalbhen CL, Demos TC, Lonchyna VA: Aortobronchial fistula occurring after coarctation repair: Findings on aortography, helical CT, and CT angiography. AJR 171:401, 1998.

84. Pearce DJ: Respiratory acidosis and subcutaneous emphysema during laparoscopic cholecystectomy. Can J Anaesth 41:314, 1994.

85. Liu SY, Leighton T, Davis I, et al: Prospective analysis of cardiopulmonary responses to laparoscopic cholecystectomy. J Laparoendosc Surg 1:241, 1991.

85a. Lantz PE, Smith JD: Fatal carbon dioxide embolism complicating attempted laparoscopic cholecystectomy—case report and literature review. J Forensic Sci 39:1468, 1994.

85b. Tarnoff M, Moncure M, Jones F, et al: The value of routine posttracheostomy chest radiography. Chest 113:1647, 1998.

86. Nesbitt JC, Carrasco H: Expandable stents. Chest Surg Clin North Am 6:305, 1996.

87. Hauck RW, Romer W, Schulz C, et al: Ventilation perfusion scintigraphy and lung function testing to assess metal stent efficacy. J Nucl Med 38:1584, 1997.

88. Wilson GE, Walshaw MJ, Hind CR: Treatment of large airway obstruction in lung cancer using expandable metal stents inserted under direct vision via the fibreoptic bronchoscope. Thorax 51:248, 1996.

89. Hauck RW, Lembeck RM, Emslander HP, et al: Implantation of Accuflex and Strecker stents in malignant bronchial stenoses by flexible bronchoscopy. Chest 112:134, 1997.

90. Takamori S, Fujita H, Hayashi A, et al: Expandable metallic stents for tracheobronchial stenoses in esophageal cancer. Ann Thorac Surg 62:844, 1996.

91. Subramanian V, Anstead M, Cottrill CM, et al: Tetralogy of Fallot with absent pulmonary valve and bronchial compression: Treatment with endobronchial stents. Pediatr Cardiol 18:237, 1997.

92. Sacco O, Fregonese B, Oddone M, et al: Severe endobronchial obstruction in a girl with relapsing polychondritis: Treatment with Nd YAG laser and endobronchial silicon stent. Eur Respir J 10:494, 1997.

93. Watanabe Y, Murakami S, Oda M, et al: Treatment of bronchial stricture due to endobronchial tuberculosis. World J Surg 21:480, 1997.

94. Moser NJ, Woodring JH, Wolf KM, et al: Management of postpneumonectomy syndrome with a bronchoscopically placed endobronchial stent. South Med J 87:1156, 1994.

95. Wilson IC, Hasan A, Healey M, et al: Healing of the bronchus in pulmonary transplantation. Eur J Cardiothorac Surg 10:521, 1996.

96. Higgins R, McNeil K, Dennis C, et al: Airway stenoses after lung transplantation: Management with expanding metal stents. J Heart Lung Transplant 13:774, 1994.

97. Redington AN, Somerville J: Stenting of aortopulmonary collaterals in complex pulmonary atresia. Circulation 94:2479, 1996.

98. Hijazi ZM, al-Fadley F, Geggel RL, et al: Stent implantation for relief of pulmonary artery stenosis: Immediate and short-term results. Cathet Cardiovasc Diagn 38:16, 1996.

99. Abdulhamed JM, Alyousef SA, Mullins C: Endovascular stent placement for pulmonary venous obstruction after Mustard operation for transposition of the great arteries. Heart 75:210, 1996.

100. Haskal ZJ, Soulen MC, Huettl EA, et al: Life-threatening pulmonary emboli and cor pulmonale: Treatment with percutaneous pulmonary artery stent placement. Radiology 191:473, 1994.

101. Clark SC, Levine AJ, Hasan A, et al: Vascular complications of lung transplantation. Ann Thorac Surg 61:1079, 1996.

102. Hramiec JE, Haasler GB: Tracheal wire stent complications in malacia: Implications of position and design. Ann Thorac Surg 63:209, 1997.

103. Remacle M, Lawson G, Minet M, et al: Endoscopic treatment of tracheal stenosis using the carbon dioxide laser and the Gianturco stent: Indications and results. Laryngoscope 106:306, 1996.

104. Hendra KP, Saukkonen JJ: Erosion of the right mainstem bronchus by an esophageal stent. Chest 110:857, 1996.

105. Erasmus JJ, Goodman PC: Focal pulmonary edema: A complication of endovascular stent dilatation of pulmonary artery stenoses. Am J Roentgenol 165:821, 1995.

106. Brown DL, MacIsaac AI, Topol EJ: Pulmonary hemorrhage after intracoronary stent placement. J Am Coll Cardiol 24:91, 1994.

107. Khanavkar B, Stern P, Alberti W, et al: Complications associated with brachytherapy alone or with laser in lung cancer. Chest 99:1062, 1991.

108. Gustafson G, Vicini F, Freedman L, et al: High dose rate endobronchial brachytherapy in the management of primary and recurrent bronchogenic malignancies. Cancer 75:2345, 1995.

109. Speiser BL, Spratling L: Radiation bronchitis and stenosis secondary to high dose rate endobronchial irradiation. Int J Radiat Oncol Biol Phys 25:589, 1993.

110. McCaughan JS Jr, Hawley PC, LaRosa JC, et al: Photodynamic therapy to control life-threatening hemorrhage from hereditary hemorrhagic telangiectasia. Lasers Surg Med 19:492, 1996.

111. Lam S: Photodynamic therapy of lung cancer. Thorax 48:469, 1993.

112. Edell ES, Cortese DA, McDougall JC: Ancillary therapies in the management of lung cancer: Photodynamic therapy, laser therapy, and endobronchial prosthetic devices. Mayo Clin Proc 68:685, 1993.

113. Smith SGT, Bedwell J, MacRobert AJ, et al: Experimental studies to assess the potential of photodynamic therapy for the treatment of bronchial carcinomas. Thorax 48:474, 1993.

114. Lam S: Photodynamic therapy of lung cancer. Thorax 48:469, 1993.

115. Temeck BK, Pass HI: Esophagopleural fistula: A complication of photodynamic therapy. South Med J 88:271, 1995.

116. Cavaliere S, Venuta F, Foccoli P, et al: Endoscopic treatment of malignant airway obstructions in 2,008 patients. Chest 110:1536, 1996.

117. Krawtz S, Mehta AC, Wiedemann HP, et al: Nd-YAG laser-induced endobronchial burn: Management and long-term follow-up. Chest 95:916, 1989.

118. Leading article: Traumatic perforation of oesophagus. BMJ 1:524, 1972.

119. Scholl DG, Tsai SH: Esophageal perforation following the use of the esophageal obturator airway. Radiology 122:315, 1977.

120. Stark P: Radiology of thoracic trauma. Invest Radiol 25:1265, 1990.

121. Stark P, Phillips JM: Rupture of the esophagus as a complication of Sengstaken-Blakemore tube. Radiology 25:76, 1985.

122. Nygaard SD, Berger HA, Fick RB: Chylothorax as a complication of oesophageal sclerotherapy. Thorax 47:134, 1992.

123. Deslauriers J: History of surgery for emphysema. Semin Thorac Cardiovasc Surg 8:43, 1996.

124. Perelman MI, Strelzov VP: Surgery for pulmonary tuberculosis. World J Surg 21:457, 1997.

125. Treasure RL, Seaworth BJ: Current role of surgery in *Mycobacterium tuberculosis*. Ann Thorac Surg 59:1405, 1995.

126. Peppas G, Molnar TF, Jeyasingham K, et al: Thoracoplasty in the context of current surgical practice. Ann Thorac Surg 56:903, 1993.

127. Barker WL: Thoracoplasty. Chest Surg Clin North Am 4:593, 1994.

128. Horowitz MD, Otero M, Thurer RJ, et al: Late complications of plombage. Ann Thorac Surg 53:803, 1992.

129. Light RW: Pleural Diseases. Philadelphia, Lea & Febiger, 1983.

130. Case records of the Massachusetts General Hospital. Weekly clinicopathological exercises. Case 38-1983. Empyema 40 years after a thoracoplasty. N Engl J Med 309:715, 1983.

131. Martin A, Capron F, Liguory-Brunaud MD, et al: Epstein-Barr virus-associated primary malignant lymphomas of the pleural cavity occurring in longstanding pleural chronic inflammation. Hum Pathol 25:1314, 1994.

132. Vigneswaran WT, Ramasastry SS: Paraffin plombage of the chest revisited. Ann Thorac Surg 62:1837, 1996.

133. Ashour M, Campbell IA, Umachandran V, et al: Late complication of plombage thoracoplasty. Thorax 40:394, 1985.

134. Sultan M, Kelly ME, Hilliard G, et al: Complications of plombage in a Cuban exile. J Fla Med Assoc 81:815, 1994.

135. Harland RW, Sharma M, Rosenzweig DY: Lung carcinoma in a patient with Lucite sphere plombage thoracoplasty. Chest 103:1295, 1993.

136. Thompson JR, Entin SD: Primary extraskeletal chondrosarcoma: A report of a case arising in conjunction with extrapleural Lucite ball plombage. Cancer 23:936, 1969.

137. Millikan JS, Moore EE, Steiner E, et al: Complications of tube thoracostomy for acute trauma. Am J Surg 140:738, 1980.

138. Daly RC, Mucha P, Pairolero PC, et al: The risk of percutaneous chest tube thoracostomy for blunt thoracic trauma. Ann Emerg Med 14:865, 1985.

139. Miller KS, Sahn SA: Chest tubes: Indications, technique, management and complications. Chest 91:258, 1987.

140. Dalbec DL, Krome RL: Thoracostomy. Emerg Med Clin North Am 4:441, 1986.

141. Miller KS, Sahn SA: Chest tubes: Indications, technique, management and complications. Chest 91:258, 1987.

142. Maurer JR, Friedman PJ, Wing VW: Thoracostomy tube in an interlobar fissure: Radiologic recognition of a potential problem. Am J Roentgenol 139:1155, 1982.

143. Stark DD, Federle MP, Goodman PC: CT and radiographic assessment of tube thoracostomy. Am J Roentgenol 141:253, 1983.

144. Webb WR, LaBerge JM: Radiographic recognition of chest tube malposition in the major fissure. Chest 85:81, 1984.

145. Stark DD, Federle MP, Goodman PC: CT and radiographic assessment of tube thoracostomy. Am J Roentgenol 141:253, 1983.

146. Mirvis SE, Tobin KD, Kostrubiak I, et al: Thoracic CT in detecting occult disease in critically ill patients. Am J Roentgenol 148:685, 1987.

147. Cameron EW, Mirvis SE, Shanmuganathan K, et al: Computed tomography of malpositioned thoracostomy drains: A pictorial essay. Clin Radiol 52:187, 1997.

148. Curtin JJ, Goodman LR, Quebbeman EJ, et al: Thoracostomy tubes after acute chest injury: Relationship between location in a pleural fissure and function. Am J Roentgenol 163:1339, 1994.

149. Fraser RS: Lung perforation complicating tube thoracostomy: Pathologic description of three cases. Hum Pathol 19:518, 1988.

150. Gilsanz V, Cleveland RH: Pleural reaction to thoracotomy tube. Chest 74:167, 1978.

151. Fein AB, Godwin JD, Moore AV, et al: Systemic artery-to-pulmonary vascular shunt: A complication of closed-tube thoracostomy. Am J Roentgenol 140:917, 1983.

152. Lurus AG, Cowen RL, Eckert JF: Systemic-pulmonary arteriovenous fistula following closed-tube thoracotomy. Radiology 92:1296, 1969.

153. Hirsch M, Maroko I, Gueron M, et al: Systemic-pulmonary arteriovenous fistula of traumatic origin: A case report. Cardiovasc Intervent Radiol 6:160, 1983.

154. Bertino RE, Wesbey GE, Johnson RJ: Horner syndrome occurring as a complication of chest tube placement. Radiology 164:745, 1987.

155. Pingleton SK, Jeter J: Necrotizing fasciitis as a complication of tube thoracostomy. Chest 83:925, 1983.

156. Stahly TL, Tench WD: Lung entrapment and infarction by chest tube suction. Radiology 122:307, 1977.

157. Neff CC, Mueller PR, Ferrucci JT Jr, et al: Serious complications following transgression of the pleural space in drainage procedures. Radiology 152:335, 1984.

158. Nichols DM, Cooperberg PL, Golding RH, et al: The safe intercostal approach? Pleural complications in abdominal interventional radiology. Am J Roentgenol 141:1013, 1984.

159. Samelson SL, Ferguson MK: Empyema following percutaneous catheter drainage of upper abdominal abscess. Chest 102:1612, 1992.

160. Valentine RJ, Turner WW: Pleural complications of nasoenteric feeding tubes. JPEN 8:450, 1984.

161. Hendry PJ, Akyurekl Y, McIntyre R, et al: Bronchopleural complications of nasogastric feeding tubes. Crit Care Med 14:892, 1986.

162. Ghahremani GG, Gould RJ: Nasoenteric feeding tubes: Radiographic detection of complications. Dig Dis Sci 31:574, 1986.

163. Miller KS, Tomlinson JR, Sahn SA: Pleuropulmonary complications of enteral tube feedings: Two reports, review of the literature and recommendations. Chest 86:230, 1985.

164. Woodall BH, Winfield DF, Bisset GS: Inadvertent tracheobronchial placement of feeding tubes. Radiology 165:727, 1987.

165. Wiener MD, Garay SM, Leitman BS, et al: Imaging of the intensive care unit patient. Clin Chest Med 12:169, 1991.

166. Stark P: Inadvertent nasogastric tube insertion into the tracheobronchial tree: A hazard of new high-residual volume cuffs. Radiology 142:239, 1982.

167. Miller WT: Inadvertent tracheobronchial placement of feeding tubes (letter to the editor). Radiology 167:875, 1988.

168. Hand RW, Kempster M, Levy JH, et al: Inadvertent transbronchial insertion of narrow-bore feeding tubes into the pleural space. JAMA 251:2396, 1984.

169. Grossman TW, Duncavage JA, Dennison B, et al: Complications associated with a narrow bore nasogastric tube. Ann Otol Rhinol Laryngol 93(5 Pt 1):460, 1984.

170. Woodall BH, Winfield DF, Bisset GS III: Inadvertent tracheobronchial placement of feeding tubes. Radiology 165:727, 1987.

171. Roubenoff R, Ravich WJ: Pneumothorax due to nasogastric feeding tubes: Report of four cases, review of the literature, and recommendations for prevention. Arch Intern Med 149:184, 1989.

172. Twigg HL, Buckley CE: Complications of endotracheal intubation. Am J Roentgenol 109:452, 1970.

173. Conrardy PA, Goodman LR, Laing F, et al: Alteration of endotracheal tube position: Flexion and extension of the neck. Crit Care Med 4:7, 1976.

174. Goodman LR, Conrardy PA, Laing F, et al: Radiographic evaluation of endotracheal tube position. Am J Roentgenol 127:433, 1976.

175. Smith GM, Reed JC, Choplin RH: Radiographic detection of esophageal malpositioning of endotracheal tubes. Am J Roentgenol 154:23, 1990.

176. Abbey NC, Green DE, Cicale MJ: Massive tracheal necrosis complicating endotracheal intubation. Chest 95:459, 1989.

177. Stark P: Imaging of tracheobronchial injuries. J Thorac Imaging 10:206, 1995.

178. Sutera PT, Smith CE: Asystole during direct laryngoscopy and tracheal intubation. J Cardiothorac Vasc Anesth 8:79, 1994.

179. Shneerson J: Transtracheal oxygen delivery. Thorax 47:57, 1992.

180. Heimlich HJ, Carr GC: Transtracheal catheter technique for pulmonary rehabilitation. Ann Otol Rhinol Laryngol 94:502, 1985.

181. Fletcher EC, Nickeson D, Costarangos-Galarza C: Endotracheal mass resulting from a transtracheal oxygen catheter. Chest 93:438, 1988.

182. Borer H, Frey M, Keller R: Ulcerous tracheitis and mucus ball formation: A nearly fatal complication of a transtracheal oxygen catheter. Respiration 63:400, 1996.

182a. Wechsler RJ, Spirn PW, Conant EF, et al: Thrombosis and infection caused by thoracic venous catheters: Pathogenesis and imaging findings. Am J Roentgenol 160:467, 1993.

183. Scott WL: Complications associated with central venous catheters: A survey. Chest 94(6):1221, 1988.

184. Fletcher JP, Little JM: Subclavian vein catheterisation for parenteral nutrition. Ann R Coll Surg Engl 70:150, 1988.

185. Clarke DE, Raffin TA: Infectious complications of indwelling long-term central venous catheters. Chest 97:966, 1990.

186. Duntley P, Siever J, Korwes ML, et al: Vascular erosion by central venous catheters: Clinical features and outcome. Chest 101:1633, 1992.

187. Dunbar RD, Mitchell R, Lavine M: Aberrant locations of central venous catheters. Lancet 1:711, 1981.

188. Langston CS: The aberrant central venous catheter and its complications. Radiology 100:55, 1971.

188a. Hoshal VL Jr, Ause RG, Hoskins PA: Fibrin sleeve formation on indwelling subclavian central venous catheters. Arch Surg 102:353, 1971.

188b. Ahmed N, Payne RF: Thrombosis after central venous cannulation. Med J Aust 1:217, 1976.

189. Brismar B, Hardstedt C, Jacobson S: Diagnosis of thrombosis by catheter phlebography after prolonged central venous catheterization. Ann Surg 194:779, 1981.

190. Horattas MC, Wright DJ, Fenton AH, et al: Changing concepts of deep venous thrombosis of upper extremity: Report of a series and review of the literature. Surgery 104:561, 1988.

191. Hill SL, Berry RE: Subclavian vein thrombosis: A continuing challenge. Surgery 108:1, 1990.

192. Warden GD, Wilmore DW, Pruitt BA Jr: Central venous thrombosis: Hazard of medical process. J Trauma 13:620, 1973.

193. Natu SS, Sequeira JC, Weitzman AF: An improved technique for axillary phlebography. Radiology 142:529, 1982.

194. Falk RL, Smith DF: Thrombosis of upper extremity thoracic inlet veins: Diagnosis with duplex Doppler sonography. Am J Roentgenol 149:677, 1987.

195. Yedlicka JW Jr, Cormier MG, Gray R, et al: Computed tomography of superior vena cava obstruction. J Thorac Imaging 2:72, 1987.

196. Hansen ME, Spritzer CE, Sostman HD: Assessing the patency of mediastinal and thoracic inlet veins: Value of MR imaging. Am J Roentgenol 155:1177, 1990.

197. Press OW, Ramsey PG, Larson EB, et al: Hickman catheter infections in patients with malignancies. Medicine 63:189, 1984.

198. Maggs PR, Schwaber JR: Fatal bilateral pneumothoraces complicating subclavian vein catheterization. Chest 71:552, 1977.

199. Dronen S, Thompson B, Nowak R, et al: Subclavian vein catheterization during cardiopulmonary resuscitation. JAMA 247:3227, 1982.

200. Shiloni E, Meretyk S, Weiss Y: Tension haemothorax: An unusual complication of central vein catheterization. Injury 16:385, 1985.

201. Mitchell A, Steer HW: Late appearance of pneumothorax after subclavian vein catheterization: An anaesthetic hazard. BMJ 281:1339, 1980.

202. Chute E, Cerrs FB: Late development of hydrothorax and hydromediastinum in patients with central venous catheters. Crit Care Med 10:868, 1982.

203. Damtew B, Lewandowski B: Hydrothorax, hydromediastinum and pericardial effusion: A complication of intravenous alimentation. Can Med Assoc J 130:1573, 1984.

204. Tocino IM, Watanabe A: Impending catheter perforation of superior vena cava: Radiographic recognition. Am J Roentgenol 146:487, 1986.

205. Topaz O, Sharon M, Rechavia E, et al: Traumatic internal jugular vein cannulation. Ann Emerg Med 16:1394, 1987.

206. Tapson JS, Uldall PR: Fatal hemothorax caused by a subclavian hemodialysis catheter: Thoughts on prevention. Arch Intern Med 144:1685, 1984.

207. McGoon MD, Benedetto PW, Greene BM: Complications of percutaneous central venous catheterization: A report of two cases and review of the literature. Johns Hopkins Med 145:1, 1979.

208. LaPenna R, Whinnery C: An unusual complication of subclavian vein catheterization for total parenteral nutrition. Postgrad Med 64:171, 1978.

209. Kotozoglou T, Mambo N: Fatal retropleural hematoma complicating internal jugular vein catheterization: A case report. Am J Forensic Med Pathol 4:125, 1983.

210. Molinari PS, Belani KG, Buckley JJ: Delayed hydrothorax following percutaneous central venous cannulation. Acta Anaesthesiol Scand 28:493, 1984.

211. Usselman JA, Seat SG: Superior caval catheter displacement causing bilateral pleural effusions. Am J Roentgenol 133:738, 1979.

212. Brennan MF, Sugarbaker PH, Moore FD: Venobronchial fistula: A rare complication of central venous catheterization for parenteral hyperalimentation. Arch Surg 106:871, 1973.

213. Demey HE, Colemont LJ, Hartoko TJ, et al: Venopulmonary fistula: A rare complication of central venous catheterization. J Parenter Enteral Nutr 11:580, 1987.

214. Norman WJ, Moule NJ, Walrond ER: Lung abscess: A complication of malposition of a central venous catheter. Br J Radiol 47:498, 1974.

215. Paskin DL, Hoffman WS, Tuddenham WJ: A new complication of subclavian vein catheterization. Ann Surg 179:266, 1974.

216. Johnson CL, Lazarchick J, Lynn HB: Subclavian venipuncture: Preventable complications. Report of two cases. Mayo Clin Proc 45:712, 1970.

217. Flanagan JP, Gradisar IA, Gross RJ, et al: Air embolus: A lethal complication of subclavian venipuncture. N Engl J Med 281:488, 1969.

218. Woodring JH, Fried AM: Nonfatal venous air embolism after contrast-enhanced CT. Radiology 167:405, 1988.

219. Hunt R, Hunter TB: Cardiac tamponade and death from perforation of the right atrium by a central venous catheter (letter to the editor). Am J Roentgenol 151:1250, 1988.

220. Rossleigh MA: Unusual complication of intravenous catheterisation. Med J Aust 1:236, 1982.

221. Kappes S, Towne J, Adams M, et al: Perforation of the superior vena cava: A complication of subclavian dialysis. JAMA 249:2232, 1983.

222. Weiner P, Sznajder I, Plavnick L, et al: Unusual complication of subclavian vein catheterization. Crit Care Med 12:538, 1984.

223. Amesbury S, Vargish T, Hall J: An unusual complication of central venous catheterization. Chest 105:905, 1994.

224. Ciment LM, Rotbart A, Galbut RN: Contralateral effusions secondary to subclavian venous catheters: Report of two cases. Chest 83:926, 1983.

225. Milam MG, Sahn SA: Horner's syndrome secondary to hydromediastinum: A complication of extravascular migration of a central venous catheter. Chest 94:1093, 1988.

226. Swan HJC, Ganz W, Forrester J, et al: Catheterization of the heart in man with use of a flow-directed balloon-tipped catheter. N Engl J Med 283:447, 1970.
227. Goodman DJ, Rider AK, Billingham ME, et al: Thromboembolic complications with the indwelling balloon-tipped pulmonary arterial catheter. N Engl J Med 291:777, 1974.
228. Foote GA, Schabel SI, Hodges M: Pulmonary complications of the flow-directed balloon-tipped catheter. N Engl J Med 290:927, 1974.
229. McLoud TC, Putman CE: Radiology of the Swan-Ganz catheter and associated pulmonary complications. Radiology 116:19, 1975.
230. Katz JD, Cronau LH, Barash PG, et al: Pulmonary artery flow-guided catheters in the perioperative period: Indications and complications. JAMA 237:2832, 1977.
231. Hannan AT, Brown M, Bigman O: Pulmonary artery catheter-induced hemorrhage. Chest 85:128, 1984.
232. Dieden JD, Friloux LA III, Renner JW: Pulmonary artery false aneurysms secondary to Swan-Ganz pulmonary artery catheters. Am J Roentgenol 149:901, 1987.
233. Davis SD, Neithamer CD, Schreiber TS, et al: False pulmonary artery aneurysm induced by Swan-Ganz catheter: Diagnosis and embolotherapy. Radiology 164:741, 1987.
234. Ferretti GR, Thony F, Link KM, et al: False aneurysm of the pulmonary artery induced by a Swan-Ganz catheter: Clinical presentation and radiologic management. Am J Roentgenol 167:941, 1996.
235. O'Toole JD, Wurtzbacher JJ, Wearner NE, et al: Pulmonary-valve injury and insufficiency during pulmonary-artery catheterization. N Engl J Med 301:1167, 1979.
236. Hartung EJ, Ender J, Sgouropoulou S, et al: Severe air embolism caused by a pulmonary artery introducer sheath. Anesthesiology 80:1402, 1994.
237. Michel L, Marsh HM, McMichan JC, et al: Infection of pulmonary artery catheters in critically ill patients. JAMA 245:1032, 1981.
238. Vicente Rull JR, Loza Aquirre J, de la Puerta E: Thrombocytopenia induced by pulmonary artery flotation catheters: A prospective study. Intensive Care Med 10:29, 1984.
239. Boyd KD, Thomas SJ, Gold J, et al: A prospective study of complications of pulmonary artery catheterizations in 500 consecutive patients. Chest 84:245, 1983.
240. Katz JD, Cronau LH, Barash PG, et al: Pulmonary artery flow-guided catheters in the perioperative period: Indications and complications. JAMA 237:2832, 1977.
241. Chun GMH, Ellestad MH: Perforation of the pulmonary artery by a Swan-Ganz catheter. N Engl J Med 284:1041, 1971.
242. Shin MS, Ho K-J: Cavitary pulmonary lesions complicating use of flow-directed balloon-tipped catheters in two cases. Am J Roentgenol 132:650, 1979.
243. Kearney TJ, Shabot MM: Pulmonary artery rupture associated with the Swan-Ganz catheter. Chest 108:1349, 1995.
244. Fraser RS: Catheter-induced pulmonary artery perforation: Pathologic and pathogenic features. Hum Pathol 18:1246, 1987.
245. Stone JG, Khambatta HJ, McDaniel DD: Catheter-induced pulmonary arterial trauma: Can it always be averted? J Thorac Cardiovasc Surg 86:146, 1983.
246. Rosenblum SE, Ratliff NB, Shirey EK, et al: Pulmonary artery dissection induced by a Swan-Ganz catheter. Cleve Clin Q 51:671, 1984.
247. Dieden JD, Friloux LA III, Renner JW: Pulmonary artery false aneurysms secondary to Swan-Ganz pulmonary artery catheters. Am J Roentgenol 149:901, 1987.
248. Davis SD, Neithamer CD, Schreiber TS, et al: False pulmonary artery aneurysm induced by Swan-Ganz catheter: Diagnosis and embolotherapy. Radiology 164:741, 1987.
249. Cooper JP, Jackson J, Walker JM: False aneurysm of the pulmonary artery associated with cardiac catheterisation. Br Heart J 69:188, 1993.
250. Guttentag AR, Shepard J-AO, McLoud TC: Catheter-induced pulmonary artery pseudoaneurysm: The halo sign on CT. Am J Roentgenol 158:637, 1992.
251. Forman MB, Obel IWP: Pulmonary haemorrhage following Swan-Ganz catheterization in a patient without severe pulmonary hypertension. S Afr Med J 58:329, 1980.
252. Timsit J-F, Farkas J-C, Boyer J-M, et al: Central vein catheter–related thrombosis in intensive care patients: Incidence, risk factors, and relationship with catheter-related sepsis. Chest 114:207, 1998.
253. Pellegrini RV, Marcelli GD, DiMarco RF, et al: Swan-Ganz catheter induced pulmonary hemorrhage. J Cardiovasc Surg 28:646, 1987.
254. Rubin SA, Puckett RP: Pulmonary artery—Bronchial fistula: A new complication of Swan-Ganz catheterization. Chest 75:515, 1979.
255. Kron IL, Piepgrass W, Carabello B, et al: False aneurysm of the pulmonary artery: A complication of pulmonary artery catheterization. Ann Thorac Surg 33:629, 1982.
256. Urschel JD, Myerowitz PD: Catheter-induced pulmonary artery rupture in the setting of cardiopulmonary bypass. Ann Thorac Surg 56:585, 1993.
257. Kirton OC, Varon AJ, Henry RP, et al: Flow-directed, pulmonary artery catheter-induced pseudoaneurysm: Urgent diagnosis and endovascular obliteration. Crit Care Med 20:1178, 1992.
258. Tooker J, Huseby J, Butler J: The effect of Swan-Ganz catheter height on the wedge pressure-left atrial pressure relationship in edema during positive-pressure ventilation. Am Rev Respir Dis 117:721, 1978.
259. Shasby DM, Dauber IM, Pfister S, et al: Swan-Ganz catheter location and left atrial pressure determine the accuracy of the wedge pressure when positive end expiratory pressure is used. Chest 80:666, 1981.
260. Brown BG, Goldfarb D, Topaz SR, et al: Diastolic augmentation by intra-aortic balloon: Circulatory hemodynamics and treatment of severe acute left ventricular failure in dogs. J Thorac Cardiovasc Surg 53:789, 1967.
261. Hyson EA, Ravin CE, Kelley MJ, et al: Intra-aortic counterpulsation balloon: Radiographic considerations. Am J Roentgenol 128:915, 1977.
262. Ravin CE, Putman CE, McLoud TC: Hazards of the intensive care unit. Am J Roentgenol 126:423, 1976.
263. Steiner RM, Tegtmeyer CJ, Morse D, et al: The radiology of cardiac pacemakers. Radiographics 6(3):373, 1986.
264. Grier D, Cook PG, Hartnell GG: Chest radiographs after permanent pacing. Are they really necessary? Clin Radiol 42:244, 1990.
265. Bejvan SM, Ephron JH, Takasugi JE, et al: Imaging of cardiac pacemakers. Am J Roentgenol 169:1371, 1997.
266. Goodman LR, Almassi GH, Troup PJ, et al: Complications of automatic implantable cardioverter defibrillators: Radiographic CT and echocardiographic evaluation. Radiology 170:447, 1989.
267. Verheyden CN, Price L, Lynch DJ, et al: Implantable cardioverter defibrillator patch erosion presenting as hemoptysis. J Cardiovasc Electrophysiol 5:961, 1994.
268. Dasgupta A, Mehta AC, Rick TW, et al: Erosion of implantable cardioverter defibrillator patch electrode into airways. An unusual cause of recurrent hemoptysis. Chest 113:252, 1998.

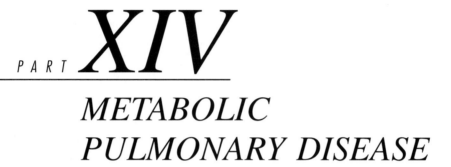

PART XIV

METABOLIC
PULMONARY DISEASE

Metabolic Pulmonary Disease

The diseases covered in this chapter comprise a heterogeneous group based on their generally accepted, or suspected, metabolic or endocrine pathogenesis. Many are rare and are associated with no or only mild clinical and functional abnormalities.

PULMONARY CALCIFICATION AND OSSIFICATION

Abnormal calcification may occur in normal tissue (metastatic calcification) or in tissue that is degenerating or dead (dystrophic calcification). The latter form is by far the more common and in the lung is usually associated with foci of remote granulomatous inflammation. Dystrophic calcification may also occur in fibrous tissue resulting from many underlying disorders, in which case there may be bone formation in addition to the deposition of calcium salts. These abnormalities are also discussed in Chapter 18 (*see* page 463).

Metastatic Calcification

Metastatic calcification typically occurs in patients who have hypercalcemia, usually associated with chronic renal failure and secondary hyperparathyroidism[1, 2] and less often with multiple myeloma;[3, 4] it has also been reported following kidney[5] and liver[6, 7] transplantation. The abnormality is especially common in patients undergoing maintenance hemodialysis.[8] For example, in one prospective study of 31 such patients, of whom 15 died, 9 (60%) had histologic evidence of calcification at autopsy.[2] In another investigation of 23 patients on long-term dialysis, 14 (61%) had pulmonary uptake on technetium 99m (^{99m}Tc)-diphosphonate scanning;[1] radiographic evidence of calcification was absent in all 23 patients.

Pathologically, metastatic calcification is characterized by the presence of strong hematoxylin (purple) staining in the alveolar septa and the walls of small pulmonary vessels and bronchi (Fig. 68–1).[2, 9] Under the light microscope, the calcium deposits usually appear discontinuous, although in very severe cases the parenchyma may be extensively involved. Alveolar septa may show a mild to moderate degree of fibrosis;[2] adjacent air spaces are typically unaffected. X-ray diffraction analysis has shown the deposits to consist of whitlockite $[(CaMg)_3 (PO_4)_2]$.[2] If necessary, the presence of the calcium-phosphate mixture can be confirmed with the von Kossa stain or calcium stains such as alizarin red.

On both radiographs and HRCT scans (Fig. 68–2), metastatic pulmonary calcification may be manifested as numerous 3- to 10-mm-diameter calcified nodules or, more

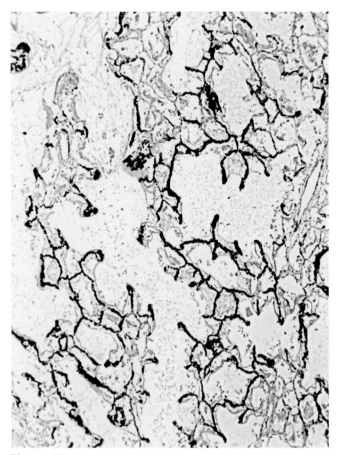

Figure 68–1. Metastatic Pulmonary Calcification. The section shows extensive deposition of calcium phosphate (stained black) in alveolar septa. The tissue was from the upper lobe of a patient with chronic renal failure; no corresponding radiographic abnormality was detected.

commonly, as fluffy and poorly defined nodular opacities mimicking air-space nodules.[10–13] When coalescent, the nodular opacities seen on the radiograph may be misdiagnosed as pulmonary edema or pneumonia.[14–16] The calcific nature of the opacities in these situations can be readily confirmed by scanning with bone imaging agents such as ^{99m}Tc-diphosphonate[17] or by HRCT.[11, 12] HRCT may also demonstrate calcification of arteries in the chest wall or, less commonly, of the pulmonary arteries, superior vena cava, or myocardium (*see* Fig. 68–2).[11–13] Occasionally, foci of subcutaneous vascular calcification mimic pulmonary lesions on the radiograph.[18] In one case, previously existing large pulmonary nodules became calcified.[19] Radiographically apparent calcification may develop over several days or weeks.[10, 20]

The abnormality shows a predilection for apical and subapical lung zones, a feature attributable to regional differences in the pulmonary physiology.[21] Because there is a much higher ventilation-perfusion ratio at the apex than at the base of the lung, the local milieu at the former site has a higher partial pressure of oxygen (Po_2), a lower partial pressure of carbon dioxide (Pco_2), and a higher pH; thus, it has been estimated that the pH at the apex of the normal lung is roughly 7.50, versus 7.39 at the base.[22] The relative alkalinity favors the precipitation of calcium salts.

As indicated previously, few patients in whom metastatic calcification is demonstrable pathologically show evi-

dence of its presence on radiographs.[2, 23] For example, in a study of nine patients who had metastatic calcification at autopsy, only one had positive findings on the chest radiograph;[2] this patient had extremely high tissue levels of calcium. In another review of the chest radiographs and CT scans of seven patients who had biopsy-proven disease, calcification was evident on radiographs in only two cases and on CT scans in four.[12] On magnetic resonance (MR) imaging, calcification is usually associated with a reduction in signal intensity or a signal void. In one case, it resulted in a hyperintense signal on T1-weighted spin-echo images.[24]

Clinical manifestations of metastatic calcification are typically absent, although patients have rarely been reported to develop respiratory failure.[25] Pulmonary function abnormalities—primarily a decrease in the carbon monoxide diffusing capacity (D_{LCO})—have also been found in patients undergoing dialysis and in experimental animals by several groups of investigators.[1, 2, 26] Decreases in vital capacity and Pao_2 have also been found in some studies,[2] and there is experimental evidence that the effects of calcification may be complicated by an elevation in pulmonary artery pressure.[26] In patients in whom the serum calcium levels become normal following therapy for the underlying cause of hypercalcemia, clinical and radiologic evidence of pulmonary calcification may regress.[4, 27]

Dendriform Pulmonary Ossification

Dendriform pulmonary ossification (also known as idiopathic disseminated pulmonary ossification or ossifying pneumonitis) is a rare and distinctive form of diffuse pulmonary ossification.[28–30] As the name suggests, it is characterized by branching, often tubular foci of bone, commonly containing prominent cores of adipose tissue (Fig. 68–3). Despite the branching, an association with airways or vessels usually cannot be identified, and it is unclear in exactly what anatomic location the ossification occurs. A lower-lobe predominance is common. The pathogenesis is unclear; however, many cases have been associated with underlying interstitial fibrosis, most often idiopathic pulmonary fibrosis (Fig. 68–4),[31, 33] and occasionally with long-standing busulfan treatment,[34] amyloidosis, cystic fibrosis, and asbestosis.[36] It has been suggested that the process may involve metaplasia of fibroblasts into osteoblasts;[30, 37] however, apparent transition between areas of fibrosis and active bone formation can be identified only rarely. In some instances, a transition from cartilage to bone can be seen.[28]

The majority of patients are asymptomatic, and the abnormality is discovered most often in older persons at autopsy or incidentally on radiographs taken during investigation of an unrelated condition. The ossific nature of the process may not be recognized radiographically, the abnormality being interpreted solely as interstitial fibrosis.[28] If suspected, it can be definitively diagnosed by bone scanning[38] or HRCT.[39] The condition can progress slowly over years or remain unchanged.[37]

PULMONARY ALVEOLAR PROTEINOSIS

Pulmonary alveolar proteinosis (PAP), also called alveolar lipoproteinosis and pulmonary alveolar phospholip-

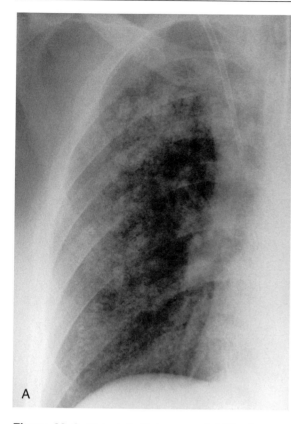

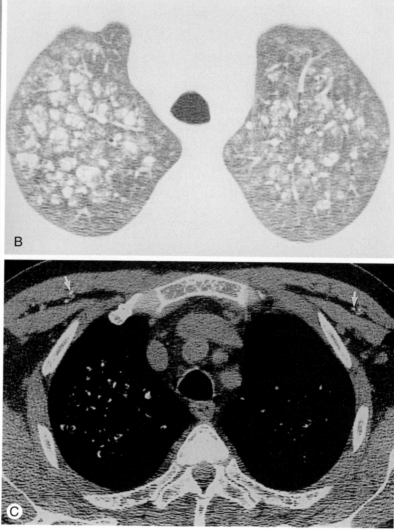

Figure 68–2. Metastatic Pulmonary Calcification. A close-up view of the right lung from a posteroanterior chest radiograph *(A)* in a 42-year-old patient who had chronic renal failure shows poorly defined nodular opacities involving mainly the upper lobe. Similar findings were present in the left lung. A hemodialysis catheter is in place. An HRCT scan through the lung apices *(B)* shows nodular areas of increased attenuation. Soft tissue windows *(C)* demonstrate the presence of calcification within the opacities. Vascular calcification in the chest wall is also evident *(arrows).*

idosis,[40] is an uncommon disease characterized by the accumulation of abundant protein- and lipid-rich material resembling surfactant within the parenchymal air spaces.[41–43] Although the disease occurs predominantly in patients between the ages of 20 and 50 years, very young children constitute a subgroup at increased risk.[44–46] There is a male-to-female predominance of about 2 to 4:1.[43]

Etiology and Pathogenesis

The etiology and pathogenesis of PAP are poorly understood. However, the bulk of evidence suggests an abnormality of surfactant production, metabolism or clearance by type II alveolar cells and macrophages. For this reason, the disease is included in this chapter, although it is possible that factors other than, or in addition to, those involved with surfactant metabolism may be important in pathogenesis. In fact, the pathologic pattern characteristic of PAP is seen in a variety of settings in both humans and experimental animals, suggesting that multiple factors may be involved in the pathogenesis and that the histologic and biochemical findings characteristic of the disease may represent a final common

pathway of a number of pulmonary insults. These settings include the following:

1. An immunocompromised state, especially lymphopenia, thymic aplasia, and immunoglobulin deficiency in infants and children[46, 47] and lymphoma and leukemia in adults.[49–51] Occasional cases also have been reported in patients who have acquired immunodeficiency syndrome (AIDS)[52] or autoimmune connective tissue diseases.[53] Although it has been suggested that the drugs used in the therapy of some of these conditions may be responsible for the proteinosis,[54] a more attractive hypothesis is that the underlying immunodeficiency is associated with malfunction of alveolar macrophages that in turn leads to the accumulation of the abnormal intra-alveolar material *(see* farther on).

2. Rarely, in infants and young children without evidence of underlying systemic disease[46, 55, 56] or who have autosomal recessive lysinuric protein intolerance.[57] Some of these children are siblings with a history of consanguinity[56, 59] and/or an inherited deficiency of surfactant protein B.[60–62] Despite abundant intra-alveolar phospholipid, typical myelin structures do not form in these infants.[63–66] In some cases, the deficiency is only partial as a result of heterozy-

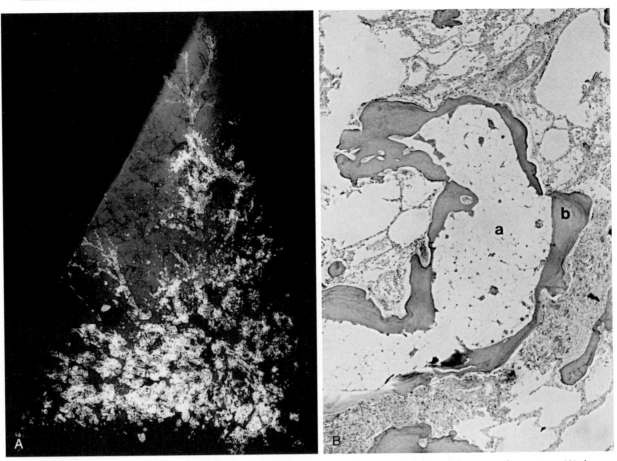

Figure 68–3. Dendriform Pulmonary Ossification. A radiograph of a 1-cm thick slice of left lower lobe removed at autopsy *(A)* shows extensive foci of calcification, some clearly branching and tubular in appearance. A section *(B)* shows an irregularly shaped fragment of bone (b) with abundant adipose tissue (a) in its central portion (responsible for the tubular pattern on the specimen radiograph). Despite the branching appearance on the radiograph, no definite association of the bone fragments with airways or vessels could be identified. The patient was a 72-year-old man with unknown respiratory history. *(B, ×60.)*

gosity, in which case the affected infant may benefit from glucocorticoid therapy.[67]

3. In experimental animals following exposure to a variety of airborne dusts, including aluminum powder, silica,[68–70] and fiberglass,[71] and in humans exposed to a high concentration of silicon dioxide (acute silicoproteinosis; *see* page 2390)[72] or titanium.[73] The early stage of the disease process in animals is manifested by the presence of extruded lamellar bodies from type II pneumocytes;[68] these are phagocytosed by alveolar macrophages that enlarge and undergo degenerative changes, ultimately releasing a fine granular substance resembling that found in human alveolar proteinosis.

4. In association with infection by a variety of microorganisms, especially *Nocardia, Aspergillus,* and *Cryptococcus* species;[42, 59] other agents such as cytomegalovirus,[74] *Mycobacterium tuberculosis,* nontuberculous mycobacteria,[75] *Pneumocystis carinii,*[76] *Histoplasma capsulatum, Candida* species, *Mucorales* species, and herpesvirus have been reported less frequently.[42] It has been suggested that the organisms themselves may be the cause of the proteinosis,[42, 74] and in fact, in some cases, the condition appears to undergo remission following antibiotic therapy.[77] Nevertheless, it seems more likely that the presence of such microorganisms is the result of underlying immune deficiency, immunosup-

pressive therapy, and/or the presence of a favorable growth environment provided by the intra-alveolar proteinaceous material.

As the foregoing discussion suggests, an abnormality of surfactant production, metabolism, or clearance (or a combination of these) has been strongly implicated in the pathogenesis of PAP. Many investigators have attempted to confirm and elaborate upon this hypothesis. One line of study has concerned the nature of the intra-alveolar material itself. The results of a number of ultrastructural,[78–80] immunochemical,[81] and biochemical[82–84] investigations have confirmed that it resembles surfactant or a component thereof (including surfactant proteins A,[85] C,[86] and D[87]). Most investigators have found that the material obtained from tissue and lung washings is qualitatively similar to that obtained in normal persons. However, some workers have described lipoproteins that differ from those in normal alveolar secretions and that may have different functional properties.[82, 88–90] In addition, the specific components of the fluid may not be the same in different persons who have the disease; for example, in a comparison of the bronchoalveolar lavage (BAL) fluid from two patients, one who recovered completely and one who required repeated alveolar lavage, glycosaminoglycans were found only in the one who had refractory disease.[84]

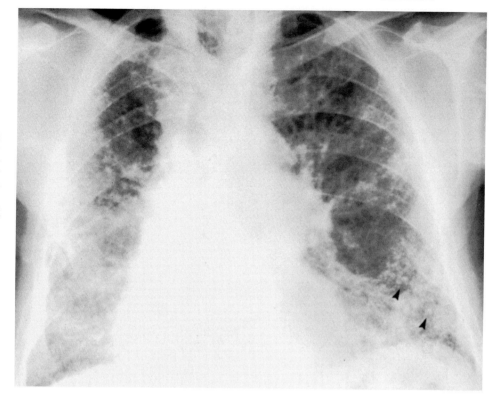

Figure 68–4. Interstitial Calcification (Ossification) Associated with Idiopathic Pulmonary Fibrosis. A posteroanterior chest radiograph discloses a nodular and reticulonodular pattern throughout both lungs with considerable lower zonal predominance. Many of the nodular opacities in the left lower lobe *(arrowheads)* are of sufficient density to suggest calcification. Biopsy of the left lung in this 72-year-old man disclosed foci of mature bone and idiopathic pulmonary fibrosis.

Thus, good evidence exists that the material accumulating within the alveoli in PAP is derived from type II pneumocytes and that it represents surfactant or a component thereof. There is still considerable uncertainty, however, about the cause of its accumulation. A theoretical possibility is that an overproduction of surfactant by hyperplastic or abnormally stimulated type II pneumocytes is responsible; however, the results of clinical and experimental studies have generally failed to detect evidence of enhanced lipid synthesis.[91–94] Corresponding to clinical observations, the development of proteinosis-like disease in immunodeficient mice suggests that an interaction between T lymphocytes and alveolar macrophages or epithelial cells may be important;[95, 96] however, the details of this potential interaction are unclear.

The results of a number of experiments have provided evidence of abnormal macrophage function and structure,[57, 97, 98] implying that this cell is particularly important in disease pathogenesis. However, the basis for these abnormalities is again unclear. Although it has been suggested that underlying immunodeficiency may be involved,[42] the rarity of PAP compared with the relatively common occurrence of immunodeficiency states indicates that other factors are implicated. The results of an experimental model involving mice deficient in the gene for granulocyte-macrophage colony–stimulating factor (GM-CSF) suggest that a lack of this substance may be an important factor.[99] It is also possible that inhaled materials are responsible for alveolar macrophage damage, a hypothesis that might explain the development of PAP following exposure to silica and other inorganic dusts. An understanding of the underlying cause of macrophage dysfunction is made more difficult by *in vitro*[100–102] and animal[68] studies in which the phagocytic function of alveolar macrophages has been shown to be suppressed by the lipoproteinaceous debris itself; this suggests that once the condition has begun, a feedback mechanism may act to perpetuate and possibly worsen the abnormality.

Pathologic Characteristics

At autopsy, the lungs are firm, and cut sections show patchy or diffuse consolidation; a viscous, yellowish fluid may ooze from the cut surface.[42] The normal architecture is preserved unless there is superimposed infection. Microscopically, the walls of transitional airways and alveoli are usually normal or at most slightly thickened by a lymphocytic infiltrate;[103, 104] rarely, interstitial fibrosis (sometimes severe) has been described.[56, 105–107] The alveoli are filled with fine granular material that stains eosinophilic with hematoxylin and eosin and pink or light purple with periodic acid–Schiff (PAS) stain (Fig. 68–5); on frozen section, the material may be basophilic.[108] In some cases, the air spaces are filled with abundant cholesterol crystals.[109] Acicular (needle-shaped) crystals and laminated bodies believed to be cellular fragments are also commonly present. Intact and apparently degenerating macrophages are usually evident within the granular material but are usually not abundant; small aggregates may be evident focally at the border between normal and affected lung. Ultrastructural investigation shows the intra-alveolar material to consist of amorphous granular debris containing numerous, relatively discrete osmiophilic granules or lamellar bodies, some of which resemble tubular myelin (Fig. 68–6).[35, 78–80]

Although enlargement of lymph nodes is typically not seen, either radiographically or pathologically, a case has been reported in which proteinaceous material was identified in a supraclavicular lymph node.[110]

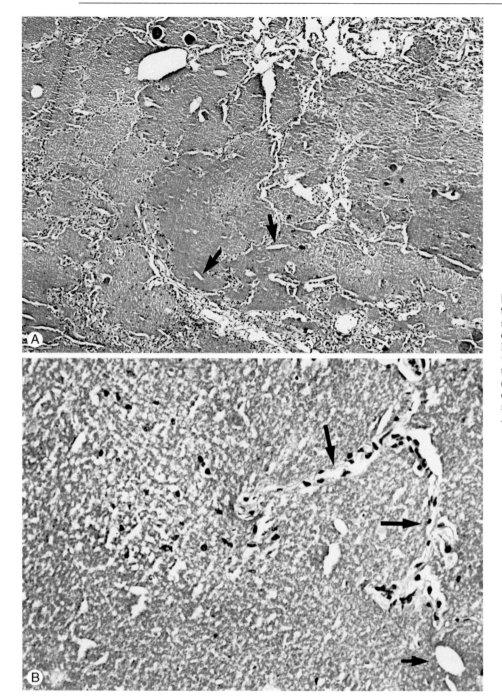

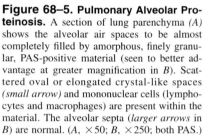

Figure 68–5. Pulmonary Alveolar Proteinosis. A section of lung parenchyma *(A)* shows the alveolar air spaces to be almost completely filled by amorphous, finely granular, PAS-positive material (seen to better advantage at greater magnification in *B*). Scattered oval or elongated crystal-like spaces *(small arrow)* and mononuclear cells (lymphocytes and macrophages) are present within the material. The alveolar septa *(larger arrows in B)* are normal. (*A*, ×50; *B*, ×250; both PAS.)

Radiologic Manifestations

The classic radiographic pattern consists of bilateral and symmetric areas of air-space consolidation with a vaguely nodular appearance and in a predominantly perihilar distribution (Fig. 68–7).[41, 111–113] This appearance was seen at some time in all 27 patients included in the first description of PAP in 1958.[41] In patients who have less severe disease, the radiographic findings may consist of ground-glass opacities rather than consolidation.[114] The parenchymal abnormalities range in extent from poorly defined nodular opacities or patchy areas of confluence involving mainly the lower lung zones to diffuse consolidation throughout both lungs.[112, 113, 115]

Differentiation from edema of cardiac origin can be made by the absence of cardiac enlargement or the lack of upper-lobe vessel distention, Kerley B lines, or pleural effusions. Occasionally, the parenchymal involvement is asymmetric or unilateral.[40, 112, 116] In some patients, a linear interstitial pattern can be seen superimposed on the areas of consolidation or ground-glass opacities; rarely, it is the predominant or only abnormality seen on the radiograph.[112, 117]

Conventional 7- to 10-mm-collimation CT scans demonstrate bilateral areas of consolidation with poorly defined margins (Fig. 68–8).[112] HRCT is superior to both conventional CT and chest radiography in the assessment of the pattern and distribution of abnormalities[112, 115] and may dem-

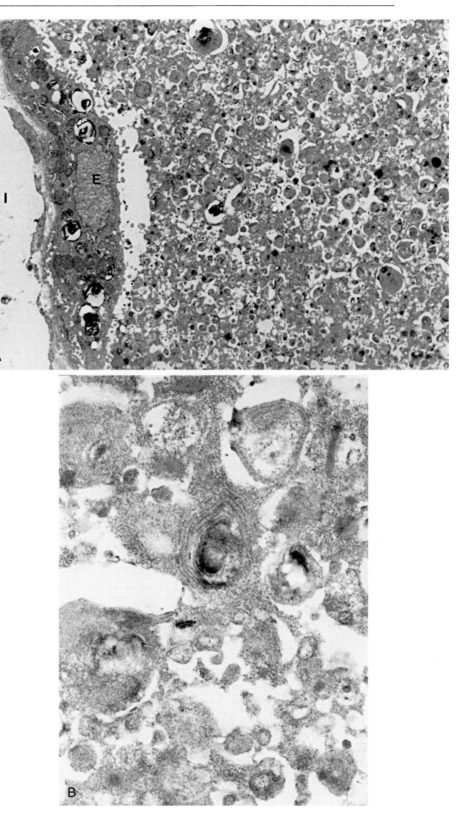

Figure 68–6. Pulmonary Alveolar Proteinosis. A transmission electron micrograph *(A)* shows a type II pneumocyte (E) overlying a somewhat fibrotic interstitium (I). The adjacent alveolar air space is filled with numerous, variably electron-dense bodies; at greater magnification *(B)*, some can be seen to have distinct lamellations resembling those seen in the normal type II cell osmiophilic body. *(A, ×9,500; B, ×56,000.)*

onstrate lesions even when the radiograph is normal.[116] The predominant abnormality consists of areas of ground-glass attenuation, although consolidation may also be present (particularly in the dorsal lung regions).[112, 113, 115] The distribution of disease is variable: most commonly it is random, but sometimes it is predominantly central or peripheral.[112, 115]

The areas of ground-glass attenuation often have sharply defined straight and angulated margins, giving them a geographic appearance.[115] The sharp margination usually reflects lobular or lobar boundaries.

In the majority of cases, a fine linear pattern forming polygonal shapes measuring 3 to 10 mm in diameter can be

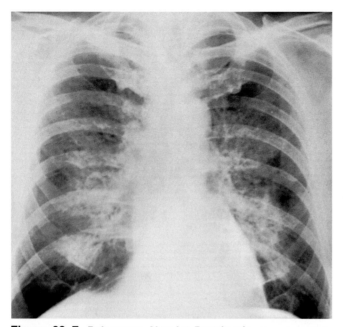

Figure 68–7. Pulmonary Alveolar Proteinosis. A posteroanterior chest radiograph reveals air-space consolidation with a vaguely nodular appearance involving the mid and lower lung zones. The disease possesses a "butterfly" pattern of distribution, the peripheral zones of the lungs being spared. The patient was a 65-year-old man who had a 5-month history of dry cough and dyspnea.

seen superimposed on the areas of ground-glass attenuation (Fig. 68–9).[114, 115] This combination gives an appearance that has been described as "crazy-paving"; in one study, this pattern was seen in all six patients.[115] The linear pattern was seen only in the areas of ground-glass attenuation or consolidation and was not apparent on the chest radiograph;[115] histologic assessment of open-lung biopsy specimens demonstrated septal edema. Apparent thickening of interlobular septa also may be seen at HRCT in patients who have normal septa pathologically, an effect that is presumably related to accumulation of lipoprotein in the air spaces adjacent to the septa.[118] It should be noted that the crazy-paving appearance can also be seen in a variety of other conditions, including bronchioloalveolar carcinoma,[119] lipid pneumonia, pulmonary hemorrhage, hydrostatic and permeability pulmonary edema, and bacterial pneumonia.[58, 120]

Resolution usually is complete radiographically but can occur asymmetrically and in a patchy fashion; occasionally, new foci of air-space consolidation develop in areas not previously affected.[121, 122] Resolution also may be associated with manifestations of bronchial obstruction, including segmental atelectasis and obstructive overinflation.[122] In fact, one case has been described in which bullae developed and were associated with subsequent spontaneous pneumothorax.[123] Neither lymph node enlargement nor pleural effusion occurs at any stage of PAP. The overall extent of disease and the degree of parenchymal opacification on the chest radiograph and HRCT scan correlate with the impairment in DLCO and with the severity of hypoxemia.[114]

Clinical Manifestations

Approximately one third of patients who have PAP are asymptomatic. The remainder manifest a variety of symptoms, the most frequent being shortness of breath on exertion that is usually slowly progressive in severity and unassociated with orthopnea; rarely, disease is fulminant.[124] Cough is often present; it is usually dry but may be associated with the expectoration of "chunky" gelatinous material that may take the form of a bronchial cast (Fig. 68–10). Hemoptysis occurs rarely.[125] Fatigue, weight loss, and pleuritic pain are evident in some patients.[41] A low-grade fever is said to develop at the onset of the illness in approximately 50% of patients;[41] although it may be a manifestation of the proteinosis, it should suggest the possibility of concomitant infection. Fine or coarse crackles sometimes can be heard on auscultation; in some patients, they have been found to disappear following BAL and recur with exacerbations of the disease.[126] Clubbing of the fingers and toes is not uncommon.[59, 127]

Laboratory Findings and Diagnosis

Laboratory investigation reveals a normal or slightly elevated white blood cell count and, not uncommonly, polycythemia. Hyperglobulinemia is present in a minority of patients.[41] Occasionally, immunoglobulin A (IgA) levels have been decreased in serum,[59, 82] and IgG, IgA, and IgM levels have been increased in BAL fluid.[82, 83] An increase in the level of serum lactate dehydrogenase is common.[128, 129] Analyses of BAL fluid and serum have shown an increase in some tumor markers such as carcinoembryonic antigen (CEA),[130] Lewis group antigen and squamous cell carcinoma antigen,[131] and in surfactant proteins A[85, 132] and D.[133] The degree of elevation of many of these substances seems to reflect the severity of disease.

Pulmonary function studies can be completely normal or can reveal a reduction in diffusing capacity,[134] vital capacity, and pulmonary compliance. Hypoxemia is caused by ventilation-perfusion inequality and intrapulmonary shunt[135, 136] and may be associated with pulmonary hypertension.[137] The results of follow-up function studies of patients managed successfully with BAL correlate well with clinical improvement.[138, 139]

The diagnosis of PAP should be strongly suspected when a chest radiograph reveals a pattern consistent with pulmonary edema in a patient who does not have clinical evidence of heart failure. It has been suggested that the diagnosis can be confirmed by the finding of an elevated level of surfactant protein A in sputum;[140] however, because sputum production is often slight, analysis of BAL fluid has been a more common diagnostic procedure. Features of BAL fluid suggestive of the diagnosis include:[141, 141a] (1) a grossly opaque or milky effluent; (2) relatively few inflammatory cells, including alveolar macrophages; (3) large acellular eosinophilic bodies in a diffuse background of granular basophilic material; (4) positive PAS staining of the proteinaceous material; (5) elevated levels of surfactant proteins; and (6) characteristic ultrastructural features. Although it is often possible to demonstrate one or more of these abnormalities, it is sometimes necessary to confirm the diagnosis by tissue examination, in which case transbronchial biopsy is often sufficient.[142]

Natural History and Prognosis

Analysis of cases documented in the literature before the widespread use of therapeutic BAL shows the disease to

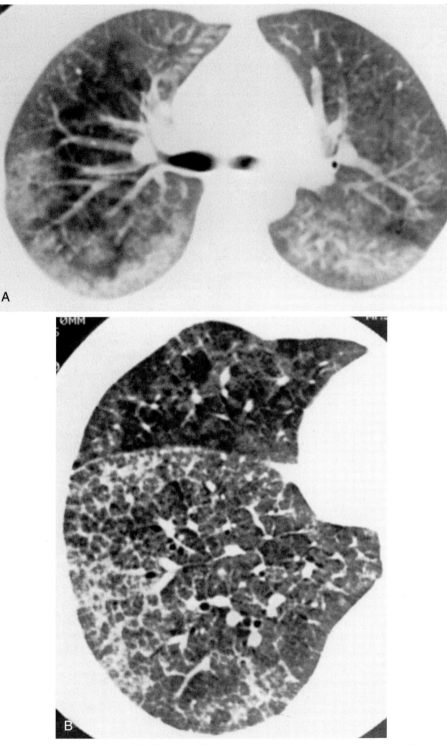

Figure 68–8. Pulmonary Alveolar Proteinosis: CT Manifestations in Two Patients. In the first patient, a 39-year-old woman, a CT scan with 10-mm collimation *(A)* reveals extensive bilateral air-space opacities with peripheral anatomic predominance, at least in the right lung. This appearance is consistent with virtually any diffuse air-space filling process, including alveolar proteinosis. In the second patient, a 44-year-old man, an HRCT scan *(B)* shows patchy areas of ground-glass attenuation and multiple polygonal lines.

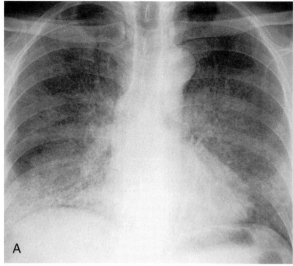

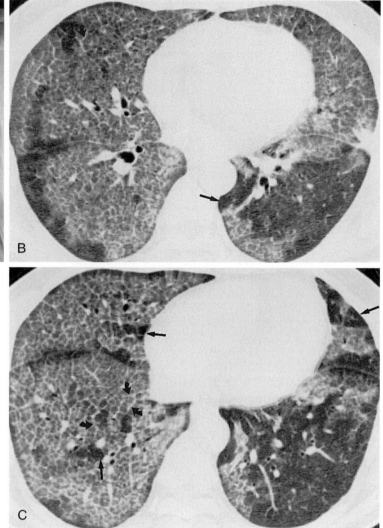

Figure 68–9. Pulmonary Alveolar Proteinosis. A posteroanterior chest radiograph *(A)* in a 49-year-old patient demonstrates bilateral areas of consolidation with a faintly nodular pattern involving mainly the mid and lower lung zones. HRCT scans *(B and C)* demonstrate extensive bilateral areas of ground-glass attenuation and a superimposed fine linear pattern forming polygonal arcades *(curved arrows)*. Note the sharp demarcation between normal and abnormal parenchyma *(straight arrows)*, a feature that usually reflects lobular boundaries. (Courtesy of Dr. Jim Barrie, University of Alberta Medical Centre.)

have been fatal in about one third of patients, death resulting either from respiratory failure caused by the proteinosis or from superimposed infection.[125, 143–146] Irrigation of the tracheobronchial tree by BAL is an effective therapeutic procedure that can be life-saving (Fig. 68–11) and has greatly improved the prognosis.[126, 147] Some patients do not require more than one or two procedures,[148, 149] whereas a few require whole-lung lavage repeated semiannually or annually.[45, 126, 134] The condition has been documented to recur following lung transplantation.[151]

In one prospective study published in 1984 in which 23 patients were followed over a period of 15 years, spontaneous remission without treatment was observed in 24%, and progressive dyspnea and decrease in pulmonary function requiring BAL in the remainder;[45] there were no deaths or opportunistic infections during the period of observation. In cases of spontaneous remission, it is thought that the intra-alveolar material is partly expectorated and partly phagocytosed and removed by the lymphatics.[121] When such remission occurs, it is usually permanent;[127] however, a patient has been described who had a relapse 18 years after the primary episode.[152] Rarely, the disease is associated with interstitial fibrosis of sufficient severity to cause pulmonary insufficiency and death.[105]

AMYLOIDOSIS

Although originally considered to represent a single substance, amyloid is now known to consist of several proteins, each of which resembles the others morphologically but is distinctive biochemically.[150, 153] Ultrastructurally, amyloid appears as a twisted array of nonbranching fibrils 7.5 to 10 nm in diameter; examination by x-ray crystallography shows them to be arranged as beta-pleated sheets, regardless of their chemical composition. Light microscopic examination demonstrates amorphous material that is pink with hematoxylin and eosin staining, violet-red with crystal violet staining (as a manifestation of metachromasia), and red with Congo red staining (the last also showing apple-green birefringence with polarization microscopy).

Because of its great variety of clinical and pathologic manifestations, amyloidosis has been classified in several ways.[154] The traditional division has been into four major forms depending on the underlying clinical features: (1) *primary amyloidosis*, in which no associated disease is recognized or in which there is an underlying plasma cell disorder (most commonly multiple myeloma); (2) *secondary amyloidosis*, in which there is an identifiable underlying chronic inflammatory abnormality such as tuberculosis,

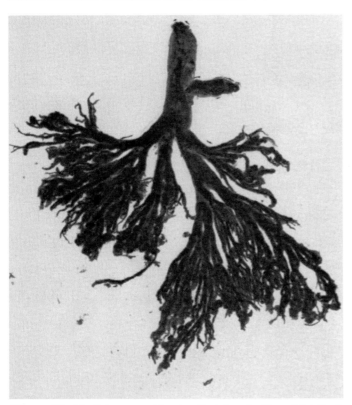

Figure 68–10. Pulmonary Alveolar Proteinosis: Bronchial Cast Formation. The specimen is a cast of the right lower lobe bronchial tree that was expectorated by a a 57-year-old woman who gave a 5-year history of dyspnea and several episodes of expectoration of bronchial casts similar to the one illustrated. Open-lung biopsy showed characteristic features of pulmonary alveolar proteinosis. Despite repeated bronchoalveolar lavage, her symptoms progressed and she died of respiratory failure 1 year later. (Courtesy of Dr. R. Chapela and Dr. R. Sansores, National Respiratory Disease Institute of Mexico.)

bronchiectasis, rheumatoid disease, syphilis, or certain neoplasms such as Hodgkin's disease; (3) *familial amyloidosis*, a relatively uncommon form that may be localized to a specific tissue such as nerve; and (4) so-called *senile amyloidosis*, which affects many organs and tissues and is usually seen in persons older than 70 years of age. A subdivision of amyloidosis into localized (i.e., within a single organ or tissue) and generalized forms is also common.

It has also been proposed that amyloidosis is better classified on the basis of the specific protein of which the amyloid is composed.[153] Over 15 such proteins have been identified, of which several have been implicated in respiratory disease. The most important in this respect are *amyloid L* (AL) and *amyloid A* (AA). AL is related to the deposition of immunoglobulin light chains and is thus usually associated with abnormal plasma cell function, either localized to the lungs or as part of a systemic disease such as multiple myeloma or macroglobulinemia. AA is related to a protein derived from a serum acute phase reactant (SAA) synthesized in the liver. The latter can be formed in several settings, including:

- chronic inflammatory disease, such as connective tissue disease (particularly rheumatoid disease but also other conditions such as systemic lupus erythematosus[155]), infection (primarily tuberculosis but occasionally caused by other

organisms such as *Coxiella burnetii*[156]), bronchiectasis, Crohn's disease, ulcerative colitis, and heroin abuse
- certain neoplasms, such as renal cell carcinoma[157] and Hodgkin's disease
- familial Mediterranean fever[158]

Other precursor proteins of amyloid include *transthyretin* (prealbumin, ATTR), a serum protein that normally transports thyroxine and that is associated with heart and pulmonary deposits in so-called senile amyloidosis;[159] *beta₂-microglobulin* (β_2M), a normal serum protein that is often increased in chronic renal failure;[160] and *endocrine-related amyloid* (AE), derived from local hormone deposition in the stroma of some neuroendocrine tumors of the lung and other organs.[161–163]

Although these classifications are helpful in understanding the underlying nature of amyloidosis, from the point of view of diagnosis and the clinical consequences of thoracic involvement, it is often more useful to consider the anatomic location of disease. According to this concept, three major patterns of amyloid deposition can occur in the lower respiratory tract: tracheobronchial, nodular parenchymal, and diffuse parenchymal (interstitial). Although these patterns can occur in combination,[164, 165] in most cases the amyloid is deposited predominantly in one site, thus providing some rationale for a discussion on this basis. In addition to airway and pulmonary parenchymal disease, amyloidosis can also affect the pleura (Fig. 68–12),[166, 167] pulmonary arteries,[159] hilar[168–170] and mediastinal lymph nodes,[171, 172] and the diaphragm (in some cases associated with respiratory failure).[173, 174]

When considering a diagnosis of thoracic amyloidosis, it must be remembered that pleuropulmonary disease caused by such abnormalities as chronic tuberculosis, bronchiectasis, lung abscess, chronic aspergillosis,[175] rheumatoid pleuritis,[176] extrinsic allergic alveolitis,[177] and cystic fibrosis[178–180] can result in amyloidosis; rarely, this secondary phenomenon can alter the course and/or radiographic or pathologic appearance of the underlying pulmonary abnormality.

Pathogenesis

A detailed description of the basic pathogenetic features of amyloidosis is beyond the scope of this text; however, certain specific features related to pulmonary disease deserve mention. With the exception of "senile"-type amyloid, which is composed of transthyretin,[153, 181] most (albeit not all[182, 183]) localized deposits of amyloid in the lungs consist of AL,[184–187] often the lambda III subgroup.[188] In the great majority of these cases, there is no evidence of systemic immunologic disease (such as multiple myeloma or Waldenström's macroglobulinemia) or serologic immunoglobulin abnormality.[184, 186] Thus, it has been speculated that local immunoglobulin deposition, possibly related to either overproduction or impaired clearance secondary to a chronic inflammatory process, may be responsible for the amyloid accumulation.[186] Immunohistochemical and gene rearrangement studies of some pulmonary amyloid nodules have also shown evidence of clonal plasma cell expansion, suggesting a localized neoplastic process.[48]

The presence of clusters of plasma cells adjacent to localized deposits of amyloid in some cases supports both

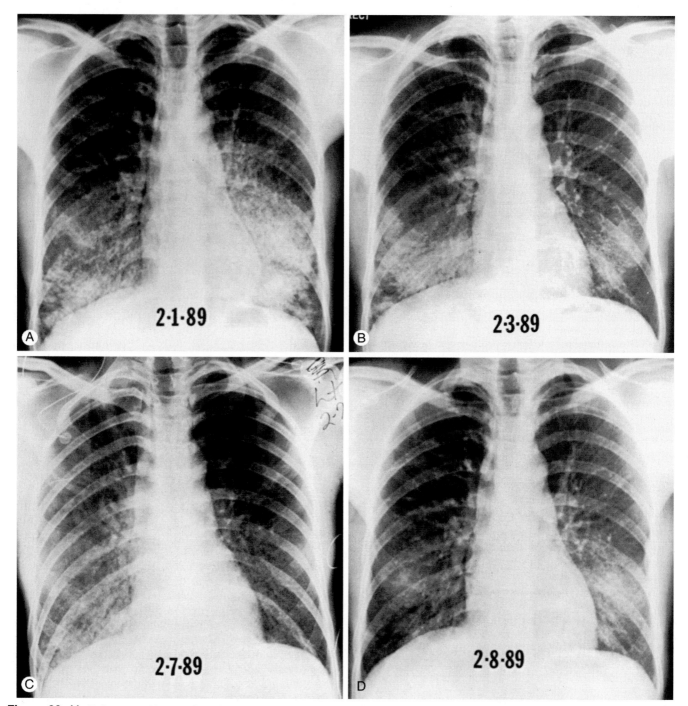

Figure 68–11. Pulmonary Alveolar Proteinosis: Response to Bronchoalveolar Lavage. A posteroanterior radiograph *(A)* of this 29-year-old woman with known alveolar proteinosis reveals extensive bilateral patchy air-space opacities with middle and lower zonal predominance. Approximately 1 month later, a repeat radiograph 24 hours following left lung lavage *(B)* shows almost complete clearing of the left-sided opacities. Four days later, a radiograph obtained immediately following right lung lavage *(C)* reveals marked worsening of the opacities throughout this lung, caused by the presence of lavage fluid within lung parenchyma. Twenty-four hours later *(D)*, the fluid had been absorbed and the right lung was almost normal in appearance.

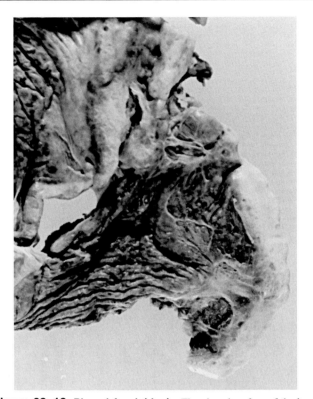

Figure 68–12. Pleural Amyloidosis. The pleural surface of the lower lobe and parts of the upper lobe are partially covered by creamy white plaques and thin strands, shown on histologic examination to be composed of amyloid. (The wrinkled structure at the base of the lower lobe is an adherent hemidiaphragm).

inflammatory and neoplastic concepts.[189] Typically, the cytoplasm of the plasma cells in such cases reacts with antiserum directed toward immunoglobulin light chain or Bence Jones protein (or both), whereas adjacent amyloid reacts with AL antiserum, suggesting that the plasma cells produce and secrete immunoglobulin light chains or Bence Jones protein that undergoes proteolysis to protein AL.[189]

Pathologic Characteristics

The pathologic characteristics of the various forms of pulmonary amyloidosis have been well described in both the older[164, 190] and more recent[159, 184, 185, 191] literature.

Airway involvement occurs most commonly in the trachea and proximal bronchi. Although there is overlap, it is usually manifested in one of two ways:[154, 184, 186, 187] a localized tumor-like nodule or (more commonly) multiple discrete or confluent plaques that cause distortion of the airway wall and stenosis of its lumen. Histologically, the amyloid is situated in the subepithelial interstitial tissue and often surrounds tracheobronchial ducts and acini, some of which may show secondary atrophy (Fig. 68–13). Calcification, ossification, and foreign body giant cell reaction may be present but are probably less common than in the nodular form of parenchymal disease;[185] however, ossification is so severe in some patients that the disease can be confused with tracheobronchopathia osteochondroplastica.[192] Plasma cells and lymphocytes are present in variable numbers between foci of amyloid deposition.

The parenchymal nodules of localized pulmonary amy-

loidosis can be solitary or multiple and usually are fairly well defined. Grossly, they have a grayish-brown, waxy appearance and may be firm or quite hard, depending on the extent of associated calcification or ossification. At the periphery of the nodule, amyloid is often present in the alveolar interstitium only; however, in the central regions, normal parenchymal structure is usually inapparent as a result of the presence of a mass of amyloid, typically containing numerous multinucleated giant cells and variable numbers of lymphocytes and plasma cells (Fig. 68–14). The presence of amyloid in the tunica media of blood vessels, both within and immediately adjacent to the main mass, is common.

In diffuse interstitial disease, amyloid is present in the media of small (and occasionally medium-sized) blood vessels and in the parenchymal interstitium (Fig. 68–15). In the latter site, it is situated in relation to endothelial and epithelial basement membranes and can appear in a uniform and more or less linear pattern or as multiple small nodules;[165] in early disease, it may be manifested as no more than a slight thickening of the alveolar septal basement membrane (Fig. 68–16). Inflammatory cells (multinucleated giant cells, plasma cells, and lymphocytes) and ossification or calcification are typically absent.

As indicated, vascular involvement is common in each of these forms of amyloidosis. It is also not infrequent in senile amyloidosis, particularly when the heart is also affected;[159] in the latter circumstance, the sole site of amyloid deposition is usually the vessels. In all situations, the amyloid is usually most prominent in the media of small to medium-sized pulmonary arteries (Fig. 68–17); involvement of the lymphatics is also common.[193]

Amyloidosis may be confused histologically with disease associated with light chain deposition. In this abnormality, kappa or lambda light chains produced in association with a plasma cell dyscrasia are deposited in tissue but fail to polymerize into the beta-pleated sheet typical of amyloid; extracellular deposits are thus formed that are histologically similar to but ultrastructurally and histochemically different from amyloid. Although most often identified in the kidneys, such deposits also have been reported in the lungs, either as an isolated finding[194, 195] or admixed with typical amyloid deposits.[196]

Radiologic Manifestations

In the tracheobronchial form of amyloidosis, focal or diffuse (Fig. 68–18) thickening of the wall (Fig. 68–19) or a localized intraluminal nodule may occasionally be seen on the radiograph or CT scan.[197–199] More common radiographic features include general accentuation of bronchovascular markings associated with overinflation, and atelectasis or obstructive pneumonitis. The latter may involve a segment, a lobe, or an entire lung.[200–202]

Nodular parenchymal amyloidosis is manifested by solitary or, less commonly, multiple nodules usually ranging from 0.5 to 5 cm in diameter (Fig. 68–20).[185, 199, 203] Calcification is seldom evident on the radiograph[204] but is seen in 20% to 50% of nodules on CT scans.[198, 203, 205, 206] Rarely, the nodules are cavitated.[184, 207] Occasionally, cystic changes are seen adjacent to the nodules (Fig. 68–20). The nodules occur most commonly in the lower lobes and typically are located

Text continued on page 2716

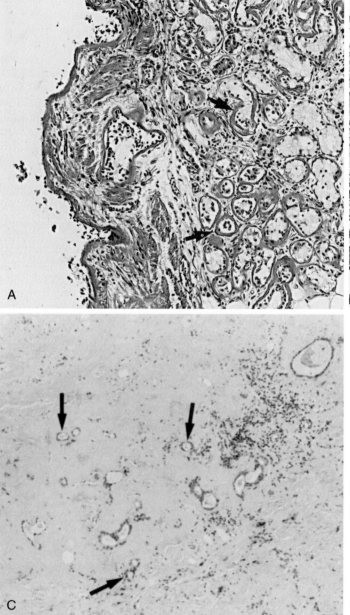

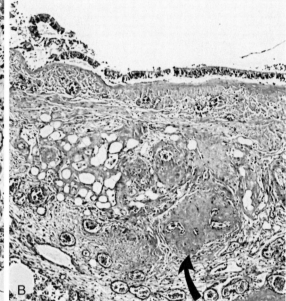

Figure 68–13. Amyloidosis: Bronchial Wall Involvement. Sections show mild *(A)*, moderate *(B)*, and marked *(C)* amyloidosis of the bronchial wall. In *A*, there is a slight thickening of the tissue adjacent to the bronchial gland acini *(arrows)*. Small nodules of amyloid *(arrow)* are evident in *B* as well as thickening of the lamina propria and tissue between fat cells. In *C*, there is marked amyloid deposition associated with significant bronchial gland atrophy (residual acini are indicated by arrows). *(A,* ×100; *B,* ×50; *C,* ×60.)

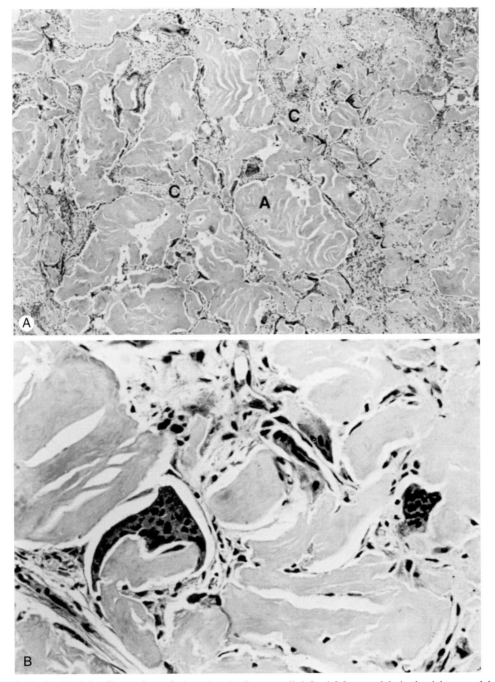

Figure 68–14. Amyloidosis: Nodular Parenchymal. A section *(A)* from a well-defined 2.5-cm nodule in the right upper lobe of an asymptomatic 60-year-old man shows abundant amyloid (A) separated by a small amount of connective tissue (C) containing plasma cells, occasional lymphocytes, and rather numerous multinucleated giant cells. The last-named are seen to better advantage in a magnified view *(B)*. (A, ×40; B, ×275.)

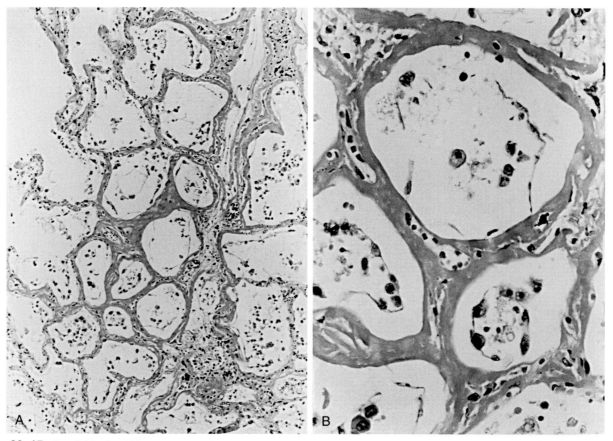

Figure 68–15. Amyloidosis: Diffuse Interstitial. Sections show mild to moderate thickening of the alveolar septal interstitium by amyloid. Its location between the capillary wall and alveolar epithelial surface can be clearly seen in *B*.

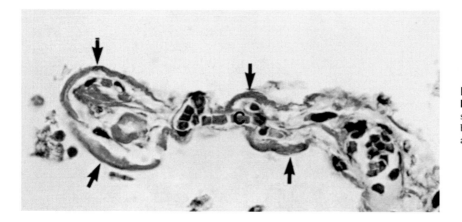

Figure 16–16. Amyloidosis: Early Interstitial Involvement. A magnified view of an alveolar septum shows several very thin deposits of amyloid situated between the capillary lumen (C) and the overlying alveolar epithelium *(arrows)*. (×600.)

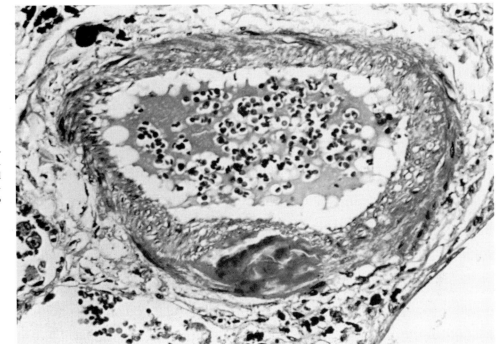

Figure 68–17. Amyloidosis: Pulmonary Arterial. A section of a muscular pulmonary artery reveals focal amyloid deposition in the media. This was an incidental finding in an 87-year-old man who also had left atrial amyloidosis. (×250.)

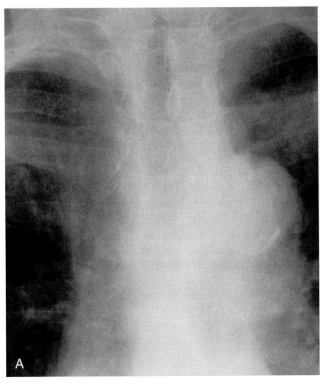

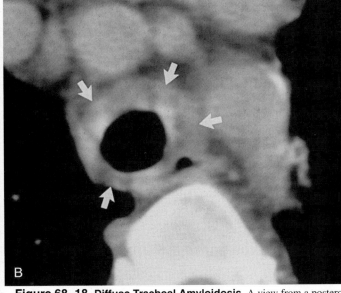

Figure 68–18. Diffuse Tracheal Amyloidosis. A view from a posteroanterior chest radiograph *(A)* demonstrates irregular narrowing of the trachea. A CT scan immediately above the level of the aortic arch *(B)* demonstrates marked circumferential thickening of the trachea *(arrows).* On CT and at bronchoscopy the entire trachea was abnormal. The diagnosis of diffuse tracheal amyloidosis was proven by endoscopic biopsy.

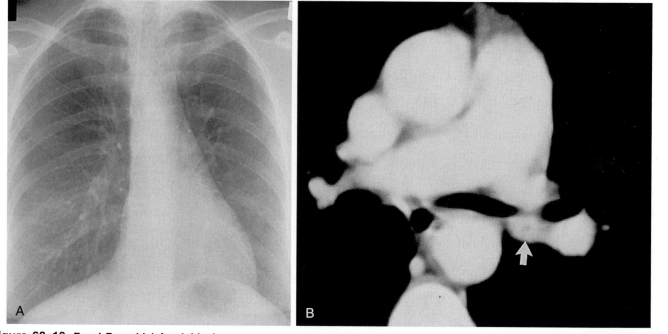

Figure 68–19. Focal Bronchial Amyloidosis. A posteroanterior chest radiograph *(A)* in a 51-year-old woman demonstrates slight loss of volume and decreased vascularity of the left lung. An intravenous contrast-enhanced CT scan *(B)* demonstrates an enhancing soft tissue nodule *(arrow)* that has caused partial obstruction of the left upper and left lower lobe bronchi and led to reflex vasoconstriction. The lesion was resected surgically and shown to be composed of amyloid.

peripherally.[185, 203] Disease usually progresses slowly over several years, with a slight increase in size of the nodules and the development of additional nodules.[207, 208] A case has been described in which a homogeneous mass measuring several centimeters in diameter and situated at the apex of the left lung was associated with destruction of the first rib, thus simulating a Pancoast tumor.[209] Obstructive bronchial amyloidosis and peripheral parenchymal disease occasion-

ally occur concomitantly.[200, 201] A combination of lymphoid interstitial pneumonitis and amyloid nodules that had irregular margins and cystic changes on HRCT has also been reported.[209a]

Diffuse interstitial disease is rarely seen in primary pulmonary amyloidosis, being present in only 6 of 48 cases in one study[185] and in none of 55 in another.[199] The radiographic findings consist of a diffuse, linear interstitial pattern or, less commonly, air-space consolidation or a small nodular pattern (Fig. 68–21).[185, 210, 211] HRCT in one case revealed a linear interstitial pattern, small nodules, and patchy areas of consolidation involving mainly the subpleural regions of the lower lung zones;[210] several of the small nodules contained calcific foci.

In patients who have systemic amyloidosis associated with pulmonary parenchymal involvement, the radiographic findings consist of a reticular, nodular, or reticulonodular pattern that may be diffuse or involve mainly the lower lobes.[199] The nodules may be small, mimicking miliary tuberculosis, or measure up to 2.5 cm in diameter.[203] Unilateral or bilateral pleural effusions may be seen and occasionally constitute the only abnormality evident on the chest radiograph (Fig. 68–22).[199] In a review of the HRCT findings in 12 patients who had systemic amyloidosis with thoracic involvement, the most common abnormality was hilar and mediastinal lymphadenopathy, present in 9 patients (75%).[203] Punctate calcifications were present within the enlarged nodes in 3 of the 9 patients. Diffuse lung involvement was present in 8 patients (66%). The parenchymal abnormalities consisted of multiple small nodules, interlobular septal thickening, irregular lines giving a reticular pattern, and areas of ground-glass attenuation or consolidation. Punctate calcification was seen in some of the nodules and areas of consoli-

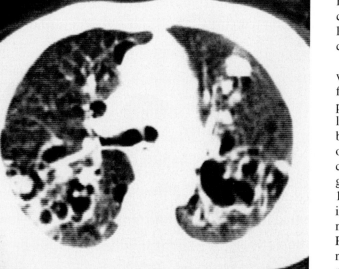

Figure 68–20. Amyloidosis: Nodular Parenchymal. A CT scan at the level of the carina reveals multiple nodules and cystic spaces. The patient was an elderly woman who complained of dyspnea.

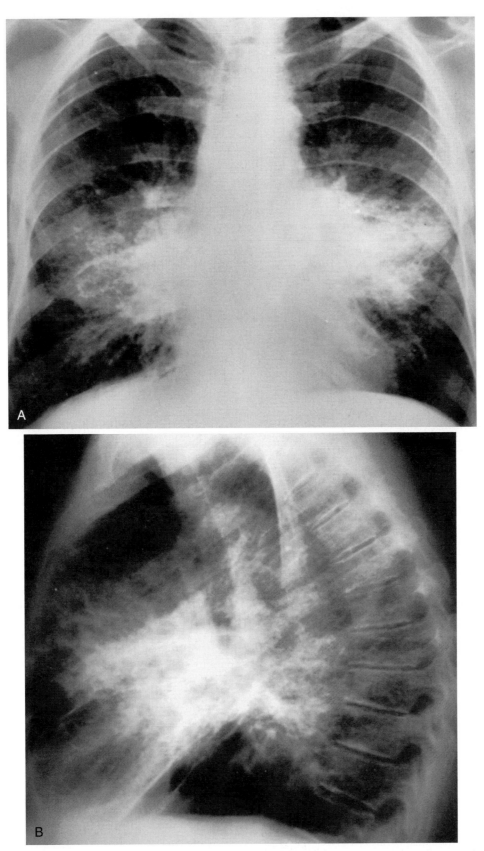

Figure 68–21. Diffuse Parenchymal Amyloidosis. Posteroanterior *(A)* and lateral *(B)* radiographs reveal fairly large, poorly defined inhomogeneous opacities in the medial and central portions of both lungs that possess a "butterfly" distribution. The lungs are otherwise normal. Possible hilar lymph node enlargement cannot be evaluated because of contiguity of the parenchymal disease. Open lung biopsy showed typical interstitial amyloid.

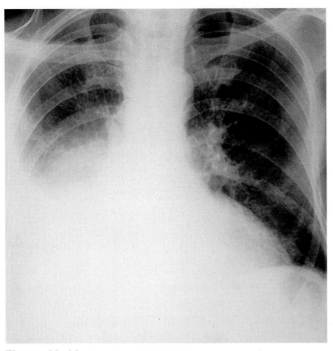

Figure 68–22. Pleural Amyloidosis. A posteroanterior chest radiograph in a 53-year-old man with systemic amyloidosis demonstrates right pleural effusion. The diagnosis of pleural amyloidosis was confirmed by biopsy and at autopsy (*see* Fig. 68–12).

dation (Fig. 68–23). The abnormalities frequently had a predominantly basilar and peripheral distribution.

Clinical Manifestations

The plaquelike form of tracheobronchial amyloidosis can cause progressive dyspnea or symptoms that simulate asthma;[212, 213] hemoptysis[202, 212] and recurrent bronchitis and pneumonia are common.[202, 214] Laryngeal amyloidosis is frequently associated with hoarseness,[215, 216] and involvement of the tongue (leading to macroglossia) can cause obstructive sleep apnea.[217] Occasional cases of combined upper and lower airway disease have been described.[218] Discrete tracheal and endobronchial "tumors" seldom cause symptoms and are usually discovered incidentally at bronchoscopy; however, as indicated previously, they can be large enough to cause airway obstruction, atelectasis, and bronchiectasis.[216, 219] Other symptoms and signs depend on the volume of lung affected and whether infection is present. Some patients who have familial amyloidotic polyneuropathy have been shown to have airway hyper-responsiveness, possibly on the basis of amyloid deposition in airway autonomic nerves.[220]

Patients who have the nodular parenchymal form of amyloidosis are usually asymptomatic,[185, 221, 222] the lesion being discovered on a screening chest radiograph; rarely, the nodules are extensive and large enough to cause respiratory symptoms and even respiratory failure.[223] A patient has been described in whom multinodular deposits of amyloid compressed small bronchi, causing bronchiectasis and fatal hemorrhage.[224] An unusual case apparently complicated by an arteriovenous fistula has also been documented.[225] New lesions occasionally have been reported to appear following surgical excision of nodules;[223] whether this represents the effect of inadequate resection or the development of independent lesions is unclear. The majority of patients have no evidence of extrathoracic disease (either amyloidosis or otherwise); however, nodules have been reported in patients who had Sjögren's syndrome[182] or Crohn's disease.[183]

Diffuse interstitial amyloidosis is commonly accompanied by dyspnea and may be associated with respiratory insufficiency.[184, 185, 226] Although dyspnea may be secondary to pulmonary disease itself, it is important to remember that this manifestation may be related to cardiac amyloidosis. Associated pulmonary vascular amyloidosis has been reported to be complicated by hypertension[227] and repeated hemoptysis (the latter ascribed to medial dissection of pulmonary arteries[228]). Diffuse interstitial amyloidosis is most often seen as part of multisystem disease (primary amyloidosis), in which circumstance AL is typically present and may be associated with multiple myeloma.[229] Rarely, AA protein has been shown to be responsible.[230] Pulmonary function tests may show evidence of restriction and impaired gas transfer.[231]

Diagnosis

Biopsy of rectal tissue or of subcutaneous abdominal fat may be required to confirm the diagnosis. When disease is localized to the lungs, transbronchial biopsy,[232] open-lung biopsy, or transthoracic needle aspiration[233] usually yields diagnostic tissue; rarely, amyloid has been identified in bronchial brushing specimens.[232] Excessive bleeding following transbronchial biopsy has been reported in some patients.[234] Bronchoscopy reveals irregular-shaped nodules or plaques with an intact mucous membrane.[212, 235]

Circulating and tissue-bound monoclonal light chains, more often lambda than kappa, are frequently present in patients who have primary amyloidosis.[185, 215, 236–238] In other patients, including those who have secondary disease, nonspecific immunoglobulin abnormalities may be observed, with serum levels of IgA, IgG, and IgM either increased or decreased. In the 5% to 10% of patients who have multiple myeloma and amyloidosis, IgG (less commonly IgA) monoclonal gammopathy is invariable.[239, 240]

Natural History and Prognosis

The prognosis of patients who have nodular parenchymal amyloidosis is generally good: in most cases, the nodules remain stationary in size or grow slowly and cause no symptoms;[241] spontaneous regression has also been described.[242] By contrast, progression of disease is frequent in the tracheobronchial and diffuse interstitial forms of disease. Bronchoscopic or surgical excision of localized airway deposits may provide relief of obstruction; however, recurrence is common, and approximately 30% of patients have been reported to die of the disease.[202] The natural history and prognosis of disease in patients who have diffuse interstitial pulmonary involvement may reflect the presence of amyloid elsewhere in the body, particularly the heart and kidneys; however, many affected persons die of respiratory failure.[221] In one series of 35 patients, the median survival time after diagnosis was only 16 months.[229]

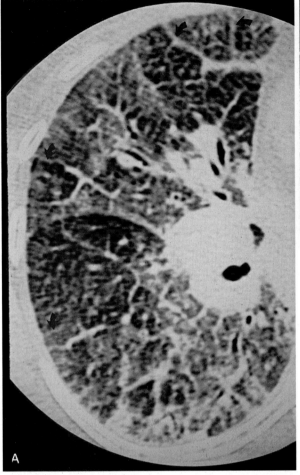

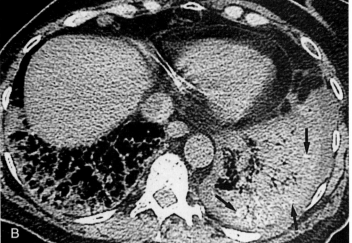

Figure 68–23. Diffuse Interstitial Amyloidosis. A magnified view of the right hemithorax from an HRCT scan *(A)* demonstrates diffuse interlobular septal thickening *(curved arrows)* as well as irregular opacities, areas of ground-glass attenuation, and right hilar lymphadenopathy. An HRCT scan through the level of the right hemidiaphragm photographed at soft tissue windows *(B)* shows interlobular septal thickening in the right lower lobe and extensive left lower lobe consolidation. Punctate areas of calcification *(arrows)* within the consolidated left lower lobe and a small left pleural effusion are also evident. The patient was a 69-year-old woman who had primary systemic amyloidosis. (From Pickford HA, Swensen SJ, Utz JP: Thoracic cross-sectional imaging of amyloidosis. Am J Roentgenol 168:351, 1997. Courtesy of Dr. Stephen Swensen, Mayo Clinic, Rochester, MN.)

PULMONARY ALVEOLAR MICROLITHIASIS

Pulmonary alveolar microlithiasis is a rare disease characterized by the presence of innumerable tiny calculi ("calcispherytes") within alveolar air spaces. An early treatise on the subject, published in 1957, was based on 26 cases collected from many centers throughout the world.[243] Approximately 300 cases had been published by 1997;[244–246] the authors of reviews of the Turkish[247] and Italian[246] literature in 1993 and 1997, respectively, found a total of 100 cases in these countries.

Although the disease can occur at any age—having been identified in premature stillborn twins[248] and in an 80-year-old woman[249]—the majority of reported cases have been in patients between the ages of 20 and 50 years.[247] In Japan[250] and Italy,[246] however, the peak incidence has been found to be in the first and second decades of life, respectively. Some investigators have documented a predilection for men[244, 247] or women;[246] however, most have found no sex predominance.[243, 247]

Etiology and Pathogenesis

The etiology and pathogenesis of pulmonary alveolar microlithiasis are unknown. Hypothetical mechanisms that have been invoked include an inborn error of metabolism, an unusual response to an unspecified pulmonary insult, an immune-mediated reaction to various irritants, and an acquired abnormality of calcium or phosphorus metabolism.

A familial occurrence has been noted in approximately half the reported cases,[243, 246, 247, 251] and, as indicated previously, the abnormality has been documented in twins.[248] Although these observations suggest a genetic factor such as an inborn error of metabolism, familial cases have been restricted almost entirely to siblings, suggesting that environmental factors may also be important. Circumstantial evidence in support of this hypothesis comes from a report of a family of seven siblings in which the disease developed in the four sisters who lived together but not in the three who had left home at an early age.[251] A history of occupational or environmental dust exposure is generally lacking;[247] however, there have been reports of the disease in a patient who was strongly addicted to the inhalation of snuff containing over 9% calcium,[253] in a patient who had occupational exposure to mica (although no mica was evident in samples of her lung tissue),[254] and in four patients exposed to sand particles in the desert.[254a]

The findings in several case reports suggest that an acquired metabolic disturbance may be involved in the pathogenesis of the disease. For example, although the microliths are almost invariably confined to the lungs, one patient had multiple urinary calculi[255] and another had calcific deposits in his sympathetic ganglia (histologically) and gonads (radiographically).[256] In addition, in one patient with milk-alkali syndrome, microliths appeared to form secondary to mineralization of desquamated epithelial cells.[257] Despite these observations, the finding that serum calcium and phosphorus levels are generally normal suggests that a systemic metabolic abnormality is not likely to be involved in most cases.[258, 259] The condition has been found to develop in a renal transplant recipient,[260] suggesting the possibility of an immunologic abnormality in pathogenesis; however, the number of such cases is so small that a coincidental association cannot be excluded.

Because calcium salts are more soluble in an acid medium and are more easily precipitated from alkaline solutions, it has been postulated that microliths may result from some undefined alteration in alveolar epithelial secretions that promotes alkalinity at the alveolar interface and thus predisposes to the deposition or precipitation of calcium phosphate within the alveoli.[243, 259] Scintigraphy with ^{99m}Tc-diphosphonate has shown uptake of the tracer by microliths,[261] suggesting the presence of an active metabolic exchange across the alveolocapillary membrane.

Pathologic Characteristics

Grossly, the lungs are firm to hard and may be very difficult to cut. The surface of individual slices may be gritty and have a fine granular appearance somewhat resembling that in intravenous talcosis (Fig. 68–24). On histologic examination, microliths range in size from about 250 to 750 μm in diameter and are located almost invariably within alveolar air spaces.[244, 254] Nevertheless, evidence suggests that they are formed in the alveolar walls, possibly in association with type II cells,[248] and are subsequently extruded into the adjacent air spaces.[262] Occasionally, microliths are present outside the alveolar lumen in bronchial wall or fibrotic interstitium;[249] rarely, they are found in extrapulmonary sites.[256, 263]

Individual microliths are round, oval, or irregular in shape and have a concentric laminated appearance (*see* Fig. 68–24), often with a PAS-positive central core.[265–267] In one scanning electron microscopic study, they were found to be globular or irregular in shape and to have a granular or rough outer surface.[266] Chemical analysis and energy-dispersive x-ray microanalysis have shown them to be composed principally of calcium phosphate.[244, 254, 263, 268] Some investigators have found evidence of a noncalcified stage before the development of the typical dense calcification.[249, 250]

In the early stages of the disease, the alveolar walls are normal;[243] eventually, interstitial fibrosis develops (*see* Fig. 68–24), sometimes associated with multinucleated giant cell formation.[263] Blebs and bullae are often present, particularly

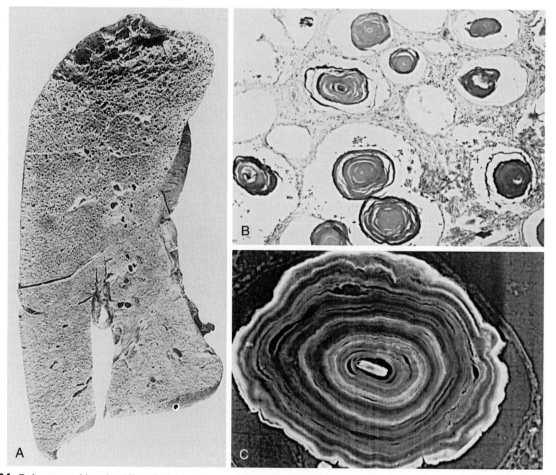

Figure 68–24. Pulmonary Alveolar Microlithiasis. The cut surface of a midsagittal lung slice *(A)* has fine granular appearance from apex to base. A section *(B)* shows interstitial fibrosis and several laminated microliths within the residual air spaces. An electron micrograph of one of the microliths *(C)* shows a central particulate nidus surrounded by concentric layers of calcium phosphate. (From Moran CA, et al: Pulmonary alveolar microlithiasis: A clinicopathologic and chemical analysis of seven cases. Arch Pathol Lab Med 121:607, 1997.)

in the lung apices;[243, 251, 255] how these relate to the presence of microliths is unclear.

Microliths should not be confused with corpora amylacea, which are also round, laminated bodies present in the alveolar air spaces of many persons. These bodies are mostly 50 to 200 μm in diameter and are often surrounded by one or more alveolar macrophages (Fig. 68–25); most contain a central birefringent particle. Unlike microliths, corpora amylacea are strongly PAS-positive and contain little or no calcium; the results of some investigations suggest that they are related to amyloid, possibly the β₂M component.[269, 270] The etiology and pathogenesis of these bodies are unclear. Some investigators have found evidence that they may form on inhaled spores of *Lycopodium clavatum*.[271] Others have suggested that they may result from aggregation and compaction of degenerated alveolar macrophages[270] or surfactant apoprotein.[272] Corpora amylacea are fairly common, having been documented in about 0.5%[271] to 4%[273] of routine autopsies. They are of no clinical or radiologic significance.

Radiologic Manifestations

No other pulmonary disease has a radiographic pattern as characteristic and diagnostic as that of alveolar microlithiasis. Although considerable variation occurs from patient to patient, depending on the severity of affliction, the fundamental pattern is one of a very fine micronodulation diffusely involving both lungs (Fig. 68–26).[244, 275, 276] Regardless of the effect of superimposition or summation of shadows, individual deposits are usually identifiable as very sharply defined nodules measuring less than 1 mm in diameter. The overall density is greater over the lower than the upper zones. The opacities may be so numerous as to appear confluent, in which circumstance a normally exposed chest radiograph shows the lungs as almost uniformly white, often with total obliteration of the mediastinal and diaphragmatic contours; however, use of an overexposed radiographic technique usually reveals the underlying pattern to better advantage. In most cases, chest radiographs obtained up to 20

to 30 years previously, sometimes in early childhood, are abnormal.[244, 274] Radiographs from asymptomatic relatives of an index case may also show characteristic manifestations of the disease.[275]

Occasionally, radiographic changes consist of a reticular pattern or septal lines superimposed on the characteristic "sandstorm" appearance.[276, 277] Other findings that may be seen include bullae in the lung apices, a zone of increased lucency between the lung parenchyma and the ribs (known as a black pleural line), and pleural calcification.[251, 278, 279] Calcification in the pericardium has also been described in a 13-year-old child.[280]

The HRCT manifestations of pulmonary alveolar microlithiasis consist of calcific nodules measuring 1 mm or less in diameter, sometimes confluent, and distributed predominantly along the cardiac borders and dorsal portions of the lower lung zones (Fig. 68–27).[281–283] The higher attenuation in the dorsal portion of the lungs persists when scans are obtained with the patient in the prone position.[282] Calcific interlobular septal thickening is also commonly seen (Fig. 68–27).[118, 281, 283] Correlation of HRCT findings with pathologic specimens has shown that this apparent thickening is the result of a high concentration of microliths in the periphery of the secondary lobules, rather than calcification of the septa themselves.[118, 281] Other features seen on HRCT scans include apical bullae and thin-walled subpleural cysts.[282] Correlation of HRCT with radiographic findings has shown that the black pleural line mentioned previously can be caused either by subpleural cysts along the costal and mediastinal pleura[282] or by a layer of extrapleural fat.[264] The cysts and the apical bullae are also presumably the cause of the recurrent pneumothoraces that occur in some patients.[282, 284, 285]

Magnetic resonance (MR) imaging performed in one patient showed increased signal intensity on T1-weighted images and "slight hypointensity" on T2-weighted images in the areas that had the largest concentration of microliths.[264] However, MR imaging showed little or no signal in areas with relatively few microliths on HRCT.

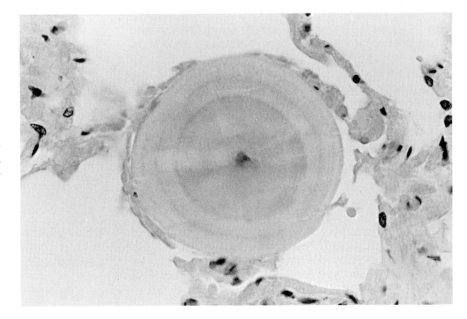

Figure 68–25. Corpus Amylacea. A highly magnified view of an alveolar air space shows a round laminated structure with an irregularly shaped central particle.

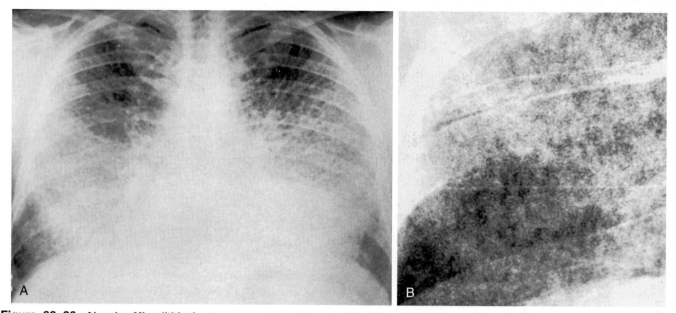

Figure 68–26. Alveolar Microlithiasis. A posteroanterior radiograph *(A)* of this 40-year-old asymptomatic man reveals a remarkably uniform opacification of both lungs. On close scrutiny *(B)*, this can be seen to be produced by a multitude of tiny, discrete opacities of calcific density. Pulmonary function test results were normal except for a reduction in residual volume of 800 ml, representing the displacement of pulmonary volume by the calcispherytes.

Clinical Manifestations

Many patients are asymptomatic when the disease is first discovered,[243] the diagnosis often being made on the basis of the typical radiographic pattern seen on a screening chest film or on a film obtained in an individual whose sibling is known to have the disease. Symptoms may be absent even when the chest radiograph reveals the lungs to be almost solid and white, with little visible air-containing parenchyma. In fact, this lack of association between radiologic and clinical findings is more striking in pulmonary alveolar microlithiasis than in any other condition.

The most common symptom of pulmonary alveolar microlithiasis is dyspnea on exertion.[243, 251, 286] Cough develops in some patients;[287] although it is typically nonproductive, some patients have been reported to produce microliths.[261] Chest pain is uncommon;[247] hemoptysis is rare. Pectus excavatum and hypertrophic pulmonary osteoarthropathy have been present in some patients.[247] Physical examination is usually unrevealing, except in the late stages, when breath sounds may be decreased, particularly at the lung bases. As the disease progresses, respiratory insufficiency may develop, associated with cyanosis, clubbing of the fingers, and evidence of pulmonary hypertension.[289]

Pulmonary Function Tests

Results of pulmonary function studies vary considerably from case to case, depending upon both the extent of replacement of alveolar air by microliths and the presence or absence of interstitial fibrosis. The principal finding may be a reduction in residual volume caused by the physical presence of calculi in the pulmonary air spaces.[290] In one investigation of five patients who had this abnormality, all also had an increased alveolar-arterial oxygen gradient;[290] the arterial oxygen saturation at rest and the diffusing capacity were decreased in only two. Other investigators have found decreased vital capacity, diffusing capacity, and arterial Po_2, with low dynamic compliance and high maximal inspiratory pressures.[259] In another series of eight patients, most values for lung volumes were on the low side of predicted normal.[244] Mild to moderate pulmonary hypertension has been detected in some patients.[291]

Diagnosis and Natural History

The diagnosis of pulmonary alveolar microlithiasis usually can be made with confidence from the classic radiographic pattern and the striking radiologic-clinical dissociation. Values for chemical analysis of blood are invariably within the normal range.[243] Microliths can be identified in sputum, BAL fluid,[268, 292, 293] and transbronchial biopsy specimens.[245, 294] Open-lung biopsy is seldom, if ever, indicated.

It has been suggested that in many patients, the microliths continue to form and perhaps increase in size as the disease progresses, rather than appearing as a single massive deposit at one time.[243] In a follow-up study of three sisters who had the disease, a definite increase in micronodularity was observed in two;[243] there was no obvious change in the other. We have studied two brothers with the disease in whom extensive radiographic changes were stationary for 30 years. When disease does progress, it may do so very slowly; cases have been reported in which respiratory failure and death ensued after a period as long as 40 years.[254]

LIPID STORAGE DISEASE

Gaucher's Disease

The underlying abnormality in Gaucher's disease is a deficiency of beta-glucosidase, the enzyme that catabolizes glucosylceramide. The deficiency is inherited in autosomal

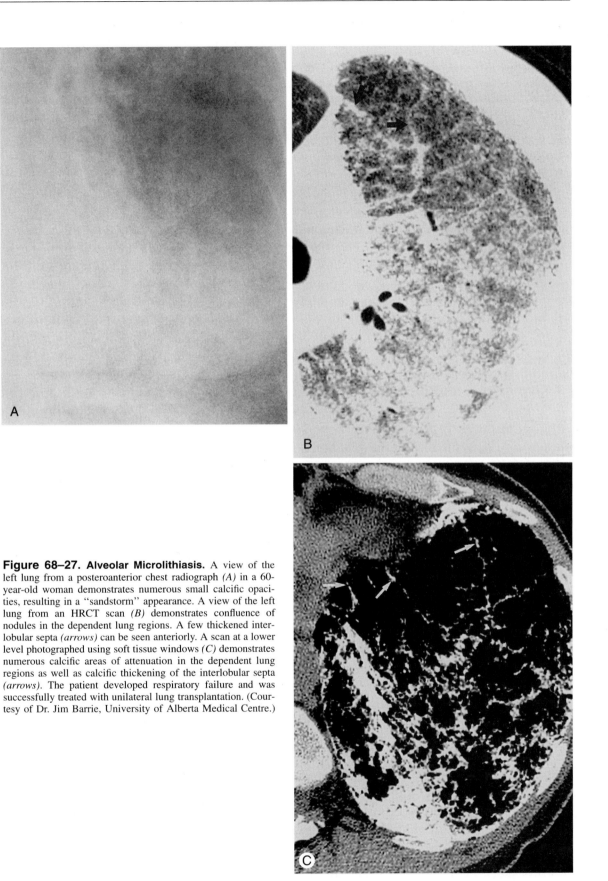

Figure 68–27. Alveolar Microlithiasis. A view of the left lung from a posteroanterior chest radiograph *(A)* in a 60-year-old woman demonstrates numerous small calcific opacities, resulting in a "sandstorm" appearance. A view of the left lung from an HRCT scan *(B)* demonstrates confluence of nodules in the dependent lung regions. A few thickened interlobular septa *(arrows)* can be seen anteriorly. A scan at a lower level photographed using soft tissue windows *(C)* demonstrates numerous calcific areas of attenuation in the dependent lung regions as well as calcific thickening of the interlobular septa *(arrows)*. The patient developed respiratory failure and was successfully treated with unilateral lung transplantation. (Courtesy of Dr. Jim Barrie, University of Alberta Medical Centre.)

recessive fashion and leads to an accumulation of glucosyl-ceramide in various cells, resulting in striated, PAS-positive inclusions that resemble wrinkled tissue paper (Gaucher cells). These cells are particularly prominent in the liver, spleen, lymph nodes, bones, and, in the infantile form of the disease, the brain. Clinically and radiologically significant involvement of other tissues and organs, including the lungs, occurs uncommonly. The majority of patients are female, and more than 95% are Ashkenazi Jews.

Three varieties of the disease are recognized: (1) a neurologic (or infantile) type that manifests in infants and is fatal before the age of 2 years, (2) a visceral (or juvenile) type that becomes clinically apparent between the age of 6 months and early adolescence and is associated with rapid enlargement of the liver and spleen and death from intercurrent infection or a hemorrhagic diathesis, and (3) an osseous (or adult) type that usually develops in late adolescence or adulthood and is characterized by splenomegaly and bone involvement. Patients who have the osseous type can survive into old age.

Although pulmonary involvement can occur in all three forms of the disease,[295] few cases have been reported; for example, in a review of the literature in 1975, only 10 cases were found in which pulmonary disease of any form could be demonstrated.[296] Despite this, pulmonary involvement may be more common than is generally appreciated; in one investigation of 95 patients who had the adult form of disease, approximately two thirds had pulmonary function abnormalities (most commonly, reduced functional residual capacity [FRC] and DLCO); 17% had radiographic abnormalities.[297] There is evidence that an increased risk for pulmonary disease is associated with homozygosity for the L444P mutation.[297a]

Histologically, Gaucher cells are found predominantly in the alveolar interstitium and adjacent air spaces;[298–300] they can be few in number or so numerous that the underlying lung structure is difficult to appreciate. Bone marrow emboli containing Gaucher cells derived from pathologic fractures or bone infarcts occasionally can be identified in pulmonary vessels.[295] The cells should not be confused with "pseudo-Gaucher cells," which have been seen in a variety of hematologic diseases as well as in rare cases of pulmonary mycobacterial infection.[301]

Radiographic manifestations consist of a reticulonodular or miliary pattern affecting both lungs diffusely (Fig. 68–28).[300] Lytic lesions, occasionally seen in the ribs, represent foci of bone involvement.

Clinically significant pulmonary involvement is usually manifested by dyspnea; pulmonary hypertension (apparently related to the presence of Gaucher cells in the pulmonary capillaries)[295, 302] and respiratory failure have also been described.[298, 299] Gaucher cells can be detected in BAL fluid.[303] Elevated levels of serum angiotensin-converting enzyme (ACE) have been documented in some patients,[304] a finding that may be interpreted as evidence of sarcoidosis. One unusual case has been reported in which Gaucher's disease was complicated by fatal pulmonary amyloidosis.[305]

Niemann-Pick Disease

Niemann-Pick disease is caused by an inherited deficiency in the production of sphingomyelinase. This results in the deposition of the ceramide phospholipid sphingomyelin in the liver, spleen, lung, bone marrow, and brain. Several clinical variants have been described that are defined by age at onset and predominant organs affected. Many patients die in infancy or childhood; however, some survive into adulthood, occasionally presenting with the first manifestations of their disease at that time.[306]

Pathologically, aggregates of large multivacuolated cells (NP cells) are present in the parenchyma of many organs, particularly the brain, spleen, liver, bone marrow, and lymph nodes. In the lungs, NP cells appear to be most numerous in the alveoli.[307] Histiocytes containing fine and coarse granules that stain deep blue with May-Grünwald-Giemsa stain ("sea-blue histiocytes") have been detected in some patients, most often in bone marrow but occasionally the lung.[307, 308]

Radiographic manifestations consist of a diffuse reticulonodular pattern (Fig. 68–29);[306, 307, 309] the nodules measure from 1 to 2 mm in diameter and are associated with linear strands that have been said to create a honeycomb pattern.[309] One case has been described of a 23-year-old woman who had a fine reticular pattern involving the lower lung zones;[288] HRCT demonstrated interlobular septal thickening and centrilobular areas of ground-glass attenuation. Hepatomegaly and peripheral lymph node enlargement are common; pulmonary involvement may be asymptomatic or severe enough to cause respiratory failure.[310]

Fabry's Disease

Fabry's disease (angiokeratoma corporis diffusum universale) is caused by an inherited deficiency of α-galactosidase A, the enzyme responsible for metabolizing ceramide trihexoside. The deficiency results in the accumulation of a number of glycolipids in endothelial, muscle, and mesenchymal cells in several organs and tissues including the skin, kidneys, and heart. The initial clinical presentation is usually in the form of red spots in the skin and is followed 5 to 10 years later by the development of renal and myocardial failure.

Although some authors have expressed skepticism about the validity of reports of lung involvement in Fabry's disease,[311] occasional well-documented cases suggest that it does indeed occur.[312] However, in most affected persons the functional significance of such involvement is unclear. In one study of seven patients who had Fabry's disease, evidence was found of air-flow obstruction of severity out of proportion to the smoking history;[313] the authors suggested that the physiologic abnormality may have been caused by airway narrowing secondary to glycolipid accumulation, demonstrated in biopsy specimens of airway epithelial cells. Another group of investigators described a woman whose clinical presentation suggested multiple pulmonary thromboemboli and whose chest radiograph revealed a slight accentuation of lung markings;[314] because of a history of several episodes of hemoptysis, it was thought likely that the changes were caused by multiple angiomas in the tracheobronchial tree similar to those that were present in the skin.

G$_{M1}$ Gangliosidosis

G$_{M1}$ gangliosidosis is caused by a deficiency of beta-galactosidase and is characterized by the accumulation in

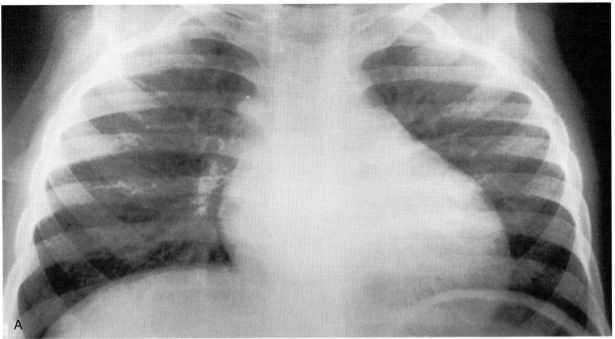

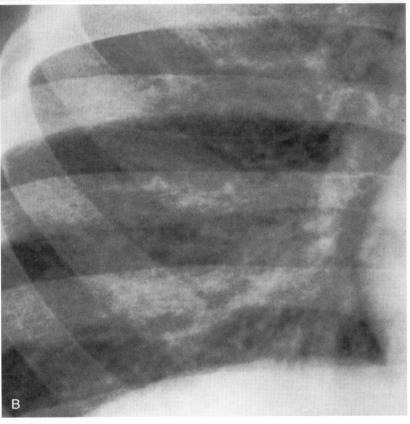

Figure 68–28. Gaucher's Disease. A posteroanterior radiograph *(A)* and a magnified view of the right lower zone *(B)* reveal a fine reticular pattern throughout both lungs without anatomic predominance. There are no other abnormalities. Although the lung volume is small, this could be a technical aberration. (Courtesy of Dr. J. S. Dunbar.)

various organs of histiocytes containing a monocyaloganglioside. The condition usually affects infants or young children and is manifested principally by mental retardation, sometimes with hepatosplenomegaly and skeletal abnormalities. In the occasional patient in whom pulmonary disease has been identified, aggregates of foamy macrophages similar to those of Niemann-Pick disease have been found predominantly within alveoli.[315] Miliary "shadows" have been described on chest radiographs, and the condition has been said to cause respiratory insufficiency.[315]

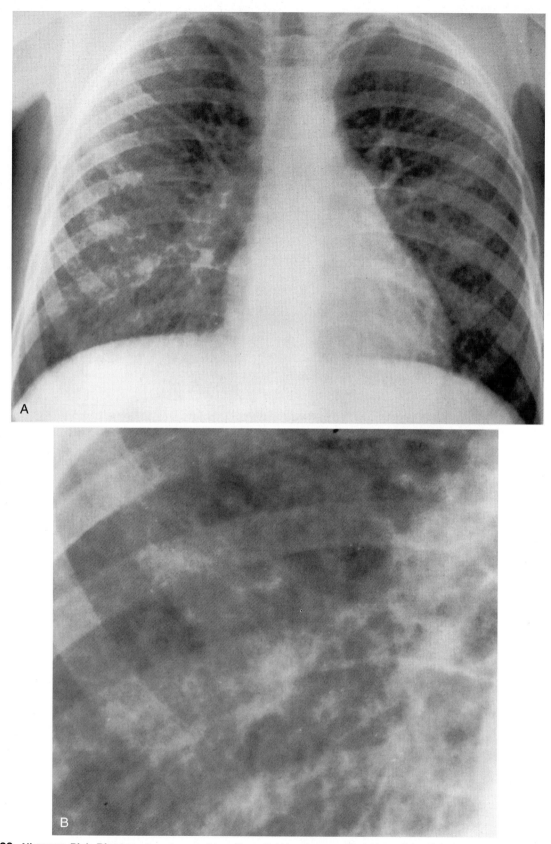

Figure 68–29. Niemann-Pick Disease. A posteroanterior radiograph *(A)* and a magnified view of the right lower lung zone *(B)* reveal a coarse reticular pattern throughout both lungs without anatomic predominance. The pattern indicates diffuse interstitial lung disease. There are no other findings. (Courtesy of Dr. J. S. Dunbar.)

Hermansky-Pudlak Syndrome

The Hermansky-Pudlak syndrome is an inherited condition characterized by tyrosinase-positive oculocutaneous albinism, a defect in platelet function, and the accumulation of ceroid pigment in macrophages throughout the body.[316, 317] The mode of inheritance is autosomal recessive. The disease is uncommon, approximately 200 cases having been reported by 1985.[317] It has been documented most often in persons from Puerto Rico and southern Holland.[318, 319]

Ceroid is a complex chromolipid, the origin and chemical structure of which are incompletely understood. It is recognized histologically as a brown pigment that is PAS-positive, diastase-resistant, and acid-fast and that shows brilliant yellow-orange fluorescence when viewed under ultraviolet light. Ultrastructurally, the pigment is finely granular or (less commonly) whorled and is found most often in membrane-bound vacuoles.[317] The latter finding and other observations suggest that the ceroid is stored within lysosomes, thus representing a possible enzymatic defect;[317, 320, 321] however, the nature of such a defect is unknown.

Involvement of the pulmonary interstitium has been documented in a number of reports.[319, 320, 322, 323] Histologically, it consists of variably severe parenchymal fibrosis, similar to idiopathic pulmonary fibrosis, associated with variable numbers of ceroid-laden macrophages. The pathogenetic relationship between the macrophages and the fibrosis is unclear. In one study of pulmonary inflammatory cells obtained by BAL from patients who had the syndrome, superoxide production by stimulated alveolar macrophages was increased compared with normal;[322] the authors speculated that ceroid-laden macrophages may be more responsive to exogenous stimuli and that subsequent release of toxic oxygen metabolites may cause the pulmonary fibrosis. In another BAL investigation, immunoassay for platelet-derived growth factor showed a sixfold increase in physiologically normal patients who had the syndrome compared with controls, suggesting to the authors that it might be involved in the development of subsequent fibrosis.[324]

Radiographic manifestations of pulmonary disease range from a fine reticulation to a coarse reticulonodular pattern with honeycombing.[325–327] The abnormalities may be diffuse or involve mainly the lower or upper lung zones.[325–327] In some cases, bullae and bronchiectasis are seen involving mainly the upper lung zones.[325] HRCT scans in some patients who have advanced pulmonary involvement demonstrate diffuse interstitial abnormalities with reticular changes and honeycombing; in one patient the honeycombing had a predominantly peripheral distribution[327] and in another it involved mainly the medullary portion of the lungs.[252]

In addition to the abnormal skin pigmentation and ocular signs, patients complain of progressive dyspnea and appear to be susceptible to infection and a bleeding tendency. Some patients develop granulomatous colitis similar to that in Crohn's disease.[316, 320] Pulmonary function studies reveal a restrictive pattern; hypoxemia at rest is characteristic.

Erdheim-Chester Disease

Erdheim-Chester disease is a rare abnormality characterized by the deposition of lipid-laden macrophages in a variety of tissues, particularly the bones. Although traditionally considered to be a lipid storage disease, the possibility that it may represent a primary macrophage disorder has also been considered.[327a] Pulmonary involvement was documented in 13 patients in a 1998 review;[327a] mediastinal fibrosis and pleural thickening or effusion have also been reported.[327a] The radiologic manifestations of pulmonary disease are best appreciated on HRCT and consist most commonly of interlobular septal thickening, subpleural micronodules, and areas of ground-glass attenuation.[328b] Clinical manifestations include dyspnea and cough. A restrictive defect can be seen on pulmonary function testing, and some patients have hypoxemia. Progression to respiratory failure and death has been seen in a number of patients.

Miscellaneous Lipid Storage Diseases

Krabbe's disease (globoid leukodystrophy) is a rare lipid storage disease characterized by cerebral accumulation of sphingolipid and corresponding neurologic symptoms. Pulmonary disease has been reported rarely.[328]

Rare cases have been reported in which ceroid-laden macrophages have accumulated within alveolar air spaces in the absence of evidence of significant extrathoracic disease.[329, 330] The etiology, pathogenesis, and natural history of the condition *(idiopathic pulmonary ceroidosis)* are unknown. Some cases have been associated with mild interstitial fibrosis, dyspnea, and pulmonary function abnormalities.

Cerebrotendinous xanthomatosis is a lipid storage disease inherited in autosomal recessive fashion that is associated with a deficiency of the mitochondrial enzyme sterol 27-hydroxylase. Granuloma-like aggregates of foamy macrophages and free cholesterol have been found in the lung parenchyma and pleura.[331] A single case has been reported in a patient who also had lymphangioleiomyomatosis.[332]

GLYCOGEN STORAGE DISEASE

Involvement of thoracic structures other than the heart is only rarely detectable either clinically or radiologically in glycogen storage disease. However, aggregates of intra-alveolar foamy macrophages containing glycogen-like material have been noted in some patients and can cause respiratory dysfunction and radiographic abnormalities.[333]

Pompe's disease (acid maltase deficiency) is a type II glycogen storage disease characterized by the accumulation of glycogen in skeletal muscle and a variety of visceral organs. Although the condition usually affects infants and is fatal, occasional cases with onset in adulthood have been reported.[334] Involvement of the diaphragm and respiratory muscles of the chest wall in these persons can cause dyspnea and respiratory failure.[334]

MUCOPOLYSACCHARIDE STORAGE DISEASES

In mucopolysaccharide storage disorders, deficient activity of lysosomal enzymes involved in the catabolism of glycosaminoglycans causes disease that predominantly affects the skeletal, cardiovascular, and central nervous systems. Patients with some of these metabolic disorders die in childhood or adolescence, whereas others with conditions such as Hurler's, Hunter's, and Morquio's syndromes may survive into adulthood. Respiratory complications include kyphoscoliosis, respiratory failure, susceptibility to pulmonary infection, and airway obstruction, sometimes accompanied by sleep apnea.[335]

MISCELLANEOUS METABOLIC ABNORMALITIES

Lipoid Proteinosis

Lipoid proteinosis is a rare familial disorder originally considered to be a disease of the skin and the mucous membranes of the oral cavity and larynx,[336] but now recognized to be a generalized abnormality that can affect many organ systems, including the lungs.[337] It has an autosomal recessive pattern of transmission. Pathologically, the condition is characterized by the deposition in affected tissues of an amorphous eosinophilic material that consists of lipid and glycoproteins.[338] Pulmonary involvement has been reported to be characterized by its presence in alveolar septa.[339] A reticulonodular radiographic pattern throughout both lungs resulting in diffuse interstitial pulmonary fibrosis has been reported.[337]

Patients characteristically are seen for the first time by either the dermatologist (with a presentation of markedly thickened eyelids) or the otolaryngologist (with a presentation of chronic hoarseness). Pulmonary symptoms are rare.[339]

Familial Retardation of Growth, Renal Aminoaciduria, and Cor Pulmonale

The rare and unusual combination of familial retardation of growth, renal aminoaciduria, and cor pulmonale has been associated with abnormal skeletal musculature. In one study of three affected children, the left lung was found to be smaller than normal and was the site of atelectasis and recurrent infection involving the basilar segments;[340, 341] arterial P_{CO_2} was elevated and P_{O_2} was diminished, indicative of an "alveolar hypoventilation syndrome" that was considered to be caused by deficient musculature.

Nasu-Hakola Disease

Nasu-Hakola disease is a rare abnormality characterized by peculiar membranocystic structures in systemic adipose tissue and leukoencephalopathy in the brain. A single case has been reported in which the microcystic structures were also present in alveolar septa.[342]

Vegetable Wax Storage Disease

We are aware of a single remarkable case of an asymptomatic 55-year-old man who had diffuse micronodular disease evident on chest radiographs. The abnormality was shown at autopsy to be the result of an interstitial granulomatous inflammatory reaction to an acicular substance identified by spectrometry as hydrocarbon consistent with vegetable cuticle;[343] the origin of the material was believed to be ingested apples and Brussels sprouts, which the patient had consumed excessively!

PULMONARY ABNORMALITIES IN SYSTEMIC ENDOCRINE DISEASE

Diabetes Mellitus

The most common and serious pulmonary complication of diabetes mellitus is infection. Disease caused by organisms such as *M. tuberculosis, Mucorales* species, *Staphylococcus aureus*, and a variety of gram-negative bacteria appears to have an increased incidence;[344–346] there is also evidence that infection caused by some agents (e.g., *Streptococcus pneumoniae, Legionella* species, gram-negative organisms, and influenza virus) may be associated with increased morbidity and mortality.[344, 345] A number of cases of adult respiratory distress syndrome (ARDS) apparently unassociated with pulmonary infection have also been reported in patients who have diabetes, usually in the setting of ketoacidosis.[347–349]

A number of investigators have attempted to identify intrinsic pathologic abnormalities in the lungs. One group measured the thickness of the alveolar epithelial and capillary basement membranes in diabetic patients and age-matched controls;[350] they found both measurements to be significantly greater in the diabetics, although the increased thickness was much less than that observed in the basement membranes of muscle and renal tubules. Similar thickening has been found in the basement membrane underlying bronchial epithelium.[351] In one autopsy investigation of 61 diabetic patients, foci of nodular fibrosis were found that the authors considered to be characteristic of the disease.[352] In another autopsy study of 339 diabetic patients, 20 (6%) were found to have perivascular "xanthogranulomas" consisting of aggregates of multinucleated giant cells and foamy histiocytes;[353] in a control group of 156 nondiabetic individuals, only 3 were similarly affected. Although the fundamental nature of this abnormality is unclear, the most likely explanation may be prior hemorrhage; whatever the cause, it appears to have no functional or radiographic significance. Another group of investigators found the degree of muscularization of small pulmonary arteries, measured morphometrically, to be significantly greater in preterm infants of mothers who had diabetes mellitus than in age-matched controls;[354] they speculated that this might be related to an *in utero* increase in smooth muscle growth promoters such as insulin and that the abnormality may contribute to the pulmonary hypertension and respiratory difficulty observed in some newborns of diabetic mothers.

A variety of pulmonary function abnormalities, some hypothesized to be related to the vascular changes just described, have also been reported in patients who have either insulin-dependent or non–insulin-dependent diabetes mellitus. The most consistent finding is a reduction in D_{LCO};[355–357] some investigators have found this to be related to the presence of renal disease,[355] the duration of the diabetes,[357] or posture (i.e., supine rather than sitting).[358] Other reported abnormalities include reductions (usually mild) in lung elastic recoil,[359] forced vital capacity (FVC), FEV₁[355] and pulmonary capillary blood volume.[359] The threshold for cough in response to inhaled citric acid has been found to be higher in diabetics who have autonomic neuropathy than in non-neuropathic control diabetic patients, suggesting impairment of the vagal innervation of the bronchial tree.[360] No relation between the presence of diabetes and respiratory muscle strength was found in the study of elderly patients by the Cardiovascular Health Study Research Group in Seattle.[361]

Hypopituitarism and Acromegaly

Investigations in both experimental animals[362] and humans[363, 364] suggest that growth hormone exerts an important influence on lung structure. Functional abnormalities have also been demonstrated in patients who have either hypopituitarism or growth hormone excess, i.e., acromegaly. Hypopituitarism has been found to be associated with a restrictive type of ventilatory impairment, total lung capacity being approximately 75% of normal.[363] By contrast, patients who have acromegaly have large lungs with a total lung capacity greater than that in matched controls by 25% or more.[35, 365–367] This larger lung capacity appears to be more frequent in men than in women,[367] suggesting a possible influence of sex hormones. Another relatively common finding in patients who have acromegaly is upper airway obstruction, associated in some patients with sleep apnea and significant nocturnal hypoxemia.[368, 369] Abnormal small airway function has also been described by some[370] but not all[367] investigators. A decrease in inspiratory or expiratory muscle force and an increase in respiratory frequency were detected in one study of 10 patients.[371]

Hypothyroidism

Abnormal accumulations of fluid have been found in the pericardial and pleural spaces in patients who have myxedema in the absence of cardiovascular, renal, or other causes of fluid retention.[372, 373] The mechanism has been hypothesized to be related to abnormal fluid and protein transport across the capillary wall.[374] Patchy air-space disease has been described as well; in one study, it was presumed to be edema, although there was no dyspnea or cardiomegaly.[375]

Hypoxemia and reduced lung volumes also can occur in patients who have myxedema, usually in association with obesity and hypoventilation and often with coma.[376–379] However, some of these patients are not obese, and their blood gas values have been shown to return to normal with thyroid therapy despite little or no change in body weight.[380, 381] In one investigation of 14 patients whose myxedema was inadequately treated, histologic examination revealed the presence of amorphous eosinophilic material in relation to pulmonary capillaries and small pulmonary veins in 4;[382] the author suggested that this material consisted of mucopolysaccharides and that its presence might explain the hypoxemia detected in some patients. Other abnormalities reported to occur in patients who have myxedema include depressed respiratory drive[383] and sleep apnea.[384] It has also been speculated that there may be an association of hypothyroidism with idiopathic pulmonary hemorrhage[385] and pulmonary arterial hypertension.[386]

Hyperthyroidism

Pulmonary function studies in some patients who have hyperthyroidism have shown a decrease in vital capacity and an increase in minute ventilation during exercise.[387] Some investigators have also found evidence of inspiratory and expiratory muscle weakness,[388, 389] an increase in hypoxic and hypercarbic ventilatory drive,[390] and pulmonary artery hypertension.[391]

Hyperparathyroidism

Hypercalcemia associated with hyperparathyroidism can result in diffuse metastatic calcification of the lungs (*see* page 2699). Although usually detectable only by histologic examination, it is sometimes severe enough to be visible radiologically and rarely causes symptoms.

Klinefelter's Syndrome

Klinefelter's syndrome is an inherited endocrine syndrome characterized by small testes, azoospermia, gynecomastia, elevated urinary gonadotropins, and (often) eunuchoid skeletal proportions. Affected persons are said to be prone to bronchitis, bronchiectasis, and asthma. In one investigation of 24 patients who had the disorder, 4 were found to have asthma, 4 chronic cough, 2 an obstructive defect, and 11 reduced FRC;[392] the last-named was attributed to chest wall abnormality, because the lungs were considered to be normal.

REFERENCES

1. Faubert PF, Shapiro WB, Porush JG, et al: Pulmonary calcification in hemodialyzed patients detected by technetium-99m diphosphate scanning. Kidney Int 18:95, 1980.
2. Conger JD, Hammond WS, Alfrey AC, et al: Pulmonary calcification in chronic dialysis patients. Ann Intern Med 83:330, 1975.
3. Kempf K, Capesius P, Mugel JL: Un cas de calcinose pulmonaire au cours d'une myélomatose diffuse. J Radiol Electrol Med Nucl 53:861, 1972.
4. Weber CK, Friedrich JM, Merkle E, et al: Reversible metastatic pulmonary calcification in a patient with multiple myeloma. Ann Hematol 72:329, 1996.
5. Breitz HB, Sirotta PS, Nelp WB, et al: Progressive pulmonary calcification complicating successful renal transplantation. Am Rev Respir Dis 136:1480, 1987.
6. Munoz SJ, Nagelberg SB, Green PJ, et al: Ectopic soft tissue calcium deposition following liver transplantation. Hepatology 8:476, 1988.
7. Raisis IP, Park CH, Yang SL, et al: Lung uptake of technetium-99m phosphate compounds after liver transplantation. Clin Nucl Med 13:188, 1988.
8. Parfitt AM, Massry SG, Winfield AC, et al: Disordered calcium and phosphorus metabolism during maintenance hemodialysis. Correlation of clinical, roentgenographic and biochemical changes. Am J Med 51:319, 1971.
9. Bestetti-Bosisio M, Cotelli F, Schiaffino E, et al: Lung calcification in long-term dialysed patients: A light and electronmicroscopic study. Histopathology 8:69, 1984.
10. Sanders C, Frank MS, Rostand SG, et al: Metastatic calcification of the heart and lungs in end-stage renal disease: detection and quantification by dual-energy digital chest radiography. Am J Roentgenol 149:881, 1987.
11. Johkoh T, Ikezoe J, Nagareda T, et al: Case report. Metastatic pulmonary calcification: Early detection by high-resolution CT. J Comput Assist Tomogr 17:471, 1993.
12. Hartman TE, Müller NL, Primack SL, et al: Metastatic pulmonary calcification in patients with hypercalcemia: Findings on chest radiographs and CT scans. Am J Roentgenol 162:799, 1994.
13. Greenberg S, Suster B: Metastatic pulmonary calcification: Appearance on high resolution CT. J Comput Assist Tomogr 18:497, 1994.
14. Mootz JR, Sagel SS, Roberts TH: Roentgenographic manifestations of pulmonary calcifications. Radiology 107:55, 1973.
15. Neff M, Yakin S, Gupta S, et al: Extensive metastatic calcification of the lung in an azotemic patient. Am J Med 56:103, 1974.
16. Firooznia H, Pudlowski R, Golimbu C, et al: Diffuse interstitial calcification of the lungs in chronic renal failure mimicking pulmonary edema. Am J Roentgenol 129:1103, 1977.
17. Rosenthal DI, Chandler HL, Azizi F, et al: Uptake of bone imaging agents by diffuse pulmonary metastatic calcification. Am J Roentgenol 129:871, 1977.
18. Jolles H, Johnson AC, Ell SR: Subcutaneous calcifications masquerading as pulmonary lesions in long-term hemodialysis. Review of nodular pulmonary opacities in the population undergoing hemodialysis. Chest 88:234, 1985.
19. Chinn DH, Gamsu G, Webb WR, et al: Calcified pulmonary nodules in chronic renal failure. Am J Roentgenol 137:402, 1981.
20. Margolin RJ, Addison TE: Hypercalcemia and rapidly progressive respiratory failure. Chest 86:767, 1984.
21. Jost RG, Sagel SS: Metastatic calcification in the lung apex. Am J Roentgenol 133:1188, 1979.
22. West JB: Regional Differences in the Lung. New York Academic Press, 1977, p 239.
23. Murris-Espin M, Lacassagne L, Didier A, et al: Metastatic pulmonary calcification after renal transplantation. Eur Respir J 10:1925, 1997.
24. Taguchi Y, Fuyuno G, Shioya S, et al: MR appearance of pulmonary metastatic calcification. J Comput Assist Tomogr 20:38, 1996.
25. Mootz JR, Sagel SS, Roberts TH: Roentgenographic manifestations of pulmonary calcifications: A rare cause of respiratory failure in chronic renal disease. Radiology 107:55, 1973.
26. Akmal M, Barndt RR, Ansari AN, et al: Excess PTH in CRF induces pulmonary calcification, pulmonary hypertension and right ventricular hypertrophy. Kidney Int 47:158, 1995.
27. Hwang GJ, Lee JD, Park CY, et al: Reversible extraskeletal uptake of bone scanning in primary hyperparathyroidism. J Nucl Med 37:469, 1996.
28. Jones RW, Roggli VL: Dendriform pulmonary ossification. Report of two cases with unique findings. Am J Clin Pathol 91:398, 1989.
29. Ndimbie OK, Williams CR, Lee MW: Dendriform pulmonary ossification. Arch Pathol Lab Med 111:1062, 1987.
30. Muller KM, Friemann J, Stichnoth E: Dendriform pulmonary ossification. Path Res Prac 168:163, 1980.
31. Mendeloff J: Disseminated nodular pulmonary ossification in the Hamman-Rich lung. Am Rev Respir Dis 103:269, 1971.
32. Genereux G: Personal communication, 1973.
33. Gevenois PA, Abehsera M, Knoop C, et al: Disseminated pulmonary ossification in end-stage pulmonary fibrosis: CT demonstration. Am J Roentgenol 162:1303, 1994.
34. Kuplic JB, Higley CS, Niewoehner DE: Pulmonary ossification associated with long-term busulfan therapy in chronic myeloid leukemia. Case report. Am Rev Respir Dis 106:759, 1972.
35. Mikami T, Yamamoto Y, Yokoyama M, et al: Pulmonary alveolar proteinosis: Diagnosis using routinely processed smears of bronchoalveolar lavage fluid. J Clin Pathol 50:981, 1997.
36. Joines RW, Roggli VL. Dendriform pulmonary ossification. Am J Clin Pathol 91:398, 1989.
37. Pear BL: Idiopathic disseminated pulmonary ossification. Radiology 91:746, 1969.
38. Jiminez JM, Casey SO, Citron M, et al: Calcified pulmonary metastases from medullary carcinoma. Comput Med Imag Graph 19:325, 1995.
39. Gevenois PA, Abehsera M, Knoop C, el al: Disseminated pulmonary ossification in end-stage pulmonary fibrosis: CT demonstration. Am J Roentgenol 162:1303, 1994.
40. Prakash UBS, Barham SS, Carpenter HA, et al: Pulmonary alveolar phospholipoproteinosis: Experience with 34 cases and a review. Mayo Clin Proc 62:499, 1987.
41. Rosen SH, Castleman B, Liebow AA: Pulmonary alveolar proteinosis. N Engl J Med 58:1123, 1958.
42. Bedrossian CWM, Luna MA, Conklin RH, et al: Alveolar proteinosis as a consequence of immunosuppression. A hypothesis based on clinical and pathologic observations. Hum Pathol 11:527, 1980.
43. Wang BM, Stern EJ, Schmidt RA, et al: Diagnosing pulmonary alveolar proteinosis. A review and an update. Chest 111:460, 1997.
44. McCook TA, Kirks DR, Merton DF, et al: Pulmonary alveolar proteinosis in children. Am J Roentgenol 137:1023, 1981.
45. Kariman K, Kylstra JA, Spook A: Pulmonary alveolar proteinosis: Prospective clinical experience in 23 patients for 15 years. Lung 162:223, 1984.
46. Mahut B, Delacourt C, Scheinmann P, et al: Pulmonary alveolar proteinosis: Experience with eight pediatric cases and a review. Pediatrics 97:117, 1996.
47. Colón AR, Lawrence RD, Mills SD, et al: Childhood pulmonary alveolar proteinosis (PAP). Am J Dis Child 121:481, 1971.
48. Ihling C, Weirich G, Gaa A, et al: Amyloid tumors of the lung—an immunocytoma? Pathol Res Pract 192:446, 1996.
49. Green D, Dighe P, Ali NO, et al: Pulmonary alveolar proteinosis complicating chronic myelogenous leukemia. Cancer 46:1763, 1980.
50. Carnovale R, Zornoza J, Goldman AM, et al: Pulmonary alveolar proteinosis: Its association with hematologic malignancy and lymphoma. Radiology 122:303, 1977.
51. Cordonnier C, Fleury-Feith J, Escudier E, et al: Secondary alveolar proteinosis is a reversible cause of respiratory failure in leukemic patients. Am J Respir Crit Care Med 149:788, 1994.
52. Liu AT, Miedzinski LJ, Vallieres E, et al: Pulmonary alveolar proteinosis in an AIDS patient without concurrent pulmonary infection. Can Respir J 2:183, 1995.
53. Samuels MP, Warner J: Pulmonary alveolar lipoproteinosis complicating juvenile dermatomyositis. Thorax 43:939, 1988.
54. Aymard J-P, Gyger M, Lavallee R, et al: A case of pulmonary alveolar proteinosis complicating chronic myelogenous leukemia. Cancer 53:954, 1984.
55. Knight DP, Knight JA: Pulmonary alveolar proteinosis in the newborn. Arch Pathol Lab Med 109:529, 1985.
56. Teja K, Cooper PH, Squires JE, et al: Pulmonary alveolar proteinosis in four siblings. N Engl J Med 305:1390, 1981.
57. Parto K, Kallajoki M, Aho H, et al: Pulmonary alveolar proteinosis and glomerulonephritis in lysinuric protein intolerance: Case reports and autopsy findings of four pediatric patients. Hum Pathol 25:400, 1994.
58. Johkoh T, Itoh H, Müller NL, et al: Crazy-paving appearance at thin-section CT: Spectrum of disease and pathologic findings. Radiology 1999; in press.
59. Webster JR, Battifora H, Furey C, et al: Pulmonary alveolar proteinosis in 2 siblings with decreased immunoglobulin-A. Am J Med 69:786, 1980.
60. deMello DE, Heyman S, Phelps DS, et al: Ultrastructure of lung in surfactant protein B deficiency. Am J Respir Cell Mol Biol 11:230, 1994.
61. deMello DE, Nogee LM, Heyman S, et al: Molecular and phenotypic variability in the congenital alveolar proteinosis syndrome associated with inherited surfactant protein B deficiency. J Pediatr 125:43, 1994.
62. de la Fuente AA, Voorhout WF, deMello DE: Congenital alveolar proteinosis in the Netherlands: A report of five cases with immunohistochemical and genetic studies on surfactant apoproteins. Pediatr Pathol Lab Med 17:221, 1997.
63. deMello DE, Heyman S, Phelps DS, Hamvas A, Nogee L, Cole S, Colten HR. Ultrastructure of lung in surfactant protein B deficiency. Am J Respir Cell Mol Biol 11:230, 1994.
64. Hamvas A, Cole FS, deMello DE, et al: Surfactant protein B deficiency: Antenatal diagnosis and prospective treatment with surfactant replacement. J Pediatr 125:356, 1994.
65. deMello DE, Nogee LM, Heyman S, et al: Molecular and phenotypic variability in the congenital alveolar proteinosis syndrome associated with inherited surfactant protein B deficiency. J Pediatr 125:43, 1994.
66. Nogee LM, Garnier G, Dietz HC, et al: A mutation in the surfactant protein B gene responsible for fatal neonatal respiratory disease in multiple kindreds. J Clin Invest 93:1860, 1994.
67. Ballard PL, Nogee LM, Beers MF, et al: Partial deficiency of surfactant protein B in an infant with chronic lung disease. Pediatrics 96:1046, 1995.
68. Corrin B, King E: Pathogenesis of experimental pulmonary alveolar proteinosis. Thorax 25:230, 1970.
69. Gross P, deTreville RTP: Alveolar proteinosis. Its experimental production in rodents. Arch Pathol 86:255, 1968.

70. Heppleston AG, Wright NA, Stewart JA: Experimental alveolar lipo-proteinosis following the inhalation of silica. J Pathol 101:293, 1970.
71. Lee KP, Barras CE, Griffith FD, et al: Pulmonary response to glass fiber by inhalation exposure. Lab Invest 40:123, 1979.
72. Buechner HA, Ansari A: Acute silico-proteinosis. A new pathologic variant of acute silicosis in sandblasters, characterized by histologic features resembling alveolar proteinosis. Dis Chest 55:274, 1969.
73. Keller CA, Frost A, Cagle PT, et al: Pulmonary alveolar proteinosis in a painter with elevated pulmonary concentrations of titanium. Chest 108:277, 1995.
74. Ranchod M, Bissell M: Pulmonary alveolar proteinosis and cytomegalovirus infection. Arch Pathol Lab Med 103:139, 1979.
75. Witty LA, Tapson VF, Piantadosi CA: Isolation of mycobacteria in patients with pulmonary alveolar proteinosis. Medicine 73:103, 1994.
76. Van Nhieu JT, Vojtek A-M, Bernaudin J-F, et al: Pulmonary alveolar proteinosis associated with Pneumocystis carinii: Ultrastructural identification in bronchoalveolar lavage in AIDS and immunocompromised non-AIDS patients. Chest 98:801, 1990.
77. Gumpert BC, Nowacki MR, Amundson DE: Pulmonary alveolar lipoproteinosis. Remission after antibiotic treatment. West J Med 161:66, 1994.
78. Costello JF, Moriarty DC, Branthwaite MA: Diagnosis and management of alveolar proteinosis: The role of electron microscopy. Thorax 30:121, 1975.
79. Heppleston AG, Young AE: Alveolar lipo-proteinosis: An ultrastructural comparison of the experimental and human forms. J Pathol 107:107, 1972.
80. Gilmore LB, Talley FA, Hook GE: Classification and morphometric quantitation of insoluble materials from the lungs of patients with alveolar proteinosis. Am J Pathol 133:252, 1988.
81. Singh G, Katyal SL: Surfactant apoprotein in nonmalignant pulmonary disorders. Am J Pathol 101:51, 1980.
82. Bell DY, Hook GER: Pulmonary alveolar proteinosis: Analysis of airway and alveolar proteins. Am Rev Respir Dis 119:979, 1979.
83. Ito M, Takeuchi N, Ogura T, et al: Pulmonary alveolar proteinosis: Analysis of pulmonary washings. Br J Dis Chest 72:313, 1978.
84. Satoh K, Arai H, Yoshida T, et al: Glycosaminoglycans and glycoproteins in bronchoalveolar lavage fluid from patients with pulmonary alveolar proteinosis. Inflammation 7:347, 1983.
85. Honda Y, Takahashi H, Shijubo N, et al: Surfactant protein-A concentration in bronchoalveolar lavage fluids of patients with pulmonary alveolar proteinosis. Chest 103:496, 1993.
86. Suzuki Y, Shen HQ, Sato A, et al: Analysis of fused-membrane structures in bronchoalveolar lavage fluid from patients with alveolar proteinosis. Am J Respir Cell Mol Biol 12:238, 1995.
87. Crouch E, Persson A, Chang D: Accumulation of surfactant protein D in human pulmonary alveolar proteinosis. Am J Pathol 142:241, 1993.
88. Sahu S, DiAugustine RP, Lynn WS: Lipids found in pulmonary lavage of patients with alveolar proteinosis and in rabbit lung lamellar organelles. Am Rev Respir Dis 114:177, 1976.
89. Hattori A, Kuroki Y, Katoh T, et al: Surfactant protein A accumulating in the alveoli of patients with pulmonary alveolar proteinosis: Oligomeric structure and interaction with lipids. Am J Respir Cell Mol Biol 14:608, 1996.
90. Hattori A, Kuroki Y, Takahashi H, et al: Immunoglobulin G is associated with surfactant protein A aggregate isolated from patients with pulmonary alveolar proteinosis. Am J Respir Crit Care Med 155:1785, 1997.
91. Ramirez J, Harlan WR Jr: Pulmonary alveolar proteinosis. Nature and origin of alveolar lipid. Am J Med 45:502, 1968.
92. Ramirez J: Pulmonary alveolar proteinosis. Treatment by massive bronchopulmonary lavage. Arch Intern Med 119:147, 1967.
93. Huffman JA, Hull WM, Dranoff G, et al: Pulmonary epithelial cell expression of GM-CSF corrects the alveolar proteinosis in GM-CSF–deficient mice. J Clin Invest 97:649, 1996.
94. Alberti A, Luisetti M, Braschi A, et al: Bronchoalveolar lavage fluid composition in alveolar proteinosis. Early changes after therapeutic lavage. Am J Respir Crit Care Med 154:817, 1996.
95. Warner T, Balish E: Pulmonary alveolar proteinosis: A spontaneous and inducible disease in immunodeficient germ-free mice. Am J Pathol 146:1017, 1995.
96. Jennings VM, Dillehay DI, Webb SK, et al: Pulmonary alveolar proteinosis in SCID mice. Am J Respir Cell Mol Biol 13:297, 1995.
97. Gonzalez-Rothi FJ, Harris JO: Pulmonary alveolar proteinosis: Further evaluation of abnormal alveolar macrophages. Chest 90:656, 1986.
98. Golde DW, Territo M, Finley TN, et al: Defective lung macrophages in pulmonary alveolar proteinosis. Ann Intern Med 85:304, 1976.
99. Stanley E, Lieschke GJ, Grail D, et al: Granulocyte/macrophage colony-stimulating factor–deficient mice show no major perturbation of hematopoiesis but develop a characteristic pulmonary pathology. Proc Natl Acad Sci U S A 91:5592, 1994.
100. Gonzalez-Rothi RJ, Harris JO: Pulmonary alveolar proteinosis. Further evaluation of abnormal alveolar macrophages. Chest 90:656, 1986.
101. Muller-Quernheim J, Schopf RE, Benes P, et al: A macrophage-suppressing 40-kD protein in a case of pulmonary alveolar proteinosis. Klin Wochenschr 65:893, 1987.
102. Nugent KM, Pesanti EL: Macrophage function in pulmonary alveolar proteinosis. Am Rev Respir Dis 127:780, 1983.
103. Spencer H: Pathology of the Lung: Excluding Pulmonary Tuberculosis. London–New York, Pergamon Press, 1962.
104. Divertie MB, Brown AL Jr, Harrison EG Jr: Pulmonary alveolar proteinosis. Two cases studied by electron microscopy. Am J Med 40:351, 1966.
105. Hudson AR, Halprin GM, Miller JA, et al: Pulmonary interstitial fibrosis following alveolar proteinosis. Chest 65:700, 1974.
106. Kaplan AI, Sabin S: Case report: Interstitial fibrosis after uncomplicated pulmonary alveolar proteinosis. Postgrad Med 61:263, 1977.
107. Clague HW, Wallace AC, Morgan WKC: Pulmonary interstitial fibrosis associated with alveolar proteinosis. Thorax 38:865, 1983.
108. Corsello BF, Choi H: Basophilic staining in pulmonary alveolar proteinosis. Report of three cases. Arch Pathol Lab Med 108:68, 1984.
109. Sato K, Takahashi H, Amano H, et al: Diffuse progressive pulmonary interstitial and intra-alveolar cholesterol granulomas in childhood. Eur Respir J 9:2419, 1996.
110. Sieracki JC, Horn RC Jr, Kay S: Pulmonary alveolar proteinosis: Report of three cases. Ann Intern Med 51:728, 1959.
111. Preger L: Pulmonary alveolar proteinosis. Radiology 92:1291, 1969.
112. Godwin JD, Müller NL, Takasugi JE. Pulmonary alveolar proteinosis: CT findings. Radiology 169:609, 1988.
113. Wang BM, Stern EJ, Schmidt RA, et al: Diagnosing pulmonary alveolar proteinosis: A review and an update. Chest 111:460, 1997.
114. Lee KN, Levin DL, Webb WR, et al: Pulmonary alveolar proteinosis: High-resolution CT, chest radiographic, and functional correlations. Chest 111:989, 1997.
115. Murch CR, Carr DH: Computed tomography appearances of pulmonary alveolar proteinosis. Clin Radiol 40:240, 1989.
116. Zimmer WE, Chew FS. Pulmonary alveolar proteinosis. Am J Roentgenol 161:26, 1993.
117. Miller PA, Ravin CE, Smith GJW, et al: Pulmonary alveolar proteinosis with interstitial involvement. Am J Roentgenol 137:1069, 1981.
118. Kang EY, Grenier P, Laurent F, Müller NL: Interlobular septal thickening: patterns at high-resolution computed tomography. J Thorac Imaging 11:260, 1996.
119. Tan RT, Kuzo RS: High-resolution CT findings of mucinous bronchioloalveolar carcinoma: A case of pseudopulmonary alveolar proteinosis. Am J Roentgenol 168:99, 1997.
120. Franquet T, Giménez A, Bordes R, et al: The crazy-paving pattern in exogenous lipoid pneumonia: CT-pathologic correlation. Am J Roentgenol 170:315, 1998.
121. Ramirez J: Pulmonary alveolar proteinosis. A roentgenologic analysis. Am J Roentgenol 92:571, 1964.
122. Greenspan RH: Chronic disseminated alveolar diseases of the lung. Semin Roentgenol 2:77, 1967.
123. Anton HC, Gray B: Pulmonary alveolar proteinosis presenting with pneumothorax. Clin Radiol 18:428, 1967.
124. Ito K, Iwabe K, Okai T, et al: Rapidly progressive pulmonary alveolar proteinosis in a patient with chronic myelogenous leukemia. Intern Med 33:710, 1994.
125. Kroeker EJ, Korfmacher S: Pulmonary alveolar proteinosis. Report of case with application of a special sputum examination as an aid to diagnosis. Am Rev Respir Dis 87:416, 1963.
126. Rogers RM, Levin DC, Gray BA, et al: Physiologic effects of bronchopulmonary lavage in alveolar proteinosis. Am Rev Respir Dis 118:255, 1978.
127. Jay SJ: Pulmonary alveolar proteinosis: Successful treatment with aerosolized trypsin. Am J Med 66:348, 1979.
128. Martin RJ, Rogers RM, Myers NM: Pulmonary alveolar proteinosis: Shunt fraction and lactic acid dehydrogenase concentration as aids to diagnosis. Am Rev Respir Dis 117:1059, 1978.
129. Hoffman RM, Rogers RM: Serum and lavage lactate dehydrogenase isoenzymes in pulmonary alveolar proteinosis. Am Rev Respir Dis 143:42, 1991.
130. Fujishima T, Honda Y, Shijubo N, et al: Increased carcinoembryonic antigen concentrations in sera and bronchoalveolar lavage fluids of patients with pulmonary alveolar proteinosis. Respiration 62:317, 1995.
131. Hirakata Y, Kobayashi J, Sugama Y, et al: Elevation of tumour markers in serum and bronchoalveolar lavage fluid in pulmonary alveolar proteinosis. Eur Respir J 8:689, 1995.
132. Honda Y, Kuroki Y, Shijubo N, et al: Aberrant appearance of lung surfactant protein A in sera of patients with idiopathic pulmonary fibrosis and its clinical significance. Respiration 62:64, 1995.
133. Honda Y, Kuroki Y, Matsuura E, et al: Pulmonary surfactant protein D in sera and bronchoalveolar lavage fluids. Am J Respir Crit Care Med 152:1860, 1995.
134. Selecky PA, Wasserman K, Benfield JR, et al: The clinical and physiological effects of whole-lung lavage in pulmonary alveolar proteinosis: A ten-year experience. Ann Thorac Surg 24:451, 1977.
135. Fraimow W, Cathcart RT, Taylor RC: Physiologic and clinical aspects of pulmonary alveolar proteinosis. Ann Intern Med 52:1177, 1960.
136. Snider TH, Wilner FM, Lewis BM: Cardiopulmonary physiology in a case of pulmonary alveolar proteinosis. Ann Intern Med 52:1318, 1960.
137. Oliva PB, Vogel JHK: Reactive pulmonary hypertension in alveolar proteinosis. Chest 58:167, 1970.
138. Yeh SD, White DA, Stover-Pepe DE, et al: Abnormal gallium scintigraphy in pulmonary alveolar proteinosis (PAP). Clin Nucl Med 12:294, 1987.
139. Ramirez J, Campbell GD: Pulmonary alveolar proteinosis. Endobronchial treatment. Ann Intern Med 63:429, 1965.
140. Masuda T, Shimura S, Sasaki H, et al: Surfactant apoprotein-A concentration in sputum for diagnosis of pulmonary alveolar proteinosis. Lancet 337:580, 1991.
141. Mermolja M, Rott T, Debeljak A: Cytology of bronchoalveolar lavage in some rare pulmonary disorders: pulmonary alveolar proteinosis and amiodarone pulmonary toxicity. Cytopathology 5:9, 1994.
141a. Sosolik RC, Gammon RR, Julius CJ, et al: Pulmonary alveolar proteinosis. A

report of two cases with diagnostic features in bronchoalveolar lavage specimens. Acta Cytol 42:377, 1998.

142. Rubinstein I, Mullen JB, Hoffstein V: Morphologic diagnosis of idiopathic pulmonary alveolar lipoproteinosis revisited. Arch Intern Med 148:813, 1988.

143. Oka S, Shiraishi K, Ogata K, et al: The course of the first case in Japan of pulmonary alveolar proteinosis. Am Rev Respir Dis 93:608, 1966.

144. Plenk HP, Swift SA, Chambers WL, et al: Pulmonary alveolar proteinosis—a new disease? Radiology 74:928, 1960.

145. Nicholas JJ, Auchincloss JH Jr, Rudolph L: Pulmonary alveolar proteinosis. A case with improvement after a short course of endobronchial instillations of heparin. Ann Intern Med 62:358, 1965.

146. Davidson JM, MacLeod WM: Pulmonary alveolar proteinosis. Br J Dis Chest 63:13, 1969.

147. Du Bois RM, McAllister WA, Branthwaite MA: Alveolar proteinosis: Diagnosis and treatment over a 10-year period. Thorax 38:360, 1983.

148. Wilson JW, Rubinfeld AR, White A, et al: Alveolar proteinosis treated with a single bronchial lavage. Med J Aust 145:158, 1986.

149. Busque L: Pulmonary lavage in the treatment of alveolar proteinosis. Can Anaesth Soc J 24:380, 1977.

150. Westermark P: The pathogenesis of amyloidosis. Understanding general principles. Am J Pathol 152:1125, 1998.

151. Parker LA, Novotny DB: Recurrent alveolar proteinosis following double lung transplantation. Chest 111:1457, 1997.

152. Wilson DO, Rogers RM: Prolonged spontaneous remission in a patient with untreated pulmonary alveolar proteinosis. Am J Med 82:1014, 1987.

153. Kisilevsky R: Biology of disease. Amyloidosis: A familiar problem in the light of current pathogenetic developments. Lab Invest 49:381, 1983.

154. Editorial: Amyloid and the lower respiratory tract. Thorax 38:84, 1983.

155. Nomura S, Kumagai N, Kanoh T, et al: Pulmonary amyloidosis associated with systemic lupus erythematosus. Arthritis Rheum 29:68, 1986.

156. Kayser K, Wiebel M, Schulz V, et al: Necrotizing bronchitis, angiitis, and amyloidosis associated with chronic Q fever. Respiration 62:114, 1995.

157. Vanatta PR, Silva FG, Taylor WE, et al: Renal cell carcinoma and systemic amyloidosis: Demonstration of AA protein and review of the literature. Hum Pathol 14:195, 1983.

158. Meyerhoff J: Familial Mediterranean fever: Report of a large family, review of the literature, and discussion of the frequency of amyloidosis. Medicine 59:66, 1980.

159. Smith RRL, Hutchins GM, Moore GW, et al: Type and distribution of pulmonary parenchymal and vascular amyloid. Correlation with cardiac amyloidosis. Am J Med 66:96, 1979.

160. Fernandez-Alonso J, Rios-Camacho C, Valenzuela-Castano A, et al: Mixed systemic amyloidosis in a patient receiving long term haemodialysis. J Clin Pathol 47:560, 1994.

161. Gordon HW, Miller R Jr, Mittman C: Medullary carcinoma of the lung with amyloid stroma: A counterpart of medullary carcinoma of the thyroid. Hum Pathol 4:431, 1973.

162. Bretherton-Watt D, Ghatei MA, Bloom SE, et al: Islet amyloid polypeptide-like immunoreactivity in human tissue and endocrine tumors. J Clin Endocrinol Metab 76:1072, 1993.

163. Abe Y, Utsunomiya H, Tsutsumi Y: Atypical carcinoid tumor of the lung with amyloid stroma. Acta Pathol Jpn 42:286, 1992.

164. Whitwell F: Localized amyloid infiltrations of the lower respiratory tract. Thorax 8:309, 1953.

165. Monreal FA: Pulmonary amyloidosis: Ultrastructural study of early alveolar septal deposits. Hum Pathol 15:388, 1984.

166. Kavuru MS, Adamo JP, Ahmad N, et al: Amyloidosis and pleural disease. Chest 98:20, 1990.

167. Knapp MJ, Roggli VL, Kim J, et al: Pleural amyloidosis. Arch Pathol Lab Med 112:57, 1988.

168. Hsiu J-G, Stitik FP, D'Amato NA, et al: Primary amyloidosis presenting as a unilateral hilar mass. Report of a case diagnosed by fine needle aspiration biopsy. Acta Cytol 30:55, 1986.

169. Thompson PJ, Jewkes J, Corrin B, et al: Primary bronchopulmonary amyloid tumour with massive hilar lymphadenopathy. Thorax 38:153, 1983.

170. Desai RA, Mahajan VK, Benjamin S, et al: Pulmonary amyloidoma and hilar adenopathy. Rare manifestations of primary amyloidosis. Chest 76:170, 1979.

171. Melato M, Antonutto G, Falconieri G, et al: Massive amyloidosis of mediastinal lymph nodes in a patient with multiple myeloma. Thorax 38:151, 1983.

172. Osnoss KL, Harrell DD: Isolated mediastinal mass in primary amyloidosis. Chest 78:786, 1980.

173. Streeten EA, de la Monte SM, Kennedy TP: Amyloid infiltration of the diaphragm as a cause of respiratory failure. Chest 89:760, 1986.

174. Santiago RM, Scharnhorst D, Ratkin G, et al: Respiratory muscle weakness and ventilatory failure in AL amyloidosis with muscular pseudohypertrophy. Am J Med 83:175, 1987.

175. Winter JH, Milroy R, Stevenson RD, et al: Secondary amyloidosis in association with *Aspergillus* lung disease. Br J Dis Chest 80:400, 1986.

176. Smith FB, Brown RB, Maguire G, et al: Localized pleural microdeposition of type A amyloid in a patient with rheumatoid pleuritis. Histologic distinction from pleural involvement in systemic amyloidosis. Am J Clin Pathol 99:261, 1993.

177. Orriols R, Aliaga JL, Rodrigo MJ, et al: Localized alveolar-septal amyloidosis with hypersensitivity pneumonitis. Lancet 339:1261, 1992.

178. Travis WD, Castile R, Vawter G, et al: Secondary (AA) amyloidosis in cystic fibrosis. A report of three cases. Am J Clin Pathol 85:419, 1986.

179. Michalsen H, Storrøsten OT, Lindboe CF: Generalized amyloidosis in cystic fibrosis. Eur J Respir Dis 66:306, 1985.

180. McGlennen RC, Burke BA, Dehner LP: Systemic amyloidosis complicating cystic fibrosis. A retrospective pathologic study. Arch Pathol Lab Med 110:879, 1986.

181. Pitkänen P, Westermark P, Cornwell GG III: Senile systemic amyloidosis. Am J Pathol 117:391, 1984.

182. Wong BC, Wong KL, Ip MS, et al: Sjögren's syndrome with amyloid A presenting as multiple pulmonary nodules. J Rheumatol 21:165, 1994.

183. Beer TW, Edwards CW: Pulmonary nodules due to reactive systemic amyloidosis (AA) in Crohn's disease. Thorax 48:1287, 1993.

184. Cordier JF, Loire R, Brune J: Amyloidosis of the lower respiratory tract. Clinical and pathologic features in a series of 21 patients. Chest 90:827, 1986.

185. Hui AN, Koss MN, Hochholzer L, et al: Amyloidosis presenting in the lower respiratory tract. Clinicopathologic, radiologic, immunohistochemical, and histochemical studies on 48 cases. Arch Pathol Lab Med 110:212, 1986.

186. Da Costa P, Corrin B: Amyloidosis localized to the lower respiratory tract: Probable immunoamyloid nature of the tracheobronchial and nodular pulmonary forms. Histopathology 9:703, 1985.

187. Toyoda M, Ebihara Y, Kato H, et al: Tracheobronchial al amyloidosis: Histologic, immunohistochemical, ultrastructural, and immunoelectron microscopic observations. Hum Pathol 24:970, 1993.

188. Miura K, Shirasawa H: Lamba III subgroup immunoglobulin light chains are precursor proteins of nodular pulmonary amyloidosis. Am J Clin Pathol 100:561, 1993.

189. Masuda C, Mohri S, Nakajima H: Histopathological and immunohistochemical study of amyloidosis. Br J Dermatol 119:33, 1988.

190. Prowse CB: Amyloidosis of the lower respiratory tract. Thorax 13:308, 1958.

191. Chen KTK: Amyloidosis presenting in the respiratory tract. Pathol Ann 24:253, 1989.

192. Jones AW, Chatterji AN: Primary tracheobronchial amyloidosis with tracheobronchopathia osteoplastica. Br J Dis Chest 71:268, 1977.

193. Kaiserling E, Krober S: Lymphatic amyloidosis, a previously unrecognized form of amyloid deposition in generalized amyloidosis. Histopathology 24:215, 1994.

194. Kijner CH, Yousem SA: Systemic light chain deposition disease presenting as multiple pulmonary nodules. A case report and review of the literature. Am J Surg Pathol 12:405, 1988.

195. Linder J, Vollmer RT, Croker BP, et al: Systemic kappa light-chain deposition: An ultrastructural and immunohistochemical study. Am J Surg Pathol 7:85, 1983.

196. Stokes MB, Jagirdar J, Burchstin O, et al: Nodular pulmonary immunoglobulin light chain deposits with coexistent amyloid and nonamyloid features in an HIV-infected patient. Mod Pathol 10:1059, 1997.

197. Kwong JS, Müller NL, Miller RR: Diseases of the trachea and main-stem bronchi: Correlation of CT with pathologic findings. Radiographics 12:645, 1992.

198. Urban BA, Fishman EK, Goldman SM, et al: CT evaluation of amyloidosis: Spectrum of disease. RadioGraphics 13:1295, 1993.

199. Utz JP, Swensen SJ, Gertz MA: Pulmonary amyloidosis: The Mayo Clinic experience from 1980 to 1993. Ann Intern Med 124:407, 1996.

200. Cotton RE, Jackson JW: Localized amyloid "tumours" of the lung simulating malignant neoplasms. Thorax 19:97, 1964.

201. Mosetitsch W: Amyloid "tumoren" der lungen. [Amyloid tumors of the lungs.] Fortschr Roentgenstr 94:579, 1961.

202. Rubinow A, Celli BR, Cohen AS, et al: Localized amyloidosis of the lower respiratory tract. Am Rev Respir Dis 118:603, 1978.

203. Pickford HA, Swensen SJ, Utz JP: Thoracic cross-sectional imaging of amyloidosis. Am J Roentgenol 168:351, 1997.

204. Bhate DV: Case of the spring season: Diffuse primary amyloidosis with nodular calcified lung lesions. Semin Roentgenol 14:81, 1979.

205. Ayuso MC, Gilabert R, Bombi JA, et al: CT appearance of localized pulmonary amyloidosis. J Comput Assist Tomogr 3:197, 1987.

206. Mata JM, Caceres J, Senac JP, et al: General case of the day. Radiographics 11:716, 1991.

207. Gross BH, Felson B, Birnberg FA: The respiratory tract in amyloidosis and the plasma cell dyscrasias. Semin Roentgenol 21:113, 1986.

208. Tamura K, Nakajima N, Makino S, et al: Primary pulmonary amyloidosis with multiple nodules. Eur J Radiol 8:128, 1988.

209. Gibney RTN, Connolly TP: Pulmonary amyloid nodule simulating Pancoast tumor. J Can Assoc Radiol 35:90, 1984.

209a. Desai SR, Nicholson AG, Stewart S, et al: Benign pulmonary lymphocytic infiltration and amyloidosis: Computed tomographic and pathological features in three cases. J Thorac Imaging 12:215, 1997.

210. Graham CM, Stern EJ, Finkbeiner WE, et al: High-resolution CT appearance of diffuse alveolar septal amyloidosis. Am J Roentgenol 158:265, 1992.

211. Morgan RA, Ring NJ, Marshall AJ: Pulmonary alveolar-septal amyloidosis — an unusual radiographic presentation. Respir Med 86:345, 1992.

212. Prowse CB, Elliott RIK: Diffuse tracheo-bronchial amyloidosis: A rare variant of a protean disease. Thorax 18:326, 1963.

213. Brown J: Primary amyloidosis. Clin Radiol 15:358, 1964.

214. Hodge DS, Anderson WR, Tsai SH: Primary diffuse bronchial amyloidosis. Arch Pathol Lab Med 101:615, 1977.

215. Michaels L, Hyams VJ: Amyloid in localized deposits and plasmacytomas of the respiratory tract. J Pathol 128:29, 1979.

216. Simpson GT 2nd, Strong MS, Skinner M, et al: Localized amyloidosis of the head and neck and upper aerodigestive and lower respiratory tracts. Ann Otol Rhinol Laryngol 93:374, 1984.

217. Carbone JE, Barker D, Stauffer JL: Sleep apnea in amyloidosis. Chest 87:401, 1985.
218. Schulz C, Hauck RW, Nathrath WB, et al: Combined amyloidosis of the upper and lower respiratory tract. Respiration 62:163, 1995.
219. Flemming AFS, Fairfax AJ, Arnold AG, et al: Treatment of endobronchial amyloidosis by intermittent bronchoscopic resection. Br J Dis Chest 74:183, 1980.
220. Kawano O, Kohrogi H, Ando Y, et al: Bronchial hyperreactivity in patients with familial amyloidotic polyneuropathy and autonomic neuropathy. Am J Respir Crit Care Med 155:1465, 1997.
221. Lee S-C, Johnson HA: Multiple nodular pulmonary amyloidosis. A case report and comparison with diffuse alveolar-septal pulmonary amyloidosis. Thorax 30:178, 1975.
222. Moldow RE, Bearman S, Edelman MH: Pulmonary amyloidosis simulating tuberculosis. Am Rev Respir Dis 105:114, 1972.
223. Laden SA, Cohen ML, Harley RA: Nodular pulmonary amyloidosis with extrapulmonary involvement. Hum Pathol 15:594, 1984.
224. Lee AB, Bogaars HA, Passero MA: Nodular pulmonary amyloidosis. A cause of bronchiectasis and fatal pulmonary hemorrhage. Arch Intern Med 143:603, 1983.
225. Kamei K, Kusumoto K, Suzuki T: Pulmonary amyloidosis with pulmonary arteriovenous fistula. Chest 96:1435, 1989.
226. Celli BR, Rubinow A, Cohen AS, et al: Patterns of pulmonary involvement in systemic amyloidosis. Chest 74:543, 1978.
227. Shiue S-T, McNally DP: Pulmonary hypertension from prominent vascular involvement in diffuse amyloidosis. Arch Intern Med 148:687, 1988.
228. Road JD, Jacques J, Sparling JR: Diffuse alveolar septal amyloidosis presenting with recurrent hemoptysis and medial dissection of pulmonary arteries. Am Rev Respir Dis 132:1368, 1985.
229. Utz JP, Swensen SJ, Gertz MA: Pulmonary amyloidosis. The Mayo Clinic experience from 1980 to 1993. Ann Intern Med 124:407, 1996.
230. Planes C, Kleinknecht D, Brauner M, et al: Diffuse interstitial lung disease due to AA amyloidosis. Thorax 47:323, 1992.
231. Crosbie WA, Lewis ML, Ramsay ID, et al: Pulmonary amyloidosis with impaired gas transfer. Thorax 27:625, 1972.
232. Kline LR, Dise CA, Ferro TJ, et al: Diagnosis of pulmonary amyloidosis by transbronchial biopsy. Am Rev Respir Dis 132:191, 1985.
233. Dundore PA, Aisner SC, Templeton PA, et al: Nodular pulmonary amyloidosis: Diagnosis by fine-needle aspiration cytology and a review of the literature. Diagn Cytopathol 9:562, 1993.
234. Strange C, Heffner JE, Collins BS, et al: Pulmonary hemorrhage and air embolism complicating transbronchial biopsy in pulmonary amyloidosis. Chest 92:367, 1987.
235. Kamberg S, Loitman BS, Holtz S: Amyloidosis of the tracheobronchial tree. N Engl J Med 266:587, 1962.
236. Wakasa K, Sakurai M, Koezuka I, et al: Primary tracheobronchial amyloidosis. A case report and review of reported cases. Acta Pathol Jpn 34:145, 1984.
237. Jimenez C, Vital C, Merlio JP, et al: Plasmacytoma and gastric amyloidosis associated with nodular pulmonary amyloidosis. Ann Pathol 8:155, 1988.
238. Cathcart ES, Ritchie RF, Cohen AS, et al: Immunoglobulins and amyloidosis. An immunologic study of sixty-two patients with biopsy-proved disease. Am J Med 52:93, 1972.
239. Kyle RA: Multiple myeloma. Review of 869 cases. Mayo Clin Proc 50:29, 1975.
240. Morgan JE, McCaul DS, Rodriquez FH, et al: Pulmonary immunologic features of alveolar septal amyloidosis associated with multiple myeloma. Chest 92:704, 1987.
241. Eisenberg R, Sharma OP: Primary pulmonary amyloidosis. An unusual case with 14 years' survival. Chest 89:889, 1986.
242. Hof DG, Rasp FL: Spontaneous regression of diffuse tracheobronchial amyloidosis. Chest 76:237, 1979.
243. Sosman MC, Dodd GD, Jones WD, et al: The familial occurrence of pulmonary alveolar microlithiasis. Am J Roentgenol 77:947, 1957.
244. Prakash UBS, Barham SS, Rosenow EC III, et al: Pulmonary alveolar microlithiasis. A review including ultrastructural and pulmonary function studies. Mayo Clin Proc 58:290, 1983.
245. Miro JM, Moreno A, Coca A, et al: Pulmonary alveolar microlithiasis with an unusual radiological pattern. Br J Dis Chest 76:91, 1982.
246. Mariotta S, Guidi L, Papale M, et al: Pulmonary alveolar microlithiasis: Review of Italian reports. Eur J Epidemiol 13:587, 1997.
247. Ucan ES, Keyf AI, Aydilek R, et al: Pulmonary alveolar microlithiasis: Review of Turkish reports. Thorax 48:171, 1993.
248. Caffrey PR, Altman RS: Pulmonary alveolar microlithiasis occurring in premature twins. J Pediatr 66:758, 1965.
249. Sears MR, Chang AR, Taylor AJ: Pulmonary alveolar microlithiasis. Thorax 26:704, 1971.
250. Kino T, Kohara Y, Tsuji S: Pulmonary alveolar microlithiasis. A report of two young sisters. Am Rev Respir Dis 105:105, 1972.
251. Gómez GE, Lichtemberger E, Santamaria A, et al: Familial pulmonary alveolar microlithiasis: Four cases from Colombia, S.A. Is microlithiasis also an environmental disease? Radiology 72:550, 1959.
252. Shimizu K, Matsumoto T, Miura G, et al: Hermansky-Pudlak syndrome with diffuse pulmonary fibrosis: Radiologic-pathologic correlation. J Comput Assist Tomogr 22:249, 1998.
253. Chinachoti N, Tangchai P: Pulmonary alveolar microlithiasis associated with the inhalation of snuff in Thailand. Dis Chest 32:687, 1957.
254. Moran CA, Hochholzer L, Hasleton PS, et al: Pulmonary alveolar microlithiasis.

A clinicopathologic and chemical analysis of seven cases. Arch Pathol Lab Med 121:607, 1997.
254a. Nouh MS: Is the desert lung syndrome (nonoccupational dust pneumoconiosis) a variant of pulmonary alveolar microlithiasis? Respiration 55:122, 1989.
255. Badger TL, Gottlieb L, Gaensler EA: Pulmonary alveolar microlithiasis, or calcinosis of the lungs. N Engl J Med 253:709, 1955.
256. Coetzee T: Pulmonary alveolar microlithiasis with involvement of the sympathetic nervous system and gonads. Thorax 25:637, 1970.
257. Portnoy LM, Amadeo B, Hennigar GR: Pulmonary alveolar microlithiasis. An unusual case (associated with milk-alkali syndrome). Am J Clin Pathol 41:194, 1964.
258. Greenberg MJ: Miliary shadows in the lungs due to microlithiasis alveolaris pulmonum. Thorax 12:171, 1957.
259. O'Neill RP, Cohn JE, Pellegrino ED: Pulmonary alveolar microlithiasis—a family study. Ann Intern Med 67:957, 1967.
260. Richardson J, Slovis B, Miller G, et al: Development of pulmonary alveolar microlithiasis in a renal transplant recipient. Transplantation 59:1056, 1995.
261. Brown ML, Swee RG, Olson RJ, et al: Pulmonary uptake of 99mTc-diphosphonate in alveolar microlithiasis. Am J Roentgenol 131:703, 1978.
262. Bab I, Rosenmann E, Ne'eman Z, et al: The occurrence of extracellular matrix vesicles in pulmonary alveolar microlithiasis. Virchows Arch [Pathol Anat] 391:357, 1981.
263. Barnard NJ, Crocker PR, Blainey AD, et al: Pulmonary alveolar microlithiasis. A new analytical approach. Histopathology 11:639, 1987.
264. Hoshino H, Koba H, Inomata S-I, et al: Pulmonary alveolar microlithiasis: High-resolution CT and MR findings. J Comput Assist Tomogr 22:245, 1998.
265. Tao L-C: Microliths in sputum specimens and their relationship to pulmonary alveolar microlithiasis. Am J Clin Pathol 69:482, 1978.
266. Kawakami M, Sato S, Takishima T: Electron microscopic studies on pulmonary alveolar microlithiasis. Tohoku J Exp Med 126:343, 1978.
267. Hawass ND, Noah MS: Pulmonary alveolar microlithiasis. Eur J Respir Dis 69:199, 1986.
268. Pracyk JB, Simonson SG, Young SL, et al: Composition of lung lavage in pulmonary alveolar microlithiasis. Respiration 63:254, 1996.
269. Rocken C, Linke RP, Saeger W: Corpora amylacea in the lung, prostate and uterus. A comparative and immunohistochemical study. Pathol Res Pract 192:998, 1996.
270. Dobashi M, Yuda F, Narabayashi M, et al: Histopathological study of corpora amylacea pulmonum. Histol Histopathol 4:153, 1989.
271. Hollander DH, Hutchins GM: Central spherules in pulmonary corpora amylacea. Arch Pathol Lab Med 102:629, 1978.
272. Akino T, Mizumoto M, Shimizu H, et al: Pulmonary corpora amylacea contain surfactant apoprotein. Path Res Pract 186:687, 1990.
273. Michaels L, Levene C: Pulmonary corpora amylacea. J Pathol 74:49, 1957.
274. Thind GS, Bhatia JL: Pulmonary alveolar microlithiasis. Br J Dis Chest 72:151, 1978.
275. Helbich TH, Wojnarovsky C, Wunderbaldinger P, et al: Pulmonary alveolar microlithiasis in children: Radiographic and high-resolution CT findings. Am J Roentgenol 168:63, 1997.
276. Balikian JP, Fuleihan FJD, Nucho CN: Pulmonary alveolar microlithiasis: Report on 5 cases with special reference to roentgen manifestations. Am J Roentgenol 103:509, 1968.
277. Sosman MC, Dodd GD, Jones WD, et al: The familial occurrence of pulmonary alveolar microlithiasis. Am J Roentgenol 77:947, 1957.
278. Cheong WY, Wang YT, Tan LKA, et al: Pulmonary alveolar microlithiasis. Australas Radiol 32:401, 1988.
279. Felson B: The roentgen diagnosis of disseminated pulmonary alveolar diseases. Semin Roentgenol 2:3, 1967.
280. Varma BN: Pulmonary alveolar microlithiasis in a child of thirteen years. Br J Dis Chest 57:213, 1963.
281. Cluzel P, Grenier P, Bernadac P, et al: Pulmonary alveolar microlithiasis: CT findings. J Comput Assist Tomogr 15:938, 1991.
282. Korn MA, Schurawitzki H, Klepetko W, et al: Pulmonary alveolar microlithiasis: Findings on high-resolution CT. Am J Roentgenol 158:981, 1992.
283. Melamed JW, Sostman HD, Ravin CE: Interstitial thickening in pulmonary alveolar microlithiasis: An underappreciated finding. J Thorac Imaging 9:126, 1994.
284. Waters MH: Microlithiasis alveolaris pulmonum. Tubercle 41:276, 1960.
285. Winzelberg GG, Boller M, Sachs M, et al: CT evaluation of pulmonary alveolar microlithiasis. J Comput Assist Tomogr 8:1029, 1984.
286. Drinković I, Strohal K, Sabljica B: Mikrolithiasis alveolaris pulmonum. [Pulmonary alveolar microlithiasis.] Fortschr Roentgenstr 97:180, 1962.
287. Turktas I, Saribas S, Balkanci F: Pulmonary alveolar microlithiasis presenting with chronic cough. Postgrad Med J 69:70, 1993.
288. Ferretti GR, Lantuejoul S, Brambilla E, et al: Pulmonary involvement in Niemann-Pick disease subtype B: CT findings. J Comput Assist Tomogr 20:990, 1996.
289. Stamatis G, Zerkowski HR, Doetsch N, et al: Sequential bilateral lung transplantation for pulmonary alveolar microlithiasis. Ann Thorac Surg 56:972, 1993.
290. Fuleihan FJD, Abboud RT, Balikian JP, et al: Pulmonary alveolar microlithiasis: Lung function in five cases. Thorax 24:84, 1969.
291. Brown J, Leon W, Felton C: Hemodynamic and pulmonary studies in pulmonary alveolar microlithiasis. Am J Med 77:176, 1984.
292. Chalmers AG, Wyatt J, Robinson PJ: Computed tomographic and pathological findings in pulmonary alveolar microlithiasis. Br J Radiol 59:408, 1986.

293. Palombini BC, Porto NS, Wallau CV, et al: Bronchopulmonary lavage in alveolar microlithiasis (letter). Anaesth Intensive Care 6:265, 1978.

294. Cale WF, Petsonk EL, Boyd CB: Transbronchial biopsy of pulmonary alveolar microlithiasis. Arch Intern Med 143:358, 1983.

295. Smith RRL, Hutchins GM, Sack GH Jr, et al: Unusual cardiac, renal and pulmonary involvement in Gaucher's disease. Interstitial glucocerebroside accumulation, pulmonary hypertension and fatal bone marrow embolization. Am J Med 65:352, 1978.

296. Wolson AH: Pulmonary findings in Gaucher's disease. Am J Roentgenol 123:712, 1975.

297. Kerem E, Elstein D, Abrahamov A, et al: Pulmonary function abnormalities in type I Gaucher disease. Eur Respir J 9:340, 1996.

297a. Santamaria F, Parenti G, Guidi G, et al: Pulmonary manifestations of Gaucher disease. An increased risk for L444P homozygotes? Am J Respir Crit Care Med 157:985, 1998.

298. Schneider EL, Epstein CJ, Kaback MJ, et al: Severe pulmonary involvement in adult Gaucher's disease. Report of three cases and review of the literature. Am J Med 63:475, 1977.

299. Peters SP, Lee RE, Glew RH: Gaucher's disease: A review. Medicine 56:425, 1977.

300. Jackson DC, Simon G: Unusual bone and lung changes in a case of Gaucher's disease. Br Med J 38:698, 1965.

301. Links TP, Karrenbeld A, Steensma JT, et al: Fatal respiratory failure caused by pulmonary infiltration by pseudo-Gaucher cells. Chest 101:265, 1992.

302. Roberts WC, Fredrickson DS: Gaucher's disease of the lung causing severe pulmonary hypertension with associated acute pericarditis. Circulation 35:783, 1967.

303. Carson KF, Williams CA, Rosenthal DL, et al: Bronchoalveolar lavage in a girl with Gaucher's disease. A case report. Acta Cytol 38:597, 1994.

304. Lieberman J, Beutler E: Elevation of serum angiotensin-converting enzyme in Gaucher's disease. N Engl J Med 294:1442, 1976.

305. Hrebicek M, Zeman J, Musilova J, et al: A case of type I Gaucher disease with cardiopulmonary amyloidosis and chitotriosidase deficiency. Virchows Arch 429:305, 1996.

306. Long RG, Lake BD, Pettit JE, et al: Adult Niemann-Pick disease. Its relationship to the syndrome of the sea-blue histiocyte. Am J Med 62:627, 1977.

307. Crocker AC, Farber S: Niemann-Pick disease: A review of eighteen patients. Medicine 37:1, 1958.

308. Gogus S, Gocmen A, Kocak N, et al: Lipidosis with sea-blue histiocytes. Report of two siblings with lung involvement. Turk J Pediatr 36:139, 1994.

309. Lachman R, Crocker A, Schulman J, et al: Radiological findings in Niemann-Pick disease. Radiology 108:659, 1973.

310. Niggemann B, Rebien W, Rahn W, et al: Asymptomatic pulmonary involvement in 2 children with Niemann-Pick disease type B. Respiration 61:55, 1994.

311. Bartimmo EE Jr, Guisan M, Moser KM: Pulmonary involvement in Fabry's disease: A reappraisal. Follow-up of a San Diego kindred and review of the literature. Am J Med 53:755, 1972.

312. Bagdade JD, Parker F, Ways PO, et al: Fabry's disease. A correlative clinical, morphologic, and biochemical study. Lab Invest 18:681, 1968.

313. Rosenberg DM, Ferrans VJ, Fulmer JD, et al: Chronic airflow obstruction in Fabry's disease. Am J Med 68:898, 1980.

314. Parkinson JE, Sunshine A: Angiokeratoma corporis diffusum universale (Fabry) presenting as suspected myocardial infarction and pulmonary infarcts. Am J Med 31:951, 1961.

315. Matsumoto T, Matsumori H, Taki T, et al: Infantile GM_1-gangliosidosis with marked manifestation of lungs. Acta Pathol Jpn 29:269, 1979.

316. Garay SM, Gardella JE, Fazzini EP, et al: Hermansky-Pudlak syndrome. Pulmonary manifestations of a ceroid storage disorder. Am J Med 66:737, 1979.

317. Schinella RA, Greco MA, Garay SM, et al: Hermansky-Pudlak syndrome: A clinicopathologic study. Hum Pathol 16:366, 1985.

318. DePinho RA, Kaplan KL: The Hermansky-Pudlak syndrome. Report of three cases and review of pathophysiology and management considerations. Medicine 64:192, 1985.

319. Hoste P, Willems J, Devriendt J, et al: Familial diffuse interstitial pulmonary fibrosis associated with oculocutaneous albinism. Report of two cases with a family study. Scand J Respir Dis 60:128, 1979.

320. Takahashi A, Yokoyama T: Hermansky-Pudlak syndrome with special reference to lysosomal dysfunction. A case report and review of the literature. Virchows Arch [Pathol Anat] 402:247, 1984.

321. Sakuma T, Monma N, Satodate R, et al: Ceroid pigment deposition in circulating blood monocytes and T lymphocytes in Hermansky-Pudlak syndrome: An ultrastructural study. Pathol Int 45:866, 1995.

322. Rankin JA: Hermansky-Pudlak syndrome and interstitial lung disease: Report of a case with lavage findings. Am Rev Respir Dis 130:138, 1984.

323. Reynolds SP, Davies BH, Gibbs AR: Diffuse pulmonary fibrosis and the Hermansky-Pudlak syndrome: clinical course and postmortem findings. Thorax 49:617, 1994.

324. Harmon KR, Witkop CJ, White JG, et al: Pathogenesis of pulmonary fibrosis: Platelet-derived growth factor precedes structural alterations in the Hermansky-Pudlak syndrome. J Lab Clin Med 123:617, 1994.

325. Leitman BS, Balthazar EJ, Garay SM, et al: The Hermansky-Pudlak syndrome: Radiographic features. J Can Assoc Radiol 37:41, 1986.

326. Reynolds SP, Davies BH, Gibbs AR: Diffuse pulmonary fibrosis and the Hermansky-Pudlak syndrome: Clinical course and postmortem findings. Thorax 49:617, 1994.

327. Horowitz ID: Dyspnea in a 30-year-old Hispanic man with albinism. Chest 108:1158, 1995.

327a. Devouassoux G, Lantuejoul S, Chatelain P, et al: Erdheim-Chester disease. A primary macrophage cell disorder. Am J Respir Crit Care Med 157:650, 1998.

327b. Remy-Jardin M, Remy J, Gosselin B, et al: Pulmonary involvement in Erdheim-Chester disease: High-resolution CT findings. Eur Radiol 3:389, 1993.

328. Clarke JTR, Ozere RL, Krause VW: Early infantile variant of Krabbe globoid cell leucodystrophy with lung involvement. Arch Dis Child 56:640, 1981.

329. Sastre J, Renedo G, González Mangado N, et al: Pulmonary ceroidosis. Chest 91:281, 1987.

330. Takahashi K, Hakozaki H, Kojima M: Idiopathic pulmonary ceroidosis. Acta Pathol Jpn 28:301, 1978.

331. Schimschock JR, Alvord ECJ, Swanson PD: Cerebrotendinous xanthomatosis: Clinical and pathological studies. Arch Neurol 18:688, 1968.

332. Dormans TP, Verrips A, Bulten J, et al: Pulmonary lymphangioleiomyomatosis and cerebrotendinous xanthomatosis: Is there a link? Chest 112:273, 1997.

333. Caplan H: A case of endocardial fibro-elastosis with features of glycogen-storage disease. J Pathol Bact 76:77, 1958.

334. Lightman NI, Schooley RT: Adult-onset acid maltase deficiency. Case report of an adult with severe respiratory difficulty. Chest 72:250, 1977.

335. Semenza GL, Pyeritz RE: Respiratory complications of mucopolysaccharide storage disorders. Medicine 67:209, 1988.

336. Hardcastle SW, Rosenstrauch WJ: Lipoid proteinosis. A case report. S Afr Med J 66:273, 1984.

337. Weidner WA, Wenzl JE, Swischuk LE: Roentgenographic findings in lipoid proteinosis: A case report. Am J Roentgenol 110:457, 1970.

338. Shore RN, Howard BV, Howard WJ, et al: Lipoid proteinosis: demonstration of normal lipid metabolism in cultured cells. Arch Dermatol 110:591, 1974.

339. Caplan RM: Visceral involvement in lipoid proteinosis. Arch Dermatol 95:149, 1967.

340. Rowley PT, Mueller PS, Watkin DM, et al: Familial growth retardation, renal aminoaciduria and cor pulmonale. I. Description of a new syndrome, with case reports. Am J Med 31:187, 1961.

341. Rosenberg LE, Mueller PS, Watkin DM: A new syndrome: Familial growth retardation, renal aminoaciduria and cor pulmonale. II. Investigation of renal function, amino acid metabolism and genetic transmission. Am J Med 31:205, 1961.

342. Yagishita S, Ito Y, Sakai H, et al: Membranocystic lesions of the lung in Nasu-Hakola disease. Virchows Arch 408:211, 1985.

343. Duboucher C, Rocchiccioli F, Lageron A, et al: Diffuse storage of vegetal wax hydrocarbons of dietary origin. Pathologic and chemical findings in a case. Arch Pathol Lab Med 113:423, 1989.

344. Koziel H, Koziel MJ: Pulmonary complications of diabetes mellitus. Pneumonia. Infect Dis Clin North Am 9:65, 1995.

345. Pablos-Mendez A, Blustein J, Knirsch CA: The role of diabetes mellitus in the higher prevalence of tuberculosis among Hispanics. Am J Public Health 87:574, 1997.

346. Loukides S, Polyzogopoulos D: The effect of diabetes mellitus on the outcome of patients with chronic obstructive pulmonary disease exacerbated due to respiratory infections. Respiration 63:170, 1996.

347. Russel J, Follansbee S, Matthay MA: Adult respiratory distress syndrome complicating diabetic ketoacidosis. West J Med 135:148, 1981.

348. Powner D, Snyder JV, Grenwich A: Altered pulmonary capillary permeability recovering from diabetic ketoacidosis. Chest 68:253, 1975.

349. Young MC: Simultaneous acute cerebral and pulmonary edema complicating diabetic ketoacidosis. Diabetes Care 18:1288, 1995.

350. Vracko R, Thorning D, Huang TW: Basal lamina of alveolar epithelium and capillaries: Quantitative changes with aging and in diabetes mellitus. Am Rev Respir Dis 120:973, 1979.

351. Watanabe K, Senju S, Toyoshima H, et al: Thickness of the basement membrane of bronchial epithelial cells in lung diseases as determined by transbronchial biopsy. Respir Med 91:406, 1997.

352. Farina J, Furio V, Fernandez-Acenero MJ, et al: Nodular fibrosis of the lung in diabetes mellitus. Virchows Arch 427:61, 1995.

353. Reinilä A: Perivascular xanthogranulomatosis in the lungs of diabetic patients. Arch Pathol Lab Med 100:542, 1976.

354. Colpaert C, Hogan J, Stark AR, et al: Increased muscularization of small pulmonary arteries in preterm infants of diabetic mothers: A morphometric study in noninflated, noninjected, routinely fixed lungs. Pediatr Pathol Lab Med 15:689, 1995.

355. Innocenti F, Fabbri A, Anichini R, et al: Indications of reduced pulmonary function in type 1 (insulin-dependent) diabetes mellitus. Diabetes Res Clin Pract 25:161, 1994.

356. Strojek K, Ziora D, Sroczynski JW, et al: Pulmonary complications of type one (insulin-dependent) diabetic patients. Diabetologia 35:1173, 1992.

357. Mori H, Okubo M, Okamura M, et al: Abnormalities of pulmonary function in patients with non-insulin-dependent diabetes mellitus. Intern Med 31:189, 1992.

358. Fuso L, Cotroneo P, Basso S, et al: Postural variations of pulmonary diffusing capacity in insulin-dependent diabetes mellitus. Chest 110:1009, 1996.

359. Sandler M, Bunn AE, Stewart RI: Cross-section study of pulmonary function in patients with insulin-dependent diabetes mellitus. Am Rev Respir Dis 135:223, 1987.

360. Vianna LG, Gilbey SG, Barnes NC, et al: Cough threshold to citric acid in diabetic patients with and without autonomic neuropathy. Thorax 43:569, 1988.

361. Enright PL, Kronmal RA, Manolio TA, et al: Respiratory muscle strength in the

elderly. Correlates and reference values. Cardiovascular Health Study Research Group. Am J Respir Crit Care Med 149:430, 1994.

362. Brody JS, Buhain WJ: Hormonal influence on post-pneumonectomy lung growth in the rat. Respir Physiol 19:344, 1973.
363. De Troyer A, Desir D, Copinschi G: Regression of lung size in adults with growth hormone deficiency. Q J Med (New Series 49) 195: 329, 1980.
364. Donnelly PM, Grunstein RR, Peat JK, et al: Large lungs and growth hormone: an increased alveolar number? Eur Respir J 8:938, 1995.
365. Siafakas NM, Sigalas J, Filaditaki B, et al: Small airway function in acromegaly. Bull Eur Physiopathol Respir 23:329, 1987.
366. Harrison BD, Millhouse KA, Harrington M: Lung function in acromegaly. Q J Med 47:517, 1978.
367. Brody JS, Fisher AB, Gocmen A, et al: Acromegalic pneumomegaly: Lung growth in the adult. J Clin Invest 49:1051, 1970.
368. Trotman-Dickenson B, Weetman AP, Hughes JM: Upper airway obstruction and pulmonary function in acromegaly: Relationship to disease activity. Q J Med 79:527, 1991.
369. Murrant NJ, Gatland DJ: Respiratory problems in acromegaly. J Laryngol Otol 104:52, 1990.
370. Kitabara LM: Airway difficulties associated with anesthesia in acromegaly. Br J Anaesth 43:1187, 1971.
371. Iandelli I, Gorini M, Duranti R, et al: Respiratory muscle function and control of breathing in patients with acromegaly. Eur Respir J 10:977, 1997.
372. Schneierson SJ, Katz M: Solitary pleural effusion due to myxedema. JAMA 168:1003, 1958.
373. Brown SD, Brashear RE, Schnute RB: Pleural effusion in a young woman with myxedema. Arch Intern Med 143:1458, 1983.
374. Parving HH, Hansen JM, Nielsen SL, et al: Mechanisms of edema formation in myxedema—increased protein extravasation and relative slow lymphatic drainage. N Engl J Med 301:460, 1979.
375. Sadiq MA, Davies JC: Unusual lung manifestations of myxoedema. Br J Clin Pract 31:224, 1977.
376. Forester CF: Coma in myxedema. Report of a case and review of the world literature. Arch Intern Med 111:734, 1963.
377. Menendez CE, Rivlin RS: Thyrotoxic crisis and myxedema coma. Med Clin North Am 57:1463, 1973.
378. Weg John C, Calverly JR, Johnson C: Hypothyroidism and alveolar hypoventilation. Arch Intern Med 115:302, 1965.
379. Wilson WR, Bedell GN: The pulmonary abnormalities in myxedema. J Clin Invest 39:42, 1960.
380. Massumi RA, Winnacker JJ: Severe depression of the respiratory center in myxedema. Am J Med 36:876, 1964.
381. Domm BM, Vassalo CL: Myxedema coma with respiratory failure. Am Rev Respir Dis 107:842, 1973.
382. Naeye RL: Capillary and venous lesions in myxedema. Lab Invest 12:465, 1963.
383. Ingar SH, Woebar KA: The thyroid gland. *In* Wilson JB, Foster DW (eds): Williams' Textbook of Endocrinology. 7th ed. Philadelphia, WB Saunders, 1974, pp 95–232.
384. Orr WC, Males JL, Imes NK: Myxedema and obstructive sleep apnea. Am J Med 70:1060, 1981.
385. Bouros D, Panagou P, Arseniou P, et al: Idiopathic pulmonary haemosiderosis and autoimmune hypothyroidism: Bronchoalveolar lavage findings after cimetidine treatment. Respir Med 89:307, 1995.
386. Badesch DB, Wynne KM, Bonvallet S, et al: Hypothyroidism and primary pulmonary hypertension: An autoimmune pathogenetic link? Ann Intern Med 119:44, 1993.
387. Stein M, Kimball P, Johnson RL: Pulmonary function in hyperthyroidism. J Clin Invest 40:348, 1961.
388. Siafakas NM, Milona A, Salesiotou V, et al: Respiratory muscle strength in hyperthyroidism before and after treatment. Am Rev Respir Dis 146:1025, 1992.
389. McElvaney GN, Wilcox PG, Fairbran MS, et al: Respiratory muscle weakness and dyspnea in thyrotoxic patients. Am Rev Respir Dis 141:1221, 1990.
390. Zwillich CW, Matthay MA, Potts DE, et al: Thyrotoxicosis: Comparison of effects of thyroid ablation and beta-adrenergic ventilatory control. J Clin Endocrinol Metab 46:491, 1978.
391. Thurnheer R, Jenni R, Russi EW, et al: Hyperthyroidism and pulmonary hypertension. J Intern Med 242:185, 1997.
392. Huseby JS, Petersen D: Pulmonary function in Klinefelter's syndrome. Chest 80:31, 1981.

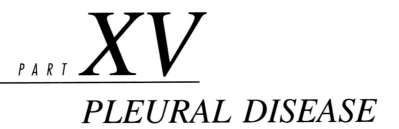

PART *XV*

PLEURAL DISEASE

CHAPTER 69

Pleural Effusion

GENERAL FEATURES OF PLEURAL EFFUSION

Pleural effusion is an accumulation of fluid* in the pleural space that results when homeostatic forces that control the flow in and out of the space are disrupted.[1] Although its precise incidence is unknown, it has been estimated that approximately 1 million people develop the abnormality each year in the United States.[2]

The physiology of pleural fluid accumulation is discussed in detail in Chapter 6 (*see* page 168). Briefly, fluid usually enters the pleural space from the systemic microvasculature, which, in humans, supplies both the parietal and visceral pleura. Under normal circumstances, the main flow is from the parietal pleura; however, in pulmonary edema, movement of fluid from the lung interstitium into the pleural space may be important. An *exudative effusion* may result from disease of the pleural surface itself or from injury in the adjacent lung, whereas a *transudative effusion* generally results from alterations in the systemic circulation that influence the movement of fluid into and out of the pleural space. In experimental studies of hydrostatic and permeability pulmonary edema, pleural effusion develops when the amount of extravascular lung water has reached a certain level for a certain amount of time.[3] Fluid flow across the visceral pleura becomes greater than the capacity of the parietal pleural lymphatics to clear it. When the lung is injured, such as in pneumonia or infarction, associated exudative effusions probably are also derived in part from the fluid in the pulmonary interstitium.[4] The identification of fluid as a transudate or an exudate is useful, as this indicates whether the fluid results from increased hydrostatic pressure or decreased osmotic pressure, or from increased permeability.[4]

Effusion may occur by itself or in association with abnormalities of the lungs, mediastinum, or chest wall; in the former situation, diagnosis of a specific etiology may

---

*The character of fluid in the pleural space—transudate, exudate, pus, blood, chyle, or any combination of these—is seldom, if ever, discernible radiographically; therefore, "increase in pleural fluid" and not "pleural effusion" should be the correct term for reporting these radiographic appearances. Because it is in common usage, however, the term *pleural effusion* is used here. Where appropriate, the precise terms *hydrothorax* (for serous effusions, either transudate or exudate), *pyothorax, hemothorax,* and *chylothorax* are employed.

prove difficult, even following bacteriologic, biochemical, and pathologic investigations. However, when it occurs as part of a complex of radiologic changes, other important clues may be available to permit diagnosis. For example, when effusion accompanies enlargement of the heart or multiple rib fractures, it is reasonable to conclude that it is the result of cardiac decompensation or chest wall trauma, respectively. Similarly, an absent breast shadow or an elevated hemidiaphragm suggests the possibility of metastatic carcinoma or subphrenic disease. Often, however, an effusion constitutes one facet of a complex of radiologic signs that tries the diagnostic skills of the physician. In fact, even after careful evaluation, the etiology remains undetermined in as many as 25% of effusions in some series.[5]

Because the differential diagnosis of pleural effusion varies according to the presence or absence of associated disease in the lungs, mediastinum, diaphragm, or chest wall, the approach to differential diagnosis must be along different lines when effusion is the sole abnormality and when one or more of these structures is affected. With this in mind, it is important to note that underlying pulmonary or mediastinal disease is not always detectable on initial radiographs; large effusions may mask parenchymal shadows or mediastinal masses, and these may become evident only when fluid has been removed or when other imaging procedures render the underlying lung or mediastinal structures visible.

When considering the etiology of an effusion, it is important to remember that some are multifactorial. For example, the transformation of a transudate into an exudate following the treatment of heart failure may indicate the presence of underlying thromboembolic disease or malignancy.[6] Occasionally, such a change in fluid character is the result of aggressive diuresis.[7, 8] Conceivably, a borderline transudate could meet criteria for an exudative effusion after the patient assumes a sitting position if the initial values originated from a sample drawn while the patient was in the supine position.[9] This "postural sedimentary effect" may be related to the molecular weight of certain fluid constituents.

Uncommonly, bilateral pleural effusions have a different etiology, a situation known as *Contarini's condition* in reference to the 95th doge of Venice who died in 1625 with orthopnea, foul-smelling sputum, cardiac arrhythmia, and clear pleural fluid on one side and pus on the other.[10] Several examples of this unusual combination have been reported in the more recent literature;[10, 11] as in the original description, there is usually empyema on one side and effusion secondary to fluid overload or congestive heart failure on the other (Fig. 69–1).

This chapter is concerned with the diagnosis and differential diagnosis of diseases of the pleura. The radiographic signs of pleural disease (*see* page 563), the use of imaging in the detection of loculated effusion (*see* page 579), and the analysis of cell number and type in pleural fluid (*see* page 343) have been discussed elsewhere. Before reviewing the specific causes of pleural effusion—of which there are many (Table 69–1)—the general features of clinical and pulmonary function disturbances, the findings on biochemical analysis of pleural fluid, and the means of investigation are summarized briefly.

Clinical Manifestations

Pleural pain that is sharp, localized, and exacerbated by inspiration is a frequent manifestation of "dry" pleurisy (*see*

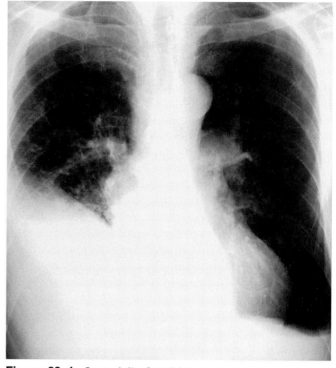

Figure 69–1. Contarini's Condition. A 74-year-old man presented with a 1-week history of fever and progressive shortness of breath. A posteroanterior chest radiograph demonstrates moderate-sized right and small sized left pleural effusions. The upper margin of the right effusion has a convex contour consistent with loculation. Localized areas of atelectasis and consolidation in the right lower lobe and mild increase in size of the upper lobe vessels are also evident. Aspiration of fluid from the right pleural space revealed an empyema; cultures grew *Pasteurella multocida.* The left pleural effusion was a transudate secondary to cardiac decompensation; cultures were negative.

page 385), but it often diminishes when effusion develops. In some cases, the pain is not accentuated by breathing and is felt as a dull ache. The parietal pleura is innervated by branches of the intercostal nerves; thus, pleural pain usually is well localized, although it may be referred to the abdomen. When the phrenic nerve endings are irritated by inflammation of the diaphragmatic pleura, the pain may be felt in the shoulder. Dry cough may be seen and can become productive if there is associated pneumonia. Dyspnea is common and may be severe, as a result of either compromise of respiratory reserve by the effusion or concomitant pulmonary parenchymal or vascular disease. The mediastinal displacement that occurs in tension hydrothorax can cause respiratory distress, dysphagia, engorged neck veins, a tender liver, and edema of the lower extremities;[12] thoracentesis is characteristically followed by immediate relief of symptoms and signs. Approximately 15% of patients who have pleural effusions are asymptomatic.[13] A number of conditions are associated with pleural effusions in the absence of chest-related symptoms, including recent childbirth or abdominal surgery, asbestos-related effusion, uremia, malignancy, and tuberculosis.

Physical examination reveals dullness or flatness on percussion and a decrease or an absence of breath sounds. Although the latter are usually absent when effusion is large, at times they persist; in this situation, they may sound distant

Table 69–1. PLEURAL EFFUSION—ETIOLOGY

ETIOLOGY	SELECTED REFERENCE(S)
PLEUROPULMONARY INFECTION	See text
Mycobacterium tuberculosis	
Nontuberculous bacteria	
Actinomyces and *Nocardia* species	
Fungi	
Parasites	
Viruses, *Mycoplasma,* and Rickettsiae	
PLEUROPULMONARY MALIGNANCY	See text
Pulmonary carcinoma	
Metastatic neoplasm to pleura and mediastinal lymph nodes	
Lymphoma	
Leukemia	
CONNECTIVE TISSUE DISEASE	See text
Systemic lupus erythematosus	
Rheumatoid disease	
Others	
ASBESTOS	319
DRUGS	
See Table 69–3, page 2756	
HEART FAILURE	See text
TRAUMA	
Penetrating and nonpenetrating injury	
Coronary artery bypass procedures	
Pulmonary resection	
Esophageal rupture	
Intravascular therapeutic or monitoring devices	
Abdominal surgery	
Subarachnoid-pleural fistula	697
METABOLIC AND ENDOCRINE DISEASE	
Myxedema	611
Diabetes mellitus	698
Amyloidosis	699, 700
SKELETAL DISEASE	
Neoplasms	
Langerhans' cell histiocytosis	701
Spondylitis	702, 751
Gorham's disease	703
LIVER DISEASE	
Cirrhosis	504, 510
Biliary tract fistula	521
Transplantation	523a
KIDNEY DISEASE	See text
Dialysis	
Urinoma	
Nephrotic syndrome	
Acute glomerulonephritis	
Uremia	
PANCREATIC DISEASE	
Acute pancreatitis	551
Chronic pancreatitis with pleuropancreatic fistula	564
GYNECOLOGIC TUMORS	
Ovary, uterus, fallopian tube	See text
Ovarian hyperstimulation syndrome	752
GASTROINTESTINAL TRACT	
Gastric/duodenal–pleural fistula	602
Diaphragmatic hernia	488
Idiopathic inflammatory bowel disease	605
MISCELLANEOUS CAUSES	
Subphrenic abscess	See text
Lymphatic hypoplasia	See text
Dressler's syndrome	See text
Familial paroxysmal polyserositis	See text
Rupture of silicon gel mammoplasty device	704
Systemic cholesterol embolization	705
Extramedullary hematopoiesis	753
IDIOPATHIC	706

and/or be bronchial in type. In one study of 21 patients who had protracted unilateral pleural effusion, examination showed edema of the ipsilateral chest wall in 13, all of whom proved to have either empyema or a malignant effusion.[14] Another rare cause of ipsilateral chest wall "edema" is thoracentesis (Fig. 69–2).

Pulmonary Function Tests

The results of pulmonary function studies in patients who have pleural effusion depend on the presence and the nature of underlying pulmonary disease and are so variable that little information of value is available. In the absence of pulmonary disease, the effects of pleural effusion on pulmonary function reflect the combination of a space-occupying process and a reduction in lung volume as a consequence of relaxation atelectasis. The former results in reduction of all subdivisions of lung volume, including total lung capacity, functional residual capacity, and vital capacity; despite this, ventilatory ability may be little impaired when the other lung is normal and there is no pleural pain inhibiting chest movement.[15] In a canine model of pleural effusion, dynamic elastance and resistance of the lung have been shown to increase significantly without change in these parameters in the chest wall.[16]

Depending on the amount of fluid and, therefore, on the degree of ipsilateral pulmonary collapse, diffusing capacity may be moderately diminished, although it often remains within the predicted normal range. Blood gas tensions also may be normal; arterial oxygen saturation usually is unaffected, even with a major degree of passive atelectasis, because regional perfusion diminishes in response to the reduction in regional ventilation. Arterial P_{CO_2} may decrease if unilateral pulmonary collapse results in hyperventilation but otherwise remains unaffected. Arterial oxygen saturation can fall significantly in the lateral decubitus position when the hemithorax with the pleural effusion is dependent, a phenomenon that can also occur in the presence of parenchymal consolidation.[17, 18] However, when care is taken to study patients who have only effusion, there is usually little difference between measurements taken when the effusion side or the normal side is down.[5]

The slight but significant increase in PaO_2 and lung volumes and the decrease in $P(A-a)O_2$ that occur in some patients following thoracentesis are insufficient to explain the relief of dyspnea that is commonly experienced. This improvement may result from a reduction in the size of the thoracic cage that allows the inspiratory muscles to operate on a more advantageous portion of their length-tension curve.[19, 20] In some patients, thoracentesis results in hypoxemia, presumably as a result of the development of reexpansion pulmonary edema (*see* page 2001).[21]

Biochemical Findings

Knowledge of the biochemical characteristics of a pleural effusion can greatly aid in the determination of its etiology. The most useful substances for evaluation are protein, lactate dehydrogenase (LDH), glucose, and hydrogen ion (pH) (Table 69–2).

The measurement of protein and LDH concentrations in pleural fluid and the comparison of these with the values in serum have proved invaluable in making an accurate

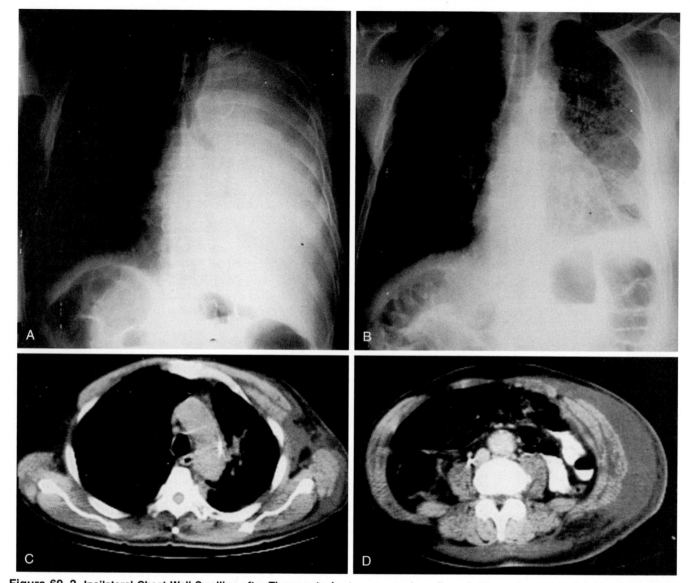

Figure 69–2. Ipsilateral Chest Wall Swelling after Thoracentesis. A posteroanterior radiograph *(A)* reveals a massive left pleural effusion; note the markedly depressed left hemidiaphragm. Thoracentesis was attempted, but only 50 ml of straw-colored fluid could be removed. Despite this, a radiograph obtained following thoracentesis *(B)* shows virtually no fluid remaining in the pleural space; however, a marked increase in the thickness of the left chest wall has occurred. CT scans at the level of the aortic arch *(C)* and upper abdomen *(D)* show a marked increase in the volume of soft tissue in the left chest wall and abdomen that was caused by drainage of pleural fluid through the needle tract created for thoracentesis. The cause of the effusion was metastatic adenocarcinoma from the bowel.

distinction between transudative and exudative effusions.[22] In a prospective study of 150 effusions, Light and colleagues determined that there were three biochemical characteristics that separated one from the other:[23] (1) a fluid-to-serum protein ratio greater than 0.5, (2) a pleural fluid LDH greater than 200 IU, and (3) a fluid-to-serum LDH ratio greater than 0.6. All but 1 of the 103 clinically diagnosed exudates had at least one of these characteristics, whereas only 1 of the 47 transudates had any. Simultaneous measurement of both protein and LDH levels had better differential diagnostic value than did the measurement of either one.

Applying the criteria used by Light and colleagues prospectively to patients who had carefully defined causes of effusion, another group found them to be 95% accurate for identifying exudates.[24] Neither modification of the criteria[24] nor measurement of other biochemical substances has

significantly improved on these results.[25–31] The use of a cut-off value for LDH of 45% of the upper limits of a laboratory's normal serum LDH to define an exudate and the elimination of the absolute pleural fluid LDH value have not been found to diminish the diagnostic accuracy.[32] Although not practiced widely, the use of a pleural LDH value greater than 200 IU per liter and a pleural cholesterol value greater than 45 mg per dl allows diagnosis of an exudate without the need for simultaneous blood measurements and at a lower cost.[30, 33] It has also been suggested that the presence of a difference in the albumen content of 12 gm per liter between the serum and pleural fluid is useful for the recognition of a transudative effusion in patients who have congestive heart failure and have been treated with diuretics;[29] however, larger studies are required to confirm this hypothesis.[32]

Glucose levels in transudative pleural effusions are normal.[34] The levels in tuberculous or neoplastic effusions may be normal or low.[34, 35] Very low values for pleural fluid glucose have been found in patients who have tuberculosis or rheumatoid arthritis;[34, 36, 37] in fact, values below 1.4 mmol per liter should prompt consideration of these diagnoses. However, very low glucose contents have also been reported in neoplastic pleural effusions; for example, in one review of 88 such effusions, it was less than 1.4 mmol in 8.[38] Such low values have been related to the presence of very large collections of fluid.[34, 38]

A variety of factors determine the pH of pleural fluid. Acid can be produced in the fluid or in the pleura itself by the anaerobic metabolism of glucose by bacteria and leukocytes (with the production of CO_2 and lactate) as well as directly by tumor cells and red blood cells. Pleural fluid does not have the buffering capacity of blood, so that small changes in H^+ concentration are more apparent.[39] In one study of 183 patients who had simultaneous blood and pleural fluid pH determination, all 36 transudates were found to have a pH above 7.30;[39] 46 of 147 exudates had a pH less than 7.30 in the presence of a normal blood pH. The 46 patients who had pleural fluid acidosis but not acidemia had empyema, malignancy, connective tissue disease, hemothorax, tuberculosis, or esophageal rupture; the lowest observed pH (6.00) occurred in a patient who had esophageal rupture, presumably as a result of contamination of the pleural fluid by gastric fluid. Thus, the measurement of pH is not helpful in distinguishing malignant from benign effusions.[40]

Pleural effusion, usually left-sided and sometimes hemorrhagic,[41] is present in 5% to 15% of patients who have acute pancreatitis.[34] In one investigation of 38 such patients, elevated amylase values were found in 37.[42] The amylase content is greater in the pleural effusion than in blood serum in patients who have esophageal perforation,[43] probably because of contamination by saliva.[44]

Chylothorax should be suspected when the gross appearance of the effusion is cloudy or milky. The fat content exceeds 4 gm per liter, and the protein content is almost invariably greater than 30 gm per liter. In some cases, effusions related to tuberculosis or rheumatoid disease contain high levels of cholesterol and may resemble chylothorax (pseudochylous effusion).[45] Reduced pleural fluid complement has been reported in systemic lupus erythematosus and rheumatoid arthritis.[46] A high level of hyaluronic acid in pleural fluid suggests the diagnosis of mesothelioma.[47, 48] Some workers have found pleural fluid levels of lysozyme (as well as pleural fluid-to-blood ratios of this enzyme) to be helpful in identifying empyema and tuberculous pleural effusion.[49]

Thoracentesis, Thoracoscopy, and Pleural Biopsy

Thoracentesis is often the first diagnostic test performed in patients who have pleural effusion of unknown etiology;[22] it also serves to drain pleural fluid for the relief of dyspnea. When performed by relatively inexperienced operators, complications are surprisingly common.[50] Although many of these are minor, pneumothorax developed in 15 of 129 patients (12%) in one series;[50] pain at the site of thoracentesis was experienced by many of the patients. When a diagnostic procedure is performed, 30 to 50 ml of fluid should be withdrawn. The fluid should be examined for its gross appearance and odor. Unless being performed solely for the separation of exudate from transudate, the analysis of the sample should include determination of white blood cell count and differential, red blood cell count, Gram and acid-fast stains, and culture. A sample for cytologic evaluation also should be obtained in most patients. As indicated previously, a variety of other tests may be appropriate in other circumstances, depending on the clinical impression.

Although an appreciation of clinical, radiologic, and laboratory findings results in an etiologic diagnosis in many patients who have pleural effusion, sometimes this remains unclear even after extensive diagnostic evaluation, including thoracentesis. In this situation, invasive diagnostic procedures are often necessary, the usual sequence of events following thoracentesis being closed biopsy, followed (if necessary) by thoracoscopic or open biopsy. The latter procedures frequently yield a diagnosis. For example, in one review of 28 patients who had pleural effusion of unknown etiology (out of a consecutive series of 110 patients subjected to needle biopsy), a definitive diagnosis was obtained following thoracotomy in 16 (57%).[51] In another study of 102 patients who underwent thoracoscopic biopsy for effusion that defied diagnosis despite less invasive studies, including closed pleural biopsy, a definitive diagnosis was established in 95;[17] 42 had malignancy and 53 had benign pleural disease. No information was available concerning distinguishing clinical features of these two groups of patients; however, on the basis of this evidence and our own experience, we consider that a pleural effusion of uncertain etiology that persists for longer than 1 or 2 weeks warrants complete investigation. Despite this, 25% to 30% of pleural effusions do not recur, and follow-up indicates a benign outcome.[2, 52–57]

PLEURAL EFFUSION CAUSED BY INFECTION

Pleural infection invariably produces an exudative effusion (i.e., with a protein content greater than 3 gm per 100 ml). The inflammatory reaction results in increased capillary permeability, causing protein loss from capillaries; in addition, reabsorption of fluid by the lymphatics may be impaired as a result of inflammatory exudate on the pleural surface and fibrous thickening of the pleura itself.[58] By far the most common etiologic agents are bacteria.

Mycobacteria

As with pulmonary disease, the vast majority of cases of pleural mycobacterial infection are caused by *M. tuberculosis*; only occasional cases are related to non-tuberculous mycobacteria, either as a manifestation of primary disease or in association with reactivation.[59, 60]

Epidemiology

The frequency of tuberculosis as a cause of pleural effusion depends on the prevalence of tuberculosis in the population studied. Where the disease is common, it may be the most frequent cause of pleural effusion or empyema.[61–66] For example, in one study of 127 patients who were investi-

Table 69–2. CHARACTERISTICS OF PLEURAL EFFUSIONS OF DIFFERENT ETIOLOGY

	TRANSUDATE	MALIGNANCY	TUBERCULOSIS	NONTUBERCULOUS PARAPNEUMONIC	RHEUMATOID DISEASE
Clinical	Signs and symptoms of congestive heart failure, cirrhosis, or nephrosis (hypoproteinemia)	Older patient; poor health prior to effusion; known primary malignancy	Acute onset or indolent with fever, cough and chest pain	Signs and symptoms of respiratory infection	History of arthritis ± subcutaneous rheumatoid nodules ±
Gross Appearance	Clear, straw-colored ("serous")	Serous → often sanguineous	Serous → occasionally sanguineous	Serous → sanguineous turbid (pus)	Serous → turbid or yellow-green
Microscopic Examination	0	Cytology positive, 40–87% higher with multiple samples, cell block + smears	Smear rarely positive for organisms	May or may not be + for organisms	0
Cell Count + Differential	85% RBC count < 10,000 mm³; majority WBC count < 1000 mm³	40% > 100,000 RBC/mm³; WBC 1,000 to 10,000, usually mononuclears predominant	In majority small lymphocytes predominant. Polymorphonuclear leukocytes may predominate initially. Rarely > 5% mesothelial cells	Polymorphonuclear predominant; 10,000/mm³ and left shift	Mononuclear cells predominant
Culture	0	0	Fluid positive in 15%	May or may not be positive	0
Protein	75% < 3 gm; pleural fluid/serum protein ratio < 0.5	90% > 3 gm; pleural fluid/serum protein ratio > 0.5	90% > 3 gm; pleural fluid/serum protein ratio > 0.5	> 3 gm; pleural fluid/ serum protein ratio > 0.5	> 3 gm; pleural fluid/ serum protein ratio > 0.5
Lactic Acid Dehydrogenase (LDH)	Pleural fluid/serum LDH ratio < 0.6	Pleural fluid/serum LDH ratio > 0.6	Pleural fluid/serum LDH ratio > 0.6	Pleural fluid/serum LDH ratio > 0.6; LDH level greater than 1,000 IU/ml suggests complicated effusion (empyema)	Pleural fluid/serum LDH ratio > 0.6
Glucose	> 60 mg/dl	May be < 60 mg/dl; lower levels associated with poor prognosis	May be < 60 mg/dl	May be < 60 mg/dl; lower levels suggest complicated effusion (empyema)	83% < 50 mg/dl; 63% < 20 mg/dl
pH	Equal to or higher than blood pH	15% have pH < 7.20; low pH associated with poor prognosis	May be less than 7.20	May be < 7.20; lower pH suggests complicated pleural effusion (empyema)	May be < 7.20
Other	Associated with pulmonary venous hypertension	Lung and breast are most common sites of primary tumor	Tuberculin skin test usually positive. Adenosine deaminase levels may be helpful in diagnosis	Foul-smelling fluid with anaerobic organisms	Reduced complement; high rheumatoid factor (higher than serum titer); may have high cholesterol level

gated for pleural effusion in Rwanda, tuberculosis was identified as the cause in 110 (86%).[64] The prevalence of human immunodeficiency virus (HIV) infection in this population is also likely to have been important in explaining this high figure; among the 98 patients tested for HIV-1-antibody, 82 were positive! In another prospective study from Tanzania, 112 of 118 patients who had pleural effusion had tuberculosis.[66] This disease has also been found to be the most common cause of pleural effusion in a study of 642 patients from Spain (occurring in 25% of cases)[62] and in 253 young immigrants in Saudi Arabia, accounting for 35% of the population studied.[67]

Tuberculous effusion is much less common in "developed" countries such as the United States, Canada, and parts of Europe. For example, in one investigation of 102 patients from Montreal who underwent thoracoscopy after pleural fluid analysis and closed pleural needle biopsy had proved inconclusive, only 3 had tuberculosis.[68] In another study of 171 adults who had pleural effusion evaluated in Prague, 11 (6%) had the disease.[69] Overall, only about 1,000 cases of pleural tuberculosis are reported annually in the United

States.[70] Despite these observations, the results of a study of Greek Army recruits from 1965 to 1993 suggest that the incidence of pleural tuberculosis might be underestimated.[70a] In this investigation, many of the patients who had tuberculous effusion were identified during screening radiography at enrollment and might otherwise never have come to medical attention. Although the incidence decreased after 1980 coincident with the institution of BCG vaccination, it remained well above the rate in the general population.

In regions in which exposure to tuberculosis is common, tuberculous effusion occurs most often in young people.[71] However, where tuberculosis is less prevalent, infection and associated pleural disease develop more commonly when the patient is middle-aged or elderly. Several reports illustrate these observations. In the Spanish series cited previously, 69% of the 111 patients who had pleural tuberculosis were younger than 40 years of age;[62] in the study from Rwanda, the mean age was 34 years old.[64] In another investigation from Alabama, the median age of 70 patients who had tuberculous pleurisy was 47 years;[72] half had evidence of simultaneous parenchymal disease on the chest radio-

Table 69–2. CHARACTERISTICS OF PLEURAL EFFUSIONS OF DIFFERENT ETIOLOGY *Continued*

SYSTEMIC LUPUS ERYTHEMATOSUS	PULMONARY EMBOLISM	FUNGAL INFECTION	TRAUMATIC	CHYLOUS	CHYLIFORM
Known SLE ± young women	Predisposing factors: postoperative, immobilized, venous disease	Exposure in endemic area	History of trauma—fractured ribs	History of trauma (25%) or malignancy (50%)	Usually chronic effusions
Serous → occasionally sanguineous	Serous → often sanguineous	Serous → occasionally sanguineous	Sanguineous	Turbid whitish; turbid supernatant with centrifugation	Turbid whitish; turbid supernatant with centrifugation; clears with ethyl alcohol
0	0	May or may not be + for organisms	0	Fat droplets	Cholesterol crystals
Mononuclear or polymorphonuclear cells predominant	Mononuclear or polymorphonuclear cells predominant; RBC < 10,000 in 30%, RBC > 100,000 in 20%	Mononuclear or polymorphonuclear cells predominant	RBC predominant	Mononuclear cells predominant	Variable
0	0	May or may not be positive	0	0	0
> 3 gm; pleural fluid/serum protein ratio > 0.5 Pleural fluid/serum LDH ratio > 0.6	> 3 gm; pleural fluid/serum protein ratio > 0.5 Pleural fluid/serum LDH ratio > 0.6	> 3 gm; pleural fluid/serum protein ratio > 0.5 Pleural fluid/serum LDH ratio > 0.6	> 3 gm; pleural fluid/serum protein ratio > 0.5 Pleural fluid/serum LDH ratio > 0.6	> 3 gm; pleural fluid/serum protein ratio > 0.5 Pleural fluid/serum LDH ratio > 0.6	> 3 gm; pleural fluid/serum protein ratio > 0.5 Pleural fluid/serum LDH ratio > 0.6
> 60 mg/dl	> 60 mg/dl	> 60 mg/dl	> 60 mg/dl	> 60 mg/dl	May be < 60 mg/dl depending on etiology
> 7.20	> 7.20	?	May be < 7.20 with hemothorax	> 7.20	May be < 7.20 depending on etiology
Reduced complement detectable; antinuclear antibody and LE cells	Source of emboli may or may not be apparent	Uncommon cause of pleural effusion	—	Pleural fluid triglyceride usually > 110 mg/dl; cholesterol level is low	Triglycerides are low; cholesterol level may be high

graph. Other workers have estimated that up to 80% of patients who have tuberculous pleural effusion have concomitant pulmonary tuberculosis.[71]

Pathogenesis

Tuberculous pleural effusion is believed to result from rupture of subpleural foci of necrosis into the adjacent pleural space.[73, 74] Although such foci usually cannot be seen on conventional chest radiographs, they have been documented pathologically[73] and on CT scans.[75] Several investigators have demonstrated T lymphocytes in tuberculous pleural fluid that are specifically sensitized to purified protein derivative (PPD).[76–79] Such activated lymphocytes, as well as macrophages, produce cytokines such as interleukin-2 (IL-2), IL-1, tumor necrosis factor-alpha (TNF-α), IL-12, IL-10, IL-6, and interferon-gamma (IFN-γ) that participate in the production and regulation of the local inflammatory process.[80–86] Most of the lymphocytes are of the CD4 type.[87] Lymphocyte activation can occur in the pleura of some patients who fail to react to cutaneous PPD, a fact that is explained by the presence in the circulation of suppressor cells that inhibit response in the skin; these suppressor cells are apparently lacking in the pleural fluid.[76]

Clinical Manifestations

The clinical presentation of tuberculous pleural effusion is acute in about two thirds of patients and relatively indolent in the remainder.[70, 88] Symptoms of chest pain, cough, breathlessness, fever, and prostration may suggest the diagnosis of acute pneumonia.[67, 89, 90] Weight loss and weakness are seen in some patients.[2] Occasionally, effusion occurs in critically ill patients as part of a polyserositis associated with pericardial effusion and ascites.[71]

Classically, tuberculous effusion associated with acute symptoms and the absence of radiographically evident parenchymal lung disease has been felt to represent primary infection. Generally, this clinical and radiologic constellation has been seen in children and young adults.[70, 83] By contrast, tuberculous effusion that is associated with an indolent course and with parenchymal lung disease on the chest radiograph has been seen more frequently in older patients and has been considered to be a manifestation of postprimary (reactivation) infection.[70, 83] However, such a clear-cut distinction between primary and postprimary disease cannot always be made with certainty. On the one hand, parenchymal lung disease resulting from reactivation may be obscured by the presence of the effusion;[73, 75] on the other, primary tuberculosis occurring in immunologically naive or debilitated older patients may have an indolent clinical course.[70]

Diagnosis

Tuberculous pleural effusion is almost invariably unilateral and seldom massive. Thoracentesis typically yields clear, straw-colored fluid containing more than 3 gm of protein per 100 ml of fluid. If the aspirate is bloody or serosanguineous, a tuberculous etiology is unlikely. Lymphocytes predominate, typically accounting for 70% or more of the total white blood cell count; on preparations examined cytologically, they can appear to be the only cell type, a finding that may result in a mistaken diagnosis of lymphoma.[91] The percentage and absolute numbers of T lymphocytes of predominantly CD4$^+$ type are higher than in the blood;[87, 92] by contrast, the percentage and number of B lymphocytes are significantly lower.[77, 78, 93] Natural killer cells are much more evident in tuberculous than in carcinomatous pleural effusions;[94] however, like T lymphocytes, their quantification is not useful in the differential diagnosis. Although polymorphonuclear leukocytes may be fairly numerous during the early stage of the disease, it is reasonable to assume that effusions containing more than 50% of these cells are of a nontuberculous etiology. Eosinophils rarely are present in significant numbers, unless there is an associated pneumothorax, a complication that may have been caused by an earlier thoracentesis.

A variety of other pleural fluid abnormalities have been investigated for potential use in the diagnosis of tuberculous effusion. Some investigators have stated that the diagnosis is unlikely if the percentage of mesothelial cells is higher than 5%;[95, 96] however, any inflammatory process affecting the pleura can be associated with a reduction in the number of mesothelial cells in pleural fluid, and numerous mesothelial cells have been found in some patients who have pleural tuberculosis.[97] Other workers have proposed that a determination of macrophage size can be helpful in diagnosis;[96] in their experience, macrophages are considerably smaller in tuberculous effusion than in effusion associated with malignancy or heart failure.

Pleural fluid glucose content can be low in tuberculous effusion; however, this can also be seen in bacterial pneumonia, rheumatoid disease, and pulmonary carcinoma. In fact, the majority of patients who have effusions of tuberculous etiology have pleural fluid glucose levels above 3.3 mmol per liter.[74] It has been reported that intravenous infusion of glucose increases glucose levels in tuberculous effusions but not in those of rheumatoid origin,[98] a curious finding that is remembered by all and utilized by none in our experience. In a small series of patients, the level of lysozyme in pleural fluid was shown to be useful in distinguishing tuberculous from nontuberculous effusions,[99] the concentration being significantly higher in the former presumably because of secretion from epithelioid cells.

The level of adenosine deaminase (ADA), a marker of lymphocyte activation, has been reported to be increased in tuberculous pleural effusions by several groups of investigators;[100–105] however, there is some overlap with effusions of other origin,[104, 106–108] particularly those of rheumatoid disease.[108] Simultaneous determination of ADA and pleural fluid/serum lysozyme ratio has been recommended as a more sensitive and specific biochemical approach to diagnosis,[109, 110] as has combining measurement of ADA level with pleural fluid lymphocyte to neutrophil ratio.[107, 111, 112] In one study of 472 consecutive pleural effusions in which a ratio of greater than 0.75 was used for the latter and a cut-off level of 50 U per liter for ADA, tuberculosis was identified with a sensitivity of 88% and a specificity of 95%;[107] the combined measures had a positive predictive value of 95% and a negative predictive value of 88%. Another group examined pleural fluid ADA, lysozyme, and INF-γ levels as well as pleural-to-serum ADA and pleural-to-serum lysozyme ratios in 405 pleural effusions (including 91 caused by tuberculosis);[105] a pleural fluid ADA level of greater than 47 U per liter had a sensitivity of 100% and a specificity of 95% for the diagnosis of tuberculosis, whereas pleural fluid interferon levels greater than 140 pg/ml had a sensitivity of 94% and specificity of 92%; a pleural-to-serum lysozyme ratio of 1.1 or greater had a specificity of 90%. In another study of pleural fluid INF-γ in 388 patients, the final diagnosis was tuberculosis in 73, some of whom were immunocompromised;[113] using a cut-off of 3.7 U/ml, the test had a sensitivity of 99% and a specificity of 98% for the diagnosis of tuberculosis.

Although the results of these and other studies[114, 115] suggest that these markers may prove to be useful, definitive diagnosis of pleural tuberculosis requires the identification of mycobacteria by microscopy or culture of pleural fluid or tissue. The incidence of positive culture from pleural fluid is surprisingly low, being found in only 15% of proven cases;[2] by contrast, cultures of biopsy specimens are positive in 55% to 80%.[99, 116] Image-guided pleural biopsies can be useful in obtaining diagnostic tissue in patients who have small effusions.[117] Granulomatous inflammation can be identified in pleural biopsy specimens in about 60% to 90% of patients who have proven tuberculosis;[118, 119] given the rarity of other conditions that cause granulomatous pleuritis, this finding is virtually diagnostic of the disease in the appropriate clinical setting.

A number of investigators have attempted to identify organisms in pleural fluid by polymerase chain reaction;[120–124] although the sensitivity and specificity of the test have been very good in some small studies,[122, 123] some have shown false-positive results in patients who have malignant effusion[121, 124] or have shown poor sensitivity.[120, 124] Thus, at the present time this procedure remains an investigational tool. Other unproven diagnostic techniques include the identification by enzyme-linked immunosorbent assay of a variety of antibodies in pleural fluid,[125–127] the measurement of pleural fluid neopterin (a marker of macrophage activation) by radioimmunoassay,[128] and the measurement of pleural fluid CA50 (to distinguish malignant from tuberculous effusion).[129]

A diagnosis of tuberculous pleural effusion should be considered when there is a predominantly lymphocytic response in the pleural fluid of a patient who has a positive PPD.[130] However, a negative PPD reaction does not exclude the diagnosis, and the skin test should be repeated in any patient suspected of having tuberculosis whose initial reaction is negative.

Natural History

The natural history of tuberculous pleuritis and effusion is usually complete absorption of fluid and apparently complete restoration of the patient's health to normal (although some degree of pleural fibrosis may be evident pathologically or radiologically). However, the likelihood of the subsequent development of pulmonary tuberculosis is high; for example, in one prechemotherapy follow-up study of 141 military personnel who had presented with pleural effusion and a positive PPD, 92 (65%) subsequently developed some form of tuberculosis.[131] Thus, the long-term prognosis in patients who have tuberculous pleurisy is determined by its recognition and the initiation of effective therapy.

Bacteria Other than Mycobacteria

In 1981, it was estimated that parapneumonic pleural effusion* occurred in approximately 40% of the 1.2 million cases of bacterial pneumonia annually in the United States;[137] of these, tube thoracostomy was required for drainage in about 10%. It is likely that the complication is more common than these figures suggest, because its presence is frequently unrecognized as a result of the small amount of fluid; i.e., it is likely that the recorded incidence of parapneumonic effusion would increase sharply if radiographs were obtained in the lateral decubitus position in all cases (Fig. 69–3). This supposition was borne out by the results of a prospective evaluation of 203 patients who had acute bacterial pneumonia on whom bilateral decubitus radiographs were obtained within 72 hours of the onset of the pneumonia;[138] 90 patients (44%) were found to have radiographically demonstrable pleural effusion. Parapneumonic effusions usually are serous exudates that resolve spontaneously.[138]

The incidence of empyema is about 0.5 to 0.8 per thousand admissions to hospital;[132] the complication is acquired in hospital in about one third of these cases. In an acutely ill but debilitated group of New York City patients hospitalized for pneumonia, the incidence of nontuberculous bacterial empyema was almost 7%.[139]

Pathogenesis and Pathologic Characteristics

Pleural effusion of nontuberculous bacterial origin is characterized by a predominance of polymorphonuclear leukocytes; in a few patients, the fluid is grossly cloudy or frankly purulent (empyema). Although the majority of empyemas are secondary to spread from a pneumonic focus in the adjacent lung,[140–143] many other mechanisms are possible, including extension from the perimandibular space, infection via the mediastinum or across the diaphragm (e.g., from a

---

*A parapneumonic effusion is defined as a pleural effusion associated with pneumonia; it may be infected or uninfected. Although some have considered any infection in the pleural space to be empyema,[132] we and others feel the term is better reserved for cases in which infection is associated with frank pus in the pleural space.[133–136]

subphrenic abscess), inadvertent contamination of the pleural space during thoracotomy or following an intravenous drug abuser's attempt to inject the cervical veins, rupture of the esophagus or an intrathoracic stomach, and trauma (*see* farther on).[132, 144] Rare cases appear to be related to seeding of the pleural space during bacteremia.[145–147] Empyema that develops in the context of pneumonia can occur by direct extension of pneumonia to the pleura, by rupture of a subpleural abscess into the pleural space (Fig. 69–4), or by the formation of a bronchopleural fistula following necrosis of lung tissue.[132]

The initial response to bacteria in the pleural space is an exudative inflammatory reaction in which there is a thin fluid containing few leukocytes.[134] Under the influence of a variety of chemotactic cytokines released by activated mesothelial cells,[148, 149a–c] this is followed by the accumulation of large numbers of neutrophils and fibrin (Fig. 69–5).[132] At this stage, the pleural surface may be covered by a shaggy white exudate several millimeters thick (Fig. 69–6); if untreated, the empyema may drain spontaneously through the chest wall (empyema necessitans).[132] Organization of the exudate may result in a fibrous pleural "peel" that can measure as much as 2 cm in thickness.

Microbiology

As in the bacterial pneumonias, the organisms responsible for empyema vary with the host's state of health. In "developed" countries, about two thirds of cases are generally attributed to aerobic bacteria;[132, 142, 143] anaerobic bacteria with or without associated aerobic infection are responsible for the remainder.[151–154] However, higher estimates of the frequency of anaerobes have been reported in studies in which the microbiology has been performed by research laboratories that specialize in the identification of anaerobic organisms.[132] In these reports, up to 75% of empyemas have been the result of anaerobic or mixed aerobic-anaerobic infections,[153, 155] leading some investigators to conclude that anaerobes (with or without coexistent aerobes) are the most common cause of empyema.[70] The most frequently encountered anaerobic bacteria are *Fusobacterium nucleatum*; *Bacteroides melaninogenicus*; *Bacteroides fragilis*; anaerobic and microaerophilic gram-positive cocci; *Clostridia*; and catalase-negative, non–spore-forming, gram-positive bacteria.[155]

Among the aerobic organisms, *Staphylococcus aureus* and enteric gram-negative bacilli are important pathogens,[141, 156–158] particularly in the post-trauma setting. The same organisms, as well as anaerobic bacteria, are a common cause of empyema in HIV-positive drug abusers.[150] *Streptococcus pneumoniae* is also an important cause in some series;[158, 159] in one review of 123 patients who had pneumococcal pneumonia diagnosed on the basis of sputum smears and radiographic appearance, 14 (11%) were found to have effusion or empyema.[160] Pleural effusion was identified in 19 of 20 patients who had acute β-hemolytic streptococcal pneumonia in a military population.[161] *S. aureus* is a frequent cause of pneumonia with parapneumonic effusion or empyema in patients who have the acquired immunodeficiency syndrome (AIDS), accounting for 53% of community-acquired pneumonias in this population in one series.[162] In infants and young children, empyema is also very common in association with staphylococcal pneumonia, being observed in ap-

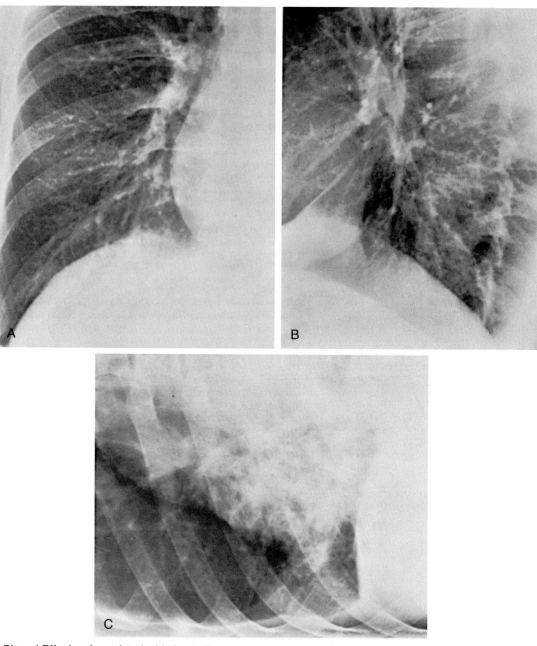

Figure 69–3. Pleural Effusion Associated with Acute Bronchopneumonia. Detail views of the lower half of the right lung from posteroanterior *(A)* and lateral *(B)* radiographs reveal inhomogeneous consolidation of all basal segments of the right lower lobe. Note that the parenchymal abnormality extends from the hilum to the diaphragmatic pleural surface in strict segmental distribution. Although no pleural effusion is evident on these radiographs exposed in the erect position, a lateral decubitus view *(C)* shows a small free pleural effusion extending along the lateral chest wall.

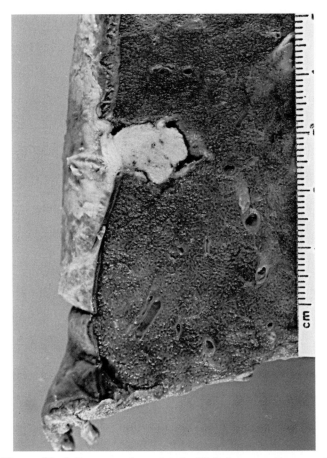

Figure 69–4. Empyema Associated with Pulmonary Abscess. A slice of lower lobe shows a focus of necrotic lung (part sequestrum, part abscess) related to infection by an unidentified organism. The infection has extended from the lung into the pleural space, where it appears as a creamy white exudate lining the pleural surface (empyema).

proximately 90% of patients in several series.[163–167] In these individuals, the radiographic appearance characteristically progresses from minimal to extensive involvement within a few hours; the underlying bronchopneumonia can be partly or completely obscured by the effusion, which can be massive. *Haemophilus influenzae* is also a common cause of empyema in children[168, 169] and is responsible for effusion in approximately 50% of adults who have *H. influenzae* pneumonia.[170–172]

Most cases of *Klebsiella-Enterobacter-Serratia* infection occur in elderly hospitalized patients whose antibacterial defense has been compromised by major medical or surgical illnesses. As discussed previously, pneumonia caused by *Klebsiella* usually develops in alcoholic or otherwise debilitated patients and is rarely hospital-acquired;[173] empyema frequently complicates acute pneumonia caused by these organisms. Radiographic features of associated necrotizing pneumonia, occasionally with gangrene or lung abscess, can be appreciated in the CT examinations of such patients.[174] Other hospital-acquired gram-negative pneumonias that are associated with a high incidence of empyema include those caused by *Escherichia coli*[74, 175–177] and *Pseudomonas aeruginosa*.[74, 178]

Pneumonia caused by *Francisella tularensis* is associated with pleural effusion in 25% to 50% of patients;[179–182]

the diagnosis can be suspected from a history of contact with animals and can be confirmed by a rise in specific serum agglutinins or positive culture of the organism from sputum or pleural fluid. *Proteus* pneumonia has been reported to cause empyema in which an elevated pH is believed to be related to ammonia production by the organism.[183] Although it was once thought that pleural effusion is not a prominent manifestation of legionnaires' pneumonia,[184] in two series the incidence was approximately 50%.[185, 186] In one case report, pleuropericarditis was the only apparent manifestation of infection.[187] Other bacterial infections in which empyema is a frequent complication include those caused by *Bacillus anthracis*, *Pseudomonas mallei*, *Salmonella* species,[188, 189] and *Brucella* species.[190–192] Uncommon causes are *Yersinia pestis*, *Morganella morganii*,[193] *Yersinia enterocolitica*,[194] *Neisseria meningitidis*, *Campylobacter fetus*,[195] *Bartonella henselae*,[196] *Listeria monocytogenes*,[197] *Streptococcus viridans*,[197a] and *Tropheryma whippleii* (the organism associated with Whipple's disease).[198]

Not uncommonly, pus aspirated from the pleural cavity in patients who have empyema is sterile on culture. Although this may reflect the administration of antimicrobial drugs before admission, it is more likely to be caused by a failure to culture pleural fluid anaerobically.[155] In these circumstances, the etiologic agent may be determined by counterimmunoelectrophoresis, because soluble bacterial antigens can persist in body fluids after organisms no longer can be isolated.[199] Identification of pneumococcal antigen by latex agglutination has also provided a rapid means of identification of the responsible pathogen.[200]

Clinical and Radiologic Manifestations

Although most patients who have empyema are febrile and have blood neutrophilia, the compromised host[139] and patients receiving corticosteroid therapy[201, 202] can be afebrile and have a normal white blood cell count. Patients who have aerobic bacterial pneumonia and effusion usually have an acute onset of chest pain, fever, cough, and sputum, whereas symptoms are more indolent in patients who have anaerobic infection.[2]

In the vast majority of cases of empyema, there are no radiologic findings that permit the identification of a specific etiology, diagnosis being made by isolation of the organism from the pleural fluid. An exception is infection by the gas-forming bacteria *Clostridium perfringens* and *B. fragilis* in which pneumonia and pleural effusion may be associated with gas in the soft tissues of the chest wall or in the pleural space (pyopneumothorax).

Prognosis and Natural History

Uninfected parapneumonic effusions clear spontaneously and do not alter the prognosis of pneumonia. By contrast, pleural effusions that require drainage or thoracotomy are associated with an increased morbidity and mortality.[168, 169, 203, 204] The prognosis also varies with the age of the patient, the presence or absence of underlying disease,[205, 206] and the specific organism responsible for the empyema. Empyema in children usually responds to simple closed drainage,[168, 207] whereas hospital-acquired empyema in the elderly is associated with considerable morbidity and high mortality.[208, 209] Loculation of pleural fluid always indicates

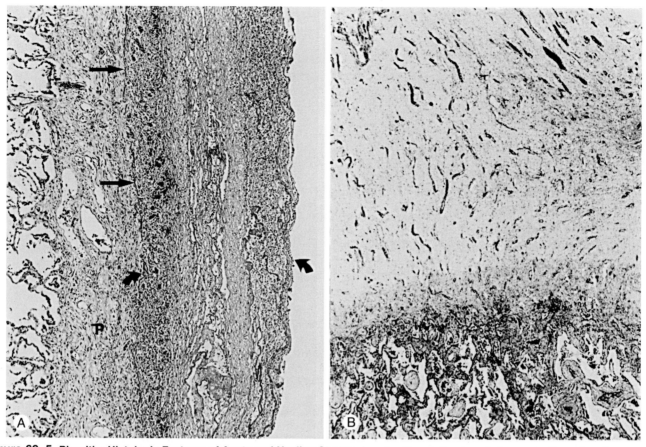

Figure 69–5. Pleuritis: Histologic Features of Acute and Healing Stages. A section through the visceral pleura and adjacent lung from a patient who had staphylococcal empyema *(A)* shows an acute fibrinous exudate *(between curved arrows)*. The pleura itself (P) is moderately thickened as a result of edema and a proliferation of mesenchymal cells. Note the thin layer of granulation tissue adjacent to the external elastic lamina *(straight arrows)*. A section from another patient who had been treated for empyema for several weeks *(B)* shows marked thickening of the pleura by loose fibrous tissue containing numerous vessels.

an exudate (albeit not necessarily empyema).[210] Occasionally a loculated empyema is situated adjacent to a pocket of sterile parapneumonic effusion; such pockets were shown by one group of investigators to contain complement breakdown products, alerting them to the presence of a contiguous empyema.[211]

In many series, failure to drain the empyema adequately has been associated with an increase in morbidity and mortality.[137, 156, 159, 204, 209, 212, 213] Although it would be highly desirable to be able to identify patients who require an invasive therapeutic procedure and to know which procedure to employ, there is unfortunately no consensus concerning these issues.[214] The lack of consensus may be related to the lack of clarity and consistency in published reports; in part, this has to do with definitions applied to parapneumonic effusions.

Several classifications of parapneumonic effusion have been proposed.[134, 135] At one extreme are patients who have a small amount of pleural fluid in association with pneumonia (less than 10 mm thick on lateral decubitus films) and do not require thoracentesis unless the volume of effusion increases following initiation of antibiotic therapy.[138] At the other extreme are patients who have "complicated empyema"[134, 135] that is characterized by the presence of frank pus, multiple loculations, and grossly thickened pleura; most of these patients require surgical decortication.[133–135] Between

these two extremes are patients who have larger parapneumonic effusions without evidence of infection or patients who have effusions that are infected. The latter may drain freely or be loculated, and may be serous or consist of frank pus; they have been managed by antibiotic therapy,[136] tube thoracostomy,[133] intrapleural installation of thrombolytics,[215, 216] surgery,[134, 135, 217] or a combination of these procedures.[133]

The measurement of pleural fluid pH, LDH, and glucose has been used to try to identify the need for drainage of parapneumonic effusion that is not purulent at the time of thoracentesis.[218, 219] (One group has also used the presence of IL-1β to separate parapneumonic from infected effusions.[220]) It has been said that effusions having a pH less than 7.0, an LDH greater than 1000 IU per liter, and a glucose less than 2.2 mmol per liter require surgical drainage,[218] because if left untreated they can be expected to develop rapidly into loculated collections of pus.[219] However, this view may not be entirely valid. In one retrospective review of 91 patients undergoing thoracentesis for "neutrophilic effusion," 43 met one of the biochemical criteria for surgical drainage listed previously (including 9 who had empyema) and 48 did not.[218] Only 21 of the first group had immediate drainage of the effusion; half the remainder eventually required tube thoracostomy, decortication, or both, and half did not. Of the 48 patients not meeting any of the criteria, 7 eventually required surgical intervention.

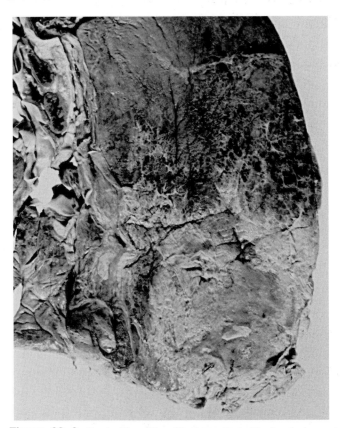

Figure 69–6. Acute Pleuritis with Empyema. The basal pleura at the medial aspect of the left lower lobe is covered by a shaggy, creamy white exudate typical of an acute purulent pleuritis. The pleural space contained approximately 1 liter of pus; postmortem culture grew pure *Staphylococcus aureus.*

The authors of a meta-analysis of studies of the utility of pleural fluid chemical analysis for identifying parapneumonic effusions requiring drainage pointed out that many of the studies had serious limitations.[219] These included small sample size, variability of decision thresholds for each of the tests, inappropriate use of indeterminate pH values of 7.1 to 7.3 to identify effusions requiring drainage, differences in definitions, failure to appropriately blind the investigators, opportunities for verification bias, and failure to consider individual patient features that make a poor prognosis effusion more or less likely. Within these limitations, pH was the test that performed the best in patients who did not have frank empyema. A pH of less than 7.21 suggested that observation was inappropriate and that tube thoracostomy for drainage of the fluid was required.

Although a detailed discussion of the management of empyema is beyond the scope of this text, we agree with those workers who state that one should not rely *solely* on laboratory results in decision making in this clinical setting;[218] clinical judgment and serial observation have important roles in the evaluation of such patients.

Actinomyces and *Nocardia* Species

Pleural diseases caused by these organisms can be considered together, because their radiologic characteristics are identical. Pulmonary involvement is an almost invariable accompaniment, usually in the form of acute nonsegmental homogeneous air-space pneumonia and often accompanied by abscess formation. The infection extends into the pleura, producing empyema; from here, it may transgress the parietal pleura to affect the chest wall, with rib destruction and subcutaneous abscess formation.[221] In one series of 15 cases, pleural effusion in the form of either empyema or pleural "thickening" was observed in 12 patients and chest wall involvement in 9.[222] Although this course is typical of the diseases caused by these organisms, it may also occur in other infections such as blastomycosis, cryptococcosis, and tuberculosis.

The manifestations of chest wall involvement include a soft tissue mass and osteomyelitis or periostitis of the ribs; the former was seen in almost half the patients with this type of involvement in one series,[222] sometimes without radiographically apparent pulmonary disease.[223, 224] Periosteal proliferation along the ribs may have a peculiar wavy configuration.[222] Although pulmonary nocardiosis is usually associated with empyema, chest wall involvement is less commonly seen in *Nocardia* infection than in patients who are infected with *Actinomyces.*[225] Identification of either *Actinomyces* or *Nocardia* species from pleural fluid or a chest wall abscess is necessary for positive diagnosis.

Fungi

Pleural effusion caused by fungi is uncommon;[241] for example, in one series of 100 patients who had primary pulmonary infection with *Histoplasma capsulatum*, only 2 had the complication.[226] Effusion has been reported to occur in about 7% of symptomatic patients who have primary *Coccidioides immitis* infection;[227] the effusion may be associated with erythema nodosum and peripheral blood eosinophilia (rarely pleural fluid eosinophilia). In addition, hydropneumothorax can develop when a coccidioidal cavity ruptures into the pleural space, a complication said to occur in 1% to 5% of patients who have chronic cavitary disease.[74]

Effusions caused by *Blastomyces dermatitidis* and *Cryptococcus neoformans* are usually associated with acute air-space pneumonia.[228–230] The reporting of nine patients who had AIDS-associated cryptococcal pleural effusion, with[231, 232] or without[231, 233, 234] pneumonia, suggests that the complication may be more common in this group than in the nonimmunosuppressed host. Isolation of the fungus or, in the case of *Cryptococcus*, detection of antigen in the pleural fluid[229, 229a] is essential for definitive diagnosis.

Pleural invasion by *Aspergillus* species occurs most commonly in two clinical situations: (1) as a late complication of thoracoplasty for tuberculosis, often in association with a bronchopleural fistula;[74, 235] or (2) as a complication of resectional surgery.[236, 237] In the latter situation, it can be caused by either direct infection of the pleural space or extension of organisms from an aspergilloma that forms in a bronchial stump.[238, 239] The infection can develop rapidly in the pleural cavity after an operative procedure; a characteristic finding is the lack of any tendency to form pus. When infection is caused by *Aspergillus niger*, the effusion may be black.[70] *Aspergillus terreus*[240] and other species[241] have rarely been reported in the pleural effusion of immunocompromised hosts. Pleural effusion caused by *Aspergillus* species has also been seen in some patients who have allergic bronchopulmonary aspergillosis.[70]

In one study of eight patients who underwent CT scans of the chest for evaluation of pulmonary zygomycosis, five had pleural effusion in association with a variety of parenchymal abnormalities;[242] direct extension of infection into the pleural space likely accounts for some cases.[241] Other fungal infections reported to cause pleural effusion include sporotrichosis[241] and candidiasis.[241] Pleural effusion may also accompany *Pneumocystis carinii* infection in patients who are severely immunocompromised (particularly those who have AIDS).[243, 244]

Viruses, *Mycoplasma*, and Rickettsiae

Radiographic demonstration of pleural effusion in viral and *Mycoplasma* pneumonia was formerly considered rare.[245–247] However, in one series of 59 patients who had serologically proven *Mycoplasma*, viral, or cold agglutinin-positive pneumonia, 12 (20%) developed pleural effusion.[248] (In 4 cases, this required examination in the lateral decubitus position, a procedure that was not performed in studies reporting a low incidence of effusion.) The overall incidence of effusion in this series was roughly the same in *Mycoplasma* pneumonia (6 of 29), influenza pneumonia (1 of 4), and pneumonia associated with elevated cold agglutinin titers (4 of 19); however, it occurred in only 1 of 7 cases of adenovirus pneumonia. In two other series of patients who had acute *Mycoplasma* pneumonia, small effusions were noted in 4 of 20 cases (25%)[249] and in 9 of 48 cases (19%).[250]

Combined pleural effusion and pericarditis have been reported in influenza A infection.[251] In a review of the chest radiographs of 59 patients who had infectious mononucleosis, 3 (5%) were found to have pleural effusion.[252] Effusion has also been described in a patient who had pneumonia and a mononucleosis-like syndrome caused by cytomegalovirus,[240] in a single immunocompromised host who had herpes simplex type 2 infection,[253] in 3% of patients who had Lassa fever,[254] in occasional patients who have acute Q fever pneumonia (sometimes with eosinophilia),[255–257] and (rarely) in patients who have viral hepatitis.[74] Pleural effusion, large in some cases, is said to be a common accompaniment of the acute pneumonia of "atypical measles."[258]

Parasites

Entamoeba histolytica. Pleuropulmonary involvement in amebiasis is almost invariably secondary to liver abscess, with transmission of the infection into the thorax by direct extension through the diaphragm into the pleural space and eventually into the lung.[259] It is said to occur in 15% to 20% of patients who have liver involvement.[260, 261] In one series of 153 patients who had pleuropulmonary amebiasis described in 1936, 27 (18%) presented with empyema that extended from liver abscesses.[262] In a 1997 review of 88 patients who had extension of hepatic amebiasis into the pleural cavity, all had symptoms and signs that could be attributed to liver abscesses;[263] the clinical course ran from 3 days to 8 months (average, 71 days) before the onset of

pleural complications. Chest radiographs revealed total or near-total opacification of the right hemithorax with a shift of the mediastinum to the left. On thoracentesis, the color of the fluid ranged from clear to dark brown, green, or yellow. The clinical picture of rupture into the pleural cavity consisted of the abrupt onset of sharp, tearing lower thoracic pain or worsening of the already present right upper quadrant pain, frequently radiating to the ipsilateral shoulder; rapidly progressing dyspnea was common.

The effusion usually is serofibrinous. When the infestation extends into lung parenchyma, the pulmonary lesion may cavitate, providing communication between the bronchial tree and the liver abscess. In this situation, fluid of typical "chocolate sauce" appearance may be expectorated. Identification of fragments of liver parenchyma in fluid specimens should suggest the diagnosis. Occasionally, the pleural space becomes secondarily infected, with the development of frank empyema.

In addition to right-sided pleural effusion, radiography commonly reveals elevation and fixation of the right hemidiaphragm and consolidation of the right lower lobe with or without abscess formation. This combination of findings should suggest the diagnosis, especially in a patient from an area endemic for amebiasis whose liver is enlarged; the differential diagnosis includes subphrenic abscess of other etiology.

Paragonimus westermani. The route of entry of this organism into the thorax is also through the diaphragm, during which time effusion may be apparent.[263a] The complication may also be seen in patients who have chronic pulmonary paragonimiasis.[271, 271a] Radiographically detectable pleural effusion was seen rarely in one study of 100 Nigerian patients who had pulmonary paragonimiasis;[264] in this comprehensive study, only 1 case of free pleural effusion was noted and that was in the form of empyema from which *Paragonimus* ova were recovered. Pleural thickening was apparent in 4 other cases. By contrast, the authors of a more recent study from Korea reported pleural lesions in 43 of 71 patients (61%);[265] among them, 12 had bilateral pleural effusions or pneumothoraces. Pleural fluid may show eosinophilia, a low sugar level, a low pH, and high protein and LDH;[265a] ova are seen in some cases.[271]

Echinococcus granulosus. Pleural effusion is uncommon in hydatid disease, being observed in only 3 of 100 cases in one series.[266] It occurs when a pulmonary hydatid cyst ruptures into the pleural space rather than into the lung or bronchial tree. Because air also is present in most cases, the radiographic appearance is that of a hydropneumothorax. Daughter cysts floating on the surface of the fluid produce irregularities of the fluid surface, creating the "water lily" sign or "sign of the camalote" (Fig. 69–7). A partly or wholly collapsed cyst may be visible in the pulmonary parenchyma, in some cases associated with "solid" cysts. Hooklets or fragments of exo- or endocyst may be identified in samples of fluid obtained by thoracentesis.

Miscellaneous Parasites. Empyema caused by *Trichomonas* species has been reported following esophageal surgery.[267] Filariasis was the cause of pleural effusion in one case report;[268] pleural biopsy revealed microfilariae, and appropriate therapy led to resolution of the effusion. Effusion has also been described in association with infestation by

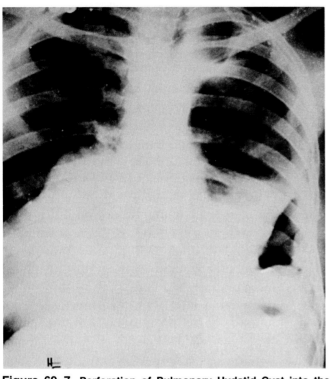

Figure 69–7. Perforation of Pulmonary Hydatid Cyst into the Pleural Space. A posteroanterior radiograph reveals a left hydropneumothorax, the surface of the fluid being irregular as a result of the presence of collapsed membranes (the sign of the camalote). A large hydatid cyst is present in the right lung. (Courtesy of Dr. Manuel Gonzalez Maseda, Uruguay, and Dr. Luis Suarez Halty, Rio Grande, Brazil.)

visceral larva migrans (toxocariasis),[269, 270] *Strongyloides stercoralis,*[270a] and *Dracunculus medinensis.*[272]

PLEURAL EFFUSION CAUSED BY IMMUNOLOGIC DISEASE

Among the connective tissue diseases, systemic lupus erythematosus (SLE) and rheumatoid disease are the most important causes of pleural effusion. In patients who have other disorders, such as progressive systemic sclerosis,[272a] dermatomyositis, and Sjögren's syndrome, effusion more commonly results from other causes (e.g., heart failure) than from the primary disease. To the extent that pleural disease is found in these last disorders, it is discussed in Chapter 39.

Systemic Lupus Erythematosus

Clinical involvement of the pleura occurs during the course of SLE in up to 70% of patients and is the presenting manifestation in 5%.[143] Patients typically have pleuritic pain accompanied by dyspnea, cough, and fever.[273] Effusions are generally bilateral and small to moderate in size but may be unilateral, massive, or both.[274, 275] The importance of distinguishing pleural effusion secondary to direct involvement of the pleura by SLE from that associated with lupus-induced renal disease has been emphasized;[276] the former characteristically is accompanied by pain and splinting, whereas the serous effusions related to kidney disease are

painless. It is important to remember that a new effusion also may be the result of pulmonary infarction or infection or of heart failure.

Effusions related to lupus pleuritis are generally serous or serosanguineous and invariably exudative.[273, 277] The cell count ranges from several hundred to 15,000/μl; it may be predominantly neutrophilic at the onset of pleuritis, but it becomes lymphocytic with time.[273] In a case report of drug-induced lupus, neutrophilia was so marked as to suggest a diagnosis of empyema.[278] Despite occasional reports to the contrary,[273] the glucose level is generally greater than 3.3 mmol per liter and the pH greater than 7.3.

A variety of studies have been undertaken in an attempt to identify specific substances in the fluid that confirm a diagnosis of SLE-associated effusion. A review of published data indicates a very high specificity for the finding of LE cells in cytology specimens,[279, 280] with false positives being reported in only one instance.[281] The reported sensitivity for the presence of antinuclear antibodies (ANA) has been quite variable and is apparently dependent on sample preparation and observer skill. However, although these antibodies are occasionally seen in pleural fluid of other etiologies,[275] the finding of a titer of 160 or greater, a pleural fluid-to-serum ANA ratio greater than 1, or a homogeneous immunofluorescence pattern strongly support the diagnosis of lupus effusion.[273, 282] These observations are important in diagnosis, because lower titers of ANA may be seen in the fluid of patients who have SLE and effusions of other etiologies. Although low levels of complement and high levels of immune complexes are often seen in effusions associated with SLE, these findings lack sufficient specificity to have diagnostic importance.[279] Similarly, the findings on pleural biopsy lack specificity, and this procedure is generally reserved for clinical situations in which a cause other than SLE is suspected.

The most common associated radiologic finding is enlargement of the cardiopericardial silhouette, which is said to occur in 35% to 50% of patients.[283, 284] This enlargement is usually nonspecific in character and minimal to moderate in degree. It has been ascribed to pericardial effusion, endocarditis, or myocarditis or to the effects of hypertension, renal disease, or anemia. Variation in heart size usually takes place over a period of weeks but may occur with startling abruptness; in the latter situation, pericardial effusion is the most likely cause. When cardiac enlargement is associated with bilateral pleural effusion, the diagnosis of lupus serositis should be strongly considered, particularly in young women.

Rheumatoid Disease

As discussed previously (*see* page 1443), pleural abnormalities are probably the most frequent manifestation of rheumatoid disease in the thorax;[285] pleuritis and pleural effusion are the most common of these. For unknown reasons, pleural effusion in association with rheumatoid disease has a strong predilection for men,[273, 286–290] despite the fact that rheumatoid arthritis occurs predominantly in women. Middle-aged patients are most often affected, the average age of 52 years in one large series being identical to that usually reported for rheumatoid arthritis as a whole.[287] In contrast to patients who have rheumatoid arthritis unassociated with pleural effusion, those who have the complication have a high frequency of HLA-B8 and Dw3 antigens and multiple intrathoracic manifestations of rheumatoid disease.[291]

The pleural fluid is an exudate with a high protein content and is pale yellow to yellowish-green. Characteristically, the glucose content is very low; it has been estimated that levels lower than 30 mg per 100 ml are found in 70% to 80% of patients.[292] These values are found despite normal blood sugar levels and do not rise following intravenous infusion of glucose.[287, 290, 293–296] The development of these biochemical abnormalities can occur fairly rapidly; for example, in one investigation, a change from normal values to a glucose of 20 mg/dl occurred over an interval of 6 days.[297] Once the low values develop, pleural fluid does not appear to revert to normal.[297] A low glucose level should suggest the diagnosis when the fluid is nonpurulent, contains no bacteria on smear and culture, and shows no malignant cells on cytologic examination, especially if the possibility of tuberculosis has been reasonably excluded by other diagnostic studies.

A variety of other biochemical abnormalities can be seen in rheumatoid pleural effusion. Lactate dehydrogenase may be increased to a level much higher than in the serum.[294, 295, 298] The titer of rheumatoid factor also tends to be high and often exceeds the level found in blood.[275] Despite this, an elevated level of rheumatoid factor in pleural fluid does not necessarily imply rheumatoid disease, because this is present in an appreciable number of patients who have other causes of effusion.[299] In some patients, complement levels in pleural fluid are decreased,[300, 301] and immune complexes are found at higher levels than in the serum.[302] Measurement of complement components and its activation products may be useful in distinguishing rheumatoid effusion from effusion associated with malignancy or tuberculosis; in the former, levels of SC5b-9 are higher than 2 AU/mL, and the ratio of C4d/C4 is higher than in effusions of the latter two.[302a]

Rheumatoid pleural effusion usually has a protein content greater than 40 gm per liter and may have a milky appearance as a result of a high concentration of cholesterol and other fats, a nonspecific finding that may be seen in any chronic pleural effusion.[292, 303] This so-called chyliform effusion must be differentiated from a true chylous effusion caused by leakage from the thoracic duct, a complication that has been reported in a patient who had rheumatoid disease associated with obstruction of the central lymphatics by amyloid.[304] The level of ADA in the pleural fluid relative to that in the blood also has been found to be increased in rheumatoid effusion, suggesting local synthesis; however, this finding lacks specificity.[305] High levels of IL-2 also may be seen; although the same finding has been noted in patients who have tuberculous pleurisy,[306] high values have been reported to distinguish rheumatoid effusion from that associated with SLE.[306]

Cytologic examination of aspirated fluid may reveal the presence of cells that contain elongated vesicular nuclei, irregularly shaped multinucleated giant cells, and clumps of amorphous material (Fig. 69–8); this appearance is probably caused by rupture of rheumatoid nodules into the pleural space and is highly suggestive of a rheumatoid etiology of the effusion.[307, 308] As indicated previously, cells in the pleu-

ral fluid are predominantly lymphocytes, although polymorphonuclear leukocytes are found in abundance in some cases.[295] Some investigators have suggested that the finding of "rheumatoid arthritis" cells is evidence of a rheumatoid etiology.[296, 298] These cells consist of leukocytes, usually polymorphonuclear, whose cytoplasm contains dense black granules about 0.5 to 1.5 μm in diameter that are believed to be lipid. They can be produced experimentally by the intrapleural injection of antigen into previously immunized mice, suggesting that immunologic factors are involved in their formation.[309] However, similar cells have been found in tuberculous[310] and malignant[309] pleural effusions, indicating that they are not specific for rheumatoid disease.

Pleural effusion of rheumatoid etiology is much more likely to occur in patients who have subcutaneous nodules than in those who do not[295, 298, 311] and has a tendency to remain relatively unchanged radiographically for many months or even years.[287, 312, 313] In one review of 25 cases, 23 were unilateral (14 on the right and 9 on the left).[287]

The effusion may be entirely unsuspected because of lack of symptoms,[312] as was the case in approximately 50% of patients in one series.[287] Occasionally, it develops abruptly and is associated with pain and fever.[314] As the amount of fluid increases, so does the likelihood of dyspnea; rarely, the effusion is so massive that it is associated with respiratory failure.[315] The effusion may antedate clinical evidence of rheumatoid arthritis[286, 287, 293, 311] or may occur when joint disease is only mild;[316] in many cases, it is associated with episodic exacerbations of arthritis[287, 295] and in some with pericarditis. The effusion can be transient, persisting, or relapsing.[275] When chronic, it may lead to fibrothorax requiring decortication.[275]

Empyema occurs with increased frequency in patients who have rheumatoid disease.[317] The most plausible explanation is impaired host defense, perhaps most commonly related to corticosteroid therapy.[317] The complication should be distinguished from the sterile effusion that results from the exudation of white blood cells and debris into the pleural space following rupture of rheumatoid nodules located in the subpleural parenchyma.[275]

PLEURAL EFFUSION CAUSED BY ASBESTOS

Benign asbestos pleural effusion is probably more common than is generally recognized.[318, 319] Estimates of its prevalence and incidence in an asbestos-exposed population have been derived from a study of 1,134 exposed workers and 717 control subjects.[319] Benign asbestos effusion was defined by (1) a history of exposure to asbestos, (2) confirmation of the presence of effusion by radiographs or thoracentesis, (3) lack of other disease associated with pleural effusion, and (4) absence of malignant tumor within 3 years. Thirty-four benign effusions were found among the exposed workers (3%) compared with no unexplained effusions among the control subjects. This contrasts with a reported history of symptomatic benign pleural effusion in only 20 (0.7%) of 2,815 insulation workers.[320] In another study, the incidence of asbestos exposure was compared in 64 consecutive men who had idiopathic pleural effusions and 129 randomly sampled age-matched controls who did not have effu-

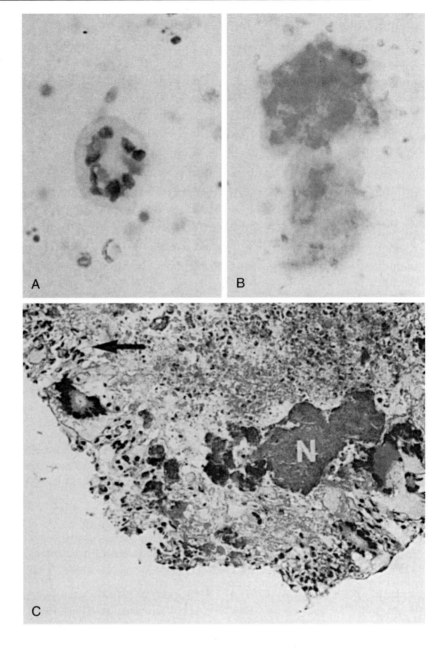

Figure 69–8. Rheumatoid Pleural Effusion: Cytologic Appearance. Highly magnified views of a filter preparation of pleural fluid show a multinucleated giant cell and scattered mononuclear cells *(A)* and an irregular fragment of more or less amorphous, acellular material *(B)*. Taken together, these findings are highly suggestive of a rheumatoid etiology. A histologic section of a closed pleural biopsy specimen from the same patient *(C)* shows that the likely origin of the material seen on the filter preparation is a fairly typical necrobiotic nodule composed of necrotic material (N), epithelioid histiocytes *(arrow),* and multinucleated giant cells. *(A and B,* Papanicolaou, ×450; *C,* hematoxylin-eosin, ×130.)

sions;[321] asbestos exposure was significantly more frequent in men who had "idiopathic" effusions than in controls.

The pathogenesis of benign asbestos effusion is uncertain; however, interactions between asbestos fibers and mesothelial or inflammatory cells, or both, are presumably important. In one study of rabbit mesothelial cells, investigators found that stimulation with crocidolite asbestos fiber resulted in the production of a protein that had chemotactic activity for neutrophils.[322] In another *in vitro* model using human mesothelial cells, exposure to asbestos fiber led to the release of the neutrophil chemotactic cytokine IL-8, an effect that was in part mediated by IL-1α.[323] The induction of antioxidants in human mesothelial cells exposed to asbestos fiber suggests that asbestos has an oxidant (and presumably deleterious) action on those cells.[324] In a rat model, intratracheal instillation of crocidolite has been shown to be associated with activation of leukocytes, including macrophages, lymphocytes, eosinophils, and mast cells, resulting

in damage to mesothelial cells.[325] Biopsy specimens from human patients often show an organizing fibrinous exudate.

The development of benign asbestos effusion appears to be dose-related, the latency period being shorter than that for other asbestos-related disorders;[319] it is probably the most common abnormality during the first 20 years after exposure. Most patients who have asbestos-related pleural effusion are asymptomatic;[326, 327] however, chest pain has been found to occur in about one third of patients in some studies.[319] Persistent pleuritic pain associated with intermittent pleural friction rubs has been described in some patients.[328] Others have fever suggesting infection.[319] Effusions are usually smaller than 500 ml and persist from 2 weeks to 6 months;[329, 330] they are recurrent in 15% to 30% of cases.[329, 330] Occasional cases are associated with the development of round atelectasis (*see* page 2430).[331]

In most patients, the fluid is a sterile serous or blood-tinged exudate. The differential diagnosis must include tuberculosis and mesothelioma. Large effusions are more likely to be caused by mesothelioma;[332] a bloody effusion, although typical of malignancy, may be benign in the setting of asbestos exposure. Differentiation from tuberculosis can be made with confidence only if biopsy and culture results are negative. Follow-up has shown that some workers are left with blunting of the costophrenic angle and diffuse pleural thickening, with consequent deleterious effects on lung function.[320]

PLEURAL EFFUSION CAUSED BY DRUGS

Many drugs have been reported to cause pleural effusion (Table 69–3).[332a] Some, such as bromocriptine, methysergide, and dantrolene sodium, appear to affect the pleura almost selectively.[333] Since the original description in 1981 of the pleuropulmonary manifestations of long-term bromo-

Table 69–3. DRUG CAUSES OF PLEURAL EFFUSION

DRUG	SELECTED REFERENCE(S)
Drug-Induced Lupus Syndrome	
Hydralazine	
Procainamide	
Isoniazid	
Phenytoin and other anticonvulsants	723
Quinidine	
Methyldopa	
Chlorpromazine	
Sulfasalazine	
Beta-adrenoreceptor blocking agents (acebutolol, labetalol, pindolol, propranolol)	707–716
Drugs That Affect the Pleural Space Selectively	
Bromocriptine	
Methysergide	
Dantrolene sodium	333
Drugs That Affect the Pleural Space Nonselectively	
Chemotherapeutic Agents	
Bleomycin	717
Mitomycin-C	718, 719
Busulfan	720
Melphalan	721
Cytosine arabinoside	722
Methotrexate	724, 725
Biologic Response Modifiers	
Interleukin-2	726
Granulocyte-macrophage colony-stimulating factor	727
Antibiotics	
Nitrofurantoin	728
Minocycline	729, 730
Metronidazole	2
Antiarrhythmia Drugs	
Amiodarone	731
Miscellaneous Drugs	
Acyclovir	732
Propylthiouracil	733
Minoxidil	723
Ergotamine	2
Ethchlorvynol	2

criptine treatment for Parkinson's disease,[334] more than 20 such cases have been described in the literature. The onset varies from 9 months to 4 years after initiation of therapy;[335, 336] in most cases, the effusion is lymphocyte-predominant and resolves following withdrawal of the drug. This medication has a chemical structure similar to methysergide, an ergot drug used in the treatment of migraine and also well known as a cause of pleural effusion and fibrosis.[337] Similar changes have been seen in a patient treated with cabergoline,[338] a long-acting ergot derivative also used in the treatment of Parkinson's disease.

Dantrolene sodium is a long-acting skeletal muscle relaxant used in the treatment of spastic neurologic disorders. Sterile exudative pleural and pericardial effusions have been described in occasional patients after long-term therapy with this drug; in one study, the effusions were associated with eosinophilia in both pleural fluid and peripheral blood and resolved on cessation of medication.[339] Dantrolene sodium is structurally similar to nitrofurantoin, which also causes eosinophilia and pleural effusion, but usually after a shorter period of treatment.[340, 341] Additional information concerning drug-induced pleural disease is found in Chapters 39 and 63 (*see* pages 1432 and 2537).

PLEURAL EFFUSION CAUSED BY NEOPLASMS

General Characteristics

The most common cause of exudative pleural effusion is malignancy.[52, 70, 74] For example, in one series of 83 patients who had pleural exudates, malignancy was the etiology in 64 (77%).[52] Although most common in patients who have clinical features indicating a primary extrapleural tumor, effusion may be the first manifestation of malignancy or the first evidence of disease recurrence; in one series of 96 patients who had neoplastic involvement of the pleura, the presence of pleural effusion was the abnormality that led to the diagnosis of carcinoma in 44 (46%).[342]

The results of several reviews indicate that the major causes of malignant pleural effusion are pulmonary, breast, ovarian, and gastric carcinoma and lymphoma;[74, 342–345] in fact, pulmonary carcinoma, breast carcinoma, and lymphoma account for 75% of all malignant pleural effusions.[346] An additional important, although relatively infrequent, cause of malignant pleural effusion is mesothelioma (*see* page 2807). In one series, malignancies manifesting with pleural effusion represented 32 of 459 (7%) carcinomas of the lung, 20 of 645 (3%) neoplasms of the breast, 9 of 303 (3%) carcinomas of the ovary, and 7 of 195 (4%) carcinomas of the stomach.[342] Approximately 90% of the lung, breast, and ovarian malignant effusions were on the same side as the primary lesions.[342] Regardless of primary site, bilateral pleural involvement in metastatic carcinoma is frequently associated with hepatic metastases.[347]

The importance of cancer as a cause of pleural effusion is also illustrated by an analysis of the etiology of bilateral effusions associated with normal heart size; of 78 such cases in one investigation, 35 (45%) were related to cancer (19 metastatic carcinoma, 13 lymphoma, and 3 primary pulmonary carcinoma);[348] of these 35 patients, 13 (37%) showed no other radiographic abnormality of the thorax.

The pathogenesis of pleural effusion in malignancy is multifactorial.[74, 349] Possible mechanisms include (1) tumor invasion of the pleura, stimulating an inflammatory reaction associated with capillary fluid leak; (2) tumor invasion of the pulmonary or pleural lymphatics and bronchopulmonary, hilar, and/or mediastinal lymph nodes, hindering the return of lymphatic fluid to the circulation; (3) bronchial obstruction by a carcinoma, creating an increased negative intrapleural pressure, thus increasing transudation; (4) hypoproteinemia in debilitated patients, leading to increased transudation; (5) infection associated with obstructive pneumonitis, resulting in a parapneumonic effusion; and (6) a drug reaction, radiation therapy, or deposition of immune complexes related to circulating tumor antigens, causing increased pleural capillary permeability.[350]

It is important to note that pleural involvement by carcinoma does not necessarily result in effusion; in a detailed autopsy report of 52 patients who had pleural metastases (29 from the lung, 9 from the breast, 4 from the pancreas, 5 from the stomach, and 5 miscellaneous), effusions were found in only 31 patients (60%).[347] The effusions bore no relation to the extent of pleural involvement by metastases; in fact, fluid appeared to accumulate principally as a result of neoplastic infiltration of mediastinal lymph nodes. It should be emphasized that mediastinal nodes may be affected by metastatic neoplasm and thereby create lymphatic obstruction and resultant pleural effusion without convincing evidence of their enlargement on conventional chest radiographs; in such cases, CT may reveal enlarged nodes. Further support for a close link between lymphatic obstruction and pleural effusion was provided by the observation that effusions did not develop with metastatic sarcomas, tumors that seldom spread via the lymphatics. In another study of 78 patients who underwent "curative" resection for pulmonary carcinoma in whom there was no gross evidence of pleural tumor involvement, lavage of the pleural space was performed before lung manipulation and after resection and the fluid evaluated cytologically;[351] 14% of the patients had a positive lavage cytology, including 6 of 53 (11%) who had Stage I carcinoma.

The diagnosis of carcinoma as the etiology of pleural effusion may be strongly suspected from the chest radiograph, the manifestation being one of either primary pulmonary carcinoma or nodular or reticulonodular opacities characteristic of metastatic carcinoma. Tension hydrothorax also has been reported as a result of extensive neoplastic involvement of the pleura, apparently related to impaired lymphatic drainage and hypoproteinemia;[352] in the case reported, the clinical picture was similar to that of "tension" pneumothorax, and the fluid was found to be under high pressure on thoracentesis. Radiologically, tension hydrothorax may be diagnosed by the presence of marked contralateral shift of the mediastinum and inversion of the diaphragm (Fig. 69–9). It can be confirmed by ultrasonography, CT, or magnetic resonance imaging.[325a–c]

In the absence of radiologic findings or symptoms such as hemoptysis or a very large effusion, bronchoscopy is likely to be fruitless;[353–355] for example, in one study of 28 patients who had effusion of unknown cause and no diagnosis after thoracentesis and pleural biopsy, fiberoptic bronchoscopy demonstrated carcinoma in only 1 patient, despite a subsequent diagnosis of pulmonary malignancy in 7.[353] Of 17 patients in the same series who had a malignant pleural effusion associated with an unknown primary and no evidence of a mass or atelectasis, bronchoscopy revealed a carcinoma in only 2 of the 5 patients who were ultimately shown to have pulmonary carcinoma. The role of fiberoptic bronchoscopy was also evaluated in another investigation of 115 patients who had pleural effusion in whom pulmonary carcinoma was considered a possible cause;[354] this diagnosis was confirmed in 6 of 12 patients who had hemoptysis, 8 of 12 who had a mass or infiltrate, and 11 of 25 who had atelectasis. Sixty-six patients had an isolated cytology-negative effusion: in 7 of the 18 patients who had massive effusion, cancer was detected bronchoscopically; in 47 of the remaining 48 patients, bronchoscopy was nondiagnostic.

Pleural effusions associated with malignancy are almost invariably exudates;[354a] those that meet exudative criteria by the LDH level but not by the protein level are usually malignant.[74] When a malignant effusion is a transudate, the patient almost invariably has a concomitant disorder that could explain the findings.[356] Although lymphocytes predominate, polymorphonuclear leukocytes are frequent. Eosinophils are uncommon, being seen in only 4 of 84 malignant effusions in one series.[357] A minority of effusions are grossly bloody (9 of the 31 cases in one series).[347] The great majority have normal glucose levels and a pH above 7.30;[74, 342] those that have glucose levels below 3.3 mmol per liter and a pH below 7.30 are more likely to be large, to have a positive cytologic examination, and to be associated with a poor prognosis.[74, 358–360] Rare cases have been reported in which the pleural "fluid" was predominantly mucin derived from an adenocarcinoma, analogous to pseudomyxoma peritonei.[361]

The incidence of a positive cytologic examination in patients who have malignant pleural effusion ranges from about 35% to 85%, with most investigators reporting a value of about 50% (see page 344). As a diagnostic procedure, cytologic examination of pleural fluid gives a higher yield than closed pleural biopsy, although these procedures are complementary.[343, 362, 363] The distinction between benign and malignant cells can be difficult, and many studies have been undertaken to identify potential markers for differential diagnosis. Techniques include immunohistochemistry, electron microscopy, cytogenetic analysis, flow cytometry, and a variety of molecular biologic applications; the diagnostic utility of some of these techniques is discussed in Chapters 14 (see page 345) and 72 (see page 2816).[364–367]

There have also been many attempts to differentiate between benign and malignant effusions on the basis of soluble substances in pleural fluid.[129, 368–380, 380a] In the majority of these, considerable overlap has been found in the levels of these markers in the two forms of effusion; moreover, most of the data have not been prospectively validated. In some instances, the sensitivity and specificity are improved by using different cut-off levels; for example, setting a high level for CEA raises the specificity to almost 100%, with the expected sacrifice of sensitivity.

When pleural fluid persists and cytologic and other analyses are negative for malignancy, open pleural biopsy or thoracoscopy with biopsy may be required for diagnosis. When technically feasible, thoracoscopy is the procedure of choice (see page 371).[381] The successful use of fiberoptic pleuroscopy for the diagnosis of malignancy in the evalua-

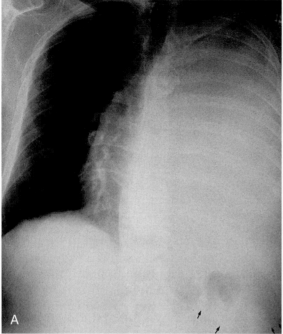

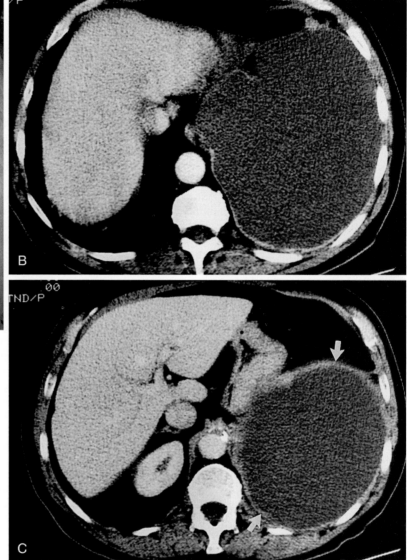

Figure 69–9. Tension Pleural Effusion. A posteroanterior chest radiograph *(A)* in a 69-year-old man demonstrates opacification of the left hemithorax as a result of a large pleural effusion. The effusion is associated with considerable contralateral shift of the mediastinum, widening of the spaces between the ribs, and inversion of the posterior aspect of the left hemidiaphragm *(arrows)*, indicating that it is under tension. (The inversion was easier to visualize on the original radiograph than on the figure.) A CT scan at the level of the dome of the right hemidiaphragm *(B)* also shows a large left pleural effusion. A CT scan at a more caudad level *(C)* demonstrates pleural fluid central to the left hemidiaphragm *(arrows)*, a characteristic finding of inversion. Note the presence of abundant intraperitoneal fat anterior to the inverted left hemidiaphragm, which provides the soft tissue contrast that allows visualization of the inverted posterior aspect of the hemidiaphragm on the chest radiograph. A cytologic examination of the pleural fluid revealed adenocarcinoma. The primary tumor was in the left lung.

tion of exudative effusion of unknown etiology has been described in a small number of patients.[382]

Pulmonary Carcinoma

Pleural involvement is evident in about 5% to 15% of patients who have primary pulmonary carcinoma at the time they first seek medical attention.[342, 383, 384] During the course of the disease, at least 50% of patients who have disseminated carcinoma develop the complication.[74] Effusion associated with these neoplasms is nearly always associated with radiographically demonstrable pulmonary abnormalities. Rarely, radiographic evidence of disease apart from the effusion is subtle, such as a hilar mass or, perhaps more frequently, a diminutive peripheral carcinoma associated with mediastinal and hilar lymph node enlargement. In such cases, CT may be required for definitive identification of the tumor. A high index of suspicion may allow a presumptive diagnosis, although differentiation from lymphoma may be impossible without histologic or cytologic examination.

The documentation of malignant cells in pleural fluid or biopsy specimens of patients who have proven pulmonary carcinoma is generally regarded as evidence of inoperability and is associated with a very poor prognosis; for example, in one series of 96 patients, 54% were dead within 1 month and 84% within 6 months.[342] In fact, the prognosis is very poor in patients who have pulmonary carcinoma and pleural effusion even in the absence of demonstrable direct pleural involvement. In one investigation of 21 patients who had a pulmonary carcinoma and a cytologically negative ipsilateral pleural effusion, only 5 appeared to have potentially resectable disease following thoracoscopy;[385] none of the 5 was resectable at thoracotomy as a result of direct mediastinal tumor invasion. In another series of 21 similar patients, 17 were found to have extrapulmonary spread of the disease at thoracotomy.[386]

Metastatic Nonpulmonary Carcinoma

As previously stated, the major extrathoracic primary sites associated with malignant pleural effusion are breast, ovary, and stomach,[342] with the breast being the most common. About 7% of patients who have malignant pleural effusion have an unknown primary tumor at the time of initial diagnosis.[70] The effusion is usually unilateral in breast carcinoma; for example, in one review of 105 cases, 90% were evident on one side only (50% ipsilateral and 40% contralateral).[387] This rough equality of ipsilateral and contralateral effusion has not been the experience of all investigators; in other series that included a total of 162 cases, 129 (80%) were ipsilateral.[388, 389] If this incidence of ipsilaterality is accepted, it obviously indicates that spread is most often via the lymphatics rather than the bloodstream, a conclusion that has been supported in an autopsy study.[390] Contiguous spread through the chest wall to the parietal pleura is extremely rare.[347] Direct spread is also rare in patients who have other primary carcinomas, such as those of liver[391] and pancreas.[392]

Although bilateral pleural effusion was found in only 10% of the 105 patients who had breast carcinoma and effusion in the study cited previously,[387] it must be considered among the major causes of this relatively uncommon manifestation of malignancy. In one review of 78 cases of bilateral pleural effusion associated with normal heart size, 35 (45%) were caused by cancer, the major site of origin being the breast.[348] This manifestation of pleural malignancy is often associated with metastases in the liver, from which the pleural tumor is probably derived.[347]

There is evidence that the location of pleural metastases varies with the site of the primary tumor. For example, in one thoracoscopic study of 85 patients who had breast carcinoma, tumors on the same side as the effusion were found to be associated with metastases on the costal pleura, whereas contralateral ones were more likely to have tumor on the mediastinal pleura.[393] Some investigators have found visceral pleural metastases more likely to be associated with pulmonary carcinoma and inferior mediastinal and diaphragmatic locations with extrapulmonary primaries.[394]

The incidence of pleural effusion in patients who have metastatic carcinoma of the breast is higher when pulmonary lymphatic involvement is present. In a retrospective study of 365 consecutive autopsies of patients who died from breast carcinoma, pleural effusion was recorded in 52 (60%) of the 87 patients who had lymphangitic spread compared with 42% of those who did not.[395] This observation supports the hypothesis that lymphatic obstruction is important in the pathogenesis of effusion in metastatic cancer.[347] The cytologic features of breast carcinoma cells in pleural fluid have been described in several reports.[396, 397]

The mean lag time between the diagnosis of the primary tumor and the identification of effusion was approximately 42 months in one series[387] and 22 months in another;[388] the range was from 1 month to as long as 23 years after diagnosis of the primary tumor. As with pulmonary carcinoma, the development of malignant pleural effusion associated with an extrapulmonary primary source carries a dismal prognosis, especially if there is evidence for metastases elsewhere;[397a] in such cases, death usually occurs within a year and often within months.[388, 398]

Hodgkin's Disease and Non-Hodgkin's Lymphoma

About 10% of malignant pleural effusions are the result of lymphoma.[70] At the time of diagnosis, pleural effusion as the sole radiographic finding is rare in Hodgkin's disease but somewhat more common in non-Hodgkin's lymphoma.[70] Although there are some differences in the incidence of pleural effusion and of pulmonary and mediastinal abnormalities between these forms of lymphoma, the general pattern is similar. Primary pleural lymphoma is rare but has been reported in patients who have chronic pyothorax associated with a monoclonal expansion of Epstein-Barr virus–infected cells[399] and in association with herpesvirus 8 infection and effusions in the pericardium or peritoneum ("primary effusion lymphoma").[400, 401]

Pleural effusion in lymphoma can be the result of a variety of mechanisms, including impaired lymphatic drainage as a result of mediastinal lymph node or thoracic duct obstruction, pleural or pulmonary infiltration by tumor,[70] venous obstruction, pulmonary infection, or radiation therapy.[402] The relative contribution of each of these mechanisms to the development of effusion in Hodgkin's disease is unclear. In one study of 50 patients with Hodgkin's disease, pleural effusion was found in approximately 25%, almost all of whom had enlarged mediastinal lymph nodes;[403] the investigators concluded that the effusions were the result of lymphatic obstruction. By contrast, in another study of 154 patients, pleural effusion was observed in 44 (28%) without any convincing evidence that even massive enlargement of lymph nodes severely obstructed lymph flow.[404] In a third series, pleural effusion was observed in only 3 of 61 patients who had mediastinal lymph node enlargement;[405] however, the effusion disappeared after irradiation of the mediastinal nodes in 2 patients. Similarly, mediastinal lymph node enlargement was found in 48% and pleural fluid in only 16% of 335 patients who had Hodgkin's disease in another review.[406] In yet another investigation of patients who had Hodgkin's disease, 16% had had pleural effusions during the course of the disease, although 29% had pleural involvement at autopsy.[406] Overall, these studies suggest that in most patients who have Hodgkin's disease, neither direct pleural involvement nor mediastinal node involvement alone is sufficient to explain the development of pleural effusion.

Enlarged mediastinal lymph nodes were described in 30% and pleural effusion in 20% in a study of patients who had non-Hodgkin's lymphoma; however, no correlation was found between the two.[407] Pleural effusion was the sole radiographic manifestation of non-Hodgkin's lymphoma in the chest in 19 patients in another series;[408] 17 had evidence of direct pleural involvement by tumor. Both these studies support the contention that direct involvement of the pleura is the usual cause of effusion in non-Hodgkin's lymphoma.

Pleural fluid associated with lymphoma is usually serous or serosanguineous.[409] Protein concentration has been reported to range from 0.8 to 6.2 gm per 100 ml in patients who have Hodgkin's disease.[410] The finding of bloody fluid suggests direct pleural involvement, whereas the finding of a transudate is more indicative of impaired lymphatic drainage. Uncommonly, chylothorax results from obstruction of the thoracic duct.

The cytologic diagnosis of lymphoma in pleural fluid specimens can be difficult, particularly in small lymphocytic (well-differentiated) tumors; as indicated previously, cytologically atypical lymphocytes can be present in tuberculous effusions, resulting in an appearance that can be mistaken for lymphoma.[91] Despite this, some investigators have reported a high degree of accuracy in diagnosis and even in classification of types of lymphoma by this means.[411] Immunohistochemical analysis can be helpful in determining the nature of an effusion in difficult cases,[412] as can the techniques using "neural network" technology[413] and computerized interactive morphometry analysis.[414]

Leukemia

As a radiographic abnormality, pleural effusion in leukemia is second in frequency only to mediastinal lymph node enlargement and is identified in up to 25% of patients.[415] The effusion is usually unilateral. It is probably caused by leukemic infiltration of the pleura in no more than 5% of cases,[416] the majority being secondary to cardiac failure or infection.[415, 416] General or local pleural thickening simulating plaques may be caused by leukemic infiltration.[417] Chylothorax has been described rarely as a complication of chronic lymphocytic leukemia.[418] Cytochemical and immunocytochemical studies of cells obtained from the fluid may be helpful in diagnosis.[419–421]

Multiple Myeloma

Pleural effusion in multiple myeloma is uncommon.[422–425] Destructive lesions in one or more ribs are frequently accompanied by soft tissue masses that typically protrude into the thorax and indent the pleura and lung. The ribs may be expanded, a finding that is almost pathognomonic of the disease. Destructive lesions also may be apparent in the shoulder girdle or thoracic spine. Despite the characteristic appearance of these chest wall abnormalities, a similar radiographic appearance can occur with a variety of primary and metastatic neoplasms.

The pleural exudate is probably caused in many cases by direct infiltration by neoplastic cells.[422] A high level of the specific paraprotein produced by the tumor cells can sometimes be identified in pleural fluid.[423, 426] Curiously, 80% of myelomatous effusions are related to IgA multiple myeloma.[427] A mediastinal plasmacytoma with extension to the pleura and secondary effusion has been described in one patient.[428]

Miscellaneous Lymphoreticular Disorders

Pleural effusion is not uncommon in Waldenström's macroglobulinemia and can occur in the absence of parenchymal disease.[429, 430] A gamma peak is found in the serum by protein electrophoresis; lymphocytes and a high level of immunoglobulin M can be identified in the pleural fluid.[430] Pleural effusion also has been reported in two patients who had alpha chain disease.[431] Castleman's disease (giant lymph node hyperplasia) has been associated with pleural effusion in occasional patients.[432, 433]

PLEURAL EFFUSION CAUSED BY THROMBOEMBOLI

As a radiographic manifestation of thromboembolic disease, pleural effusion is as common as parenchymal consolidation.[434–437] In a review of the radiographic findings of 1,063 patients who underwent pulmonary angiography for suspected pulmonary thromboembolism (PTE) in the PIOPED trial, 35% of 383 patients who were diagnosed as having PTE had pleural effusion on the side of the embolism.[438] Pleural effusions were present in 74% of patients who had pleural-based areas of increased opacity. However, the prevalence of effusions or of pleural-based areas of increased opacity was not significantly different from that in the 680 patients who did not have PTE.[438] In a prospective study of 62 patients who had PTE and effusion, radiographic evidence of infarction was found in only half.[439] In another series of 10 patients who had bilateral pleural effusion caused by PTE, the effusion was the only manifestation of disease in 7.[347]

As might be expected, effusion is often associated with pulmonary infarction. In some cases, the parenchymal shadow is diminutive or hidden by the fluid, confusing the diagnostic possibilities to such an extent that an embolic episode will be suggested only if there is a high index of suspicion.[440, 441] The amount of pleural fluid is frequently small but may be abundant and is most often unilateral;[74, 439, 442, 443] when predominantly infrapulmonary, it may be mistaken for hemidiaphragmatic elevation.[442] The effusion usually develops and absorbs synchronously with the infarct but sometimes appears later and clears sooner.[444]

Some consider that analysis of the pleural fluid is not helpful in diagnosis, because it can have the features of either a transudate or an exudate and is grossly bloody in only a minority of cases.[74] We concur that transudates can occur but suspect that in most, if not all, such cases they are caused by clinically unrecognized heart failure. We also feel that in a patient suspected on clinical grounds of having PTE, a bloody pleural effusion is strong confirmatory evidence for associated infarction. Supporting this assertion are the results of a study of 26 patients in whom thoracentesis was performed early in the course of the disease;[439] the effusion was bloody in 15 of 18 patients (83%) who had radiographic evidence of infarction but in only 3 of the 8 (38%) who did not have a parenchymal abnormality.

The pulmonary manifestations of thromboembolism and infarction are varied. However, the combination of diaphragmatic elevation, basal pulmonary opacity of almost any type (but usually homogeneous), and a small pleural effusion constitutes a triad of radiologic signs that are highly suggestive of the diagnosis. Patients who have effusions that progress during therapy should be evaluated for recurrent PTE, secondary infection, or pleural hemorrhage secondary to anticoagulation.[70]

PLEURAL EFFUSION CAUSED BY CARDIAC FAILURE

One of the most common forms of pleural effusion is that associated with an increase in hydrostatic pressure in the pulmonary venous circulation.[445] Although it occurs most commonly with cardiac decompensation, it has also been documented in about 60% of patients who have constrictive pericarditis, for which it may be the presenting clinical finding.[446–448] The fluid is usually a transudate.

There has been considerable controversy as to whether

the development of hydrothorax in cardiac decompensation is the result of left-sided heart failure alone or whether right-sided failure must contribute to the development of effusion or even be its sole cause. This issue was addressed in a study of 37 patients who had congestive heart failure, using ultrasound to document the presence or absence of effusion and obtaining simultaneous hemodynamic measurements from a pulmonary artery catheter.[449] Pleural effusions were found in 19 patients (51%); although the pulmonary artery wedge pressure was significantly higher (24 mm Hg) in patients who had effusion than in those who didn't (17 mm Hg), mean pulmonary artery pressures were also higher in the same individuals. Thus, a contributory role for an elevated right heart pressure in the pathogenesis of effusion could not be excluded. The investigators then examined a group of 18 patients who had pulmonary artery hypertension and normal left ventricular function; none of these patients had pleural effusion. Thus, the presence of effusion in patients who have pulmonary hypertension should suggest an additional diagnosis, left-sided heart failure being among the many considerations.[449] Animal experiments performed by the same investigators led to the conclusion that effusion could form by two possible mechanisms:[449] flow of interstitial edema into the pleural space or increase in the hydrostatic pressure in the microcirculation of the visceral pleura, thereby causing leakage into the pleural space. Overall, it seems reasonable to conclude that although left-sided heart failure plays a predominant role in the development of pleural effusion, a contribution of increased hydrostatic pressure in the systemic circulation cannot be excluded; however, it is very unlikely to be the sole cause.

Hydrothorax in congestive heart failure is most often bilateral; for example, almost 90% of patients in one autopsy study were found to have bilateral effusions.[450] For unknown reasons, unilateral effusion is more prone to be right-sided than left-sided; in fact, if an effusion is confined to the left hemithorax, a cause other than heart failure should be sought.[445] Associated clinical and radiologic evidence of cardiac enlargement, with or without pulmonary venous hypertension, makes the diagnosis obvious in most cases. A radiologic finding peculiar to hydrothorax associated with congestive heart failure is the so-called phantom tumor, in which fluid tends to localize (not loculate) in an interlobar pleural fissure (Fig. 69–10). For unknown reasons, these "disappearing tumors" occur most frequently in the minor fissure.

PLEURAL EFFUSION CAUSED BY TRAUMA

As might be expected, pleura effusion secondary to trauma is most often caused by an accumulation of blood; occasionally, it is chyle (following rupture of the thoracic duct [*see* page 2634]) or cerebrospinal fluid, or is serosanguineous in nature.

Hemothorax is a common manifestation of both penetrating and nonpenetrating trauma (*see* page 2623); for example, in one review of 100 children who had experienced blunt chest trauma from motor vehicle accidents, effusion was seen in 58.[451] Blood may originate in vessels within the chest wall, diaphragm, lung, or mediastinum. The importance of the site of hemorrhage in relation to the size of a

hemothorax has been emphasized:[452] when bleeding occurs from a systemic vessel in the chest wall, diaphragm, or mediastinum, the hemothorax tends to increase despite the quantity of blood present; by contrast, when the blood comes from the pulmonary vasculature, the expanding hemothorax compresses the lung, with resultant pulmonary tamponade that may produce hemostasis. Although hemorrhage may result from laceration of the parietal or visceral pleura by fractured ribs, it can also occur (with or without associated pneumothorax) in closed chest trauma without fracture. Hemothorax commonly complicates traumatic rupture of the aorta and is almost invariably left-sided;[453] as a result, care should be taken not to attribute effusion erroneously to left-sided rib fracture. This complication may also be the presenting sign of painless dissecting thoracic aortic aneurysm.[454]

When blood enters the pleural space, it coagulates rapidly; however, the clot may become defibrinated, leaving the fluid indistinguishable radiologically from effusion of any other cause.[452, 453] At other times, loculation may occur early, increasing the difficulty of needle drainage. Empyema complicating hemothorax is usually caused by *S. aureus*. By contrast, empyema that complicates serous effusions or pneumothorax in traumatized patients is usually caused by hospital-acquired gram-negative organisms; chest tube thoracostomy may be responsible for the infection in some cases.[154]

Rupture of the esophagus following closed chest trauma is rare and results in changes localized to the mediastinum and pleura.[453] Of considerably greater frequency is the rupture that occurs spontaneously following severe vomiting (Boerhaave's syndrome) or as a complication of esophagoscopy or gastroscopy,[455] overzealous dilation of a stricture or achalasia, disruption of the suture line following esophageal resection and anastomosis, or passage of an esophageal obturator airway by paramedical personnel during cardiopulmonary resuscitation.[456] "Spontaneous" rupture has also been described in a patient who had severe herpes simplex esophagitis.[457] Pleural effusion or hydropneumothorax is a frequent complication of esophageal perforation from any of these causes. Although almost always left-sided, rare cases of right-sided effusion have been documented.[458] Identification of ingested material in pleural fluid is diagnostic. The level of pleural fluid amylase (derived from the salivary glands) is raised in most,[459] but not all,[460, 461] patients. The pH of the effusion is reduced.[74] In the majority of cases, the site of rupture can be identified precisely (although sometimes with considerable difficulty) by ingestion of radiographic contrast material.

Small exudative effusions sometimes develop following endoscopic sclerotherapy of esophageal varices, presumably as a result of inflammation of the mediastinal parietal pleura.[462] This complication was identified following 31 of 65 sclerotherapy sessions in one review of 30 patients;[463] the episodes were associated with more pain and a greater volume of sclerosant in the patients who did not develop effusion.

The most common pleural effusion of "traumatic" etiology is that caused by thoracotomy (*see* page 2661). Chest radiographs 2 or 3 days after thoracotomy usually show no fluid, because the pleural space is effectively drained. Following removal of the drainage tube, however, a small

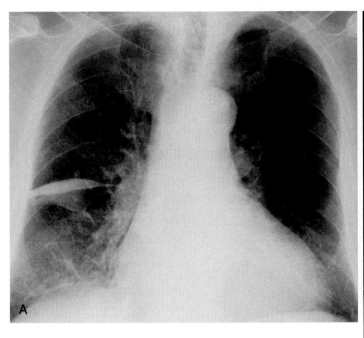
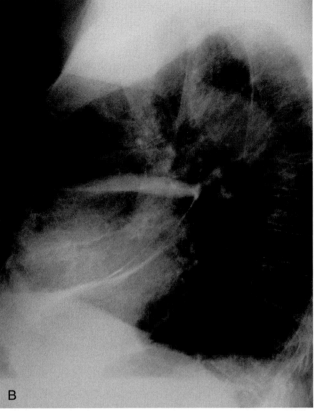

Figure 69–10. Focal Interlobar Pleural Effusions in Cardiac Decompensation. Posteroanterior *(A)* and lateral *(B)* chest radiographs demonstrate localized effusions within the right major and minor interlobar fissures. The patient was a 75-year-old who had left ventricular failure and pulmonary edema secondary to myocardial infarction.

amount of fluid often appears, only to disappear quite quickly during convalescence. Minimal pleural thickening may remain. Empyema can develop shortly after lung resection or can be delayed for several months; it is usually the result of a bronchopleural fistula. In one series of 75 patients who had empyema of varied etiology, approximately 15% developed the complication after pneumonectomy and 4% after lobectomy.[464] In four of nine cases of late onset empyema that appeared at least 3 months after surgery, the radiographic demonstration of gas in a previously opaque hemithorax led to the diagnosis of fistulas (one bronchial, two esophageal, and the fourth both bronchial and esophageal);[465] in the remaining five cases, the presence of empyema was established only following the development of empyema necessitans.

Pleural effusion is also very common after myocardial revascularization procedures, occurring in up to 90% of patients.[466, 467] The accumulation of fluid in larger than expected amounts may be attributable to a variety of causes, including poor positioning of the drainage tube, hemorrhage from an intercostal vessel, or infection (empyema). Hemorrhage from intercostal vessels is occasionally an important complication in patients undergoing heart-lung transplantation.[468]

Malpositioning of percutaneous central venous and Swan-Ganz catheters can cause perforation of a vessel, either at the time of insertion or some time later as a result of gradual erosion of a relatively thin-walled intrathoracic vessel by the catheter tip.[469] Depending on the vessel involved and on the reason for catheter insertion (monitoring of pressure or hyperalimentation), the result may be mediastinal hemorrhage, hemothorax,[470] pneumothorax, massive hydro-

thorax,[426, 471] or extrapleural hematoma.[472–475] In patients receiving hyperalimentation, the infusion of toxic or potentially toxic solutions obviously increases the hazard. Similarly, right pleural effusion has been described following the migration of a ventriculoperitoneal shunt into the pleural space.[476]

An uncommon cause of pleural effusion is subarachnoid-pleural fistula, usually secondary to accidental trauma;[477–479] rarely, such a fistula follows surgery[480] or is related to a paraspinal neurogenic tumor.[481] The diagnosis can be made by myelography,[482, 483] radionuclide myelography,[484, 485] or CT with injection of contrast into the subarachnoid space or pleural fluid.[486] One case has been described in which a combination of subarachnoid-pleural fistula and chylothorax followed trauma.[487]

Radiographic evidence of a left pleural effusion in a patient who has a history suggesting a traumatic diaphragmatic hernia should alert the physician to the likelihood of this etiology; the presence of intestinal loops within the hemithorax virtually confirms the diagnosis. Because fluid seldom accumulates in the pleural space in the absence of bowel strangulation (it leaks through the diaphragmatic rent), a pleural effusion should alert the physician to the presence of vascular compromise.[488] An unusual cause of hemothorax following severe trauma has been reported in which a lacerated spleen herniated into the thorax through a traumatically ruptured diaphragm.[489] Splenic arteriography revealed the ruptured spleen within the left hemithorax and showed extravasation of contrast medium into the pleural space. We have seen a similar case (Fig. 69–11). An association also has been reported between recurrent left-sided pleural effusion and silent splenic hematomas following trauma.[490]

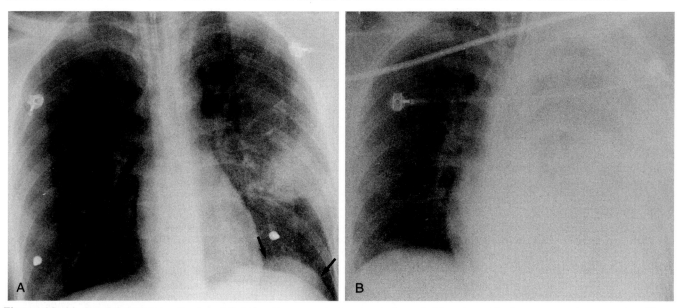

Figure 69–11. Hemothorax from Ruptured Spleen. An anteroposterior chest radiograph *(A)* performed in the emergency department in a 20-year-old man following a motor vehicle accident demonstrates a focal area of consolidation in the left lung as a result of pulmonary contusion and a curvilinear soft tissue opacity *(arrows)* immediately above the level of the left hemidiaphragm. The patient deteriorated rapidly following admission. A chest radiograph performed 2 hours later *(B)* demonstrates almost complete opacification of the left hemithorax with contralateral shift of the mediastinum. At surgery the patient was shown to have a traumatic tear of the left hemidiaphragm with a large left hemothorax secondary to laceration of the herniated spleen.

Radiographically demonstrable pleural effusion following radiation therapy to the thorax is uncommon.[491–493] However, fairly extensive thickening of the pleura may be seen both radiologically and pathologically.[491, 494] Pleural effusion can also develop in the absence of radiation pleuritis 1 to 2 years after intensive mediastinal irradiation as a result of mediastinal fibrosis.[70]

Although trauma (including thoracotomy) is by far the most common cause of hemothorax, "spontaneous" intrapleural bleeding can occur from a variety of causes. If Light's definition of hemothorax as fluid with a hematocrit of more than 50% that of blood is accepted, some malignancies involving the pleura can result in hemothorax rather than serosanguineous effusion.[74, 495] Additional rare causes include rib tumors such as chondrosarcoma and osteochondroma,[496] anticoagulation,[497, 498] endometriosis *(see* page 2767), hemophilia,[499] neurofibromatosis,[500] aspergillosis, and extramedullary hematopoiesis.[501, 502]

PLEURAL EFFUSION RELATED TO DISEASE OF ABDOMINAL ORGANS

A variety of intra-abdominal or pelvic disorders are associated with pleural effusion. The pathogenesis is complex and varies according to the particular disease examined; it can be related to secondary effects on cardiac function, changes in plasma oncotic pressure, or production of ascites or secretions that are transferred through diaphragmatic lymphatics or deficiencies into the pleural space. As discussed elsewhere *(see* page 250), lymphatic channels are present in the diaphragm that can transport particulate matter and fluid from the peritoneum to the pleural space, those of the right side being larger and able to carry more fluid than those of the left;[503, 504] flow appears always to be from the peritoneum to the pleura, never in the reverse direction.[504, 505]

Although it is likely that some fluid transfer occurs by way of these lymphatic channels, anatomic defects within the diaphragm also appear to be involved in fluid passage.[506, 507] An example of the potential importance of this route was provided in one study of eight patients who had pleural effusion and cirrhotic ascites and who underwent video thoracoscopy.[508] Diaphragmatic defects were identified in six patients; their closure led to resolution of pleural effusion in all. By contrast, effusion persisted in the two patients in whom no defect was identified. (Presumably, these two patients had transfer of pleural fluid via lymphatics or had diaphragmatic defects that were not successfully identified at the time of surgery.) Ultrafast gradient echo magnetic resonance imaging and intraperitoneal contrast enhancement have also been used to demonstrate diaphragmatic defects in this clinical setting.[509] Other arguments in favor of defects accounting for pleural effusion in patients who have ascites include the observation that pneumothorax frequently complicates induced pneumoperitoneum and the demonstration of such defects at autopsy.[510]

The development of small pleural effusions is common after abdominal surgery. For example, in one study of 200 patients in whom radiographs were obtained in the right and left lateral decubitus positions 48 to 72 hours after surgery, pleural effusions were demonstrated in 97 (49%);[511] the thickness was less than 4 mm in 50 patients, 4 to 10 mm in 26, and greater than 10 mm in 21. The incidence of effusion was higher following surgery on the upper abdomen, in patients who had postoperative atelectasis on the side on which the surgery was performed, and in patients who had free abdominal fluid. Thoracentesis was carried out on 20 of the 97 patients; in 16, the fluid had the characteristics of an exudate. All but one of the effusions resolved spontaneously, the exception being an effusion associated with staphylococcal infection. In another review of 128 patients who underwent upper abdominal surgery and were assessed by chest radiography in the posteroanterior and lateral positions, 89 had effusions in the postoperative period;[512] all resolved in the absence of specific therapy.

Liver and Biliary Tract

A large pleural effusion in a patient who has cirrhosis and no evidence of primary pulmonary or cardiac disease has been termed *hepatic hydrothorax*.[510] In a review of 200 consecutive patients who had cirrhosis associated with ascites, 12 (6%) were found to have this complication.[506] The effusion was right-sided in 8 patients, bilateral in 2, and left-sided in 2. A similar right-sided predominance has been reported by other investigators.[513–515]

There are several potential mechanisms for the development of pleural effusion in patients who have cirrhosis, including hypoproteinemia, azygos hypertension, and transfer of peritoneal fluid to the pleural cavity via lymphatics or diaphragmatic defects.[58] It is likely that the last of these is the most important.[513, 516] Some cases of effusion have been reported in the absence of ascites;[515, 517–519] however, in one such instance, intraperitoneal injection of an isotope was followed by its appearance in the pleural effusion, suggesting that the pleural fluid was peritoneal in origin.[518] Right-sided pleural effusion is also common following hepatectomy,[520] a complication that can be prevented by placing a fibrin sealant over the severed hepatic ligaments.

Bile-containing pleural effusion developed in one patient following percutaneous cholangiography;[521] the effusion resolved with biliary tract decompression. A single patient has been described who developed right-sided pleural effusion secondary to erosion of the right hemidiaphragm by gallstones, which had been spilled during a previous laparoscopic cholecystectomy.[522] In another patient, penetrating trauma caused a biliary-pleural fistula, which was manifested as a massive right-sided effusion.[523] Right-sided or bilateral pleural effusions also have been reported following liver transplantation;[523a, 524] postoperative mechanical ventilation appears to prevent this complication.[510, 524]

Kidney

Dialysis. Because ascites may be associated with pleural effusion, it might be reasonable to anticipate that peritoneal dialysis would sometimes lead to hydrothorax, and several such cases have been reported.[525–527] On one occasion, the fluid was sufficient in amount to cause tension hydrothorax.[528] Patients receiving long-term hemodialysis may also develop pleural effusion,[529, 530] the fluid often being serosanguineous as a consequence of the use of heparin during the procedure. Although some investigators have attributed the effusion to the hemodialysis itself,[529, 530] it is possible that in many, if not all, cases, it is a complication of renal failure. For example, in one study of 100 patients who were receiving hemodialysis and were observed over 3 months, 21 were found to develop pleural effusion.[531] Heart failure was considered to be the cause in 46% of these patients, and the remaining cases were attributed to uremia, atelectasis, or infection; no effusion was felt to be a complication of dialysis *per se*.

Hydronephrosis and Urinoma. The association of urinary tract obstruction and the development of unilateral or bilateral pleural effusion has been described by many investigators.[532–539] The majority of published reports attribute the source of the urine collection in the thorax to retroperitoneal collections of urine (urinomas). The latter form as a result of extravasation of urine from the urinary tract secondary to obstruction in the renal pelvis, ureters, bladder, or urethra. The diagnosis of urinothorax is made by the demonstration of a level of creatinine in pleural fluid that is higher than in the blood.[534, 536, 537, 540] The fluid may be a transudate because of the low protein content of urine.[540] Surgical drainage of the retroperitoneal urinoma results in rapid clearing of the effusion.

Nephrotic Syndrome. Pleural effusion is common in patients who have the nephrotic syndrome; for example, in one study of 52 patients, it was observed in 21 (40%).[541] The principal mechanism is diminution in the plasma osmotic pressure. The fluid is usually a transudate; empyema[542] or chylothorax in association with chylous ascites[543] has been described occasionally. The nephrotic syndrome is associated with a relatively high incidence of atypical location of pleural effusion, most commonly in the infrapulmonary space;[544] for example, in one review of 19 patients who had pleural effusion associated with the nephrotic syndrome and acute glomerulonephritis, the effusion was infrapulmonary in 10.[541] The reasons underlying this feature are obscure. Clearly, the fact that the effusion is a transudate is not significant, because a wide variety of fluids (including blood) sometimes behave similarly. Because of the increased risk of thrombosis in patients who have the nephrotic syndrome, it is particularly important to exclude thromboembolic disease as a cause of the effusion in these individuals.[545]

Acute Glomerulonephritis. The incidence of pleural effusion in association with acute glomerulonephritis is fairly high; in one study of 76 children, it was observed in 42.[546] The effusion may be associated with a variety of pulmonary changes, including segmental or lobar atelectasis, pneumonia, and pulmonary edema.[547] It has been postulated that these effusions are related to alterations in extracellular fluid volume;[547] however, the exclusion of concurrent infection was not documented.

Uremia. Both the pericardium and the pleura may become inflamed in patients who have uremia. In fact, fibrinous pleuritis has been demonstrated in about 20% of uremic patients at autopsy.[548] The fluid is an exudate that contains high levels of protein and LDH;[549, 550] it also frequently contains blood, possibly as a result of the anticoagulation used during hemodialysis.[529, 530] Affected patients sometimes complain of pain, and friction rubs frequently are heard on auscultation.[550] If the patient is receiving long-term hemodialysis, the effusion usually clears slowly.

Pancreas

Acute or chronic pancreatitis is sometimes associated with pleural effusion, often without radiographic evidence of other intrathoracic abnormality. When associated with acute pancreatitis, it is a marker of severe disease and relatively poor prognosis.[551–553] Effusions are predominantly left-sided; for example, in one review of 31 cases, it was on the left in 21, on the right in 3, and bilateral in 7.[554] In another series of 80 cases, 48 (60%) were left-sided, 24 (30%) were right-sided, and 8 (10%) were bilateral.[555] In the majority of patients who have acute pancreatitis, symptoms are present that suggest an acute upper abdominal disorder; however, in some the clinical presentation can be confused with a primary or parapneumonic pleural effusion.[556, 557] A minority of patients develop an intra-abdominal abscess that only becomes apparent 2 to 3 weeks after the acute episode, the abscess being responsible for the pleural effusion.[74, 556]

Chronic pancreatitis is associated with pleural effusion even more often than the acute disease.[558–564] The effusion is often recurrent, and symptoms frequently direct attention to the thorax rather than the abdomen. In many cases, the patient has a history of heavy alcohol consumption that has been responsible for the pancreatitis. In one review of 113 patients who had pancreatitis-related pleural effusion (almost all of whom had alcohol-related disease), abdominal symptoms were identified in only 24% and pulmonary symptoms in 68%.[564] Duct disruption can lead to the creation of a pancreaticopleural fistula, with or without pseudocyst formation.[565, 566] The fistulous tract can also communicate with the peritoneal cavity (causing ascites),[567] the mediastinum (resulting in bilateral pleural effusions and sometimes pericarditis),[561, 568, 569] and (occasionally) a bronchus.[563, 570]

The pleural fluid in both acute and chronic pancreatitis has the characteristics of an exudate and is sometimes serosanguineous or frankly bloody.[557–559, 571] In acute pancreatitis, the effusion is more likely to be slight or moderate in amount and bloody,[74, 557] whereas in chronic pancreatitis it tends to be serous, massive, and recurrent.[558, 559, 572, 573] The amylase content is characteristically very high and is almost invariably higher than that of the serum.[499, 558, 562, 563, 574] However, an elevated level of pleural fluid amylase can be found also in esophageal perforation,[459] in some parapneumonic effusions,[575] and in association with some neoplasms,[576] including carcinoma of the pancreas[577] and lung.[575, 578] A patient has been described who had chronic pancreatitis and pleural fluid eosinophilia.[579]

With proper positioning, the pancreaticopleural fistula in either acute or chronic pancreatitis can be demonstrated by endoscopic retrograde cholangiopancreatography or CT;[557, 560–563, 574, 580–582] the latter technique appears to be more sensitive,[582] although endoscopic retrograde cholangiopancreatography permits a precise evaluation of the ductal morphology that is indispensable for proper surgical management.[583] Three cases have been reported in which pleural calcification occurred in association with pancreatitis, the calcification being bilateral and basal in location and curvilinear in configuration;[584] there was no history of asbestos exposure.

Ovary

In 1934, Salmon[585] described the association of pleural effusion with benign pelvic tumors in a report that antedated by 3 years the results of a study by Meigs and Cass[586] of seven cases of ovarian fibromas associated with ascites and hydrothorax. This relationship between pleural effusion and ovarian tumors (Meigs-Salmon syndrome) is now known to be associated with a wide variety of primary neoplasms, including fibroma, thecoma, granulosa cell tumor, Brenner's tumor, cystadenoma, germ cell tumors, and even adenocarci-

noma;[587–591] occasionally, extraovarian pelvic tumors such as uterine leiomyomas[592, 593] and fallopian tube carcinoma[594] have been implicated. It is believed that the tumor size rather than the specific histologic type is the most important pathogenetic factor.[74] Supporting this hypothesis are the results of a 1945 review, in which almost 40% of ovarian neoplasms measuring more than 6 cm in diameter were associated with ascites;[595] however, hydrothorax occurred in only 2% to 3% of these cases.

The effusions vary widely in amount and may be massive; they occur more frequently on the right side but may be left-sided or bilateral. Although usually a transudate, the fluid occasionally contains blood.[592] Removal of the pelvic tumor is usually followed by disappearance of the ascites and hydrothorax. The syndrome has been seen in some patients with benign tumors in whom the serum showed elevation of CA-125, a tumor marker strongly associated with ovarian carcinoma.[596, 597]

Pleural effusion is commonly present in the ovarian hyperstimulation syndrome, a postovulatory complication seen in patients receiving exogenous gonadotropins for induction of ovulation.[598] The syndrome has two main components: (1) sudden bilateral ovarian enlargement, readily recognized by ultrasound; and (2) an acute shift of intravascular fluid into the third space.[598] The majority of patients present within 2 weeks after receiving human chorionic gonadotropin. Clinical symptoms include abdominal distention and discomfort, nausea, vomiting, and shortness of breath. Radiologic manifestations include unilateral or bilateral pleural effusion (Fig. 69–12) and, less commonly, pericardial effusion or hydrostatic pulmonary edema;[598–601] adult respiratory distress syndrome occurs rarely.

Gastrointestinal Tract

Perforation of an abdominal viscus can lead to pleural effusion, usually as a consequence of a subphrenic abscess;

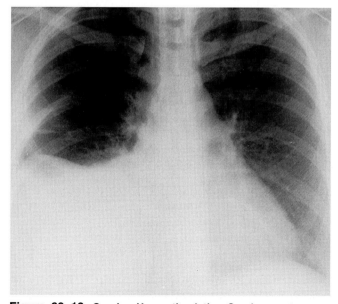

Figure 69–12. Ovarian Hyperstimulation Syndrome. A posteroanterior chest radiograph in a 30-year-old woman performed 3 weeks after *in vitro* fertilization demonstrates a large subpulmonic right pleural effusion. Ultrasound demonstrated bilateral enlarged cystic ovaries and a small amount of free intraperitoneal fluid.

occasionally a gastric or duodenal ulcer communicates directly with the pleural cavity through the diaphragm, resulting in an effusion that can contain a high bilirubin level or be grossly bilious.[602, 603] Pleural effusion rarely occurs in idiopathic inflammatory bowel disease (Crohn's disease or ulcerative colitis), in which case it may represent a manifestation of a multisystem immunologic disorder.[604, 605]

Subphrenic Abscess

Small pleural effusions are often found in association with acute subphrenic infection; for example, in one study of 47 patients, they were observed in 37 (79%).[606] Associated findings include elevation and restriction of movement of the ipsilateral hemidiaphragm (95% in the previously mentioned series) and basal linear atelectasis or pneumonitis (79%). This combination of findings should strongly suggest the diagnosis, especially in the postoperative period after laparotomy or following rupture of a hollow abdominal viscus.

Subphrenic abscess secondary to infection of abdominal viscera, with or without perforation, is often unappreciated.[74, 607] The diagnosis should be considered in any patient who has pleural effusion and who has recently undergone abdominal surgery or whose effusion has a high neutrophilic leukocyte count. Most patients have fever, leukocytosis, and abdominal pain; upper abdominal tenderness is generally present but is not invariable. The effusions are usually negative on culture and probably result from diaphragmatic inflammation; however, this is not necessarily the case.[608] The diagnosis can be confirmed by ultrasound or CT-guided aspiration of the fluid collection.[609, 609a, b]

Two patients who had subphrenic abscess have been reported who had recently undergone major abdominal surgery and were suspected of having pulmonary thromboembolism;[609] in each case, a pulmonary angiogram showed a hemidiaphragm clearly outlined by contrast medium, a phenomenon that was believed to be caused by hyperperfusion as a consequence of subdiaphragmatic inflammation.

MISCELLANEOUS CAUSES OF PLEURAL EFFUSION

Myxedema

Although most pleural effusions in patients who have hypothyroidism have cardiovascular, renal, or other causes,[610] occasionally they occur in the absence of an etiology other than myxedema.[611] There is no distinctive radiographic characteristic. The effusions are not inflammatory and biochemically are usually borderline between exudates and transudates.[610]

Lymphatic Hypoplasia

Pleural effusion is occasionally associated with hypoplasia of the lymphatic system. In some cases, the clinical presentation is that of Milroy's disease (congenital lymphedema);[612] in others, the effusion is associated with lymphedema of an extremity, yellow nails, and (sometimes)

bronchiectasis (*see* page 2284).[613, 614] The pleural fluid characteristically has a high protein content. Two siblings who had this syndrome have been described in whom pleural effusion was associated with hypogammaglobulinemia and episodes of lymphopenia.[615] Recurrent pleural effusion also has been reported in a patient who had protein-losing enteropathy, malabsorption, mosaic warts, and generalized lymphatic hypoplasia.[616]

Dressler's Syndrome

The postpericardiectomy or postmyocardial infarction syndrome, known eponymously as Dressler's syndrome, is characterized by chest pain, fever, and pericardial and pleural effusion. Dressler estimated the incidence to be 3% to 4% of patients following myocardial infarction,[617] and it is probable that the incidence is even higher following surgical procedures that affect the pericardium.[74] In the era of thrombolytic therapy, the incidence following myocardial infarction seems to be decreasing; for example, in one study of 210 patients who were given thrombolytic therapy for this reason, only 1 developed the syndrome in the following 3 weeks.[618] In patients who have infarction, the syndrome is particularly apt to occur in the presence of transmural myocardial damage with epicardial extension.[619]

The pathogenesis is unknown but is suspected to be the result of an immunologic reaction. The findings of low pleural fluid complement and a high pleural/serum antimyocardial antibody ratio in a single patient support this hypothesis.[620]

In one retrospective study of 35 patients who had the syndrome (21 patients following cardiac surgery and 14 after myocardial infarction), the onset of symptoms occurred, on average, 20 days after the injury.[621] The major clinical findings were chest pain (91%), fever (66%), pericardial rub (63%), dyspnea (57%), crackles (51%), pleural rub (46%), and leukocytosis (49%). The chest radiograph was abnormal in 94% of the patients; pleural effusion was present in 83%, parenchymal opacities in 74%, and an enlarged cardiopericardial silhouette in 49%. Analysis of pleural fluid was performed on 16 samples from 12 patients and revealed a bloody exudate with a pH greater than 7.40. The syndrome can recur several years after the initial episode.[622]

Familial Paroxysmal Polyserositis

Familial paroxysmal polyserositis (familial Mediterranean fever, recurrent hereditary polyserositis) is a rare cause of paroxysmal attacks of painful pleural effusion.[623] It occurs predominantly in Sephardic Jews, Arabs, Turks, and Armenians, although it has been described in the Chuetas of Mallorca,[624] Ashkenazim,[625] and (rarely) in Japanese.[626] The disease is transmitted in an autosomal recessive fashion in most affected families.[627] The responsible gene has been mapped to chromosome 16 and designated MEFV;[628, 629] it encodes for a protein called *pyrin* (marenostrin) that may be a transcription factor regulating genes involved in the suppression of inflammation.[629a] The actual cause of the precipitation of attacks is unknown.

In one large study of 175 Arabs who had the disease,

the most common manifestation was peritonitis (94%), followed by arthritis (34%) and pleuritis (32%).[623] An erysipelas-like rash and pericarditis are less frequent manifestations.[630] Pulmonary atelectasis has been reported in one patient,[631] with response to colchicine and recurrence on cessation of medication. Seventy-five per cent to 80% of the attacks of pleuritis are associated with arthritis and arthralgia, usually involving the large joints; joint pain typically lasts for 12 to 24 hours and occasionally for as long as 3 days. Fever, sometimes as high as 40° C (104° F), persists for 12 to 48 hours. Remissions may last for months to years. Despite the recurrent disability, the prognosis is apparently excellent in most cases.[632, 633]

Endometriosis

The presence of endometrial tissue within the thorax is uncommon, only about 110 cases having been documented in the English literature by 1996.[634] In the majority, the abnormal tissue is located in the visceral or parietal pleura and is discovered after the development of pneumothorax or hemothorax; in approximately 15% of cases, a patient presents with recurrent hemoptysis or is found to have a nodule on a screening chest radiograph, indicating involvement of the pulmonary parenchyma (*see* page 1375).[634]

Pathogenesis

Although metaplasia of pleural mesothelial and submesothelial connective tissue into endometrial tissue has been hypothesized to be a mechanism for the development of thoracic endometriosis,[635] more widely believed theories involve embolization via the pulmonary arteries and migration from the peritoneum across the diaphragm.[634] It is possible that both mechanisms are operative, one for pulmonary parenchymal disease and the other for pleural involvement.

It has been shown in experimental animal studies that endometrial tissue injected intravenously can survive and proliferate within pulmonary vessels and adjacent parenchyma.[636] Fragments of decidua have occasionally been identified within the lungs of postpartum women,[637, 638] and it is conceivable that glands as well as stromal tissue could occasionally be transported during labor or surgical trauma. Support for this mechanism was provided by one review of 65 patients who had pleuropulmonary endometriosis in which all those who had parenchymal involvement had a history of at least one spontaneous vaginal delivery or gynecologic operation.[639] There is also experimental evidence that the endometrial cells in foci of endometriosis differ from normal endometrial cells in their ability to invade tissue and in the expression of molecules that mediate invasion, such as E-cadherin;[640] this suggests that these cells might be able to directly penetrate vascular spaces.

It is also likely that endometrial tissue can migrate from the pelvic peritoneum to the pleura through developmental defects in the diaphragm (*see* page 2763).[639, 641] Such defects measure up to several millimeters in diameter and have been identified in approximately 33% of patients who have pleural endometriosis.[641] They are said to be more frequent on the right,[639] suggesting a possible explanation for the large preponderance of cases on this side. It has also been speculated

that this unusual laterality is related to the pattern of peritoneal fluid flow—down the left paravertebral gutter into the pelvis and up the right paravertebral gutter to the hemidiaphragm and liver.[639] Support for this mechanism of transport is provided by the results of the review of 65 patients cited previously;[639] although the right hemithorax was affected in 93% of the 54 patients who had pleural involvement, this laterality was present in only 64% of those considered to have parenchymal disease, suggesting that the latter is influenced by pulmonary blood flow and the former by transdiaphragmatic transport. It should be pointed out, however, that some investigators have found evidence that diaphragmatic defects might be the result of erosion of the diaphragm by necrotic and sloughed endometrium.[641]

Pathologic Characteristics

Grossly, pleural endometriosis appears as multiple (occasionally single) bluish-purple nodules ranging from 1 mm to several centimeters in diameter. As indicated previously, the right pleural cavity is affected in the vast majority of cases. Nodules can be present on either the visceral or the parietal pleura, or both; when on the costal parietal surface, concomitant diaphragmatic involvement is not infrequent. Cystic change may be evident, especially in the larger nodules.[642, 643] In some cases, the lung parenchyma is involved by direct extension from an initial focus in the pleura.

Microscopically, the diagnosis is confirmed by the presence of round or irregular glandular spaces admixed with typical endometrial stroma; hemosiderin-laden macrophages related to previous hemorrhage are often present. In some patients who have a clear-cut history of pleural endometriosis, only fibrosis is identified on pathologic examination, suggesting necrosis and healing of the affected foci. Endometrial cells and tissue have occasionally been identified in transthoracic needle aspiration specimens.[644]

Radiologic Manifestations

The radiographic manifestations are those of pneumothorax or hemothorax; pleural nodules are only rarely visible.[639, 645] In one case, CT and ultrasound demonstrated soft tissue nodules in the pleural and peritoneal cavities, as well as localized defects in the right hemidiaphragm.[645a]

Clinical Manifestations

Most women who have thoracic endometriosis are between 20 and 40 years of age, the mean age at diagnosis in one literature review being 35.[634] Pleural involvement usually manifests itself as catamenial pneumothorax (about 75% of cases) or hemothorax (about 15%).[634] The main symptoms are shoulder or chest pain and dyspnea.[635] These appear within 72 hours of the onset of menses and are typically recurrent; for example, in 63 cases in one review, the number of episodes of pneumothorax ranged from 2 to 42 (average, 14).[635] A minority of patients have hydropneumothorax or hemoptysis (the latter implying concomitant pulmonary parenchymal involvement).[634] A single case of pneumomediastinum unassociated with pneumothorax has been documented.[646] There is evidence that disease may be exacerbated by therapy with the gonadotropin-releasing hormone analogue leuprolide acetate.[647] One case has also been reported of a woman who had recurrent spontaneous pneumothorax related temporally to both sexual intercourse and menses;[648] the investigators hypothesized that the pneumothorax was the result of transtubal and transdiaphragmatic passage of air rather than endometriosis.

CHYLOTHORAX

Chylothorax is the presence of lymphatic fluid in the pleural space resulting from obstruction or disruption of the thoracic duct or one of its major divisions.[649] (The lymphatic drainage of the small intestine [chyle] is carried entirely by the thoracic duct; thus, chylothorax can occur only with obstruction or laceration of this duct. Lesions that obstruct the right lymphatic duct or pulmonary lymphatics can cause pleural effusion but never chylothorax.[650]) The fluid is characteristically "milky" in appearance, although not all milky effusions are chylous in nature[409, 651] and not all chylous effusions are milky.[652] A *chyliform* effusion results from degeneration of malignant and other cells in pleural fluid. A *pseudochylous* effusion results from the presence of cholesterol crystals and occurs most commonly in tuberculosis, rheumatoid disease, and the nephrotic syndrome. Because the separation of pseudochylous and chyliform effusions serves little useful purpose, we designate them both as chyliform.

Chylous effusions are high in neutral fat and fatty acid but low in cholesterol, whereas chyliform effusions are low in neutral fat and high in cholesterol and lecithin.[651] The simultaneous analysis of fasting samples of serum and pleural fluid by lipoprotein electrophoresis readily distinguishes between the two.[653] In an analysis of 141 patients who had chylous effusions based on the presence of chylomicrons, the gross appearance indicated chylothorax in only 50%;[652] however, triglyceride levels in the fluid readily differentiated almost all chylous from serous effusions.

Chyliform pleural fluid is uncommon; in one review of 53 nontraumatic effusions of high lipid content, only 6 (11%) were of this type. As indicated, they have a milky appearance similar to that of chylothorax and may contain some triglycerides;[654, 655] cholesterol crystals probably derive from breakdown products of blood cells and can be readily identified on smear. Patients who have chyliform effusions are often asymptomatic, although a patient may give a history indicative of the cause of the effusion; rheumatoid disease and tuberculosis are the most commonly associated diseases.[74, 655] Chyliform pleural effusions secondary to paragonimiasis have been reported in three immigrants to the United States.[656]

There are numerous causes of chylothorax (Table 69–4). In a review of 143 cases derived from five series, the most common were neoplasm and trauma, the former being responsible twice as often as the latter.[74] Lymphoma is the most common neoplasm,[658] being the cause in about 75% of patients who have malignancy.[74, 659] However, pulmonary carcinoma and metastatic cancer from virtually every organ in the body have been reported to obstruct the thoracic duct and cause chylothorax (Fig. 69–13). In the presence of cancer, the effusion is often bilateral and is usually accompa-

Table 69–4. CHYLOTHORAX—ETIOLOGY

ETIOLOGY	SELECTED REFERENCE(S)
NEOPLASIA	
Metastatic carcinoma	
Lymphoma/leukemia	657, 659
Kaposi's sarcoma	
PENETRATING OR NONPENETRATING THORACIC INJURY	665
SURGERY	
Sclerotherapy of esophageal varices	681
Thoracic	667, 734
Abdominal	677, 678
Neck	679, 680
CONGENITAL ANOMALIES	
Congenital lymphangiectasis	688
Noonan's syndrome	690
Jaffe-Campanacci syndrome	735
Adams-Oliver syndrome	736
46 XY/46 XX mosaicism	737
MISCELLANEOUS	
Pancreatitis	738
Tuberculous spondylitis or lymphadenitis	739–741
Chronic sclerosing mediastinitis	742
Subclavian vein thrombosis	743
Sarcoidosis	744, 745
Severe heart failure	746
Retrosternal goiter	747
Behçet's syndrome	748
Gorham's syndrome	703, 749
Lymphangioleiomyomatosis	
Thoracic aortic aneurysm	750
Castleman's disease	754
Cirrhosis	755

nied by chylous ascites;[660–662] sometimes it occurs spontaneously.[663, 664]

Even when the thoracic duct is blocked by neoplasm, chylous effusion tends to be very uncommon, almost certainly as a result of the presence of collaterals between the thoracic duct and the right posterior intercostal lymphatics and of the opening up of pre-existing lymphovenous channels.[650] In such circumstances, there may be a developmental or acquired deficiency of one or both of these channels of communication allowing chylothorax to occur. Chyle may reflux from an obstructed thoracic duct by two routes—the left posterior intercostal lymphatics to the parietal pleural lymphatics and the left bronchomediastinal trunk to lymphatics of the pulmonary parenchyma and visceral pleura. From either the visceral or parietal lymphatics, chyle then extravasates into the pleural cavity.

Trauma is the second most common cause of chylothorax, most episodes being related to surgery and some to penetrating or nonpenetrating thoracic injury.[665–667] Because the thoracic duct crosses to the left of the spine between the fifth and the seventh thoracic vertebrae, disruption tends to cause right-sided chylothorax when the lower portion is affected and left-sided disease when the upper half is involved. Once the thoracic duct has been disrupted, chyle can leak into the mediastinum and thence into the pleural cavity, either because of damage to the parietal pleura by the initial trauma or because the pleura breaks down under the pressure of the mediastinal fluid collection. Because of its anatomic course, the thoracic duct is particularly vulnerable to trau-

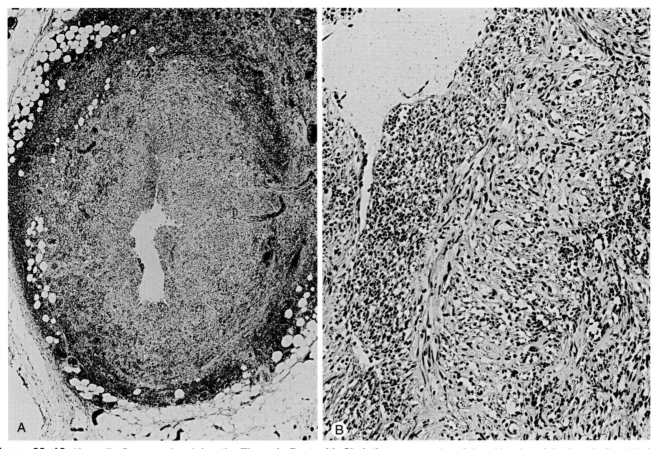

Figure 69–13. Kaposi's Sarcoma Involving the Thoracic Duct with Chylothorax. A section of the midportion of the thoracic duct *(A)* shows marked thickening of its wall and narrowing of its lumen by a neoplasm that extends into the adjacent adipose tissue. A magnified view *(B)* shows the tumor to consist of fascicles of spindle-shaped cells in a pattern typical of Kaposi's sarcoma. The patient was a 43-year-old man with acquired immunodeficiency syndrome who developed bilateral chylothorax and chyloperitoneum. The pleural and peritoneal cavities were free of tumor at autopsy. Although occasional mediastinal lymph nodes contained Kaposi's sarcoma, this was small in amount and the major focus of obstruction to lymph flow was felt to be the thoracic duct.

matic injury during surgery on the vertebral column[668, 669] or on the left hemithorax near the hilum. Postoperative chylothorax also occurs as a complication of cardiac surgery, particularly in children who have congenital heart disease[670–673] and less commonly in adults undergoing aortocoronary bypass.[674, 675] Sometimes, surgical intervention below the diaphragm[676–678] or in the neck[679, 680] results in unilateral or bilateral chyle accumulation; rarely, it has been associated with sclerotherapy of esophageal varices.[681]

Congenital defects in the lymphatic vessels are relatively infrequent causes of chylothorax;[682–684] although usually seen in neonates and infants, they have been described in adults in association with congenital lymphedema[685, 686] or localized lymphangiectasia.[687, 688] Generalized lymphatic dysplasia is a serious condition that is usually fatal.[684] The association of chylothorax with Noonan's syndrome is likely attributable to some kind of outlet obstruction to the thoracic duct as well as to other lymphatic or lymphaticovenous abnormalities.[689, 690]

Radiographic findings are no different from those of pleural effusion of nonchylous etiology. Occasionally, chylothorax can be diagnosed on CT by the presence of attenuation values as low as −17 HU as a result of the presence of fat; however, in the majority of patients the high protein content leads to higher attenuation values that are indistinguishable from those of pleural effusions of other etiology.[691] Although usually free fluid, loculated collections may result in a masslike appearance (chyloma).[692] Lymphangiography has an important role in the investigation of patients who have chylothorax[693, 694] and has been shown to be superior to CT.[695] The abnormalities that can be identified with this examination have been described in detail.[650] In one study of 12 patients who had chylothorax or chylous ascites following surgery, bipedal lymphangiography showed abnormalities in 7 cases, including 5 who had leaks from the thoracic duct, 1 who had a lymphocele in a nephrectomy bed, and 1 who had obstructed intestinal lymphatic vessels after thoracotomy.[695]

Clinical features of chylothorax are no different from those of pleural effusion of other etiologies. Persistent or recurrent chylous effusions lead to the depletion of lymphocytes and the appearance of immature forms in the peripheral circulation; these findings should not be confused with those of lymphoma.[696] The prognosis of chylothorax is generally good, with the exception of patients in whom it is caused by neoplasm, in which case it is usually a late manifestation of disease.[657, 664]

REFERENCES

1. Andrews CO, Gora ML: Pleural effusions: Pathophysiology and management. Ann Pharmacother 28:894, 1994.
2. Light RW: Pleural diseases. Dis Mon 38:261, 1992.
3. Wiener-Kronish JP, Broaddus VC: Interrelationship of pleural and pulmonary interstitial liquid. Ann Rev Physiol 55:209, 1993.
4. Broaddus VC, Light RW: What is the origin of pleural transudates and exudates? Chest 102:658, 1992.
5. Kennedy L, Sahn SA: Noninvasive evaluation of the patient with a pleural effusion. Chest Surg Clin North Am 4:451, 1994.
6. Pleural effusion. BMJ 3:192, 1975.
7. Shinto RA, Light RW: Effects of diuresis on the characteristics of pleural fluid in patients with congestive heart failure. Am J Med 88:230, 1990.
8. Chakko SC, Caldwell SH, Sforza PP: Treatment of congestive heart failure. Its effect on pleural fluid chemistry. Chest 95:798, 1989.
9. Brandstetter RD, Velazquez V, Viejo C, et al: Postural changes in pleural fluid constituents. Chest 105:1458, 1994.
10. Kutty CP, Varkey B: "Contarini's condition": Bilateral pleural effusions with markedly different characteristics. Chest 74:679, 1978.
11. Lawton F, Blackledge G, Johnson R: Co-existent chylous and serous pleural effusions associated with ovarian cancer: A case report of Contarini's syndrome. Eur J Surg Oncol 11:177, 1985.
12. DeSouza R, Lipsett N, Spagnolo SV: Mediastinal compression due to tension hydrothorax. Chest 72:782, 1977.
13. Smyrnios NA, Jederlinic PJ, Irwin RS: Pleural effusion in an asymptomatic patient. Spectrum and frequency of causes and management considerations. Chest 97:192, 1990.
14. Naschitz JE, Yeshurun D: Unilateral chest wall edema in carcinomatous pleurisy. Respiration 47:73, 1985.
15. Gilmartin JJ, Wright AJ, Gibson GJ: Effects of pneumothorax or pleural effusion on pulmonary function. Thorax 40:60, 1985.
16. Dechman G, Sato J, Bates JH: Effect of pleural effusion on respiratory mechanics, and the influence of deep inflation, in dogs. Eur Respir J 6:219, 1993.
17. Sonnenblick M, Melzer E, Rosin AJ: Body positional effect on gas exchange in unilateral pleural effusion. Chest 83:784, 1983.
18. Neagley SR, Zwillich CW: The effect of positional changes on oxygenation in patients with pleural effusions. Chest 88:714, 1985.
19. Estenne M, Yernault JC, De Troyer A: Mechanism of relief of dyspnea after thoracocentesis in patients with large pleural effusions. Am J Med 74:813, 1983.
20. Wang JS, Tseng CH: Changes in pulmonary mechanics and gas exchange after thoracentesis on patients with inversion of a hemidiaphragm secondary to large pleural effusion. Chest 107:1610, 1995.
21. Brandstetter RD, Cohen RP: Hypoxemia after thoracentesis. A predictable and treatable condition. JAMA 242:1060, 1979.
22. Sokolowski JW, Burgher LW, Jones FL Jr, et al: American Thoracic Society: Guidelines for thoracentesis and needle biopsy of the pleura. Am Rev Respir Dis 140:257, 1989.
23. Light RW, MacGregor MI, Luchsinger PC, et al: Pleural effusions: The diagnostic separation of transudates and exudates. Ann Intern Med 77:507, 1972.
24. Vives M, Porcel JM, Vicenta de Vara C, et al: A study of Light's criteria and possible modifications for distinguishing exudative from transudative pleural effusions. Chest 109:1503, 1996.
25. Roth BJ, O'Meara TF, Cragun WH: The serum-effusion albumin gradient in the evaluation of pleural effusions. Chest 98:546, 1990.
26. Meisel S, Shamiss A, Thaler M, et al: Pleural fluid to serum bilirubin concentration ratio for the separation of transudates from exudates. Chest 98:141, 1990.
27. Hamm H, Brohan U, Bohmer R, et al: Cholesterol in pleural effusions. Chest 92:296, 1987.
28. Valdes L, Pose A, Suarez J, et al: Cholesterol: A useful parameter for distinguishing between pleural exudates and transudates. Chest 99:1097, 1991.
29. Burgess LJ, Maritz FJ, Taljaard JJF: Comparative analysis of the biochemical parameters used to distinguish between pleural transudates and exudates. Chest 107:1604, 1995.
30. Costa M, Quiroga T, Cruz E: Measurement of pleural fluid cholesterol and lactate dehydrogenase. Chest 108:1260, 1995.
31. Garcia-Pachhon E, Padilla-Navas I, Sanchez JF, et al: Pleural fluid to serum cholinesterase ratio for the separation of transudates and exudates. Chest 110:97, 1996.
32. Heffner JE, Brown LK, Barbieri CA, et al: Diagnostic value of tests that discriminate between exudative and transudative pleural effusions. Chest 11:970, 1997.
33. Antony VB, Holm KA: Testing the waters: Differentiating transudates from exudates. Chest 108:1191, 1995.
34. Light RW, Ball WC Jr: Glucose and amylase in pleural effusions. JAMA 225:257, 1973.
35. Glenert: Sugar levels in pleural effusions of different etiologies. Acta Tuberc Scand 42:222, 1962.
36. Barber LM, Mazzadi L, Deakins DD, et al: Glucose level in pleural fluid as a diagnostic aid. Dis Chest 31:680, 1957.
37. Carr DT, Mayne JG: Pleurisy with effusion in rheumatoid arthritis, with reference to the low concentration of glucose in pleural fluid. Am Rev Respir Dis 85:345, 1962.
38. Berger HW, Maher G: Decreased glucose concentration in malignant pleural effusions. Am Rev Respir Dis 103:427, 1971.
39. Good JT Jr, Taryle DA, Maulitz RM, et al: The diagnostic value of pleural fluid pH. Chest 78:55, 1980.
40. Funahashi A, Sarkar TK, Kory RC: Measurements of respiratory gases and pH of pleural fluid. Am Rev Respir Dis 108:1266, 1973.
41. Hammarsten JF, Honska WL Jr, Limes BJ: Pleural fluid amylase in pancreatitis and other diseases. Am Rev Respir Dis 79:606, 1959.
42. Kaye MD: Pleuropulmonary complications of pancreatitis. Thorax 23:297, 1968.
43. Abbott OA, Mansour KA, Logan WD Jr, et al: Atraumatic so-called "spontaneous" rupture of the esophagus. A review of 47 personal cases with comments on a new method of surgical therapy. J Thorac Cardiovasc Surg 59:67, 1970.
44. Sherr HP, Light RW, Merson MH, et al: Origin of pleural fluid amylase in esophageal rupture. Ann Intern Med 76:985, 1972.
45. Roy PH, Carr DT, Payne WS: The problem of chylothorax. Mayo Clin Proc 42:457, 1967.
46. Hunder GG, McDuffie FC, Hepper NGG: Pleural fluid complement in systemic lupus erythematosus and rheumatoid arthritis. Ann Intern Med 76:357, 1972.
47. Tacquet A, Biserte F, Havez R, et al: Biochemical criteria in the diagnosis of pleural mesothelioma. Lille Med 10:146, 1965.
48. Harington JS, Wagner JC, Smith M: The detection of hyaluronic acid in pleural fluids of cases with diffuse pleural mesotheliomas. Br J Exp Pathol 44:81, 1963.
49. Klockars M, Pettersson T, Riska H, et al: Pleural fluid lysozyme in human disease. Arch Intern Med 139:73, 1979.
50. Collins TR, Sahn SA: Thoracentesis: Clinical value, complications, technical problems, and patient experience. Chest 91:817, 1987.
51. Black LF: Pleural effusions. Mayo Clin Proc 56:201, 1981.
52. Storey DD, Dines DE, Coles DT: Pleural effusion. A diagnostic dilemma. JAMA 236:2183, 1976.
53. Gunnels JJ: Perplexing pleural effusion. Chest 74:390, 1978.
54. Hirsch A, Ruffie P, Nebut M, et al: Pleural effusion: Laboratory tests in 300 cases. Thorax 34:106, 1979.
55. Ryan CJ, Rodgers RF, Unni KK, et al: The outcome of patients with pleural effusion of indeterminate cause at thoracotomy. Mayo Clin Proc 56:145, 1981.
56. Bartter T, Santarelli R, Akers SM, et al: The evaluation of pleural effusion. Chest 106:1209, 1994.
57. Ferrer JS, Munoz XG, Orriols RM, et al: Evolution of idiopathic pleural effusions. Chest 109:1508, 1996.
58. Black LF: The pleural space and pleural fluid. Mayo Clin Proc 47:493, 1972.
59. Okada Y, Ichinose Y, Yamaguchi K, et al: *Mycobacterium avium-intracellulare* pleuritis with massive pleural effusion. Eur Respir J 8:1428, 1995.
60. Igari H, Kikuchi N: Nontuberculous mycobacterium pulmonary infection with pleural effusion caused by *Mycobacterium kansasii*. Kekkaku 68:527, 1993.
61. Sinzobahamvya N, Bhakta HP: Pleural exudate in a tropical hospital. Eur Respir J 2:145, 1989.
62. Valdes L, Alvarez D, Valle JM, et al: The etiology of pleural effusions in an area with high incidence of tuberculosis. Chest 109:158, 1996.
63. Mteta KA: Thoracic empyema in Dar es Salaam, Tanzania. East Afr Med J 71:684, 1994.
64. Batungwanayo J, Taelman H, Allen S, et al: Pleural effusion, tuberculosis and HIV-1 infection in Kigali, Rwanda. AIDS 7:73, 1993.
65. Elliott AM, Halwiindi B, Hayes RJ, et al: The impact of human immunodeficiency virus on presentation and diagnosis of tuberculosis in a cohort study in Zambia. J Trop Med Hyg 96:1, 1993.
66. Richter C, Perenboom R, Swai AB, et al: Diagnosis of tuberculosis in patients with pleural effusion in an area of HIV infection and limited diagnostic facilities. Trop Geogr Med 46:293, 1994.
67. al-Quorain A, Larbi EB, Satti MB, et al: Tuberculous pleural effusion in the eastern province of Saudi Arabia. Trop Geogr Med 46:298, 1994.
68. Menzies R, Charbonneau M: Thoracoscopy for the diagnosis of pleural disease. Ann Intern Med 114:271, 1991.
69. Marel M, Stastny B, Melinová L, et al: Diagnosis of pleural effusions. Chest 107:1598, 1995.
70. Sahn SA: The pleura. Am Rev Respir Dis 138:184, 1988.
70a. Bouros D, Demoilipoulos J, Panagou P, et al: Incidence of tuberculosis in Greek armed forces from 1965–1993. Respiration 62:336, 1995.
71. Ellner JJ, Barnes PF, Wallis RS, et al: The immunology of tuberculous pleurisy. Semin Respir Infec 3:335, 1988.
72. Seibert AF, Haynes J Jr, Middleton R, et al: Tuberculous pleural effusion. Chest 99:883, 1991.
73. Stead WW, Eichenholz A, Stauss HK: Operative and pathologic findings in twenty-four patients with syndrome of idiopathic pleurisy with effusion, presumably tuberculous. Am Rev Respir Dis 71:473, 1955.
74. Light RW: Pleural Diseases. Philadelphia, Lea & Febiger, 1983.
75. Hulnick DH, Naidich DP, McCauley DI: Pleural tuberculosis evaluated by computed tomography. Radiology 149:759, 1983.
76. Ellner JJ: Pleural fluid and peripheral blood lymphocyte function in tuberculosis. Ann Intern Med 89:932, 1978.
77. Shimokata K, Kawachi H, Kishimoto H, et al: Local cellular immunity in tuberculous pleurisy. Am Rev Respir Dis 126:822, 1982.
78. Fujiwara H, Tsuyuguchi I: Frequency of tuberculin-reactive T-lymphocytes in

pleural fluid and blood from patients with tuberculous pleurisy. Chest 89:530, 1986.

79. Lorgat F, Keraan MM, Ress SR: Cellular immunity in tuberculous pleural effusions: Evidence of spontaneous lymphocyte proliferation and antigen-specific accelerated responses to purified protein derivative. Clin Exp Immunol 90:215, 1992.

80. Shimokata K, Saka H, Murate T, et al: Cytokine content in pleural effusion. Chest 99:1103, 1991.

81. Kurasawa T, Shimokata K: Cooperation between accessory cells and T lymphocytes in patients with tuberculous pleurisy. Chest 100:1046, 1991.

82. Ribera E, Ocāna I, Martinez-Vazquez JM, et al: High level of interferon gamma in tuberculous pleural effusion. Chest 93:308, 1988.

83. Antoiskis D, Amin K, Barnes PF: Pleuritis as a manifestation of reactivation tuberculosis. Am J Med 89:447, 1990.

84. Zhang M, Gately MK, Wang E, et al: Interleukin 12 at the site of disease in tuberculosis. J Clin Invest 93:1733, 1994.

85. Barnes PF, Lu S, Abrams JS, et al: Cytokine production at the site of disease in human tuberculosis. Infect Immun 61:3482, 1993.

86. Yokoyama A, Maruyama M, Ito M, et al: Interleukin 6 activity in pleural effusion. Its diagnostic value and thrombopoietic activity. Chest 102:1055, 1992.

87. Gambon-Deza F, Pacheco CM, Cerda MT, et al: Lymphocyte populations during tuberculosis infection: V beta repertoires. Infect Immun 63:1235, 1995.

88. Levine H, Szanto PB, Cugell DW: Tuberculous pleurisy—an acute illness. Arch Intern Med 122:329, 1968.

89. Korzeniewska-Kosela M, Krysl J, Muller N, et al: Tuberculosis in young adults and the elderly. A prospective comparison study. Chest 106:28, 1994.

90. Sibley JC: A study of 200 cases of tuberculous pleurisy with effusion. Am Rev Tuberc 62:314, 1950.

91. Spieler P: The cytologic diagnosis of tuberculosis in pleural effusions. Acta Cytol 23:374, 1979.

92. Lucivero G, Pierucci G, Bonomo L: Lymphocyte subsets in peripheral blood and pleural fluid. Eur Respir J 1:337, 1988.

93. Pettersson T, Klockars M, Hellström PE, et al: T and B lymphocytes in pleural effusions. Chest 73:49, 1978.

94. Okubo Y, Nakata M, Kuroiwa Y, et al: NK cells in carcinomatous and tuberculous pleurisy. Phenotypic and functional analyses of NK cells in peripheral blood and pleural effusion. Chest 92:500, 1987.

95. Hurwitz S, Leiman G, Shapiro C: Mesothelial cells in pleural fluid: TB or not TB? S Afr Med J 57:937, 1980.

96. Guzman J, Costabel U, Bross KJ, et al: Macrophage size determinations in the diagnosis of tuberculous effusions. Anal Quant Cytol Histol 10:371, 1988.

97. Lau KY: Numerous mesothelial cells in tuberculous pleural effusions. Chest 96:438, 1989.

98. Dodson WH, Hollingsworth JW: Pleural effusion in rheumatoid arthritis. Impaired transport of glucose. N Engl J Med 275:1337, 1966.

99. Klockars M, Pettersson T, Riska H, et al: Pleural fluid lysozyme in tuberculous and non-tuberculous pleurisy. BMJ 1:1381, 1976.

100. Piras MA, Gakis C, Budroni M, et al: Adenosine deaminase activity in pleural effusions: An aid to differential diagnosis. BMJ 2:1751, 1978.

101. Pettersson T, Ojala K, Weber TH: Adenosine deaminase in the diagnosis of pleural effusions. Acta Med Scand 215:299, 1984.

102. Bānales JL, Pineda PR, Fitzgerald M, et al: Adenosine deaminase in the diagnosis of tuberculous pleural effusions. Chest 99:355, 1991.

103. Burgess LJ, Maritz FJ, Le Roux I, et al: Use of adenosine deaminase as a diagnostic tool for tuberculous pleurisy. Thorax 50:672, 1995.

104. Valdes L, Alvarez D, San Jose E, et al: Value of adenosine deaminase in the diagnosis of tuberculous pleural effusions in young patients in a region of high prevalence of tuberculosis. Thorax 50:600, 1995.

105. Valdes L, San Jose E, Alvarez D, et al: Diagnosis of tuberculous pleurisy using the biologic parameters adenosine deaminase, lysozyme, and interferon gamma. Chest 103:458, 1993.

106. Pettersson T, Nyberg P, Norstrom D, et al: Similar pleural fluid findings in pleuropulmonary tularemia and tuberculous pleurisy. Chest 109:572, 1996.

107. Burgess LJ, Maritz FJ, Le Roux I, et al: Combined use of pleural adenosine deaminase with lymphocyte/neutrophil ratio. Increased specificity for the diagnosis of tuberculous pleuritis. Chest 109:414, 1996.

108. Očana I, Ribera E, Martinez-Vázquez JM, et al: Adenosine deaminase activity in rheumatoid pleural effusion. Ann Rheum Dis 47:394, 1988.

109. Fontan Bueso J, Verea Hernando H, Garcia-Buela JP, et al: Diagnostic value of simultaneous determination of pleural adenosine deaminase and pleural lysozyme/serum lysozyme ratio in pleural effusions. Chest 93:303, 1988.

110. Villena V, Navarro-Gonzalvez JA, Garcia-Benayas C, et al: Rapid automated determination of adenosine deaminase and lysozyme for differentiating tuberculous and nontuberculous pleural effusions. Clin Chem 42:218, 1996.

111. De Oliveira HG, Rossatto ER, Prolla JC: Pleural fluid adenosine deaminase and lymphocyte proportion: Clinical usefulness in the diagnosis of tuberculosis. Cytopathology 5:27, 1994.

112. Bandres Gimeno R, Abal Arca J, Blanco Perez J, et al: Adenosine deaminase activity in the pleural effusion. A study of 64 cases. Arch Bronconeumol 30:8, 1994.

113. Villena V, Lopez-Encuentra A, Echave-Sustaeta J, et al: Interferon-gamma in 388 immunocompromised and immunocompetent patients for diagnosing pleural tuberculosis. Eur Respir J 9:2635, 1996.

114. Soderblom T, Nyberg P, Teppo AM, et al: Pleural fluid interferon-gamma and tumour necrosis factor-alpha in tuberculous and rheumatoid pleurisy. Eur Respir J 9:1652, 1996.

115. Orphanidou D, Gaga M, Rasidakis A, et al: Tumour necrosis factor, interleukin-1 and adenosine deaminase in tuberculous pleural effusion. Respir Med 90:95, 1996.

116. Levine H, Metzger W, Lacera D, et al: Diagnosis of tuberculous pleurisy by culture of pleural biopsy specimen. Arch Intern Med 126:269, 1970.

117. Mueller PR, Saini S, Simeone JF, et al: Image-guided pleural biopsies: Indications, technique, and results in 23 patients. Radiology 169:1, 1988.

118. Scerbo J, Keltz H, Stone DJ: A prospective study of closed pleural biopsies. JAMA 218:377, 1971.

119. Kirsch CM, Kroe M, Azzi RL, et al: The optimal number of pleural biopsy specimens for a diagnosis of tuberculous pleurisy. Chest 112:702, 1997.

120. de Lassence A, Lecossier D, Pierre C, et al: Detection of mycobacterial DNA in pleural fluid from patients with tuberculous pleurisy by means of the polymerase chain reaction: Comparison of two protocols. Thorax 47:265, 1992.

121. de Wit D, Maartens G, Steyn L: A comparative study of the polymerase chain reaction and conventional procedures for the diagnosis of tuberculous pleural effusion. Tuber Lung Dis 73:262, 1992.

122. Querol JM, Minguez J, Garcia-Sanchez E, et al: Rapid diagnosis of pleural tuberculosis by polymerase chain reaction. Am J Respir Crit Care Med 152:1977, 1995.

123. Hayashi M, Nagai A, Kobayashi K, et al: Utility of polymerase chain reaction for diagnosis of tuberculous pleural effusion. Nippon Kyobu Shikkan Gakkai Zasshi 33:253, 1995.

124. Shi HZ, Li CQ, Long XM: Polymerase chain reaction for the diagnosis of tuberculous pleural effusion. Chung Hua Chieh Ho Ho Hu Hsi Tsa Chih 17:286, 1994.

125. Murate T, Mizoguchi K, Amano H, et al: Antipurified-protein-derivative antibody in tuberculous pleural effusions. Chest 97:670, 1990.

126. Gupta S, Kumari S, Banwalikar JN, et al: Diagnostic utility of the estimation of mycobacterial antigen A60 specific immunoglobulins IgM, IgA and IgC in the sera of cases of adult human tuberculosis. Tuber Lung Dis 76:418, 1995.

127. Caminero JA, Rodriguez de Castro F, Carrillo T, et al: Diagnosis of pleural tuberculosis by detection of specific IgG anti-antigen 60 in serum and pleural fluid. Respiration 60:58, 1993.

128. Baganha MF, Mota-Pinto A, Pego MA, et al: Neopterin in tuberculous and neoplastic pleural fluids. Lung 170:155, 1992.

129. Yang SZ, Ji SQ: Serum and pleural fluid levels of CA50 in malignant and tuberculous effusions. Respir Med 88:27, 1994.

130. Mestitz P, Pollard AC: The diagnosis of tuberculosis pleural effusion. Br J Dis Chest 53:86, 1959.

131. Roper WH, Waring JJ: Primary serofibrinous pleural effusion in military personnel. Am Rev Respir Dis 71:616, 1955.

132. Bartlett JG: Bacterial infections of the pleural space. Semin Respir Infec 3:308, 1988.

133. Sahn SA: Management of complicated parapneumonic effusions. Am Rev Respir Dis 148:813, 1993.

134. Light RW: A new classification of parapneumonic effusions and empyema. Chest 108:299, 1995.

135. Wells FC: Empyema thoracis: What is the role of surgery? Respir Med 84:97, 1990.

136. Berger HA, Morganroth ML: Immediate drainage is not required for all patients with complicated parapneumonic effusions. Chest 97:731, 1990.

137. Light RW: Management of parapneumonic effusions. Arch Intern Med 141:1339, 1981.

138. Light RW, Girard WM, Jenkinson SG, et al: Parapneumonic effusions. Am J Med 69:507, 1980.

139. Vianna NJ: Nontuberculous bacterial empyema in patients with and without underlying diseases. JAMA 215:69, 1971.

140. LeMense GP, Strange C, Sahn SA: Empyema thoracis. Therapeutic management and outcome. Chest 107:1532, 1995.

141. Smith JA, Mullerworth MH, Westlake GW, et al: Empyema thoracis: 14 year experience in a teaching center. Ann Thorac Surg 51:39, 1991.

142. Ali I, Unruh H: Management of empyema thoracis. Ann Thorac Surg 50:355, 1990.

143. Alfageme I, Mūnoz F, Pēna N, et al: Empyema of the thorax in adults. Etiology, microbiologic findings and management. Chest 103:839, 1993.

144. Steenhuis LH, Tjon A, Tham RT, et al: Bochdalek hernia: A rare cause of pleural empyema. Eur Respir J 7:204, 1994.

145. Braman SS, Donat WE: Explosive pleuritis. Manifestations of group A beta-hemolytic streptococcal infection. Am J Med 81:723, 1986.

146. Bennett MR, Fiehler PC, Weinbaum DL: Occult pneumococcal bacteremia and empyema without preceding pulmonary parenchymal involvement. South Med J 80:774, 1987.

147. Streifler J, Pitlik S, Dux S, et al: Spontaneous bacterial pleuritis in a patient with cirrhosis. Respiration 46:382, 1984.

148. Broaddus VC, Hébert CA, Vitangcol RV, et al: Interleukin-8 is a major chemotactic factor in pleural liquid of patients with empyema. Am Rev Respir Dis 146:825, 1992.

149. Antony VB, Hott JW, Kunkel SL, et al: Pleural mesothelial cell expression of C-C (monocyte chemotactic peptide) and C-X-C (interleukin 8) chemokines. Am J Respir Cell Mol Biol 12:581, 1995.

149a. Marie C, Losser M-R, Fitting C, et al: Cytokines and soluble cytokine receptors in pleural effusions from septic and nonseptic patients. Am J Respir Crit Care Med 156:1515, 1997.

149b. Mohammed KA, Nasreen N, Ward MJ, et al: Macrophage inflammatory protein-

1 alpha C-C chemokine in parapneumonic pleural effusions. J Lab Clin Med 132:202, 1998.

149c. Segura RM, Alegre J, Varela E, et al: Interleukin-8 and markers of neutrophil degranulation in pleural effusions. Am J Respir Crit Care Med 157:1565, 1998.

150. Borge JH, Michavila IA, Mendez JM, et al: Thoracic empyema in HIV-infected patients. Chest 113:732, 1998.

151. Delikaris PG, Conlan AA, Abramor E, et al: Empyema thoracis: A prospective study on 73 patients. S Afr Med J 65:47, 1984.

152. Mavroudis C, Symmonds JB, Minagi H, et al: Improved survival in management of empyema thoracis. J Thorac Cardiovasc Surg 82:49, 1981.

153. Varkey B, Rose HD, Kutty CPK, et al: Empyema thoracis during a 10-year period: Analysis of 72 cases and comparison to a previous study (1952 to 1967). Arch Intern Med 141:1771, 1981.

154. Caplan ES, Hoyt NJ, Rodriguez A, et al: Empyema occurring in the multiple traumatized patient. J Trauma 24:785, 1984.

155. Bartlett JG, Gorbach SL, Thadepalli H, et al: Bacteriology of empyema. Lancet 1:338, 1974.

156. Cham CW, Haq SM, Rahamim J: Empyema thoracis: A problem with late referral? Thorax 48:925, 1993.

157. Hughes CE, Van Scoy RE: Antibiotic therapy of pleural empyema. Semin Respir Infec 6:94, 1991.

158. Brook I, Frazier EH: Aerobic and anaerobic microbiology of empyema. A retrospective review in two military hospitals. Chest 103:1502, 1993.

159. Ashbaugh DG: Empyema thoracis. Factors influencing morbidity and mortality. Chest 99:1162, 1991.

160. Brewin A, Arango L, Hadley WK, et al: High-dose penicillin therapy and pneumococcal pneumonia. JAMA 230:409, 1974.

161. Welch CC, Tombridge TL, Baker WJ, et al: Beta-hemolytic streptococcal pneumonia: Report of an outbreak in a military population. Am J Med Sci 242:157, 1961.

162. Gil Suay V, Cordero PJ, Martinez E, et al: Parapneumonia effusions secondary to community-acquired bacterial pneumonia in human immunodeficiency virus–infected patients. Eur Respir J 8:1934, 1995.

163. Hendren WH III, Haggerty RJ: Staphylococcal pneumonia in infancy and childhood: Analysis of seventy-five cases. JAMA 168:6, 1958.

164. Dines DE: Diagnostic significance of pneumatocele of the lung. JAMA 204:1169, 1968.

165. Meyers HI, Jacobsen G: Staphylococcal pneumonia in children and adults. Radiology 72:665, 1959.

166. Schultze G: Unusual roentgen manifestations of primary staphylococcal pneumonia in infants and young children. Am J Roentgenol 81:290, 1959.

167. Huxtable KA, Tucker AS, Wedgwood RJ: Staphylococcal pneumonia in childhood. Long-term follow-up. Am J Dis Child 108:262, 1964.

168. McLaughlin FJ, Goldmann DA, Rosenbaum DM, et al: Empyema in children: Clinical course and long-term follow-up. Pediatrics 73:587, 1984.

169. Fajardo JE, Chang MJ: Pleural empyema in children: A nationwide retrospective study. South Med J 80:593, 1987.

170. Wallace RJ Jr, Musher DM, Martin RR: *Haemophilus influenzae* pneumonia in adults. Am J Med 64:87, 1978.

171. Berk SL, Holtsclaw SA, Wiener SL, et al: Nontypeable *Haemophilus influenzae* in the elderly. Arch Intern Med 134:537, 1982.

172. Stratton CW, Hawley HB, Horsman TA, et al: *Haemophilus influenzae* pneumonia in adults: Report of five cases caused by ampicillin-resistant strains. Am Rev Respir Dis 121:595, 1980.

173. Steinhauer BW, Eickhoff TC, Kislak JW, et al: The *Klebsiella-Enterobacter-Serratia* division: Clinical and epidemiologic characteristics. Ann Intern Med 65:1180, 1966.

174. Moon WK, Im JG, Yeol KM, et al: Complications of *Klebsiella* pneumonia: CT evaluation. J Comput Assist Tomogr 19:176, 1995.

175. Tillotson JR, Lerner AM: Pneumonias caused by gram-negative bacilli. Medicine 45:65, 1966.

176. Unger JD, Rose HD, Unger GF: Gram-negative pneumonia. Radiology 107:283, 1973.

177. Tillotson JR, Lerner AM: Characteristics of pneumonias caused by *Escherichia coli.* N Engl J Med 277:115, 1967.

178. Iannini PB, Claffey T, Quintiliani R: Bacteremic *Pseudomonas* pneumonia. JAMA 230:558, 1974.

179. Miller RP, Bates JH: Pleuropulmonary tularemia. A review of 29 patients. Am Rev Respir Dis 99:31, 1969.

180. Overholt EL, Tigertt WD: Roentgenographic manifestations of pulmonary tularemia. Radiology 74:758, 1960.

181. Dennis JM, Boudreau RP: Pleuropulmonary tularemia: Its roentgen manifestations. Radiology 68:25, 1957.

182. Ivie JM: Roentgenological observations on pleuropulmonary tularemia. Am J Roentgenol 74:466, 1955.

183. Pine JR, Hollman JL: Elevated pleural fluid pH in *Proteus mirabilis* empyema. Chest 84:109, 1983.

184. Swartz MN: Clinical aspects of legionnaires' disease. Ann Intern Med 90:492, 1979.

185. Kirby BD, Snyder KM, Meyer RD, et al: Legionnaires' disease: Report of sixty-five nosocomially acquired cases and review of the literature. Medicine 59:188, 1980.

186. Kroboth FJ, Yu VL, Reddy SC, et al: Clinicoradiographic correlation with the extent of legionnaires' disease. Am J Roentgenol 141:263, 1983.

187. Torrus Tendero D, Gutierrez Fernandez J, Diez Ruiz A, et al: Pleuropericarditis

as the only manifestation of *Legionella pneumophila* infection. Arch Bronconeumol 31:249, 1995.

188. Weiss W, Eisenberg GM, Flippin HF: *Salmonella* pleuropulmonary disease. Am J Med Sci 233:487, 1957.

189. Hahne OH: Lung abscess due to *Salmonella typhi.* Am Rev Respir Dis 89:566, 1964.

190. García-Rodriguez JA, García-Sanchez JE, Muñoz Bellido JL, et al: Review of pulmonary brucellosis: A case report on brucellar pulmonary empyema. Diagn Microbiol Infect Dis 11:53, 1988.

191. Papiris SA, Maniati MA, Haritou A, et al: Brucella haemorrhagic pleural effusion. Eur Respir J 7:1369, 1994.

192. Kerem E, Diav O, Navon P, et al: Pleural fluid characteristics in pulmonary brucellosis. Thorax 49:89, 1994.

193. Isobe H, Motomura K, Kotou K, et al: Spontaneous bacterial empyema and peritonitis caused by *Morganella morganii.* J Clin Gastroenterol 18:87, 1994.

194. Clarridge J, Roberts C, Peters J, et al: Sepsis and empyema caused by *Yersinia enterocolitica.* J Clin Microbiol 17:936, 1983.

195. Nadir A, Wright HI, Nadir F, et al: *Campylobacter fetus* presenting as a septic pleural effusion: A case report. J Okla State Med Assoc 87:267, 1994.

196. Whitman BW, Krafte-Jacobs B: Cat-scratch disease associated with pleural effusions and encephalopathy in a child. Respiration 62:171, 1995.

197. Hood S, Liddel G, Baxter RH: *Listeria monocytogenes:* A rare cause of pleural effusion in a patient with congestive heart failure. Scott Med J 42:18, 1997.

197a. Jerng J-S, Hsueh P-R, Teng L-J, et al: Empyema thoracis and lung abscess caused by viridans streptococci. Am J Respir Crit Care Med 156:1508, 1997.

198. Pollock JJ: Pleuropulmonary Whipple's disease. South Med J 78:216, 1985.

199. Coonrod JD, Wilson HD: Etiologic diagnosis of intrapleural empyema by counterimmunoelectrophoresis. Am Rev Respir Dis 113:637, 1976.

200. Boersma WG, Lowenberg A, Holloway Y, et al: Rapid detection of pneumococcal antigen in pleural fluid of patients with community acquired pneumonia. Thorax 48:160, 1993.

201. Jones FL Jr, Blodgett RC Jr: Empyema in rheumatic pleuropulmonary disease. Ann Intern Med 74:665, 1971.

202. Sahn SA, Lakshminarayan S, Char DC: "Silent" empyema in patients receiving corticosteroids. Am Rev Respir Dis 107:873, 1973.

203. Jess P, Brynitz S, Friis Møller A: Mortality in thoracic empyema. Scand J Thorac Cardiovasc Surg 18:85, 1984.

204. Muskett A, Burton NA, Karwande SV, et al: Management of refractory empyema with early decortication. Am J Surg 156:529, 1988.

205. Forty J, Yeatman M, Wells FC: Empyema thoracis: A review of a 4½ year experience of cases requiring surgical treatment. Respir Med 84:147, 1990.

206. Pothula V, Krellenstein DJ: Early aggressive surgical management of parapneumonic empyemas. Chest 105:832, 1994.

207. LeBlanc KA, Tucker WY: Empyema of the thorax. Surg Gynecol Obstet 158:66, 1984.

208. Wehr CJ, Adkins RB Jr: Empyema thoracis: A ten-year experience. South Med J 79:171, 1986.

209. Mayo P: Early thoracotomy and decortication for nontuberculous empyema in adults with and without underlying disease. A twenty-five year review. Am Surg 51:230, 1985.

210. Himelman RB, Callen PW: The prognostic value of loculations in parapneumonic pleural effusions. Chest 90:852, 1986.

211. Lew PD, Perrin LH, Waldvogel FA, et al: Loculated pleural empyema: Identification of complement breakdown products in contiguous sterile pleural fluid. Scand J Infect Dis 14:225, 1982.

212. Hoover EL, Hsu HK, Ross MJ, et al: Reappraisal of empyema thoracis. Surgical intervention when the duration of illness is unknown. Chest 90:511, 1986.

213. Iioka S, Sawamura K, Mori T, et al: Surgical treatment of chronic empyema. A new one-stage operation. J Thorac Cardiovasc Surg 90:179, 1985.

214. Strange C, Sahn SA: The clinician's perspective on parapneumonic effusions and empyema. Chest 103:259, 1993.

215. Henke CA, Leatherman JW: Intrapleurally administered streptokinase in the treatment of acute loculated nonpurulent parapneumonic effusions. Am Rev Respir Dis 145:680, 1992.

216. Pollak JS, Passik CS: Intrapleural urokinase in the treatment of loculated pleural effusions. Chest 105:868, 1994.

217. Orringer MB: Thoracic empyema—back to basics. Chest 93:901, 1988.

218. Poe RH, Marin MG, Israel RH, et al: Utility of pleural fluid analysis in predicting tube thoracostomy/decortication in parapneumonic effusion. Chest 100:963, 1991.

219. Heffner JE, Brown LK, Barbieri C, et al: Pleural fluid chemical analysis in parapneumonic effusions. Am J Respir Crit Care Med 151:1700, 1995.

220. Silva-Mejias C, Gamboa-Anttinolo F, Lopez-Cortes LF, et al: Interleukin-1β in pleural fluids of different etiologies. Chest 108:942, 1995.

221. Murray JF, Finegold SM, Froman S, et al: The changing spectrum of nocardiosis. A review and presentation of nine cases. Am Rev Respir Dis 83:315, 1961.

222. Flynn MW, Felson B: The roentgen manifestations of thoracic actinomycosis. Am J Roentgenol 110:707, 1970.

223. Harvey JC, Cantrell JR, Fisher AM: Actinomycosis: Its recognition and treatment. Ann Intern Med 46:868, 1957.

224. Coodley EL, Yoshinaka R: Pleural effusion as the major manifestation of actinomycosis. Chest 106:1615, 1994.

225. Neu HC, Silva M, Hazen E, et al: Necrotizing nocardial pneumonitis. Ann Intern Med 66:274, 1967.

226. Curry FJ, Wier JA: Histoplasmosis: A review of one hundred consecutively hospitalized patients. Am Rev Tuberc 77:749, 1958.

227. Lonky SA, Catanzaro A, Moser KM, et al: Acute coccidioidal pleural effusion. Am Rev Respir Dis 114:681, 1976.
228. Arora NS, Oblinger MJ, Feldman PS: Chronic pleural blastomycosis with hyperprolactinemia, galactorrhea, and amenorrhea. Am Rev Respir Dis 120:451, 1979.
229. Young EJ, Hirsh DD, Fainstein V, et al: Pleural effusions due to *Cryptococcus neoformans*: A review of the literature and report of two cases with cryptococcal antigen determinations. Am Rev Respir Dis 121:743, 1980.
229a. Fukuchi M, Mizushima Y, Kobayashi M: Cryptococcal pleural effusion in a patient receiving long-term corticosteroid therapy for rheumatoid arthritis. Int Med 37:534, 1998.
230. Failla PJ, Cerise FP, Karam GH, et al: Blastomycosis: Pulmonary and pleural manifestations. South Med J 88:405, 1995.
231. Mauri M, Fernandez Sola A, Capdevila JA, et al: Pleural cryptococcosis in patients with human immunodeficiency virus infection. Med Clin 106:380, 1996.
232. Friedman EP, Miller RF, Severn A, et al: Cryptococcal pneumonia in patients with the acquired immunodeficiency syndrome. Clin Radiol 50:756, 1995.
233. Garcia Garcia JC, Baloira Villar A, Anibarro Garcia L, et al: Pleural effusion as the only manifestation of cryptococcosis in an AIDS patient. Arch Bronconeumol 30:166, 1994.
234. de Lalla F, Vaglia A, Franzetti M, et al: Cryptococcal pleural effusion as first indictor of AIDS: A case report. Infection 21:192, 1993.
235. Case records of the Massachusetts General Hospital. Weekly clinicopathological exercises. Case 38–1983. Empyema 40 years after a thoracoplasty. N Engl J Med 309:715, 1983.
236. Monod O, Dieudonné P, Tardieu P: Les aspergilloses pulmonaires post-opératoires. (Postoperative pulmonary aspergillosis.) J Fr Med Chir Thorac 18:579, 1964.
237. Meredith HC, Corgan BM, McLaulin B: Pleural aspergillosis. Am J Roentgenol 130:164, 1978.
238. Sawasaki H, Horie K, Yamada M, et al: Bronchial stump aspergillosis. Experimental and clinical study. J Thorac Cardiovasc Surg 58:198, 1969.
239. Parry MF, Coughlin FR, Zambetti FX: *Aspergillus* empyema. Chest 81:768, 1982.
240. Desselle BC, Bozeman PM, Patrick CC: Diagnostic utility of thoracentesis for neutropenic children with cancer. Clin Infect Dis 21:887, 1995.
241. Lambert RS, George RB: Fungal disease of the pleura: Clinical manifestations, diagnosis, and treatment. Semin Respir Infec 3:343, 1988.
242. Jamadar DA, Kazerooni EA, Daly BD, et al: Pulmonary zygomycosis: CT appearance. J Comput Assist Tomogr 19:733, 1995.
243. Schaumberg TH, Schnapp LM, Taylor KG, et al: Diagnosis of *Pneumocystis carinii* infection in HIV-seropositive patients by identification of *P. carinii* in pleural fluid. Chest 103:1890, 1993.
244. Horowitz ML, Schiff M, Samuels J, et al: *Pneumocystis carinii* pleural effusion. Pathogenesis and pleural fluid analysis. Am Rev Respir Dis 148:232, 1993.
245. George RB, Ziskind M, Rasch JR, et al: *Mycoplasma* and adenovirus pneumonias. Comparison with other atypical pneumonias in a military population. Ann Intern Med 65:931, 1966.
246. Rytel MW: Primary atypical pneumonia: Current concepts. Am J Med Sci 247:84, 1964.
247. Rosmus HH, Paré JAP, Masson AM, et al: Roentgenographic patterns of acute *Mycoplasma* and viral pneumonitis. J Can Assoc Radiol 19:74, 1968.
248. Fine NL, Smith LR, Sheedy PF: Frequency of pleural effusions in *Mycoplasma* and viral pneumonias. N Engl J Med 283:790, 1970.
249. Lambert HP: *Mycoplasma pneumoniae* infections. J Clin Pathol 21(Suppl 2):52, 1968.
250. Putnam CE, Curtis AM, Simeone JF, et al: *Mycoplasma* pneumonia. Clinical and roentgenographic patterns. Am J Roentgenol 124:417, 1975.
251. Proby CM, Hackett D, Gupta S, et al: Acute myopericarditis in influenza A infection. Q J Med 60:887, 1986.
252. Lander P, Palayew MJ: Infectious mononucleosis—a review of chest roentgenographic manifestations. J Can Assoc Radiol 25:303, 1974.
253. Trudo FJ, Gopez EV, Gupta PK, et al: Pleural effusion due to herpes simplex type II infection in an immunocompromised host. Am J Respir Crit Care Med 155:371, 1997.
254. McCormick JB, King IJ, Webb PA, et al: A case-control study of the clinical diagnosis and course of Lassa fever. J Infect Dis 155:445, 1987.
255. Johnson JE III, Perry JE, Fekety FR, et al: Laboratory-acquired Q fever: A report of 50 cases. Am J Med 41:391, 1966.
256. Ramos HS, Hodges RE, Meroney WH: Q fever: Report of a case simulating lymphoma. Ann Intern Med 47:1030, 1957.
257. Murphy PP, Richardson SG: Q fever pneumonia presenting as an eosinophilic pleural effusion. Thorax 44:228, 1989.
258. Gokeirt JG, Beamish WE: Altered reactivity to measles virus in previously vaccinated children. Can Med Assoc J 103:724, 1970.
259. Delahaye RP, Pannier R, Laaban J, et al: Les aspects radiologiques des localisations thoraciques de l'amibase: 17 observations metropolitaines. (Radiologic aspects of thoracic amebiasis: 17 metropolitan observations.) J Radiol Electrol Med Nucl 48:173, 1967.
260. Webster BH: Pleuropulmonary amebiasis. A review with an analysis of ten cases. Am Rev Respir Dis 81:683, 1960.
261. Daniels AC, Childress ME: Pleuropulmonary amebiasis. Calif Med 85:369, 1956.
262. Ochsner A, DeBakey M: Pleuropulmonary complications of amebiasis. An analysis of 153 collected and 15 personal cases. J Thorac Surg 5:225, 1936.
263. Ibarra-Perez C, Selman-Lama M: Diagnosis and treatment of amebic "empyema." Report of eighty-eight cases. Am J Surg 134:283, 1977.
263a. Pachucki CT, Levandowski RA, Brown VA, et al: American paragonimiasis treated with praziquantel. N Engl J Med 311:582, 1984.
264. Ogakwu M, Nwokolo C: Radiological findings in pulmonary paragonimiasis as seen in Nigeria. A review based on one hundred cases. Br J Radiol 46:699, 1973.
265. Im JG, Whang HY, Kim WS, et al: Pleuropulmonary paragonimiasis: Radiologic findings in 71 patients. Am J Roentgenol 159:39, 1992.
265a. Romeo DP, Pollock JJ: Pulmonary paragonimiasis: Diagnostic value of pleural fluid analysis. South Med J 79:241, 1986.
266. Rakower J, Miwidsky H: Hyatid pleural disease. Am Rev Respir Dis 90:623, 1964.
267. Miller MJ, Leith DE, Brooks JR, et al: *Trichomonas* empyema. Thorax 37:384, 1982.
268. Arora VK, Gowrinath K: Pleural effusion due to lymphatic filariasis. Indian J Chest Dis Allied Sci 36:159, 1994.
269. Herry I, Philippe B, Hennequin C, et al: Acute life-threatening toxocaral tamponade. Chest 112:1692, 1997.
270. Jeanfaivre T, Cimon B, Tolstuchow N, et al: Pleural effusion and toxocariasis. Thorax 51:106, 1996.
270a. Goyal SB: Intestinal strongyloidiasis manifesting as eosinophilic pleural effusion. South Med J 91:768, 1998.
271. Uchida K, Sekiguchi S, Doi Y, et al: Pulmonary paragonimiasis with pleural effusion containing *Paragonimus* ova: Sonographical appearance of pleural effusion. Intern Med 34:1178, 1995.
271a. Minh V-D, Engle P, Greenwood JR, et al: Pleural paragonimiasis in a southeast Asian refugee. Am Rev Respir Dis 124:186, 1981.
272. Pancholia AK, Jain SM: Pleural effusion due to dracunculosis. Indian J Chest Dis Allied Sci 27:122, 1985.
272a. Lee YH, Ji JD, Shim JJ, et al: Exudative pleural effusion and pleural leukocytoclastic vasculitis in limited scleroderma. J Rheum 25:1006, 1998.
273. Good JT Jr, King TE, Antony VB, et al: Lupus pleuritis: Clinical features and pleural fluid characteristics with special references to pleural fluid antinuclear antibodies. Chest 84:714, 1983.
274. Bouros D, Panagou P, Papandreou L, et al: Massive bilateral pleural effusion as the only first presentation of systemic lupus erythematosus. Respiration 59:173, 1992.
275. Joseph JJ, Sahn SA: Connective tissue disease and the pleura. Chest 104:262, 1993.
276. Levin DC: Proper interpretation of pulmonary roentgen changes in systemic lupus erythematosus. Am J Roentgenol 111:510, 1971.
277. Winslow WA, Ploss LN, Loitman B: Pleuritis in systemic lupus erythematosus: Its importance as an early manifestation in diagnosis. Ann Intern Med 49:70, 1958
278. Smith PR, Nacht R: Drug-induced lupus pleuritis mimicking pleural space infection. Chest 101:268, 1992.
279. Orens JB, Martinez FJ, Lynch III JP: Pleuropulmonary manifestations of systemic lupus erythematosus. Rheum Dis Clin North Am 20:159, 1994.
280. Naylor B: Cytological aspects of pleural, peritoneal and pericardial fluids from patients with systemic lupus erythematosus. Cytopathology 3:1, 1992.
281. Greis M, Atay Z: Cytomorphologic concomitant reactions in malignant pleural effusions. Pneumologie 1:263, 1990.
282. Khare V, Baethge B, Lang S, et al: Antinuclear antibodies in pleural fluid. Chest 106:866, 1994.
283. Bulgrin JG, Dubois EL, Jacobson G: Chest roentgenographic changes in systemic lupus erythematosus. Radiology 74:42, 1960.
284. Gould DM, Daves ML: A review of roentgen findings in systemic lupus erythematosus (SLE). Am J Med Sci 235:596, 1958.
285. Wiedemann HP, Matthay RA: Pulmonary manifestations of the collagen vascular diseases. Clin Chest Med 10:677, 1989.
286. Ward R: Pleural effusion and rheumatoid disease. Lancet 2:1336, 1961.
287. Carr DT, Mayne JG: Pleurisy with effusion in rheumatoid arthritis, with reference to the low concentration of glucose in pleural fluid. Am Rev Respir Dis 85:345, 1962.
288. Walker WC, Wright V: Rheumatoid pleuritis. Ann Rheum Dis 26:467, 1967.
289. Petty TL, Wilkins M: The five manifestations of rheumatoid lung. Dis Chest 49:75, 1966.
290. Dodson WH, Hollingsworth JW: Pleural effusion in rheumatoid arthritis. Impaired transport of glucose. N Engl J Med 275:1337, 1966.
291. Hakala M, Tiilikainen A, Hameenkorpi R, et al: Rheumatoid arthritis with pleural effusion includes a subgroup with autoimmune features and HLA-B8, Dw3 association. Scand J Rheumatol 15:290, 1986.
292. Lillington GA, Carr DT, Mayne JG: Rheumatoid pleurisy with effusion. Arch Intern Med 128:764, 1971.
293. Grossman LA, Kaplan HJ, Ownby FD, et al: Acute pericarditis: With subsequent clinical rheumatoid arthritis. Arch Intern Med 109:665, 1962.
294. Stengel BF, Watson RA, Darling RJ: Pulmonary rheumatoid nodule with cavitation and chronic lipid effusion. JAMA 198:1263, 1966.
295. Campbell GD, Ferrington E: Rheumatoid pleuritis with effusion. Dis Chest 53:521, 1968.
296. Berger HW, Seckler SG: Pleural and pericardial effusions in rheumatoid disease. Ann Intern Med 64:1291, 1966.
297. Sahn SA, Kaplan RL, Maulitz RM, et al: Rheumatoid pleurisy: Observations on the development of low pleural fluid pH and glucose level. Arch Intern Med 140:1237, 1980.
298. Mays EE: Rheumatoid pleuritis: Observations in eight cases and suggestions for making the diagnosis in patients without the "typical findings." Dis Chest 53:202, 1968.

299. Levine H, Szanto M, Grieble HG, et al: Rheumatoid factor in nonrheumatoid pleural effusions. Ann Intern Med 69:487, 1968.
300. Ganda OB, Caplan HH: Rheumatoid disease without joint involvement. JAMA 228:338, 1974.
301. Hunder GG, McDuffie FC, Hepper NGG: Pleural fluid complement in systemic lupus erythematosus and rheumatoid arthritis. Ann Intern Med 76:357, 1972.
302. Kanok JM, Steinberg P, Cassidy JT, et al: Serum IgE levels in patients with selective IgA deficiency. Ann Allergy 41:220, 1978.
302a. Salomaa E-R, Viander M, Saaresranta T, et al: Complement components and their activation products in pleural fluid. Chest 114:723, 1998.
303. Pleural effusion in rheumatoid arthritis (editorial). Lancet 1:480, 1972.
304. Baim S, Samuelson CO, Ward JR: Rheumatoid arthritis, amyloidosis, and chylous effusions. Arthritis Rheum 22:182, 1979.
305. Pettersson T, Ojala K, Weber TH: Adenosine deaminase in the diagnosis of pleural effusions. Acta Med Scand 215:299, 1984.
306. Pettersson T, Soderblom T, Nyberg P, et al: Pleural fluid soluble interleukin 2 receptor in rheumatoid arthritis and systemic lupus erythematosus. J Rheum 21:1820, 1994.
307. Naylor B: The pathognomonic cytologic picture of rheumatoid pleuritis. The 1989 Maurice Goldblatt Cytology Award Lecture. Acta Cytol 34:465, 1990.
308. Nosanchuk JS, Naylor B: A unique cytologic picture in pleural fluid from patients with rheumatoid arthritis. Am J Clin Pathol 50:330, 1968.
309. Faarup P, Faurschou P: Rheumatoid arthritis cells in experimental pleuritis in mice. Acta Pathol Microbiol Immunol Scand 93:209, 1985.
310. Faurschou P, Faarup P: Granulocytes containing cytoplasmic inclusions in human tuberculous pleuritis. Scand J Respir Dis 54:341, 1973.
311. Pleurisy and rheumatoid arthritis. BMJ 2:1, 1968.
312. Locke CB: Rheumatoid lung. Clin Radiol 14:43, 1963.
313. Lee PR, Sox HC, North FS, et al: Pleurisy with effusion in rheumatoid arthritis. Arch Intern Med 104:634, 1959.
314. Torrington KG: Rapid appearance of rheumatoid pleural effusion. Chest 73:409, 1978.
315. Pritikin JD, Jensen WA, Yenokida GG, et al: Respiratory failure due to a massive rheumatoid pleural effusion. J Rheum 17:673, 1990.
316. Schools GS, Mikkelsen WM: Rheumatoid pleuritis. Arthritis Rheum 5:369, 1962.
317. Jones FL Jr, Blodgett RC Jr: Empyema in rheumatic pleuropulmonary disease. Ann Intern Med 74:665, 1971.
318. Robinson BWS, Musk AW: Benign asbestos pleural effusion: Diagnosis and course. Thorax 36:896, 1981.
319. Epler GR, McCloud TC, Gaensler EA: Prevalence and incidence of benign asbestos pleural effusion in a working population. JAMA 247:617, 1982.
320. Lilis R, Lerman Y, Selikoff IJ: Symptomatic benign pleural effusions among asbestos insulation workers: Residual radiographic abnormalities. Br J Industr Med 45:443, 1988.
321. Martensson G, Hagberg S, Pettersson K, et al: Asbestos pleural effusion: A clinical entity. Thorax 42:646, 1987.
322. Antony VB, Owen CL, Hadley KJ: Pleural mesothelial cells stimulated by asbestos release chemotactic activity for neutrophils in vitro. Am Rev Respir Dis 139:199, 1989.
323. Griffith DE, Miller EJ, Gray LD, et al: Interleukin-1–mediated release of interleukin-8 by asbestos-stimulated human pleural mesothelial cells. Am J Respir Cell Mol Biol 10:245, 1994.
324. Janssen YMW, Marsh JP, Absher MP, et al: Oxidant stress responses in human pleural mesothelial cells exposed to asbestos. Am J Respir Crit Care Med 149:795, 1994.
325. Li XY, Lamb D, Donaldson K: Mesothelial cell injury caused by pleural leukocytes from rats treated with intratracheal instillation of crocidolite asbestos or Corynebacterium parvum. Environ Res 64:181, 1994.
326. Smith KW: Pulmonary disability in asbestos workers. AMA Arch Ind Health 12:198, 1955.
327. Gaenslor EA, Kaplan AI: Asbestos pleural effusion. Am Intern Med 74:178, 1971.
328. Miller A: Chronic pleuritic pain in four patients with asbestos induced pleural fibrosis. Br J Ind Med 47:147, 1990.
329. Robinson BWS, Musk AW: Benign asbestos pleural effusion: Diagnosis and course. Thorax 36:896, 1981.
330. Hillerdal G: Non-malignant asbestos pleural disease. Thorax 36:669, 1981.
331. Smith LS, Schillaci RF: Rounded atelectasis due to acute exudative effusion. Spontaneous resolution. Chest 85:830, 1984.
332. Mysterious pleural effusion (editorial). Lancet 1:1226, 1982.
332a. Antony VB: Drug-induced pleural disease. Clin Chest Med 19:331, 1998.
333. Jurivich DA: Iatrogenic pleural effusions. South Med J 81:1417, 1988.
334. Rinne UK: Pleuropulmonary changes during long-term bromocriptine treatment for Parkinson's disease. Lancet 1:44, 1981.
335. McElvaney NG, Wilcox PG, Churg A, et al: Pleuropulmonary disease during bromocriptine treatment of Parkinson's disease. Arch Intern Med 148:2231, 1988.
336. Kinnunen E, Viljanen A: Pleuropulmonary involvement during bromocriptine treatment. Chest 94:1034, 1988.
337. Gefter WB, Epstein DM, Bonavita JA, et al: Pleural thickening caused by Sansert and Ergotrate in the treatment of migraine. Am J Roentgenol 135:375, 1980.
338. Frans E, Dom R, Demedts M: Pleuropulmonary changes during treatment of Parkinson's disease with a long-acting ergot derivative, cabergoline. Eur Resp J 5:263, 1992.
339. Petusevsky ML, Faling LJ, Rocklin RE, et al: Pleuropericardial reaction to treatment with dantrolene. JAMA 242:2772, 1979.
340. Holmberg L, Boman G, Bottiger LE, et al: Adverse reactions to nitrofurantoin: Analysis of 921 reports. Am J Med 69:733, 1980.
341. Aronchick JM, Gefter WB: Drug-induced pulmonary disorders. Semin Roentgenol 30:18, 1995.
342. Chernow B, Sahn SA: Carcinomatous involvement of the pleura: An analysis of 96 patients. Am J Med 63:695, 1977.
343. Hsu C: Cytologic detection of malignancy in pleural effusion: A review of 5,255 samples from 3,811 patients. Diagn Cytopathol 3:8, 1987.
344. Johnston WW: The malignant pleural effusion. A review of cytopathologic diagnoses of 584 specimens from 472 consecutive patients. Cancer 56:905, 1985.
345. Ruckdeschel JC: Management of malignant pleural effusions. Semin Oncol 22:58, 1995.
346. Vargas FS, Teixeira LR: Pleural malignancies. Curr Opin Pulm Med 2:335, 1996.
347. Meyer PC: Metastatic carcinoma of the pleura. Thorax 21:437, 1966.
348. Rabin CB, Blackman NS: Bilateral pleural effusion. Its significance in association with a heart of normal size. J Mt Sinai Hosp 24:45, 1957.
349. Treatment of malignant effusions (editorial). Lancet 1:198, 1981.
350. Andrews BS, Arora NS, Shadforth MF, et al: The role of immune complexes in the pathogenesis of pleural effusions. Am Rev Respir Dis 124:115, 1981.
351. Kjellberg SI, Dresler CM, Goldberg M: Pleural cytologies in lung cancer without pleural effusions. Ann Thorac Surg 64:941, 1997.
352. Rabinov K, Stein M, Frank H: Tension hydrothorax—an unrecognized danger. Thorax 21:465, 1966.
352a. Subramanyam BR, Raghavendra BN, Lefleur RS: Sonography of the inverted right hemidiaphragm. Am J Roentgenol 136:1004, 1981.
352b. Halvorsen RA, Redyshin PJ, Korobkin M, et al: Ascites or pleural effusion? CT differentiation: Four useful criteria. Radiographics 6:135, 1986.
352c. Müller NL: Imaging of the pleura. Radiology 186:297, 1993.
353. Feinsilver S, Barrows AA, Braman SS: Fiberoptic bronchoscopy and pleural effusion of unknown origin. Chest 90:517, 1986.
354. Poe RH, Levy PC, Israel RH, et al: Use of fiberoptic bronchoscopy in the diagnosis of bronchogenic carcinoma. A study of patients with idiopathic pleural effusions. Chest 105:1663, 1994.
354a. Assi Z, Caruso JL, Herndon J, et al: Cytologically proved malignant pleural effusions. Chest 113:1302, 1998.
355. Chang SC, Perng RP: The role of fiberoptic bronchoscopy in evaluating the causes of pleural effusions. Arch Intern Med 149:855, 1989.
356. Aschi M, Golish J, Eng P, et al: Transudative malignant pleural effusions: Prevalence and mechanisms. South Med J 91:23, 1998.
357. Kuhn M, Fitting JW, Leuenberger P: Probability of malignancy in pleural fluid eosinophilia. Chest 96:992, 1989.
358. Berger HW, Maher G: Decreased glucose concentration in malignant pleural effusions. Am Rev Respir Dis 103:427, 1971.
359. Sahn SA, Good JT Jr: Pleural fluid pH in malignant effusions. Diagnostic, prognostic, and therapeutic implications. Ann Intern Med 108:345, 1988.
360. Rodriguez-Panadero F, Lopez-Mejias J: Survival time of patients with pleural metastatic carcinoma predicted by glucose and pH studies. Chest 95:320, 1989.
361. Radosavljevic G, Nedeljkovic B, Kacar V: Pseudomyxoma of the pleural and peritoneal cavities. Thorax 48:94, 1993.
362. Salyer WR, Eggleston JC, Erozan YS: Efficacy of pleural needle biopsy and pleural fluid cytopathology in the diagnosis of malignant neoplasm involving the pleura. Chest 67:536, 1975.
363. Irani DR, Underwood RD, Johnson EH, et al: Malignant pleural effusions. A clinical cytopathologic study. Arch Intern Med 147:1133, 1987.
364. Falor WH, Ward RM, Brezler MR: Diagnosis of pleural effusions by chromosome analysis. Chest 81:193, 1982.
365. Falor WH, Ward RM, Brezler MR: Diagnosis of pleural effusions by chromosome analysis. Chest 81:193, 1982.
366. Høstmark J, Vigander T, Skaarland E: Characterization of pleural effusions by flow-cytometric DNA analysis. Eur J Respir Dis 66:315, 1985.
367. Huang MS, Tsai MS, Hwang JJ, et al: Comparison of nucleolar organiser regions and DNA flow cytometry in the evaluation of pleural effusion. Thorax 49:1152, 1994.
368. Siri A, Carnemolla B, Raffanti S, et al: Fibronectin concentrations in pleural effusions of patients with malignant and nonmalignant diseases. Cancer Lett 22:1, 1984.
369. Niwa Y, Kishimoto H, Shimokata K: Carcinomatous and tuberculous pleural effusions. Comparison of tumor markers. Chest 87:351, 1985.
370. Tamura S, Nishigaki T, Moriwaki Y, et al: Tumor markers in pleural effusion diagnosis. Cancer 61:298, 1988.
371. Shimokata K, Totani Y, Nakanishi K, et al: Diagnostic value of cancer antigen 15–3 (CA15–3) detected by monoclonal antibodies (115D8 and DF3) in exudative pleural effusions. Eur Respir J 1:341, 1988.
372. Yinnon A, Konijn AM, Link G, et al: Diagnostic value of ferritin in malignant pleural and peritoneal effusions. Cancer 62:2564, 1988.
373. Delpuech P, Desch G, Fructus F: Fibronectin is unsuitable as a tumor marker in pleural effusions. Clin Chem 35:166, 1989.
374. Iguchi H, Hara N, Miyazaki K, et al: Elevation of sialyl stage-specific mouse embryonic antigen levels in pleural effusion in patients with adenocarcinoma of the lung. Cancer 63:1327, 1989.
375. Menard O, Dousset B, Jacob C, et al: Improvement of the diagnosis of the cause of pleural effusion in patients with lung cancer by simultaneous quantification of carcinoembryonic antigen (CEA) and neuron-specific enolase (NSE) pleural levels. Eur J Cancer 29:1806, 1993.
376. Takahashi K, Sone S, Kimura S, et al: Phenotypes and lymphokine-activated

killer activity of pleural cavity lymphocytes of lung cancer patients without malignant effusion. Chest 103:1732, 1993.

377. Yang PC, Luh KT, Kuo SH, et al: Immunocytochemistry and ELISA quantitation of mucin for diagnosis of malignant pleural effusions. Am Rev Respir Dis 146:1571, 1992.

378. Imecik O, Ozer F: Diagnostic value of sialic acid in malignant pleural effusions. Chest 102:1819, 1992.

379. Shijobo N, Tsutahara S, Hirasawa M, et al: Pulmonary surfactant protein A in pleural effusions. Cancer 69:2905, 1992.

380. Garcia-Pachon E, Padilla-Navas I, Dosda D, et al: Elevated level of carcinoembryonic antigen in nonmalignant pleural effusions. Chest 111:643, 1997.

380a. Salama G, Miedouge M, Rouzaud P, et al: Evaluation of pleural CYFRA 21-1 and carcinoembryonic antigen in the diagnosis of malignant pleural effusions. Br J Cancer 77:472, 1998.

381. Kendall SW, Bryan AJ, Large SR, et al: Pleural effusions: Is thoracoscopy a reliable investigation? A retrospective review. Respir Med 86:437, 1992.

382. Robinson GR, Gleeson K: Diagnostic flexible fiberoptic pleuroscopy in suspected malignant pleural effusions. Chest 107:424, 1995.

383. Emerson GL, Emerson MS, Sherwood CE: The natural history of carcinoma of the lung. J Thorac Cardiovasc Surg 37:291, 1959.

384. Cohen S, Hossain MS-A: Primary carcinoma of the lung. A review of 417 histologically proved cases. Dis Chest 49:67, 1966.

385. Rodriguez Panadero F: Lung cancer and ipsilateral pleural effusion. Ann Oncol 6:25, 1995.

386. Brinkman GL: The significance of pleural effusion complicating otherwise operable bronchogenic carcinoma. Dis Chest 36:152, 1959.

387. Fentiman IS, Millis R, Sexton S, et al: Pleural effusion in breast cancer: A review of 105 cases. Cancer 47:2087, 1981.

388. Raju RN, Kardinal CG: Pleural effusion in breast carcinoma: Analysis of 122 cases. Cancer 48:2524, 1981.

389. Banerjee AK, Willetts I, Robertson JF, et al: Pleural effusion in beast cancer: A review of the Nottingham experience. Eur J Surg Oncol 20:33, 1994.

390. Thomas JM, Redding WH, Sloane JP: The spread of breast cancer: Importance of the intrathoracic lymphatic route and its relevance to treatment. Br J Cancer 40:540, 1979.

391. DeVita VT, Trujillo NP, Blackman AH, et al: Pulmonary manifestations of primary hepatic carcinoma. Am J Med Sci 250:428, 1965.

392. Ward P: Pulmonary and oesophageal presentations of pancreatic carcinoma. Br J Radiol 37:27, 1964.

393. Cantó-Armengod A: Macroscopic characteristics of pleural metastases arising from the breast and observed by diagnostic thoracoscopy. Am Rev Respir Dis 142:616, 1990.

394. Cantó A, Ferrer G, Romagosa V, et al: Lung cancer and pleural effusion. Clinical significance and study of pleural metastatic locations. Chest 87:649, 1985.

395. Goldsmith HS, Bailey HD, Callahan EL, et al: Pulmonary lymphangitic metastases from breast carcinoma. Arch Surg 94:483, 1967.

396. Danner DE, Gmelich JT: A comparative study of tumor cells from metastatic carcinoma of the breast in effusions. Acta Cytol 19:509, 1975.

397. Ashton PR, Hollingsworth AS Jr, Johnston WW: The cytopathology of metastatic breast cancer. Acta Cytol 19:1, 1975.

397a. Poe RH, Qazi R, Israel RH, et al: Survival of patients with pleural involvement by breast carcinoma. Am J Clin Oncol 6:523, 1983.

398. Dieterich M, Goodman SN, Rojas-Corona RR, et al: Multivariate analysis of prognostic features in malignant pleural effusions from breast cancer patients. Acta Cytol 38:945, 1994.

399. Ibuka T, Fukayama M, Hayashi Y, et al: Pyothorax-associated pleural lymphoma. A case evolving from T-cell-rich lymphoid infiltration to overt B-cell lymphoma in association with Epstein-Barr virus. Cancer 73:738, 1994.

400. Cesarman E, Knowles DM: Kaposi's sarcoma–associated herpesvirus: A lymphotropic human herpesvirus associated with Kaposi's sarcoma, primary effusion lymphoma, and multicentric Castleman's disease. Semin Diagn Pathol 14:54, 1997.

401. Gaidano G, Pastore C, Gloghini A, et al: Human herpesvirus type-8 (HHV-8) in hematopoietic neoplasia. Leuk Lymphoma 24:257, 1997.

402. Rodriguez-Garcia JL, Fraile G, Moreno MA, et al: Recurrent massive pleural effusion as a late complication of radiotherapy in Hodgkin's disease. Chest 100:1165, 1991.

403. Stolberg HO, Patt NL, MacEwen KF, et al: Hodgkin's disease of the lung: Roentgenologic-pathologic correlation. Am J Roentgenol 92:96, 1964.

404. Fisher AMH, Kendall B, Van Leuven BD: Hodgkin's disease. A radiological survey. Clin Radiol 13:115, 1962.

405. Martin JJ: The Nisbet Symposium: Hodgkin's disease. Radiological aspects of the disease. Australas Radiol 11:206, 1967.

406. Vieta JD, Craver LF: Intrathoracic manifestations of the lymphomatoid diseases. Radiology 37:138, 1941.

407. Molander DW, Pack GT: Treatment of lymphosarcoma. In Pack GT, Ariel IM (eds): Treatment of Cancer and Allied Diseases. Vol 9. 2nd ed. Lymphomas and Related Diseases. New York, Harper & Row, 1964, pp 131–167.

408. Gelikoglu F, Teirstein AS, Krellenstein DJ, et al: Pleural effusion in non-Hodgkin's lymphoma. Chest 101:1357, 1992.

409. Bruneau R, Rubin P: The management of pleural effusions and chylothorax in lymphoma. Radiology 85:1085, 1965.

410. Wong F, Grace WJ, Rottino A: Pleural effusions, ascites, pericardial effusions and edema in Hodgkin's disease. Am J Med Sci 246:678, 1963.

411. Spriggs AI, Vanhegan RI: Cytological diagnosis of lymphoma in serous effusions. J Clin Pathol 34:1311, 1981.

412. Spieler P, Kradolfer D, Schmid U: Immunocytochemical characterization of lymphocytes in benign and malignant lymphocyte-rich serous effusions. Virchows Arch 409:211, 1986.

413. Truong H, Morimoto R, Walts AE, et al: Neural networks as an aid in the diagnosis of lymphocyte-rich effusions. Anal Quant Cytol Histol 17:48, 1995.

414. Walts AE, Svidler R, Tolmachoff T, et al: Lymphoid-rich effusions. Diagnosis by morphometry using the CAS 200 system. Am J Clin Pathol 101:526, 1994.

415. Hartweg H: Das röntgenbild des thorax bei den chronischen leukosen. (The roentgenogram of the thorax in chronic leukoses.) Fortschr Roentgenstr 92:477, 1960.

416. Green RA, Nichols NJ: Pulmonary involvement in leukemia. Am Rev Respir Dis 80:833, 1959.

417. Siegel MJ, Shackelford GD, McAlister WH: Pleural thickening: An unusual feature of childhood leukemia. Radiology 138:367, 1981.

418. Zimhony O, Davidovitch Y, Shtalrid M: Chronic lymphocytic leukemia complicated by chylothorax. J Intern Med 235:375, 1994.

419. Yam LT: Granulocytic sarcoma with pleural involvement. Identification of neoplastic cells with cytochemistry. Acta Cytol 29:63, 1985.

420. Janckila AJ, Yam LT, Li C-Y: Immunocytochemical diagnosis of acute leukemia with pleural involvement. Acta Cytol 29:67, 1985.

421. Krause JR, Dekker A: Hairy cell leukemia (leukemic reticuloendotheliosis) in serous effusions. Acta Cytol 22:80, 1978.

422. Kapadia SB: Cytological diagnosis of malignant pleural effusion in myeloma. Arch Pathol Lab Med 101:534, 1977.

423. Shoenfeld Y, Pick AI, Weinberger A, et al: Pleural effusion—presenting sign in multiple myeloma. Respiration 36:160, 1978.

424. Hughes JC, Votaw ML: Pleural effusion in multiple myeloma. Cancer 44:1150, 1979.

425. Kamal MK, Williams E, Poskitt TR: IgD myeloma with malignant pleural effusion. South Med J 80:657, 1987.

426. Favis E, Kerman H, Shildecker W: Multiple myeloma manifested as a problem in the diagnosis of pulmonary disease. Am J Med 28:323, 1960.

427. Rodriguez JN, Pereira A, Martinez JC, et al: Pleural effusion in multiple myeloma. Chest 105:622, 1994.

428. Pacheco A, Perpina A, Escribano L, et al: Pleural effusion as first sign of extramedullary plasmacytoma. Chest 102:296, 1992.

429. Winterbauer RH, Riggins RCK, Griesman FA, et al: Pleuropulmonary manifestations of Waldenström's macroglobulinemia. Chest 66:368, 1974.

430. Teo SK, Lee SK: Recurrent pleural effusion in Waldenström's macroglobulinemia. BMJ 2:607, 1978.

431. Kumar PV, Esfahani FN, Tabei SZ, et al: Cytopathology of alpha chain disease involving the central nervous system and pleura. Acta Cytol 32:902, 1988.

432. Reynolds SP, Gibbs AR, Weeks R, et al: Massive pleural effusion: An unusual presentation of Castleman's disease. Eur Respir J 5:1150, 1992.

433. Blankenship ME, Rowlett J, Timby JW, et al: Giant lymph node hyperplasia (Castleman's disease) presenting with chylous pleural effusion. Chest 112:1132, 1997.

434. Williams JR, Wilcox WC: Pulmonary embolism: Roentgenographic and angiographic considerations. Am J Roentgenol 89:333, 1963.

435. Wiener SN, Edelstein J, Charms BL: Observations on pulmonary embolism and the pulmonary angiogram. Am J Roentgenol 98:859, 1966.

436. Stein GN, Chen JT, Goldstein F, et al: The importance of chest roentgenography in the diagnosis of pulmonary embolism. Am J Roentgenol 81:255, 1959.

437. Kaye J, Cohen G, Sandler A, et al: Massive pulmonary embolism without infarction. Br J Radiol 31:326, 1958.

438. Worsley DF, Alavi A, Aronchick JM, et al: Chest radiographic findings in patients with acute pulmonary embolism: Observations from the PIOPED study. Radiology 189:133, 1993.

439. Bynum LJ, Wilson JE III: Radiographic features of pleural effusions in pulmonary embolism. Am Rev Respir Dis 117:829, 1978.

440. Fleischner FG: Pulmonary embolism. Can Med Assoc J 78:653, 1958.

441. Torrance DJ Jr: Roentgenographic signs of pulmonary artery occlusion. Am J Med Sci 237:651, 1959.

442. Fleischner FG: Roentgenology of the pulmonary infarct. Semin Roentgenol 2:61, 1967.

443. Fleischner FG: Pulmonary embolism. Clin Radiol 13:169, 1962.

444. Figley MM, Gerdes AJ, Ricketts HJ: Radiographic aspects of pulmonary embolism. Semin Roentgenol 2:389, 1967.

445. Logue RB, Rogers JV Jr, Gay BB Jr: Subtle roentgenographic signs of left heart failure. Am Heart J 65:464, 1963.

446. Cornell SH, Rossi NP: Roentgenographic findings in constrictive pericarditis. Analysis of 21 cases. Am J Roentgenol 102:301, 1968.

447. Plum GE, Bruwer AJ, Clagett OT: Chronic constrictive pericarditis: Roentgenologic findings in 35 surgically proved cases. Mayo Clin Proc 32:555, 1957.

448. Tomaselli G, Gamsu G, Stulbarg MS: Constrictive pericarditis presenting as pleural efusion of unknown origin. Arch Intern Med 149:201, 1989.

449. Wiener-Kronish J, Matthay MA: Pleural effusions associated with hydrostatic and increased permeability pulmonary edema. Chest 93:852, 1988.

450. Race GA, Scheifley CH, Edwards JE: Hydrothorax in congestive heart failure. Am J Med 22:83, 1957.

451. Roux P, Fisher RM: Chest injuries in children: An analysis of 100 cases of blunt chest trauma from motor vehicle accidents. J Pediatr Surg 27:551, 1992.

452. Reynolds J, Davis JT: Injuries of the chest wall, pleura, pericardium, lungs, bronchi and esophagus. Radiol Clin North Am 4:383, 1966.

453. Williams JR, Bonte FJ: The Roentgenologic Aspect of Nonpenetrating Chest Injuries. Springfield, Ill, Charles C Thomas, 1961.

454. Gandelman G, Barzilay N, Krupsky M, et al: Left hemorrhagic effusions. Chest 106:636, 1994.

455. Traumatic perforation of oesophagus. BMJ 1:524, 1972.

456. Scholl DG, Tsai SH: Esophageal perforation following the use of the esophageal obturator airway. Radiology 122:315, 1977.

457. Cronstedt JL, Bouchama A, Hainau B, et al: Spontaneous esophageal perforation in herpes simplex esophagitis. Am J Gastroenterol 87:124, 1992.

458. Levy F, Mysko WK, Kelen GD: Spontaneous esophageal perforation presenting with right-sided pleural effusion. J Emerg Med 13:321, 1995.

459. Abbott OA, Mansour KA, Logan WD Jr, et al: Atraumatic so-called "spontaneous" rupture of the esophagus. A review of 47 personal cases with comments on a new method of surgical therapy. J Thorac Cardiovasc Surg 59:67, 1970.

460. Faling LJ, Pugatch RD, Robbins AH: Case report: The diagnosis of unsuspected esophageal perforation by computed tomography. Am J Med Sci 281:31, 1981.

461. Rudin JS, Ellrodt AG, Phillips EH: Low pleural fluid amylase associated with spontaneous rupture of the esophagus. Arch Intern Med 143:1034, 1983.

462. Edling JE, Bacon BR: Pleuropulmonary complications of endoscopic variceal sclerotherapy. Chest 99:1252, 1991.

463. Bacon BR, Bailey-Newton RS, Connors AF Jr: Pleural effusions after endoscopic variceal sclerotherapy. Gastroenterology 88:1910, 1985.

464. de la Rocha AG: Empyema thoracis. Surg Gynecol Obstet 155:839, 1982.

465. Kerr WF: Late-onset post-pneumonectomy empyema. Thorax 32:149, 1977.

466. Vargas FS, Cukier A, Hueb W, et al: Relationship between pleural effusion and pericardial involvement after myocardial revascularization. Chest 105: 1748, 1994.

467. Peng MJ, Vargas FS, Cukier A, et al: Postoperative pleural changes after coronary revascularization. Chest 101:327, 1992.

468. Tazelaar HD, Yousem SA: The pathology of combined heart-lung transplantation: An autopsy study. Hum Pathol 19:1403, 1988.

469. Hart U, Ward DR, Gillilian R, et al: Fatal pulmonary hemorrhage complicating Swan-Ganz catheterization. Surgery 91:24, 1982.

470. Carbone K, Gimenez LF, Rogers WH, et al: Hemothorax due to vena caval erosion by a subclavian dual-lumen dialysis catheter. South Med J 80:795, 1987.

471. Rudge CJ, Bewick M, McColl I: Hydrothorax after central venous catheterization. BMJ 3:23, 1973.

472. Usselman JA, Seat SG: Superior caval catheter displacement causing bilateral pleural effusions. Am J Roentgenol 133:738, 1979.

473. Paskin DL, Hoffman WS, Tuddenham WJ: A new complication of subclavian vein catheterization. Ann Surg 179:266, 1974.

474. Knight L, Tobin J Jr, L'Heureux P: Hydrothorax: A complication of hyperalimentation with radiologic manifestations. Radiology 111:693, 1974.

475. Holt S, Kirkham N, Myrescough E: Haemothorax after subclavian vein cannulation. Thorax 32:101, 1977.

476. Meeker DP, Barnett GH: Right pleural effusion due to a migrating ventriculoperitoneal shunt. Cleve Clin J Med 61:144, 1994.

477. Lovaas ME, Castillo RG, Deutschman CS: Traumatic subarachnoid-pleural fistula. Neurosurgery 17:650, 1985.

478. Beutel EW, Roberts JD, Langston HT, et al: Subarachnoid-pleural fistula. J Thorac Cardiovasc Surg 80:21, 1980.

479. Peter JC, Rode H: Traumatic subarachnoid-pleural fistula: Case report and review of the literature. J Trauma 34:303, 1993.

480. Qureshi MM, Roble DC, Gindin RA, et al: Subarachnoid-pleural fistula. Case report and review of the literature. J Thorac Cardiovasc Surg 91:238, 1986.

481. Qureshi MM, Roble DC, Gindin A, et al: Subarachnoid-pleural fistula. J Thorac Cardiovasc Surg 91:238, 1986.

482. Cantu RC: Value of myelography in thoracic spinal cord injuries. Int Surg 56:23, 1971.

483. Pollack IIF, Pang D, Hall WA: Subarachnoid-pleural and sub-arachnoid-mediastinal fistulae. Neurosurgery 26:519, 1990.

484. DePinto D, Payne T, Kittle CF: Traumatic subarachnoid-pleural fistula. Ann Thorac Surg 25:477, 1978.

485. Beutel EW, Roberts JD, Langston HT, et al: Subarachnoid-pleural fistula. J Thorac Cardiovasc Surg 80:21, 1980.

486. Hicken P, Martin J, Hakanson S: Computed tomography demonstration of subarachnoid-pleural fistula. J Can Assoc Radiol 41:222, 1990.

487. Azambuja PC, Fragomeni LS: Traumatic chylothorax associated with subarachnoid-pleural fistula. Thorax 36:699, 1981.

488. Aronchick JM, Epstein DM, Gefter WB, et al: Chronic traumatic diaphragmatic hernia: The significance of pleural effusion. Radiology 168:675, 1988.

489. Tempero SJ, Bookstein JJ: Angiographic demonstration of a ruptured spleen causing hemothorax. Case report. J Can Assoc Radiol 24:78, 1973.

490. Koehler PR, Jones R: Association of left-sided pleural effusions and splenic hematomas. Am J Roentgenol 135:851, 1980.

491. Lougheed MN, Maguire GH: Irradiation pneumonitis in the treatment of carcinoma of the breast. J Can Assoc Radiol 11:1, 1960.

492. Bachman AL, Macken K: Pleural effusions following supervoltage radiation for breast carcinoma. Radiology 72:699, 1959.

493. Whitcomb ME, Schwarz MI: Pleural effusion complicating intensive mediastinal radiation therapy. Am Rev Respir Dis 103:100, 1971.

494. Deeley TJ: The effects of radiation on the lungs in the treatment of carcinoma of the bronchus. Clin Radiol 11:33, 1960.

495. Bevelaqua FA, Valensi Q, Hulnick D: Epithelioid hemangioendothelioma. A rare tumor with variable prognosis presenting as a pleural effusion. Chest 93:665, 1988.

496. Harrison NK, Wilkinson J, O'Donohue J, et al: Osteochondroma of the rib: An unusual cause of haemothorax. Thorax 49:618, 1994.

497. Rostand RA, Feldman RL, Block ER: Massive hemothorax complicating heparin anticoagulation for pulmonary embolus. South Med J 70:1128, 1977.

498. Kollef MH, Gronski TJ: Hemothorax and an abdominal hematoma after treatment of ischemic cardiomyopathy with warfarin. Heart Lung 23:125, 1994.

499. Wilimas JA, Presbury G, Orenstein D, et al: Hemothorax and hemomediastinum in patients with hemophilia. Acta Haematol 73:176, 1985.

500. Brady DB, Bolan JC: Neurofibromatosis and spontaneous hemothorax in pregnancy: Two case reports. Obstet Gynecol 63(3 Suppl):35S, 1984.

501. Kupferschmid JP, Shahian DM, Villanueva AG: Massive hemothorax associated with intrathoracic extramedullary hematopoiesis involving the pleura. Chest 103:974, 1993.

502. Smith PR, Manjoney DL, Teitcher JB, et al: Massive hemothorax due to intrathoracic extramedullary hematopoiesis in a patient with thalassemia intermedia. Chest 94:658, 1988.

503. Lemon WS, Higgins GM: Lymphatic absorption of particulate matter through the normal and paralyzed diaphragm: An experimental study. Am J Med Sci 178:536, 1929.

504. Johnston RF, Loo RV: Hepatic hydrothorax. Studies to determine the source of the fluid and report of thirteen cases. Ann Intern Med 61:385, 1964.

505. Meigs JV: Pelvic tumors other than fibromas of the ovary with ascites and hydrothorax. Obstet Gynecol 3:471, 1954.

506. Stanley NN, Williams AJ, Dewar CA, et al: Hypoxia and hydrothoraces in a case of liver cirrhosis: Correlation of physiological, radiographic, scintigraphic, and pathological findings. Thorax 32:457, 1977.

507. Lieberman FL, Peters RL: Cirrhotic hydrothorax—further evidence that an acquired diaphragmatic defect is at fault. Arch Intern Med 125:114, 1970.

508. Mouroux J, Perrin C, Venissac N, et al: Management of pleural effusion of cirrhotic origin. Chest 109:1093, 1996.

509. Urhahn R, Gunther RW: Transdiaphragmatic leakage of ascites in cirrhotic patients: Evaluation with ultrafast gradient echo MR imaging and intraperitoneal contrast enhancement. Magn Reson Imaging 11:1067, 1993.

510. Alberts WM, Salem AJ, Solomon DA, et al: Hepatic hydrothorax—cause and management. Arch Intern Med 151:2383, 1991.

511. Light RW, George RB: Incidence and significance of pleural effusion after abdominal surgery. Chest 69:621, 1976.

512. Nielsen PH, Jepsen SB, Olsen AD: Postoperative pleural effusion following upper abdominal surgery. Chest 96:1133, 1989.

513. Verreault J, Lepage S, Bisson G, et al: Ascites and right pleural effusion: Demonstration of a peritoneopleural communication. J Nucl Med 27:1706, 1986.

514. Noseda A, Adler M, Ketelbant P, et al: Massive vitamin A intoxication with ascites and pleural effusion. J Clin Gastroenterol 7:344, 1985.

515. Frazer IH, Lichtenstein M, Andrews JT: Pleuroperitoneal effusion without ascites. Med J Aust 2:520, 1983.

516. Mouroux J, Perrin C, Venissac N, et al: Management of pleural effusion of cirrhotic origin. Chest 109:1093, 1996.

517. Amemiya T, Nishi K, Ohmori T, et al: A case of liver cirrhosis presenting with right pleural fluid without ascites. Nippon Kyobu Shikkan Gakkai Zasshi 32:796, 1994.

518. Daly JJ, Potts JM, Gordon L, et al: Scintigraphic diagnosis of peritoneo-pleural communication in the absence of ascites. Clin Nucl Med 19:892, 1994.

519. Haitjema T, de Maat CE: Pleural effusion without ascites in a patient with cirrhosis. Neth J Med 44:207, 1994.

520. Uetsuji S, Komada Y, Kwon AH, et al: Prevention of pleural effusion after hepatectomy using fibrin sealant. Int Surg 79:135, 1994.

521. Pisani RJ, Zeller FA: Bilious pleural effusion following liver biopsy. Chest 98:1535, 1990.

522. Neumeyer DA, LoCicero J, Pinkston P: Complex pleural effusion associated with a subphrenic gallstone phlegmon following laparoscopic cholecystectomy. Chest 109:284, 1996.

523. Bamberger PK, Stojadinovic A, Shaked G, et al: Biliary-pleural fistula presenting a massive pleural effusion after thoracoabdominal penetrating trauma. Surgery 62:1662, 1996.

523a. Olutola PS, Hutton L, Wall WJ: Pleural effusion following liver transplantation. Radiology 157:594, 1985.

524. Matsumata T, Kanematsu T, Okudaira Y, et al: Postoperative mechanical ventilation preventing the occurrence of pleural effusion after hepatectomy. Surgery 102:493, 1987.

525. Rudnick MR, Coyle JF, Beck LH, et al: Acute massive hydrothorax complicating peritoneal dialysis, report of 2 cases and a review of the literature. Clin Nephrol 12:38, 1979.

526. Lepage S, Bisson G, Verreault J, et al: Massive hydrothorax complicating peritoneal dialysis. Isotopic investigation (peritoneopleural scintigraphy). Clin Nucl Med 18:498, 1993.

527. Otsuka M, Kawai S, Fukunaga M, et al: Confirmation of dialysate leakage by intraperitoneal administration of radioactive colloid. Radiat Med 10:253, 1992.

528. Varon J, Gonzalez JM, Sternbach GL, et al: Tension hydrothorax: A rare complication of continuous cyclical peritoneal dialysis. J Emerg Med 12:155, 1994.

529. Galen MA, Steinberg SM, Lowrie EG, et al: Hemorrhagic pleural effusion in patients undergoing chronic hemodialysis. Ann Intern Med 82:359, 1975.

530. Berger HW, Rammohan G, Neff MS, et al: Uremic pleural effusion—a study in 14 patients on chronic dialysis. Ann Intern Med 82:362, 1975.

531. Jarratt ML, Sahn SA: Pleural effusions in hospitalized patients receiving long-term hemodialysis. Chest 108:470, 1995.

532. Corriere JN Jr, Miller WT, Murphy JJ: Hydronephrosis as a cause of pleural effusion. Radiology 90:79, 1968.

533. Barek LB, Cigtay OS: Urinothorax—an unusual pleural effusion. Br J Radiol 48:685, 1975.
534. Baron RL, Stark DD, McClennan BL, et al: Intrathoracic extension of retroperitoneal urine collections. Am J Roentgenol 137:37, 1981.
535. Leung FW, Williams AJ, Oill PA: Pleural effusion associated with urinary tract obstruction: Support for a hypothesis. Thorax 36:632, 1981.
536. Shanes JG, Senior RM, Stark DD, et al: Pleural effusion associated with urinary tract obstruction. Thorax 37:160, 1982.
537. Stark DD, Shanes JG, Baron RL, et al: Biochemical features of urinothorax. Arch Intern Med 142:1509, 1982.
538. Nusser RA, Culhane RH: Recurrent transudative effusion with an abdominal mass. Urinothorax. Chest 90:263, 1986.
539. Weiss Z, Shalev E, Zuckerman H, et al: Obstructive renal failure and pleural effusion caused by the gravid uterus. Acta Obstet Gynecol Scand 65:187, 1986.
540. Miller KS, Wooten S, Sahn SA: Urinothorax: A cause of low pH transudative pleural effusions. Am J Med 85:448, 1988.
541. Cavina C, Vichi G: Radiological aspects of pleural effusions in medical nephropathy in children. Ann Radiol Diag 31:163, 1958.
542. Frew AJ, Higgins RM: Empyema and mesangiocapillary glomerulonephritis with nephrotic syndrome. Br J Dis Chest 82:93, 1988.
543. Moss R, Hinds S, Fedullo AJ: Chylothorax: A complication of the nephrotic syndrome. Am Rev Respir Dis 140:1436, 1989.
544. Dunbar JS, Favreau M: Infrapulmonary pleural effusion with particular reference to its occurrence in nephrosis. J Can Assoc Radiol 10:24, 1959.
545. Llach F, Arieff AL, Massry SG: Renal vein thrombosis and nephrotic syndrome: A prospective study of 36 adult patients. Ann Intern Med 83:8, 1975.
546. Kirkpatrick JA Jr, Fleisher DS: The roentgenographic appearance of the chest in acute glomerulonephritis in children. J Pediatr 64:492, 1964.
547. Holzel A, Fawcitt J: Pulmonary changes in acute glomerulonephritis in childhood. J Pediatr 57:695, 1960.
548. Hopps HC, Wissler RW: Uremic pneumonitis. Am J Pathol 31:261, 1955.
549. Gilbert L, Ribot S, Frankel H, et al: Fibrinous uremic pleuritis—surgical entity. Chest 67:53, 1975.
550. Nidus BD, Matalon R, Cantacuzino D, et al: Uremic pleuritis—a clinicopathological entity. N Engl J Med 281:255, 1969.
551. Maringhini A, Ciambra M, Patti R, et al: Ascites, pleural, and pericardial effusions in acute pancreatitis. A prospective study of incidence, natural history, and prognostic role. Dig Dis Sci 41:848, 1996.
552. Lankisch PG, Droge M, Becher R: Pleural effusions: A new negative prognostic parameter for acute pancreatitis. Am J Gastroenterol 89:1849, 1994.
553. Gumaste V, Singh V, Dave P: Significance of pleural effusion in patients with acute pancreatitis. Am J Gastroenterol 87:871, 1992.
554. Hammarsten JF, Honska WL Jr, Limes BJ: Pleural fluid amylase in pancreatitis and other diseases. Am Rev Respir Dis 79:606, 1959.
555. Kaye MD: Pleuropulmonary complications of pancreatitis. Thorax 23:297, 1968.
556. Falk A, Gustafsson L, Gamklou R: Silent pancreatitis. Report of 4 cases of acute pancreatitis with atypical symptomatology. Acta Chir Scand 150:341, 1984.
557. Belfar HL, Radecki PD, Friedman AC, et al: Pancreatitis presenting as pleural effusions: Computed tomography demonstration of pleural space extension of pancreatitis exudate. J Comput Tomogr 11:184, 1987.
558. Dewan NA, Kinney WW, O'Donohue WJ Jr: Chronic massive pancreatic pleural effusion. Chest 85:497, 1984.
559. Bedingfield JA, Anderson MC: Pancreatopleural fistula. Pancreas 1:283, 1986.
560. Bronner MH, Marsh WH, Stanley JH: Pancreaticopleural fistula: Demonstration by computed tomography and endoscopic retrograde cholangiopancreatography. J Comput Tomogr 10:167, 1986.
561. Louie S, McGahan JP, Frey C, et al: Pancreatic pleuropericardial effusions. Fistulous tracts demonstrated by computed tomography. Arch Intern Med 145:1231, 1985.
562. Becx MC, van den Berg W, Bruggink ED, et al: Relapsing pleural exudate complicating chronic pancreatitis. Neth J Med 34:88, 1989.
563. Izbicki JR, Wilker DK, Waldner H, et al: Thoracic manifestations of internal pancreatic fistulas: Report of five cases. Am J Gastroenterol 84:265, 1989.
564. Uchiyama T, Suzuki T, Adachi A, et al: Pancreatic pleural effusion: Case report and review of 113 cases in Japan. Am J Gastroenterol 87:387, 1992.
565. Williams SGJ, Bhupalan A, Zureikat N, et al: Pleural effusions associated with pancreaticopleural fistula. Thorax 48:867, 1993.
566. Burgess NA, Moore HE, Williams JO, et al: A review of pancreatico-pleural fistula in pancreatitis and its management. HPB Surg 5:79, 1992.
567. Gertsch P, Marquis C, Diserens H, et al: Chronic pancreatic pleural effusions and ascites. Int Surg 69:145, 1984.
568. Lee DH, Shin DH, Kim TH, et al: Mediastinal pancreatic pseudocyst with recurrent pleural effusion. Demonstration by endoscopic retrograde cholangiopancreatogram and subsequent computed tomography scan. J Clin Gastroenterol 14:68, 1992.
569. Zeilender S, Turner MA, Glauser FL: Mediastinal pseudocyst associated with chronic pleural effusions. Chest 97:1014, 1990.
570. Cooper CB, Bardsley PA, Rao SS, et al: Pleural effusions and pancreaticopleural fistulae associated with asymptomatic pancreatic disease. Br J Dis Chest 82:315, 1988.
571. Tewari SC, Jayaswal R, Chauhan MS, et al: Bilateral recurrent haemorrhagic pleural effusion in asymptomatic chronic pancreatitis. Thorax 44:824, 1989.
572. Liedberg G, Lindmark G, Struwe I: Pleural effusion with dyspnea as the presenting symptom in chronic pancreatitis. A case report. Acta Chir Scand 149:209, 1983.

573. Anderson WJ, Skinner DB, Zuidema GD, et al: Chronic pancreatic pleural effusions. Surg Gynecol Obstet 137:827, 1973.
574. Rotman N, Fagniez PL: Chronic pancreaticopleural fistulas. Arch Surg 119:1204, 1984.
575. Joseph J, Viney S, Beck P, et al: A prospective study of amylase-rich pleural effusions with special reference to amylase isoenzyme analysis. Chest 102:1455, 1992.
576. Kramer MR, Saldana MJ, Cepero RJ, et al: High amylase levels in neoplasm-related pleural effusion. Ann Intern Med 110:567, 1989.
577. Sankarankutty M, Baird JL, Dowse JA, et al: Adenocarcinoma of the pancreas with massive pleural effusion. Br J Clin Pract 32:294, 1978.
578. Kramer MR, Saldana MJ, Cepero RJ, et al: High amylase levels in neoplasm-related pleural effusion. Ann Int Med 110:567, 1989.
579. Yamaguchi S, Kawashima A, Honda T, et al: A case of chronic pancreatitis with eosinophilic pleural effusion. Nippon Kyobu Shikkan Gakkai Zasshi 33:660, 1995.
580. Strimlan CV, Turbiner EH: Pleuropericardial effusions associated with chest and abdominal pain. Chest 81:493, 1982.
581. Ihse I, Lindström E, Evander A, et al: The value of preoperative imaging techniques in patients with chronic pancreatic pleural effusions. Int J Pancreatol 2:269, 1987.
582. McCarthy S, Pellegrini CA, Moss AA, et al: Pleuropancreatic fistula: Endoscopic retrograde cholangiopancreatography and computed tomography. Am J Roentgenol 142:1151, 1984.
583. Iglesias JI, Cobb J, Levey J, et al: Recurrent left pleural effusion in a 44-year-old woman with a history of alcohol abuse. Chest 110:547, 1996.
584. Bydder GM, Kreel L: Pleural calcification in pancreatitis demonstrated by computed tomography. J Comput Assist Tomogr 5:161, 1981.
585. Salmon VJ: Benign pelvic tumors associated with ascites and pleural effusion. J Mt Sinai Hosp 1:169, 1934.
586. Meigs JV, Cass JW: Fibroma of the ovary with ascites and hydrothorax. With a report of seven cases. Am J Obstet Gynecol 33:249, 1937.
587. Carson SA, Mazur MT: Atypical endometrioid cystadenofibroma with Meigs' syndrome: Ultrastructure and S-phase fraction. Cancer 49:472, 1982.
588. Mokrohisky JF: So-called "Meigs' syndrome" associated with benign and malignant ovarian tumors. Radiology 70:578, 1958.
589. Amr SS, Hassan AA: Struma ovarii with pseudo-Meigs' syndrome: Report of a case and review of the literature. Eur J Obstet Gynecol Reprod Biol 55:205, 1994.
590. Young RH: New and unusual aspects of ovarian germ cell tumors. Am J Surg Pathol 17:1210, 1993.
591. Aoshima M, Tanaka H, Takahashi M, et al: Meigs' syndrome due to Brenner tumor mimicking lupus peritonitis in a patient with systemic lupus erythematosus. Am J Gastroenterol 90:657, 1995.
592. Handler CE, Fray RE, Snashall PD: Atypical Meigs' syndrome. Thorax 37:396, 1982.
593. Terada S, Suzuki N, Uchide K, et al: Uterine leiomyoma associated with ascites and hydrothorax. Gynecol Obstet Invest 33:54, 1992.
594. Chen FC, Fink RL, Jolly H: Meigs' syndrome in association with a locally invasive adenocarcinoma of the fallopian tube. Aust N Z J Surg 65:761, 1995.
595. Dockery MB: Ovarian neoplasms. A collective review of the recent literature. Int Abstr Surg 81:179, 1945.
596. Siddiqui M, Toub DB: Cellular fibroma of the ovary with Meigs' syndrome and elevated CA-125. A case report. J Reprod Med 40:817, 1995.
597. Timmerman D, Moerman P, Vergote I: Meigs' syndrome with elevated serum CA 125 levels: Two case reports and review of the literature. Gynecol Oncol 59:405, 1995.
598. Pride SM, James CSJ, Yuen BH: The ovarian hyperstimulation syndrome. Semin Reprod Endocrin 8:247, 1990.
599. Kingsland C, Collins JV, Rizk B, et al: Ovarian hyperstimulation presenting as acute hydrothorax after in vitro fertilization. Am J Obstet Gynecol 161:381, 1989.
600. Shulman D, Sherer D, Bellin B: Pulmonary edema in the ovarian hyperstimulation syndrome. N Z Med J 101:643, 1988.
601. Zosmer A, Katz Z, Lancet M, et al: Adult respiratory distress syndrome complicating ovarian hyperstimulation syndrome. Fertil Steril 47:524, 1987.
602. Brandstetter RD, Klass SC, Gutherz P, et al: Pleural effusion due to communicating gastric ulcer. N Y State J Med 85:706, 1985.
603. Daee SA, Wagner R, Boneval H: Bilious pleural effusion. An unusual consequence of gastrointestinal perforation. Md State Med J 31:54, 1982.
604. Rosenbaum AJ, Murphy PJ, Engel JJ: Pleurisy during the course of ulcerative colitis. J Clin Gastroenterol 5:517, 1983.
605. Patwardhan RV, Heilpern RJ, Brewster AC, et al: Pleuropericarditis: An extraintestinal complication of inflammatory bowel disease. Report of three cases and review of literature. Arch Intern Med 43:94, 1983.
606. Miller WT, Talman EA: Subphrenic abscess. Am J Roentgenol 101:961, 1967.
607. Buscaglia AJ: Empyema due to splenic abscess with *Salmonella newport*. JAMA 240:1990, 1978.
608. Ballantyne KC, Sethia B, Reece IJ, et al: Empyema following intra-abdominal sepsis. Br J Surg 71:723, 1984.
609. Mueller PR, Simeone JF, Butch RJ, et al: Percutaneous drainage of subphrenic abscess: Review of 62 patients. Am J Roentgenol 147:1237, 1986.
609a. Van Gansbeke D, Matos C, Gelin M, et al: Percutaneous drainage of subphrenic abscesses. Br J Radiol 62:127, 1989.
609b. Philips RL: Computed tomography and ultrasound in the diagnosis and treatment of liver abscesses. Australas Radiol 38:165, 1994.

610. Gottehrer A, Roa J, Stanford GG, et al: Hypothyroidism and pleural effusions. Chest 98:1130, 1990.
611. Schneierson SJ, Katz M: Solitary pleural effusion due to myxedema. JAMA 168:1003, 1958.
612. Hurwitz PA, Pinals DJ: Pleural effusion in chronic hereditary lymphedema (Nonne, Milroy, Meige's disease). Report of two cases. Radiology 82:246, 1964.
613. Morandi U, Golinelli M, Brandi L, et al: "Yellow nail syndrome" associated with chronic recurrent pericardial and pleural effusions. Eur J Cardiothorac Surg 9:42, 1995.
614. Jiva TM, Poe RH, Kallay MC: Pleural effusion in yellow nail syndrome: Chemical pleurodesis and its outcome. Respiration 61:300, 1994.
615. Siegelman SS, Heckman BH, Hasson J: Lymphedema, pleural effusions and yellow nails: Associated immunologic deficiency. Dis Chest 56:114, 1969.
616. Ross JD, Reid KDG, Ambujakshan VP, et al: Recurrent pleural effusion, protein-losing enteropathy, malabsorption, and mosaic warts associated with generalized lymphatic hypoplasia. Thorax 26:119, 1971.
617. Dressler W: The post-myocardial infarction syndrome. Arch Intern Med 103:28, 1959.
618. Shahar A, Hod H, Barabash GM, et al: Disappearance of a syndrome: Dressler's syndrome in the era of thrombolysis. Cardiology 85:255, 1994.
619. Wen JY, Baughman KL: The Dressler syndrome. Johns Hopkins Med J 148:179, 1981.
620. Kim S, Sahn SA: Postcardiac injury syndrome. Chest 109:570, 1996.
621. Stelzner TJ, King TE Jr, Antony VB, et al: The pleuropulmonary manifestations of the postcardiac injury syndrome. Chest 84:383, 1983.
622. Domby WR, Whitcomb ME: Pleural effusion as a manifestation of Dressler's syndrome in the distant post-infarction period. Am Heart J 96:243, 1978.
623. Barakat MH, Karnik AM, Majeed HW, et al: Familial Mediterranean fever (recurrent hereditary polyserositis) in Arabs—a study of 175 patients and review of the literature. Q J Med 60:837, 1986.
624. Buades J, Ben-Chetrit E, Levy M: Familial Mediterranean fever in the "Chuetas" of Mallorca—origin in inquisition? Isr J Med Sci 31:497, 1995.
625. Daniels M, Shohat T, Brenner-Ullman A, et al: Familial Mediterranean fever: High gene frequency among the non-Ashkenazic and Ashkenazic Jewish populations in Israel. Am J Med Genet 55:311, 1995.
626. Takahashi M, Ebe T, Kohara T, et al: Periodic fever compatible with familial Mediterranean fever. Intern Med 31:893, 1992.
627. Yuval Y, Hemo-Zisser M, Zemer D, et al: Dominant inheritance in two families with familial Mediterranean fever. Am J Med Genet 57:455, 1995.
628. Shohat M, Fischel-Ghodsian N, Rotter JI, et al: The gene for familial Mediterranean fever is mapped to 16p 13.3-p13.1 with evidence for homogeneity. Adv Exp Med Biol 371:901, 1995.
629. Aksentijevich I, Gruberg L, Pras E, et al: Evidence for linkage of the gene causing familial Mediterranean fever to chromosome 17q in non-Ashkenazi Jewish families: Second locus or type I error? Hum Genet 91:527, 1993.
629a. Babior BM, Matzner Y: The familial Mediterranean fever gene—cloned at last. N Engl J Med 337:1548, 1997.
630. Dabestani A, Noble LM, Child JS, et al: Pericardial disease in familial Mediterranean fever: An echocardiographic study. Chest 81:592, 1982.
631. Brauman A, Gilboa Y: Recurrent pulmonary atelectasis as a manifestation of familial Mediterranean fever. Arch Intern Med 147:378, 1987.
632. Mancini JL: Familial paroxysmal polyserositis, phenotype I (familial Mediterranean fever). A rare cause of pleurisy. A case report and review of the literature. Am Rev Respir Dis 107:461, 1973.
633. Siegal S: Familial paroxysmal polyserositis. Am J Med 36:893, 1964.
634. Joseph J, Sahn SA: Thoracic endometriosis syndrome: New observations from an analysis of 110 cases. Am J Med 100:164, 1996.
635. Karpel JP, Appel D, Merav A: Pulmonary endometriosis. Lung 163:151, 1985.
636. Hobbs JE, Bortnick AR: Endometriosis of the lungs. Am J Obstet Gynecol 40:832, 1940.
637. Park WW: The occurrence of decidual tissue within the lung: Report of a case. J Pathol Bacteriol 67:563, 1954.
638. Hartz PH: Occurrence of decidua like tissue in the lung (report of a case). Am J Clin Pathol 26:48, 1956.
639. Foster DC, Stern JL, Buscema J, et al: Pleural and parenchymal pulmonary endometriosis. Obstet Gynecol 58:552, 1981.
640. Gaetje R, Kotzian S, Herrmann G, et al: Nonmalignant epithelial cells, potentially invasive in human endometriosis, lack the tumor suppressor molecule E-cadherin. Am J Pathol 150:461, 1997.
641. Slasky BS, Siewers RD, Lecky JW, et al: Catamenial pneumothorax: The roles of diaphragmatic defects and endometriosis. Am J Roentgenol 138:639, 1982.
642. Jelihovsky T, Grant AF: Endometriosis of the lung. Thorax 23:434, 1968.
643. Assor D: Endometriosis of the lung. Am J Clin Pathol 57:311, 1972.
644. Granberg I, Willems JS: Endometriosis of lung and pleura diagnosed by aspiration biopsy. Acta Cytol 21:295, 1977.
645. Yamazaki S, Ogawa J, Koide S, et al: Catamenial pneumothorax associated with endometriosis of the diaphragm. Chest 77:107, 1980.
645a. Im J-G, Kang HS, Choi BI, et al: Pleural endometriosis: CT and sonographic findings. Am J Roentgenol 148:523, 1987.
646. Shahar J, Angelillo VA: Catamenial pneumomediastinum. Chest 90:776, 1986.
647. Margolis MT, Thoen LD, Mercer LJ, et al: Hemothorax after Lupron therapy of a patient with pleural endometriosis—a case report and literature review. Int J Fertil Menopausal Stud 41:53, 1996.
648. Müller NL, Nelems B: Postcoital catamenial pneumothorax: A case report. Am Rev Respir Dis 134:803, 1986.

649. Miller JI Jr: Diagnosis and management of chylothorax. Chest Surg Clin North Am 6:139, 1996.
650. Schulman A, Fataar S, Dalrymple R, et al: The lymphographic anatomy of chylothorax. Br J Radiol 51:420, 1978.
651. Latner AL: Cantarow and Trumper Clinical Biochemistry. 7th ed. Philadelphia, WB Saunders, 1975.
652. Staats BA, Ellefson RD, Budahn LL, et al: The lipoprotein profile of chylous and nonchylous pleural effusions. Mayo Clin Proc 55:700, 1980.
653. Seriff NS, Cohen ML, Samuel P, et al: Chylothorax: Diagnosis by lipoprotein electrophoresis of serum and pleural fluid. Thorax 32:98, 1977.
654. Sassoon CS, Light RW: Chylothorax and pseudochylothorax. Clin Chest Med 6:163, 1985.
655. Hillerdal G: Chyliform (cholesterol) pleural effusion. Chest 88:426, 1985.
656. Johnson JR, Falk A, Iber C, et al: Paragonimiasis in the United States: A report of 9 cases in Hmong immigrants. Chest 82:168, 1982.
657. Mares DC, Mathur PN: Medical thoracoscopic talc pleurodesis for chylothorax due to lymphoma. Chest 114:731, 1998.
658. Strausser JL, Flye MW: Management of nontraumatic chylothorax. Ann Thorac Surg 31:520, 1981.
659. Ampil FL, Burton GV, Hardjasudarma M, et al: Chylous effusion complicating chronic lymphocytic leukemia. Leuk Lymphoma 10:507, 1993.
660. Segal R, Waron M, Reif R, et al: Chylous ascites and chylothorax as presenting manifestations of stomach carcinoma. Isr J Med Sci 22:897, 1986.
661. Quinonez A, Halabe J, Avelar F, et al: Chylothorax due to metastatic prostatic carcinoma. Br J Urol 63:325, 1989.
662. Tani K, Ogushi F, Sone S, et al: Chylothorax and chylous ascites in a patient with uterine cancer. Jpn J Clin Oncol 18:175, 1988.
663. Schmidt A: Chylothorax. Review of 5 years' cases in the literature and report of a case. Acta Chir Scand 118:5, 1959.
664. Macfarlane JR, Holman CW: Chylothorax. Am Rev Respir Dis 105:287, 1972.
665. Dulchavsky SA, Ledgerwood AM, Lucas CE: Management of chylothorax after blunt chest trauma. J Trauma 28:1400, 1988.
666. Nguyen DM, Shum-Tim D, Dobell AR, et al: The management of chylothorax/chylopericardium following pediatric cardiac surgery: A 10 year experience. J Card Surg 10:302, 1995.
667. Haniuda M, Nishimura H, Kobayashi O, et al: Management of chylothorax after pulmonary resection. J Am Coll Surg 180:537, 1995.
668. Fine PG, Bubela C: Chylothorax following celiac plexus block. Anesthesiology 63:454, 1985.
669. Nakai S, Zielke K: Chylothorax—a rare complication after anterior and posterior spinal correction. Report of six cases. Spine 11:830, 1986.
670. Higgins CB, Reinke RT: Postoperative chylothorax in children with congenital heart disease. Clinical and roentgenographic features. Radiology 119:409, 1976.
671. Kaul TK, Bain WH, Turner MA, et al: Chylothorax: Report of a case complicating ductus ligation through a median sternotomy, and review. Thorax 31:610, 1976.
672. Verunelli F, Giorgini V, Luisi VS, et al: Chylothorax following cardiac surgery in children. J Cardiovasc Surg 24:227, 1983.
673. Fairfax AJ, McNabb WR, Spiro SG: Chylothorax: A review of 18 cases. Thorax 41:880, 1986.
674. Zakhour BJ, Drucker MH, Franco AA: Chylothorax as a complication of aortocoronary bypass. Two case reports and a review of the literature. Scand J Thorac Cardiovasc Surg 22:93, 1988.
675. Smith JA, Goldstein J, Oyer PE: Chylothorax complicating coronary artery bypass grafting. J Cardiovasc Surg 35:307, 1994.
676. Kostiainen S, Meurala H, Mattila S, et al: Chylothorax. Clinical experience in nine cases. Scand J Thorac Cardiovasc Surg 17:79, 1983.
677. Muns G, Rennard SI, Floreani AA: Combined occurrence of chyloperitoneum and chylothorax after retroperitoneal surgery. Eur Respir J 8:185, 1995.
678. Cespedes RD, Peretsman SJ, Harris MJ: Chylothorax as a complication of radical nephrectomy. J Urol 150:1895, 1993.
679. Jabbar AS, al-Abdulkareem A: Bilateral chylothorax following neck dissection. Head Neck 17:69, 1995.
680. La Hei ER, Menzie SJ, Thompson JF: Right chylothorax following left radical neck dissection. Aust N Z J Surg 63:77, 1993.
681. Nygaard SD, Berger HA, Fick RB: Chylothorax as a complication of oesophageal sclerotherapy. Thorax 47:134, 1992.
682. Koffler H, Papile L-A, Burstein RL: Congenital chylothorax: Two cases associated with maternal polyhydramnios. Am J Dis Child 132:638, 1978.
683. Petres RE, Redwine FO, Cruikshank DP: Congenital bilateral chylothorax: Antepartum diagnosis and successful intrauterine surgical management. JAMA 248:1360, 1982.
684. Smeltzer DM, Stickler GB, Fleming RE: Primary lymphatic dysplasia in children: Chylothorax, chylous ascites, and generalized lymphatic dysplasia. Eur J Pediatr 145:286, 1986.
685. Pauwels R, Oomen C, Huybrechts W, et al: Chylothorax in adult age in association with congenital lymphedema. Eur J Respir Dis 69:285, 1986.
686. Bresser P, Kromhout JG, Reekers JA, et al: Chylous pleural effusion associated with primary lymphedema and lymphangioma-like malformations. Chest 103:1916, 1993.
687. Wilmshurst PT, Burnie JP, Turner PR, et al: Chylopericardium, chylothorax, and hypobetalipoproteinaemia. BMJ 293:483, 1986.
688. Canil K, Fitzgerald P, Lau G: Massive chylothorax associated with lyphangiomatosis of the bone. J Pediatr Surg 29:1186, 1994.
689. Noonan JA, Walters LR, Reeves JT: Congenital pulmonary lymphangiectasia. Am J Dis Child 120:314, 1970.

690. Sailer M, Unsinn K, Fink C, et al: Pulmonary lymphangiectasis with spontaneous chylothorax bei Noonan-syndrome. Klin Padiatr 207:302, 1995.
691. Sullivan KL, Steiner RM, Wexler RJ: Lymphaticopleural fistula: Diagnosis by computed tomography. J Comput Assist Tomogr 8:1005, 1984.
692. Milano S, Maroldi R, Vezzoli G, et al: Chylothorax after blunt chest trauma: An unusual case with a long latent period. Thorac Cardiovasc Surg 42:187, 1994.
693. Freundlich IM: The role of lymphangiography in chylothorax. A report of six nontraumatic cases. Am J Roentgenol 125:617, 1975.
694. Ngan H, Fok M, Wong J: The role of lymphography in chylothorax following thoracic surgery. Br J Radiol 61:1032, 1988.
695. Sachs PB, Zelch MG, Rice TW, et al: Diagnosis and localization of laceration of the thoracic duct: Usefulness of lymphangiography and CT. Am J Roentgenol 157:703, 1991.
696. Camiel MR, Benninghoff DL, Alexander LL: Chylous effusions, extravasation of lymphographic contrast material, hypoplasia of lymph nodes and lymphocytopenia. Chest 59:107, 1971.
697. Sarwal V, Suri RK, Sharma OP, et al: Traumatic subarachnoid-pleural fistula. Ann Thorac Surg 62:1622, 1996.
698. Chertow BS, Kadzielawa R, Burger AJ: Benign pleural effusions in long-standing diabetes mellitus. Chest 99:1108, 1991.
699. Kavuru MS, Adamo JP, Ahmad M, et al: Amyloidosis and pleural disease. Chest 98:20, 1990.
700. Graham DR, Ahmad D: Amyloidosis with pleural involvement. Eur Respir J 1:571, 1988.
701. Pappas CA, Rheinlander HF, Stadecker MJ: Pleural effusion as a complication of solitary eosinophilic granuloma of the rib. Hum Pathol 11:675, 1980.
702. Horn BR, Byrd RB: Simulation of pleural disease by disk space infection. Chest 74:575, 1978.
703. Feigl D, Seidel L, Marmor A: Gorham's disease of the clavicle with bilateral pleural effusions. Chest 79:242, 1981.
704. Hirmand H, Hoffman LA, Smith JP: Silicone migration to the pleural space associated with silicone-gel augmentation mammaplasty. Ann Plastic Surg 32:645, 1994.
705. Kolef MH, McCormack MT, Kristo DA, et al: Pleural effusion in patients with systemic cholesterol embolization. Chest 103:792, 1993.
706. Buchanan DR, Johnston IDA, Kerr IH, et al: Cryptogenic bilateral fibrosing pleuritis. Br J Dis Chest 82:186, 1988.
707. Dupont A, Six R: Lupus-like syndrome induced by methyldopa. BMJ 285:693, 1982.
708. Harrington TM, Davis DE: Systemic lupus-like syndrome induced by methyldopa therapy. Chest 79:696, 1981.
709. McCraken M, Benson EA, Hickling P: Systemic lupus erythematosus induced by aminoglutethimide. BMJ 281:1254, 1980.
710. Hughes GRV: Hypotensive agents, beta-blockers, and drug-induced lupus. BMJ 284:1358, 1982.
711. Record NB Jr: Acebutolol-induced pleuropulmonary lupus syndrome. Ann Intern Med 95:326, 1981.
712. West SG, McMahon M, Protanova JP: Quinidine-induced lupus erythematosus. Ann Intern Med 100:840, 1984.
713. Price EJ, Venables PJ: Drug-induced lupus. Drug Safety 112:283, 1995.
714. Laversuch CJ, Collins DA, Charles PJ, et al: Sulphasalazine-induced autoimmune abnormalities in patients with rheumatic disease. Br J Rheum 344:435, 1995.
715. Sato-Matsumura KC, Koizumi H, Matsumura T, et al: Lupus erythematosus–like syndrome induced by thiamazole and propylthiouracil. J Dermatol 21:501, 1994.
716. Drory VE, Korczyn AD: Hypersensitivity vasculitis and systemic lupus erythematosus induced by anticonvulsants. Clinic Neuropharm 16:19, 1993.
717. Yousem S, Lifson J, Colby T: Chemotherapy-induced eosinophilic pneumonia. Relation to bleomycin. Chest 88:103, 1985.
718. Orwoll ES, Kiessling PJ, Patterson JR: Interstitial pneumonia from mitomycin. Ann Intern Med 89:352, 1978.
719. Castro M, Veeder MH, Mailliard JA, et al: A prospective study of pulmonary function in patients receiving mitomycin. Chest 109:939, 1996.
720. Smalley RV, Wall RL: Two cases of busulfan toxicity. Ann Intern Med 64:154, 1966.
721. Major PP, Laurin S, Bettez P: Pulmonary fibrosis following therapy with melphalan: Report of two cases. Can Med Assoc J 123:197, 1980.
722. Tjon A, Tham RTO, Peters WG, et al: Pulmonary complications of cytosine-arabinoside therapy: Radiographic findings. Am J Roentgenol 149:23, 1987.
723. Thompson J, Chengappa KN, Good CB, et al: Hepatitis, hyperglycemia, pleural effusion, eosinophilia, hematuria and proteinuria occurring early in clozapine treatment. Int Clin Psychopharmacol 13:95, 1998.
724. Kreisman H, Wolkove N: Pulmonary toxicity of antineoplastic therapy. Sem Oncol 19:508, 1992.
725. Twohig KJ, Matthay RA: Pulmonary effects of cytotoxic agents other than bleomycin. Clin Chest Med 11(1):31, 1990.
726. Vogelzang PJ, Bloom SM, Mier JW, et al: Chest roentgenographic abnormalities in IL-2 recipients. Chest 101:746, 1992.
727. Seebach J, Speich R, Fehr J, et al: GM-CSF–induced eosinophilic pneumonia. Br J Haematol 90:963, 1995.
728. Murray MJ, Kronenberg R: Pulmonary reactions simulating cardiac pulmonary edema caused by nitrofurantoin. N Engl J Med 273:1185, 1965.
729. Bando T, Fujimura M, Noda Y, et al: Minocycline-induced pneumonitis with bilateral hilar lymphadenopathy and pleural effusion. Intern Med 33:177, 1994.
730. Osanai S, Fukuzawa J, Akiba Y, et al: Minocycline-induced pneumonia and pleurisy—a case report. Nippon Kyobu Shikkan Gakkai Zasshi 30:322, 1992.
731. McNeil KD, Firouz-Abadi A, Oliver W, et al: Amiodarone pulmonary toxicity—three unusual manifestations. Aust N Z J Med 22:14, 1992.
732. Pusateri DW, Muder RR: Fever, pulmonary infiltrates and pleural effusion following acyclovir therapy for herpes zoster ophthalmicus. Chest 98:754, 1990.
733. Middleton KL, Santella R, Couser JI Jr: Eosinophilic pleuritis due to propylthiouracil. Chest 103:955, 1993.
734. Zaidenstein R, Cohen N, Dishi V, et al: Chylothorax following median sternotomy. Clin Cardiol 19:910, 1996.
735. Kotzot D, Stoss H, Wagner H, et al: Jaffe-Campanacci syndrome: Case report and review of literature. Clin Dysmorphol 3:328, 1994.
736. Farrell SA, Warda LJ, LaFlair P, et al: Adams-Oliver syndrome: A case with juvenile chronic myelogenous leukemia and chylothorax. Am J Med Genet 47:1175, 1993.
737. Fryns JP, Moerman P: 46,XY/46XX mosaicism and congenital pulmonary lymphangiectasis with chylothorax. Am J Med Genet 47:934, 1993.
738. Goldfarb JP: Chylous effusions secondary to pancreatitis: Case report and review of the literature. Am J Gastroenterol 79:133, 1984.
739. Menzies R, Hidvegi R: Chylothorax associated with tuberculous spondylitis. J Can Assoc Radiol 39:238, 1988.
740. Vennera MC, Moreno R, Cot J, et al: Chylothorax and tuberculosis. Thorax 38:694, 1983.
741. Anton PA, Rubio S, Casan P, et al: Chylothorax due to *Mycobacterium tuberculosis*. Thorax 50:1019, 1995.
742. Bristo LD, Mandal AK, Oparah SS, et al: Bilateral chylothorax associated with sclerosing mediastinitis. Int Surg 68:273, 1983.
743. Van Veldhuizen PJ, Taylor S: Chylothorax: A complication of a left subclavian vein thrombosis. Am J Clin Oncol 19:99, 1996.
744. Lengyel RJ, Shanley DJ: Recurrent chylothorax associated with sarcoidosis. Hawaii Med J 54:817, 1995.
745. Jarman PR, Whyte MK, Sabroe I, et al: Sarcoidosis presenting with chylothorax. Thorax 50:1324, 1995.
746. Villena V, De Pablo A, Martin-Escribano P: Chylothorax and chylous ascites due to heart failure. Eur Respir J 8:1235, 1995.
747. Delgado C, Martin M, de la Portilla F: Retrosternal goiter associated with chylothorax. Chest 106:1924, 1994.
748. Cöplü L, Emri S, Selcuk ZT, et al: Life threatening chylous pleural and pericardial effusion in a patient with Behçet's syndrome. Thorax 47:64, 1992.
749. Tie MLH, Poland GA, Rossenow EC III: Chylothorax in Gorhams' syndrome: A common complication of a rare disease. Chest 105:208, 1994.
750. Gil-Suay V, Martinez-Moragon E, de Diego A, et al: Chylothorax complicating a thoracic aortic aneurysm. Eur Respir J 10:737, 1997.
751. Bass SN, Ailani RK, Shekar R, et al: Pyogenic vertebral osteomyelitis presenting as exudative pleural effusion: A series of five cases. Chest 114:642, 1998.
752. Wood N, Edozien L, Lieberman B: Symptomatic unilateral pleural effusion as a presentation of ovarian hyperstimulation syndrome. Hum Reprod 13:571, 1998.
753. Garcia-Riego A, Cuinas C. Vilanova JJ, Ibarrola R: Extramedullary hematopoietic effusions. Acta Cytol 42:1116, 1998.
754. Blankenship ME, Rowlett J, Timby JW, et al: Giant lymph node hyperplasia (Castleman's disease) presenting with chylous pleural effusion. Chest 112:1132, 1997.
755. Romero S, Martin C, Hernandez L, et al: Chylothorax in cirrhosis of the liver: Analysis of its frequency and clinical characteristics. Chest 114:154, 1998.

Pneumothorax

The presence of air within the pleural space, or pneumothorax, is one of the more common forms of thoracic disease. It is caused most often by trauma, either accidental or iatrogenic. In the absence of such a history, it is traditionally referred to as spontaneous: in this situation, it can be either primary (unassociated with clinical or radiographic evidence of significant pulmonary disease) or secondary (in which such disease is present). Pneumothorax can also occur secondary to pneumomediastinum, air tracking from that location into the pleural space through the mediastinal pleura. In this situation, there is evidence that the most likely sites of rupture are small areas just above the root of the left lung and at the junction with the pericardium.[1]

This chapter is concerned predominantly with the epidemiology, etiology, pathogenesis, and clinical manifestations of spontaneous pneumothorax; radiologic signs were discussed in detail in Chapter 21 (*see* page 563).

EPIDEMIOLOGY

Primary spontaneous pneumothorax occurs most commonly in men in the third and fourth decades of life.[2–4] Although the male-to-female predominance varies in different studies—from as low as 2:1[5] to as high as 15:1[6]—most investigators have found a ratio of about 4:1 or 5:1.[7–10]

In a study from Olmsted County, Minnesota, 318 patients were identified in whom a diagnosis of pneumothorax or pneumomediastinum was made during a 25-year period from 1950 to 1974.[10] Of these episodes, 75 were attributed to accidental trauma and 102 to iatrogenic causes. In the remaining 141 patients, the pneumothorax was spontaneous; 77 were considered to have primary spontaneous pneumothorax and 64 secondary disease. The age-adjusted incidence of primary pneumothorax was 7.4 per 100,000 men per year and 1.2 per 100,000 women per year (male-to-female predominance, 6.2:1); the incidence of secondary spontaneous pneumothorax was 6.3 per 100,000 men per year and 2.0 per 100,000 women per year (male-to-female predominance, 3.2:1). In another epidemiologic study of 15,204 individuals from Stockholm, Sweden, the annual incidence of first spontaneous pneumothorax was somewhat higher, 18 per 100,000 in men and 6 per 100,000 in women.[11]

A familial incidence of spontaneous pneumothorax has been described by several groups of investigators.[12–17] In one family of 23 members, 6 had repeated episodes;[14] the risk appeared to be related to the presence of HLA haplotype A2, B40, and the alpha$_1$-antitrypsin phenotype M1M2. In another study, a familial tendency was found to be more likely in women than in men.[18] Two modes of inheritance have been suggested for these familial cases:[19] (1) an autosomal dominant gene with incomplete penetrance (50% in males and about 20% in females) and (2) more than one gene, with some cases inherited as an X-linked recessive disorder and others as an autosomal dominant trait with incomplete penetrance.

ETIOLOGY AND PATHOGENESIS

Primary Spontaneous Pneumothorax

The primary form of spontaneous pneumothorax appears to be caused by rupture of an air-containing space within or immediately deep to the visceral pleura. These spaces may be a *bulla* (defined as a sharply demarcated region of emphysema greater than 1 cm in diameter [Fig. 70–1])[20] or a *bleb* (a focal gas-containing space situated entirely within the pleura). In fact, although often referred to as blebs, it is likely that most of the air-containing spaces associated with pneumothorax are in fact bullae. CT scans demonstrate focal areas of emphysema in more than 80% of patients who have spontaneous pneumothorax, even in lifelong nonsmokers.[7–9] These areas are situated predominantly in the peripheral regions of the apex of upper lobes and are seen as localized areas of low attenuation measuring 3 mm or more in diameter that may or may not be delineated by thin walls (Fig. 70–2).[8] In patients in whom emphysema is not apparent on CT, it is often evident at surgery or pathologic examination.[21] In one study in which of 116 consecutive patients who had undergone thoracotomy for recurrent or persistent primary or secondary pneumothorax, emphy-

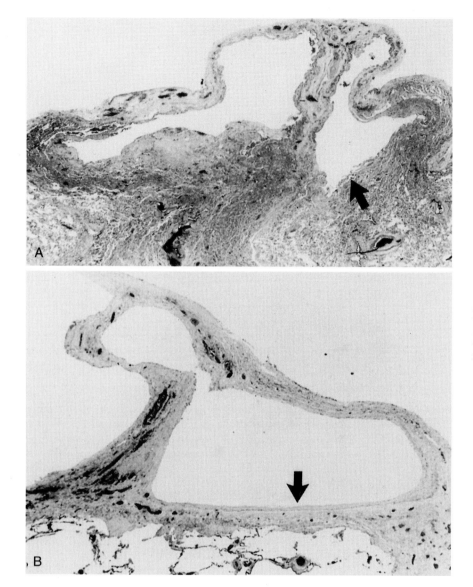

Figure 70–1. Blebs and Bullae: Pathologic Distinction. Lung tissue resected from an individual with spontaneous pneumothorax *(A)* shows two cystic spaces lined by fibrous tissue. Although these spaces appear to be largely within the pleura, one *(arrow)* is in direct contact with lung parenchyma, indicating that it represents a bulla. A section of lung from another patient *(B)* shows a similar cystic space, in this instance completely surrounded by pleura *(arrow)* indicating that it is a bleb. *(A,* ×12; *B,* ×18.)

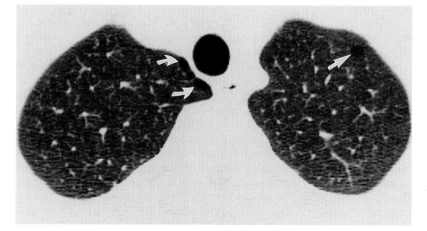

Figure 70–2. Localized Emphysema in a Non-smoker. HRCT scan in an 18-year-old man demonstrates small subpleural bullae in the right lung apex *(curved arrows)* and a localized area of emphysema in the left lung apex *(straight arrow)*. The patient was a lifelong nonsmoker who had previously undergone chest tube drainage for recurrent right pneumothorax. The emphysema and bullae could not be visualized on the chest radiograph even in retrospect.

sema with bulla formation was identified histologically in 93 patients (80%), emphysema without bulla formation in 13 (11%), isolated bullae or blebs in 2 patients each, and other pulmonary or pleural abnormalities in 6 (5%).[21] Seventy-four patients had irregular emphysema, 26 had paraseptal emphysema, 4 had mixed irregular and centrilobular or paraseptal emphysema, and 2 had unclassifiable emphysema.[21] In lifelong nonsmokers, the areas of emphysema often measure less than 1 cm in diameter.

The pathogenesis of blebs usually is attributed to the dissection of air from ruptured alveoli through interstitial tissue into the fibrous layer of visceral pleura, where it accumulates in the form of a "cyst."[22, 23] The mechanism is analogous to that postulated to occur in the development of mediastinal emphysema.[24, 25] Theoretically, alveolar rupture may be the result of check-valve obstruction of a small airway, leading to distention of distal air spaces. Such airway obstruction could have several causes, including recent or remote infection and accumulation of intraluminal mucus. Support for this obstructive hypothesis is provided by the high incidence of cigarette smoking in patients with spontaneous pneumothorax, tobacco smoke clearly being associated with increased mucus production.[5, 11, 26] In addition, in one study of 11 nonsmokers who had healed spontaneous pneumothorax, findings on ventilation-perfusion scintigraphy suggested the presence of airway obstruction.[27]

The mechanisms behind the formation of bullae are less clear than those of blebs. Most speculation has centered around the possibility of regional damage to the apical portion of the lung, related either to ischemia or to the greater distending forces on apical alveoli caused by more negative pleural pressure.[28] In support of both of these mechanisms are the pathologic and radiologic identification of apical bullae in many patients with spontaneous pneumothorax and the clinical observation that primary spontaneous pneumothorax shows a predilection for tall, thin men.[29–31] For example, in one series, an increased incidence of primary spontaneous pneumothorax was found with increased height and reached more than 200 per 100,000 person-years for people 76 inches (193 cm) tall or more.[29] Some investigators have measured chest dimensions in young adults with spontaneous pneumothorax and concluded that, on average, the men had longer chests and greater height-to-width ratios than matched controls, whereas the women had a diminished anteroposterior diameter only.[32]

An intrinsic abnormality of connective tissue resulting in an increased tendency to bulla or bleb formation is probably also important in some people. For example, spontaneous pneumothorax is a well-known complication in patients who have Marfan's syndrome[33, 34] or Ehlers-Danlos syndrome;[35] it also shows a strong association with mitral valve prolapse, especially in people who have an abnormal body build.[36]

Bullae can be recognized on the radiograph as localized areas of radiolucency measuring 1 cm or more in diameter. They are more likely to be identified when they cause an irregular outline of the visceral pleura, a finding most easily appreciated in the presence of pneumothorax (Fig. 70–3). Even in the latter situation, however, bullae are often not identifiable on conventional chest radiographs.[37, 38] By contrast, they can be seen on CT in most patients.[7, 8, 21] For example, in one study, evidence of emphysema was seen on CT in 16 of 20 (80%) patients with spontaneous pneumotho-

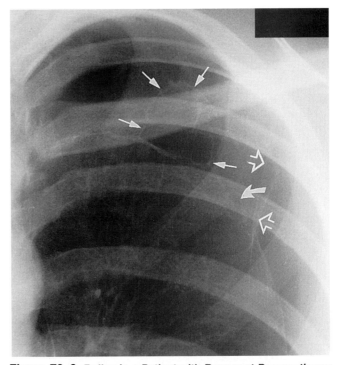

Figure 70–3. Bullae in a Patient with Recurrent Pneumothorax. A view of the left upper chest from a posteroanterior radiograph in a 17-year-old man who had recurrent pneumothorax shows large bullae *(straight arrows)*. Irregularity of the margins of the visceral pleura as a result of subpleural bullae *(curved arrow)* and adhesions between the visceral and parietal pleura *(open arrows)* are also evident. The patient was a 3-pack-year smoker.

rax.[7] In another investigation, in which the conventional CT findings in 27 lifelong nonsmokers who had previous spontaneous pneumothorax were compared with those in 10 nonsmoking controls, localized areas of emphysema were identified in 22 (81%) of the patients and in none of the controls.[8] The emphysema involved mainly the upper lobes and the peripheral rather than the central lung region; in patients with unilateral pneumothorax, the ipsilateral lung was predominantly or exclusively affected. In none of the patients was the emphysema evident on chest radiograph.[8]

In a third study, conventional 10-mm collimation CT was compared with chest radiography in 35 patients who had primary spontaneous pneumothorax.[39] Localized emphysema with or without bulla formation was identified on CT in 31 of 35 patients (89%) and on the radiograph in 15 of 35 (43%). Abnormalities were detected in the lung ipsilateral to the pneumothorax on 28 of 35 (80%) CT scans and on 11 of 35 (31%) chest radiographs, and in the contralateral lung on 23 of 35 (66%) CT scans and on 4 of 35 (11%) chest radiographs. In most cases, the abnormalities consisted of a few localized areas of emphysema ($n < 5$) measuring less than 2 cm in diameter.

The immediate cause of rupture of a bleb or bulla is often unknown. It is clearly not related to exertional effort because most patients are at rest when the pneumothorax occurs.[40] Localized areas of emphysema distend with decrease in atmospheric pressure (e.g., with increasing altitude during flight[41] and with rapid surfacing after diving[42, 43]), and this mechanism may be important in some cases. In one comprehensive study, a change in atmospheric pressure was chronologically correlated with the development of pneumothorax.[44] It has also been postulated that the mechanical stress to which the apex of the lung is subjected with

increasing lung height causes rupture of apical bullae in addition to acting as a mechanism in their formation.[45, 46]

Secondary Spontaneous Pneumothorax

The pathogenesis of secondary spontaneous pneumothorax is multifactorial. Many cases are associated with the formation of subpleural cystic spaces related to diffuse interstitial fibrosis or emphysema; rupture of one of these is likely the immediate cause of pneumothorax in many cases. As might be expected from a knowledge of the pathogenesis of emphysema and interstitial fibrosis, patient height is not nearly as important a factor in the secondary as in the primary form.[29] The most common concurrent condition in patients who have secondary spontaneous pneumothorax is chronic obstructive pulmonary disease (COPD); presumably reflecting this association, the incidence of pneumothorax increases with age.[29] The mechanism of cyst or bulla rupture in secondary spontaneous pneumothorax is probably also multifactorial. Local airway obstruction caused by pneumonia, mucous plugs, or bronchoconstriction may be important. In addition, many episodes occur during artificial ventilation used as therapy for the underlying disease, and this is undoubtedly a factor (*see* farther on).

Numerous conditions have been associated with secondary spontaneous pneumothorax; the list given in Table 70–1

Table 70–1. SECONDARY SPONTANEOUS PNEUMOTHORAX

CAUSE	SELECTED REFERENCES
Developmental Disease	
Congenital cystic adenomatoid malformation	21
Connective Tissue Disease	
Lymphangioleiomyomatosis	120, 121
Tuberous sclerosis	122, 123
Neurofibromatosis	124
Marfan's syndrome	33, 34
Ehlers-Danlos syndrome	125
Mitral valve prolapse	36
Infection	
Fungal pneumonia (particularly *Pneumocystis carinii* pneumonia patients with the acquired immunodeficiency syndrome [AIDS])	47, 126–130
Hydatid disease	131
Bacterial pneumonia	47
Neoplasms	
Primary pulmonary carcinoma	132
Carcinoid tumor	133
Mesothelioma	21, 47
Metastatic carcinoma	134
Metastatic sarcoma	135–137
Metastatic germ cell tumors	138
Drugs and Toxins	
Chemotherapy for malignancy	47, 139, 140
Paraquat poisoning	141
Hyperbaric oxygen therapy	142
Radiation therapy	143, 144, 144a
Aerosolized pentamidine therapy in patients with AIDS	145
Immunologic Disease	
Wegener's granulomatosis	146
Idiopathic pulmonary hemorrhage	147
Idiopathic pulmonary fibrosis	21, 47
Langerhans' cell histiocytosis	47, 148
Sarcoidosis	47, 149, 150
Chronic Obstructive Pulmonary Disease	
Asthma	47, 151
Emphysema	7, 8, 152
Cystic fibrosis	153
Pneumoconiosis	
Silicoproteinosis	154
Berylliosis	155
Bauxite pneumoconiosis	156
Vascular Disease	
Pulmonary infarction	157, 158
Metabolic Disease	
Pulmonary alveolar proteinosis	159
Intra-abdominal Disease	
Gastropleural fistula	160, 161
Colopleural fistula	162

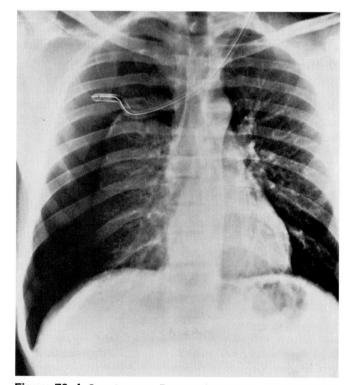

Figure 70–4. Spontaneous Pneumothorax Associated with Pulmonary Sarcoidosis. A posteroanterior radiograph reveals a large right pneumothorax. A chest tube has been introduced, but the lung is still collapsed to less than 50% of its normal volume. Although the left lung looks normal on this radiograph, within the next few weeks, widespread interstitial disease developed that proved to be sarcoidosis following pathologic study. The patient was a 24-year-old man who had no symptoms referable to his chest other than those related to the spontaneous pneumothorax.

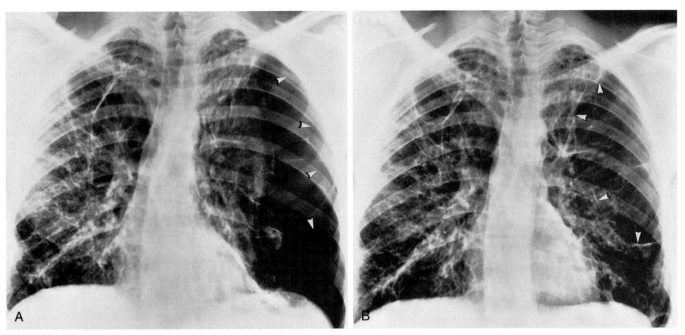

Figure 70–5. Spontaneous Pneumothorax Associated with Diffuse Bullae. A posteroanterior radiograph *(A)* reveals a left pneumothorax. Both lungs contain a multitude of small and large thin-walled bullae, several of which have failed to collapse because of air trapping *(arrowheads)*. A chest tube was promptly inserted and the pneumothorax evacuated. After removal of the chest tube 4 days later *(B)*, the pneumothorax is no longer evident. The bullae that failed to collapse at the time of the pneumothorax are again indicated by arrowheads.

is by no means complete. In some cases, the pneumothorax is the first manifestation of the disease (Fig. 70–4). Examples of the complication associated with emphysema (Fig. 70–5), lymphangioleiomyomatosis (Fig. 70–6), mesothelioma (Fig. 70–7), acute bacterial pneumonia (Fig. 70–8), and congenital cystic adenomatoid malformation (Fig. 70–9) are given for illustrative purposes.

The prevalence of the various causes of pneumothorax has been assessed in two studies of 116 and 120 patients.[21, 47] In the first, emphysema with or without bullae was identi-fied in the resected specimens in 106 of the 116 patients (91%) (Fig. 70–10), isolated bullae or blebs in 2 patients each, and other etiologies in 6 (5%).[21] The pathologic diagnoses in the patients without emphysema, bullae, or blebs included mesothelioma (in 2 patients) and metastatic angiosarcoma from the breast, subpleural fibrosis, interstitial fibrosis with honeycombing, and congenital cystic adenomatoid malformation (in 1 patient each).

In a second retrospective study of 120 patients with spontaneous pneumothorax admitted to the hospital, 31

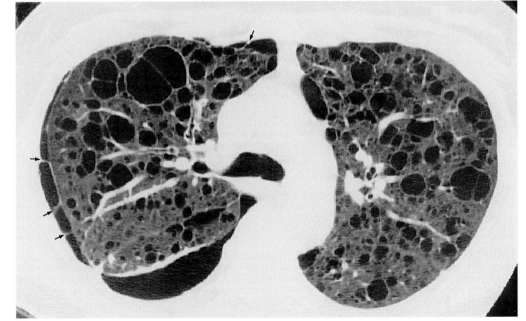

Figure 70–6. Pneumothorax Associated with Lymphangioleiomyomatosis. An HRCT scan in a 40-year-old woman demonstrates a small right pneumothorax and numerous cystic lesions with well-defined walls, characteristic of lymphangioleiomyomatosis. Pleural adhesions *(arrows)* related to recurrent pneumothorax can be seen on the right.

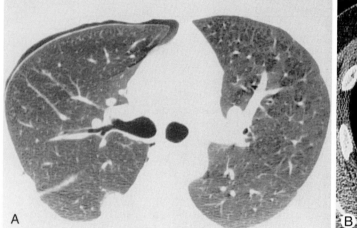

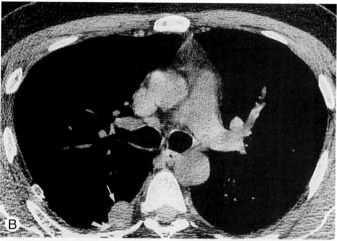

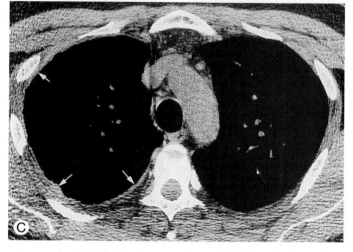

Figure 70–7. Pneumothorax Associated with Mesothelioma.
An HRCT scan *(A)* in a 37-year-old man demonstrates a small right pneumothorax. Soft tissue windows *(B* and *C)* demonstrate localized areas of pleural thickening *(straight arrows)*. At one level, there is evidence of soft tissue extension into the extrapleural fat *(curved arrow)*. At thoracotomy, this was shown to represent a malignant mesothelioma. The underlying lung parenchyma was normal. The patient had no history of exposure to asbestos.

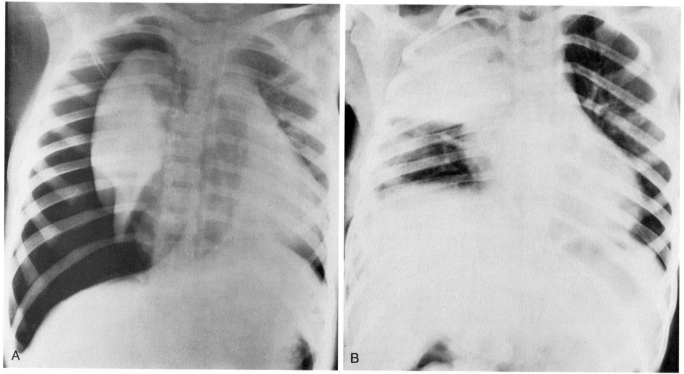

Figure 70–8. Spontaneous Pneumothorax Associated with Pneumonia. This 6-year-old girl was admitted to the hospital following a 2-day history of acute respiratory illness and the abrupt onset 2 hours before of severe right-sided chest pain and shortness of breath. An anteroposterior radiograph *(A)* demonstrates a large right pneumothorax associated with marked shift of the mediastinum to the left and depression of the right hemidiaphragm, an appearance consistent with the presence of "tension." A chest tube was promptly inserted and the pneumothorax drained. A radiograph obtained 24 hours later *(B)* demonstrates homogeneous consolidation of the right upper lobe. The patient was diagnosed as having acute staphylococcal pneumonia. (Courtesy of St. Joseph's General Hospital, Blind River, Ontario.)

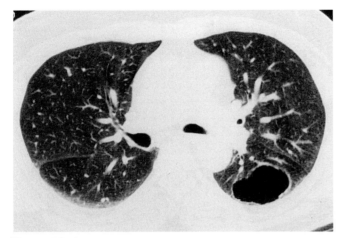

Figure 70–9. Congenital Cystic Adenomatoid Malformation. An HRCT scan in a 62-year-old patient with recurrent left pneumothorax demonstrates a 4- × 3-cm diameter cystic lesion with a well-defined smooth wall in the superior segment of the left lower lobe. The patient had been a lifelong nonsmoker. The lesion was shown to represent congenital cystic adenomatoid malformation following surgical excision.

(26%) had localized areas of emphysema, bullae, or blebs; 12 (10%) had COPD; 32 (27%) had the acquired immunodeficiency syndrome (AIDS); and 45 (37%) had other underlying lung diseases.[47] Twenty-five (78%) of the patients with AIDS had *Pneumocystis carinii* pneumonia, and the remaining 7 had infection by *Mycobacterium tuberculosis* or nontuberculous mycobacteria. The diagnoses in the 45 patients with underlying lung disease other than AIDS, emphysema, or COPD included pneumonia, carcinoma, asthma, tuberculosis, Langerhans' cell histiocytosis (LCH), sarcoidosis, idiopathic pulmonary fibrosis, Job's syndrome, drug-induced lung disease, and immunologically mediated connective tissue disease.

In addition to the numerous diseases associated with pneumothorax listed in Table 70–1, several specific disease processes and forms of pneumothorax deserve more detailed comment.

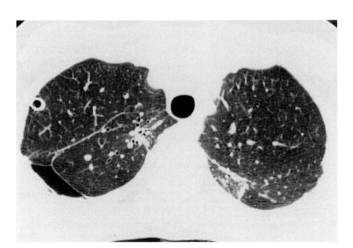

Figure 70–10. Pneumothorax with Irregular Emphysema. An HRCT scan in a 23-year-old woman shows a small right pneumothorax with a chest tube in place. Localized areas of scarring, presumed to be the result of previous tuberculosis, are present in both upper lobes. Although no emphysematous lesions were seen on HRCT, a wedge resection specimen of the right lung apex showed irregular emphysema.

Bilateral Pneumothorax

In the study of 120 patients with pneumothorax cited previously, bilateral pneumothoraces occurred in 2% of patients with underlying emphysema or COPD, 34% of patients with AIDS, and 11% of patients with other underlying lung diseases (Fig. 70–11).[47] In another series of 298 patients, 12 (4%) developed simultaneous bilateral spontaneous pneumothorax;[48] in 7 of these, it was secondary to underlying lung disease, including LCH, lymphangioleiomyomatosis, metastatic osteosarcoma, Hodgkin's disease, mesothelioma, cystic fibrosis, and miliary tuberculosis. The relatively high frequency of abnormalities other than localized areas of emphysema or bullae in patients with simultaneous bilateral pneumothorax has also been observed by other investigators;[49, 50] 19 of 56 patients (34%) with simultaneous bilateral spontaneous pneumothorax described in the literature by 1994 had underlying pulmonary disease other than emphysema.[48]

Pneumothorax *Ex Vacuo*

Pneumothorax *ex vacuo* is an uncommon condition seen in patients experiencing lobar collapse secondary to acute bronchial obstruction.[51, 52] Such collapse results in a sudden increase in negative intrapleural pressure adjacent to the affected lobe, which leads to focal accumulation of gas originating in ambient tissues and blood. The complication is recognized by the presence of a crescentic gas collection between the visceral pleural surface of the atelectatic lobe and the chest wall or hemidiaphragm. Four of the five reported cases involved the right upper lobe and one the right middle and lower lobes.[51, 52] Characteristically, the pneumothorax resolves after relief of the obstruction and resolution of the atelectasis.

Catamenial Pneumothorax

The term *catamenial pneumothorax* refers to the development of pneumothorax at the time of menstruation. The complication can probably develop by several mechanisms. It is likely that some cases are the result of migration of air directly through the vagina, uterus, and fallopian tubes into the peritoneal cavity and thence through diaphragmatic fenestrations into the pleural space.[53] In support of this mechanism are the occasional cases in which diagnostic pneumoperitoneum has been associated with pneumothorax, the observation that air can be found within the peritoneum in postpartum women carrying out exercises in the knee-chest position,[54] the presence of concurrent pneumoperitoneum and catamenial pneumothorax in one patient,[55] and the observation that tubal ligation cures the condition in some patients.[56] It is clear, however, that intraperitoneal migration of air cannot be the sole mechanism of catamenial pneumothorax because diaphragmatic defects are not present in all affected individuals. For example, in one study of 18 patients with catamenial pneumothorax who were subjected to thoracotomy, defects were identified in only 3.[57] Even more convincing in this regard is a report of recurrent catamenial pneumothorax in eight patients who had undergone hysterectomy.[54]

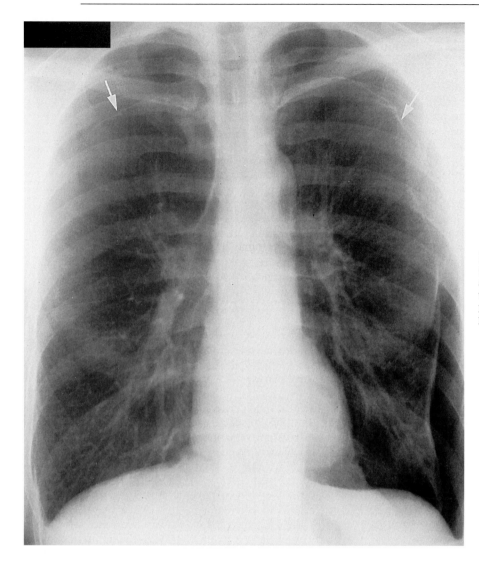

Figure 70–11. Spontaneous Bilateral Pneumothorax. A posteroanterior chest radiograph in a 25-year-old man demonstrates bilateral pneumothoraces. Note the irregular outline of the visceral pleura related to subpleural bullae *(arrows)*. The patient was a 5-pack-year smoker.

Another, probably more frequent, mechanism for catamenial pneumothorax is related to pleural endometriosis. Clinical or pathologic evidence of pelvic endometriosis is present in 20% to 60% of patients with catamenial pneumothorax,[58, 59] and diaphragmatic or pleural endometrial implants have been demonstrated at thoracotomy in about 25% to 35% of patients.[60, 61] The presence of endometrial tissue within the thorax is uncommon; only about 120 cases were documented by 1996.[58, 62, 63] In most cases, the abnormal tissue is located in the visceral or parietal pleura and is discovered after the development of pneumothorax or hemothorax; in about 10% to 15% of cases, a patient presents with recurrent hemoptysis or is found to have an asymptomatic nodule on a screening chest radiograph, indicating involvement of the pulmonary parenchyma.[63]

Several mechanisms may be responsible for the development of pleural endometriosis.[62–65] As discussed previously *(see* page 1375), it is likely that many cases of parenchymal endometriosis are the result of embolization of endometrial tissue through the pulmonary arteries, and it is possible that this mechanism may also be involved in some cases of pleural disease. It has also been hypothesized that

metaplasia of pleural mesothelial and submesothelial connective tissue into endometrial tissue may be responsible for the disease in some cases.[62]

Another, perhaps more likely, explanation is regurgitation of endometrial tissue through the fallopian tubes or its release into the peritoneal cavity from foci of peritoneal endometriosis, followed by migration to the pleura through diaphragmatic sinuses.[65, 66] The fundamental nature of these sinuses is uncertain. Stomas that connect with lymphatics are present normally on both surfaces of the diaphragm in the parietal pleura and peritoneum *(see* page 250). These are only 4 to 12 μm in diameter, however, and would permit the passage only of individual or very small clusters of cells; whether such small collections would be capable of proliferating into macroscopic foci of endometrial tissue has not been established. A more plausible route is the diaphragmatic fenestrations that measure up to several millimeters in diameter and have been identified in about 33% of patients with pleural endometriosis.[66] They are said to be more frequent on the right,[65] suggesting a possible explanation for the large preponderance of cases on this side. It has also been speculated that this unusual laterality is the result of the normal pattern of peritoneal fluid flow—down the left paravertebral gutter into the pelvis and up the right paravertebral gutter to the hemidiaphragm and liver.[65]

Although it is possible that the diaphragmatic fenestrae represent developmental defects (a hypothesis supported by the observation of familial catamenial pneumothorax[67]), their intimate association with endometrial tissue has suggested to some investigators that they are instead secondary to necrotic and sloughed endometrium.[66] It has also been hypothesized that necrosis of endometrial tissue on the visceral pleura during menses might result in the formation of an air leak between the lung and pleura, thus causing pneumothorax.[58, 66] Some investigators have also suggested a role for prostaglandin $F_{2\alpha}$–mediated vasospasm and bronchoconstriction.[68] According to these workers, this substance is present in menstrual debris of some women and has been shown to have these effects on the lungs; they speculated that rupture of parenchyma damaged by local vasoconstriction rather than necrosis of endometrial tissue might be the source of the air leak.

Grossly, pleural endometriosis appears as multiple (occasionally single) bluish purple nodules ranging from 1 mm to several centimeters in diameter on the visceral or parietal pleura or both; when on the parietal surface, associated diaphragmatic involvement is not infrequent. Cystic changes may be evident, especially in the larger nodules.[64, 69] In some cases, lung parenchyma is involved by direct extension from an initial focus in the pleura. Microscopic examination shows the presence of round or irregularly shaped glandular spaces admixed with typical endometrial stroma; hemosiderin-laden macrophages are often present. Decidualization of stromal cells may occur during pregnancy and can result in an increase in the size of nodules.[70] In some patients with a clear-cut history of pleural endometriosis, only fibrosis is identified on pathologic examination, suggesting necrosis and healing of the affected foci. Endometrial tissue has occasionally been identified in transthoracic needle aspiration specimens.[71]

The radiologic manifestations are typically those of pneumothorax, hemothorax, or pleural effusion;[58, 72] pleural nodules are visible rarely.[65, 73] About 85% to 90% of cases occur on the right side, 5% on the left, and 5% bilaterally.[58] One patient has been described in whom pleural endometriosis was demonstrated by CT and ultrasonography;[74] the abnormal tissue was shown to extend into the pleural space through defects in the diaphragm.

The main symptoms are shoulder or chest pain and dyspnea.[62] They usually appear within 72 hours of the onset of menses and are typically recurrent; for example, in the 63 cases in one review, the number of episodes of pneumothorax ranged from 2 to 42 (average, 14).[62] Symptoms are absent between menstruations.[58, 60, 75] A single case of catamenial pneumomediastinum unassociated with pneumothorax has been documented.[76]

The Valsalva Maneuver and Pneumothorax

The Valsalva maneuver has resulted in pneumomediastinum and pneumothorax during emesis,[47] coughing,[77] and, perhaps most commonly, during pregnancy and labor.[9, 78–81] Smoking of marijuana and cocaine, possibly associated with

the use of a prolonged Valsalva maneuver to augment the "high," have also been associated with these complications in drug users.[77, 82–85] However, a more frequent mechanism for the production of pneumothorax in addicts is needle puncture while mainlining into neck veins (*see* farther on).

Traumatic Pneumothorax

As indicated previously, trauma is probably the most common cause of pneumothorax. Of the 318 cases described in one series, it was the responsible mechanism in 177 (56%);[29] it was iatrogenic in 102 cases and noniatrogenic in 75. In a second study of 196 patients seen over a 5-year period, iatrogenic pneumothorax was seen in 106 (54%) and spontaneous pneumothorax in 90.[86] Traumatic pneumothorax can be caused by direct communication of the pleural space with the atmosphere through chest wall puncture or by disruption of the proximal tracheobronchial tree or the visceral pleura.

With the increasing use of invasive diagnostic procedures, iatrogenic pneumothorax is likely to be even more common in the future, although most cases are of little clinical significance. A variety of investigative and biopsy procedures can be complicated by pneumothorax (Table 70–2). In a review of 106 cases, 35 (33%) were related to transthoracic needle aspiration biopsy, 30 (28%) to thoracentesis, 23 (22%) to subclavian vein catheterization, 7 (7%) to positive-pressure ventilation, and 11 (10%) to miscellaneous causes.[86] Two of the 106 patients died as a result of the pneumothorax.

Patients being assisted by artificial ventilation are also at risk for the development of pneumothorax, particularly when inspiratory pressures are used.[87] The incidence of the complication in these situations has been estimated to be between 0.5% and 15%, depending on the duration of ventilation and the nature of the underlying disease.[88] Alveolar rupture is more likely to occur when very high peak-inspira-

Table 70–2. IATROGENIC CAUSES OF PNEUMOTHORAX

PROCEDURE	SELECTED REFERENCES
Biopsy Procedures	
Transthoracic needle aspiration	86, 163, 164
Transbronchial biopsy	165
Transtracheal biopsy	86
Colonoscopy	166
Liver biopsy	86
Fine-needle aspiration of breast	167
Therapeutic Procedures	
Thoracentesis	86
Central venous catheterization	168, 169
Feeding tube insertion	170, 171
Positive-pressure ventilation	86
Tracheal intubation	172, 173
Pacemaker insertion	86
Electromyographic electrode insertion	174
Acupuncture	18, 175
Percutaneous nephrolithotomy	176, 177
Use of a voice box prosthesis	178

tory pressures are employed to ventilate patients with severely obstructed airways or noncompliant lungs; in such circumstances, pneumothorax (sometimes associated with pneumomediastinum or pneumoperitoneum) may be a terminal event. Attempted cardiopulmonary resuscitation has also been associated with an increased risk of pneumothorax at autopsy.[87]

Noniatrogenic traumatic pneumothorax can result from either penetrating or nonpenetrating chest injury. There need not be radiologic evidence of rib fracture, in which circumstances the likely pathogenesis is an abrupt increase in intrathoracic pressure that results in interstitial emphysema and tracking of air to the visceral pleura. It is likely that this is also the mechanism behind pneumomediastinum and subcutaneous emphysema, conditions that frequently accompany pneumothorax in these circumstances. When rib fractures are present, the likely mechanism is laceration of the visceral pleura by rib fragments; in this situation, hemothorax can be expected as a concomitant finding.

One unusual mechanism of traumatic pneumothorax has been recognized in drug addicts whose peripheral veins are thrombosed and who use the internal jugular vein to inject drugs directly. In some areas, this procedure has been responsible for a significant increase in the incidence of pneumothorax.[89–91] For example, in a study from the Detroit Receiving Hospital of 525 cases of pneumothorax seen over a 2-year period, 113 (22%) were associated with drug abuse.[89] Not infrequently, this complication is bilateral, presumably as a result of sequential insertion of needles.[92–94]

PATHOLOGIC CHARACTERISTICS

Pathologic characteristics of the pleura and subpleural lung parenchyma in patients who have pneumothorax clearly depend to some extent on the presence and type of underlying disease. As indicated previously, it is our experience that the most common abnormality of lung excised from patients with primary spontaneous pneumothorax is one or more foci of emphysema, usually 0.5 to 1.5 cm in diameter and located adjacent to fibrotic pleura (see Fig. 70–1, page 2782); true blebs (i.e., entirely intrapleural cystic spaces) are uncommon. Like bullae, the latter are usually isolated abnormalities measuring 0.5 to 1.5 cm in diameter; in patients who have undergone vigorous ventilatory support, they may be associated with the presence of air cysts in the peribronchovascular and interlobular interstitial tissue (Fig. 70–12).[95] Histologic examination of these interstitial cysts may reveal the presence of multinucleated giant cells, representing a tissue manifestation of the reaction to air.[95, 96]

The most common pathologic findings in patients who have secondary spontaneous pneumothorax are emphysematous bullae and cystic spaces associated with interstitial fibrosis. One group described subpleural cystic spaces in patients with cystic fibrosis that appeared to be the result of localized bronchiectasis ("bronchiectatic cysts");[96] although there was often a zone of compressed, fibrotic lung between the cyst wall and the pleura, the authors suggested that their rupture might sometimes be the mechanism of pneumothorax in these patients.

Histologic examination of pleura excised at thoracotomy in the therapy of pneumothorax often reveals characteristic changes believed to represent a reaction to the presence

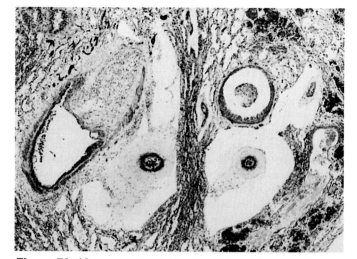

Figure 70–12. Interstitial Emphysema. The section shows the interstitial tissue surrounding two bronchioles and their accompanying pulmonary arteries to be expanded by irregularly shaped spaces that *in vivo* contained air. The section is from a neonate who had had positive-pressure ventilatory support for several days before death. (×35.)

of air.[97, 98] These consist of a fibrinous exudate within and adjacent to which are large numbers of mononuclear cells (probably mostly macrophages) and eosinophils, and occasional multinucleated giant cells (Fig. 70–13). A similar reaction can be seen in the mediastinum in pneumomediastinum.[99] This eosinophilic pleuritis resembles the inflammatory infiltrate of Langerhans' cell histiocytosis (LCH), a condition known to have an increased incidence of spontaneous pneumothorax and with which it should not be confused;[100] the presence or absence of the characteristic parenchymal histologic changes of LCH should suffice to make the pathologic distinction. It must be remembered, however, that eosinophilic pleuritis and LCH can coexist.[98] Infiltration of the walls of pulmonary parenchymal vessels by eosinophils can also be seen in some cases.[101]

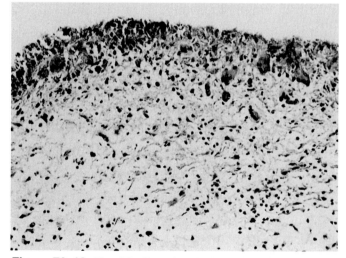

Figure 70–13. Pleuritis Associated with Pneumothorax. A section of parietal pleura removed at thoracotomy for spontaneous pneumothorax shows it to be thickened by loose fibroblastic tissue and a cellular infiltrate composed of histiocytes, multinucleated giant cells, and numerous smaller inflammatory cells, many of which are eosinophils. (×200.)

CLINICAL MANIFESTATIONS

Chest pain and dyspnea, either alone or in combination, are the classic symptoms of spontaneous pneumothorax; pain was the sole complaint of 69% of 72 patients in one series.[4] Dyspnea, which can be severe, may disappear within 24 hours regardless of whether the collapsed lung undergoes partial re-expansion. The major physical sign of pneumothorax is a decrease or absence of breath sounds despite normal or increased resonance on percussion. However, this may be difficult to detect, particularly in patients who have a small pneumothorax or who have underlying emphysema.

Hamman's sign, originally considered to be caused by pneumomediastinum, is now thought to be associated much more frequently with a left pneumothorax. The sign results from the presence of gas in close contact with the heart and has been described as a variety of "clicks" and "whoops" that occur throughout the entire cardiac cycle; the sounds are influenced by the respiratory phase and the position of the patient.[102, 103] In some cases, the sounds disappear completely when the patient is moved from the left to the right lateral decubitus position.

Unusual clinical manifestations of pneumothorax include ptosis (as a result of extension of subcutaneous emphysema),[104] pneumocephalus (secondary to tension pneumothorax associated with a comminuted fracture of the thoracic spine),[105] and recurrent pneumopericardium (in association with pleuropericardial defect[106]).

Occasionally, inspired air becomes trapped in a pleural space, presumably on the basis of a bronchopleural check-valve mechanism, leading to a tension pneumothorax (*see* page 589). Immediate recognition of this complication is essential because affected patients rapidly become severely hypoxic and acidotic and often die.[108, 109] In one series of 3,500 autopsies, unsuspected tension pneumothorax was found in 12 patients;[87] 10 of these had been supported by mechanical ventilators, and 9 had undergone cardiopulmonary resuscitation.

Pleural effusion coincident with pneumothorax appears to occur less frequently than might be anticipated. For example, in one series of 72 patients, fluid was found in only 19 (26%) before diagnostic or therapeutic manipulation;[4] of the 15 effusions aspirated, 11 were serous and 4 were bloody. Spontaneous hemopneumothorax is especially rare; of 228 cases of spontaneous pneumothorax seen over a 10-year period in one study, hemopneumothorax was observed in only 5 patients (2%).[110] According to the authors of this report, bleeding results from the rupture or tearing of fibrovascular adhesions between the parietal and visceral layers of pleura as the lung collapses. Pneumothorax is a major cause of an eosinophilic effusion.[98, 111]

PULMONARY FUNCTION TESTS

The effect of pneumothorax on pulmonary function depends largely on its size, although reduction in lung volumes and flow rates can also be influenced at least partly by pleural pain. In one study of 12 patients who had spontaneous pneumothorax, 9 were found to have a P_{O_2} below 80 mm Hg.[112] In another study of three young men who had pneumothoraces ranging in size from 25% to 40%, the lung with the pneumothorax showed uniform airway closure at low lung volumes.[113]

PROGNOSIS AND NATURAL HISTORY

The frequency of recurrence of spontaneous pneumothorax on the same side is surprisingly high, amounting to roughly 30% in most reported series.[2, 29, 38, 114] In about 10% of cases, spontaneous pneumothorax develops subsequently on the contralateral side.[2, 114] The complication of re-expansion pulmonary edema[115, 116] that may occur after removal of air in patients with pneumothorax is discussed in Chapter 51 (*see* page 2001).

At long-term follow-up, patients who are subjected to unilateral pleurodesis for pneumothorax have normal pulmonary function[117] or, at most, mild restriction.[118] However, they show a change in regional lung ventilation manifested by distribution of boluses of xenon more to the apex and less to the base on the operated than on the unoperated side.[117] In addition, an assessment of diaphragmatic motion using ultrasonography has shown a measurable reduction in excursion of the sclerosed hemithorax.[119]

REFERENCES

1. Riemann R, Jakse R: Pneumothorax nach mediastinalemphysem: Über den ort und den mechanismus der pleuraruptur. Acta Anat 128:115, 1986.
2. Smith WG, Rothwell PPG: Treatment of spontaneous pneumothorax. Thorax 17:342, 1962.
3. Hyde L: Benign spontaneous pneumothorax. Ann Intern Med 56:746, 1962.
4. Lindskog GE, Halasz NA: Spontaneous pneumothorax: A consideration of pathogenesis and management with review of seventy-two hospitalized cases. Arch Surg 75:693, 1957.
5. Primrose WR: Spontaneous pneumothorax: A retrospective review of aetiology, pathogenesis and management. Scott Med J 29:15, 1984.
6. Chan TB, Tan WC, Tech PC: Spontaneous pneumothorax in medical practise in a general hospital. Ann Acad Med Singapore 14:457, 1985.
7. Lesur O, Delorme N, Fromaget JM, et al: Computed tomography in the etiologic assessment of idiopathic spontaneous pneumothorax. Chest 98:341, 1990.
8. Bense L, Lewander R, Eklund G, et al: Nonsmoking, non-alpha1-antitrypsin deficiency-induced emphysema in nonsmokers with healed spontaneous pneumothorax, identified by computed tomography of the lungs. Chest 103:433, 1993.
9. Andrivet P, Kjedaini K, Teboul JL, et al: Spontaneous pneumothorax: Comparison of thoracic drainage vs immediate or delayed needle aspiration. Chest 108:335, 1995.
10. Melton LJ III, Hepper NGG, Offord KP: Incidence of spontaneous pneumothorax in Olmsted County, Minnesota: 1950 to 1974. Am Rev Respir Dis 120:1379, 1979.
11. Bense L, Eklund G, Wiman LG: Smoking and the increased risk of contracting spontaneous pneumothorax. Chest 92:1009, 1987.
12. Wilson WG, Aylsworth AS: Familial spontaneous pneumothorax. Pediatrics 64:172, 1979.
13. Pierce JA, Suarez B, Reich T: More on familial spontaneous pneumothorax. Chest 78:263, 1980.
14. Sharpe IK, Ahmad M, Braun W: Familial spontaneous pneumothorax and HLA antigens. Chest 78:264, 1980.
15. Sugiyama Y, Maeda H, Yotsumoto H, et al: Familial spontaneous pneumothorax. Thorax 41:969, 1986.
16. Rashid A, Sendi A, Al-Kadhimi A, et al: Concurrent spontaneous pneumothorax in identical twins. Thorax 41:971, 1986.
17. Gibson GJ: Familial pneumothoraces and bullae. Thorax 32:88, 1977.
18. Nakamura H, Konishiike J, Sugamura A, et al: Epidemiology of spontaneous pneumothorax in women. Chest 89:378, 1986.
19. Abolnik IZ, Lossos IS, Zlotogora J, et al: On the inheritance of primary spontaneous pneumothorax. Am J Med Genet 40:155, 1991.
20. Lichter I, Gwynne JF: Spontaneous pneumothorax in young subjects. Thorax 26:409, 1971.
21. Jordan KG, Kwong JS, Flint J, Müller NL: Surgically treated pneumothorax: Radiologic and pathologic findings. Chest 111:280, 1997.
22. Grimes OF, Farber SM: Air cysts of the lung. Surg Gynecol Obstet 113:720, 1961.
23. Feraru F, Morrow CS: Surgery of subpleural blebs: Indications and contraindications. Am Rev Respir Dis 79:577, 1959.
24. Macklin MT, Macklin CC: Malignant interstitial emphysema of the lungs and mediastinum as an important occult complication in many respiratory diseases and other conditions: An interpretation of the clinical literature in the light of laboratory experiment. Medicine 23:281, 1944.
25. Cooley JC, Gillespie JB: Mediastinal emphysema: Pathogenesis and management. Report of a case. Dis Chest 49:104, 1966.
26. Jansveld CAF, Dijkman JH: Primary spontaneous pneumothorax and smoking. BMJ 4:559, 1975.
27. Bense L, Hedenstierna G, Lewander R, et al: Regional lung function of nonsmokers with healed spontaneous pneumothorax: A physiologic and emission radiologic study. Chest 90:352, 1986.
28. Leading article: Spontaneous pneumothorax and apical lung disease. BMJ 4:573, 1971.
29. Melton LJ III, Hepper NGG, Offord KP: Influence of height on the risk of spontaneous pneumothorax. Mayo Clin Proc 56:678, 1981.
30. Kawakami Y, Irie T, Kamishima K: Stature, lung height, and spontaneous pneumothorax. Respiration 43:35, 1982.
31. West JB: Distribution of mechanical stress in the lung, a possible factor in localisation of pulmonary disease. Lancet 1:839, 1971.
32. Peters RM, Peters BA, Benirschke SK, et al: Chest dimensions in young adults with spontaneous pneumothorax. Ann Thorac Surg 25:193, 1978.
33. Hall JR, Pyeritz RE, Dudgeon DL, et al: Pneumothorax in the Marfan syndrome: Prevalence and therapy. Ann Thorac Surg 37:500, 1984.
34. Lipton RA, Greenwald RA, Seriff NS: Pneumothorax and bilateral honeycombed lung in Marfan syndrome: Report of a case and review of the pulmonary abnormalities in this disorder. Am Rev Respir Dis 104:924, 1971.
35. Smit J, Alberts C, Balk AG: Pneumothorax in the Ehlers-Danlos syndrome: Consequence or coincidence? Scand J Respir Dis 59:239, 1978.
36. Margaliot SZ, Barzilay J, Bar-David M, et al: Spontaneous pneumothorax and mitral valve prolapse. Chest 89:93, 1986.
37. Inouye WY, Berggren RB, Johnson J: Spontaneous pneumothorax: Treatment and mortality. Dis Chest 51:67, 1967.
38. Ruckley CV, McCormack RJM: The management of spontaneous pneumothorax. Thorax 21:139, 1966.
39. Mitlehner W, Friedrich M, Dissmann W: Value of computer tomography in the detection of bullae and blebs in patients with primary spontaneous pneumothorax. Respiration 59:221, 1992.
40. Bense L, Wiman LG, Hedenstierna G: Onset of symptoms in spontaneous pneumothorax: Correlations to physical activity. Eur J Respir Dis 71:181, 1987.
41. Dermksian G, Lamb LE: Spontaneous pneumothorax in apparently healthy flying personnel. Ann Intern Med 51:39, 1959.
42. Rose DM, Jarczyk PA: Spontaneous pneumoperitoneum after scuba diving. JAMA 239:223, 1978.
43. Saywell WR: Submarine escape training, lung cysts and tension pneumothorax. Br J Radiol 62:276, 1989.
44. Scott GC, Berger R, McKean HE: The role of atmospheric pressure variation in the development of spontaneous pneumothoraces. Am Rev Respir Dis 139:659, 1989.
45. West J: Distribution of mechanical stress in the lung, a possible factor in localisation of pulmonary disease. Lancet 1:839, 1971.
46. Vawter DL, Matthews FL, West JB: Effect of shape and size of lung and chest wall on stresses in the lung. J Appl Physiol 39:9, 1975.
47. Wait MA, Estrera A: Changing clinical spectrum of spontaneous pneumothorax. Am J Surg 164:528, 1992.
48. Graf-Deuel E, Knoblauch A: Simultaneous bilateral spontaneous pneumothorax. Chest 105:1142, 1994.
49. Pettersson GB, Gatzinsky P, Selin K: A case of total bilateral spontaneous pneumothorax. Scand J Thorac Cardiovasc Surg 17:175, 1983.
50. Donovan PJ: Bilateral spontaneous pneumothorax: A rare entity. Ann Emerg Med 16:1277, 1987.
51. Woodring JH, Baker MD, Stark P: Pneumothorax ex vacuo. Chest 110:1102, 1996.
52. Berdon WE, Dee GJ, Abramson ST, et al: Localized pneumothorax adjacent to a collapsed lobe: A sign of bronchial obstruction. Radiology 150:691, 1984.
53. Maurer ER, Schaal JA, Mendez FL: Chronic recurrent spontaneous pneumothorax due to endometriosis of the diaphragm. JAMA 168:2013, 1958.
54. Soderberg CH Jr, Dahlquist EH Jr: Catamenial pneumothorax. Surgery 79:236, 1976.
55. Downey DB, Towers MJ, Poon PY, et al: Pneumoperitoneum with catamenial pneumothorax. Am J Roentgenol 155:29, 1990.
56. Müller NL, Nelems B: Postcoital catamenial pneumothorax: Report of a case not associated with endometriosis and successfully treated with tubal ligation. Am Rev Respir Dis 134:803, 1986.
57. Lillington GA, Mitchell SP, Wood GA: Catamenial pneumothorax. JAMA 219:1328, 1972.
58. Shiraishi T: Catamenial pneumothorax: A report of a case and review of the Japanese and non-Japanese literature. Thorac Cardiovasc Surg 39:304, 1991.
59. Balasingham S, Arulkumaran S, Nadarajah K, et al: Catamenial pneumothorax. Aust N Z J Obstet Gynecol 26:88, 1986.
60. Schoenfeld A, Ziv E, Zeelel Y, et al: Catamenial pneumothorax: A literature review and report of an unusual case. Obstet Gynecol Surv 41:20, 1986.
61. Carter EJ, Ettensohn DB: Catamenial pneumothorax. Chest 98:713, 1990.
62. Karpel JP, Appel D, Merav A: Pulmonary endometriosis of the lung. Lung 163:151, 1985.
63. Joseph J, Sahn SA: Thoracic endometriosis syndrome: New observations from an analysis of 110 cases. Am J Med 100:164, 1996.
64. Jelihovsky T, Grant AF: Endometriosis of the lung. Thorax 23:434, 1968.
65. Foster DC, Stern JL, Buscema J, et al: Pleural and parenchymal pulmonary endometriosis. Obstet Gynecol 58:552, 1981.
66. Slasky BS, Siewers RD, Lecky JW, et al: Catamenial pneumothorax: The roles of diaphragmatic defects and endometriosis. Am J Roentgenol 138:639, 1982.
67. Hinson JM, Brigham KL, Daniell J: Catamenial pneumothorax in sisters. Chest 80:634, 1981.
68. Rossi NP, Goplerud CP: Recurrent catamenial pneumothorax. Arch Surg 109:173, 1974.
69. Assor D: Endometriosis of the lung. Am J Clin Pathol 57:311, 1972.
70. Lattes R, Shepard F, Tovell H, et al: A clinical and pathologic study of endometriosis of the lung. Surg Gynecol Obstet 103:552, 1956.
71. Granberg I, Willems JS: Endometriosis of lung and pleura diagnosed by aspiration biopsy. Acta Cytol 21:295, 1977.
72. Van Schil PE, Vercauteren SR, Vermeire PA, et al: Catamenial pneumothorax caused by thoracic endometriosis. Ann Thorac Surg 62:585, 1996.
73. Yamazaki S, Ogawa J, Koide S, et al: Catamenial pneumothorax associated with endometriosis of the diaphragm. Chest 77:107, 1980.
74. Im J-G, Kang HS, Choi BI, et al: Pleural endometriosis: CT and sonographic findings. Am J Roentgenol 148:523, 1987.
75. Brown RC: A unique case of catamenial pneumothorax (letter to editor). Chest 95:1368, 1989.
76. Shahar H, Angelillo VA: Catamenial pneumomediastinum. Chest 90:776, 1986.
77. Birrer RB, Calderon J: Pneumothorax, pneumomediastinum, and pneumopericardium following Valsalva's maneuver during marijuana smoking. NY State J Med 84:619, 1984.
78. Najafi JA, Guzman LG: Spontaneous pneumothorax in labor. Am J Obstet Gynecol 129:463, 1977.
79. Najafi JA, Guzman LG: Spontaneous pneumothorax in labor: Case report. Milit Med 143:341, 1978.

80. Bending JJ: Spontaneous pneumothorax in pregnancy and labour. Postgrad Med J 58:711, 1982.
81. Farrell SJ: Spontaneous pneumothorax in pregnancy: A case report and review of the literature. Obstet Gynecol 62(3 Suppl):43s, 1983.
82. Shesser R, Davis C, Edelstein S: Pneumomediastinum and pneumothorax after inhaling alkaloidal cocaine. Ann Emerg Med 10:213, 1981.
83. Weiner MD, Putman CE. Pain in the chest in a user of cocaine. JAMA 258:2087, 1987.
84. Eurman DW, Potash HI, Eyler WR, et al: Chest pain and dyspnea related to "crack" cocaine smoking: Value of chest radiography. Radiology 172:459, 1989.
85. Haim DY, Lippmann ML, Goldberg SK, et al: The pulmonary complications of crack cocaine: A comprehensive review. Chest 107:233, 1995.
86. Despars JA, Sassoon CSH, Light RW: Significance of iatrogenic pneumothoraces. Chest 105:1147, 1994.
87. Ludwig J, Kienzle GD: Pneumothorax in a large autopsy population: A study of 77 cases. Am J Clin Pathol 70:24, 1978.
88. Albelda SM, Gefter WB, Kelley MA, et al: Ventilator-induced subpleural air cysts: Clinical, radiographic, and pathologic significance. Am Rev Respir Dis 127:360, 1983.
89. Douglass RE, Levison MA: Pneumothorax in drug abusers: An urban epidemic? Am Surg 52:377, 1986.
90. Wisdom K, Nowak RM, Richardson HH, et al: Alternate therapy for traumatic pneumothorax in "pocket shooters." Ann Emerg Med 15:428, 1986.
91. Lewis JW Jr, Groux N, Elliot JP Jr, et al: Complications of attempted central venous injections performed by drug abusers. Chest 78:613, 1980.
92. Cohen HL, Cohen SW: Spontaneous bilateral pneumothorax in drug addicts. Chest 86:645, 1984.
93. Savitt D, Oblinger P, Levy RC: Bilateral pneumothorax in an intravenous drug abuser. J Emerg Med 2:405, 1985.
94. Zorc TG, O'Donnell AE, Holt RW, et al: Bilateral pneumothorax secondary to intravenous drug abuse. Chest 93:645, 1988.
95. Brewer LL, Moskowitz PS, Carrington CB, et al: Pneumatosis pulmonalis: A complication of the idiopathic respiratory distress syndrome. Am J Pathol 95:171, 1979.
96. Tomashefski JF, Bruce M, Stern RC, et al: Pulmonary air cysts in cystic fibrosis: Relation of pathologic features to radiologic findings and history of pneumothorax. Hum Pathol 16:253, 1985.
97. Askin FB, McCann BG, Kuhn C: Reactive eosinophilic pleuritis: A lesion to be distinguished from pulmonary eosinophilic granuloma. Arch Pathol Lab Med 101:187, 1977.
98. McDonnell TJ, Crouch EC, Gonzalez JG: Reactive eosinophilic pleuritis: A sequela of pneumothorax in pulmonary eosinophilic granuloma. Am J Clin Pathol 91:107, 1989.
99. Halíček F, Rosai J: Histioeosinophilic granulomas in the thymuses of 29 myasthenic patients. A complication of pneumomediastinum. Hum Pathol 15:1137, 1984.
100. Lacronique J, Roth C, Battesti J-P, et al: Chest radiographic features of pulmonary histiocytosis X: A report based on 50 adult cases. Thorax 37:104, 1982.
101. Luna E, Tomashefski JF Jr, Brown D, et al: Reactive eosinophilic pulmonary vascular infiltration in patients with spontaneous pneumothorax. Am J Surg Pathol 18:195, 1994.
102. Roelandt J, Willems J, van der Hauwaert LG, et al: Clicks and sounds (whoops) in left-sided pneumothorax: A clinical and phonocardiographic study. Dis Chest 56:31, 1969.
103. Desser KB, Benchimol A: Clicks secondary to pneumothorax confounding diagnosis of mitral valve prolapse. Chest 71:523, 1977.
104. Widder D: Ptosis associated with iatrogenic pneumothorax: A false lateralizing sign. Arch Intern Med 142:145, 1982.
105. McCall CS, Nguyen TQ, Vines FS, et al: Pneumocephalus secondary to tension pneumothorax associated with comminuted fracture of the thoracic spine. Neurosurgery 19:120, 1986.
106. Bogaert MG, van der Straeten M: Relapsing spontaneous pneumopericardium and pneumothorax with proven pleuropericardial defect: A case report. Scand J Respir Dis 60:17, 1979.
107. No reference cited.
108. Peatfield RC, Edwards PR, Johnson NM: Two unexpected deaths from pneumothorax. Lancet 1:356, 1979.
109. Woodruff WW III, Gamba JL, Putman CE, et al: Chronic tension pneumothorax presumably due to a "ball valve" bronchopleural fistula. South Med J 79:510, 1986.
110. Abyholm FE, Storen G: Spontaneous haemopneumothorax. Thorax 28:376, 1973.
111. Adelman M, Albelda SM, Gottlieb J, et al: Diagnostic utility of pleural fluid eosinophilia. Am J Med 77:915, 1984.
112. Norris RM, Jones JG, Bishop JM: Respiratory gas exchange in patients with spontaneous pneumothorax. Thorax 23:427, 1968.
113. Anthonisen NR: Regional lung function in spontaneous pneumothorax. Am Rev Respir Dis 115:873, 1977.
114. Hickok DF, Ballenger FP: The management of spontaneous pneumothorax due to emphysematous blebs. Surg Gynecol Obstet 120:499, 1965.
115. Yamazaki S, Ogawa J, Shohzu A, et al: Pulmonary blood flow to rapidly re-expanded lung in spontaneous pneumothorax. Chest 81:118, 1982.
116. Pavlin DJ, Raghu G, Rogers TR, et al: Reexpansion hypotension: A complication of rapid evacuation of prolonged pneumothorax. Chest 89:70, 1986.
117. Fleetham JA, Forkert L, Clarke H, et al: Regional lung function in the presence of pleural symphysis. Am Rev Respir Dis 122:33, 1980.
118. Lange P, Mortensen J, Groth S: Lung function 22–35 years after treatment of idiopathic spontaneous pneumothorax with talc poudrage or simple drainage. Thorax 43:559, 1988.
119. Loring SH, Kurachek SC, Wohl ME: Diaphragmatic excursion after pleural sclerosis. Chest 95:374, 1989.
120. Graham ML, Spelsberg TC, Dines DE, et al: Pulmonary lymphangiomyomatosis: With particular reference to steroid-receptor assay studies and pathologic correlation. Mayo Clin Proc 59:3, 1984.
121. Müller NL, Chiles C, Kullnig P: Pulmonary lymphangiomyomatosis: Correlation of CT with radiographic and functional findings. Radiology 175:335, 1990.
122. Babcock TL, Snyder BA: Spontaneous pneumothorax associated with tuberous sclerosis. J Thorac Cardiovasc Surg 83:100, 1982.
123. Castro M, Shepherd CW, Gomez MR, et al: Pulmonary tuberous sclerosis. Chest 107:189, 1995.
124. Torrington KG, Ashbaugh DG, Stackle EG: Recklinhausen's disease. Occurence with intrathoracic vagal neurofibroma and contralateral spontaneous pneumothorax. Arch Intern Med 143:568, 1983.
125. Cohen S, Hossain MS-A: Primary carcinoma of the lung. A review of 417 histologically proved cases. Dis Chest 49:67, 1966.
126. Torre D, Martegani R, Speranza F, et al: Pulmonary cryptococcosis presenting as pneumothorax in a patient with AIDS. Clin Infect Dis 21:1524, 1995.
127. Haber K, Freundlich IM: Spontaneous pneumothorax with unusual manifestations. Chest 65:675, 1974.
128. Edelstein G, Levitt RG: Cavitary coccidioidomycosis presenting as spontaneous pneumothorax. Am J Roentgenol 141:533, 1983.
129. McClellan MD, Miller SB, Parsons PE, et al: Pneumothorax with *Pneumocystis carinii* pneumonia in AIDS: Incidence and clinical characteristics. Chest 100:1224, 1991.
130. Goodman PC, Daley C, Minagi H: Spontaneous pneumothorax in AIDS patients with *Pneumocystis carinii* pneumonia. Am J Roentgenol 147:29, 1986.
131. Bakir F, Al-Omeri MM: Echinococcal tension pneumothorax. Thorax 24:547, 1969.
132. Khan F, Seriff NS: Pneumothorax. A rare presenting manifestation of lung cancer. Am Rev Respir Dis 108:1397, 1973.
133. Wagner RB, Knox GS: Pneumothorax: An unusual manifestation of a bronchial carcinoid. Md Med J 39:263, 1990.
134. Michelassi PL, Sbragia S: Clinicoradiological considerations on 2 cases of spontaneous pneumothorax, apparently idiopathic, secondary to pulmonary metastases. Ann Radiol Diag 33:39, 1960.
135. Smevik B, Klepp O: The risk of spontaneous pneumothorax in patients with osteogenic sarcoma and testicular cancer. Cancer 49:1734, 1982.
136. Janetos GP, Ochsner SF: Bilateral pneumothorax in metastatic osteogenic sarcoma. Am Rev Respir Dis 88:73, 1963.
137. D'Angio GJ, Iannaccone G: Spontaneous pneumothorax as a complication of pulmonary metastases in malignant tumors of childhood. Am J Roentgenol 86:1092, 1961.
138. Slasky BS, Deutsch M: Germ cell tumors complicated by pneumothorax. Urology 22,:39, 1983.
139. Lote K, Dahl O, Vigander T: Pneumothorax during combination chemotherapy. Cancer 47:1743, 1981.
140. Lesser JE, Carr D: Fatal pneumothorax following bleomycin and other cytotoxic drugs. Cancer Treat Rep 69:344, 1985.
141. Chen KW, Wu MH, Huang JJ, et al: Bilateral spontaneous pneumothoraces, pneumopericardium, pneumomediastinum, and subcutaneous emphysema: A rare presentation of paraquat intoxication. Ann Emerg Med 23: 1132,1994.
142. Murphy DG, Sloan EP, Hart RG, et al: Tension pneumothorax associated with hyperbaric oxygen therapy. Am J Emerg Med 9:176, 1991.
143. Twiford TW Jr, Zornoza J, Libshitz HI: Recurrent spontaneous pneumothorax after radiation therapy to the thorax. Chest: 73:387, 1978.
144. Pezner RD, Horak DA, Sayegh HO, et al: Spontaneous pneumothorax in patients irradiated for Hodgkin's disease and other malignant lymphomas. Int J Radiat Oncol Biol Phys 18:193, 1990.
144a. Okada M, Ebe K, Matsumoto T, et al: Ipsilateral spontaneous pneumothorax after rapid development of large thin-walled cavities in two patients who had undergone radiation therapy for lung cancer. Am J Roentgenol 170:932, 1998.
145. Metersky ML, Colt HG, Olson LK, et al: AIDS-related spontaneous pneumothorax. Risk factors and treatment. Chest 109:946, 1995.
146. Epstein DM, GEften WB, Miller WT, et al: Spontaneous pneumothorax: An uncommon manifestation of Wegener granulomatosis. Radiology 135:327, 1980.
147. Nickol KH: Idiopathic pulmonary haemosiderosis presenting with spontaneous pneumothorax. Tubercle 41:216, 1960.
148. Moore ADA, Godwin JD, Müller NL, et al: Pulmonary histiocytosis X: Comparison of radiographic and CT findings. Radiology 172:249, 1989.
149. Neitzschman HR, Ramirez J, McCarthy K: Radiology case of the month. Sudden onset of shortness of breath. Sarcoidosis, complicated by acute pneumothorax. J Louisiana State Med Soc 149:145, 1997.
150. Froudarakis ME, Bouros D, Voloudaki A, et al: Pneumothorax as a first manifestation of sarcoidosis. Chest 112:278, 1997.
151. Bierman CW: Pneumomediastinum and pneumothorax complicating asthma in children. Am J Dis Child 114:42, 1967.
152. Bense L, Eklund G, Wiman LG: Smoking and the increased risk of contracting spontaneous pneumothorax. Chest 92:1009, 1987.
153. Spector ML, Stern RC: Pneumothorax in cystic fibrosis: A 26-year experience. Ann Thorac Surg 47:204, 1989.
154. Bailey WC, Brown M, Buechner HA, et al: Silico-mycobacterial disease in sandblasters. Am Rev Respir Dis 110:115, 1974.

155. Weber AL, Stoeckle JD, Hardy HL: Roentgenologic patterns in long-standing beryllium disease. Report of 8 cases. Am J Roentgenol 93:879, 1965.

156. Shaver CG, Riddell AR: Lung changes associated with the manifestation of alumina abrasives. J Industr Hyg Toxicol 29:145, 1947.

157. Blundell JE: Pneumothorax complicating pulmonary infarction. Br J Radiol 40:226, 1967.

158. Hall FM, Salzman EW, Ellis BI, et al: Pneumothorax complicating aseptic cavitating pulmonary infarction. Chest 72:232, 1977.

159. Anton HC, Gray B: Pulmonary alveolar proteinosis presenting with pneumothorax. Clin Radiol 18:428, 1967.

160. McDonald CF, Walbaum PR, Sircus W, et al: Intrapleural perforation of peptic ulcer in association with diaphragmatic hernia. Br J Dis Chest 79:196, 1985.

161. Rotstein OD, Pruett TL, Simmons RL: Gastropleural fistula. Report of three cases and review of the literature. Am J Surg 150:392, 1985.

162. Price BA, Elliott MJ, Featherstone G, et al: Perforation of intrathoracic colon causing acute pneumothorax. Thorrax 38:959, 1983.

163. Kazerooni EA, Lim FT, Mikhail A, et al: Risk of pneumothorax in CT-guided transthoracic needle aspiration biopsy of the lung. Radiology 198:371, 1996.

164. Westcott JL, Rao N, Colley DP: Thoracic needle biopsy of small pulmonary nodules. Radiology 202:97, 1997.

165. Anders GT, Johnson JE, Bush BA, et al: Transbronchial biopsy without fluoroscopy: A seven-year perspective. Chest 94:557, 1988.

166. Schmidt G, Börsch G, Wegener M: Subcutaneous emphysema and pneumothorax complicating diagnostic colonoscopy. Dis Colon Rectum 29:136, 1986.

167. Catania S, Boccato P, Bono A, et al: Pneumothorax: A rare complication of fine needle aspiration of the breast. Acta Cytol 33:140, 1989.

168. Maggs PR, Schwaber JR: Fatal bilateral pneumothoraces complicating subclavian vein catheterization. Chest 71:552, 1977.

169. Slezak FA, Williams GB: Delayed pneumothorax: A complication of subclavian vein catheterization. J Parenter Enteral Nutr 8:571, 1984.

170. Sheffner SE, Gross BH, Birnberg FA, et al: Iatrogenic bronchopleural fistula caused by feeding tube insertion. J Can Assoc Radiol 36:52, 1985.

171. Scholten DJ, Wood TL, Thompson DR: Pneumothorax from nasoenteric feeding tube insertion. A report of five cases. Am Surg 52:381, 1986.

172. Padovan IF, Dawson CA, Henschel EO, et al: Pathogenesis of mediastinal emphysema and pneumothorax following tracheotomy (experimental approaches). Chest 66:553, 1974.

173. Biswas C, Jana N, Maitra S: Bilateral pneumothorax following tracheal intubation. Br J Anaesth 62:338, 1989.

174. Honet JE, Honet JC, Cascade P: Pneumothorax after electromyographic electrode insertion in the paracervical muscles: Case report and radiographic analysis. Arch Phys Med Rahabil 67: 601, 1986.

175. Ritter HG, Tarala R: Pneumothorax after acupuncture. BMJ 2:602, 1978.

176. Munshi CA, Bardeen-Henschel A: Hydropneumothorax after percutaneous nephrolithotomy. Anesth Analg 64:840, 1985.

177. O'Donnell A, Schoenberger C, Weiner J, et al: Pulmonary complications of percutaneous nephrostomy and kidney stone extraction. South Med J 81:1002, 1988.

178. Odland R, Adams G: Pneumothorax as a complication of tracheoesophageal voice prosthesis use. Ann Otol Rhinol Laryngol 97:537, 1988.

CHAPTER 71

Pleural Fibrosis

After effusion, fibrosis is undoubtedly the most common pleural abnormality. As with the former condition, fibrosis has numerous etiologies and is the outcome of many primary pleural diseases, as well as a potential complication of virtually every inflammatory condition that affects the lungs. In the majority of cases, the fibrosis is patchy or is localized to a single, relatively small area; in these circumstances clinical and functional abnormalities are absent, and the condition is recognized on a screening radiograph or computed tomography (CT) during the investigation of other intrathoracic disease or at autopsy. Less commonly, the fibrosis is more or less diffuse in one or both pleural cavities, in which case functional abnormalities may be apparent. Because of this important difference, the two forms are discussed separately.

LOCAL PLEURAL FIBROSIS

Healed Pleuritis

The most common cause of localized pleural fibrosis is organized fibrinous or fibrinopurulent pleuritis secondary to pneumonia. Because pleural effusions of infectious etiology are almost invariably basal, it is not surprising that this is the anatomic location of most pleural thickening of this etiology. The usual radiographic abnormality is partial obliteration or blunting of the posterior and lateral costophrenic sulci, in some cases associated with line shadows. Thickening of the pleural line may extend for a variable distance up the lateral and posterior thoracic walls, diminishing gradually toward the apex and seldom amounting to more than 1 to 2 mm in width. Obliteration of the costophrenic sulci sometimes has a radiographic appearance difficult to differentiate from that of a small pleural effusion, in which case radiography in the lateral decubitus position, ultrasound, or CT is required for clarification.

The "Apical Cap"

An "apical cap" can be defined as a curved soft tissue opacity seen on the chest radiograph at the apex of one or both hemithoraces (Fig. 71–1).[1, 2] Although the abnormality can have a number of etiologies, in most cases the cause is unknown. Such "idiopathic" caps usually measure less than 5 mm in height and have a sharply marginated smooth or undulating lower margin.[1, 2] In a review of the chest radiographs of 258 patients, a unilateral cap was seen in 11% and bilateral caps in 12%.[1] The prevalence increased with age, being identified in 6% of patients younger than 45 years and 16% of those older than 45.[1] The prevalence is similar in men and women.[1]

Pathologically, "idiopathic" apical caps consist of a combination of pleural and pulmonary parenchymal fibrosis, the latter usually predominating (Fig. 71–2).[3] Histologically, the pleura is thickened by dense, sometimes hyalinized, collagen, accompanied in some cases by small foci of mononuclear inflammatory cells. The architecture of the underlying lung parenchyma is preserved, but the air spaces are obliterated by fibrous tissue (*see* Fig. 71–2); elastic tissue in the alveolar septa is typically increased. Although focal areas of calcification or ossification can be seen, evidence of prior granulomatous inflammation and necrosis, such as seen in tuberculosis, is absent.[1, 3] The pathogenesis of the fibrosis is uncertain. In one autopsy study, an association with histologic evidence of chronic bronchitis and pulmonary artery narrowing was identified; the investigators suggested that intermittent or continuing low-grade infection combined with relative apical ischemia might be responsible for the fibrosis.[3]

As indicated, a specific cause for a cap can be identified occasionally. The abnormality is commonly present in patients who have upper lobe fibrosis secondary to tuberculosis.[4] In this situation, the cap is often larger than in the idiopathic variety, not uncommonly measuring several centimeters in thickness (Fig. 71–3).[4] In one HRCT study of 18 patients who had longstanding tuberculosis, most of the apical cap was the result of an accumulation of extrapleural fat. Where the fat and lung came in contact, a 1 to 3 mm thick rim of soft tissue was evident, presumably representing the thickened visceral and parietal pleural layers. The lung adjacent to the cap showed evidence of scarring and traction bronchiectasis. Apical caps may also be the result of pleural and subpleural fibrosis following radiation therapy for carcinoma of the breast, lung, or neck.[2, 5]

An apical cap may be confused radiologically with the

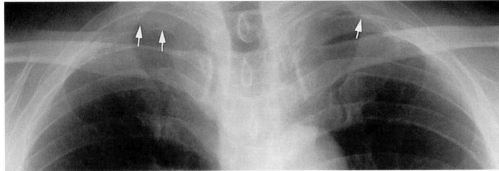

Figure 71–1. Apical Cap. A view of the upper hemithorax from a posteroanterior chest radiograph in a 72-year-old man demonstrates normal apical caps *(arrows)*.

companion shadows of the first and second ribs. Of greater importance from a differential diagnostic point of view is the early stage of an apical pulmonary carcinoma (Pancoast's tumor, Fig. 71–4). Suspicion of the latter condition should be aroused when the apical abnormality is predominantly unilateral, when there is a greater than 5 mm difference in height between right and left apical caps, when there is a focal convexity, or when sequential radiographs show progressive enlargement. Other uncommon causes of an increased apical opacity include extrapleural extension of tumor in patients who have lymphoma, mesothelioma, and dilation of the subclavian veins.[2] Apical caps that develop acutely are usually the result of the extrapleural accumulation of blood following trauma to the chest wall or thoracic aorta.[6, 7] A similar process may occur as a complication of placement of internal jugular or subclavian venous catheters.[2]

Pleural Plaques

Pleural plaques are well circumscribed foci of dense fibrous tissue that typically are located on the parietal pleura (*see* pages 2424 and 2431). The lesion is common: of 7,085 autopsies in the general population reported in 16 separate studies, they were identified in 857 (12%).[8] Because the etiology of the fibrosis is asbestos in the vast majority of cases (*see* farther on), the prevalence is influenced by the population studied and is especially high if there has been contact with an increased level of asbestos particles in the ambient air. For example, the prevalence has been found to be approximately 4% in 381 autopsies in a general urban population,[9] 8% in 862 autopsies in a general population in an asbestos-industrial region,[10] and 39% in a population in a coastal, urban, and asbestos-mining region.[11]

Etiology

The identification of pleural plaques can be regarded as highly suggestive evidence of asbestos-related disease. In several series in which they have been discovered in randomized or consecutive autopsies or at chest radiography, a history of asbestos exposure has been obtained in approximately 80% of cases.[12–14] Even without such a history, evidence of an asbestos etiology sometimes is obtained by fiber analysis of lung digests. For example, in one retrospective study in which the number of asbestos bodies in the lung at autopsy was correlated with radiologic appearances premor-

tem, radiographic features of asbestos-related disease (most often calcified and noncalcified pleural plaques) were found in eight of nine cases in which asbestos bodies exceeded 40 in number;[15] in only one of these cases had significant exposure been recognized during life. However, such findings need not reflect direct occupational exposure, as evidenced by asbestos-induced disease acquired from tremolite-contaminated soil in the Metsovo area of northwestern Greece,[16, 17] in isolated villages in Turkey,[18, 19] in Corsica,[20] and in Quebec.[21]

Pleural plaques are evident on the chest radiograph in 20% to 60% of workers exposed to high concentrations of asbestos.[8] The latency period between exposure to asbestos and development of radiologically visible plaques is approximately 15 years; for radiologically visible calcified plaques, the latency period is at least 20 years.[8, 22]

Pathologic Characteristics

Pleural plaques are usually found in the parietal pleura, where they appear as well-circumscribed foci of fibrosis that are typically ivory white in color (Fig. 71–5). Occasionally, they affect the visceral pleura.[23–25] The plaques may be smooth or nodular in contour and can measure up to 1 cm in thickness, although they usually are much thinner (*see* page 2424). They occur most commonly on the tendinous portion of the diaphragm, on the posterolateral chest wall between the seventh and tenth ribs, and on the lateral chest wall between the sixth and ninth ribs. Adhesions between visceral and parietal pleural membranes develop infrequently.[26]

Radiologic Manifestations

Radiographically, the earliest manifestation of a pleural plaque is a thin line of soft tissue density under a rib in the axillary region, usually the seventh or eighth, on one or both sides. The plaques may be very difficult to visualize, particularly when viewed *en face,* and tangential radiographs or CT scans may be necessary. Although the value of 45-degree oblique projections has been stressed by some researchers,[27, 28] other investigators have concluded that these views add little to the detection of asbestos-induced disease in exposed workers: in a series of 489 male pipefitters examined in a screening program, the oblique views represented the sole evidence of an asbestos-related radiographic abnormality in only 8 (1.6%).[29] A comparison of radio-

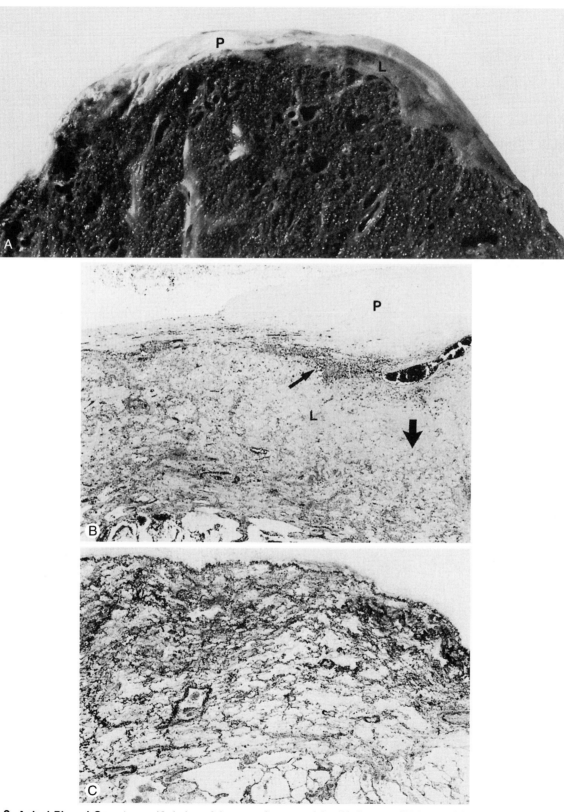

Figure 71–2. Apical Pleural Cap. A magnified view of the apex of an upper lobe *(A)* shows a mild degree of fibrosis affecting both the pleura (P) and underlying lung parenchyma (L). A section *(B)* reveals fibrosis within the pleura (P) and lung (L) associated with focal chronic inflammation *(thin arrow)*. Despite the parenchymal fibrosis, the underlying lung architecture is clearly preserved, as demonstrated in sections stained with hematoxylin-eosin *(large arrow* in *B)* and with elastic tissue stain *(C)*. *(B,* ×25; *C,* Verhoeff–van Gieson, ×25.)

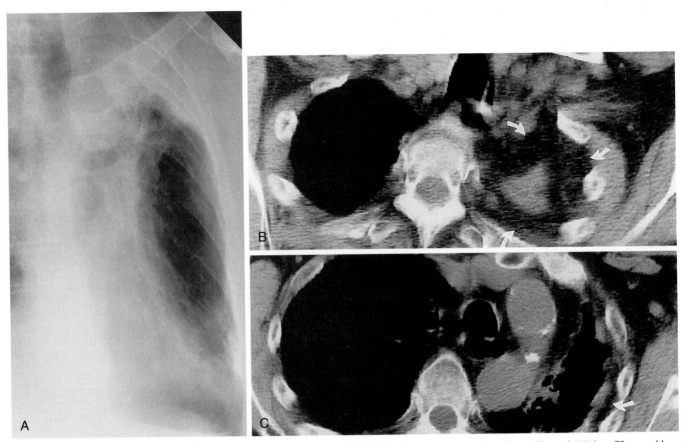

Figure 71–3. Apical Cap: Previous Tuberculosis. A view of the left hemithorax from a posteroanterior chest radiograph *(A)* in a 72-year-old man demonstrates marked loss of volume of the left upper lobe with superior retraction of the hilum. A large left apical cap is present. High-resolution CT scans *(B* and *C)* demonstrate that most of the apparent pleural thickening is due to the accumulation of extrapleural fat *(arrows)*. The patient had been treated for tuberculosis 20 years previously.

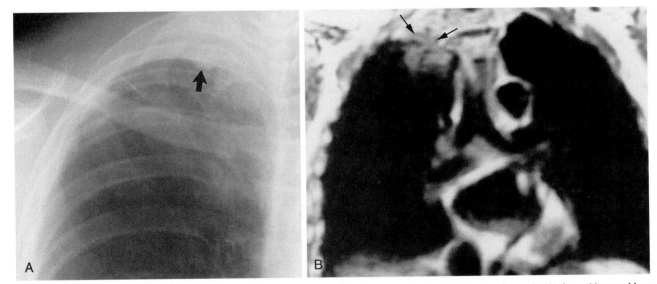

Figure 71–4. Pancoast's Tumor. A view of the right upper hemithorax from a posteroanterior chest radiograph *(A)* in a 44-year-old woman demonstrates a poorly defined right apical opacity with a focal inferior convexity *(arrow)*. Localized areas of scarring in the right upper lobe are also evident. Cardiac-gated T1-weighted (TR 706, TE 20) spin-echo coronal MR image *(B)* demonstrates tumor in the right lung apex with focal infiltration of the pleura and extrapleural soft tissues *(arrows)*. At surgery, the lesion proved to be a pulmonary carcinoma with focal chest wall invasion.

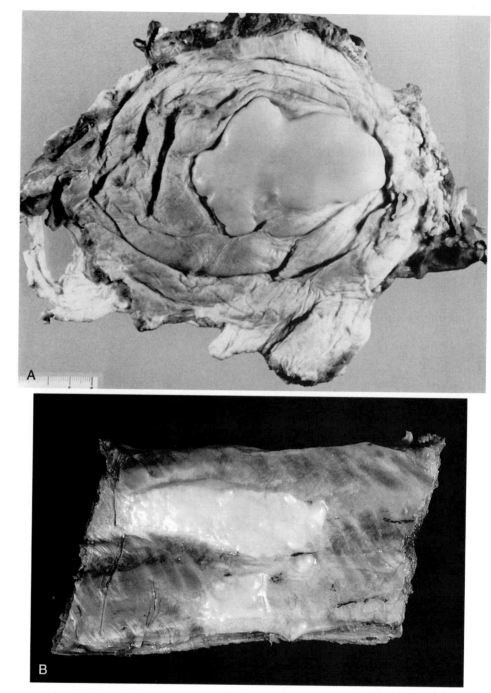

Figure 71–5. Parietal Pleural Plaques: Gross Appearance. A specimen of a hemidiaphragm *(A)* shows a smooth, pearly-white well-circumscribed area of fibrosis on the tendinous portion. A segment of two ribs *(B)* shows similar foci of fibrosis, one of which is elongated and roughly parallel to the long axis of the rib.

graphic findings during life with observations at autopsy indicates that a significant number of pleural plaques are missed on premortem radiographs.[30]

Pleural plaques are usually, but not invariably, bilateral. In a review of radiographs of 105,064 civilian and military employees of the U.S. Navy, 1,914 (1.8%) were interpreted as definitely showing pleural plaques.[31] Of these, 1,545 (81%) showed bilateral pleural plaques, 287 (15%) demonstrated only left plaques, and 82 (4%) showed only right plaques. This unexplained left-sided predominance has also been reported by others.[32, 33] The width and extent of pleural thickening and the extent of pleural plaque calcification are also frequently greater on the left than on the right (Fig.

71–6). For example, in one review of 408 patients who had asbestos-related pleural disease, the subjects were shown to be approximately 1.5 times as likely to have more severe localized pleural thickening and costal pleural calcification on the left than on the right; diaphragmatic calcification was 2.5 times as likely to be more severe on the left than on the right.[33]

The greatest problem in the diagnosis of early plaque formation lies in distinguishing plaques from normal companion shadows of the chest wall—not those that are associated with the first three ribs (because this area is rarely involved in asbestos-related disease) but those muscle and fat shadows that may be identified in as many as 75% of

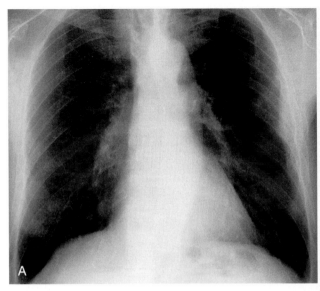

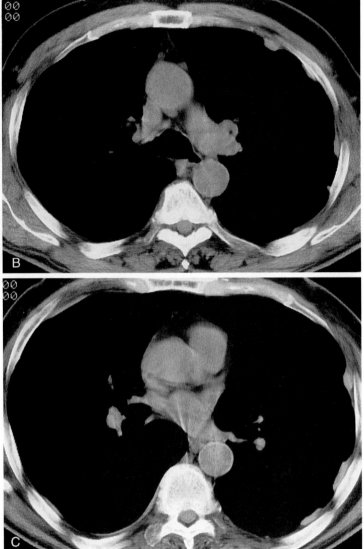

Figure 71–6. Pleural Plaques: Asymmetric Distribution.
A posteroanterior chest radiograph *(A)* in a 74-year-old shipyard
worker shows evidence of pleural plaques only on the left side.
High-resolution CT at the level of the tracheal carina *(B)* also
demonstrates only plaques on the left side. A scan through the lower
lung zones *(C)* demonstrates prominent plaques on the left side and
thin plaques on the right side.

normal posteroanterior radiographs along the convexity of
the thorax inferiorly. In fact, it is sometimes impossible to
differentiate pleural plaques from such companion shadows
with conviction. For example, in one study of 30 asbestos-
exposed patients in whom CT scans were performed because
of uncertainty as to whether the pleural changes observed
on chest radiographs were due to plaques or extrapleural fat,
the radiographic findings in 14 of the 30 patients (47%)
were shown on CT to be related to extrapleural fat (Fig.
71–7).[34] Noncalcified pleural plaques may also be difficult
to differentiate from normal diaphragmatic undulations (Fig.
71–8) and from focal postinfectious pleural thickening.

The accuracy in the diagnosis of pleural plaques on
chest radiography depends on the disease prevalence in the
sample population and the presence or absence of calcification.[13, 35, 36] In a study in which radiographic findings were
correlated with those at autopsy, the combination of bilateral
abnormalities and posterolateral pleural-based opacities at
least 5 mm thick or bilateral calcified diaphragmatic plaques
had a 100% positive predictive value for pathologically
confirmed asbestos-related plaques;[13] however, these criteria

allowed detection of only 3 of 24 (12%) plaques found at
autopsy. Using less strict criteria, similar to those recommended by the International Labor Office,[37] 11 of 24 (46%)
cases were identified; however, there were 15 (8.4%) false-
positive diagnoses.[13]

The detection of noncalcified pleural plaques on the
chest radiograph is determined mainly by plaque thickness.[38]
In one study of 402 patients from a general urban and rural
industrial region, 70 (17%) had pleural plaques at autopsy;[38]
27 (39%) of these were detected by chest radiography. None
of the plaques measuring less than 3 mm in thickness at
autopsy was detected radiographically. Overall, the sensitivity of radiography in the detection of pleural plaques in
various studies ranges from about 30% to 80% and the
specificity from 60% to 80%.[9, 13, 38, 39]

Several groups of investigators have shown that CT is
superior to chest radiography in the detection of pleural
plaques (*see* Fig. 71–6).[40–43] Normally, a 1- to 2-mm thick
stripe of soft tissue attenuation is visible on HRCT in the
intercostal spaces at the point of contact between the lung
and the chest wall.[44] This stripe (the intercostal stripe) corre-

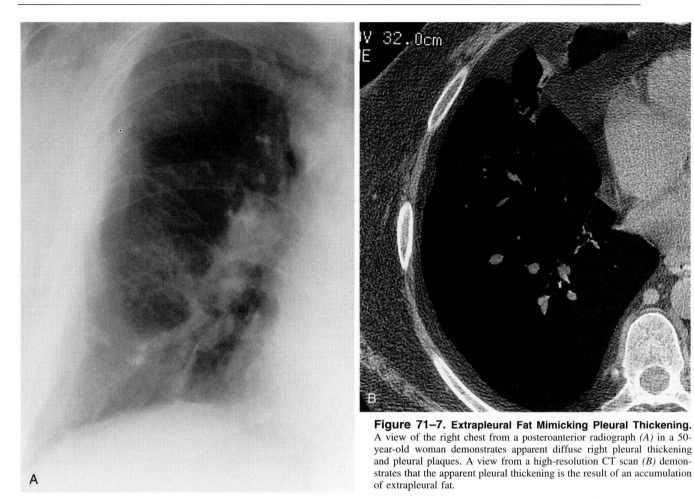

Figure 71–7. Extrapleural Fat Mimicking Pleural Thickening. A view of the right chest from a posteroanterior radiograph *(A)* in a 50-year-old woman demonstrates apparent diffuse right pleural thickening and pleural plaques. A view from a high-resolution CT scan *(B)* demonstrates that the apparent pleural thickening is the result of an accumulation of extrapleural fat.

sponds to the visceral and parietal pleura, the endothoracic fascia, and the innermost intercostal muscle. Normally, no soft tissue attenuation is seen internal to a rib or in the paravertebral regions because the intercostal muscles do not pass internally to the ribs or vertebrae and because the pleura is normally not thick enough to be seen in these locations. Pleural plaques are identified as circumscribed areas of pleural thickening, usually separated from the underlying rib and extrapleural soft tissues by a thin layer of fat. The majority of plaques are seen along the posterolateral surface of the parietal pleura in the lower thorax, with sparing of the lung apex and costophrenic angles. Occasionally, visceral pleural plaques can be identified within the interlobar fissures (Fig. 71–9).[23–25]

It is controversial whether HRCT is superior to conventional CT in the detection of pleural plaques.[40, 43, 45] In one study in which the HRCT, conventional CT, and chest radiographic findings were prospectively analyzed in 100 asbestos-exposed workers, plaques were evident on chest radiographs in 49 individuals, on conventional CT in 56, and on HRCT in 64.[40] In a second study in which HRCT was compared with conventional CT findings in 159 asbestos-exposed workers who had normal chest radiograph results, plaques were identified by both techniques in 48 patients, by HRCT alone in 1, and by conventional CT alone in 10.[43]

The frequency of radiologically detectable calcification in pleural plaques is also variable (Fig. 71–10), some investi-

gators having found calcified and noncalcified plaques in roughly equal numbers[46] and others having observed calcification in only about 20% of patients.[47] In one survey of 261 American workers exposed to asbestos in industry, none had evidence of pleural calcification,[48] whereas in Finland calcification was common;[49] this difference may be related to the variety of asbestos to which the individuals were exposed. Radiologically, calcified plaques vary from small linear or circular shadows usually situated over the diaphragmatic domes[50] to large shadows that completely encircle the lower portion of the lungs.[51] When calcification is minimal, a radiograph overexposed at maximal inspiration facilitates visibility.[52] When extensive and viewed *en face*, they may obscure or be confused with interstitial lung disease.

Clinical Manifestations

Pleural plaques do not cause symptoms. Although they also do not interfere with pulmonary function in most patients, some investigators have suggested that they are sometimes responsible for mild restriction.[53, 54] In one review of this subject, the authors concluded that (1) pleural plaques are not associated with a clinically significant reduction in pulmonary function; (2) diffuse pleural thickening, when extensive, can severely impair ventilation; and (3) when pleural lesions are responsible for reduced pulmonary func-

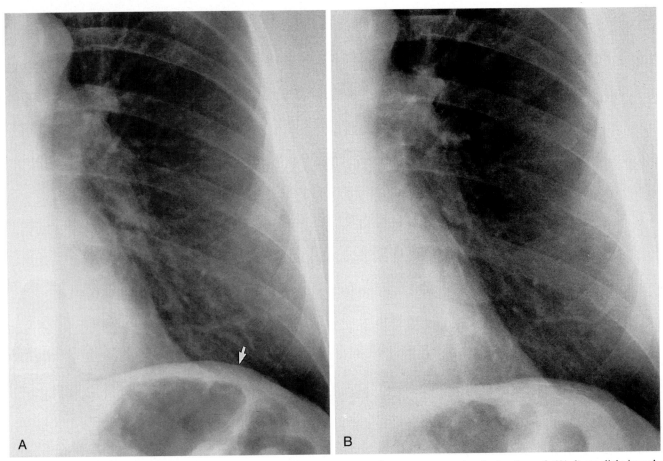

A   B

Figure 71–8. Diaphragmatic Pleural Plaque. A view of the left hemidiaphragm from a posteroanterior chest radiograph *(A)* shows slight irregularity
of the diaphragmatic contour due to a pleural plaque *(arrow).* This finding was missed prospectively. A view from a chest radiograph 4 years later *(B)*
shows calcification of the plaque. The patient was a 49-year-old man who had a history of exposure to asbestos.

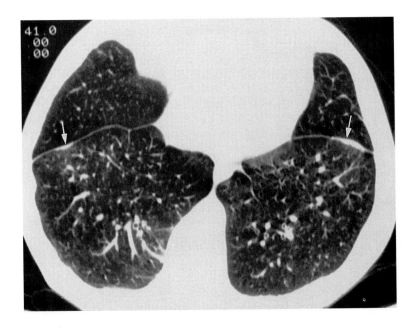

Figure 71–9. Plaques within Interlobar Fissures. A
high-resolution CT scan demonstrates pleural plaques in the right
and left major fissures *(arrows).* Curvilinear opacities in the
right paravertebral region can be seen to extend to an area of
pleural thickening. The patient was a 71-year-old man who had
previously worked in a shipyard.

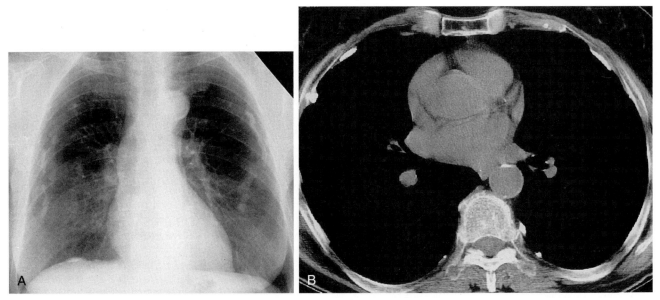

Figure 71–10. Calcified Asbestos-Related Pleural Plaques. A posteroanterior chest radiograph *(A)* and a CT scan *(B)* reveal multiple bilateral discrete calcified pleural plaques involving the costal, diaphragmatic, and paravertebral pleura. The patient was a 79-year-old man with previous occupational asbestos exposure.

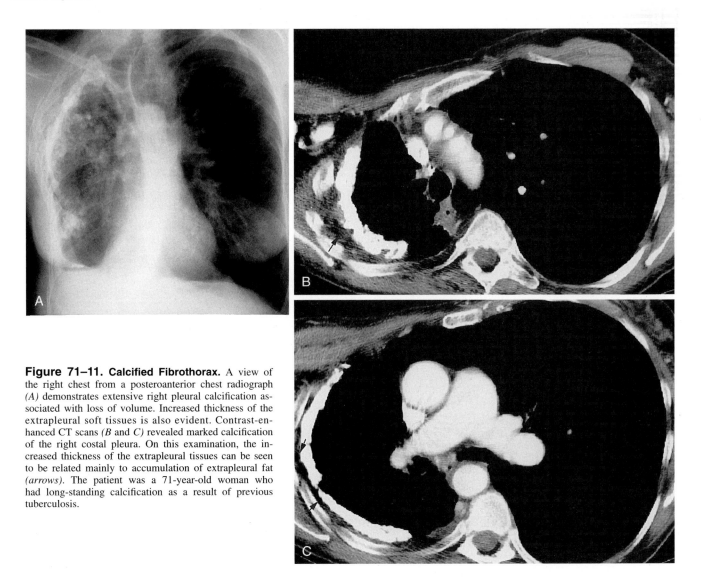

Figure 71–11. Calcified Fibrothorax. A view of the right chest from a posteroanterior chest radiograph *(A)* demonstrates extensive right pleural calcification associated with loss of volume. Increased thickness of the extrapleural soft tissues is also evident. Contrast-enhanced CT scans *(B* and *C)* revealed marked calcification of the right costal pleura. On this examination, the increased thickness of the extrapleural tissues can be seen to be related mainly to accumulation of extrapleural fat *(arrows)*. The patient was a 71-year-old woman who had long-standing calcification as a result of previous tuberculosis.

tion, the expected pattern is restriction with preserved diffusing capacity.[55]

DIFFUSE PLEURAL FIBROSIS

Radiographically, diffuse pleural thickening (fibrothorax) is considered to be present when a smooth, uninterrupted pleural opacity is seen extending over at least one fourth of the chest wall with or without obliteration of the costophrenic sulci.[56, 57] The thickness of the pleural "peel" may be as much as 2 cm or more but usually is less than 1 cm.[58] Pleural thickening is diagnosed as diffuse on CT when it extends for more than 8 cm craniocaudally and 5 cm laterally and the pleura is more than 3 mm thick.[57, 59] Depending to some extent on the severity and duration of the fibrosis, calcification may or may not be evident. Although focal or diffuse areas of increased attenuation of the pleura in fibrothorax are usually the result of calcification, occasionally a similar appearance is caused by clusters of talc following talc pleurodesis.[60] Long-standing fibrothorax is frequently associated with accumulation of extrapleural fat (Fig. 71–11).

Fibrothorax seldom affects the mediastinal pleura (Fig. 71–12).[57, 58, 61, 62] (The latter is defined as the pleura that abuts the mediastinum, the posterior extent of which is demarcated by the anterior aspect of the vertebrae; the paravertebral pleura is considered part of the costal pleura.[44, 57, 58]) For example, in one study of 16 patients who had diffuse pleural thickening related to asbestos exposure and 8 who had fibrothorax due to other causes, only 1 in each group (6% and 12.5%, respectively) had thickening of the mediastinal pleura evident on CT.[58] By comparison, thick-

ening of the mediastinal pleura was seen on CT in 8 of 11 (73%) patients who had mesothelioma and in 13 of 24 (54%) patients who had pleural metastases.

Fibrous obliteration of the pleural space develops most often following tuberculosis, empyema associated with nontuberculous bacteria, hemorrhagic effusion, and benign asbestos-related pleurisy. Less common causes include connective tissue diseases (particularly rheumatoid disease) and uremia.[63] The abnormality is a less common sequela of asbestos exposure than circumscribed plaques (*see* Fig. 71–12);[36, 40, 65, 66] for example, in a prospective study of 100 asbestos-exposed workers, pleural plaques were identified on HRCT in 64 and diffuse pleural thickening in only 7.[40] Four patients have also been reported who had disabling bilateral pleural effusions that progressed to diffuse pleural thickening; all four were human leukocyte antigen (HLA)-B44 positive, and none gave a history of asbestos exposure. The authors referred to this disorder as *cryptogenic bilateral fibrosing pleuritis.*[64]

The distribution and character of the fibrosis may yield clues to its etiology. Fibrothorax secondary to tuberculosis, nontuberculous bacterial empyema, and hemorrhagic effusion is most often unilateral, whereas in patients who have asbestos pleurisy there is usually evidence of bilateral pleural disease (either diffuse pleural thickening or pleural plaques).[57–59] Extensive calcification of the fibrothorax is seen most commonly in patients who have previous tuberculosis, empyema, or hemothorax and is uncommon in asbestos-related thickening.[24] Assessment of the underlying lungs may also be helpful. If the lung appears relatively normal, the antecedent insult was most likely traumatic hemothorax. If there is local scarring and loss of volume, the pleural change probably was the result of a remote empyema sec-

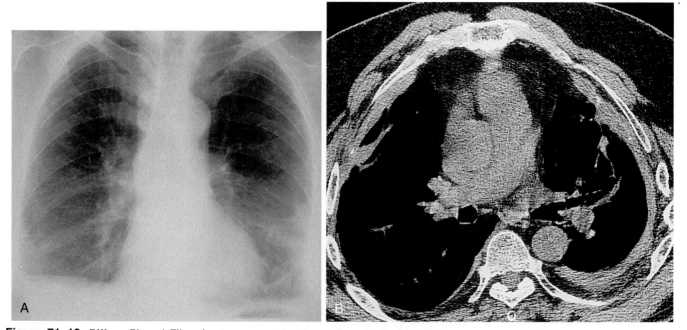

Figure 71–12. Diffuse Pleural Fibrosis. A posteroanterior chest radiograph *(A)* demonstrates extensive bilateral pleural thickening. The blunted costophrenic angles are sharply angulated rather than meniscus shaped, a finding helpful in distinguishing pleural thickening from effusion. Curved bands of increased opacity can be seen to extend from the left lung to the pleural thickening. This feature is most commonly seen with pleural thickening related to asbestos. A CT scan *(B)* reveals marked bilateral pleural thickening with small areas of calcification. Note that although there is marked thickening of the costal and paravertebral pleura, the mediastinal pleura is not affected. The patient was a 53-year-old man who had a history of exposure to asbestos.

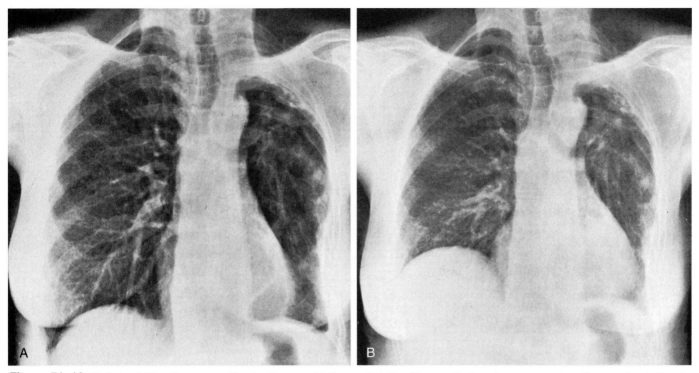

Figure 71–13. Unilateral Fibrothorax Leading to Hypoventilation and Reflex Hypoperfusion. A posteroanterior radiograph *(A)* of this 73-year-old asymptomatic woman reveals moderate thickening of the pleura over the whole of the left lung. Calcification is evident over the lower axillary lung zone. The volume of the left lung is moderately reduced and its vessel markings diminutive. A posteroanterior radiograph exposed at full expiration *(B)* shows excellent movement of the right hemidiaphragm, whereas elevation of the left hemidiaphragm has been minimal. Thus, the volume of the left lung has shown little change from inspiration to expiration, indicating hypoventilation.

ondary to *Mycobacterium tuberculosis* or some pyogenic organism.

Diffuse pleural thickening can result in marked decrease in volume of the affected hemithorax and in impaired ventilation of the underlying lung. The degree of ventilation impairment can be gauged, at least roughly, by assessing pulmonary vascularity. If the pulmonary vessels of the affected lung are smaller than those of the opposite side, it can be assumed that the reduction in perfusion has occurred in response to reduced ventilation, presumably as a result of hypoxic vasoconstriction (Fig. 71–13). If the vascularity of the two lungs is roughly symmetric, it is reasonable to assume that reflex vasoconstriction has not occurred and that ventilation is therefore preserved.

Diffuse pleural fibrosis related to asbestos exposure may cause restrictive impairment in the absence of radiologic evidence of pulmonary disease.[55, 67–69] The characteristic alteration in lung function consists of a decrease in static lung volumes, reduced transfer factor (D_{LCO}), and a normal or increased transfer coefficient (K_{CO}).[55, 69, 70] In one study, unilateral diffuse pleural fibrosis was associated with a 500-ml reduction in vital capacity.[71] In another study of 36 patients, serial measurements of lung function over a mean follow-up period of 8.9 years showed a progressive decrease in FEV_1 and FVC;[70] although there was also a progression in the thickness and extent of fibrothorax on the radiograph, there was no significant correlation between the change in lung function and the increase in radiographic score.

REFERENCES

1. Renner RR, Markarian B, Pernice NJ, et al: The apical cap. Radiology 110:569, 1974.
2. McLoud TC, Isler RJ, Novelline RA, et al: The apical cap. Am J Roentgenol 137:299, 1981.
3. Butler C II, Kleinerman J: The pulmonary apical cap. Am J Pathol 60:205, 1970.
4. Im JG, Webb WR, Han MC, et al: Apical opacity associated with pulmonary tuberculosis: High-resolution CT findings. Radiology 178:727, 1991.
5. Fennessy JJ: Irradiation damage to the lung. J Thorac Imag 2:68, 1987.
6. Marnocha KE, Maglinte DDT: Plain-film criteria for excluding aortic rupture in blunt chest trauma. Am J Roentgenol 144:19, 1985.
7. Mirvis SE, Bidwell JK, Buddemeyer EU, et al: Value of chest radiography in excluding traumatic aortic rupture. Radiology 163:487, 1987.
8. Schwartz DA: New developments in asbestos-induced pleural disease. Chest 99:191, 1991.
9. Hourihane DO, Lessof L, Richardson PC: Hyaline and calcified pleural plaques as an index of exposure to asbestos: A study of radiological and pathological features of 100 cases with a consideration of epidemiology. BMJ 1:1069, 1966.
10. Rubino GF, Scansetti G, Pira E, et al: Pleural plaques and lung asbestos bodies in the general population: An autopical and clinical-radiological survey. In Wagner JC (ed): Biological Effects of Mineral Fibres. Lyon, France, International Agency for Research on Cancer, 1980.
11. Meurman L: Asbestos bodies and pleural plaques in a Finnish series of autopsy cases. Acta Pathol Microbiol Scand 181(Suppl):1, 1966.
12. Hillerdal G: Pleural plaques in a health survey material: Frequency, development and exposure to asbestos. Scand J Respir Dis 59:257, 1978.
13. Hillerdal G, Lindgren A: Pleural plaques: Correlation of autopsy findings to radiographic findings and occupational history. Eur J Respir Dis 61:315, 1980.
14. Albelda SM, Epstein DM, Gefter WB, et al: Pleural thickening: Its significance and relationship to asbestos dust exposure. Am Rev Respir Dis 126:621, 1982.
15. MacPherson P, Davidson JK: Correlation between lung asbestos count at necropsy and radiological appearances. BMJ 1:355, 1969.
16. Constantopoulos SH, Goudevenos JA, Saratzis NA, et al: Metsovo lung: Pleural calcification and restrictive lung function in northwestern Greece. Environmental exposure to mineral fiber as etiology. Environ Res 38:319, 1985.
17. Constantopoulos SH, Saratzis NA, Kontogiannis D, et al: Tremolite whitewashing and pleural calcification. Chest 92:709, 1987.
18. Yazicioglu S, Ilcayto R, Balci K, et al: Pleural calcification, pleural mesotheliomas, and bronchial cancers caused by tremolite dust. Thorax 35:564, 1980.
19. Baris YI, Sahin AA, Erkan ML: Clinical and radiological study in sepiolite workers. Arch Environ Health 35:343, 1980.
20. Boutin C, Viallat JR, Steinbauer J, et al: Bilateral pleural plaques in Corsica: A nonoccupational asbestos exposure marker. Eur J Respir Dis 69:4, 1986.
21. Churg A, DePaoli L: Environmental pleural plaques in residents of a Quebec chrysotile mining town. Chest 94:58, 1988.
22. Fletcher DE, Edge JR: The early radiological changes in pulmonary and pleural asbestosis. Clin Radiol 21:355, 1970.
23. Rockoff SD, Kagan E, Schwartz A, et al: Visceral pleural thickening in asbestos exposure: The occurrence and implications of thickening interlobar fissures. J Thorac Imaging 2:58, 1987.
24. Friedman AC, Fiel SB, Radecki PD, et al: Computed tomography of benign pleural and pulmonary parenchymal abnormalities related to asbestos exposure. Semin Ultrasound CT MR 11:393, 1990.
25. Solomon A: Radiological features of asbestos-related visceral pleural changes. Am J Ind Med 19:339, 1991.
26. Roberts WC, Ferrans VJ: Pure collagen plaques on the diaphragm and pleura—gross, histologic and electron microscopic observations. Chest 61:357, 1972.
27. Fletcher DE, Edge JR: The early radiological changes in pulmonary and pleural asbestosis. Clin Radiol 21:355, 1970.
28. MacKenzie FAF: The radiological investigation of the early manifestations of exposure to asbestos dust. Proc R Soc Med 64:834, 1971.
29. Sherman CB, Barnhart S, Rosenstock L: Use of oblique chest roentgenograms in detecting pleural disease in asbestos-exposed workers. J Occup Med 30:681, 1988.
30. Svenes KB, Borgersen A, Haaversen O, et al: Parietal pleural plaques: A comparison between autopsy and x-ray findings. Eur J Respir Dis 69:10, 1986.
31. Withers BF, Ducatman AM, Yang WN: Roentgenographic evidence for predominant left-sided location of unilateral pleural plaques. Chest 95:1262, 1989.
32. Fisher MS: Asymmetrical changes in asbestos-related disease. J Can Assoc Radiol 36:110, 1985.
33. Hu H, Beckett L, Kelsey K, et al: The left-sided predominance of asbestos-related pleural disease. Am Rev Respir Dis 148:981, 1993.
34. Sargent EN, Boswell WD Jr, Ralls PW, et al: Subpleural fat pads in patients exposed to asbestos: Distinction from non-calcified pleural plaques. Radiology 152:273, 1984.
35. Greene R, Boggis C, Jantsch H: Asbestos-related pleural thickening: Effect of threshold criteria on interpretation. Radiology 152:569, 1984.
36. Gefter WB, Conant EF: Issues and controversies in the plain-film diagnosis of asbestos-related disorders in the chest. J Thorac Imaging 3:11, 1988.
37. Bourbeau J, Ernst P: Between- and within-reader variability in the assessment of pleural abnormality using the ILO 1980 international classification of pneumoconiosis. Am J Ind Med 14:537, 1988.
38. Svenes KB, Borgersen A, Haaversen O, et al: Parietal pleural plaques: A comparison between autopsy and x-ray findings. Eur J Respir Dis 69:10, 1986.
39. Wain SL, Roggli VL, Foster WL: Parietal pleural plaques, asbestos bodies, and neoplasia: A clinical, pathologic, and roentgenographic correlation of 25 consecutive cases. Chest 86:707, 1984.
40. Aberle DR, Gamsu G, Ray CS: High-resolution CT of benign asbestos-related diseases: Clinical and radiographic correlation. Am J Roentgenol 151:883, 1988.
41. Friedman AC, Fiel SB, Fisher MS, et al: Asbestos-related pleural disease and asbestosis: A comparison of CT and chest radiography. Am J Roentgenol 150:269, 1988.
42. Staples CA, Gamsu G, Ray CS, et al: High resolution computed tomography and lung function in asbestos-exposed workers with normal chest radiographs. Am Rev Respir Dis 139:1502, 1989.
43. Gevenois PA, de Vuyst P, Dedeire S, et al: Conventional and high-resolution CT in asymptomatic asbestos-exposed workers. Acta Radiologica 35:226, 1994.
44. Im JG, Webb WR, Rosen A, et al: Costal pleura: Appearances at high-resolution CT. Radiology 171:125, 1989.
45. Aberle DR, Gamsu G, Ray CS, et al: Asbestos-related pleural and parenchymal fibrosis: Detection with high-resolution CT. Radiology 166:729, 1988.
46. Anton HC: Multiple pleural plaques, part II. Br J Radiol 41:341, 1968.
47. Freundlich IM, Greening RR: Asbestosis and associated medical problems. Radiology 89:224, 1967.
48. Smith AR: Pleural calcification resulting from exposure to certain dusts. Am J Roentgenol 67:375, 1952.
49. Kiviluoto R: Pleural calcification as a roentgenologic sign of nonoccupational endemic anthophyllite-asbestosis. Acta Radiol (Suppl)194, 1960.
50. Solomon A: Radiology of asbestosis. Environ Res 3:320, 1970.
51. Kleinfeld M: Pleural calcification as a sign of silicatosis. Am J Med Sci 251:215, 1966.
52. Krige L: Asbestosis—with special reference to the radiological diagnosis. S Afr J Radiol 4:13, 1966.
53. Fridriksson HV, Hedenstrom H, Hillerdal G, et al: Increased lung stiffness in persons with pleural plaques. Eur J Respir Dis 62:412, 1981.
54. Hjortsberg U, Orbaek P, Aborelius M Jr, et al: Railroad workers with pleural plaques: I. Spirometric and nitrogen washout investigation on smoking and non-smoking asbestos-exposed workers. Am J Ind Med 14:635, 1988.
55. Jones RN, McLoud T, Rockoff SD: The radiographic pleural abnormalities in asbestos exposure: Relationship to physiologic abnormalities. J Thorac Imaging 3:57, 1988.
56. McLoud TC, Woods BO, Carrington CB, et al: Diffuse pleural thickening in an asbestos-exposed population. Am J Roentgenol 144:9, 1985.
57. Müller NL: Imaging of the pleura. Radiology 186:297, 1993.
58. Leung AN, Müller NL, Miller RR: CT in differential diagnosis of diffuse pleural disease. Am J Roentgenol 154:487, 1990.
59. Lynch DA, Gamsu G, Aberle DR: Conventional and high resolution computed tomography in the diagnosis of asbestos-related diseases. Radiographics 9:523, 1989.
60. Murray JG, Patz EF Jr, Erasmus JJ, et al: CT appearance of the pleural space after talc pleurodesis. Am J Roentgenol 169:89, 1997.
61. Barrett NR: The pleura, with special reference to fibrothorax. Thorax 25:515, 1970.
62. Herbert A: Pathogenesis of pleurisy, pleural fibrosis, and mesothelial proliferation. Thorax 41:176, 1986.
63. Gilbert L, Ribot S, Frankel H, et al: Fibrinous uremic pleuritis—surgical entity. Chest 67:53, 1975.
64. Buchanan DR, Johnston ID, Kerr IH, et al: Cryptogenic bilateral fibrosing pleuritis. Br J Dis Chest 82:186, 1988.
65. McLoud TC, Woods BO, Carrington CB, et al: Diffuse pleural thickening in an asbestos-exposed population: Prevalence and causes. Am J Roentgenol 144:9, 1985.
66. Bohlig H, Calavrezos A: Development, radiological zone patterns, and importance of diffuse pleural thickening in relation to occupational exposure to asbestos. Br J Ind Med 44:673, 1987.
67. Corris PA, Best JJ, Gibson GJ: Effects of diffuse pleural thickening on respiratory mechanics. Eur Respir J 1:248, 1988.
68. Picado C, Laporta D, Grassino A, et al: Mechanisms affecting exercise performance in subjects with asbestos-related pleural fibrosis. Lung 165:45, 1987.
69. Schwartz DA, Fuortes LJ, Galvin JR, et al: Asbestos-induced pleural fibrosis and impaired lung function. Am Rev Respir Dis 141:321, 1990.
70. Yates DH, Browne K, Stidolph PN, et al: Asbestos-related bilateral diffuse pleural thickening: Natural history of radiographic and lung function abnormalities. Am J Respir Crit Care Med 153:301, 1996.
71. Bourbeau J, Ernst P, Chrome J, et al: The relationship between respiratory impairment and asbestos-related pleural abnormality in an active work force. Am Rev Respir Dis 142:837, 1990.

CHAPTER 72

Pleural Neoplasms

MESOTHELIOMA

Diffuse mesothelioma is an uncommon, but increasingly recognized, malignant neoplasm derived from mesothelial cells of the pericardium, peritoneum, or pleura; rare cases apparently derived from mediastinal mesothelial cysts have also been reported.[1] Of all these sites, the pleura is by far the most common. The neoplasm is important not only because of its dismal prognosis but also because of the potential economic impact of litigation and workers' compensation.[2]

Epidemiology

Before 1960, mesothelioma was so rare that its very existence was questioned by some prominent pathologists.[3] Although it is now a well-established entity, the tumor is indeed very uncommon; for example, the overall incidence in the United States has been estimated to be only about 2 cases per million per year.[4, 5] However, incidence figures vary considerably in different geographic regions, largely reflecting the likelihood of environmental or occupational asbestos exposure. For example, incidence rates in areas that have had heavy shipbuilding activity, such as Seattle and Rotterdam, have been found to be 20[6] and 60[7] per million, respectively. There is evidence that the incidence has been increasing in the recent past (at least in men and in some geographic regions) and may not cease until the early part of the next century.[8-11]

The incidence of mesothelioma also shows a striking sex predominance, a finding largely, if not entirely, related to the increased likelihood of occupational asbestos exposure in men: it has been estimated that only about 5% of women in North America have such exposure[12] and that 85% to 90% of all mesotheliomas occur in men.[13] In groups of women who have occupational asbestos exposure, incidence rates are equivalent to those of men.[15] It is thus unlikely that gender itself is a risk factor. The vast majority of cases of mesothelioma occur in adults, the mean age at diagnosis being 60 to 65 years.[13, 16] It has been estimated that only 2% to 5% of tumors appear during adolescence or childhood.[17]

Etiology

There is good evidence that the majority of cases of mesothelioma are related to a carcinogenic effect of asbestos. However, there are some patients in whom the lung asbestos burden is relatively slight[18] or overlaps that of the general population.[19] In addition, the tumor was recognized at the turn of the century when little asbestos was being used[20] and sporadic cases occur in children too young to have had significant asbestos exposure within the usually accepted latent period.[21] Although these observations may reflect the existence of a very low threshold for asbestos-related neoplasia, other factors, including fibrous minerals such as erionite, radiation, and pleural fibrosis, have been clearly implicated in a small number of cases.[22] The possibility that hereditary, infectious, or dietary influences may be important has also been considered.

Asbestos

The close association between asbestos and mesothelioma was first reported by Wagner and colleagues in 1960.[23] Since that time, abundant evidence has been published confirming their observation,[24] and it is now clear that exposure to asbestos is by far the most important risk factor for the development of this neoplasm. (Despite this, it should be remembered that many more cases of pulmonary carcinoma have been associated with asbestos exposure than mesothelioma.[25]) The evidence in favor of a pathogenic relationship between mesothelioma and asbestos is derived from several sources.

Epidemiologic Studies and Clinical Experience Showing a Strong Relationship between Asbestos Exposure and Mesothelioma. A history of exposure to asbestos varies considerably in different series of patients who have mesothelioma,[26] a feature related in part to the particular population under study; however, it has been greater than 50% in most studies[27-35] and as high as 80% to 90% in many.[36-41] In some reports in which the number of asbestos-related cases is relatively small, the lack of association may be the result of an inadequate occupational or environmental history: it is well known that the neoplasm can develop after minimal asbestos exposure[28, 42] and many years after the initial contact (*see* farther on);[19, 43] in addition, secondary contact from a family member may be easily missed if not carefully assessed.

As indicated previously, the association between asbestos exposure and mesothelioma has generally been found to be much stronger in men than in women;[4, 38] however, in one review of 105 female patients who had the tumor, 74 (80%) of the 93 for whom information was available had a history of contact with the mineral.[44]

Epidemiologic studies show a high incidence of the tumor in individuals involved both in the mining and production of asbestos and in the numerous secondary occupations associated with its use (Table 72–1).[16, 45-47] Workers at particular risk in the latter occupations include those in the construction, oil refining, and railroad industries, insulators, garage mechanics, shipbuilders, and plumbers. As indicated previously, some occupations have been associated with an especially high risk; for example, a number of investigators have shown a dramatic clustering of cases in the vicinity of shipyards,[6, 48-51] the incidence of the tumor in such regions being as high as 6.2 per 100,000.[7] As might be expected, spraying asbestos-based insulation material has also been associated with a significantly increased risk of the disease.[52] Occupational asbestos exposure can also occur in uncommon or apparently unlikely situations. For example, exposure (and

Table 72–1. OCCUPATIONS AT RISK FOR ASBESTOS EXPOSURE: MINING, MILLING, MANUFACTURING, AND SECONDARY USES

PROCESS	PRODUCTS MADE OR USED	JOBS POTENTIALLY AT RISK
Production		
Mining		Rock mining, loading, trucking
Milling		Crushing, milling
Handling		Transport workers, dockers, loaders, those who unpack jute sacks (recently replaced with sacks that do not permit fibers to escape)
Primary Uses		
Spray insulation	Spray of fiber mixed with oil	Spray insulators (construction, shipbuilding)
Filler and grouting		
Manufacturing of		
Textiles	Cloth, curtains, lagging, protective clothing, mailbags, padding, conveyor belts	Blending, carding, spinning, twisting, winding, braiding, weaving, slurry mixing, laminating, molding, drying
Cement products	Sheets, pipes, roofing shingles, gutters, ventilation shafts, flower pots	Blending, slurry preparation, rolling, pressing, pipe cutting
"Paper" products	Millboard, roofing felt, fine-quality electrical papers, flooring felt, fillers	
Friction materials	Automotive products: gaskets, clutch plates, brake linings	
Insulation products	Pipe and boiler insulation, bulkhead linings for ships	
Applications		
Construction		
New construction	Boards and tiles; putties, caulk, paints, joint fillers; cement products (tiles, pipes, siding, shingles)	Direct: carpenters, laggers, painters, tile layers, insulation workers, sheet metal and heating equipment workers, masons
		Indirect: all other workers on construction sites, such as plumbers, welders, electricians
		Demolition workers for all of these
Repair, demolition		
Shipbuilding		
Construction	Insulation materials (boards, mattresses, cloth) for engines, hull, decks, lagging of ventilation and water pipes, cables	Laggers, refitters, strippers, steam fitters, sailmakers, joiners, shipwrights, engine fitters, masons, painters, welders, caulkers
Repair, refits	Insulation materials, as described for "Construction"	Direct: all above jobs on refits, dry dock, and other repair operations
		Indirect: maintenance fitters and repairers, electricians, plumbers, welders, carpenters
Automotive industry		
Manufacture	Gaskets, brake linings, undercoating	Installation of brake linings, gaskets, and so on
Repair	Gaskets, brake linings, undercoating	Service people, brake repairers, body repairers, auto mechanics

Modified from Becklake MR: Asbestos-related diseases of the lung and other organs: Their epidemiology and implications for clinical practice. Am Rev Respir Dis 114:187, 1976.

mesothelioma) has been documented in workers involved in the manufacture of cigarette filters[53] or gas masks,[54] in the production of jewelry,[55] and after the preparation of an asbestos-based cement product in a home basement.[56]

There is good evidence that exposure to asbestos outside the workplace is also hazardous.[41] Such contact can be secondarily related to occupation; for example, mesothelioma has been reported in wives, children, and siblings of individuals who work in asbestos plants, cement factories, or shipbuilding sites, in some cases probably after asbestos exposure during laundering of the workers' clothes.[14, 51, 57, 58] Similarly, an increased incidence of tumors has been documented in individuals who reside near factories that process asbestos, presumably as a result of an increased level of asbestos in the atmosphere.[16, 59] It has also been speculated that significant contact with asbestos may occur in office buildings or schools in which asbestos has been used for insulation, fireproofing, or acoustic control;[46] however, although occasional case reports[60] and the results of epidemiologic studies[61] have shown that asbestos-related disease (including mesothelioma) does occur in these settings, the magnitude of the problem appears to be very small.[4] Some cases of nonoccupational environmental mesothelioma are also related to the presence of asbestos in the soil, as in some regions of Greece,[62, 63] Corsica,[64] Turkey,[65] and Cyprus,[66] where significant quantities of tremolite have been found in this source.

Studies of Asbestos Burden in the Lungs of Patients with Mesothelioma. Many investigators have documented an association between an increased number of asbestos bodies and/or fibers in lung tissue and the presence of mesothelioma.[67–71] For example, in one study of 50 workers seeking compensation in Quebec, 48 had an asbestos body or total fiber count greater than the 95% confidence interval of a control population.[72] Asbestos body and fiber counts are not always elevated in the same patient. For example, in one investigation of the lungs of 18 patients who had mesothelioma in which the asbestos body counts were within normal limits, 6 were found to have an asbestos fiber burden in the upper fifth percentile of normal levels.[73]

Despite the finding of an increased number of asbestos fibers in the lungs of many patients who have malignant mesothelioma, several groups of investigators have found this number to be intermediate between those found in the general population and in patients who have asbestosis.[18, 29, 74] In one study of patients in the latter group, an increased incidence of pulmonary carcinoma was found in those with moderate to severe asbestosis and of mesothelioma in those with minimal or slight disease.[75] It has been speculated that this finding may reflect a dose relationship between asbestos burden and the development of asbestosis and lung cancer that does not exist for mesothelioma;[76, 77] this, in turn, suggests that there may be no threshold of asbestos burden below which there is no risk for the development of mesothelioma. Although this hypothesis has not been proven conclusively, some experimental evidence supports it.[78]

Experimental Studies in Animals Showing the Development of Mesothelioma after Asbestos Exposure. Diffuse mesothelioma morphologically similar to that seen in humans has been shown to develop after instillation of asbestos fibers into the pleural space[79, 80] or trachea[81] of various animals.

Mesothelioma Risk and Asbestos Fiber Type. The risk of developing mesothelioma varies considerably with the type of asbestos to which an individual is exposed. The majority of evidence indicates that the greatest risk occurs with the amphiboles crocidolite and (to a lesser extent) amosite;[71, 82–85] the risk with anthophyllite appears to be very small.[86] The importance of chrysotile has been the subject of some debate;[11, 79, 87] although the results of most studies suggest that exposure to this substance is associated with an increased risk of mesothelioma, there is substantial evidence that the risk is much smaller than that of crocidolite and amosite and may, in fact, be related to the presence of contaminating tremolite.[88–91]

The variable pathogenicity of the different types of asbestos may be related to their different physicochemical characteristics. Long straight fibers, such as those of the amphiboles, tend to be transported to the periphery of the lung, whereas the irregular curly shape of the chrysotile fiber predisposes to its deposition in the more central airways.[79] Thus, amosite and crocidolite tend to accumulate in relatively large numbers in the peripheral portions of the lung close to the pleura. There is also evidence that chrysotile fibers fragment with time and are transported out of the lung via the mucociliary escalator or lymphatics.[79, 92] Amphiboles, on the other hand, are relatively stable and remain either constant in number in an individual who is no longer exposed or continue to accumulate over the lifetime of an individual who is continually exposed. For example, in one study of workers in a Norwegian cement plant, analysis of fiber types showed approximately 92% of the fibers to be chrysotile, 3% amosite, 4% crocidolite, and 1% anthophyllite.[93] However, electron microscopic and x-ray microanalysis of lung tissue samples from workers who had died of mesothelioma or pulmonary carcinoma showed a completely inverse proportion, the percentage of chrysotile asbestos fibers ranging from 0% to 9% and of amphiboles from 76% to 99%. There is also experimental evidence that chrysotile and crocidolite fibers interact differently with chromosomes of mesothelial cells,[94] possibly reflecting a different carcinogenic potential.

Other Fibrous Minerals

Because the risk of mesothelioma appears to be closely related to the size and shape of inhaled asbestos fibers, attention has been directed to the possibility that other minerals that have the same physical characteristics as asbestos also may be pathogenic. The most clearly implicated of these minerals is erionite, a member of the zeolite group that is found in the soil of central Turkey and the western United States (*see* page 2452). Several epidemiologic[95–97] and experimental[98] studies have provided evidence implicating this substance in the production of both pleural plaques and mesothelioma. A variety of man-made fibers, including fiberglass, can also induce cancer when introduced directly into the pleural space of animals;[79, 99] however, inhalation of these substances by humans does not appear to be associated with an increased risk of mesothelioma.[100] A possible association with silica fibers in inhaled sugar cane has also been reported.[101]

Radiation

Although the findings of several reports suggest that external radiation is responsible for occasional cases of mesothelioma,[102–105] this is clearly a very uncommon event. For example, in one retrospective review of 1,000 patients who had received thoracic radiation at the M. D. Anderson Cancer Center, only 3 were considered to have developed complicating mesothelioma.[106] In another series of 251,750 women who had breast carcinoma (of whom approximately 25% had received radiotherapy) and 13,743 patients who had Hodgkin's disease (about 50% having had radiotherapy), mesothelioma developed in only 6 patients (in 2 who had breast carcinoma and radiotherapy and in 4 who had carcinoma and no radiotherapy).[107] In one review of eight cases of radiation-associated mesothelioma, the mean age at the time of diagnosis was 45 years and the average interval between radiation and diagnosis of mesothelioma was 21 years (range, 11 to 29 years).[103] Experimental evidence suggests that the risk is significantly increased when radiation is combined with asbestos exposure.[108] An increased incidence of mesothelioma (predominantly peritoneal) has also been documented in patients who have a history of exposure to Thorotrast.[109]

Infection

Simian virus 40 (SV40) is a double-stranded DNA organism of the papovavirus group that normally infects the kidneys of rhesus monkeys.[110] The virus was inadvertently transmitted to many humans in contaminated polio vaccines in the late 1950s and early 1960s. Although potential adverse effects associated with such transmission were inapparent for a long time, concern was raised when it was found that the virus has a variety of oncogenic effects in tissue culture and can induce mesotheliomas in hamsters.[111] Moreover, a number of investigators have found DNA sequences identical to those of the virus in a substantial proportion of human mesotheliomas.[112–116] The oncoprotein of the virus (SV40 large cell antigen [Tag]) has been found to bind and inactivate retinoblastoma family proteins[114] and p53,[115] suggesting that the virus may mediate oncogenesis by inactivating tumor suppressor genes. These observations provide evidence of a possible role for SV40 in the pathogenesis of mesothelioma, either by itself or as a cofactor with asbestos. However, not all investigators have been able to demonstrate evidence of the virus[117] or of associated oncogene mutations[118] in mesothelioma, and further studies are necessary before it can be concluded that SV40 has a pathogenic role in the development of the tumor.

Rare cases of mesothelioma have been documented in patients who have the acquired immunodeficiency syndrome in the absence of asbestos exposure;[119] although their number is insufficient to be certain of a true relationship, it has been postulated that the tumor may be secondary to human immunodeficiency virus or cytomegalovirus infection. Based on the observation of two cases of mesothelioma in 458 patients who had *Yersinia enterocolitica* infection, one group of investigators speculated that immunologic reactions related to the latter organism might be involved in the pathogenesis of the tumor.[120] In one investigation of 50 mesotheliomas in which *in-situ* hybridization was utilized in an attempt to detect Epstein-Barr virus–encoded RNA-1, no evidence of infection was identified in any tumor.[121]

Genetic Factors

A familial occurrence of mesothelioma has been documented by several investigators.[122–126] Although many cases are likely the result of a common source of environmental or occupational asbestos exposure,[126a] it is also possible that there is a degree of genetic susceptibility. For example, in one investigation of the first-degree relatives of 196 patients who had pathologically confirmed mesothelioma, a twofold increase for the risk of the tumor was found in asbestos-exposed men who had two or more relatives with a history of cancer.[127] In another study of 39 patients who had mesothelioma, 28 (71%) reported a parental history of cancer (most often of the gastrointestinal tract) compared with 114 of 259 (44%) in an age-matched control group.[128]

Miscellaneous Factors

Malignant neoplasms occasionally arise in relation to a chronically scarred pleura after chronic empyema or therapeutic pneumothorax for tuberculosis; although most of these are squamous cell carcinomas,[129] occasional tumors morphologically similar to mesothelioma have been described.[130] The results of one epidemiologic investigation suggest that ingestion of some carotenoid fruits and vegetables may decrease the risk of developing mesothelioma.[131] There is no evidence of a pathogenetic association between the tumor and tobacco smoke.[132, 133]

Pathogenesis

The pathogenesis of asbestos-related mesothelioma is far from clear.[79, 134] As indicated earlier, the size and shape of asbestos fibers are important determinants of carcinogenicity, those that are relatively long and thin being the most harmful.[80, 82, 135] As an example of the significance of this feature, it is possible to prepare samples of chrysotile that are long and straight (in contrast to their natural state) and that are at least as carcinogenic as amosite, both in inhalation experiments and after introduction of the fiber into the pleural space.[80] Support for the importance of this feature is derived from a study of cultured human mesothelial cells in which the presence of longer asbestos fibers was associated with an increase in the potent mesothelial mitogen epidermal growth factor.[135a] It is possible that factors associated with particle deposition or clearance are also important in determining pathogenicity.[136] Although it is unclear exactly how they emigrate from the lung, fibers have been shown to be concentrated in "black spots" (focal aggregates of carbon-laden macrophages) in the parietal pleura;[137] because there is evidence that most, if not all, mesotheliomas originate in the parietal rather than in the visceral pleura,[138] such localization may be important pathogenetically.

Instillation of asbestos into the peritoneal space of experimental animals is rapidly followed by evidence of mesothelial injury and an inflammatory reaction;[139] mesothelial hyperplasia, sometimes atypical cytologically, ensues and can remain for months after the initial asbestos contact.[140] It is possible that oxygen radical production induced by asbestos fibers may be important in the inflammatory reaction and in causing cell damage.[141] A variety of such molecules can be seen in association with asbestos, derived either directly by an iron-catalyzed reaction on the fiber surface or indirectly after phagocytosis of the fiber by macrophages.[142]

The immunologic and molecular features of mesothelioma have been reviewed by several authors.[143, 144] Tumor-derived cell lines have the capacity to produce a variety of growth factors, including platelet-derived growth factors A and B, insulin-like growth factors I and II, and transforming growth factors α and β;[143] some investigators have also found platelet-derived growth factor receptors in tumor cells, suggesting the possibility of an autocrine stimulatory effect.[145] Somewhat surprisingly, oncogene mutations described in many carcinomas appear to be absent in the majority of mesotheliomas.[118] Although a variety of chromosomal abnormalities have been identified,[146–149] including deletion of p16, trisomy 7, and anomalies of 1p21-p22 and 9p21-p22,[150–152] none is specific for the tumor. Mutations of the neurofibromatosis type 2 gene (which is located on chromosome 22) have also been noted in a substantial proportion of tumors by some investigators.[153, 154] The tumor suppressor gene WT-1, which is frequently the site of mutation in Wilms' tumor, can be identified in many mesotheliomas;[143] although the significance of this association is unclear, both tumors have occasionally been documented in the same patient.[155]

Both immunologic and inflammatory reactions are likely to be important in modifying the progression of mesothelioma. For example, it has been suggested that fibrin deposition at the advancing edge of a tumor may promote its extension locally.[145] Perhaps more importantly, various cytokines such as interferons α and γ and tumor necrosis factor-α have been shown to inhibit growth in mesothelioma cell lines.[143] In addition, cells in such preparations express abundant class I MHC molecules but few or none of class II; it has been suggested that this deficiency may contribute to an ability to escape immune surveillance.[143] It is also possible that mesothelioma cells may secrete factors such as TGF-β and interleukin-6 that may alter immune cell function locally.

Pathologic Characteristics

Although mesothelioma can present grossly as a solitary, more or less spherical intrapleural mass[156–158] or (in very early cases) as scattered, somewhat dome-shaped nodules 1 to 2 mm in diameter on the parietal surface,[159] in the vast majority of patients it appears as a plaquelike or lobulated thickening encasing a portion of the lung. In autopsy specimens, the entire lung is typically affected (Fig. 72–1).[161, 162] Discrete cystlike spaces containing gelatinous or hemorrhagic fluid can be occasionally identified within the tumor and probably represent portions of the original pleural space. Extension of the neoplasm along fissures and into adjacent tissues, such as the chest wall, diaphragm, and pericardium, is not uncommon. Although the tumor may expand in a nodular fashion into the lung (Fig. 72–2), more often it does not extend beneath the pleura (Fig. 72–3); rare tumors have been reported to infiltrate the underlying lung in a "lepidic" fashion similar to bronchioloalveolar carcinoma.[163] The tumor varies in consistency from soft and fleshy to firm or hard, the last-named virtually indistinguishable from mature fibrous tissue and typically associated with desmoplastic tumors (*see* farther on).

Very early tumors are rarely seen microscopically; they can appear as solid nodules, papilloma-like structures, or diffuse pleural thickening (Fig. 72–4). Such patterns can also be seen focally in association with more advanced neoplasms. Grossly invasive tumors can be classified histologically in three forms—epithelial, sarcomatous (mesenchymal, fibrous, or spindle-cell), and biphasic (mixed).[142] The first of these is the most common, comprising 60% to 70% of cases in most series; however, the number of mixed tumors increases as more tissue is examined.[164] The epithelial form has a variable appearance, cells being organized in papillary or tubular structures, acinar clusters, or relatively solid sheets (Fig. 72–5); although one of these patterns may predominate, combinations are frequent. Individual tumor cells are usually cuboidal or round and possess a moderate amount of eosinophilic cytoplasm (Fig. 72–6); occasionally, they have a foamy, clear, or signet ring appearance.[161, 165, 166] Nuclei are often rather uniform in size and shape, although significant pleomorphism is seen in the less differentiated forms. Nucleoli are characteristically prominent. A variant composed of small cells resembling small cell carcinoma of the lung has been described;[167] squamous differentiation is seen rarely.[168]

The sarcomatous form typically consists of spindle cells arranged haphazardly or in a fascicular or storiform pattern (Fig. 72–7). Interstitial collagen may be apparent, suggesting fibroblastic differentiation; occasionally (approximately 5% of cases in some studies[169]) this tissue is abundant, leading to the designation "desmoplastic" mesothelioma.[169, 170] Differentiation of the latter form of tumor from a benign fibrous proliferation can be difficult, particularly with small biopsy specimens or when there is mild cytologic atypia; in one case, this variant was initially misinterpreted as sclerosing mediastinitis.[171] Other forms of mesenchymal differentiation, including cartilage, bone, and fat, occur occasionally.[172–175] A rare variant of the sarcomatous form, termed *lymphohistiocytoid mesothelioma*,[176] shows an intense lymphocytic infiltrate admixed with the neoplastic cells, a pattern that can be confused with lymphoma.

As the name implies, mixed tumors consist of a combination of epithelial and mesenchymal patterns (Fig. 72–8); although the proportion of each that is necessary for such classification is arbitrary, a minimum of 10% seems reasonable. Identification of this pattern is useful, because it enables a fairly confident diagnosis of mesothelial differentiation in a malignant neoplasm located in the pleura; although other tumors are possible (e.g., pleomorphic carcinoma of the lung or synovial sarcoma of the chest wall), in practice these are rare compared with mesothelioma in tissue specimens derived from the pleura.

There are two major practical problems in the pathologic diagnosis of mesothelioma: (1) distinguishing mesothelial hyperplasia from neoplasia; and (2) distinguishing mesothelioma from metastatic carcinoma, especially adenocarcinoma. Less common but also potentially difficult are the distinction between desmoplastic mesothelioma and a reactive, fibroblast proliferation and between malignant vascular tumors (e.g., epithelioid hemangioendothelioma) and epithelial or mixed mesothelioma.[177, 178] Each of these differential diagnostic problems is particularly troublesome with the small tissue fragments commonly obtained by closed-chest pleural biopsy; however, they may also be encountered

Text continued on page 2816

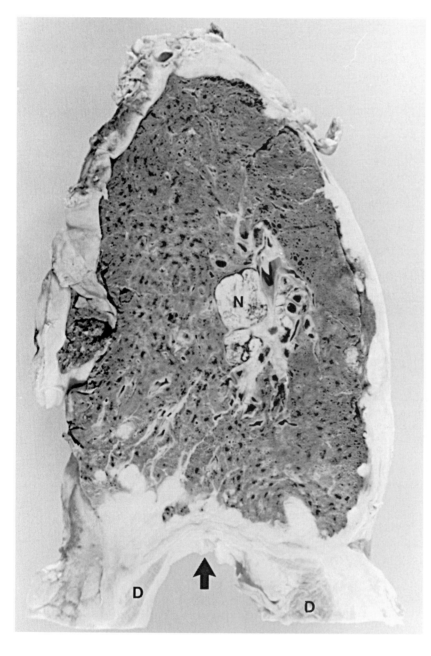

Figure 72–1. Diffuse Mesothelioma. A sagittal section of left lung shows mild to moderate thickening of the pleura over almost its entire surface; apart from mild centrilobular emphysema, the lung parenchyma is unremarkable. The tumor has extended into the adjacent hemidiaphragm (D) to involve the peritoneum *(arrow)*. Metastases are evident in peribronchial lymph nodes (N).

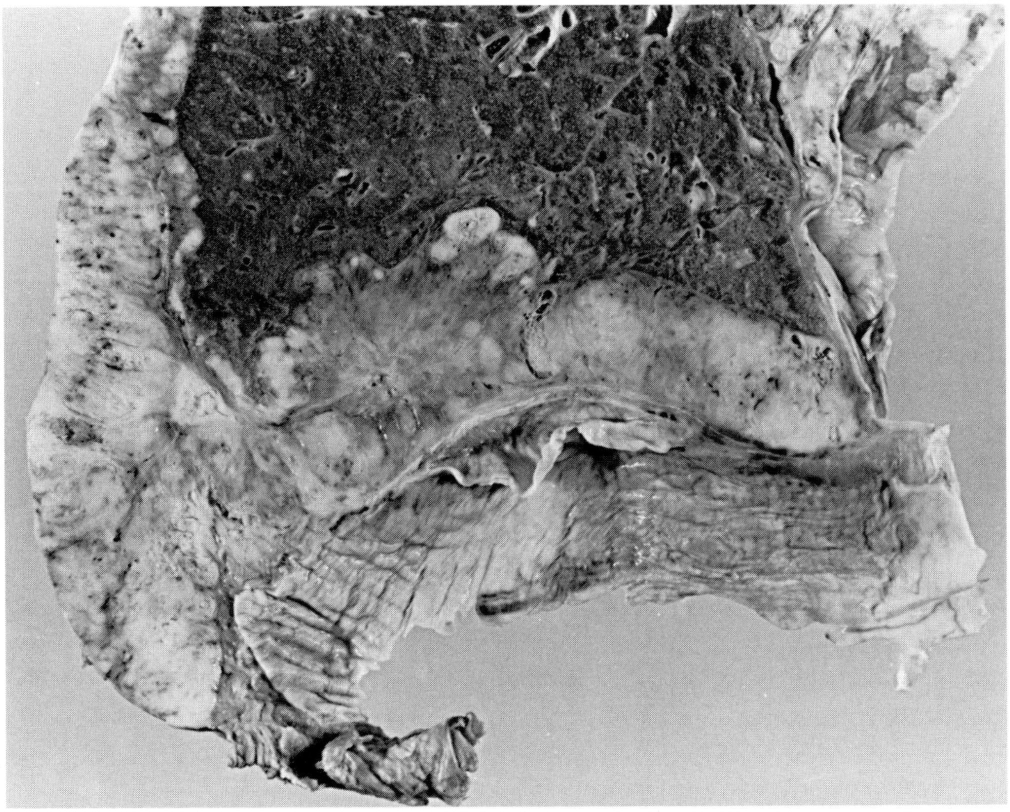

Figure 72–2. Diffuse Mesothelioma: Parenchymal Extension.
A slice of the basal aspect of a lower lobe shows marked pleural thickening by a tumor that possesses a somewhat variegated appearance. It has extended from the diaphragmatic portion of the pleura into adjacent lung parenchyma along a broad, focally somewhat nodular front.

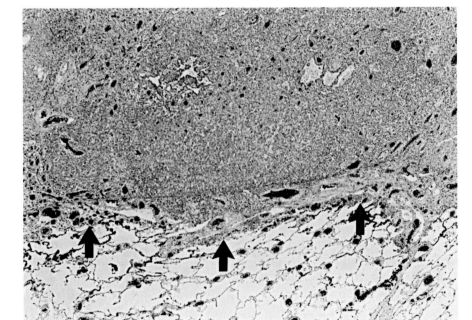

Figure 72–3. Mesothelioma. The section shows a mesothelioma composed of solid sheets of cells that extend to but do not transgress the visceral pleura *(arrows)*.

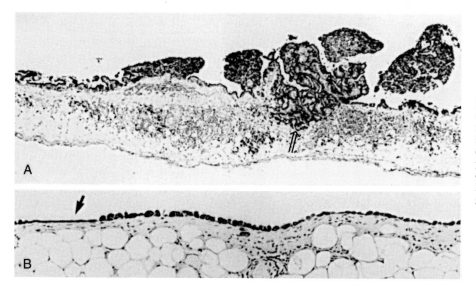

Figure 72–4. Early Mesothelioma. Sections of parietal pleura show a somewhat papillary tumor associated with focal invasion of the underlying tissue *(arrow* in *A)* and a more diffuse proliferation of neoplastic cells that causes only slight pleural thickening *(B).* (From Whitaker D, Henderson DW, Shilkin KB: The concept of mesothelioma *in situ*: Implications for diagnosis and histogenesis. Semin Diagn Pathol 9:151, 1992.)

Figure 72–5. Diffuse Mesothelioma: Epithelial Type. A section *(A)* reveals small nests of cells separated by a fibroblastic stroma and with round or elongated slitlike spaces. A section from another tumor *(B)* demonstrates multiple papillary projections (P) lined by a single layer of malignant mesothelial cells. The adjacent pleura is focally invaded *(arrows).* (A, ×100; B, ×60.)

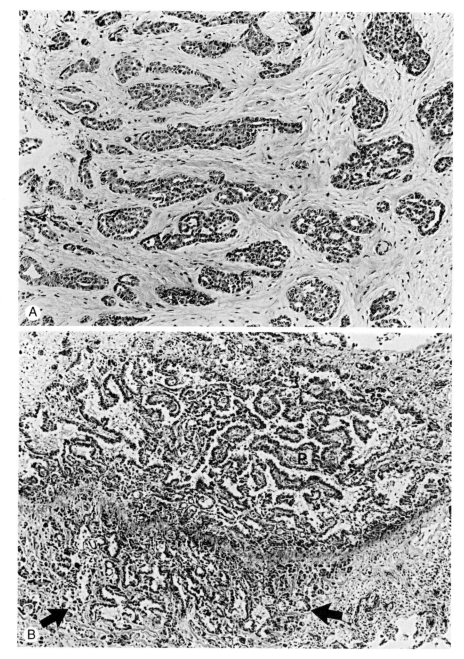

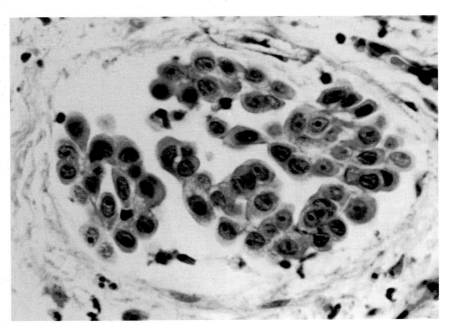

Figure 72–6. Mesothelioma: Cytologic Appearance. A magnified view of a well-differentiated epithelial mesothelioma shows several clusters of cells with moderately abundant lightly eosinophilic cytoplasm, fairly uniform round or oval nuclei, and prominent central nucleoli. (×600.)

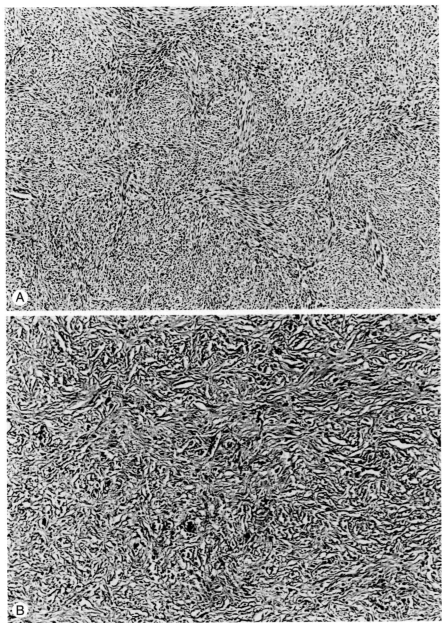

Figure 72–7. Diffuse Mesothelioma: Sarcomatous Type. A section *(A)* reveals fascicles of spindle-shaped cells arranged in an interdigitating pattern; a storiform appearance is present focally. A section of another tumor *(B)* shows moderately abundant, intercellular collagen. *(A,* ×80; *B,* ×120.)

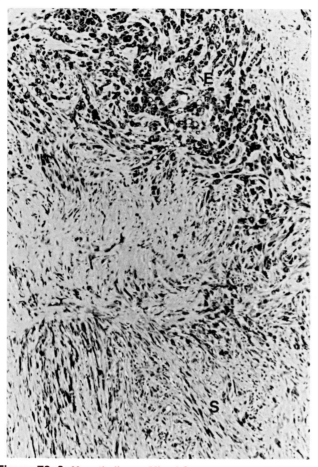

Figure 72–8. Mesothelioma: Mixed Sarcomatous and Epithelial Patterns. The section shows a combination of loose clusters of polygonal ("epithelial") cells (E) and spindle-shaped cells (S). The slide has been incubated with an antibody to low-molecular-weight keratin; a strong reaction is evident in both the epithelial and the spindle cells.

with material derived from open or thoracoscopic biopsy. These difficulties in pathologic diagnosis are reflected in the results of interobserver variability studies, in which significant disagreement in diagnosis has been documented in 5% to 15% of cases.[177, 179, 180]

Mesothelial Hyperplasia versus Neoplasia

Although there is evidence that significant mesothelial hyperplasia is infrequent in association with common pleural abnormalities,[181] it is clear that mesothelial cells can react to pleural injury by proliferating, sometimes to a marked degree. This proliferation can be associated with a variety of morphologic appearances, including simple or complex papillary projections and aggregates of cells of variable thickness covering the pleural surface (Fig. 72–9);[182, 183] occasionally, mitotic figures, cytologic atypia, and entrapment of mesothelial cell clusters in underlying fibrous tissue (*see* Fig. 72–9) can be seen.[183] Because each of these features also can be present in mesothelioma, the distinction between a reactive and a neoplastic process can be difficult, particularly if only a small amount of pleural tissue is present in a biopsy specimen. (A mistaken interpretation of carcinoma can also occur in the pleural specimens that are sometimes

obtained inadvertently by transbronchial biopsy.[184]) Although histologic criteria have been proposed to aid in the distinction between benign and malignant mesothelial proliferations,[161, 183, 185, 186] in some cases it may be impossible to be definitive. Indeed, it is possible that some cases represent examples of dysplastic mesothelium analogous to the preinvasive neoplastic process that commonly occurs in epithelia throughout the body (Fig. 72–10).[159]

In addition to simple light microscopic examination of hematoxylin-eosin–stained sections, several ancillary procedures have been investigated in an attempt to distinguish reactive from neoplastic mesothelium. The most promising has been the identification of antibodies capable of reacting specifically with neoplastic mesothelial cells;[187] among the substances examined for this property have been bcl-2, p53, P-170 glycoprotein, and the β chain of platelet-derived growth factor receptor (PDGF-R).[188–191] The most thoroughly investigated of these has been p53 protein, for which a number of investigators have found a high degree of specificity and a moderate degree of sensitivity in the identification of a neoplastic process. In five studies utilizing this antigen, a positive reaction was found in 25% to 85% of 211 mesotheliomas (specific percentages depending on the series) and none of 113 cases of mesothelial hyperplasia.[189, 192–195] In another investigation of serous fluid specimens, a positive reaction was identified in 17 of 35 malignant effusions (including 2 probable mesotheliomas) and none of 115 benign effusions.[196] Although other antigens have been studied less extensively than p53, similar results have generally been found; for example, in one investigation of PDGF-R, approximately half of 33 mesotheliomas were found to be positive as opposed to none of 35 cases of reactive mesothelium.[191]

Many other techniques have been investigated in an attempt to distinguish reactive from neoplastic mesothelial cells, with variable results. Although some of these show some differential diagnostic ability, none has been accepted as a definitive test.

Analysis of DNA Content by Flow Cytometry.[197, 198] Although the identification of an aneuploid population by this technique supports a diagnosis of malignancy, 40% to 75% of mesotheliomas have been found to be diploid in various series[160, 199–201] and the technique thus has limited sensitivity. Moreover, reactive mesothelial cells themselves have been reported to be polyploid by some investigators.[202]

Quantification of Nucleolar Organizer Regions (AgNOR). Statistically significant differences of this measure of proliferative activity have been shown between the mean values of reactive and malignant mesothelial proliferations;[203–206] however, there is overlap in individual measurements, with 20% to 30% of mesotheliomas in some studies having values within the range of reactive mesothelial cells.[204, 206] As a result, although a value greater than 3 supports a diagnosis of malignancy (the upper limit of the 95% confidence interval being approximately 1.7, 2.2, and 3.0 in three studies[203, 204, 206]), lower values must be considered indeterminate. One group of investigators found considerably less overlap in measurements of AgNOR area as opposed to absolute AgNOR count;[206a] using 0.6677 μm² as the cutoff between benign and malignant processes, they found a specificity of 100% and a sensitivity of 64% for the diagnosis of mesothelioma.

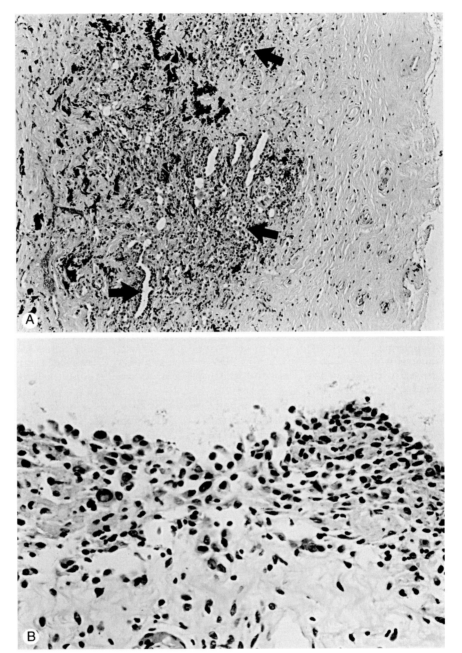

Figure 72–9. Pleuritis with Atypical Mesothelial Cells. A section of grossly thickened parietal pleura sampled at autopsy *(A)* shows a moderately severe lymphocytic infiltrate associated with small clusters of mesothelial cells *(arrows)* (the pleural surface is at the far right). Such entrapped clusters presumably develop during an episode of acute pleuritis; their presence in a small biopsy specimen, especially if cytologically atypical, can be mistaken for mesothelioma. In a 23-year-old patient who had spontaneous pneumothorax, a section of visceral pleura *(B)* shows hyperplastic mesothelial cells, focally possessing a moderate degree of cytologic atypia. *(A, ×100; B, ×300.)*

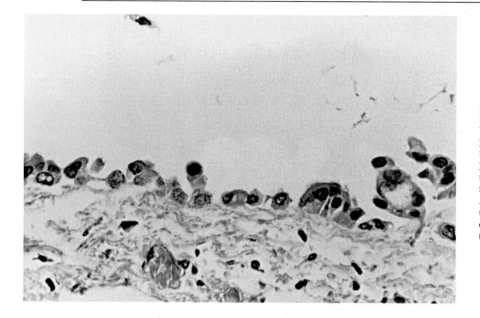

Figure 72–10. Atypical Mesothelial Hyperplasia. A magnified view of a pleural biopsy specimen shows a layer of enlarged mesothelial cells with a moderate degree of nuclear atypia. Slight piling up of cells is evident at the right. There is no significant inflammation. The patient was a 50-year-old man who had a history of asbestos exposure and an unexplained pleural effusion. There was no gross evidence of mesothelioma at thoracoscopy. Although the natural history of such a lesion is uncertain, it is likely that it represents a dysplastic change similar to that in epithelia elsewhere in the body.

Quantification of Proliferating Cell Nuclear Antigen (PCNA). In one investigation of 31 cases of mesothelioma and 33 of reactive mesothelium, the mean PCNA was 27 (standard deviation [SD] 9) for the tumor cells and 9.5 (SD 5) for reactive cells.[207] In another study, none of 11 reactive mesothelial cell proliferations had a PCNA index greater than 20.[204] A third group found 24 of 35 mesotheliomas to have between 26% and 95% cells positive, whereas the remaining 11 cases of mesothelioma and all 20 specimens of hyperplastic mesothelium had values less than 25%.[208] Thus, as with AgNOR counts, a high PCNA value is highly suggestive of malignancy; however, the overlap in values between groups limits the usefulness of the test.

Morphometric Analysis of Nuclear and Cytoplasmic Area. This has been carried out in cells derived from tissue sections[209] and from preparations of pleural fluid.[210, 211] As might be expected, reactive cells have been found to possess a significantly smaller mean area than neoplastic ones; however, there is again overlap between the two populations and the practical advantage of performing measurements in a particular case is not clear. In a somewhat similar stereologic investigation of nuclear volume, significantly higher mean values were also found in mesotheliomas than in hyperplastic mesothelial cells.[212]

Mesothelioma versus Metastatic Carcinoma

The second major problem in the pathologic diagnosis of mesothelioma lies in distinguishing it from metastatic carcinoma. This difficulty is related predominantly to the fact that epithelial forms of mesothelioma histologically resemble adenocarcinoma. In addition, some carcinomas, particularly of the lung, can spread along the pleura in a fashion grossly identical to that of mesothelioma (Fig. 72–11). The latter manifestation of disease is again usually seen with adenocarcinoma;[213, 214] however, cases of small cell carcinoma have also been reported.[215] The issue is further complicated by the observation that pulmonary carcinoma can itself be associated with atypical mesothelial hyperplasia.[216]

As with hyperplasia and neoplasia, a variety of ancillary techniques have been employed to aid in the solution of this problem, including histochemistry, immunohistochemistry, electron microscopy, and biochemical analysis.

Histochemistry. Many malignant mesothelial cells contain glycogen and thus show a positive reaction to para-amino salicylic acid (PAS),[217] a feature that is characteristic, but not diagnostic, of the neoplasm. Of greater differential diagnostic value is the reaction to PAS with diastase,[217–219] which is positive in the cytoplasm of many adenocarcinomas and almost always negative in mesothelioma.[220, 221] For example, in two series of 25[222] and 39[223] cases of adenocarcinoma the reaction was positive in 15 and 8 cases, respectively; by contrast, the reaction was negative in all 57 cases of mesothelioma. The demonstration of acid-mucopolysaccharides, specifically hyaluronic acid, within tumor cell cytoplasm is quite suggestive of mesothelioma;[219, 223–225] it can be detected by stains such as colloidal iron or alcian blue, and its presence confirmed by a negative reaction after treatment of the tissue with hyaluronidase. The use of a biotinylated probe to hyaluronic acid has been reported to be a more sensitive means of detecting the substance.[226]

Immunohistochemistry. Numerous studies have been carried out in an attempt to identify distinctive immunohistochemical features of mesothelioma and carcinoma (particularly adenocarcinoma).[227, 228] Using paraffin-embedded tissue sections, exfoliated cells in pleural effusions, and mesothelioma cell lines,[229] investigators have evaluated many antibodies, some of which have been associated with minimal or no overlap in their reaction to the two tumors (Table 72–2). The use of a panel of antibodies rather than a single antibody has consistently been shown to be most useful in diagnosis.[230–235]

The first and most extensively studied antibodies were those directed against carcinoembryonic antigen (CEA) and cytoplasmic intermediate filaments (principally keratins and vimentin). Many investigators have reported a positive reaction for CEA in adenocarcinoma (in 60% to 100% of cases) and a negative reaction in mesothelioma;[223, 231, 232, 236–239] however, the latter tumor can be positive,[237, 238] particularly with the use of a polyclonal antibody.[227, 240] Thus, depending to

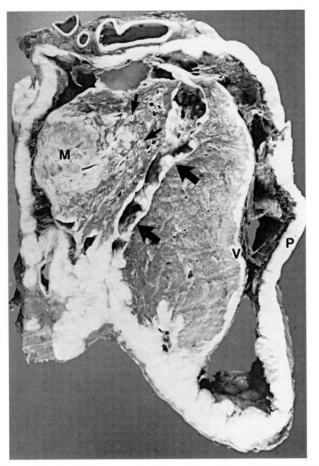

Figure 72–11. Pulmonary Carcinoma Simulating Mesothelioma. A sagittal section of a left lung shows marked thickening of both visceral (V) and parietal (P) pleura by a white tumor. The neoplasm extends into the major fissure *(large arrows)*. This appearance is highly suggestive of diffuse mesothelioma; however, a nodular mass is present in the upper lobe (M) and is associated with fairly extensive lymphangitic spread *(small arrows)*, both features being very unusual for mesothelioma. Histologic sections showed the tumor to be a mucin-secreting adenocarcinoma, considered to originate in the upper lobe.

some extent on the particular antibody utilized, it can be concluded that a clearly positive reaction for CEA is very much against a diagnosis of mesothelioma; however, because as many as 40% of adenocarcinomas show no evidence of CEA in some series, the lack of a reaction does not establish a diagnosis of mesothelioma.

The presence of a positive reaction with both low- and high-molecular-weight antikeratin antibodies is characteristic of epithelial forms of mesothelioma and is detected in virtually all tumors.[237, 238, 241, 242] A positive reaction to most keratins is also seen in many adenocarcinomas, so that its presence is of generally no differential diagnostic value; however, one group found a strong positive reaction to cytokeratin 5/6 in 33 mesotheliomas and a negative one in all but 1 of 27 pulmonary adenocarcinomas, suggesting that this particular antibody may be more discriminating.[243] The spindle cells of the mixed and sarcomatous forms of mesothelioma also often react strongly with antibodies to low-molecular-weight keratin;[244, 245] however, although this feature is useful in the differentiating these tumors from a primary or metastatic chest wall sarcoma, or from solitary

fibrous tumor of pleura, it does not exclude a reactive pleural process or pleomorphic pulmonary carcinoma.[228] Among other intermediate filaments, vimentin is positive almost always in sarcomatous tumors and occasionally in epithelial ones; desmin has also been reported to be positive in occasional cases.[246, 247]

The reaction to Leu-M1, a sugar linked to membrane proteins and lipids, has also been found to be almost always negative in mesothelioma and often positive in adenocarcinoma.[218, 248, 249] However, the reaction is often focal and may be missed in small biopsy specimens.[227] Other antibodies found to react with many carcinomas (the precise proportion varying with different antibodies and in different series) but with few mesotheliomas include pregnancy-specific glycoprotein,[236, 248] human milk fat globulin,[223, 241, 248–250] protein S-100,[236, 248, 251] human placental lactogen,[248] secretory component,[248] surfactant lipoprotein,[252] Lewis blood groups (or related antigen CA 19-9),[248, 252, 253] and a variety of miscellaneous antibodies (*see* Table 72-2).

The reaction to epithelial membrane antigen (EMA) has been found to be variable by different investigators.[223, 224, 236, 248, 254, 255] Some have noted a positive cytoplasmic reaction in a large proportion of adenocarcinomas and few mesotheliomas[256] whereas others have found a similar reaction in both tumors.[223, 224] Still other investigators have emphasized the presence of strong membranous staining as a characteristic feature of mesothelioma, related to the presence of apical microvili.[227]

A variety of antibodies have also been identified that appear to have a high sensitivity and specificity for mesothelioma, including those directed against the adhesion molecules ICAM-1, VCAM-1, and N-cadherin, thrombomodulin, Wilms' tumor susceptibility gene, calretinin, and "antimesothelial cell" antigens such as K1, AMAD-1, and ME1 (*see* Table 72–2). Additional studies are required to confirm the encouraging results related to these antibodies; however, it is likely that they or other, newly developed antibodies will supplant the more traditional ones in the near future.

Ultrastructure. The ultrastructural features of mesothelioma, especially the better differentiated epithelial forms, include[219, 257] (1) the absence of microvillous core rootlets, glycocalyceal bodies, and secretory granules (three structures that are characteristic of adenocarcinoma) and (2) the presence of intercellular desmosomes and junctional complexes, intracytoplasmic lumens (sometimes containing flocculent material thought to be hyaluronic acid), glycogen, intermediate filaments (often aggregated in a perinuclear location), and microvilli (Fig. 72–12). As might be expected, these findings are not as well seen in poorly differentiated as in well-differentiated tumors; however, other criteria suggestive of mesothelioma have been described for the former neoplasms.[258]

Of all these features just listed, the appearance of the microvilli is the most important diagnostically: in mesothelioma they are numerous and are characteristically long and thin, whereas in adenocarcinoma they are typically much less frequent and are usually short and stubby.[219, 257, 259] Several attempts have been made to quantify this subjective impression by measuring the length and width of microvilli; in general, the mean length-to-width ratio has been found to be about 10:1 in mesotheliomas and 5:1 in adenocarcinomas.[257] Microvilli are usually most prominent on the apical

Table 72–2. IMMUNOHISTOCHEMICAL FEATURES OF MESOTHELIOMA AND CARCINOMA

ANTIGEN	MESOTHELIOMA*	CARCINOMA*	SELECTED REFERENCES
Intercellular adhesion molecule-1, vascular cell adhesion molecule-1	+ + +	±	451
N-cadherin	+ + +	±	452, 453
E-cadherin	+ + +	±	450
Calretinin	+ + +	±	454–456
Wilms' tumor susceptibility gene	+ + +	±	457
K1	+ + +	±	458
ME1	+ + +	±	459
Thrombomodulin	+ + +	+	460–462
AMAD-1	+ + +	±	463
α_5, β_1-Fibronectin receptor	+ + +	+	464
HBME-1	+ + + (cell surface)	+ + (cytoplasmic)	463, 465, 466
CA 125	+ + +	+ +	466
Keratins	+ + +	+ + +	238, 242
Cytokeratin 5/6	+ + +	±	243
Parathyroid hormone–related protein	+ +	+	467
CD44H	+ +	+	468
Ber-EP4	+	+ +	233, 469, 470
MOC 31	±	+ + +	471, 472, 477
IOB3	±	+ + +	473
C-*erb* B-2 oncoprotein	±	+ +	474
Blood group–related antigens	±	+ +	233
HEA-125	±	+ +	233
Leu-M1 (CD 15)	±	+ +	233, 234
CEA	±	+ +	232–234, 240, 241
B72.3	±	+ + +	475
44-3A6	±	+ + +	476

*Frequency of positive reactions
± 0–20; + 21–40; + + 41–80; + + + 81–100
Figures are approximate and overlap occurs between different reported series depending on specific antibodies used, the length and form of tumor fixation, the subjective assessment of positivity/negativity, and the types of carcinoma studied.

cell surface where they project into empty lumens; however, they can be seen also between adjacent cells and directly interdigitating with collagen fibers of the adjacent stroma.[219, 257] Although scanning electron microscopy is not routinely performed for diagnostic purposes, microvillous features similar to those described by transmission electron microscopy can be seen by this technique.[260]

The spindle cells of the mesenchymal form of mesothelioma show few intercellular junctions, focal basal lamina, absent or occasional microvilli (usually much shorter than those in the epithelial form), abundant rough endoplasmic reticulum, and numerous randomly oriented intermediate filaments.[257] As expected, most cells of biphasic mesotheliomas show ultrastructural features that are either epithelial or mesenchymal; in addition, a variable number of cells possess intermediate (transitional) features.[257]

Biochemical Analysis of Tissue. As with the histochemical detection of hyaluronic acid in mesothelioma cells, the demonstration of this substance in tissue fragments by digestion and electrophoresis is evidence in favor of mesothelioma.[225, 261, 262] A second glycosaminoglycan, chondroitin sulfate, is also elaborated by some mesotheliomas[262, 263] and is sometimes the principal substance present;[264] its identification in tissue fragments also supports the diagnosis. Measurement of a variety of substances in tumor-associated pleural effusion has also been performed in an attempt to distinguish mesothelioma from metastatic carcinoma (*see* farther on).

Miscellaneous Investigations. One study of the reaction of various lectins (a form of nonimmune glycoprotein that binds specifically to carbohydrate groups) in mesotheliomas and pulmonary adenocarcinomas showed that the pattern of positive reactions differed in the two forms of tumor, suggesting that these substances may be useful in differential diagnosis.[265]

Radiologic Manifestations

The most common radiographic manifestation of malignant mesothelioma is unilateral sheetlike or lobulated pleural thickening encasing the entire lung (Fig. 72–13).[266–268] In one review of the radiographic findings in 25 patients, this was seen in 22 (88%);[266] additional findings included volume loss of the ipsilateral hemithorax (in 64%), extension of tumor into the major fissure (in 44%), and extension into the minor fissure (in 16%). Less commonly, the tumor is manifested as multiple masses; rarely, it presents as a solitary mass.[268] Unilateral pleural effusions are identified at presentation in 30% to 80% of cases[266, 268] and often obscure the underlying neoplasm (Fig. 72–14).

In advanced tumors, chest wall invasion may be identified on the radiograph by the presence of periosteal reaction along the ribs, rib erosion, or rib destruction.[268] Occasionally, hematogenous metastases to the lung may be seen as multiple lung nodules or masses;[268] rarely, a miliary pattern is identified.[269, 270] In two cases, the predominant radiographic finding consisted of an interstitial pattern secondary to lymphangitic spread.[271, 272]

CT is superior to conventional radiography both in the

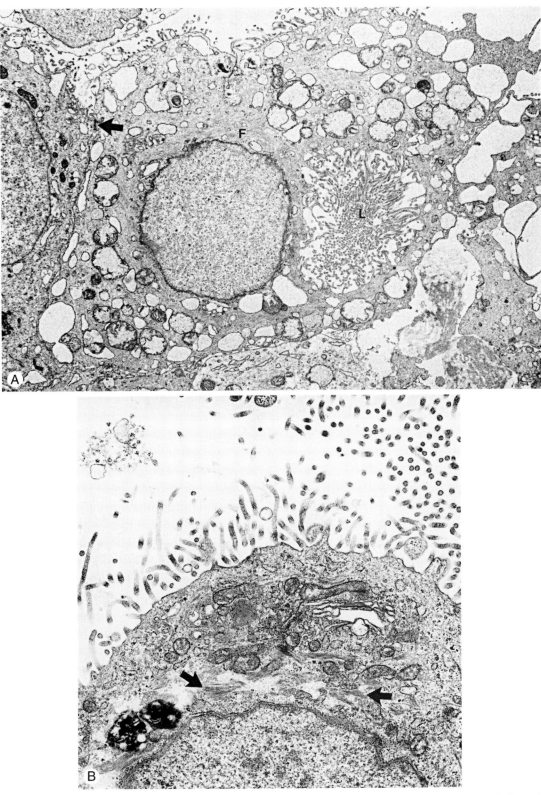

Figure 72–12. Diffuse Mesothelioma: Ultrastructure. An electron micrograph of a well-differentiated epithelial mesothelioma *(A)* shows a large cell with a more or less round nucleus and finely granular nuclear material. The cell cytoplasm contains a moderate number of intermediate filaments (F), focally in clusters adjacent to the nucleus. A poorly developed intercellular junction is evident *(arrow)*. Long, thin microvilli are present on the cell surface and are especially numerous within an intracellular lumen (L). A magnified view of another cell from the same tumor *(B)* reveals perinuclear clusters of intermediate filaments *(arrows)* and long thin surface microvilli. (*A*, ×7200; *B*, ×21,700.)

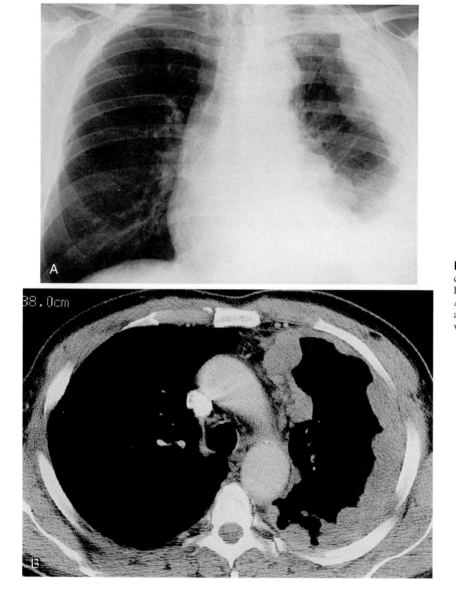

Figure 72–13. Mesothelioma. A posteroanterior chest radiograph *(A)* in a 70-year-old man shows marked, lobulated left pleural thickening encasing the entire lung. A contrast medium–enhanced CT scan *(B)* demonstrates a nodular pleural rind. The diagnosis of mesothelioma was confirmed by pleural biopsy.

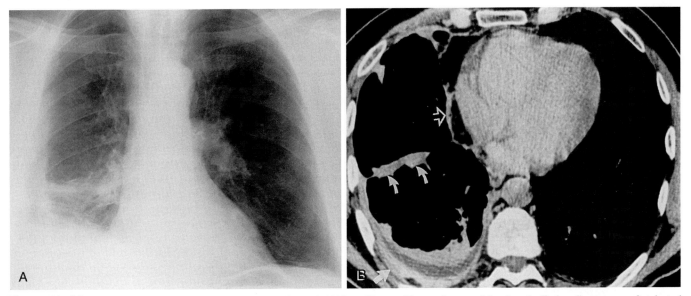

Figure 72–14. Mesothelioma. A posteroanterior chest radiograph *(A)* in a 59-year-old man shows a right pleural effusion, linear areas of atelectasis in the right lower lobe, and loss of volume of the right hemithorax. The appearance on the radiograph would be consistent with either a benign or a malignant process. A CT scan *(B)* demonstrates nodular thickening of the right parietal *(straight arrow)* and visceral pleura associated with extension of tumor into the right major fissure *(curved arrows)*. Mild thickening of the mediastinal pleura *(open arrow)* is also evident. The diagnosis of mesothelioma was proven by open pleural biopsy. The patient had been a shipyard worker.

determination of the presence and extent of mesothelioma and in the assessment of invasion of mediastinum, chest wall, and upper abdomen.[266, 273, 274] In a review of the CT manifestations in 50 patients, the most common finding consisted of pleural thickening (seen in 92%); this varied from nonspecific plaquelike lesions (in 6% of cases) to complete or nearly complete rindlike encasement of the lung (Fig. 72–15).[275] In the remaining 8% of cases, the abnormalities consisted of focal pleural masses ranging from 7 to 18 cm in diameter, all of which were associated with pleural effusion and half of which had evidence of chest

wall invasion. Extension of tumor into the minor or major interlobar fissure, manifested as thickening and/or nodularity, was seen in 86% of cases. Pleural effusion was present in 74% of patients, loss of volume of the ipsilateral hemithorax in 42%, contralateral shift of the mediastinum in 14%, lymphadenopathy in 59%, evidence of chest wall invasion in 18%, and rib involvement in 14%.

Calcification within mesothelioma is seen in approximately 10% of cases and usually represents engulfment of calcified plaques;[275] rarely, it is the result of an osteosarcomatous component (Fig. 72–16).[276] Findings suggestive of

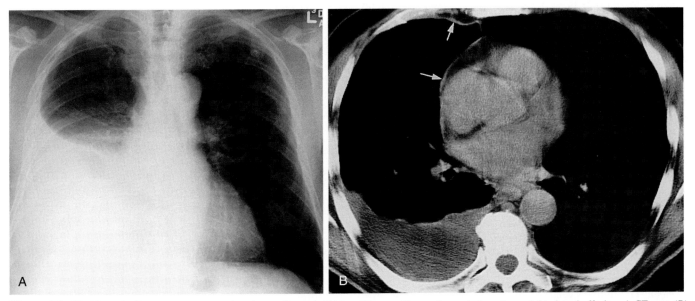

Figure 72–15. Mesothelioma. A posteroanterior chest radiograph *(A)* in a 79-year-old man demonstrates a large right pleural effusion. A CT scan *(B)* demonstrates the effusion and focal plaquelike areas of thickening involving the anterior costal and mediastinal pleura *(arrows)*. Initial biopsy of the posterior costal pleura was negative. Repeat CT-guided surgical biopsy of the anterior costal pleura was diagnostic of mesothelioma. The patient had been a shipyard worker.

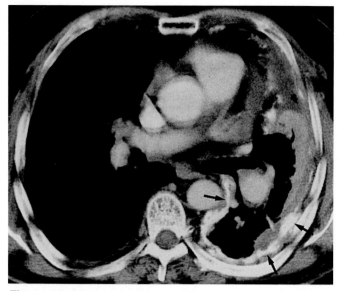

Figure 72–16. Mesothelioma. A contrast medium–enhanced CT scan in a 63-year-old man demonstrates extensive left pleural thickening associated with loss of volume of the left hemithorax. A loculated pleural effusion is present anteriorly. Note extensive calcification of the thickened left pleura *(arrows)*. At biopsy this was shown to be a mesothelioma with an osteosarcomatous component. The patient was a construction worker.

chest wall invasion include obscuration of fat planes, infiltration of intercostal muscles, periosteal reaction, and bone destruction. Features of mediastinal invasion include obliteration of fat planes, nodular pericardial thickening, and direct soft tissue extension.

Diffuse sheetlike or nodular pleural thickening identical to that of mesothelioma may be seen on CT with pleural metastasis or lymphoma but are rarely present with benign processes.[267, 277] In one CT study of 74 consecutive patients who had diffuse pleural disease, including 39 who had malignancy (11 with mesothelioma) and 35 who had benign thickening, findings most helpful in distinguishing malignant from benign disease included circumferential, mediastinal, and nodular pleural thickening (seen in 73%, 73%, and 55%, respectively, of patients who had malignant mesothelioma as compared with 0%, 12%, and 25%, respectively, of patients who had fibrothorax [Fig. 72–17]).[277] Loss of volume of the ipsilateral hemithorax, pleural plaques, and effusion were not helpful in distinguishing the two.

In one study in which the CT findings were evaluated in 34 consecutive patients who underwent surgery for mesothelioma, 10 had surgically unresectable tumors (2 with diaphragmatic invasion, 4 with chest wall invasion, and 4 with mediastinal invasion) and 24 underwent complete extrapleural pneumonectomy.[278] The sensitivity of CT was 93% for excluding chest wall involvement, 94% for excluding transdiaphragmatic extension, and 100% for excluding mediastinal involvement. The most helpful findings in assessing resectability included preservation of normal extrapleural fat for excluding chest wall invasion, a clear fat plane between the inferior diaphragmatic surface and the adjacent abdominal organs for excluding transdiaphragmatic extension, and preservation of normal mediastinal fat for exclusion of mediastinal invasion. The application of the proposed international TNM staging system (*see* farther on)

for the CT evaluation of malignant pleural mesothelioma has been reviewed.[279]

Magnetic resonance (MR) imaging is comparable or slightly superior to CT in the assessment of the morphologic features and tumor extent.[278, 280, 281] Mesothelioma has slightly greater signal intensity than the intercostal muscles on T1-weighted imaging but considerably greater signal intensity on proton-density and T2-weighted images (Fig. 72–18). In one study, all six mesotheliomas had a hyperintense signal relative to intercostal muscle on proton-density and T2-weighted images, whereas 14 of 16 benign causes of pleural thickening, including all pleural plaques and cases of fibrothorax, were isointense or hypointense.[280] The two exceptions were a case of tuberculous pleurisy and one of acute pleurisy. MR imaging is also comparable to CT in predicting tumor resectability.[278]

Preliminary results suggest that positron emission tomography (PET) imaging with 2-fluoro-2-deoxy-D-glucose (FDG) may be helpful in the assessment of patients who have suspected mesothelioma. In one investigation of 28 such patients, the uptake of FDG was significantly higher in the 24 who had biopsy-proven malignant disease (22 mesothelioma, 2 metastatic adenocarcinoma) than in the 4 who had benign disease (2 pleuritis, 1 angiolipoma, and 1 asbestos-related pleural fibrosis).[281a] However, 2 patients who had mesothelioma had mildly increased FDG uptake, and 1 who had pleuritis had markedly increased FDG uptake. Thus, FDG-PET imaging had a sensitivity of 92% (22 of 24) and a specificity of 75% (3 of 4) in detecting the presence of malignant pleural disease.

Clinical Manifestations

Patients who have pleural mesothelioma most often present with vague chest or shoulder ache or true pleuritic pain;[40, 282–284] however, a substantial number (as many as one third of individuals in some series[40]) have pleural effusion unassociated with pain. As the disease progresses, shortness of breath and a dry, sometimes hacking, cough can develop; fatigue and weight loss are common. Physical examination may reveal clubbing; retraction of the thorax and dullness on percussion are common. Occasionally, the neoplasm invades the chest wall along a needle tract used for prior thoracentesis or thoracoscopy; in this circumstance, a localized tumor may be palpated in relation to the puncture site, a finding highly suggestive of the diagnosis.

Although metastases outside the thorax are common at autopsy,[284–286] and may be widespread,[287] they are infrequently detected clinically;[285, 288, 289] they are most common in tumors that have a sarcomatous morphology.[290–292] Rarely, metastases are the initial manifestation of disease, usually in cervical[293] or axillary lymph nodes.[294] Despite these observations, as with most other malignant tumors, mesothelioma can be manifested as metastatic disease in virtually any site in the body.[295–299] Additional presentations or complications of mesothelioma include the superior vena cava syndrome,[300] the syndrome of inappropriate secretion of antidiuretic hormone,[301] achalasia,[302] systemic amyloidosis (possibly related to tumor interleukin-6 production),[303] gynecomastia (related to tumor production of human chorionic gonadotropin),[304] and a leukemoid reaction or thrombocytosis (possibly related to tumor production of granulocyte colony-stimulating factor or interleukin-6).[305–307]

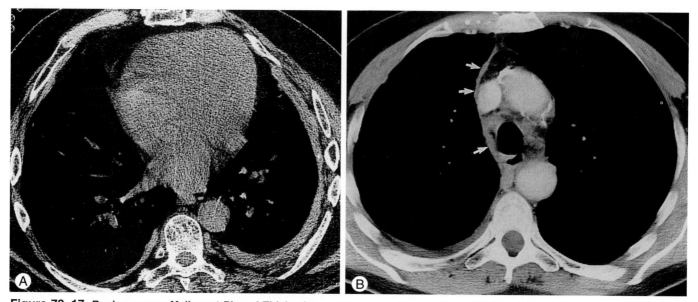

Figure 72–17. Benign versus Malignant Pleural Thickening. A CT scan in a 53-year-old man *(A)* demonstrates extensive left pleural thickening associated with loss of volume. Localized pleural plaques are present on the right side. Note that in spite of the diffuse involvement of the costal pleura, the thickening does not involve the mediastinal pleura. The diagnosis was considered to be benign asbestos-related pleural thickening; no change was seen on follow-up over 2 years. A CT scan in a 64-year-old woman *(B)* demonstrates a small right pleural effusion and thickening of the mediastinal pleura *(arrows)*. At biopsy this was shown to represent a mesothelioma. The patient had no known history of asbestos exposure.

Cardiac abnormalities are common, usually as a result of direct spread of tumor into the pericardial space. In one series of 64 patients, electrocardiographic abnormalities were present in 55 (89%) and consisted of arrhythmia (60%) and a conduction abnormality (37%).[309] Echocardiography revealed pericardial effusion in 13 patients. Cardiac invasion was found in 14 (74%) of the 19 patients who underwent autopsy; the pericardium was involved in more than half and the myocardium in over a fourth. Extension of tumor through the myocardium to form an intraluminal obstructing mass has also been reported.[309]

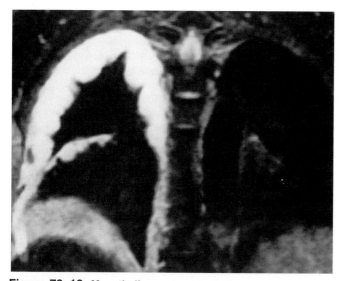

Figure 72–18. Mesothelioma. A coronal T2-weighted (TR 2118, TE 100) spin-echo MR image demonstrates diffuse nodular thickening of the right pleura associated with extension of tumor into the mediastinal pleura and right major interlobar fissure. The patient was a 37-year-old man without a history of asbestos exposure.

An occupational history of asbestos exposure may suggest the diagnosis, particularly in a patient who has an unexplained unilateral pleural effusion. Such history will usually be evident on routine questioning, because the majority of tumors occur in individuals who have jobs that are clearly associated with asbestos and the period of exposure is usually long; for example, in one study of 324 patients, the mean duration of asbestos exposure was 23 ± 14 years.[310] However, as discussed previously, some patients have only minimal exposure or have worked in occupations not easily linked to asbestos[28, 42] and careful questioning may be necessary to elicit evidence of an asbestos association. Compounding this difficulty is the latent period between exposure and the development of clinically evident disease, which is not infrequently 40 years or longer.[19, 43, 284] In one review of 1,105 cases, approximately 95% were found to have a latency period of at least 20 years;[311] the estimated median latency of the entire group was 32 years. In another review of 312 cases, the median latency was 51 years (range, 14 to 72 years).[312] An association between different occupational groups and latency period has been documented by one group of investigators, mean latency periods varying from about 30 years for insulators, 35 years for dock workers, 46 years for non–shipbuilding industry workers, 52 years for women who had domestic asbestos exposure, and 56 years for people in maritime occupations.[312]

Clinical features of asbestosis are usually absent in patients who develop mesothelioma. Rare cases have been reported of patients who have also had other definite or potential asbestos-related neoplasms, such as pulmonary carcinoma[313] and non-Hodgkin's lymphoma.[314]

Laboratory Investigation

Pleural effusion is present in the majority of patients who have mesothelioma and is often considerable in amount;[290] it may be either straw-colored or serosanguineous, in roughly equal numbers.[28] Both biochemical and cytologic examination of the fluid can be helpful in diagnosis.

Cytologic features of malignant mesothelioma cells in pleural fluid have been described by several groups of investigators.[161, 315-317] As with histologic diagnosis, problems may be encountered in distinguishing reactive from neoplastic mesothelial cells and mesothelioma from metastatic adenocarcinoma; a variety of ancillary procedures have been investigated in an attempt to overcome these problems (*see* page 2816). Despite these difficulties, some observers report a high degree of accuracy in the cytologic diagnosis of mesothelioma.[161, 318-320] Nevertheless, the overall sensitivity is probably low (e.g., 32% in one study of 29 patients[320a]), and examination of tissue specimens obtained by closed-chest needle biopsy or thoracoscopic biopsy is often necessary to establish a confident diagnosis.[321-323] In addition to pleural fluid, material may be obtained for cytologic diagnosis by fine-needle aspiration.[324] Tumor cells are rarely evident in sputum or bronchial washing specimens.[325] Cytologic examination of effusions has been advocated to be particularly useful in the follow-up of patients who have undergone extrapleural pneumonectomy.[326]

As with tissue fragments, measurement of a variety of substances in tumor-associated pleural fluid has been investigated in an attempt to distinguish between reactive and neoplastic processes and between mesothelioma and metastatic carcinoma. A low level of CEA in a malignant effusion is characteristic of mesothelioma, whereas high values are more likely to be related to metastatic carcinoma;[327-329] concomitant assay of tumor markers such as CA 15-3 has been found by some investigators to add additional discriminatory value.[330] Another group has found assessment of surfactant protein-A (SP-A) to be useful in confirming or excluding a diagnosis of pulmonary adenocarcinoma;[329] in a study of 78 effusions related to the this tumor and 10 caused by mesothelioma, SP-A levels were found to be 239 ± 140 and 16.9 ± 3.6, respectively.

Pleural fluid hyaluronate is elevated in many patients who have mesothelioma; for example, in one study of 33 patients, values greater than 100 mg/liter were identified in 23 (70%).[331] Measurement of this substance may be helpful in differential diagnosis. In one investigation of 1,610 patients who had pleural or peritoneal effusions (of which 50 were proved histologically to be the result of mesothelioma), the specificity and sensitivity for a diagnosis of mesothelioma based on assay of hyaluronic acid (using a cutoff of 75 mg/liter) were 100% and 56%, respectively;[332] however, in an additional analysis of cases from other hospitals, the investigators found the sensitivity to be considerably less. There is evidence that tumors that secrete hyaluronate have a different immunohistochemical profile from those that do not.[331] Measurement of other substances, such as the α_1-acid-glycoprotein, phosphohexose isomerase,[333] and TGF-β,[334] also has been advocated for differential diagnosis.

Prognosis and Natural History

The course of untreated mesothelioma is characterized by progressive spread of tumor over the pleural surface until the entire lung is encased. Concomitant spread to the opposite pleural and pericardial spaces and across the diaphragm into the peritoneum is not infrequent; if the patient lives long enough, involvement of the last-named tissue may result in ascites and bowel obstruction. Rare cases have been reported in which there has been apparent spread of tumor from the pleura all the way to the tunica vaginalis of the testis.[335] Although microscopic lymphangitic spread or hematogenous metastases are not uncommonly seen in the lung at autopsy, they are rarely identified during life.[336, 337] By contrast, mediastinal lymph node metastases are frequent at the time the tumor is initially identified; in one group of 89 patients undergoing staging lymph node dissections during pleurectomy, they were found in 51 (57%).[338] (Such metastases must be distinguished from the rare intranodal aggregates of hyperplastic mesothelial cells.[338a])

The prognosis of diffuse pleural mesothelioma is extremely poor: most patients die within the first year of the onset of symptoms and "long-term" survival is rare. For example, in two series of 167[339] and 114[285] patients, only 7 (2.5%) lived more than 5 years. In another review of 80 patients, the overall 2- and 5-year survival rates were 23% and 0%.[340] The median survival from the time of diagnosis varies from about 6 to 12 months in different series.[40, 284, 340-342, 342a] As with most other cancers, prognosis is related to the extent of local or distant tumor spread (Fig. 72–19);[338, 343-345] several staging systems have been described,[346] the most detailed and recent being that of the International Mesothelioma Interest Group (Table 72–3).[347] In one study of 337 patients treated with various chemotherapeutic regimens, factors associated with a better prognosis (median survival approximately 14 months) included a performance status of 0 and age younger than 49 years;[342a] patients with the worst outcome (median survival 1.4 months) had a performance status of 1 or 2 and a white blood count greater than 15.6/μl.

Most investigators have found the prognosis to be better in patients who have tumors with an epithelial rather than a sarcomatous morphology;[217, 285, 290, 343, 344, 348] some have also suggested that specific subtypes of epithelial tumor (e.g., tubulopapillary) may themselves be associated with a better outcome.[164, 349] The prognostic value of histologic type appears to be independent of stage. It is possible that the relatively good prognosis found in some of the very rare patients who have localized malignant mesothelioma is related to the combination of low stage and epithelial morphology with which these tumors are associated.[158] Some investigators have found evidence for longer survival in younger patients independent of stage and histologic type.[340, 344] Additional features that have been identified by some investigators as unfavorable prognostic factors are tumor volume greater than 100 ml (as estimated by three-dimensional CT reconstruction) and an elevated platelet count.[350]

A number of ancillary techniques have been studied in an attempt to better predict prognosis. The results of some flow cytometric investigations suggest that the outcome is better in diploid or near-diploid mesotheliomas than in aneuploid ones;[160, 199] for example, one group of investigators found the median survival from the time of diagnosis in 8 patients who had diploid tumors to be 16 months, compared with 7 months for the 11 who had aneuploid ones.[160] Assessment of cellular proliferative activity by measurement of MIB 1 index or PNCA has also been found by some investigators to be related to prognosis;[207, 350a] in one study of 31

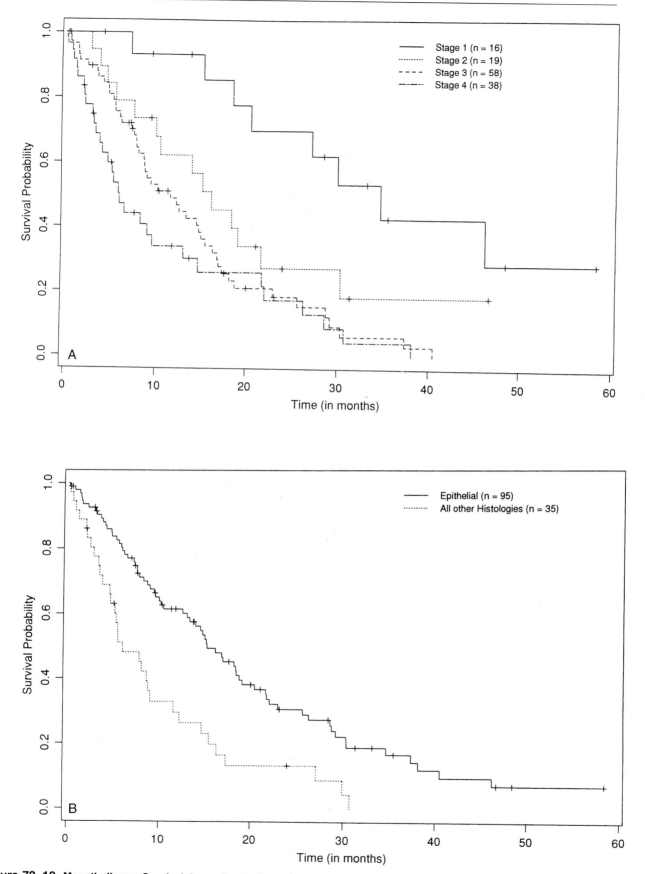

Figure 72–19. Mesothelioma: Survival According to Stage and Histologic Type. Graphs show survival curves for approximately 130 patients stratified according to stage (A) and histologic subtype (B). All patients had been treated with extrapleural pneumonectomy or pleurectomy/decortication. (From Rusch VW, Venkatramen E: The importance of surgical staging in the treatment of malignant pleural mesothelioma. J Thorac Cardiovasc Surg 111:822, 1996.)

Table 72–3. INTERNATIONAL STAGING SYSTEM FOR DIFFUSE MALIGNANT PLEURAL MESOTHELIOMA

T = Tumor
T1

　T1a　Tumor limited to the ipsilateral parietal pleura, including mediastinal and diaphragmatic portions
　　　　No involvement of the visceral pleura
　T1b　Tumor involving the ipsilateral parietal pleura, including mediastinal and diaphragmatic portions
　　　　Scattered foci of tumor also involving the visceral pleura
T2　　Tumor involving each of the ipsilateral pleural surfaces (parietal, mediastinal, diaphragmatic, and visceral pleura) with at least one of the
　　　　following features:
　　　　　　Involvement of diaphragmatic muscle
　　　　　　Confluent visceral pleural tumor (including the fissures) or extension of tumor from visceral pleura into the underlying pulmonary parenchyma
T3*　　Tumor involving all of the ipsilateral pleural surfaces (parietal, mediastinal, diaphragmatic, and visceral pleura) with at least one of the following
　　　　features:
　　　　　　Involvement of the endothoracic fascia
　　　　　　Extension into the mediastinal fat
　　　　　　Solitary, completely resectable focus of tumor extending into the soft tissues of the chest wall
　　　　　　Nontransmural involvement of the pericardium
T4†　　Tumor involving all of the ipsilateral pleural surfaces (parietal, mediastinal, diaphragmatic, and visceral) with at least one of the following
　　　　features:
　　　　　　Diffuse extension or multifocal masses of tumor in the chest wall, with or without associated rib destruction
　　　　　　Direct transdiaphragmatic extension of tumor to the peritoneum
　　　　　　Direct extension of tumor to the contralateral pleura
　　　　　　Direct extension of tumor to one or more mediastinal organs
　　　　　　Direct extension of tumor into the spine
　　　　　　Tumor extending through to the internal surface of the pericardium with or without a pericardial effusion; or tumor involving the myocardium

N = Lymph nodes
NX　　Regional lymph nodes cannot be assessed
N0　　No regional lymph node metastases
N1　　Metastases in the ipsilateral bronchopulmonary or hilar lymph nodes
N2　　Metastases in the subcarinal or the ipsilateral mediastinal lymph nodes (including the ipsilateral internal thoracic nodes)
N3　　Metastases in the contralateral mediastinal, contralateral internal thoracic, or ipsilateral or contralateral supraclavicular lymph nodes

M = Metastases
MX　　Presence of distant metastases cannot be assessed
M0　　No distant metastasis
M1　　Distant metastasis present

Stage I
　Ia　　T1a N0 M0
　Ib　　T1b N0 M0

Stage II　T2 N0 M0

Stage III　Any T3 M0
　　　　　　Any N1 M0
　　　　　　Any N2 M0

Stage IV　Any T4
　　　　　　Any N3
　　　　　　Any M1

　　*Describes locally advanced but potentially resectable tumor.
　　†Describes locally advanced but technically unresectable tumor.
　　Adapted from Rusch VW, Venkatraman E: The importance of surgical staging in the treatment of malignant pleural mesothelioma. J Thorac Cardiovasc Surg 111:815, 1996.

patients, the median survival was approximately 10 months for those who had less than 25% PNCA reactive cells and 6 months for those who had more. A higher intratumoral density of small vessels was found by one group to be associated with a shorter survival, independent of patient age and tumor histology or grade.[351]

There is little evidence that chemotherapy alone significantly alters the prognosis.[352] However, it is possible that surgery—either pleurectomy/decortication in cases of minimal disease or extrapleural pneumonectomy (en bloc excision of parietal pleura, lung, pericardium, diaphragm, and attached tumor) in more extensive tumor[353]—followed by radiation and chemotherapy may offer some benefit in selected patients.[338] For example, in one series of 120 patients who underwent these procedures, overall survival rates were 45% at 2 years and 27% at 5 years.[343] In another

review, treated patients who had negative lymph nodes and tumors with an epithelial morphology had a 5-year survival rate of 45%.[354] Unfortunately, it is not clear to what extent this relatively good survival is related to patient selection. Moreover, the surgery is not without risk, the operative mortality rate and significant morbidity rate being as high as 5% and 20%, respectively.[343, 348, 354]

MESENCHYMAL NEOPLASMS

Solitary Fibrous Tumor

This pleural tumor has been described by a variety of names, including local, fibrous, or benign mesothelioma; localized or solitary fibrous tumor; subpleural, submesothelial, or pleural fibroma; and fibrosarcoma. Among these, the relatively nonspecific *solitary fibrous tumor* is preferred for several reasons: (1) although the neoplasm is usually histologically and biologically benign, malignant forms clearly exist and in some cases the histologic distinction between the two is difficult, if not impossible; (2) the neoplasm often shows evidence of fibroblastic differentiation; and (3) the results of ultrastructural, immunohistochemical, and experimental studies suggest that the tumor originates in submesothelial connective tissue of the pleura rather than the mesothelium itself (*see* farther on). For these reasons, use of the term *mesothelioma* and of specific modifiers implying a definite benign or malignant behavior is inappropriate.

The tumor is uncommon; approximately 350 cases had been documented in the literature by 1980,[355] and an additional 223 cases were reported from the files of the Armed Forces Institute of Pathology (AFIP) in 1989.[356] It occurs slightly more often in women than in men. Although it can be seen at any age,[17] the mean age at presentation is about 50 years.[355] The etiology is unknown in the vast majority of cases; occasional tumors have developed after radiation therapy to the chest wall.[357, 358] There is no association with cigarette smoking or asbestos exposure.[355, 356]

The histogenesis of the neoplasm has been debated. On the basis of some ultrastructural[359, 360] and tissue culture[361] studies, it was initially suggested that it is derived from mesothelial cells (hence the designation benign or solitary "mesothelioma"). However, the results of additional ultrastructural and immunohistochemical investigations[362–365] have not supported this hypothesis, and most investigators now believe that the tumor originates from the submesothelial connective tissue.[356, 363–367] Histologically identical tumors have been described in the pericardium,[368] peritoneum,[369] mediastinum (*see* page 2925), lung (*see* page 1347), and a variety of other sites in the body; for purposes of the following discussion, use of the term *solitary fibrous tumor* implies a pleural origin.

Pathologic Characteristics

Sixty-five per cent to 80% of solitary fibrous tumors arise in relation to the visceral pleura.[355, 356, 371, 372] Most project into the pleural space and compress the adjacent lung to a variable degree (Fig. 72–20). Occasionally, tumors arising in the medial pleura extend into the mediastinum[370, 371] and those in a fissure extend into the pulmonary parenchyma.[355, 356] The majority are spherical or oval and well circumscribed; many are attached to the pleura by a short vascular pedicle. They can grow to a huge size, with examples up to 36 cm in diameter having been reported.[355] Cut sections often show a lobulated or whorled appearance reminiscent of a leiomyoma (Fig. 72–21). Cyst formation, calcification, hemorrhage, and necrosis can be present, especially in the larger tumors; although all can be seen in benign tumors, the presence of a significant amount of one or both of the last two should raise the possibility of malignancy.

Grossly, the tumors are usually fairly well delimited from contiguous compressed lung parenchyma or soft tissues of the chest wall or mediastinum; however, inclusions of alveolar epithelium or mesothelium are not uncommonly present between the expanding edge of the neoplasm and adjacent lung parenchyma on microscopic examination (*see*

Fig. 72–20).[356, 373, 374] Histologically, the tumor consists of haphazardly arranged or interlacing fascicles of spindle cells (Fig. 72–22), occasionally with a storiform, hemangiopericytoma-like, or neural (pallisading) pattern resembling other soft tissue tumors.[375] Between the cells is a variable amount of collagen, in some regions virtually undetectable and in others so abundant that the spindle cells themselves may be almost inapparent (*see* Fig. 72–22); focal myxoid change or fibrous tissue hyalinization are often present, particularly in larger tumors. Blood vessels are prominent in some tumors, a feature that has been associated with significant enhancement on CT.[376] The diagnosis can be strongly suggested in some cases by the appearance on fine-needle aspiration specimens.[377, 377a]

In most clinically benign tumors, nuclear atypia is minimal and mitotic figures are sparse. However, in many tumors that behave in an aggressive fashion, mitotic figures (sometimes abnormal) are more abundant and there is an appreciable degree of nuclear atypia;[356] despite this, nuclear atypia by itself does not necessarily imply an aggressive behavior (Fig. 72–23). The identification of p53 expression immunohistochemically was found by one group of investigators to be associated with nuclear atypia, recurrent tumor, and a fatal outcome.[379a] Admixed neoplastic epithelial cells are not a feature; if such cells are present, the tumor should be interpreted as a localized malignant mesothelioma of mixed type.[372]

Ultrastructural examination of solitary fibrous tumor typically reveals primitive intercellular junctions, a small amount of cytoplasmic filaments, and an absence of features usually present in tumors with mesothelial differentiation.[356] Immunohistochemical studies typically show a negative reaction for cytokeratin,[362, 363, 366, 378] and a positive one for CD34,[379, 379a] in contrast to the sarcomatous form of diffuse malignant mesothelioma in which the keratin reaction is often positive and the CD34 negative.[378–380] (However, there is evidence that CD34 positivity may be less strong or absent altogether in some malignant fibrous tumors.[379a]) Reactions for CEA, protein S-100, and epithelial membrane antigen are also invariably negative; vimentin positivity is generally present.[356, 366] Although actin positivity is sometimes present,[367] strong and extensive positive staining for desmin or muscle specific actin should raise the possibility of a smooth muscle tumor.[381] In one study of 14 tumors, a strong diffuse reaction for bcl-2 was evident in all.[382]

Radiologic Manifestations

Radiographically, solitary fibrous tumors are sharply defined, smooth, or somewhat lobulated masses of homogeneous density ranging in diameter from 1 to almost 40 cm (Fig. 72–24).[383, 384] They may be located in an interlobar fissure or adjacent to the diaphragm, mediastinum, or chest wall.[385] Small lesions (4 cm or less) typically have tapering margins and form obtuse angles with the chest wall or mediastinum, important findings in establishing the extrapulmonary nature of a thoracic mass (Fig. 72–25).[385] When a tumor is large, however, its site of origin is frequently difficult or impossible to determine on radiography or even CT (Fig. 72–26);[384, 386] in one series of six patients who had tumors ranging from 5 to 17 cm in diameter, none formed obtuse angles with the pleura with either procedure.[386] Calci-

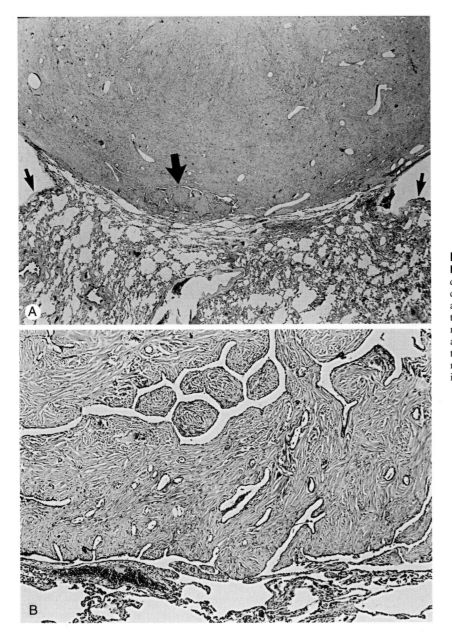

Figure 72–20. Solitary Fibrous Tumor of the Pleura. A low-power view of a small fibrous tumor discovered incidentally at autopsy *(A)* shows a well-circumscribed mass compressing, but not invading, the adjacent lung parenchyma. The tumor is clearly related to the normal pleura (*small arrows* on either side of the mass). Occasional slitlike spaces lined by a thin layer of attenuated cells are present focally at the junction of the tumor and lung parenchyma *(large arrow)*. At greater magnification *(B)*, these appear to represent mesothelial inclusions entrapped within the expanding tumor. (*A*, ×10; *B*, ×50.)

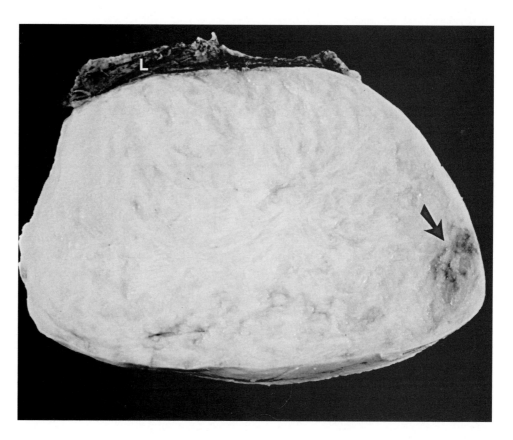

Figure 72–21. Solitary Fibrous Tumor of the Pleura. A cut section of this pleural-based tumor shows a well-circumscribed, lobulated mass compressing a small amount of attached lung parenchyma (L). There is focal hemorrhage *(arrow)* but no necrosis.

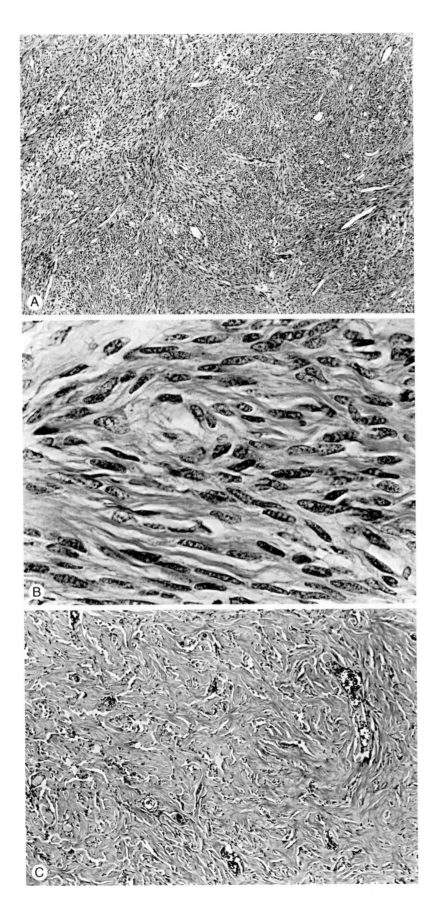

Figure 72–22. Solitary Fibrous Tumor of the Pleura. A section of a well circumscribed 5 cm tumor attached to the visceral pleura *(A)* shows interlacing fascicles of spindle cells with little intercellular collagen. A magnified view *(B)* demonstrates mild nuclear pleomorphism. A section from another tumor *(C)* shows a less cellular neoplasm with abundant intercellular collagen. (*A*, ×60; *B*, ×600; *C*, ×60.)

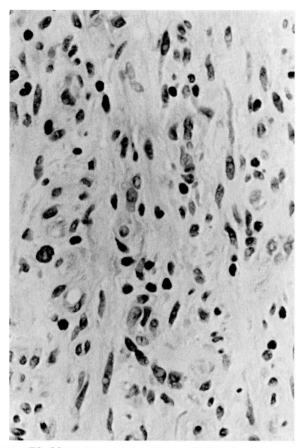

Figure 72–23. Solitary Fibrous Tumor: Cytologic Atypia. A magnified view of a section from a grossly well-circumscribed solitary fibrous tumor shows a moderate degree of nuclear atypia; mitotic figures are not evident and were sparse elsewhere in the tumor. The patient was alive and well 5 years after resection.

fication or pleural effusion were evident in 4 (7%) and 10 (17%) of 58 cases reviewed in the AFIP series.[356] The latter complication occurs more commonly in malignant than in benign tumors.[383]

A finding of considerable diagnostic value is a change in position of a pedunculated tumor with respiration, needling, or change in body position.[384, 387, 388] If the tumor originates in the visceral pleura, movement is detected by relating the position of the tumor to contiguous ribs or mediastinal structures; if origin is in the parietal pleura, movement may be related to the presence of a pedicle. Occasionally, the pedicle becomes twisted, resulting in detachment of the tumor from the pleura and the formation of a free intrapleural body.[389, 390]

Several authors have described the CT findings of fibrous pleural tumors.[386, 391–394] The vast majority of tumors larger than 5 cm in diameter have been shown to form acute or straight angles with the chest wall.[386, 392, 394] Helpful signs in determining the extrapulmonary nature of the lesion include the presence of tapering margins and displacement of adjacent lung parenchyma (see Fig. 72–25).[386, 394]

In one review of the CT manifestations in 16 patients who had tumors ranging from 4 to 17 cm in diameter, all tumors showed enhancement equal to or greater than that of muscle after intravenous administration of contrast medium.[392] Enhancement was homogeneous in 10 patients and heterogeneous in 6. A pedicle was identified in 4 patients, areas of low attenuation in 4, and calcification in 2. In another study of 9 patients, all tumors showed enhancement with intravenous contrast medium;[376] those less than 6 cm in diameter showed homogeneous enhancement, whereas larger tumors had inhomogeneous enhancement, with round or tubular areas of fluid attenuation within the mass (see Fig. 72–26). Correlation with the pathologic specimens revealed that enhancement could be explained by the vascularity of the tumor whereas the localized round or tubular areas of low attenuation were related to myxoid or cystic degeneration or hemorrhage. In a third review of 5 patients who had malignant tumors, large areas of low attenuation as a result of necrosis were present in all patients and calcification was noted in 3.[393]

MR imaging is superior to CT in determining the tissue characteristics of these tumors. With this technique, benign variants usually have a characteristic appearance of low signal intensity on both T1- and T2-weighted images, consistent with the presence of fibrous tissue.[395, 396] These characteristics allow distinction from pulmonary carcinoma, which usually has increased signal intensity on T2-weighted images. Whereas the low signal intensity is not pathognomonic for fibrous tumor, it allows a presumptive diagnosis and may obviate the need for transthoracic needle biopsy. One case has been reported of a benign fibrous tumor of the pleura that had high signal intensity on T2-weighted images, presumably related to the presence of foci of necrosis and hemorrhage.[397] High signal intensity on T2-weighted images may also be the result of myxoid degeneration (Fig. 72–27).[383] Fibrous tumors show marked increase in signal intensity after intravenous injection of gadolinium.[383, 398] MR imaging may also be helpful in determining the exact location and extent of large lesions, which may be occasionally misdiagnosed on CT as invading the mediastinum or liver (see Fig. 72–26).[393]

Clinical Manifestations

Most patients are asymptomatic;[355, 356, 374, 399] cough, chest pain, and dyspnea occur occasionally,[355] especially in association with larger tumors.[400] One particularly common finding is hypertrophic osteoarthropathy, which was seen in about one third of 350 patients identified in a literature review to 1981.[355] In fact, the association of this abnormality with solitary fibrous tumor is much stronger than with pulmonary carcinoma, and its presence in a patient with a large intrathoracic mass should suggest the diagnosis. Surgical removal of the tumor relieves the symptoms of arthropathy in most cases.[401]

Symptomatic hypoglycemia (Doege-Potter syndrome) has been documented in about 5% of patients;[400, 402] in the AFIP series, it was somewhat more common in malignant than in benign tumors (11% versus 3%) and three times more frequent in women than in men.[356] Some of these cases have been associated with the presence of insulin-like growth factor (IGF) I or II in the tumor[403, 404] and an elevated level of IGF-II in the serum.[394]

Prognosis and Natural History

The majority of solitary fibrous tumors behave in a benign fashion, with intrathoracic growth resulting in com-

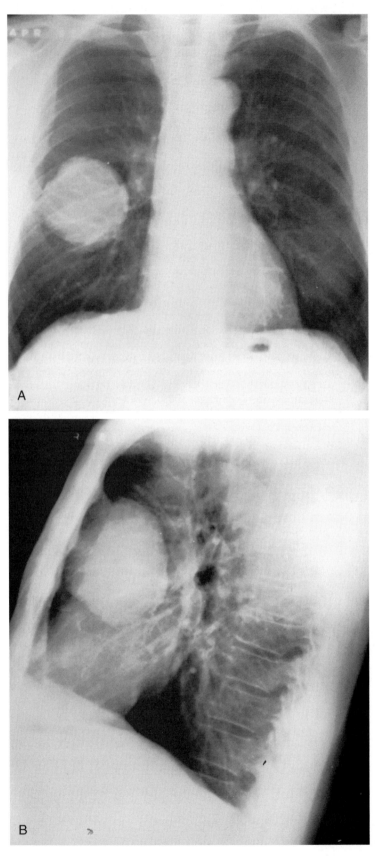

Figure 72–24. Solitary Fibrous Tumor of the Pleura. Postero-anterior *(A)* and lateral *(B)* radiographs reveal a homogeneous, somewhat lobulated mass in the anterior aspect of the right hemithorax. The relationship of the mass to the visceral pleura cannot be established from these two projections. The patient was an asymptomatic 50-year-old man.

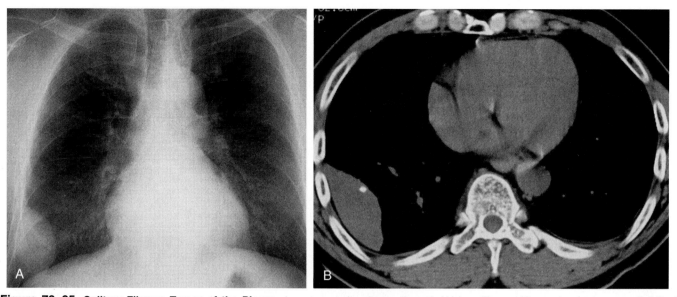

Figure 72–25. Solitary Fibrous Tumor of the Pleura. A posteroanterior chest radiograph *(A)* in a 62-year-old man demonstrates a well-defined pleural-based tumor in the right lower hemithorax. The cephalad border of the tumor tapers smoothly and forms an obtuse angle with the chest wall. A CT scan *(B)* without intravenous contrast medium enhancement demonstrates a smoothly marginated pleural-based soft tissue lesion with a focal area of calcification. The diagnosis of fibrous tumor was proven at surgical resection.

pression but not invasion of contiguous structures. Most tumors grow slowly; in one case, a 12-cm tumor was excised 20 years after it was first identified radiographically.[371] Surgical excision usually results in complete cure, particularly when the tumor possesses a well-defined pedicle; however, local recurrence can occur if initial surgery is inadequate. Tumor-related death was documented in 13% of the 350 patients reported in the literature by 1981.[355] Patients who have unresectable primary or recurrent disease usually die within 2 years as a result of extensive intrathoracic disease;[355] extrathoracic metastases are rare.

Prediction of an aggressive or benign behavior of these neoplasms can be difficult. In the AFIP series, a considerably greater proportion of malignant tumors was associated with pleural effusion and arose in the parietal pleura;[356] chest wall invasion was present in almost half the cases. Although most tumors that behave in a malignant fashion show significant cellular pleomorphism and a high mitotic rate,[405, 406] these features do not necessarily imply a bad prognosis; in the AFIP review, 32 (45%) of the patients judged to have a malignant neoplasm by light microscopic criteria were considered cured clinically.[356] Compounding the difficulty in histologic prediction is the observation that occasional tumors that have a bland histologic appearance ultimately recur. In one flow-cytometric study of 16 tumors, all were found to be diploid, including two that were recurrences;[366] however, aneuploidy has been documented in some tumors that have behaved in a malignant fashion.[405]

Miscellaneous Mesenchymal Neoplasms

In addition to localized fibrous tumors, a variety of soft tissue neoplasms have been reported to develop in the pleura. Although it is likely that some of these are derived from the submesothelial mesenchymal cells of the pleura itself and thus indeed arise in this location, it is probable that many

originate in the chest wall and simply expand into the pleural space. The most common of these is lipoma, a tumor that is usually small but can become sufficiently large to erode contiguous ribs (*see* page 3025). As with other pleural tumors, lipomas are seen on the chest radiograph as soft tissue masses that have well-defined margins where they abut the lung and poorly defined margins where they abut the chest wall. When small, they often have tapering margins and form obtuse angles with the chest wall.[407–409] CT allows a specific diagnosis by demonstrating a uniform attenuation (-50 to -100 HU) similar to that of subcutaneous fat (Fig. 72–28). A few linear strands of soft tissue attenuation may be seen related to their fibrous stroma;[409] however, when the lesion has a heterogeneous appearance with attenuation values greater than -50 HU, liposarcoma should be suspected (Fig. 72–29).[267, 409–411]

Other sarcomas that have been reported to arise in the pleura include leiomyosarcoma,[381] rhabdomyosarcoma,[412] malignant fibrous histiocytoma,[413] angiosarcoma (in some cases associated with chronic pyothorax[414]),[415, 416] epithelioid hemangioendothelioma,[178, 417] and chondrosarcoma.[418] In the absence of confirmatory immunohistochemical or ultrastructural evidence of specific differentiation, some of these (e.g., malignant fibrous histiocytoma and leiomyosarcoma) may be better regarded as variants of solitary fibrous tumor. In addition, because of the fact that some mesenchymal mesotheliomas show osseous, cartilaginous, or lipogenous differentiation, it is possible that others are simply variants of mesothelioma. Except for liposarcoma, the radiologic appearance of all these tumors is nonspecific.

Carcinosarcoma has also been reported to arise in the pleura, in some cases with a gross appearance identical to diffuse mesothelioma;[418a] in two such examples, the epithelial component showed adenosquamous and neuroendocrine features and the sarcoma a spindle cell pattern with focal osteoid formation. Such tumors must be differentiated from mixed forms of mesothelioma, which are undoubtedly much more common.

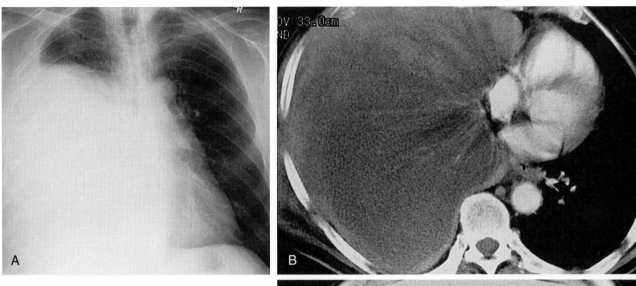

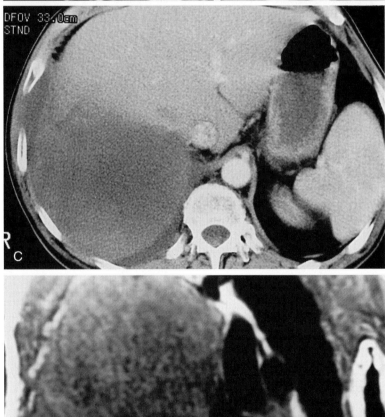

Figure 72–26. Solitary Fibrous Tumor of the Pleura. A posteroanterior chest radiograph *(A)* in a 58-year-old man demonstrates almost complete homogeneous opacification of the right hemithorax with shift of the mediastinum to the left. A right pleural effusion and multiple healing rib fractures are also evident. A CT scan performed after intravenous contrast medium enhancement *(B)* demonstrates inhomogeneous enhancement of a mass that occupies the entire right lower hemithorax. A scan at a more caudad level *(C)* shows poorly defined margins between the tumor and the liver. The possibility of transdiaphragmatic extension and invasion of the liver was considered. A T1-weighted coronal cardiac gated MR image *(D)* demonstrates low signal intensity of the mass, which, with the patient breathing quietly in the supine position, occupies the entire right hemithorax at this level. Note clear margins between the tumor and the inverted right hemidiaphragm *(arrows).* The diagnosis of fibrous tumor was made at thoracotomy; there was no evidence of diaphragmatic invasion. The resected tumor weighed approximately 4 kg.

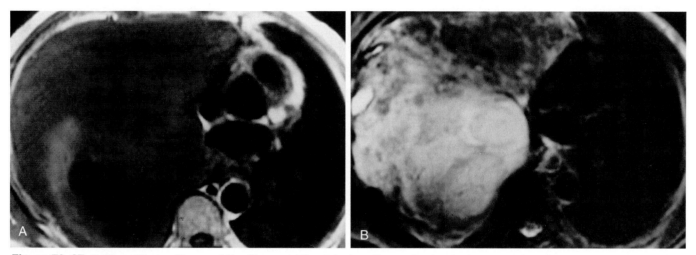

Figure 72–27. Solitary Fibrous Tumor of the Pleura. A T1-weighted, cardiac-gated, spin-echo image (TR 631, TE 17), *(A)* demonstrates a large soft tissue mass occupying the right hemithorax. Most of the tumor has a signal intensity equal to or less than that of muscle. A T2-weighted image *(B)* (TR 1400, TE 100) shows inhomogeneous hyperintensity of the tumor. At surgery this was shown to be a fibrous tumor with areas of myxoid degeneration but no necrosis.

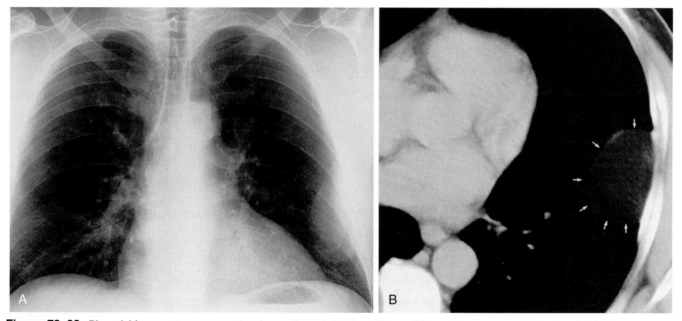

Figure 72–28. Pleural Lipoma. A posteroanterior chest radiograph *(A)* in a 50-year-old man demonstrates a pleural-based soft tissue mass. The cephalad margin of the tumor forms obtuse angles with the chest wall while the caudad aspect forms an acute angle. A CT scan *(B)* demonstrates tumor *(arrows)* with attenuation identical to that of subcutaneous fat. (Courtesy of Dr. Jim Barrie, University of Alberta, Edmonton.)

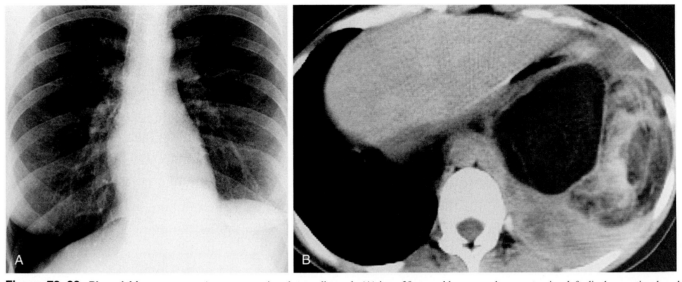

Figure 72–29. Pleural Liposarcoma. A posteroanterior chest radiograph *(A)* in a 30-year-old woman shows extensive left diaphragmatic pleural thickening. Unfortunately, no further investigation was performed at that time. A CT scan 2 years later *(B)*, at which time the chest radiograph showed considerable increase in size of the tumor, demonstrates an inhomogeneous soft tissue mass in the left lower hemithorax. The tumor contains areas with attenuation similar to that of subcutaneous fat and areas of soft tissue attenuation. The diagnosis of pleural liposarcoma was proven at thoracotomy.

LYMPHOMA

Pleural lymphoma usually occurs as part of disseminated disease and can be seen with virtually any histologic subtype;[419] rarely, it appears to be primary in this site. A history of remote tuberculous pleuritis and Epstein-Barr virus infection has been found by Japanese investigators in a number of patients who have had large cell lymphoma apparently originating in the pleura.[420, 421] Herpesvirus 8 has also been implicated in the etiology of an unusual form of primary pleural lymphoma;[422] although most affected patients have had the acquired immunodeficiency syndrome, some have been negative for human immunodeficiency virus infection.[423] In addition to a striking predilection for serosal surfaces, the lymphoma has been characterized by the absence of a tumor mass in adjacent tissues, the presence of large cells (often with immunoblastic features) on histologic examination, the absence of B-cell antigen or immunoglobulin expression (despite evidence of B-cell origin by gene rearrangement studies), frequent evidence of concomitant Epstein-Barr virus infection, and an absence of c-*myc* gene rearrangements.[424]

In the vast majority of cases, pleural lymphoma appears as a more or less diffuse or focal plaquelike thickening, rather than a localized tumor. Radiographic and CT findings consist of pleural effusion with or without pleural thickening.[277, 424a, b] In one case, the CT findings consisted of a large unilateral pleural effusion associated with inhomogeneous areas of increased attenuation and a focal area of pleural thickening;[424b] at thoracotomy, the effusion was shown to be caused by recent hemorrhage and the area of pleural thickening by lymphoma.

MISCELLANEOUS PLEURAL NEOPLASMS

Well-differentiated papillary mesothelioma is a very rare tumor that is most common in the peritoneum.[425] It is usually small (1 to 2 cm), although one example measuring 6 cm has been reported in the pleura.[426] Histologically, the tumor is composed of broad papillae lined by a layer of cytologically bland mesothelial cells. The tumors behave in a benign fashion. Another very rare benign mesothelial tumor is characterized histologically by a localized proliferation of vacuolated epithelioid cells associated with tubular spaces and a fibrous stroma (*adenomatoid tumor*). Tumors that have this morphology are usually found on the pelvic peritoneum; however, two examples have been reported as incidental findings on the pleura of patients undergoing surgery for pulmonary lesions.[427]

Squamous cell carcinoma rarely arises in the pleura, usually in association with persistent empyema that has been drained by a pleurocutaneous fistula[428] or long-standing extrapleural pneumothorax without fistula;[129, 429] in one case, it appeared to be associated with squamous metaplasia of the pleura and to develop only 5 months after the onset of empyema.[430] Primary pleural *melanoma* also has been reported,[431] although such cases must be exceedingly rare and may, in fact, represent metastasis in the absence of a documented primary tumor.

Tumors that have a histologic appearance identical to *thymoma* have occasionally been reported in the pleura;[432, 433] although some may represent neoplasia in ectopic thymic tissue, others are the result of predominant growth in the pleura after extension from a primary mediastinal tumor.[434] The tumor may present as a relatively localized mass or as a more diffuse tumor encasing the lung in a fashion similar to diffuse mesothelioma.[434a]

Neoplasms that have the histologic appearance of *desmoplastic small round cell tumor* have rarely been reported to arise in the pleura. In one study of three patients, the ages ranged from 17 to 29;[435] all presented with chest pain and pleural effusion and 2 died within 2 years. A gross appearance similar to that of diffuse mesothelioma was evident at surgery. This histologically distinctive tumor is much more common in the peritoneum; however, because of the docu-

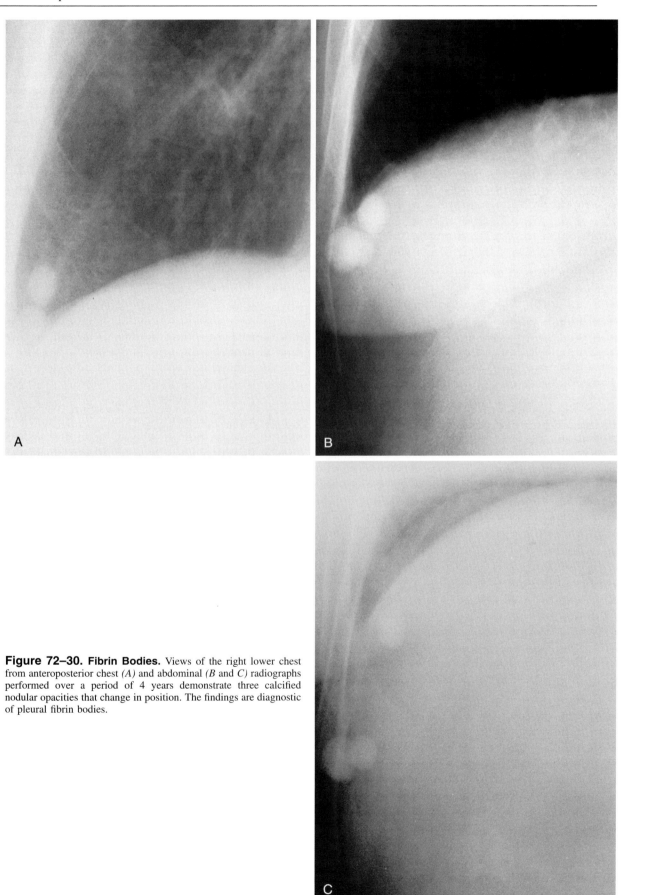

Figure 72–30. Fibrin Bodies. Views of the right lower chest from anteroposterior chest *(A)* and abdominal *(B and C)* radiographs performed over a period of 4 years demonstrate three calcified nodular opacities that change in position. The findings are diagnostic of pleural fibrin bodies.

mentation of some cases in the tunica vaginalis as well as the pleura, some have speculated that it may represent a blastomatous tumor of mesothelium in general.[435]

Pleuropulmonary blastoma is a rare malignant neoplasm that occurs in children and may originate in the pleura, lung, or mediastinum.[436, 437] As the name suggests, the histologic appearance is one of embryonic-appearing stromal cells; the prognosis is generally poor. It should not be confused with pulmonary blastoma (*see* page 1367).

PLEURAL TUMORS OF NON-NEOPLASTIC OR UNCERTAIN NATURE

Pleural *amyloidosis* is a very rare condition[438] that can present as more or less diffuse involvement, sometimes associated with effusion, or as a localized tumor-like nodule or mass (*see* page 2709).[439] There are no specific radiographic features to suggest the diagnosis.

Although oleothorax as a method of therapy for pulmonary tuberculosis was largely abandoned in the 1950s, patients are still seen occasionally in whom the instilled paraffin is visible as a mass within the pleural space. In one report, the mass increased considerably in size over time.[440]

Intrathoracic *splenosis* occurs when tissue from a traumatized spleen crosses an injured diaphragm and proliferates within the pleural space (*see* page 2643).[441, 442] The diagnosis can be confirmed by radionuclide imaging[443] and has also been made by transthoracic needle aspiration.[444]

Fibrin bodies (fibrin balls) are tumor-like accumulations of fibrin that sometimes develop in a serofibrinous pleural effusion. They may be single or multiple and are round, oval, or irregularly shaped. They are seldom more than 3 to 4 cm in diameter. They usually become evident after absorption of a pleural effusion and may disappear spontaneously and fairly rapidly[445] or remain unchanged in size, position, or shape for many years.[446] They tend to be situated near the lung base and, when viewed *en face*, can simulate a solitary pulmonary nodule. Their anatomic relationship to the pleura may be established by fluoroscopy, tangential radiography, or CT. In some cases, a specific diagnosis can be suggested radiologically by demonstrating a change in location with a change in the patient's position (Fig. 72–30).

A single case resembling *multicystic mesothelioma* has been reported to arise in the pleura.[447] This rare abnormality is far more common in the peritoneum, in which it typically occurs in young women as a multifocal, multicystic lesion; the cysts are lined by a single layer of cytologically bland mesothelial cells. In the peritoneum, the tumor commonly recurs but does not cause death.

The term *calcifying fibrous pseudotumor* was originally given to lesions located in the subcutaneous and deep soft tissue that were characterized by a mass of hyalinized collagen containing a patchy lymphoplasmacytic infiltrate and multiple foci of calcification, frequently psammoma bodies. Three examples have subsequently been reported in relation to the pleura.[448] Although said to be distinct from solitary fibrous tumor of the pleura, the abnormality clearly bears some resemblance to it and the possibility that it represents simply a "burnt-out" stage of solitary fibrous tumor has not been discounted. CT examination has shown pleural-based nodules ranging up to 12 cm in diameter with extensive areas of calcification.[449] All reported patients have been young adults.[448, 449]

REFERENCES

1. Bierhoff E, Pfeifer U: Malignant mesothelioma arising from a benign mediastinal mesothelial cyst. Gen Diagn Pathol 142:59, 1996.
2. Hoogsteden HC, Langerak AW, van der Kwast TH, et al: Malignant pleural mesothelioma. Crit Rev Oncol Hematol 25:97, 1997.
3. Willis RA: Pathology of Tumours. 3rd ed. London, Butterworths, 1960.
4. McDonald JC: Health implications of environmental exposure to asbestos. Environ Health Perspect 62:319, 1985.
5. Spirtas R, Beebe GW, Connelly RR, et al: Recent trends in mesothelioma incidence in the United States. Am J Ind Med 9:397, 1986.
6. Connelly RR, Spirtas R, Myers MH, et al: Demographic patterns for mesothelioma in the United States. J Natl Cancer Inst 78:1053, 1987.
7. Damhuis RA, van Gelder T: Malignant mesothelioma in the Rotterdam area, 1987–1989. Eur J Cancer 29A:1478, 1993.
8. Jones RD, Smith DM, Thomas PG: Mesothelioma in Great Britain in 1968–1983. Scand J Work Environ Health 14:145, 1988.
9. Huuskonen MS, Karjalainen A, Tossavainen A, et al: Asbestos and cancer in Finland. Med Lav 86:426, 1995.
10. Karjalainen A, Pukkala E, Mattson K, et al: Trends in mesothelioma incidence and occupational mesotheliomas in Finland in 1960–1995. Scand J Work Environ Health 23:266, 1997.
11. Smith AH, Wright CC: Chrysotile asbestos is the main cause of pleural mesothelioma. Am J Ind Med 30:252, 1996.
12. McDonald AD, McDonald JC: Malignant mesothelioma in North America. Cancer 46:1650, 1980.
13. Driscoll TR, Baker GJ, Daniels S, et al: Clinical aspects of malignant mesothelioma in Australia. Aust N Z J Med 23:19, 1993.
14. Roggli VL, Oury TD, Moffatt EJ: Malignant mesothelioma in women. Anat Pathol 2:147, 1997.
15. Rosler JA, Woitowitz HJ, Lange HJ, et al: Mortality rates in a female cohort following asbestos exposure in Germany. J Occup Med 36:889, 1994.
16. Begin R, Gauthier JJ, Desmeules M, et al: Work-related mesothelioma in Quebec, 1967–1990. Am J Ind Med 22:531, 1992.
17. Coffin CM, Dehner LP: Mesothelial and related neoplasms in children and adolescents: A clinicopathologic and immunohistochemical analysis of eight cases. Pediatr Pathol 12:333, 1992.
18. Roggli VL, McGavran MH, Subach J, et al: Pulmonary asbestos body counts and electron probe analysis of asbestos body cores in patients with mesothelioma: A study of 25 cases. Cancer 50:2423, 1982.
19. Mowé G, Gylseth B, Hartveit F, et al: Occupational asbestos exposure, lung-fiber concentration and latency time in malignant mesothelioma. Scand J Work Environ Health 10:293, 1984.
20. Davies D: Are all mesotheliomas due to asbestos (editorial)? BMJ 289:1164, 1984.
21. Lin-Chu M, Lee Y-J, Ho MY: Malignant mesothelioma in infancy. Arch Pathol Lab Med 113:409, 1989.
22. Peterson JT, Greenberg SD, Buffler PA: Non–asbestos-related malignant mesothelioma. Cancer 54:501, 1984.
23. Wagner JC, Sleggs CA, Marchand P: Diffuse pleural mesothelioma and asbestos exposure in the northwestern Cape Province. Br J Ind Med 7:260, 1960.
24. McDonald JC, McDonald AD: The epidemiology of mesothelioma in historical context. Eur Respir J 9:1932, 1996.
25. Liddell FD, McDonald AD, McDonald JC: The 1891–1920 birth cohort of Quebec chrysotile miners and millers: Development from 1904 and mortality to 1992. Ann Occup Hyg 41:13, 1997.
26. Rubino GF, Scansetti G, Donna A, et al: Epidemiology of pleural mesothelioma in Northwestern Italy (Piedmont). Br J Ind Med 29:436, 1972.
27. Wright GW: Asbestos and health in 1969. Am Rev Respir Dis 100:467, 1969.
28. Borow M, Couston A, Livornese L, et al: Mesothelioma following exposure to asbestos: A review of 72 cases. Chest 64:641, 1973.
29. Whitwell F, Rawcliffe RM: Diffuse malignant pleural mesothelioma and asbestos exposure. Thorax 26:6, 1971.
30. Armstrong BK, Musk AW, Baker JE, et al: Epidemiology of malignant mesothelioma in Western Australia. Med J Aust 141:86, 1984.
31. Teta MJ, Lewinsohn HC, Meigs JW, et al: Mesothelioma in Connecticut, 1955–1977: Occupational and geographic associations. J Occup Med 25:749, 1983.
32. Solomons K: Malignant mesothelioma—Clinical and epidemiological features: A report of 80 cases. S Afr Med J 66:407, 1984.
33. Edge JR, Choudhury SL: Malignant mesothelioma of the pleura in Barrow-in-Furness. Thorax 33:26, 1978.
34. Hasan FM, Nash G, Kazemi H: The significance of asbestos exposure in the diagnosis of mesothelioma: A 28-year experience from a major urban hospital. Am Rev Respir Dis 115:761, 1977.
35. Wolf KM, Piotrowski ZH, Engel JD, et al: Malignant mesothelioma with occupational and environmental asbestos exposure in an Illinois community hospital. Arch Intern Med 147:2145, 1987.
36. Churg A: Malignant mesothelioma in British Columbia in 1982. Cancer 55:672, 1985.
37. Chellini E, Fornaciai G, Merler E, et al: Pleural malignant mesothelioma in Tuscany, Italy (1970–1988): II. Identification of occupational exposure to asbestos. Am J Ind Med 21:577, 1992.
38. Spirtas R, Heineman EF, Bernstein L, et al: Malignant mesothelioma: Attributable risk of asbestos exposure. Occup Environ Med 51:804, 1994.
39. Pott F: Asbestos use and carcinogenicity in Germany and a comparison with animal studies. Ann Occup Hyg 38:589, 1994.
40. Yates DH, Corrin B, Stidolph PN, et al: Malignant mesothelioma in south east England: Clinicopathological experience of 272 cases. Thorax 52:507, 1997.
41. Howel D, Arblaster L, Swinburne L, et al: Routes of asbestos exposure and the development of mesothelioma in an English region. Occup Environ Med 54:403, 1997.
42. Chen W-J, Mottet NK: Malignant mesothelioma with minimal asbestos exposure. Hum Pathol 9:253, 1978.
43. Ferguson DA, Berry G, Jelihovsky T, et al: The Australian Mesothelioma Surveillance Program 1979–1985. Med J Aust 147:166, 1987.
44. Dawson A, Gibbs AR, Pooley FD, et al: Malignant mesothelioma in women. Thorax 48:269, 1993.
45. McDonald AD, Harper A, El-Attar OA, et al: Epidemiology of primary malignant mesothelial tumors in Canada. Cancer 26:914, 1970.
46. Huncharek M: Changing risk groups for malignant mesothelioma. Cancer 69:2704, 1992.
47. Teschke K, Morgan MS, Checkoway H, et al: Mesothelioma surveillance to locate sources of exposure to asbestos. Can J Public Health 88:163, 1997.
48. Dorward AJ, Stack BHR: Diffuse malignant pleural mesothelioma in Glasgow. Br J Dis Chest 75:397, 1981.
49. Sheers G, Coles RM: Mesothelioma risks in a naval dockyard. Arch Environ Health 35:276, 1980.
50. Kishimoto T, Okada K, Sato T, et al: Evaluation of the pleural malignant mesothelioma patients with the relation of asbestos exposure. Environ Res 48:42, 1989.
51. Dodoli D, Del Nevo M, Fiumalbi C, et al: Environmental household exposures to asbestos and occurrence of pleural mesothelioma. Am J Ind Med 21:681, 1992.
52. Oksa P, Pukkala E, Karjalainen A, et al: Cancer incidence and mortality among Finnish asbestos sprayers and in asbestosis and silicosis patients. Am J Ind Med 31:693, 1997.
53. Talcott JA, Thurber WA, Kantor AF, et al: Asbestos-associated diseases in a cohort of cigarette-filter workers. N Engl J Med 321:1220, 1989.
54. McDonald AD, McDonald JC: Mesothelioma after crocidolite exposure during gas mask manufacture. Environ Res 17:340, 1978.
55. Driscoll RJ, Mulligan WJ, Schultz D, et al: Malignant mesothelioma: A cluster in a Native American pueblo. N Engl J Med 318:1437, 1988.
56. Otte KE, Sigsgaard TI, Kjaerulff J: Malignant mesothelioma: Clustering in a family producing asbestos cement in the home. Br J Ind Med 47:10, 1990.
57. Epler GR, FitzGerald MX, Gaensler EA, et al: Asbestos-related disease from household exposure. Respiration 39:229, 1980.
58. Magnani C, Terracini B, Ivaldi C, et al: A cohort study on mortality among wives of workers in the asbestos cement industry in Casale Monferrato, Italy. Br J Ind Med 50:779, 1993.
59. Fischbein A, Rohl AN: Pleural mesothelioma and neighborhood asbestos exposure: Findings from micro-chemical analysis of lung tissue. JAMA 252:86, 1984.
60. Stein RC, Kijajewska JY, Kirkhan JB, et al: Pleural mesothelioma resulting from exposure to amosite asbestos in a building. Respir Med 83:237, 1989.
61. Oliver LC, Sprince NL, Green RE: Asbestos related disease in public school custodians. Am Rev Respir Dis 139:A211, 1989.
62. Constantopoulos SH, Malamou-Mitsi VD, Goudevenos JA, et al: High incidence of malignant pleural mesothelioma in neighbouring villages of Northwestern Greece. Respiration 51:266, 1987.
63. Langer AM, Nolan RP, Constantopoulos SH, et al: Association of Metsovo lung and pleural mesothelioma with exposure to tremolite-containing whitewash. Lancet 1:965, 1987.
64. Magee F, Wright JL, Chan N, et al: Malignant mesothelioma caused by childhood exposure to long-fiber low aspect ratio tremolite. Am J Ind Med 9:529, 1986.
65. Coplu L, Dumortier P, Demir AU, et al: An epidemiological study in an Anatolian village in Turkey environmentally exposed to tremolite asbestos. J Environ Pathol Toxicol Oncol 15:177, 1996.
66. McConnochie K, Simonato L, Mavrides P, et al: Mesothelioma in Cyprus: The role of tremolite. Thorax 42:342, 1987.
67. Roggli VL: Quantitative and analytical studies in the diagnosis of mesothelioma. Semin Diagn Pathol 9:162, 1992.
68. Gaudichet A, Janson X, Monchaux G, et al: Assessment by analytical microscopy of the total lung fibre burden in mesothelioma patients matched with four other pathological series. Ann Occup Hyg 32:213, 1988.
69. Whitwell F, Scott J, Grimshaw M: Relationship between occupations and asbestos fibre content of the lungs in patients with pleural mesothelioma, lung cancer, and other diseases. Thorax 32:377, 1977.
70. Sakai K, Hisanaga N, Huang J, et al: Asbestos and nonasbestos fiber content in lung tissue of Japanese patients with malignant mesothelioma. Cancer 73:1825, 1994.
71. Dodson RF, O'Sullivan M, Corn CJ, et al: Analysis of asbestos fiber burden in lung tissue from mesothelioma patients. Ultrastruct Pathol 21:321, 1997.
72. Dufresne A, Begin R, Churg A, et al: Mineral fiber content of lungs in patients with mesothelioma seeking compensation in Quebec. Am J Respir Crit Care Med 153:711, 1996.
73. Srebro SH, Roggli VL, Samsa GP: Malignant mesothelioma associated with low pulmonary tissue asbestos burdens: A light and scanning electron microscopic analysis of 18 cases. Mod Pathol 8:614, 1995.

74. Whitwell F, Scott J, Grimshaw M: Relationship between occupation and asbestos-fibre content of the lungs in patients with pleural mesothelioma, lung cancer, and other diseases. Thorax 32:377, 1977.

75. Wagner JC, Moncrieff CB, Coles R, et al: Correlation between fibre content of the lungs and disease in naval dockyard workers. Br J Ind Med 43:391, 1986.

76. Antman KH, Corson JM: Benign and malignant pleural mesothelioma. Clin Chest Med 6:127, 1985.

77. Mowé G, Gylseth B, Hartveit F, et al: Fiber concentration in lung tissue of patients with malignant mesothelioma: A case-control study. Cancer 56:1089, 1985.

78. Churg A, Wiggs B: Fiber size and number in amphibole asbestos-induced mesothelioma. Am J Pathol 115:437, 1984.

79. Craighead JE: Current pathogenetic concepts of diffuse malignant mesothelioma. Hum Pathol 18:544, 1987.

80. Editorial. Amosite asbestos and mesothelioma. Lancet 2:1397, 1981.

81. Humphrey EW, Ewing SL, Wrigley JV, et al: The production of malignant tumors of the lung and pleura in dogs from intratracheal asbestos instillation and cigarette smoking. Cancer 47:1994, 1981.

82. Elmes PC: Mesotheliomas, minerals, and man-made mineral fibres. Thorax 35:561, 1980.

83. Sluis-Cremer GK, Liddell FD, Logan WP, et al: The mortality of amphibole miners in South Africa, 1946–80. Br J Ind Med 49:566, 1992.

84. Murai Y, Kitagawa M: Asbestos fiber analysis in 27 malignant mesothelioma cases. Am J Ind Med 22:193, 1992.

85. Nicholson WJ, Raffn E: Recent data on cancer due to asbestos in the U.S.A. and Denmark. Med Lav 86:393, 1995.

86. Karjalainen A, Meurman LO, Pukkala E: Four cases of mesothelioma among Finnish anthophyllite miners. Occup Environ Med 51:212, 1994.

87. Stayner LT, Dankovic DA, Lemen RA: Occupational exposure to chrysotile asbestos and cancer risk: A review of the amphibole hypothesis. Am J Public Health 86:179, 1996.

88. Churg A, Wiggs B, Depaoli L, et al: Lung asbestos content in chrysotile workers with mesothelioma. Am Rev Respir Dis 130:1042, 1984.

89. McDonald JC, Armstrong B, Case B, et al: Mesothelioma and asbestos fiber type: Evidence from lung tissue analysis. Cancer 63:1544, 1989.

90. Dufresne A, Harrigan M, Masse S, et al: Fibers in lung tissues of mesothelioma cases among miners and millers of the township of Asbestos, Quebec. Am J Ind Med 27:581, 1995.

91. Elmes P: Mesotheliomas and chrysotile. Ann Occup Hyg 38:547, 1994.

92. Churg A: Asbestos fiber content of the lungs in patients with and without asbestos airways disease. Am Rev Respir Dis 127:470, 1983.

93. Gylseth B, Mowé G, Wannag A: Fibre type and concentration in the lungs of workers in an asbestos cement factory. Br J Ind Med 40:375, 1983.

94. Wang NS, Jaurand MC, Magne L, et al: The interactions between asbestos fibers and metaphase chromosomes of rat pleural mesothelial cells in culture: A scanning and transmission electron microscopic study. Am J Pathol 126:343, 1987.

95. Baris YI, Sarracci R, Simonato L, et al: Malignant mesothelioma and radiological chest abnormalities in two villages in central Turkey. Lancet 1:984, 1981.

96. Hillerdal G, Baris YI: Radiological study of pleural changes in relation to mesothelioma in Turkey. Thorax 38:443, 1983.

97. Selcuk ZT, Coplu L, Emri S, et al: Malignant pleural mesothelioma due to environmental mineral fiber exposure in Turkey: Analysis of 135 cases. Chest 102:790, 1992.

98. Wagner JC, Skidmore JW, Hill RJ, et al: Erionite exposure and mesotheliomas in rats. Br J Cancer 51:727, 1985.

99. Infante PF, Schuman LD, Dement J, et al: Fibrous glass and cancer. Am J Ind Med 26:559, 1994.

100. De Vuyst P, Dumortier P, Swaen GM, et al: Respiratory health effects of man-made vitreous (mineral) fibres. Eur Respir J 8:2149, 1995.

101. Newman RH: Fine biogenic silica fibers in sugarcane: A possible hazard. Ann Occup Hyg 30:365, 1986.

102. Austin MB, Fechner RE, Roggli VL: Pleural malignant mesothelioma following Wilms' tumor. Am J Clin Pathol 86:227, 1986.

103. Cavazza A, Travis LB, Travis WD, et al: Post-irradiation malignant mesothelioma. Cancer 77:1379, 1996.

104. Hofmann J, Mintzer D, Warhol MJ: Malignant mesothelioma following radiation therapy. Am J Med 97:379, 1994.

105. Weissmann LB, Corson JM, Neugut AI, et al: Malignant mesothelioma following treatment for Hodgkin's disease. J Clin Oncol 14:2098, 1996.

106. Shannon VR, Nesbitt JC, Libshitz HI: Malignant pleural mesothelioma after radiation therapy for breast cancer: A report of two additional patients. Cancer 76:437, 1995.

107. Neugut AI, Ahsan H, Antman KH: Incidence of malignant pleural mesothelioma after thoracic radiotherapy. Cancer 80:948, 1997.

108. Warren S, Brown CE, Chute RN, et al: Mesothelioma relative to asbestos, radiation, and methylcholanthrene. Arch Pathol Lab Med 105:305, 1981.

109. Andersson M, Wallin H, Jonsson M, et al: Lung carcinoma and malignant mesothelioma in patients exposed to Thorotrast: Incidence, histology and p53 status. Int J Cancer 63:330, 1995.

110. Stenton SC: Asbestos, Simian virus 40 and malignant mesothelioma. Thorax 52(Suppl. 3):S52, 1997.

111. Cicala C, Pompetti F, Carbone M: SV40 induces mesotheliomas in hamsters. Am J Pathol 142:1524, 1993.

112. Cristaudo A, Vivaldi A, Sensales G, et al: Molecular biology studies on mesothelioma tumor samples: Preliminary data on H-ras, p21, and SV40. J Environ Pathol Toxicol Oncol 14:29, 1995.

113. Carbone M, Pass HI, Rizzo P, et al: Simian virus 40-like DNA sequences in human pleural mesothelioma. Oncogene 9:1781, 1994.

114. De Luca A, Baldi A, Esposito V, et al: The retinoblastoma gene family pRb/p105, p107, pRb2/p130 and simian virus-40 large T-antigen in human mesotheliomas. Nat Med 3:913, 1997.

115. Carbone M, Rizzo P, Grimley PM, et al: Simian virus-40 large-T antigen binds p53 in human mesotheliomas. Nat Med 3:908, 1997.

116. Pepper C, Jasani B, Navabi H, et al: Simian virus 40 large T antigen (SV40LTAg) primer specific DNA amplification in human pleural mesothelioma tissue. Thorax 51:1074, 1996.

117. Strickler HD, Goedert JJ, Fleming M, et al: Simian virus 40 and pleural mesothelioma in humans. Cancer Epidemiol Biomarkers Prev 5:473, 1996.

118. Mor O, Yaron P, Huszar M, et al: Absence of p53 mutations in malignant mesotheliomas. Am J Respir Cell Mol Biol 16:9, 1997.

119. Behling CA, Wolf PL, Haghighi P: AIDS and malignant mesothelioma—is there a connection? Chest 103:1268, 1993.

120. Saebo A, Elgjo K, Lassen J: Could development of malignant mesothelioma be induced by *Yersinia enterocolitica* infection?. Med Hypotheses 40:275, 1993.

121. Conway EJ, Hudnall SD, Lazarides A, et al: Absence of evidence for an etiologic role for Epstein-Barr virus in neoplasms of the lung and pleura. Mod Pathol 9:491, 1996.

122. Hammar SP, Bockus D, Remington F, et al: Familial mesothelioma: A report of two families. Hum Pathol 20:107, 1989.

123. Risberg B, Nickels J, Wagermark J: Familial clustering of malignant mesothelioma. Cancer 45:2422, 1980.

124. Martensson G, Larsson S, Zettergren L: Malignant mesothelioma in two pairs of siblings: Is there a hereditary predisposing factor? Eur J Respir Dis 65:179, 1984.

125. Krousel T, Garcas N, Rothschild H: Familial clustering of mesothelioma: A report on three affected persons in one family. Am J Prev Med 2:186, 1986.

126. Dawson A, Gibbs A, Browne K, et al: Familial mesothelioma: Details of 17 cases with histopathologic findings and mineral analysis. Cancer 70:1183, 1992.

126a. Ascoli V, Scalzo CC, Bruno C, et al: Familial pleural malignant mesothelioma: Clustering in three sisters and one cousin. Cancer Lett 130:203, 1998.

127. Heineman EF, Bernstein L, Stark AD, et al: Mesothelioma, asbestos, and reported history of cancer in first-degree relatives. Cancer 77:549, 1996.

128. Huncharek M, Kelsey K, Muscat J, et al: Parental cancer and genetic predisposition in malignant pleural mesothelioma: A case-control study. Cancer Lett 102:205, 1996.

129. Willén R, Bruce T, Dahlström G, et al: Squamous epithelial cancer in metaplastic pleura following extrapleural pneumothorax for pulmonary tuberculosis. Virchows Arch (Pathol Anat Histol) 370:225, 1976.

130. Hillerdal G, Berg J: Malignant mesothelioma secondary to chronic inflammation and old scars: Two new cases and review of the literature. Cancer 55:1968, 1985.

131. Muscat JE, Huncharek M: Dietary intake and the risk of malignant mesothelioma. Br J Cancer 73:1122, 1996.

132. Hillerdal G: Malignant mesothelioma 1982: Review of 4,710 published cases. Br J Dis Chest 77:321, 1983.

133. Berry G, Newhouse ML, Antonis P: Combined effect of asbestos and smoking on mortality from lung cancer and mesothelioma in factory workers. Br J Ind Med 42:12, 1985.

134. Mossman BT: Carcinogenesis and related cell and tissue responses to asbestos: A review. Ann Occup Hyg 38:617, 1994.

135. Wagner JC: Mesothelioma and mineral fibers. Cancer 57:1905, 1986.

135a. Pache J-C, Janssen YMW, Walsh ES, et al: Increased epidermal growth factor-receptor protein in a human mesothelial cell line in response to long asbestos fibers. Am J Pathol 152:333, 1998.

136. Churg A: Deposition and clearance of chrysotile asbestos. Ann Occup Hyg 38:625, 1994.

137. Boutin C, Dumortier P, Rey F, et al: Black spots concentrate oncogenic asbestos fibers in the parietal pleura: Thoracoscopic and mineralogic study. Am J Respir Crit Care Med 153:444, 1996.

138. Boutin C, Rey F, Gouvernet J, et al: Thoracoscopy in pleural malignant mesothelioma: A prospective study of 188 consecutive patients: II. Prognosis and staging. Cancer 72:394, 1993.

139. Moalli PA, MacDonald JL, Goodglick LA, et al: Acute injury and regeneration of the mesothelium in response to asbestos fibers. Am J Pathol 128:426, 1987.

140. Friemann J, Müller KM, Pott F: Mesothelial proliferation due to asbestos and man-made fibres: Experimental studies on rat omentum. Path Res Pract 186:117, 1990.

141. Goodlick LA, Pietras LA, Kane AB: Evaluation of the causal relationship between crocidolyte asbestos-induced lipid peroxidation and toxicity to macrophages. Am Rev Respir Dis 139:1265, 1989.

142. Attanoos RL, Gibbs AR: Pathology of malignant mesothelioma. Histopathology 30:403, 1997.

143. Upham JW, Garlepp MJ, Musk AW, et al: Malignant mesothelioma: New insights into tumour biology and immunology as a basis for new treatment approaches. Thorax 50:887, 1995.

144. Bielefeldt-Ohmann H, Jarnicki AG, Fitzpatrick DR: Molecular pathobiology and immunology of malignant mesothelioma. J Pathol 178:369, 1996.

145. Langerak AW, De Laat PA, Van Der Linden-Van Beurden CA, et al: Expression of platelet-derived growth factor (PDGF) and PDGF receptors in human malignant mesothelioma *in vitro* and *in vivo*. J Pathol 178:151, 1996.

146. Xio S, Li D, Vijg J, et al: Codeletion of p15 and p16 in primary malignant mesothelioma. Oncogene 11:511, 1995.

147. Segers K, Ramael M, Singh SK, et al: Detection of numerical chromosomal

aberrations in paraffin-embedded malignant pleural mesothelioma by non-isotopic in situ hybridization. J Pathol 175:219, 1995.

148. Zeiger MA, Gnarra JR, Zbar B, et al: Loss of heterozygosity on the short arm of chromosome 3 in mesothelioma cell lines and solid tumors. Genes Chromosomes Cancer 11:15, 1994.

149. Bell DW, Jhanwar SC, Testa JR: Multiple regions of allelic loss from chromosome arm 6q in malignant mesothelioma. Cancer Res 57:4057, 1997.

150. Lee WC, Balsara B, Liu Z, et al: Loss of heterozygosity analysis defines a critical region in chromosome 1p22 commonly deleted in human malignant mesothelioma. Cancer Res 56:4297, 1996.

151. Lu YY, Jhanwar SC, Cheng JQ, et al: Deletion mapping of the short arm of chromosome 3 in human malignant mesothelioma. Genes Chromosomes Cancer 9:76, 1994.

152. Cheng JQ, Jhanwar SC, Klein WM, et al: p16 alterations and deletion mapping of 9p21-p22 in malignant mesothelioma. Cancer Res 54:5547, 1994.

153. Bianchi AB, Mitsunaga SI, Cheng JQ, et al: High frequency of inactivating mutations in the neurofibromatosis type 2 gene (NF2) in primary malignant mesotheliomas. Proc Natl Acad Sci U S A 92:10854, 1995.

154. Sekido Y, Pass HI, Bader S, et al: Neurofibromatosis type 2 (NF2) gene is somatically mutated in mesothelioma but not in lung cancer. Cancer Res 55:1227, 1995.

155. Austin MB, Fechner RE, Roggli VL: Pleural malignant mesothelioma following Wilms' tumour. Am J Clin Pathol 86:227, 1986.

156. Gotfried MH, Quan SF, Sobonya RE: Diffuse epithelial pleural mesothelioma presenting as a solitary lung mass. Chest 84:99, 1983.

157. Okike N, Bernatz PE, Woolner LB: Localized mesothelioma of the pleura: Benign and malignant variants. J Thorac Cardiovasc Surg 75:363, 1978.

158. Crotty TB, Myers JL, Katzenstein AL, et al: Localized malignant mesothelioma: A clinicopathologic and flow cytometric study. Am J Surg Pathol 18:357, 1994.

159. Whitaker D, Henderson DW, Shilkin KB: The concept of mesothelioma in situ: Implications for diagnosis and histogenesis. Semin Diagn Pathol 9:151, 1992.

160. Isobe H, Sridhar KS, Doria R, et al: Prognostic significance of DNA aneuploidy in diffuse malignant mesothelioma. Cytometry 19:86, 1995.

161. Whitaker D, Shilkin KB: Diagnosis of pleural malignant melothelioma in life—A practical approach. J Pathol 143:147, 1984.

162. Suzuki Y: Pathology of human malignant mesothelioma. Sem Oncol 8:268, 1980.

163. Wu H, Tino G, Gannon FH, et al: Lepidic intrapulmonary growth of malignant mesothelioma presenting as recurrent hydropneumothorax. Hum Pathol 27:989, 1996.

164. Johansson L, Linden CJ: Aspects of histopathologic subtype as a prognostic factor in 85 pleural mesotheliomas. Chest 109:109, 1996.

165. Martensson G, Hagmar B, Zettergren L: Diagnosis and prognosis in malignant pleural mesothelioma: A prospective study. Eur J Respir Dis 65:169, 1984.

166. Ordonez NG, Myhre M, Mackay B: Clear cell mesothelioma. Ultrastruct Pathol 20:331, 1996.

167. Mayall FG, Gibbs AR: The histology and immunohistochemistry of small cell mesothelioma. Histopathology 20:47, 1992.

168. Kwee WS, Veldhuizen RW, Golding RP, et al: Primary "adenosquamous" mesothelioma of the pleura. Virchows Arch (Pathol Anat) 393:353, 1981.

169. Wilson GE, Hasleton PS, Chatterjee AK: Desmoplastic malignant mesothelioma: A review of 17 cases. J Clin Pathol 45:295, 1992.

170. Cantin R, Al-Jabi M, McCaughey WTE: Desmoplastic diffuse mesothelioma. Am J Surg Pathol 6:215, 1982.

171. Crotty TB, Colby TV, Gay PC, et al: Desmoplastic malignant mesothelioma masquerading as sclerosing mediastinitis: A diagnostic dilemma. Hum Pathol 23:79, 1992.

172. Donna A, Betta PG: Differentiation towards cartilage and bone in a primary tumour of pleura. Further evidence in support of the concept of mesodermoma. Histopathology 10:101, 1986.

173. Yousem SA, Hochholzer L: Malignant mesotheliomas with osseous and cartilaginous differentiation. Arch Pathol Lab Med 111:62, 1987.

174. Andrion A, Mazzucco G, Bernardi P, et al: Sarcomatous tumor of the chest wall with osteochondroid differentiation. Evidence of mesothelial origin. Am J Surg Pathol 13(8):707, 1989.

175. Krishna J, Haqqani MT: Liposarcomatous differentiation in diffuse pleural mesothelioma. Thorax 48:409, 1993.

176. Henderson DW, Attwood HD, Constance TJ, et al: Lymphohistiocytoid mesothelioma: A rare lymphomatoid variant of predominantly sarcomatoid mesothelioma. Ultrastruct Pathol 12:367, 1988.

177. McCaughey WTE, Colby TV, Battifora H, et al: Diagnosis of diffuse malignant mesothelioma: Experience of a US/Canadian mesothelioma panel. Mod Pathol 4:342, 1991.

178. Lin BT, Colby T, Gown AM, et al: Malignant vascular tumors of the serous membranes mimicking mesothelioma: A report of 14 cases. Am J Surg Pathol 20:1431, 1996.

179. Andrion A, Magnani C, Betta PG, et al: Malignant mesothelioma of the pleura: Interobserver variability. J Clin Pathol 48:856, 1995.

180. Skov BG, Lauritzen AF, Hirsch F, et al: The histopathological diagnosis of malignant mesothelioma v. pulmonary adenocarcinoma: Reproducibility of the histopathological diagnosis. Histopathology 24:553, 1994.

181. Sheldon CD, Herbert A, Gallagher PJ: Reactive mesothelial proliferation: A necropsy study. Thorax 36:901, 1981.

182. Hansen RM, Caya JG, Clowry LJ Jr, et al: Benign mesothelial proliferation with effusion. Clinicopathologic entity that may mimic malignancy. Am J Med 77:887, 1984.

183. McCaughey WTE, Al-Jabi M: Differentiation of serosal hyperplasia and neoplasia in biopsies. Path Annual 1:271, 1986.

184. Chan JKC, Loo KT, Yau BKC, et al: Nodular histiocytic/mesothelial hyperplasia: A lesion potentially mistaken for a neoplasm in transbronchial biopsy. Am J Surg Pathol 21:658, 1997.

185. Herbert A, Gallagher PJ: Pleural biopsy in the diagnosis of malignant mesothelioma. Thorax 37:816, 1982.

186. Tuder RM: Malignant disease of the pleura: A histopathological study with special emphasis on diagnostic criteria and differentiation from reactive mesothelium. Histopathology 10:851, 1986.

187. Donna A, Betta PG, Robutti P: Use of antimesothelial cell antibody and computer assisted quantitative analysis for distinguishing between reactive and neoplastic serosal tissues. J Clin Pathol 40:1428, 1987.

188. Segers K, Ramael M, Singh SK, et al: Immunoreactivity for bcl-2 protein in malignant mesothelioma and non-neoplastic mesothelium. Virchows Arch 424:631, 1994.

189. Cagle PT, Brown RW, Lebovitz RM: p53 immunostaining in the differentiation of reactive processes from malignancy in pleural biopsy specimens. Hum Pathol 25:443, 1994.

190. Ramael M, van den Bossche J, Buysse C, et al: Immunoreactivity for P-170 glycoprotein in malignant mesothelioma and in non-neoplastic mesothelium of the pleura using the murine monoclonal antibody JSB-1. J Pathol 167:5, 1992.

191. Ramael M, Buysse C, van den Bossche J, et al: Immunoreactivity for the beta chain of the platelet-derived growth factor receptor in malignant mesothelioma and non-neoplastic mesothelium. J Pathol 167:1, 1992.

192. Mayall FG, Goddard H, Gibbs AR: p53 immunostaining in the distinction between benign and malignant mesothelial proliferations using formalin-fixed paraffin sections. J Pathol 168:377, 1992.

193. Ramael M, Lemmens G, Eerdekens C, et al: Immunoreactivity for p53 protein in malignant mesothelioma and non-neoplastic mesothelium. J Pathol 168:371, 1992.

194. Kafiri G, Thomas DM, Shepherd NA, et al: p53 expression is common in malignant mesothelioma. Histopathology 21:331, 1992.

195. Esposito V, Baldi A, De Luca A, et al: p53 immunostaining in differential diagnosis of pleural mesothelial proliferations. Anticancer Res 17:733, 1997.

196. Mayall F, Heryet A, Manga D, et al: p53 immunostaining is a highly specific and moderately sensitive marker of malignancy in serous fluid cytology. Cytopathology 8:9, 1997.

197. Krivinkova H, Pontén J, Blöndai T: The diagnosis of cancer from body fluids: A comparison of DNA measurement, tissue culture, scanning and transmission microscopy. Acta Pathol Microbiol Scand A 84:455, 1976.

198. Frierson HF, Mills SE, Legier JF: Flow cytometric analysis of ploidy in immunohistochemically confirmed examples of malignant epithelial mesothelioma. Am J Clin Pathol 90:240, 1988.

199. Dejmek A, Stromberg C, Wikstrom B, et al: Prognostic importance of the DNA ploidy pattern in malignant mesothelioma of the pleura. Anal Quant Cytol Histol 14:217, 1992.

200. Burmer GC, Rabinovitch PS, Kulander BG, et al: Flow cytometric analysis of malignant pleural mesotheliomas. Hum Pathol 20:777, 1989.

201. El-Naggar AK, Ordonez NG, Garnsey L, et al: Epithelioid pleural mesotheliomas and pulmonary adenocarcinomas: A comparative DNA flow cytometric study. Hum Pathol 22:972, 1991.

202. Isoda K, Hamamoto Y: Polyploid mesothelial cells in pleural fluid. Acta Pathol Jpn 33(4):733, 1983.

203. Ayres JG, Crocker JG, Skilbeck NQ: Differentiation of malignant from normal and reactive mesothelial cells by the argyrophil technique for nucleolar organiser region associated proteins. Thorax 43:366, 1988.

204. Bethwaite PB, Delahunt B, Holloway LJ, et al: Comparison of silver-staining nucleolar organizer region (AgNOR) counts and proliferating cell nuclear antigen (PCNA) expression in reactive mesothelial hyperplasia and malignant mesothelioma. Pathology 27:1, 1995.

205. Colecchia M, Leopardi O: Evaluation of AgNOR count in distinguishing benign from malignant mesothelial cells in pleural fluids. Pathol Res Pract 188:541, 1992.

206. Ribotta M, Donna A, Betta PG, et al: Quantitative analysis of nucleoli and nucleolar organizer regions in cultured primary human normal, reactive and malignant mesothelial cells. Pathol Res Pract 188:536, 1992.

206a. Wolanski KD, Whitaker D, Shilkin KB, et al: The use of epithelial membrane antigen and silver-stained nucleolar organizer regions testing in the differential diagnosis of mesothelioma from benign reactive mesotheliosis. Cancer 82:583, 1998.

207. Ramael M, Jacobs W, Weyler J, et al: Proliferation in malignant mesothelioma as determined by mitosis counts and immunoreactivity for proliferating cell nuclear antigen (PCNA). J Pathol 172:247, 1994.

208. Esposito V, Baldi A, De Luca A, et al: Role of PCNA in differentiating between malignant mesothelioma and mesothelial hyperplasia: Prognostic considerations. Anticancer Res 17:601, 1997.

209. Kwee WS, Veldhuizen RW, Golding RP, et al: Histologic distinction between malignant mesothelioma, benign pleural lesion and carcinoma metastasis. Virchows Arch (Pathol Anat) 397:287, 1982.

210. Kwee WS, Veldhuizen RW, Alons CA, et al: Quantitative and qualitative differences between benign and malignant mesothelial cells in pleural fluid. Acta Cytol 26:401, 1982.

211. Gavin FM, Gray C, Sutton J, et al: Morphometric differences between cytologically benign and malignant serous effusions. Acta Cytol 32:175, 1988.

212. Bogers J, Jacobs W, Segers K, et al: Stereological evaluation of malignant mesothelioma versus benign pleural hyperplasia. Pathol Res Pract 192:10, 1996.

213. Koss M, Travis W, Moran C, et al: Pseudomesotheliomatous adenocarcinoma: A reappraisal. Semin Diagn Pathol 9:117, 1992.

214. Harwood TR, Gracey DR, Yokoo H: Pseudomesotheliomatous carcinoma of the lung: A variant of peripheral lung cancer. Am J Clin Pathol 65:159, 1976.

215. Falconieri G, Zanconati F, Bussani R, et al: Small cell carcinoma of lung simulating pleural mesothelioma: Report of 4 cases with autopsy confirmation. Pathol Res Pract 191:1147, 1995.

216. Yokoi T, Mark EJ: Atypical mesothelial hyperplasia associated with bronchogenic carcinoma. Hum Pathol 22:695, 1991.

217. Griffiths MH, Riddell RJ, Xipell JM: Malignant mesothelioma: A review of 35 cases with diagnosis and prognosis. Pathology 12:591, 1980.

218. Warnock ML, Stoloff A, Thor A: Differentiation of adenocarcinoma of the lung from mesothelioma: Periodic acid-Schiff, monoclonal antibodies B72.3, and Leu-M1. Am J Pathol 133:30, 1988.

219. Dewar A, Valente M, Ring NP, et al: Pleural mesothelioma of epithelial type and pulmonary adenocarcinoma: An ultrastructural and cytochemical comparison. J Pathol 152:309, 1987.

220. MacDougall DB, Wang SE, Zidar BL: Mucin-positive epithelial mesothelioma. Arch Pathol Lab Med 116:874, 1992.

221. Hammar SP, Bockus DE, Remington FL, et al: Mucin-positive epithelial mesotheliomas: A histochemical, immunohistochemical, and ultrastructural comparison with mucin-producing pulmonary adenocarcinomas. Ultrastruct Pathol 20:293, 1996.

222. Kwee WS, Veldhuizen RW, Golding RP, et al: Histologic distinction between malignant mesothelioma, benign pleural lesion and carcinoma metastasis. Virchows Arch (Pathol Anat) 397:287, 1982.

223. Cibas ES, Corson JM, Pinkus GS: The distinction of adenocarcinoma from malignant mesothelioma in cell blocks of effusions: The role of routine mucin histochemistry and immunohistochemical assessment of carcinoembryonic antigen, keratin proteins, epithelial membrane antigen, and milk fat globule-derived antigen. Hum Pathol 18:67, 1987.

224. Strickler JG, Herndier BG, Rouse RV: Immunohistochemical staining in malignant mesotheliomas. Am J Clin Pathol 88:610, 1987.

225. Arai H, Kang K-Y, Sato H, et al: Significance of the quantification and demonstration of hyaluronic acid in tissue specimens for the diagnosis of pleural mesothelioma. Am Rev Respir Dis 120:529, 1979.

226. Azumi N, Underhill CB, Kagan E, et al: A novel biotinylated probe specific for hyaluronate: Its diagnostic value in diffuse malignant mesothelioma. Am J Surg Pathol 16:116, 1992.

227. Leong AS, Vernon-Roberts E: The immunohistochemistry of malignant mesothelioma. *In* Rosen PP, Fechner RE (eds): Pathology Annual Part 2. Vol 29. Norwalk, CT, Appleton & Lange, 1994, pp 157–179.

228. Sheibani K, Esteban J, Bailey A, et al: Immunopathologic and molecular studies as an aid to the diagnosis of malignant mesothelioma. Hum Pathol 23:107, 1992.

229. Zeng L, Fleury-Feith J, Monnet I, et al: Immunocytochemical characterization of cell lines from human malignant mesothelioma: Characterization of human mesothelioma cell lines by immunocytochemistry with a panel of monoclonal antibodies. Hum Pathol 25:227, 1994.

230. Grove A, Paulsen SM, Gregersen M: The value of immunohistochemistry of pleural biopsy specimens in the differential diagnosis between malignant mesothelioma and metastatic carcinoma. Pathol Res Pract 190:1044, 1994.

231. Brown RW, Clark GM, Tandon AK, et al: Multiple-marker immunohistochemical phenotypes distinguishing malignant pleural mesothelioma from pulmonary adenocarcinoma. Hum Pathol 24:347, 1993.

232. Moch H, Oberholzer M, Dalquen P, et al: Diagnostic tools for differentiating between pleural mesothelioma and lung adenocarcinoma in paraffin embedded tissue: I. Immunohistochemical findings. Virchows Arch (Pathol Anat Histopathol) 423:19, 1993.

233. Wick MR, Loy T, Mills, SE, et al: Malignant epithelioid pleural mesothelioma versus peripheral pulmonary adenocarcinoma: A histochemical, ultrastructural, and immunohistologic study of 103 cases. Hum Pathol 21:759, 1990.

234. Delahaye M, van der Ham F, van der Kwast TH: Complementary value of five carcinoma markers for the diagnosis of malignant mesothelioma, adenocarcinoma metastasis, and reactive mesothelium in serous effusions. Diagn Cytopathol 17:115, 1997.

235. Sheibani K: Increasing role of immunopathology in diagnosis of malignant mesothelioma. Hum Pathol 28:639, 1997.

236. Pfaltz M, Odermatt B, Christen B, et al: Immunohistochemistry in the diagnosis of malignant mesothelioma. Virchows Arch A 411:387, 1987.

237. Corson JM, Pinkus GS: Mesothelioma: Profile of keratin proteins and carcinoembryonic antigen: An immunoperoxidase study of 20 cases and comparison with pulmonary adenocarcinomas. Am J Pathol 108:80, 1982.

238. Holden J, Churg A: Immunohistochemical staining for keratin and carcinoembryonic antigen in the diagnosis of malignant mesothelioma. Am J Surg Pathol 8:277, 1984.

239. Ruitenbeek T, Gouw AS, Poppema S: Immunocytology of body cavity fluids. MOC-31, a monoclonal antibody discriminating between mesothelial and epithelial cells. Arch Pathol Lab Med 118:265, 1994.

240. Dejmek A, Hjerpe A: Carcinoembryonic antigen-like reactivity in malignant mesothelioma: A comparison between different commercially available antibodies. Cancer 73:464, 1994.

241. Otis CN, Carter D, Cole S, et al: Immunohistochemical evaluation of pleural mesothelioma and pulmonary adenocarcinoma: A bi-institutional study of 47 cases. Am J Surg Pathol 11(6):445, 1987.

242. Duggan MA, Masters CB, Alexander F: Immunohistochemical differentiation of malignant mesothelioma, mesothelial hyperplasia and metastatic adenocarcinoma in serous effusions, utilizing staining for carcinoembryonic antigen, keratin and vimentin. Acta Cytol 31:807, 1987.

243. Clover J, Oates J, Edwards C: Anti-cytokeratin 5/6: a positive marker for epithelioid mesothelioma. Histopathology 31:140, 1997.

244. Blobel GA, Moll R, Franke WW, et al: The intermediate filament cytoskeleton of malignant mesotheliomas and its diagnostic significance. Am J Pathol 121:235, 1985.

245. Epstein JI, Budin RE: Keratin and epithelial membrane antigen immunoreactivity in non-neoplastic fibrous pleural lesions: Implications for the diagnosis of desmoplastic mesothelioma. Hum Pathol 17:514, 1986.

246. Mayall FG, Goddard H, Gibbs AR: Intermediate filament expression in mesotheliomas: Leiomyoid mesotheliomas are not uncommon. Histopathology 21:453, 1992.

247. Hurlimann J: Desmin and neural marker expression in mesothelial cells and mesotheliomas. Hum Pathol 25:753, 1994.

248. Ordóñez NG: The immunohistochemical diagnosis of mesothelioma: Differentiation of mesothelioma and lung adenocarcinoma. Am J Surg Pathol 13(4):276, 1989.

249. Sheibani K, Battifora H, Burke JS: Antigenic phenotype of malignant mesotheliomas and pulmonary adenocarcinomas: An immunohistologic analysis demonstrating the value of Leu-M1 antigen. Am J Pathol 123:212, 1986.

250. Ghosil AK, Butler PB: Immunocytological staining reactions of anti-carcinoembryonic antigen, Ca, and anti-human milk fat globule monoclonal antibodies on benign and malignant exfoliated mesothelial cells. J Clin Pathol 40:1424, 1987.

251. Rasmussen O, Larsen KE: S-100 protein in malignant mesotheliomas. Acta Path Microbiol Immunol Scand (A) 93:199, 1985.

252. Noguchii M, Nakajima T, Hirohashi S, et al: Immunohistochemical distinction of malignant mesothelioma from pulmonary adenocarcinoma with anti-surfactant apoprotein, anti-Lewis^a, and anti-Tn antibodies. Hum Pathol 20:53, 1989.

253. Jordon D, Jagirdar J, Kaneko M: Blood group antigens, Lewis^x and Lewis^y in the diagnostic discrimination of malignant mesothelioma versus adenocarcinoma. Am J Pathol 135:931, 1989.

254. van der Kwast TH, Versnel MA, Delahaye M, et al: Expression of epithelial membrane antigen on malignant mesothelioma cells: An immunocytochemical and immunoelectron microscopic study. Acta Cytol 32:169, 1988.

255. Guzman J, Bross KJ, Würtemberger G, et al: Immunocytology in malignant pleural mesothelioma: Expression of tumor markers and distribution of lymphocyte subsets. Chest 95:590, 1989.

256. Battifora H, Kopinski MI: Distinction of mesothelioma from adenocarcinoma: An immunohistochemical approach. Cancer 55:1679, 1985.

257. Coleman M, Henderson DW, Mukherjee TM: The ultrastructural pathology of malignant pleural mesothelioma. Pathol Ann 24:303, 1989.

258. Dardick I, Al-Jabi M, McCaughey WTE: Ultrastructure of poorly differentiated diffuse epithelial mesotheliomas. Ultrastruct Pathol 7:151, 1984.

259. Warhol MJ, Corson JM: An ultrastructural comparison of mesotheliomas with adenocarcinomas of the lung and breast. Hum Pathol 16:50, 1985.

260. Jandik WR, Landas SK, Bray CK, et al: Scanning electron microscopic distinction of pleural mesotheliomas from adenocarcinomas. Mod Pathol 6:761, 1993.

261. Waxler B, Eisenstein R, Battifora H: Electrophoresis of tissue glycosaminoglycans as an aid in the diagnosis of mesotheliomas. Cancer 44:221, 1979.

262. Nakano T, Fujii J, Tamura S, et al: Glycosaminoglycan in malignant pleural mesothelioma. Cancer 57:106, 1986.

263. Kawai T, Suzuki M, Shinmei M, et al: Glycosaminoglycans in malignant diffuse mesothelioma. Cancer 56:567, 1985.

264. Iozzo RV, Goldes JA, Chen W-J, et al: Glycosaminoglycans of pleural mesothelioma: A possible biochemical variant containing chondroitin sulfate. Cancer 48:89, 1981.

265. Kawai T, Greenberg SD, Truong LD, et al: Differences in lectin binding of malignant pleural mesothelioma and adenocarcinoma of the lung. Am J Pathol 130:401, 1988.

266. Alexander E, Clark RA, Colley DP, et al: CT of malignant pleural mesothelioma. Am J Roentgenol 137:287, 1981.

267. Müller NL. Imaging of the pleura. Radiology 186:297, 1993.

268. Miller BH, Rosado-de-Christenson ML, Mason AC, et al: Malignant pleural mesothelioma: Radiologic-pathologic correlation. RadioGraphics 16:613, 1996.

269. Wechsler RJ, Rao VM, Steiner RM: The radiology of thoracic malignant mesothelioma. Crit Rev Diagn Imaging 20:283, 1983.

270. Huncharek M: Miliary mesothelioma. Chest 106:605, 1994.

271. Solomons K, Polakow R, Marchand P: Diffuse malignant mesothelioma presenting as bilateral malignant lymphangitis. Thorax 40:682, 1985.

272. Ohishi N, Oka T, Fukuhara T, et al: Extensive pulmonary metastases in malignant pleural mesothelioma: A rare clinical and radiographic presentation. Chest 110:296, 1996.

273. Rabinowitz JG, Efremidis SG, Cohen B, et al: A comparative study of mesothelioma and asbestosis using computed tomography and conventional chest radiography. Radiology 144:453, 1982.

274. Rusch VW, Godwin JD, Shuman WP: The role of computed tomography scanning in the initial assessment and the follow-up of malignant pleural mesothelioma. J Thorac Cardiovasc Surg 96:171, 1988.

275. Kawashima A, Libshitz HI: Malignant pleural mesothelioma: CT manifestations in 50 cases. AJR 155:965, 1990.

276. Raizon A, Schwartz A, Hix W, et al: Calcification as a sign of sarcomatous degeneration of malignant pleural mesotheliomas: A new CT finding. J Comput Assist Tomogr 20:42, 1996.

277. Leung AN, Müller NL, Miller RR: CT in differential diagnosis of diffuse pleural disease. AJR 154:487, 1990.

278. Patz EF Jr, Shaffer K, Piwnica-Worms, DR, et al: Malignant pleural mesothelioma: Value of CT and MR imaging in predicting resectability. AJR 159:961, 1992.

279. Patz EF Jr, Rusch VW, Heelan R: The proposed new international TNM staging system for malignant pleural mesothelioma: Application to imaging. AJR 166:323, 1996.

280. Falaschi F, Battolla L, Mascalchi M, et al: Usefulness of MR signal intensity in distinguishing benign from malignant pleural disease. AJR 166:963, 1996.

281. Lorigan JG, Libshitz HI: MR imaging of malignant pleural mesothelioma. J Comput Assist Tomogr 13:617, 1989.

281a. Bénard F, Sterman D, Smith RJ, et al: Metabolic imaging of malignant pleural mesothelioma with fluorodeoxyglucose positron emission tomography. Chest 114:713, 1998.

282. Harrison RN, Hibberd SC, Dadds JH: Malignant pleural mesothelioma at St. Mary's Hospital. Postgrad Med J 59:712, 1983.

283. Pillgram-Larsen J, Urdal L, Smith-Meyer R, et al: Malignant pleural mesothelioma: A clinical review of 19 patients. Scand J Thorac Cardiovasc Surg 18:69, 1984.

284. Tammilehto L, Maasilta P, Kostiainen S, et al: Diagnosis and prognostic factors in malignant pleural mesothelioma: A retrospective analysis of sixty-five patients. Respiration 59:129, 1992.

285. Brenner J, Sordillo PP, Magill GB, et al: Malignant mesothelioma of the pleura: Review of 123 patients. Cancer 49:2431, 1982.

286. Krumhaar D, Lange S, Hartmann C, et al: Follow-up study of 100 malignant pleural mesotheliomas. J Thorac Cardiovasc Surg 33:272, 1985.

287. Grellner W, Staak M: Multiple skeletal muscle metastases from malignant pleural mesothelioma. Pathol Res Pract 191:456, 1995.

288. Kim SB, Varkey B, Choi H: Diagnosis of malignant pleural mesothelioma by axillary lymph node biopsy. Chest 91:279, 1987.

289. Kaye JA, Wang AM, Joachim CL, et al: Malignant mesothelioma with brain metastases. Am J Med 80:95, 1986.

290. Law MR, Hodson ME, Heard BE: Malignant mesothelioma of the pleura: Relation between histological type and clinical behaviour. Thorax 37:810, 1982.

291. Harrison RN: Sarcomatous pleural mesothelioma and cerebral metastases: Case report and a review of eight cases. Eur J Respir Dis 65:185, 1984.

292. Machin T, Mashiyama ET, Henderson JAM, et al: Bony metastases in desmoplastic pleural mesothelioma. Thorax 43:155, 1988.

293. Wills EJ: Pleural mesothelioma with initial presentation as cervical lymphadenopathy. Ultrastruct Pathol 19:389, 1995.

294. Lloreta J, Serrano S: Pleural mesothelioma presenting as an axillary lymph node metastasis with anemone cell appearance. Ultrastruct Pathol 18:293, 1994.

295. Masangkay AV, Susin M, Baker R, et al: Metastatic malignant mesothelioma presenting as colonic polyps. Hum Pathol 28:993, 1997.

296. Kubota K, Furuse K, Kawahara M, et al: A case of malignant pleural mesothelioma with metastasis to the orbit. Jpn J Clin Oncol 26:469, 1996.

297. Prieto VG, Kenet B, Varghese M: Malignant mesothelioma metastatic to the skin, presenting as inflammatory carcinoma. Am J Dermatopathol 19:261, 1997.

298. Davies MJ, Ahmedzai S, Arsiwala SS, et al: Intracranial metastases from malignant pleural mesothelioma. Scand J Thorac Cardiovasc Surg 29:97, 1995.

299. Wronski M, Burt M: Cerebral metastases in pleural mesothelioma: Case report and review of the literature. J Neurooncol 17:21, 1993.

300. Ragalie GF, Varkey B, Chai H: Malignant pleural mesothelioma presenting as superior vena cava syndrome. Can Med Assoc J 128:689, 1983.

301. Siafakas NM, Tsirogiannis K, Filaditaki B, et al: Pleural mesothelioma and the syndrome of inappropriate secretion of antidiuretic hormone. Thorax 39:872, 1984.

302. Seki H, Matsumoto K, Ohmura K, et al: Malignant pleural mesothelioma presenting as achalasia. Intern Med 33:624, 1994.

303. Motoyama T, Honma T, Watanabe M, et al: Interleukin 6-producing malignant mesothelioma. Virchows Arch (Cell Pathol Incl Mol Pathol) 64:367, 1993.

304. Okamoto H, Matsuno Y, Noguchi M, et al: Malignant pleural mesothelioma producing human chorionic gonadotropin: Report of two cases. Am J Surg Pathol 16:969, 1992.

305. Rikimaru T, Ichikawa Y, Ogawa Y, et al: Production of granulocyte colony-stimulating factor by malignant mesothelioma. Eur Respir J 8:183, 1995.

306. Schmitter D, Lauber B, Fagg B, et al: Hematopoietic growth factors secreted by seven human pleural mesothelioma cell lines: Interleukin-6 production as a common feature. Int J Cancer 51:296, 1992.

307. Higashihara M, Sunaga S, Tange T, et al: Increased secretion of interleukin-6 in malignant mesothelioma cells from a patient with marked thrombocytosis. Cancer 70:2105, 1992.

308. Wadler S, Chahinian P, Slater W, et al: Cardiac abnormalities in patients with diffuse malignant pleural mesothelioma. Cancer 58:2744, 1986.

309. Walters LL, Taxy JB: Malignant mesothelioma of the pleura with extensive cardiac invasion and tricuspid orifice occlusion. Cancer 52:1736, 1983.

310. Roggli VL: Malignant mesothelioma and duration of asbestos exposure: Correlation with tissue mineral fibre content. Ann Occup Hyg 39:363, 1995.

311. Lanphear BP, Buncher CR: Latent period for malignant mesothelioma of occupational origin. J Occup Med 34:718, 1992.

312. Bianchi C, Giarelli L, Grandi G, et al: Latency periods in asbestos-related mesothelioma of the pleura. Eur J Cancer Prev 6:162, 1997.

313. Cagle PT, Wessels R, Greenberg SD: Concurrent mesothelioma and adenocarcinoma of the lung in a patient with asbestosis. Mod Pathol 6:438, 1993.

314. Tondini M, Rocco G, Travaglini M, et al: Pleural mesothelioma associated with non-Hodgkin's lymphoma. Thorax 49:1269, 1994.

315. Triol JH, Conston AS, Chandler SV: Malignant mesothelioma: Cytopathology of 75 cases seen in a New Jersey community hospital. Acta Cytol 28:37, 1984.

316. Tao L-C: The cytopathology of mesothelioma. Acta Cytol 23:209, 1979.

317. Leong AS, Stevens MW, Mukherjee TM: Malignant mesothelioma: Cytologic diagnosis with histologic, immunohistochemical, and ultrastructural correlation. Semin Diagn Pathol 9:141, 1992.

318. DiBonito L, Falconieri G, Colautti I, et al: Cytopathology of malignant mesothelioma: A study of its patterns and histological bases. Diagn Cytopathol 9:25, 1993.

319. Stevens MW, Leong AS, Fazzalari NL, et al: Cytopathology of malignant mesothelioma: A stepwise logistic regression analysis. Diagn Cytopathol 8:333, 1992.

320. Canto A, Guijarro R, Arnau A, et al: Videothoracoscopy in the diagnosis and treatment of malignant pleural mesothelioma with associated pleural effusions. Thorac Cardiovasc Surg 45:16, 1997.

320a. Renshaw AA, Dean BR, Antman KH, et al: The role of cytologic evaluation of pleural fluid in the diagnosis of malignant mesothelioma. Chest 111:106, 1997.

321. Law MR, Hodson ME, Turner-Warwick M: Malignant mesothelioma of the pleura: Clinical aspects and symptomatic treatment. Eur J Respir Dis 65:162, 1984.

322. Martensson G, Hagmar B, Zettergren L: Diagnosis and prognosis in malignant pleural mesothelioma: A prospective study. Eur J Respir Dis 65:169, 1984.

323. Boutin C, Rey F: Thoracoscopy in pleural malignant mesothelioma: A prospective study of 188 consecutive patients. I. Diagnosis. Cancer 72:389, 1993.

324. Tao L-C: Aspiration biopsy cytology of mesothelioma. Diagn Cytopathol 5:14, 1989.

325. Whitaker D, Sterrett G, Shilkin K, et al: Malignant mesothelioma cells in sputum. Diagn Cytopathol 2:21, 1986.

326. Renshaw AA, Nappi D, Swanson S, et al: Effusion cytology after extrapleural pneumonectomy for treatment of malignant mesothelioma. Am J Clin Pathol 107:206, 1997.

327. Whitaker D, Shilkin KB, Stuckey M, et al: Pleural fluid CEA levels in the diagnosis of malignant mesothelioma. Pathology 18:328, 1986.

328. Faravelli B, D'Amore E, Nosenzo M, et al: Carcinoembryonic antigen in pleural effusions. Cancer 53:1194, 1984

329. Shijubo N, Honda Y, Fujishima T, et al: Lung surfactant protein-A and carcinoembryonic antigen in pleural effusions due to lung adenocarcinoma and malignant mesothelioma. Eur Respir J 8:403, 1995.

330. Villena V, Lopez-Encuentra A, Echave-Sustaeta J, et al: Diagnostic value of CA 72-4, carcinoembryonic antigen, CA 15-3, and CA 19-9 assay in pleural fluid: A study of 207 patients. Cancer 78:736, 1996.

331. Thylen A, Levin-Jacobsen AM, Hjerpe A, et al: Immunohistochemical differences between hyaluronan- and non-hyaluronan-producing malignant mesothelioma. Eur Respir J 10:404, 1997.

332. Nurminen M, Dejmek A, Martensson G, et al: Clinical utility of liquid-chromatographic analysis of effusions for hyaluronate content. Clin Chem 40:777, 1994.

333. Martinez-Vea A, Gatell JM, Segura F, et al: Diagnostic value of tumoral markers in serous effusions: Carcinoembryonic antigen, alpha₁-acid-glycoprotein, alpha-fetoprotein, phosphohexose isomerase, and beta₂-microglobulin. Cancer 50:1783, 1982.

334. Maeda J, Ueki N, Ohkawa T, et al: Transforming growth factor-beta 1 (TGF-beta 1)- and beta 2-like activities in malignant pleural effusions caused by malignant mesothelioma or primary lung cancer. Clin Exp Immunol 98:319, 1994.

335. Ascoli V, Facciolo F, Rahimi S, et al: Concomitant malignant mesothelioma of the pleura, peritoneum, and tunica vaginalis testis. Diagn Cytopathol 14:243, 1996.

336. Ohishi N, Oka T, Fukuhara T, et al: Extensive pulmonary metastases in malignant pleural mesothelioma: A rare clinical and radiographic presentation. Chest 110:296, 1996.

337. Huncharek M: Miliary mesothelioma. Chest 106:605, 1994.

338. Rusch VW, Venkatraman E: The importance of surgical staging in the treatment of malignant pleural mesothelioma. J Thorac Cardiovasc Surg 111:815, 1996.

338a. Argani P, Rosai J: Hyperplastic mesothelial cells in lymph nodes: Report of six cases of a benign process that can simulate metastatic involvement by mesothelioma or carcinoma. Hum Pathol 29:339, 1998.

339. Chailleux E, Dabouis G, Pioche D, et al: Prognostic factors in diffuse malignant pleural mesothelioma: A study of 167 patients. Chest 93:159, 1988.

340. De Pangher Manzini V, Brollo A, Franceschi S, et al: Prognostic factors of malignant mesothelioma of the pleura. Cancer 72:410, 1993.

341. Huncharek M, Kelsey K, Mark EJ, et al: Treatment and survival in diffuse malignant pleural mesothelioma: A study of 83 cases from the Massachusetts General Hospital. Anticancer Res 16:1265, 1996.

342. Fusco V, Ardizzoni A, Merlo F, et al: Malignant pleural mesothelioma: Multivariate analysis of prognostic factors on 113 patients. Anticancer Res 13:683, 1993.

342a. Herndon JE II, Green MR, Chahinian AP, et al: Factors predictive of survival among 337 patients with mesothelioma treated between 1984 and 1994 by the cancer and leukemia group B. Chest 113:723, 1998.

343. Sugarbaker DJ, Garcia JP, Richards WG, et al: Extrapleural pneumonectomy in the multimodality therapy of malignant pleural mesothelioma: Results in 120 consecutive patients. Ann Surg 224:288, 1996.

344. Van Gelder T, Damhuis RA, Hoogsteden HC: Prognostic factors and survival in malignant pleural mesothelioma. Eur Respir J 7:1035, 1994.

345. Tammilehto L, Kivisaari L, Salminen US, et al: Evaluation of the clinical TNM staging system for malignant pleural mesothelioma: An assessment in 88 patients. Lung Cancer 12:25, 1995.

346. Rusch VW: A proposed new international TNM staging system for malignant pleural mesothelioma. From the International Mesothelioma Interest Group. Chest 108:1122, 1995.

347. Rusch VW, Venkatraman E: The importance of surgical staging in the treatment of malignant pleural mesothelioma. J Thorac Cardiovasc Surg 111:815, 1996.

348. Rice TW, Adelstein DJ, Kirby TJ, et al: Aggressive multimodality therapy for malignant pleural mesothelioma. Ann Thorac Surg 58:24, 1994.

349. Mark EJ, Shin DH: Diffuse malignant mesothelioma of the pleura: A clinicopathological study of six patients with a prolonged symptom-free interval or extended survival after biopsy and a review of the literature of long-term survival. Virchows Arch (Pathol Anat Histopathol) 422:445, 1993.

350. Pass HI, Kranda K, Temeck BK, et al: Surgically debulked malignant pleural mesothelioma: Results and prognostic factors. Ann Surg Oncol 4:215, 1997.

350a. Beer TW, Buchanan R, Matthews AW, et al: Prognosis in malignant mesothelioma related to MIB 1 proliferation index and histological subtype. Hum Pathol 29:246, 1998.

351. Kumar-Singh S, Vermeulen PB, Weyler J, et al: Evaluation of tumour angiogenesis as a prognostic marker in malignant mesothelioma. J Pathol 182:211, 1997.

352. Ong ST, Vogelzang NJ: Chemotherapy in malignant pleural mesothelioma: A review. J Clin Oncol 14:1007, 1996.

353. Sugarbaker DJ, Mentzer SJ, Strauss G: Extrapleural pneumonectomy in the treatment of malignant pleural mesothelioma. Ann Thorac Surg 54:941, 1992.

354. Sugarbaker DJ, Strauss GM, Lynch TJ, et al: Node status has prognostic significance in the multimodality therapy of diffuse, malignant mesothelioma. J Clin Oncol 11:1172, 1993.

355. Briselli M, Mark EJ, Dickerson GR: Solitary fibrous tumors of the pleura: Eight new cases and review of 360 cases in the literature. Cancer 47:2678, 1981.

356. England DM, Hochholzer L, McCarthy MJ: Localized benign and malignant fibrous tumors of the pleura. A clinicopathologic review of 223 cases. Am J Surg Pathol 13(8):640, 1989.

357. Bilbey JH, Müller NL, Miller RR, et al: Localized fibrous mesothelioma of pleura following external ionizing radiation therapy. Chest 94:1291, 1988.

358. Hill JK, Heitmiller RF, II, Askin FB, et al: Localized benign pleural mesothelioma arising in a radiation field. Clin Imaging 21:189, 1997.

359. Kawai T, Mikata A, Torikata C, et al: Solitary (localized) pleural mesothelioma: A light- and electron-microscopic study. Am J Surg Pathol 2:365, 1978.

360. Doucet J, Dardick I, Srigley JR, et al: Localized fibrous tumour of serosal surfaces: Immunohistochemical and ultrastructural evidence for a type of mesothelioma. Virchows Arch (Pathol Anat) 409:349, 1986.

361. Stout AP, Murray MR: Localized pleural mesothelioma. Arch Pathol 34:951, 1942.

362. Carter D, Otis CN: Three types of spindle cell tumors of the pleura: Fibroma, sarcoma, and sarcomatoid mesothelioma. Am J Surg Pathol 12:747, 1988.

363. Dervan PA, Tobin B, O'Connor M: Solitary (localized) fibrous mesothelioma: Evidence against mesothelial cell origin. Histopathology 10:867, 1986.

364. Hernandez FJ, Fernandez BB: Localized fibrous tumors of pleura: A light and electron microscopic study. Cancer 34:1667, 1974.

365. Said JW, Nash G, Banks-Schlegel S, et al: Localized fibrous mesothelioma: An immunohistochemical and electron microscopic study. Hum Pathol 15:440, 1984.

366. El-Naggar AK, Ro JY, Ayala AG, et al: Localized fibrous tumor of the serosal cavities. Immunohistochemical, electron-microscopic, and flow-cytometric DNA study. Am J Clin Pathol 92:561, 1989.

367. Steinetz C, Clarke R, Jacobs GH, et al: Localized fibrous tumors of the pleura: Correlation of histopathological, immunohistochemical and ultrastructural features. Path Res Pract 186:344, 1990.

368. Bortolotti U, Calabro F, Loy M, et al: Giant intrapericardial solitary fibrous tumor. Ann Thorac Surg 54:1219, 1992.

369. Young RH, Clement PB, McCaughey WTE: Solitary fibrous tumors. ('Fibrous mesotheliomas') of the peritoneum: A report of three cases and a review of the literature. Arch Pathol Lab Med 114:493, 1990.

370. Witkin GB, Rosai J: Solitary fibrous tumor of the mediastinum: A report of 14 cases. Am J Surg Pathol 13(7):547, 1989.

371. Scharifker D, Kaneko M: Localized fibrous "mesothelioma" of pleura (submesothelial fibroma): A clinicopathologic study of 18 cases. Cancer 43:627, 1979.

372. Okike N, Bernatz PE, Woolner LB: Localized mesothelioma of the pleura: Benign and malignant variants. J Thorac Cardiovasc Surg 75(3):363, 1978.

373. Yousem SA, Flynn SD: Intrapulmonary localized fibrous tumor: Intraparenchymal so-called localized fibrous mesothelioma. Am J Clin Pathol 89:365, 1988.

374. Janssen JP, Wagenaar SS, van den Bosch JM, et al: Benign localized mesothelioma of the pleura. Histopathology 9:309, 1985.

375. Moran CA, Suster S, Koss MN: The spectrum of histologic growth patterns in benign and malignant fibrous tumors of the pleura. Semin Diagn Pathol 9:169, 1992.

376. Lee KS, Im JG, Choe KO, et al: CT findings in benign fibrous mesothelioma of the pleura: Pathologic correlation in nine patients. AJR 158:983, 1992.

377. Dusenbery D, Grimes MM, Frable WJ: Fine-needle aspiration cytology of localized fibrous tumor of pleura. Diagn Cytopathol 8:444, 1992.

377a. Weynand B, Collard PH, Galant C: Cytopathological features of solitary fibrous tumor of the pleura: A study of 5 cases. Diagn Cytopathol 18:118, 1998.

378. Al-Izzi M, Thurlow NP, Corrin B: Pleural mesothelioma of connective tissue type, localized fibrous tumour of the pleura, and reactive submesothelial hyperplasia: An immunohistochemical comparison. J Pathol 158:41, 1989.

379. Flint A, Weiss SW: CD-34 and keratin expression distinguishes solitary fibrous tumor (fibrous mesothelioma) of pleura from desmoplastic mesothelioma. Hum Pathol 26:428, 1995.

379a. Yokoi T, Tsuzuki T, Yatabe Y, et al: Solitary fibrous tumour: Significance of p53 and CD34 immunoreactivity in its malignant transformation. Histopathology 32:423, 1998.

380. van de Rijn M, Lombard CM, Rouse RV: Expression of CD34 by solitary fibrous tumors of the pleura, mediastinum, and lung. Am J Surg Pathol 18:814, 1994.

381. Moran CA, Suster S, Koss MN: Smooth muscle tumours presenting as pleural neoplasms. Histopathology 27:227, 1995.

382. Chilosi M, Facchettti F, Dei Tos AP, et al: bcl-2 Expression in pleural and extrapleural solitary fibrous tumours. J Pathol 181:362, 1997.

383. Ferretti GR, Chiles C, Choplin RH, et al: Localized benign fibrous tumors of the pleura. AJR 169:683, 1997.

384. Desser TS, Stark P: Pictorial essay: Solitary fibrous tumor of the pleura. J Thorac Imaging 13:27, 1998.

385. Hutchinson WB, Friedenberg MJ: Intrathoracic mesothelioma. Radiology 80:937, 1963.

386. Dedrick CG, McLoud TC, Shepard JO, et al: Computed tomography of localized pleural mesothelioma. Am J Roentgenol 144:275, 1985.

387. Hayward RH: Migrating lung tumor. Chest 66:77, 1974.

388. Soulen MC, Greco-Hunt VT, Templeton P: Migratory chest mass. Invest Radiol 25:209, 1990.

389. Zamperlin A, Drigo R, Famulare CI, et al: A vagabond pleural pebble. Respiration 51:155, 1987.

390. Mengeot PM, Gailly CH: Spontaneous detachment of benign mesothelioma into the pleural space and removal during pleuroscopy. Eur J Respir Dis 68:141, 1986.

391. Phillips CJ, Müller NL, Miller RR, et al: Large calcified pleural-based mass in the left hemithorax. J Can Assoc Radiol 41:232, 1990.

392. Mendelson DS, Meary E, Buy JN, et al: Localized fibrous pleural mesothelioma: CT findings. Clin Imaging 15:105, 1991.

393. Saifuddin A, Da Costa P, Chalmers AG, et al: Primary malignant localized fibrous tumours of the pleura: Clinical, radiological and pathological features. Clin Radiol 45:13, 1992.

394. Fukasawa Y, Takada A, Tateno M, et al: Solitary fibrous tumor of the pleura causing recurrent hypoglycemia by secretion of insulin-like growth factor II. Pathol Int 48:47, 1998.

395. Harris GN, Rozenshtein A, Schiff MJ: Benign fibrous mesothelioma of the pleura: MR imaging findings. AJR 165:1143, 1995.

396. Ferretti GR, Chiles C, Cox JE, et al: Localized benign fibrous tumors of the pleura: MR appearance. J Comput Assist Tomogr 21:115, 1997.

397. Versluis PJ, Lamers RJS: Localized pleural fibroma: Radiological features. Eur J Radiol 18:124, 1994.

398. Padovani B, Mouroux J, Raffaelli C, et al: Benign fibrous mesothelioma of the pleura: MR study and pathologic correlation. Eur Radiol 6:425, 1996.

399. Nathan H, Seiden D: Localized fibrous mesothelioma of the pleura. Int Surg 63:161, 1978.

400. Kniznik DO, Roncoroni AJ, Rosenberg M, et al: Giant fibrous pleural mesothelioma associated with myocardial restriction and hypoglycemia: Respiration 37:346, 1979.

401. Okike N, Bernatz PE, Woolner LB: Localized mesothelioma of the pleura: Benign and malignant variants. J Thorac Cardiovasc Surg 75:363, 1978.

402. Mandal AK, Rozer MA, Salem FA, et al: Localized benign mesothelioma of the pleura associated with a hypoglycemic episode. Arch Intern Med 143:1608, 1983.

403. Sakamoto T, Kaneshige H, Takeshi A, et al: Localized pleural mesothelioma with elevation of high molecular weight insulin-like growth factor II and hypoglycemia. Chest 106:965, 1994.

404. Strfm EH, Skjfrten F, Aarseth LB, et al: Solitary fibrous tumor of the pleura: An immunohistochemical, electron microscopic and tissue culture study of a tumor producing insulin-like growth factor I in a patient with hypoglycemia. Pathol Res Pract 187:109, 1991.

405. Uzoaru I, Chou P, Reyes-Mugica M: Malignant solitary fibrous tumor of the pleura. Pediatr Pathol 14:11, 1994.

406. Hanau CA, Miettinen M: Solitary fibrous tumor: Histological and immunohistochemical spectrum of benign and malignant variants presenting at different sites. Hum Pathol 26:440, 1995.

407. Faer MJ, Burnam RE, Beck CL: Transmural thoracic lipoma: Demonstration by computed tomography. AJR 130:161, 1978.

408. Epler GR, McLoud TC, Munn CS, et al: Pleural lipoma: Diagnosis by computed tomography. Chest 90:265, 1986.

409. Buxton RC, Tan CS, Khine NM, et al: Atypical transmural thoracic lipoma: CT diagnosis. J Comput Assist Tomogr 12:196, 1988.

410. Munk PL, Müller NL: Pleural liposarcoma: CT diagnosis. J Comput Assist Tomogr 12:709, 1988.

411. Evans AR, Wolstenholme RJ, Shettar SP, et al: Primary pleural liposarcoma. Thorax 40:554, 1985.

412. Dubig JT: Solitary rhabdomyosarcoma of the pleura: Report of a case with a note on the nomenclature of pleural tumors. J Thorac Surg 37:236, 1959.

413. Rizkalla K, Ahmad D, Garcia B, et al: Primary malignant fibrous histiocytoma of the pleura: A case report and review of the literature. Respir Med 88:711, 1994.

414. Naka N, Ohsawa M, Tomita Y, et al: Angiosarcoma in Japan: A review of 99 cases. Cancer 75:989, 1995.

415. McCaughey WT, Dardick I, Barr JR: Angiosarcoma of the serous membranes. Arch Pathol Lab Med 107:304, 1983.

416. Falconieri G, Bussani R, Mirra M, et al: Pseudomesotheliomatous angiosarcoma:

A pleuropulmonary lesion simulating malignant pleural mesothelioma. Histopathology 30:419, 1997.

417. Yousem SA, Hochholzer L: Unusual thoracic manifestations of epithelioid hemangioendothelioma. Arch Pathol Lab Med 111:459, 1987.

418. Goetz SP, Robinson RA, Landas SK: Extraskeletal myxoid chondrosarcoma of the pleura: Report of a case clinically simulating mesothelioma. Am J Clin Pathol 97:498, 1992.

418a. Mayall FG, Gibbs AR: 'Pleural' and pulmonary carcinosarcomas. J Pathol 167:305, 1992.

419. Szalay F, Szathmari M, Paloczi K, et al: Immunologic and molecular biologic characterization of pleural involvement in a case of T-chronic lymphocytic leukemia. Chest 106:1283, 1994.

420. Fukayama M, Ibuka T, Hayashi Y, et al: Epstein-Barr virus in pyothorax-associated pleural lymphoma. Am J Pathol 143:1044, 1993.

421. Iuchi K, Aozasa K, Yamamoto S, et al: Non-Hodgkin's lymphoma of the pleural cavity developing from long-standing pyothorax: Summary of clinical and pathological findings in thirty-seven cases. Jpn J Clin Oncol 19:249, 1989.

422. Cesarman E, Chang Y, Moore PS, et al: Kaposi's sarcoma-associated Herpesvirus-like DNA sequences in AIDS-related body-cavity-based lymphomas. N Engl J Med 332:1186, 1996.

423. Said JW, Tasaka T, Takeuchi S, et al: Primary effusion lymphoma in women: Report of two cases of Kaposi's sarcoma like virus-associated effusion-based lymphoma in human immunodeficiency virus-negative women. Blood 88:3124, 1996.

424. Cesarman E, Knowles DM: Kaposi's sarcoma-associated herpesvirus: A lymphotropic human herpesvirus associated with Kaposi's sarcoma, primary effusion lymphoma, and multicentric Castelman's disease. Semin Diagn Pathol 14:54, 1997.

424a. Filly R, Blank N, Castellino RA: Radiographic distribution of intrathoracic disease in previously untreated patients with Hodgkin's disease and non-Hodgkin's lymphoma. Radiology 120:277, 1976.

424b. Malatskey A, Fields S, Libson E: CT appearance of primary pleural lymphoma. Comput Med Imaging Graph 13:165, 1989.

425. Daya D, McCaughey WTE: Well differentiated papillary mesothelioma of the peritoneum. Cancer 65:292, 1990.

426. Yesner R, Hurwitz A: Localized pleural mesothelioma of epithelial type. J Thorac Surg 26:325, 1953.

427. Kaplan MA, Tazelaar HD, Hayashi T, et al: Adenomatoid tumors of the pleura. Am J Surg Pathol 20:1219, 1996.

428. Rüttner JR, Heinzl S: Squamous-cell carcinoma of the pleura. Thorax 32:497, 1977.

429. Sapino A, Cavallo A, Donna A, et al: Pleural epidermoid carcinoma from displaced skin following extrapleural pneumothorax in a patient exposed to asbestos. Virchows Arch 429:173, 1996.

430. Prabhakar G, Mitchell IM, Guha T, et al: Squamous cell carcinoma of the pleura following bronchopleural fistula. Thorax 44:1053, 1989.

431. Smith S, Opipari MI: Primary pleural melanoma: A first reported case and literature review. J Thorac Cardiovasc Surg 75:827, 1978.

432. Moran CA, Travis WD, Rosado-de-Christenson M, et al: Thymomas presenting as pleural tumors: Report of eight cases. Am J Surg Pathol 16:138, 1992.

433. Shih DF, Wang JS, Tseng HH, et al: Primary pleural thymoma. Arch Pathol Lab Med 121:79, 1997.

434. Fukayama M, Maeda Y, Funata N, et al: Pulmonary and pleural thymoma: Diagnostic application of lymphocyte markers to the thymoma of unusual site. Am J Clin Pathol 89:617, 1988.

434a. Fushimi H, Tanio Y, Kotoh K: Ectopic thymoma mimicking diffuse pleural mesothelioma: A case report. Hum Pathol 29:409, 1998.

435. Parkash V, Gerald WL, Parma A, et al: Desmoplastic small round cell tumor of the pleura. Am J Surg Pathol 19:659, 1995.

436. Dehner LP: Pleuropulmonary blastoma is the pulmonary blastoma of childhood. Semin Diagn Pathol 11:144, 1994.

437. Manivel JC, Priest JR, Watterson J, et al: Pleuropulmonary blastoma: The so-called pulmonary blastoma of childhood. Cancer 62:1516, 1988.

438. Knapp MJ, Roggli VL, Kim J, et al: Pleural amyloidosis. Arch Pathol Lab Med 112:57, 1988.

439. Lundin P, Simonsson B, Winberg T: Pneumopleural amyloid tumour: Report of a case. Acta Radiol 55:139, 1961.

440. Hutton L: Oleothorax: Expanding pleural lesion. Am J Roentgenol 142:1107, 1984.

441. Jariwalla AG, Al-Nasiri NK: Splenosis pleurae. Thorax 34:123, 1979.

442. Yousem SA: Thoracic splenosis. Ann Thorac Surg 44:411, 1987.

443. Kwan AJ, Drum DE, Ahn CS, et al: Intrathoracic splenosis mimicking metastatic lung cancer. Clin Nucl Med 19:93, 1994.

444. Carlson BR, McQueen S, Kimbrell F, et al: Thoracic splenosis: Diagnosis of a case by fine needle aspiration cytology. Acta Cytol 32:91, 1988.

445. Roche G, Delanoe Y, Genevrier R: Opacités pseudo-tumorales après pleurésies sérofibrineuses de la grande cavité. (Pseudotumoral opacities after serofibrinous effusions of the pleural cavity.) J Fr Med Chir Thorac 19:789, 1965.

446. Bumgarner JR, Gahwyler M, Ward DE: Persistent fibrin bodies presenting as coin lesions. Am Rev Tuberc 72:659, 1955.

447. Ball NJ, Urbanski SJ, Green FHY, et al: Pleural multicystic mesothelial proliferation: The so-called multicystic mesothelioma. Am J Surg Pathol 14:375, 1990.

448. Pinkard NB, Wilson RW, Lawless N, et al: Calcifying fibrous pseudotumor of pleura: A report of three cases of a newly described entity involving the pleura. Am J Clin Pathol 105:189, 1996.

449. Erasmus JJ, McAdams HP, Patz EF, et al: Calcifying fibrous pseudotumor of pleura: Radiologic features in three cases. J Comput Assist Tomogr 20:763, 1996.

450. Leers MGP, Aarts MMJ, Theunissen PHMH: E-cadherin and calretinin: A useful combination of immunochemical markers for differentiation between mesothelioma and metastatic adenocarcinoma. Histopathology 32:209, 1998.

451. Ruco LP, de Laat PA, Matteucci C, et al: Expression of ICAM-1 and VCAM-1 in human malignant mesothelioma. J Pathol 179:266, 1996.

452. Peralta-Soler A, Knudsen KA, Jaurand MC, et al: The differential expression of N-cadherin and E-cadherin distinguishes pleural mesotheliomas from lung adenocarcinomas. Hum Pathol 26:1363, 1995.

453. Han AC, Peralta-Soler A, Knudsen KA, et al: Differential expression of N-cadherin in pleural mesotheliomas and E-cadherin in lung adenocarcinomas in formalin-fixed, paraffin-embedded tissues. Hum Pathol 28:84, 1997.

454. Doglioni C, Tos AP, Laurino L, et al: Calretinin: A novel immunocytochemical marker for mesothelioma. Am J Surg Pathol 20:1037, 1996.

455. Gotzos V, Vogt P, Celio MR: The calcium binding protein calretinin is a selective marker for malignant pleural mesotheliomas of the epithelial type. Pathol Res Pract 192:137, 1996.

456. Barberis MC, Faleri M, Veronese S, et al: Calretinin: A selective marker of normal and neoplastic mesothelial cells in serous effusions. Acta Cytol 41:1757, 1997.

457. Amin KM, Litzky LA, Smythe WR, et al: Wilms' tumor 1 susceptibility (WT1) gene products are selectively expressed in malignant mesothelioma. Am J Pathol 146:344, 1995.

458. Chang K, Pai LH, Pass H, et al: Monoclonal antibody K1 reacts with epithelial mesothelioma but not with lung adenocarcinoma. Am J Surg Pathol 16:259, 1992.

459. O'Hara CJ, Corson JM, Pinkus GS, et al: A monoclonal antibody that distinguishes epithelial-type malignant mesothelioma from pulmonary adenocarcinoma and extrapulmonary malignancies. Am J Pathol 136:421, 1990.

460. Ascoli V, Scalzo CC, Taccogna S, et al: The diagnostic value of thrombomodulin immunolocalization in serous effusions. Arch Pathol Lab Med 119:1136, 1995.

461. Collins CL, Ordonez NG, Schaefer R, et al: Thrombomodulin expression in malignant pleural mesothelioma and pulmonary adenocarcinoma. Am J Pathol 141:827, 1992.

462. Ordonez NG: Value of thrombomodulin in the diagnosis of mesothelioma. Histopathology 31:25, 1997.

463. Donna A, Betta PG, Chiodera P, et al: Newly marketed tissue markers for malignant mesothelioma: Immunoreactivity of rabbit AMAD-2 antiserum compared with monoclonal antibody HBME-1 and a review of the literature on so-called antimesothelioma antibodies. Hum Pathol 28:929, 1997.

464. Koukoulis GK, Shen J, Monson R, et al: Pleural mesotheliomas have an integrin profile distinct from visceral carcinomas. Hum Pathol 28:84, 1997.

465. Ascoli V, Carnovale-Scalzo C, Taccogna S, et al: Utility of HBME-1 immunostaining in serous effusions. Cytopathology 8:328, 1997.

466. Bateman AC, al-Talib RK, Newman T, et al: Immunohistochemical phenotype of malignant mesothelioma: Predictive value of CA125 and HBME-1 expression. Histopathology 30:49, 1997.

467. Clark SP, Chou ST, Martin TJ, et al: Parathyroid hormone–related protein antigen localization distinguishes between mesothelioma and adenocarcinoma of the lung. J Pathol 176:161, 1995.

468. Attanoos RL, Webb R, Gibbs AR: CD44H expression in reactive mesothelium, pleural mesothelioma and pulmonary adenocarcinoma. Histopathology 30:260, 1997.

469. Maguire B, Whitaker D, Carrello S: Monoclonal antibody Ber-EP4: Its use in the differential diagnosis of malignant mesothelioma and carcinoma in cell blocks of malignant effusions and FNA specimens. Diagn Cytopathol 10:130, 1994.

470. Sheibani K, Shin SS, Kezirian J, et al: Ber-EP4 antibody as a discriminant in the differential diagnosis of malignant mesothelioma versus adenocarcinoma. Am J Surg Pathol 15:779, 1991.

471. Edwards C, Oates SJ: OV 632 and MOC 31 in the diagnosis of mesothelioma and adenocarcinoma: An assessment of their use in formalin fixed and paraffin wax embedded material. J Clin Pathol 48:626, 1995.

472. Sosolik RC, McGaughy VR, De Young BR: Anti-MOC-31: A potential addition to the pulmonary adenocarcinoma versus mesothelioma immunohistochemistry panel. Mod Pathol 10:716, 1997.

473. Kortsik CS, Werner P, Freudenberg N, et al: Immunocytochemical characterization of malignant mesothelioma and carcinoma metastatic to the pleura: IOB3—a new tumor marker. Lung 173:79, 1995.

474. Ascoli V, Scalzo CC, Nardi F: C-erbB-2 oncoprotein immunostaining in serous effusions. Cytopathology 4:207, 1993.

475. Szpak CA, Johnston WW, Roggli V, et al: The diagnostic distinction between malignant mesothelioma of the pleura and adenocarcinoma of the lung as defined by a monoclonal antibody (B72.3). Am J Pathol 122:252, 1986.

476. Radosevich JA, Ma Y, Lee I: Monoclonal antibody 44-3A6 as a probe for a novel antigen found on human lung carcinomas with glandular differentiation. Cancer Res 45:5808, 1985.

477. Ordóñez NG: Value of the MOC-31 monoclonal antibody in differentiating epithelial pleural mesothelioma from lung adenocarcinoma. Hum Pathol 29:166, 1998.

PART XVI
MEDIASTINAL DISEASE

CHAPTER 73

Mediastinitis, Pneumomediastinum, and Mediastinal Hemorrhage

MEDIASTINITIS

Infections of the mediastinum can be acute or chronic. Acute infections are usually caused by bacteria and sometimes progress to abscess formation; they are often associated with signs and symptoms (especially retrosternal pain and fever), and many are fulminating and lethal. By contrast, chronic disease is most often the result of tuberculous or fungal infection; although chronic infections are characteristically insidious in onset and unassociated with clinical manifestations, some patients have symptoms or signs related to obstruction or compression of one or more mediastinal structures. In addition to cases of chronic mediastinitis of infectious origin, there is a group of mediastinopathies of unknown cause characterized by the accumulation of dense fibrous tissue, sometimes associated with similar deposits elsewhere in the body.

Acute Mediastinitis

Acute infections of the mediastinum are relatively uncommon. Most cases are associated with esophageal perforation,[1, 2] or with esophageal[3, 4] or cardiac[4–6] surgery. Less common causes include direct extension of infection from adjacent tissues such as the retropharyngeal space;[7–10] bones and sternoclavicular or costochondral joints;[11, 12]

lymph nodes;[13] pericardium, lungs, or pleura;[4, 12, 14] and tracheal or bronchial perforation following intubation, bronchoscopy, or penetrating trauma.[4, 14, 15] Rarely, mediastinitis is secondary to hematogenous spread of infection from an extrathoracic source, such as septic arthritis,[14] or is "spontaneous."[16]

Over 75% of cases of esophageal rupture follow diagnostic and therapeutic endoscopic procedures.[16] Such perforation most commonly results from esophagoscopy and balloon dilation,[2, 17] but may also be seen following diagnostic endoscopy without dilation,[2] insertion of an esophageal prosthesis,[18] or laser therapy.[4] Esophageal perforation may also occur in association with a necrotic esophageal carcinoma,[16] radiation esophagitis,[16] ulceration of a hiatal hernia, or penetrating or blunt trauma.[2, 12] Spontaneous perforation following a sudden rise in intraesophageal pressure (Boerhaave's syndrome) occurs most frequently following episodes of severe vomiting[2, 19] but can also develop during labor, a severe asthmatic attack, or strenuous exercise and, rarely, with no apparent cause.[12] Spontaneous rupture of the esophagus is second only to instrumentation as a cause of esophageal perforation.[2, 16] The usual site of rupture is the lower 8 cm, often adjacent to the gastroesophageal junction; typically, the tear is vertical and involves the left posterolateral wall.[19, 20] Although the usual pathogenesis of mediastinitis in all these situations is related to infection, gastric acid introduced into the mediastinum can also damage the mediastinal soft tissue and adjacent pleura and lung.[21]

In a review of the findings in 16 patients who had life-threatening acute posterior mediastinitis secondary to esophageal perforation, the perforation resulted from endoscopic procedures in 11 patients, vomiting in 4, and blunt trauma in 1.[2] Specimens of mediastinal fluid from 14 patients who underwent surgical exploration grew from 1 to 3 organisms in 6 patients, more than 3 organisms in 5 patients, and no organisms in 3; the most common organisms were *Streptococcus, Pseudomonas,* and *Candida.*[2] All three negative cultures were obtained in patients who underwent surgical exploration within 24 hours or less of perforation.

Postoperative mediastinitis occurs in approximately 0.5% to 1% of patients who have undergone median sternotomy for cardiac surgery.[5, 22] The risk of the complication is markedly increased in immunocompromised patients.[23]

Other risk factors that have been identified include diabetes, obesity, the use of bilateral internal mammary arteries for coronary artery bypass grafting, surgical re-exploration of the mediastinum, and postoperative transfusion.[5, 6, 24]

Radiologic Manifestations

The main radiographic manifestation of acute mediastinitis is widening of the mediastinum, usually more evident superiorly; typically, the abnormal region possesses a smooth, sharply defined margin (Fig. 73–1). Air may be visible within the mediastinum as well as in the soft tissues of the neck (Fig. 73–2).[25, 26] Pneumothorax or hydropneumothorax may also be evident.[26] In one study of 24 patients, distal esophageal perforation usually resulted in left hydrothorax or hydropneumothorax, whereas midesophageal perforation tended to cause pleural changes on the right.[27] Multiple abscesses may develop (Fig. 73–3).

The diagnosis can be readily confirmed by demonstrating extravasation of ingested contrast material into the mediastinum or pleural space (Fig. 73–4).[25] Esophagography can be performed safely with barium.[28] Some authors have recommended the use of water-soluble contrast agents in patients who have suspected or known esophageal perforation;[28, 29] however, small leaks may be missed using water-soluble contrast, and aspiration of this material may result in pulmonary edema.[28, 30]

CT also can be helpful both in diagnosis and in guiding percutaneous aspiration and drainage of mediastinal abscesses.[12, 31] Manifestations include esophageal thickening, obliteration of the normal fat planes, periesophageal areas of soft tissue or fluid attenuation, single or multiple abscesses, extraluminal gas, and extraluminal contrast (Fig. 73–5).[4, 12, 32–34] In one series of 12 patients with esophageal perforation, esophageal thickening was seen on the CT scan in 11 patients, extraluminal gas in 11, and pleural effusion in 9;[33]

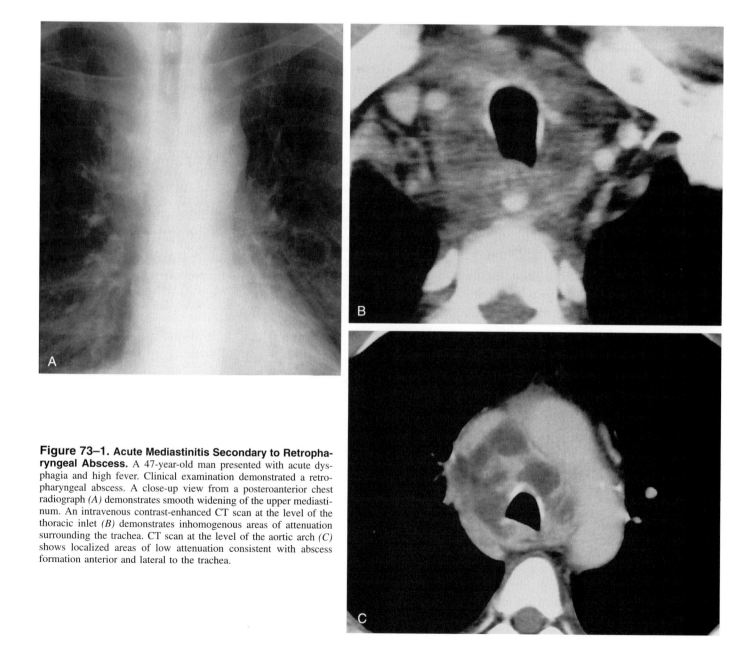

Figure 73–1. Acute Mediastinitis Secondary to Retropharyngeal Abscess. A 47-year-old man presented with acute dysphagia and high fever. Clinical examination demonstrated a retropharyngeal abscess. A close-up view from a posteroanterior chest radiograph *(A)* demonstrates smooth widening of the upper mediastinum. An intravenous contrast-enhanced CT scan at the level of the thoracic inlet *(B)* demonstrates inhomogenous areas of attenuation surrounding the trachea. CT scan at the level of the aortic arch *(C)* shows localized areas of low attenuation consistent with abscess formation anterior and lateral to the trachea.

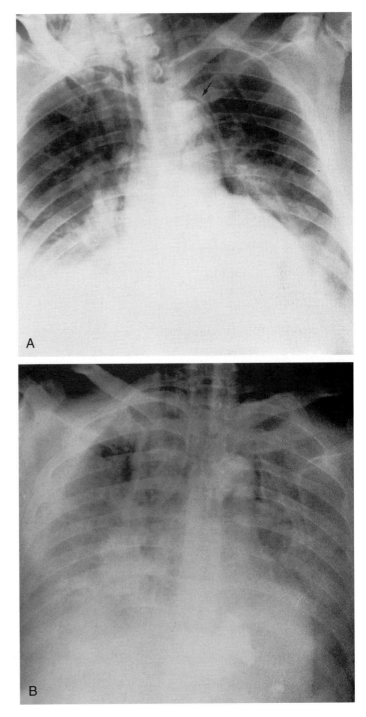

Figure 73–2. Acute Mediastinitis Secondary to Esophageal Rupture. A 41-year-old man had a surgical repair of a hiatal hernia through an abdominal approach. Several hours postoperatively, he complained of dyspnea and retrosternal pain. An anteroposterior radiograph *(A)* exposed with the patient in the supine position demonstrated lateral displacement of the left mediastinal pleura *(arrows)* related to an accumulation of gas in the mediastinum. The presence of bilateral basal opacity suggested pleural effusion; there was subcutaneous emphysema in the neck. Twelve hours later *(B),* the opacity of both lungs had increased greatly, chiefly as a result of pleural effusion. The mediastinal gas had decreased slightly, but there was still considerable subcutaneous emphysema in the neck. These changes were caused by spillage of esophageal contents into the mediastinum and pleural spaces through a tear in the esophagus near the esophagogastric junction.

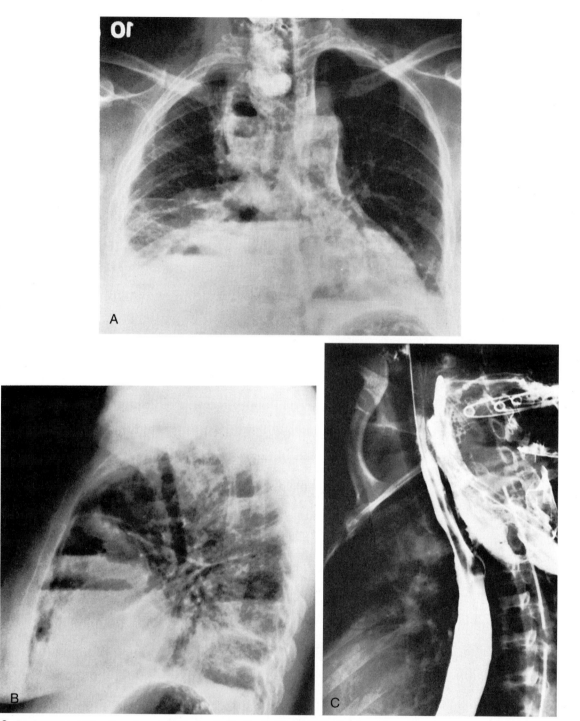

Figure 73–3. Perforation of the Esophagus with Acute Mediastinitis and Mediastinal Abscesses. A 41-year-old woman swallowed a fork and shortly thereafter developed severe retrosternal pain and fever. Three days later, posteroanterior *(A)* and lateral *(B)* radiographs exposed with the patient in the erect position reveal an irregularly widened upper mediastinum and multiple air-fluid levels within the mediastinum anteriorly and posteriorly. Bilateral pleural effusions and probable bilateral lower lobe pneumonia are evident. Several days later, barium administered by mouth opacified the whole of the esophagus but showed a large sinus tract extending into the mediastinum posteriorly *(C)*. Recovery was prolonged but complete.

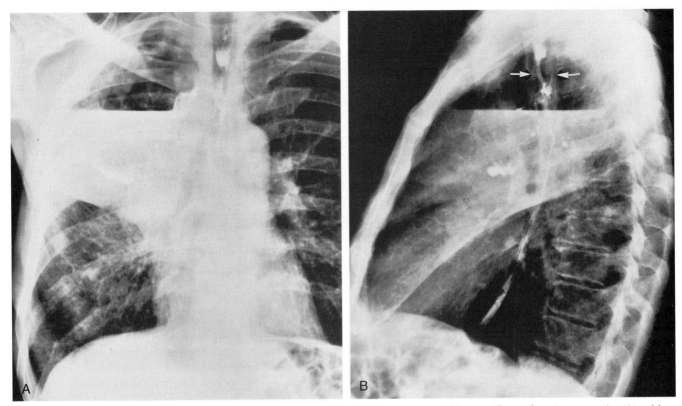

Figure 73–4. Carcinoma of the Esophagus with Perforation into the Right Lung and Abscess Formation. Posteroanterior *(A)* and lateral *(B)* radiographs reveal a large ragged cavity in the upper half of the right lung. Barium administered by mouth reveals deformity of the esophageal lumen characteristic of primary carcinoma *(arrows* in *B).* Barium has passed from the esophagus into the large lung abscess.

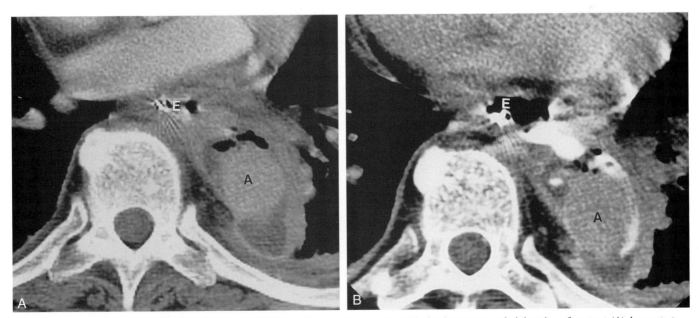

Figure 73–5. Carcinoma of the Esophagus with Perforation. A CT scan obtained after intravenous administration of contrast *(A)* demonstrates a nasogastric tube within the esophagus (E), increased soft tissue between the esophagus and the aorta (A), and localized collections of gas and fluid consistent with abscess formation. Also noted is a small left pleural effusion. A CT scan obtained after oral administration of contrast *(B)* demonstrates extravasation of contrast, confirming the presence of esophageal perforation and communication with the periaortic fluid and air collections.

the site of perforation was visible in only 2 patients. Because esophageal thickening, obliteration of fat planes, and small fluid collections are often present following surgery, it may be difficult to distinguish normal postoperative findings from those of early mediastinitis.

Clinical Manifestations

The principal symptom is retrosternal pain, often severe and abrupt in onset; radiation to the neck may occur. Chills and high fever are common, and the effects of obstruction of the superior vena cava may be seen. Physical examination of a patient who has a perforated esophagus commonly reveals subcutaneous emphysema in the soft tissues of the neck or a loud crunching or clicking sound synchronous with the heart beat on auscultation over the apex of the heart (Hamman's sign). Although suggestive of pneumomediastinum, the latter sign is not pathognomonic, being heard in some patients who have pneumothorax and occasionally in patients who have moderate elevation of the left hemidiaphragm associated with gaseous distention of the fundus of the stomach or the splenic flexure of the colon.

Prognosis and Natural History

When the diagnosis of mediastinitis is not suspected initially and treatment is not instituted promptly, the infection can progress to an abscess that in turn can rupture into the esophagus, a lung, a bronchus, or the pleural cavity. The presence of such fistulas usually can be confirmed by contrast radiographic or CT examination; microscopic examination of the pleural fluid has been reported to be useful in some cases.[35] However, iatrogenic esophageal perforation may be followed by the development of an esophagopleural fistula without radiographic or other evidence of mediastinitis.[36]

The prognosis in cases of acute mediastinitis resulting from esophageal rupture is poor.[37] In one series of 16 patients, 6 (38%) died, all of polymicrobial sepsis.[1]

Fibrosing Mediastinitis

Fibrosing mediastinitis (chronic sclerosing mediastinitis, granulomatous mediastinitis, or idiopathic mediastinal fibrosis) is a rare condition characterized by chronic inflammation and fibrosis of mediastinal soft tissues. The process is often progressive and can occur either focally or more or less diffusely throughout the mediastinum. It can cause compression and sometimes obliteration of vessels, airways, and the esophagus and result in a variety of functional and radiologic manifestations and, occasionally, death.

Etiology and Pathogenesis

A consideration of the etiology and pathogenesis of fibrosing mediastinitis is complicated to some extent by the presence of two distinct patterns of presentation: (1) more or less diffuse involvement of mediastinal tissues by inflammatory cells and fibrous tissue and (2) a relatively localized granulomatous inflammatory mass ("pseudotumor") centered on one or several lymph nodes. Some authors

consider the second form to be a separate entity (sometimes termed "mediastinal granuloma"), because it usually does not evolve to the diffuse form and because it tends to have a good prognosis.[38, 39] However, because it is the fibrotic reaction surrounding the involved nodes that results in compression of the adjacent mediastinal structures, we and others consider the localized form to be a pattern of fibrosing mediastinitis and limit the use of the term "mediastinal granuloma" to cases unassociated with significant mediastinal fibrosis (*see* page 2940).[40]

Because it is not always clear in published articles which cases represent the localized form of mediastinal granulomatous inflammation and which the diffuse fibrosing type,[41, 42] statements about the relative importance of specific organisms in the etiology of fibrosing mediastinitis are sometimes difficult to interpret. However, it is clear that infection is an important cause, at least in some geographic regions. The most frequently implicated organism is *Histoplasma capsulatum*.[73] In one review of 33 patients who had fibrosing mediastinitis, a localized pattern of disease was seen in 27 (82%) and a diffuse pattern in 6 (18%).[40] Necrotizing granulomatous inflammation was seen in 10 patients, microorganisms consistent with *H. capsulatum* were identified in 2, and both abnormalities were seen in 2. Nine patients had presumed histoplasmosis based on positive results of serologic or skin tests or on the presence of calcified granulomas or lymph nodes and negative results of skin tests for tuberculosis. Three patients had retroperitoneal fibrosis, a history of methysergide therapy, and orbital pseudotumor and 7 had no associated abnormality or evident causative factor.[40] Evidence of histoplasmosis was mostly seen in the patients who had localized disease, whereas the diffuse pattern was usually idiopathic.[40]

In geographic regions in which histoplasmosis is not endemic, tuberculosis is likely to be a more important cause of the fibrosing mediastinitis. In a review of the pathologic files of the Royal Brompton Hospital in London, only 18 cases of fibrosing mediastinitis were identified between 1970 and 1993.[42] Although no organisms or positive cultures were identified in any case, nine patients had a history of tuberculosis; three had previous mediastinal malignancy treated with chemotherapy and radiotherapy; two had autoimmune disease (rheumatoid arthritis in one and systemic lupus erythematosus in the other); one, who had previously lived in the United States, had positive serology for *Histoplasma;* and the remaining three patients had no known predisposing factors.[42] Rarely, other organisms have been implicated, including *Aspergillus* species,[43, 44] members of the group Phycomycetes,[45] *Blastomyces dermatitidis,*[46] and *Treponema pallidum.*[47]

The precise pathogenesis of the progressive mediastinal fibrosis in patients who have infection is not clear. It has been hypothesized that spillage of necrotic material from affected lymph nodes is followed by infection of the mediastinum and secondary fibrosis.[48] However, the authors of a review of the literature in 1988 failed to find evidence of such a process.[49] It has also been suggested that the disease may result from a hypersensitivity reaction to antigenic material released from the involved lymph nodes;[40, 49, 50] such a reaction would account for the paucity or lack of organisms in the fibrous tissue in the majority of cases.[40]

A second group of cases (sometimes designated *idio-*

pathic mediastinal fibrosis) shows no cultural and little or no histologic evidence of an infectious origin. This group can be substantial in size; for example, in one review of 77 patients, an infectious cause was positively established in only 3 (histoplasmosis in 2 and tuberculosis in 1).[41] Although some of these cases (perhaps the majority) may represent the end stage of chronic infection in which the organism is difficult to identify, in others the etiology and pathogenesis are undoubtedly noninfectious. Evidence for this derives from the occasional patient in whom a similar fibrotic process can be identified elsewhere,[51] including the retroperitoneal space (retroperitoneal fibrosis), the orbit ("pseudotumor of the orbit"), the thyroid (Riedel's struma), and the cecum ("ligneous perityphlitis"). The number of reported cases in which fibrosing mediastinitis has been associated with combinations of these sclerosing lesions is sufficient to indicate that the relationship is more than coincidental;[51, 52] one group has proposed the term "multifocal fibrosclerosis" to refer to these lesions.[53] The pathogenesis of this condition is probably multifactorial. A genetic effect is suggested by one report of two brothers (the offspring of a consanguineous marriage) who showed various combinations of sclerosing lesions.[53] Immunologic factors seem to be involved in some cases, as evidenced by the reports of both mediastinal and retroperitoneal fibrosis in isolated cases of systemic lupus erythematosus, rheumatoid disease, and Raynaud's phenomenon.[51] Methysergide, a drug used for the alleviation of headache, also has been clearly associated with development of the abnormality.[54, 55]

Pathologic Characteristics

Pathologically, the fibrosis tends to affect the upper half of the mediastinum, predominantly anterior to the trachea and around the hilum; more extensive lesions can extend from the brachiocephalic veins to the base of a lung.[41] Grossly, the affected tissue is typically ill defined; compression of vessels (especially the superior vena cava [SVC] and pulmonary veins), airways, and occasionally the esophagus may be apparent (Fig. 73–6). The histologic appearance varies depending on the underlying cause. In some cases—particularly those in which an infectious organism is identified—there is necrotizing granulomatous inflammation; in others, the granulomatous component is minimal in extent or absent altogether, the abnormal tissue being composed predominantly of mature fibrous tissue containing a mononuclear inflammatory cell infiltrate (Fig. 73–7). Foci of necrosis resembling those in the center of remote granulomas may or may not be seen in the latter cases.[49] The histologic differential diagnosis includes desmoplastic mesothelioma[56] and the nodular sclerosis subtype of Hodgkin's disease.[57]

Because the fibrosing process tends to compress vessels and airways in the hilar region, secondary effects on the lung are relatively common. In lobes in which the draining veins are affected, parenchymal interstitial fibrosis and pneumonitis, intra-alveolar aggregates of hemosiderin-laden macrophages, and vascular changes consistent with pulmonary hypertension may be seen.[58, 59] Occasionally, venous or arterial thrombi (or both) in various stages of organization can be identified.[60] Sometimes, these are accompanied by parenchymal infarcts. In one case, multifocal infarcts were related

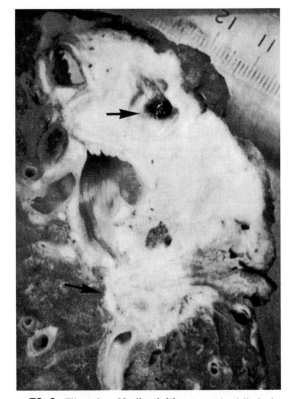

Figure 73–6. Fibrosing Mediastinitis. A poorly delimited mass of fibrous tissue can be seen in the hilar region and adjacent mediastinal tissue in this pneumonectomy specimen. The pulmonary arteries *(upper arrow)* and veins *(lower arrow)* are partly or completely obstructed. No underlying cause was apparent.

to interlobular septa, implying pulmonary venous rather than arterial obstruction as the cause.[59]

Radiologic Manifestations

As indicated previously, fibrosing mediastinitis can present as a focal mediastinal soft tissue mass or as diffuse mediastinal widening.[40] Focal lesions involve the right paratracheal region most commonly (Fig. 73–8); less often, the left paratracheal, subcarinal, or posterior mediastinal regions are affected.[61–64] Because the majority of these lesions are the result of histoplasmosis or tuberculosis, areas of calcification may be evident, particularly on CT scans, on which this feature has been identified in 60% to 90% of cases.[40, 62] In a minority of patients, parenchymal disease or bronchopulmonary lymph node enlargement suggests a pulmonary origin for the mediastinal disease. The diffuse form of disease results in extensive widening of the mediastinum, most commonly involving its upper portion; the mediastinal outline may be smooth or lobulated.[40, 61] Unlike in localized disease, calcification is rare in the diffuse form, even when it is associated with histoplasmosis.[40] When the fibrosis is methysergide-induced, the radiographic abnormalities may disappear following withdrawal of the drug.[65]

In some cases of either focal or diffuse disease, the mediastinal silhouette is normal, and the radiographic manifestations result from narrowing of the trachea or major bronchi, obstruction of pulmonary veins or arteries, or narrowing of the esophagus.[40, 64, 66] In the series of 33 patients

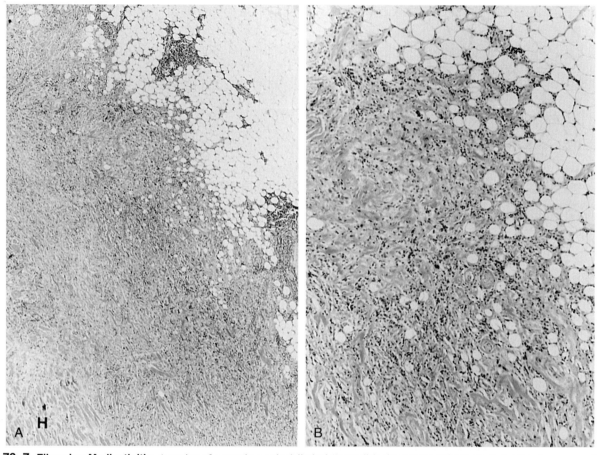

Figure 73–7. Fibrosing Mediastinitis. A section of a grossly poorly delimited "tumor" in the upper mediastinum shows it to be composed of fibrous tissue containing a variable number of lymphocytes. The "tumor" appears to invade the mediastinal adipose tissue. Inflammatory cells are more prominent at the periphery, the central portion consisting only of bands of collagen (H). The patient was a young woman who had superior vena cava syndrome. No underlying cause was identified.

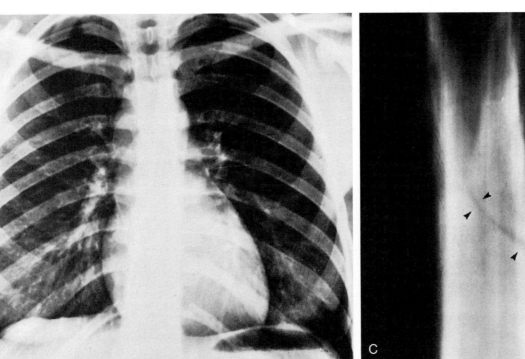

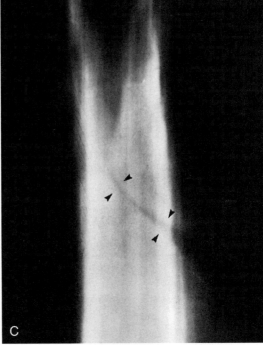

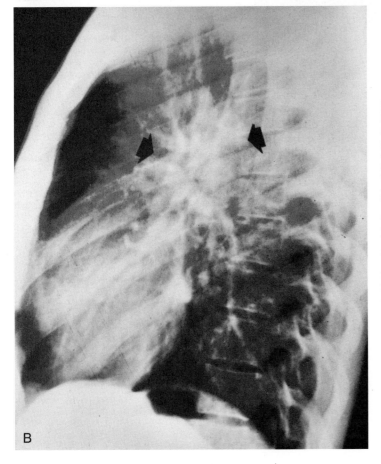

Figure 73–8. Fibrosing Mediastinitis with Involvement of Major Airways. A 19-year-old woman noted the onset of shortness of breath on exertion and recurrent wheezing episodes precipitated by physical exertion. Five months later, posteroanterior *(A)* and lateral *(B)* chest radiographs reveal a normal appearance of her lungs. A smooth, well-defined, homogeneous mass is seen in the right tracheobronchial angle, obscuring the shadow of the azygos vein. In lateral projection, the aortic window is not visualized and has apparently been obliterated. In addition, there is a suggestion of narrowing of the air column of the main bronchi. A tomogram of the carinal region in anteroposterior projection *(C)* reveals a severe degree of stenosis of the whole length of the left main bronchus *(arrowheads).* The lower 2 cm of the trachea and right main bronchus are similarly but less severely affected. Biopsies of mediastinal tissue obtained at mediastinoscopy revealed findings consistent with fibrosing mediastinitis. At right thoracotomy, a diffuse mass with ill-defined edges was found extending from the posterior wall of the superior vena cava over the trachea, into the mediastinum behind the trachea, and downward around the right upper lobe bronchus and into the mediastinum. The underlying cause was not established. (Courtesy of St. Boniface General Hospital, St. Boniface, Manitoba, Canada.)

cited previously, bronchial narrowing was evident on the radiograph or CT scan in 11 patients (33%), obstruction or narrowing of the SVC in 13 (39%), and narrowing or obstruction of the pulmonary artery in 6 (18%).[40] Bronchial narrowing most commonly affected the right main bronchus, followed in decreasing frequency by the left main bronchus, the bronchus intermedius, the right upper lobe bronchus, the left upper lobe bronchus, and the right middle lobe bronchus. Bronchial obstruction was frequently associated with obstructive pneumonitis or atelectasis or both.

Involvement of the SVC frequently results in a promi-

nent aortic nipple as a result of a dilated left superior intercostal vein.[40] Obstruction or narrowing of a pulmonary artery may result in localized areas of decreased opacification and vascularity, volume loss, or thrombosis.[40, 66] We have seen one patient in whom there was a combination of total occlusion of the left interlobar artery and compression of multiple pulmonary veins leading to interstitial pulmonary edema in all regions except the left lower lobe (Fig. 73–9). Pulmonary infarction is seen occasionally.[59, 67] A case has been described in which fibrosing mediastinitis presented initially as a predominantly posterior mediastinal mass that

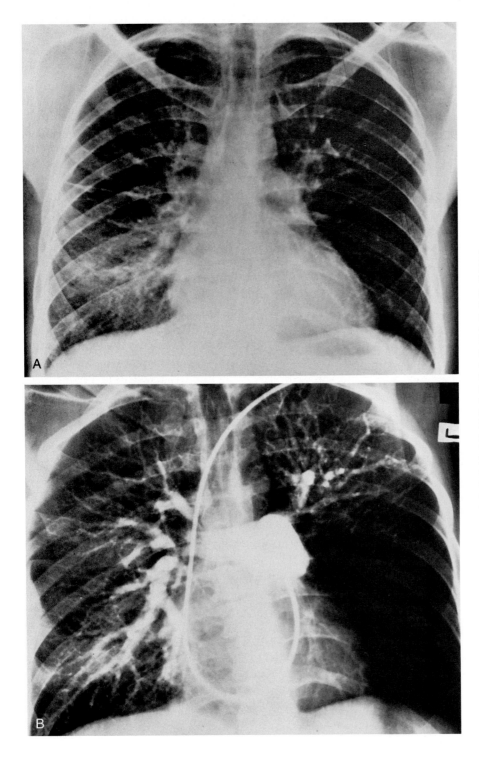

Figure 73–9. Fibrosing Mediastinitis with Encasement of Pulmonary Arteries and Veins. A posteroanterior radiograph *(A)* reveals interstitial edema throughout the right lung and left upper zone. Septal lines are present in the right costophrenic angle. A striking disparity in density of the lower half of the two lungs is observed, the left being radiolucent and oligemic. A pulmonary arteriogram *(B)* shows almost complete occlusion of the left interlobar artery with virtually no perfusion of the left lower lobe and lingula. Although there appears to be good opacification of the arteries of the right lung, the truncus anterior and interlobar arteries show concentric narrowing medial to the hilum. The venous phase of the angiogram is not available, but it is almost certain that the pulmonary veins were affected in the same manner, resulting in venous hypertension and the interstitial edema apparent on the plain radiograph. The cause of the fibrosis was *Histoplasma capsulatum* infection. (Courtesy Dr. M.J. Palayew, Jewish General Hospital, Montreal, Quebec, Canada.)

subsequently extended into continuous lung parenchyma and the retroperitoneal space.[63]

CT is performed almost routinely in the assessment of patients suspected of having fibrosing mediastinitis (Fig. 73–10).[40, 42] It allows excellent evaluation of the extent of mediastinal soft tissue infiltration and assessment of calcification, narrowing of the tracheobronchial tree, and, with the use of intravenous contrast, involvement of the pulmonary arteries, veins, and SVC (Fig. 73–11).[40, 42, 62] In the appropriate clinical context, the presence of a localized mediastinal soft tissue mass with calcification is virtually diagnostic of fibrosing mediastinitis and obviates the need for tissue sampling (Fig. 73–12).[40, 62] However, if the mass is not calcified or if there is clinical or radiologic evidence of disease progression, biopsy may be required to exclude a neoplasm.[40] Fibrosing mediastinitis associated with Riedel's struma can be recognized on CT scans by the continuity of fibrous tissue of the thyroid with the mediastinum (Fig. 73–13).

A number of other studies may be helpful in selected patients. Esophagography (barium swallow) is indicated for the assessment of esophageal obstruction. Extrinsic compression of the esophagus usually involves its supracarinal portion.[68] In one series of 29 patients, esophageal obstruction was present in 4;[61] in all cases, the radiographic appearance was distinguishable from that of carcinoma by the smooth, tapering and funnel-shaped upper and lower borders on barium swallow. Pulmonary angiography may be performed to assess the extent of pulmonary artery narrowing or the presence of pulmonary venous obstruction.[64] Scintigraphy may demonstrate decreased perfusion or, rarely, nonvisualization of one lung.[69]

Magnetic resonance (MR) imaging is comparable to CT in the assessment of tracheal or bronchial involvement and is superior to it in the assessment of vascular involvement; it has the additional advantage of not requiring the use of intravenous contrast material.[70, 71] On MR studies, fibrosing mediastinitis has heterogeneous signal intensity on T1-weighted images and, because of its fibrous content, low signal intensity on T2-weighted images.[71, 72] However, because MR imaging does not allow confident identification of calcification, it plays a limited role in diagnostic evaluation.

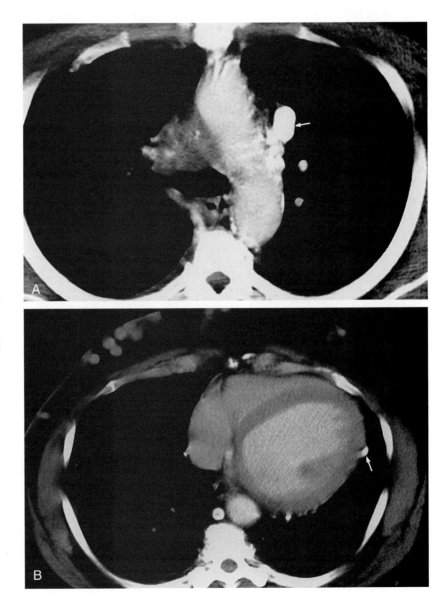

Figure 73–10. Fibrosing Mediastinitis Related to Histoplasmosis. A contrast-enhanced CT scan at the level of the aortic arch *(A)* demonstrates complete obstruction of the superior vena cava (SVC) and collateral venous circulation through the left superior intercostal vein *(arrow)*. Note foci of calcification within the right paratracheal mass consistent with previous histoplasmosis. Calcified mediastinal lymph nodes were present at several levels. A CT scan at a more caudad level *(B)* shows extensive collateral circulation through the left pericardiophrenic vein *(arrow)*, azygos vein, and chest wall veins. (Courtesy of Dr. Robert Tarver, Indiana University Medical Center, Indianapolis.)

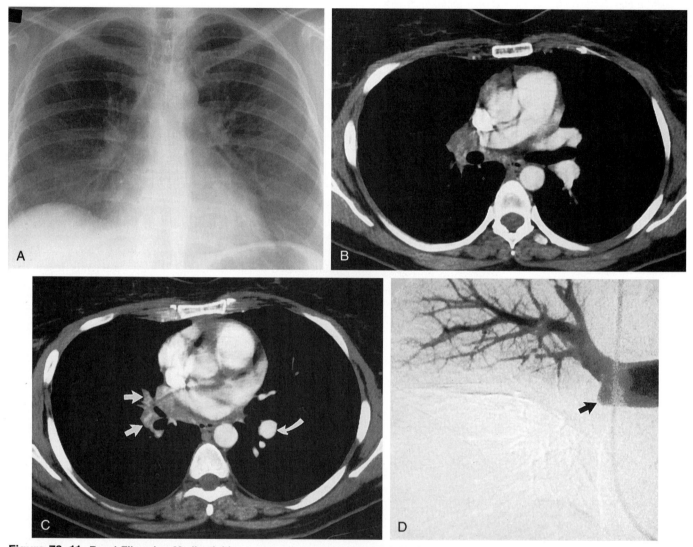

Figure 73–11. Focal Fibrosing Mediastinitis. A posteroanterior chest radiograph *(A)* from a 43-year-old woman who had progressive shortness of breath shows mild enlargement of the right hilum and slightly reduced vascularity of the right lung. Images from CT scans (5-mm collimation) with intravenous contrast enhancement *(B, C)* demonstrate a focal soft tissue mass in the right perihilar region resulting in obstruction of the right interlobular pulmonary artery. Note lack of enhancement of the right lower and middle lobe pulmonary arteries *(straight arrows)* compared with the left lower lobe artery *(curved arrows),* indicating complete vascular occlusion. A selected view of a right pulmonary angiogram *(D)* shows complete obstruction of the right interlobar artery *(arrow)* and normal flow to the right upper lobe. The diagnosis of fibrosing mediastinitis was made at thoracotomy. Extensive fibrosis around the hilum and mediastinum precluded surgical treatment. No etiologic agent was identified.

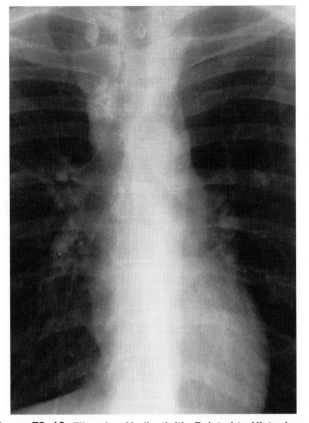

Figure 73–12. Fibrosing Mediastinitis Related to Histoplasmosis. A close-up view of the chest from a posteroanterior radiograph demonstrates enlarged and calcified right paratracheal lymph nodes. The patient presented with superior vena cava syndrome. (Courtesy of Dr. Robert Tarver, Indiana University Medical Center, Indianapolis.)

Clinical Manifestations

Symptoms and signs of fibrosing mediastinitis are quite variable depending on the extent of the fibrosis and the particular structures within the mediastinum that are affected.[73] Involvement of the SVC is probably the most common cause of clinical abnormalities and results in the typical manifestations of the SVC syndrome: giddiness, tinnitus, headache, epistaxis, hemoptysis, cyanosis, and puffiness of the face, neck, and arms.[41] The severity of these symptoms can lessen with time as collateral venous channels are developed.

Obstruction of large central pulmonary veins can cause signs of pulmonary venous hypertension and edema, sometimes associated with pulmonary arterial hypertension; however, the latter also can be caused by direct encroachment on central pulmonary arteries.[74] Such encroachment can result in recurrent, sometimes copious hemoptysis.[75–77] Despite the observation that some cases are of infectious origin, patients are rarely febrile. Additional complications result from involvement of the thoracic duct (chylothorax) and the recurrent laryngeal nerve (hoarseness).[41] Patients who have concomitant retroperitoneal fibrosis can manifest peripheral edema as a result of obstruction of the inferior vena cava or intermittent claudication secondary to aortic compression.

Definitive diagnosis usually requires histologic examination of tissue removed at mediastinoscopy or thoracot-

omy.[78] In addition to routine morphologic examination, such tissue should be cultured for mycobacteria and fungi.

The prognosis is generally good,[42] particularly in patients whose initial complaints can be relieved surgically.[73] In one study of 18 patients, 10 were alive and free of symptoms 5 to 20 years after the initial diagnosis, including three who underwent SVC bypass grafting;[42] six were lost to follow-up, and two died, one of pulmonary carcinoma and the other of Hodgkin's disease.

PNEUMOMEDIASTINUM

Pneumomediastinum (mediastinal emphysema) connotes the presence of gas in the mediastinal space. It is rare in adults and undoubtedly is most common in newborn infants, in whom it has been variously reported as occurring in 1%,[79] 0.5%,[80] and 0.04%.[81] In adults, it occurs predominantly in males during the second and third decades of life.[82]

Etiology and Pathogenesis

Gas within the mediastinum can originate from five sites: the lung, the mediastinal airways, the esophagus, the neck, and the abdominal cavity.[83] Although there is some overlap, the etiology and pathogenesis of pneumomediastinum related to each of these sites are sufficiently distinctive that they can be discussed separately.

Lung Parenchyma. Extension of gas from the air spaces of the pulmonary parenchyma into the interstitial tissues and thence into the mediastinum is the most common pathogenetic mechanism of pneumomediastinum. In most patients, the initial event is probably related to an incident that causes a sudden increase in alveolar pressure, often accompanied by airway narrowing. This results in rupture of alveoli adjacent to airways or to pulmonary arteries or veins; gas then passes into the perivascular or peribronchial interstitium and tracks through the interstitial tissue to the hilum and the mediastinum.[84–86]

Experimental evidence supporting this mechanism has been derived from studies in rabbits, in which the magnitude of tracheal pressure applied by artificial ventilation correlated directly with the frequency of development of perivascular interstitial emphysema;[87] binding the thorax of these animals also decreases the incidence of interstitial emphysema, possibly by limiting the increase in lung volume. The pathway of extension of gas from the lungs into the mediastinum has also been demonstrated in a patient who developed pneumomediastinum while receiving liquid ventilation with perfluorocarbon (PFC).[88] On chest radiographs and on CT scans, the radiopaque PFC could be seen surrounding bronchi and vessels from the lung parenchyma to the hila and extending into the mediastinum, where it surrounded the trachea, aortic arch, and descending aorta and filled the aortopulmonary window.

As well as tracking proximally into the mediastinum, gas can also extend peripherally in the interstitial tissue toward the visceral pleura and rupture into the pleural space to cause pneumothorax. This complication can also result directly from rupture of the mediastinal pleura when sufficient gas accumulates in this compartment. Mediastinal gas

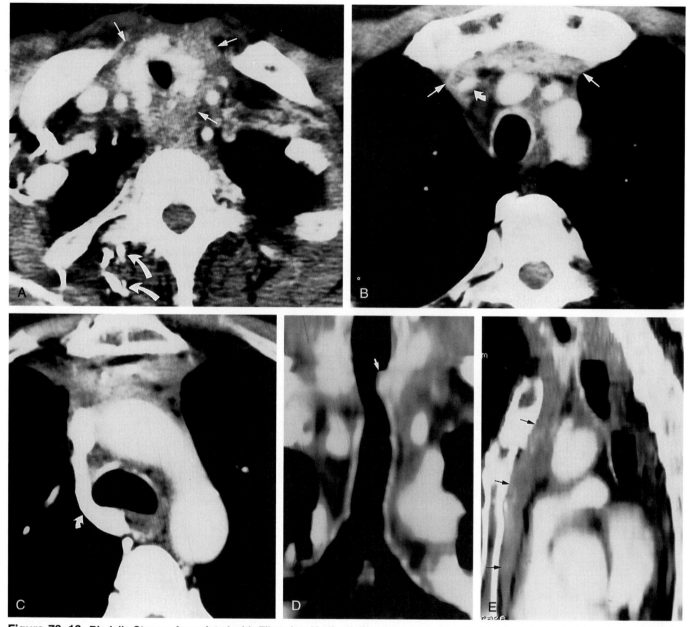

Figure 73–13. Riedel's Struma Associated with Fibrosing Mediastinitis. A contrast-enhanced CT scan at the level of the thoracic inlet *(A)* in a 74-year-old man demonstrates tracheal narrowing and an ill-defined soft tissue density *(straight arrows)* surrounding the thyroid. Note venous collateral circulation *(curved arrows)* in the chest wall. An image at the level of the great vessels *(B)* shows soft tissue *(straight arrows)* in the anterior mediastinum with associated narrowing of the right brachiocephalic vein *(curved arrow)*. An image at the level of the aortic arch *(C)* shows normal diameter of the superior vena cava, with collateral circulation from the azygos vein *(curved arrow)* bypassing the obstruction of the brachiocephalic veins. Coronal reconstruction image *(D)* demonstrates localized tracheal narrowing *(arrow)*; a sagittal reconstruction image *(E)* demonstrates the extent of anterior mediastinal soft tissue infiltration *(arrows)*. Biopsies confirmed the diagnosis of Riedel's struma with associated fibrosing mediastinitis. (Courtesy of Dr. Hiram Nogueira, Vitoria/ES, Brazil.)

may track into the neck, subcutaneous tissues, retroperitoneum, and, rarely, the peritoneal space[89] or spinal canal.[90, 91]

Although many patients who develop pneumomediastinum have no convincing evidence of pulmonary disease, an underlying abnormality is clearly present in some patients and probably constitutes an important contributory factor in the pathogenesis of the condition. For example, alveolar walls can be destroyed as a result of an associated pneumonia,[92–94] thus facilitating the passage of gas from parenchyma to interstitial tissue. Similarly, the bronchiolitis that occurs in conditions such as aspiration and some viral infections[96, 97]

may cause alveolar rupture as a result of check-valve bronchiolar obstruction and a local increase in air-space pressure. A similar mechanism may be responsible for the mediastinal emphysema reported to occur following inhalation of chlorine gas[98] and as a complication of bone marrow transplantation.[99]

In some patients a precipitating event for pneumomediastinum cannot be identified, the diagnosis being made following the discovery of subcutaneous emphysema in the soft tissues of the neck or from a chest radiograph obtained because of retrosternal discomfort;[100] however, in most the development of pneumomediastinum can be clearly related to an incident that results in a sudden rise in alveolar pressure or to a disease process in which such an incident is likely to occur. Such incidents or diseases include the following:

- deep respiratory maneuvers, such as those that occur during strenuous exercise[92, 101] or forced vital capacity breaths[102]
- Valsalva maneuvers, such as those that occur during parturition[103, 104]—a particularly common event associated with pneumomediastinum—or weight-lifting,[105] or during the smoking of marijuana[106] or cocaine[107–109]
- asthma, particularly in children[100, 110, 111] but also in adults[112, 113]
- vomiting of any cause—for example, diabetic acidosis[94, 114–116]
- artificial ventilation, particularly in patients who have obstructive pulmonary disease[117] and in those being maintained on positive end-expiratory pressure (PEEP),[118] in whom the risk of barotrauma is influenced by the maximal distending pressures, mean airway pressure, duration of ventilation, tissue fragility, surfactant depletion, secretion retention, and shear forces[119]
- closed chest trauma, in which shear forces directly disrupt alveolar walls
- a sudden drop in atmospheric pressure, such as occurs during the rapid ascent of a scuba diver or pilot

Mediastinal Airways. Rupture of the trachea or the proximal main bronchi inevitably results in pneumomediastinum. Such rupture is most often caused by trauma, usually accidental but occasionally following diagnostic instrumentation such as bronchoscopic biopsy; bronchoscopy can also result in pneumomediastinum by inducing fits of paroxysmal coughing.[120, 121] Rare cases have been reported in which pneumomediastinum has been associated with tracheal neoplasms.[122]

The Esophagus. As discussed previously, rupture of the esophagus occurs most frequently during episodes of severe vomiting[19, 123, 124] but can also develop as a result of trauma or during labor, a severe asthmatic attack, or strenuous exercise. It must be remembered that each of these events can cause pneumomediastinum in the absence of esophageal injury; because of the almost inevitable development of mediastinitis following esophageal rupture, it is obviously vital to distinguish pneumomediastinum secondary to this injury from that caused by less ominous abnormalities.[19] Occasionally, an esophageal neoplasm perforates into the mediastinum, resulting in pneumomediastinum.

The Neck. Air can track into the mediastinum along deep fascial planes as a result of trauma to the neck or following surgical procedures or dental extraction.[125, 126] In one patient, dental extraction was complicated not only by pneumomediastinum but also by pneumopericardium and pneumoperitoneum.[126]

The Abdominal Cavity. Pneumomediastinum is rarely caused by extension of gas from below the diaphragm, most often from the retroperitoneal space following perforation of a hollow abdominal viscus.[127] The reverse can also be true: pneumoperitoneum can occur as a result of progressive massive tension pneumomediastinum, the latter characteristically located both anterior and posterior to the heart;[89] in this situation, the gas may reach the extraperitoneal space via the internal mammary vessels enclosed between the sternocostal origins of the diaphragm.[128]

Pathologic Characteristics

Air within the mediastinum engenders an inflammatory reaction associated with relatively numerous eosinophils, similar to that seen in the pleura in association with pneumothorax.[129]

Radiologic Manifestations

The radiographic manifestations of pneumomediastinum consist of lucent streaks or focal bubble-like or larger collections of gas outlining the mediastinal structures.[105] In posteroanterior projection, the mediastinal pleura is seen to be displaced laterally, creating a longitudinal line shadow parallel to the heart border and separated from the heart by gas. This shadow is usually more evident on the left side (Fig. 73–14). A longitudinal gas shadow also may be identified adjacent to the thoracic aorta and around the pulmonary artery ("ring-around-the-artery" sign) (Fig. 73–15).[130] It should be noted, however, that a thin line of radiolucency can be frequently identified along the border of the heart and aortic arch. This line should not be confused with pneumomediastinum: the lateral margin of this radiolucency consists of pulmonary parenchyma rather than displaced pleura and thus represents a Mach band rather than pneumomediastinum.[131]

In some cases, pneumomediastinum is more readily identified on the lateral radiograph as lucent streaks that outline the ascending aorta, aortic arch, and pulmonary arteries.[105] Gas may also outline the sternal insertions of the diaphragm, the thymus, and the brachiocephalic veins.[83] Occasionally, the only radiographic manifestation consists of substernal gas anterior to the heart, a finding that can be seen only on the lateral radiograph.[105]

In some cases, gas from a pneumomediastinum extends between the parietal pleura and the diaphragm, or between the parietal pleura and the extrapleural tissues at the lung apex.[79, 105] Although such extrapleural gas can resemble a pneumothorax, it does not shift on radiographs exposed with the patient in different body positions.[105] Furthermore, the pleural line in this situation is not smooth, as in pneumothorax, but tends to be irregular as a result of tethering of the parietal pleural by overlying fascia.[105] This tethering is more readily detected on the CT scan than on the radiograph.[105] When the gas extends between the parietal pleura and the medial portion of the left hemidiaphragm and also outlines the descending aorta, it has a configuration that resembles a V—a finding known as the V sign of Naclerio.[105, 132]

When gas becomes interposed between the heart and diaphragm, it permits identification of the central portion of the diaphragm in continuity with the lateral portions, a finding known as the "continuous diaphragm sign" (Fig. 73–16).[133] In theory, gas within the pericardial sac should also permit visualization of the central portion of the diaphragm; however, pneumopericardium is almost always associated with pericardial fluid, thus leading to obliteration of the central portion of the diaphragm, at least on radiographs exposed with the patient in the erect position.[133] When it is

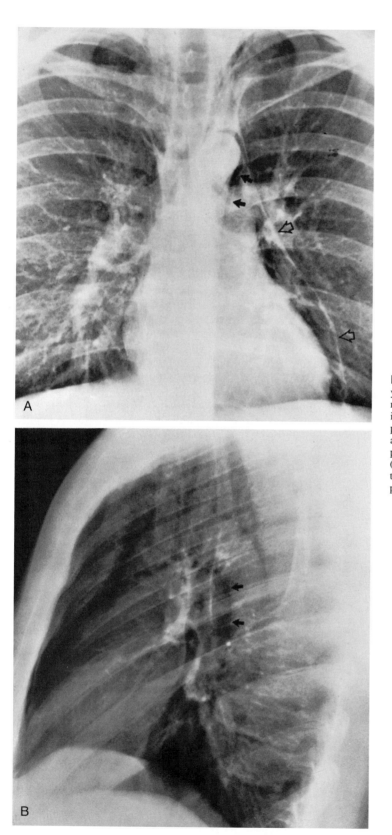

Figure 73–14. Spontaneous Pneumomediastinum. A 20-year-old man noted an abrupt onset of severe retrosternal pain. In a radiographic study performed shortly thereafter, a view of the chest in posteroanterior *(A)* projection reveals a long linear opacity roughly paralleling the left heart border *(open arrows),* representing the laterally displaced mediastinal pleura. In addition, considerable gas is present around the aortic arch and proximal descending thoracic aorta *(solid arrows* in both projections). In the lateral projection *(B),* note the gas outlining the anterior surface of the heart and the brachiocephalic vessels.

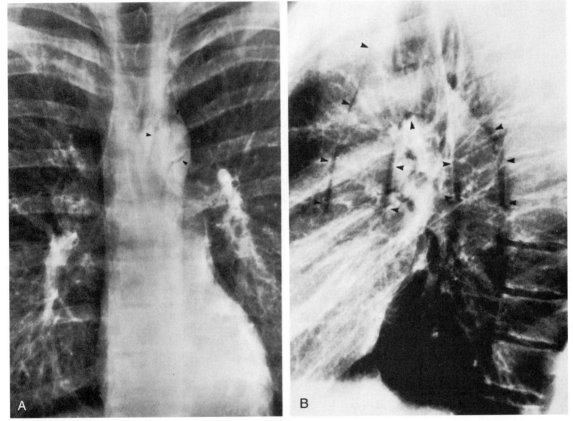

Figure 73–15. Spontaneous Pneumomediastinum. Posteroanterior *(A)* and lateral *(B)* radiographs reveal linear and curvilinear shadows of air density outlining almost all portions of the aortic arch in both projections *(arrowheads)*. In the lateral projection, the gas outlining the anterior wall of the ascending aorta extends superiorly and relates to the right innominate artery. The patient was a 20-year-old man; radiographs were exposed shortly after the abrupt onset of retrosternal chest pain. The underlying cause was not established.

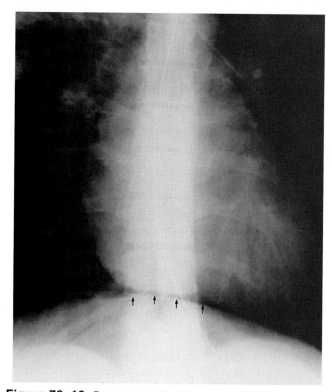

Figure 73–16. Pneumomediastinum with Continuous Diaphragm Sign. An anteroposterior chest radiograph in a 58-year-old woman demonstrates pneumomediastinum outlining the central portion of the diaphragm *(arrows)*, a finding known as the "continuous diaphragm sign." The pneumomediastinum was secondary to barotrauma related to mechanical ventilation instituted for ARDS.

not certain whether a collection of gas is within the pericardial sac or the mediastinal space, differentiation is readily established by demonstrating a change in the position of the gas in the pericardial sac on radiographs exposed with the patient in different body positions.[134] Occasionally, gas extends from the mediastinum into the extrapleural interstitial tissue in the paravertebral space or into the spinal canal

(pneumorrhachis) leading to spinal epidural emphysema (Fig. 73–17).[134a, b]

Sometimes air within the interstitial tissues of the lung ("interstitial emphysema") can be detected radiographically. Because gas in the interstitial tissues of otherwise normal lung should not be apparent because of lack of contrast, its identification requires the presence of disease in contiguous parenchyma, a feature of particular note in patients who have the adult respiratory distress syndrome. The radiographic findings include focal lucent areas giving a mottled or stippled appearance to the parenchyma, lucent bands, perivascular lucencies, and subpleural and parenchymal cysts.[135] Although these findings are often difficult to identify on radiographs, they can be readily seen on CT scans.[136] On CT scans, air also may be seen to extend along the peribronchovascular interstitium into the mediastinum (Fig. 73–18).

Pneumomediastinum resulting from either traumatic or spontaneous rupture of the esophagus is associated in many cases with hydrothorax or hydropneumothorax, usually on the left[20] but sometimes bilaterally or on the right.[25]

Clinical Manifestations

Whatever the cause of pneumomediastinum, when sufficient gas accumulates, pressure can build up and impede blood flow, particularly in low-pressure veins. Such a build-up of pressure occurs only when gas is prevented from passing into the neck—a situation particularly likely to occur in neonates. Respiratory embarrassment can also occur with the presence of large amounts of gas in the pulmonary interstitial space, which decreases pulmonary compliance.[84, 85] More frequently—and almost invariably in adults—air escapes from the mediastinum by way of the fascial planes of the great vessels into the neck and anterior chest wall, thus producing subcutaneous emphysema.

Symptoms and signs depend largely on the amount of air in the mediastinal space and on the presence or absence of associated infection. The diagnosis may be suggested by a history of abrupt onset of retrosternal pain radiating to the

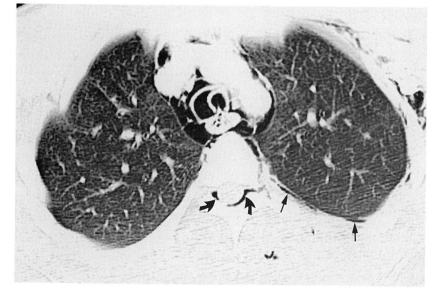

Figure 73–17. Pneumorrhachis Associated with Traumatic Pneumomediastinum. An 18-year-old man developed extensive pneumomediastinum following a snowmobile accident. A CT scan demonstrates extrapleural extension *(straight arrows)* of the pneumomediastinum and extension into the spinal canal *(curved arrows)*. Subcutaneous emphysema is also evident.

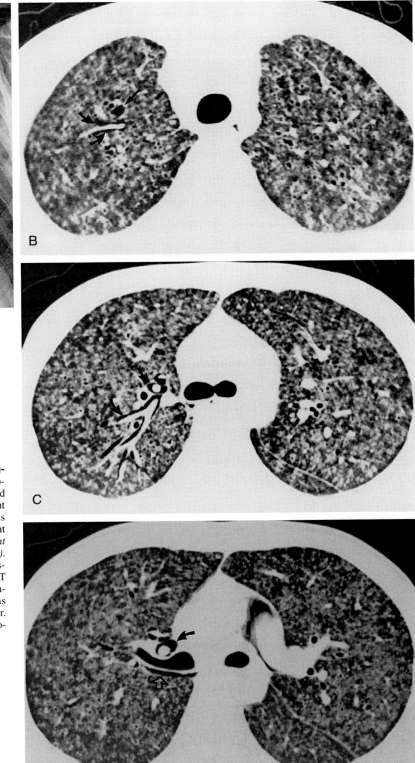

Figure 73–18. Interstitial Emphysema and Pneumomediastinum in Miliary Tuberculosis. An anteroposterior chest radiograph *(A)* in a 21-year-old man who had miliary tuberculosis demonstrates focal lucencies in the right upper lobe *(arrows)*, pneumomediastinum, and subcutaneous emphysema. HRCT scan in the region of the apical segment of the right upper lobe *(B)* shows focal lucency *(straight arrow)* and perivascular dissection of gas *(curved arrows)*. HRCT scan at a more caudad level *(C)* demonstrates perivascular gas *(curved arrows)* and pneumomediastinum. HRCT scan at the level of the right upper lobe bronchus *(D)* demonstrates peribronchial *(open arrow)* and perivascular gas *(curved arrow)* and pneumomediastinum. (Courtesy of Dr. Kun-Il Kim, Pusan National University Hospital, Pusan, Korea.)

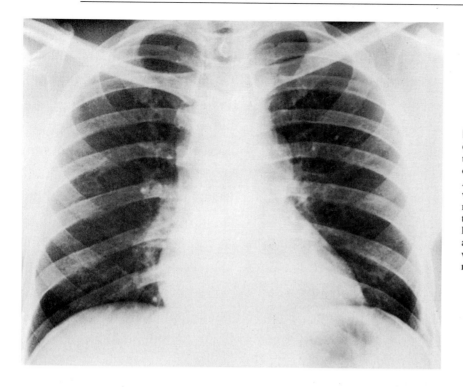

Figure 73–19. Spontaneous Mediastinal Hemorrhage. A 35-year-old hemophiliac was admitted to the hospital with evidence of recent extrathoracic hemorrhage. He had no symptoms referable to the thorax. A posteroanterior radiograph demonstrates bilateral widening of the mediastinum by a process whose lateral margins are somewhat lobulated. Involvement appears to be chiefly of the mid-mediastinal compartment. (A lateral radiograph was not helpful in localizing the abnormality.) The lesion resolved completely in 10 days without residua and was assumed to represent a spontaneous hematoma.

shoulders and down both arms, usually preceded by an event that resulted in excessive increase in intrathoracic pressure, such as a spasm of coughing, sneezing, or vomiting. The pain usually is aggravated by respiration and sometimes is worsened by swallowing. Dyspnea may be severe. Physical examination generally reveals the presence of air in the subcutaneous tissues of the neck or over the thoracic wall. Hamman's sign may be detected on auscultation over the apex of the heart. This sign, consisting of a crunching or clicking noise synchronous with the heart beat, has been estimated to occur in approximately 50% of cases; the noise is heard best when the patient is in the left lateral decubitus position.[20] Although characteristic of the condition, the sign is by no means pathognomonic.

Patients in whom air does not freely escape from the mediastinum into the neck may have engorged neck veins, a rapid, thready pulse, and significant systemic hypotension.

MEDIASTINAL HEMORRHAGE

The majority of cases of mediastinal hemorrhage result from trauma, usually of a severe nature such as that associated with an automobile accident[137–139] or vigorous cardiopulmonary resuscitation. The majority of cases result from venous bleeding.[16, 137, 139, 140] Less common causes of mediastinal hemorrhage include perforation of a vein by faulty insertion of a central venous line and migration of a central venous catheter,[16] rupture of an aortic aneurysm,[95, 141] and spontaneous hemorrhage in patients who have mediastinal tumors[142] or a coagulopathy,[142, 143] or who are undergoing chronic hemodialysis.[144] Rare causes include a sudden increase in intrathoracic pressure from sneezing, vomiting, or severe cough;[145, 146] radiation therapy;[143] and intracoronary infusion of streptokinase for coronary thrombosis.[147]

Radiologically, hemorrhage typically results in uniform,

symmetric widening of the mediastinum.[148] Local accumulation of blood in the form of a hematoma is manifested by a homogeneous mass that can project to one or both sides of the mediastinum and may be situated in any compartment (Fig. 73–19).[16, 148, 149] Hemorrhage resulting from nontraumatic rupture of the aorta often results in obscuration or a convex appearance of the aortopulmonary window and displacement of the left paraspinal interface.[95] Dissection of blood from the mediastinum in the peribronchovascular interstitial tissue can result in a radiographic pattern that simulates interstitial edema.[150] When mediastinal hemorrhage is caused by a ruptured aorta, the blood also may

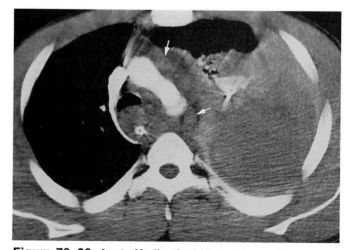

Figure 73–20. Acute Mediastinal Hemorrhage. A contrast-enhanced CT scan in a 30-year-old man demonstrates inhomogeneous areas of increased attenuation *(arrows)* in the mediastinum as a result of hemorrhage. A large left hemothorax with shift of the mediastinum to the right is also evident. A left chest tube is in place. The findings were related to traumatic tear of the aorta following a motor vehicle accident.

extend into a pleural space, usually the left only but sometimes the right as well.[139, 151]

CT is superior to plain radiography in demonstrating both the presence of mediastinal hemorrhage and the underlying cause.[138–141] Approximately 90% of acute hematomas are associated with localized areas of high attenuation as a result of the high attenuation of clotted blood (Fig. 73–20).[152, 153] These areas persist for about 72 hours; the high attenuation then gradually decreases to values similar to those for fluid secondary to lysis of the hemoglobin.[153]

The majority of cases of mediastinal hemorrhage are probably unrecognized, the amount of bleeding being insufficient to produce symptoms and signs. Retrosternal pain radiating into the back develops in some patients. Hemorrhage related to a coagulation disorder may be suspected if local symptoms are associated with evidence of bleeding elsewhere, such as into the skin or retropharyngeal space. Rarely, trauma may precipitate mediastinal hemorrhage in a person with a bleeding disorder, as reported in the case of a hemophiliac who sustained minor chest injury.[154] Hemorrhage related to a dissecting aneurysm may be associated with decreased pulsation in the arteries of the extremities. A hematoma of sufficient size and appropriate location can compress the superior vena cava.[155, 156]

REFERENCES

1. Goldstein LA, Thompson WR: Esophageal perforation: A 15 year experience. Am J Surg 143:495, 1982.
2. Burnett CM, Rosemurgy AS, Pfeiffer EA: Life-threatening acute posterior mediastinitis due to esophageal perforation. Ann Thorac Surg 49:979, 1990.
3. Larson TC III, Shuman LS, Libshitz HI, et al: Complications of colonic interposition. Cancer 56:681, 1985.
4. Carrol CL, Jeffrey B Jr, Federle MP, et al: CT evaluation of mediastinal infections. J Comput Assist Tomogr 11:449, 1987.
5. Loop FD, Lytle BW, Cosgrove DM, et al: Sternal wound complications after isolated coronary artery bypass grafting: Early and late mortality, morbidity and cost of care. Ann Surg 49:179, 1990.
6. El Oakley RM, Wright JE: Postoperative mediastinitis: Classification and management. Ann Thorac Surg 61:1030, 1996.
7. Levine TM, Wurster CF, Krespi YP: Mediastinitis occurring as a complication of odontogenic infections. Laryngoscope 96:747, 1986.
8. Laiwani AK, Kaplan MJ: Mediastinal and thoracic complications of necrotizing fasciitis of the head and neck. Head Neck 13:531, 1991.
9. Becker M, Zbären P, Hermans R, et al: Necrotizing fasciitis of the head and neck: Role of CT in diagnosis and management. Radiology 202:471, 1997.
10. Watanabe M, Ohshika Y, Aoki T, et al: Empyema and mediastinitis complicating retropharyngeal abscess. Thorax 49:1179, 1994.
11. Pollack MS: Staphylococcal mediastinitis due to sternoclavicular pyarthrosis: CT appearance. J Comput Assist Tomogr 14:924, 1990.
12. Breatnach E, Nath PH, Delany DJ: The role of computed tomography in acute and subacute mediastinitis. Clin Radiol 37:139, 1986.
13. Kushihashi T, Munechika H, Motoya H: CT and MR findings in tuberculous mediastinitis. J Comput Assist Tomogr 19:379, 1995.
14. Swensen SJ, Aughenbaugh GL, Brown LR: Chest case of the day. Am J Roentgenol 160:1318, 1993.
15. Körösj A, Halász G: Acute mediastinitis as a complication of bronchoscopy. Tuberkulózis 14:15, 1961.
16. Tocino IM, Miller MH: Mediastinal trauma and other acute mediastinal conditions. J Thorac Imag 2:79, 1987.
17. LaBerge JM, Kerlan RK Jr, Pogany AC, et al: Esophageal rupture: Complication of balloon dilatation. Radiology 157:56, 1985.
18. Chavy AL, Rougier M, Pieddeloup C, et al: Esophageal prosthesis for neoplastic stenosis. A prognostic study of 77 cases. Cancer 57:1426, 1986.
19. Rogers LF, Puig AW, Dooley BN, et al: Diagnostic considerations in mediastinal emphysema: A pathophysiologic-roentgenologic approach to Boerhaave's syndrome and spontaneous pneumomediastinum. Am J Roentgenol 115:495, 1972.
20. Gray JM, Hanson GC: Mediastinal emphysema: Aetiology, diagnosis, and treatment. Thorax 21:325, 1966.
21. Jenkins IR, Raymond R: Boerhaave's syndrome complicated by a large bronchopleural fistula. Chest 105:964, 1994.
22. Ivert T, Lindblom D, Sahni J, et al: Management of deep sternal wound infection after cardiac surgery: Hanuman syndrome. Scand J Cardiovasc Surg 25:111, 1991.
23. Karwande SV, Renlund DG, Oslen SL, et al: Mediastinitis in heart transplantation. Ann Thorac Surg 54:1039, 1992.
24. Zacharias A, Habib RH: Factors predisposing to median sternotomy complications: Deep vs superficial infection. Ann Thorac Surg 110:1173, 1996.
25. Christoforidis A, Nelson SW: Spontaneous rupture of the esophagus with emphasis on the roentgenologic diagnosis. Am J Roentgenol 78:574, 1957.
26. Appleton DS, Sandrasagra FA, Flower CDR: Perforated oesophagus: Review of twenty-eight consecutive cases. Clin Radiol 30:493, 1979.
27. Han SY, McElvein RB, Aldrete JS, et al: Perforation of the esophagus: Correlation of site and cause with plain film findings. Am J Roentgenol 145:537, 1985.
28. Gollub MJ, Bains MS: Barium sulfate: A new (old) contrast agent for diagnosis of postoperative esophageal leaks. Radiology 202:360, 1997.
29. Dodds WJ, Stewart ET, Vlymen WJ: Appropriate contrast media for evaluation of esophageal disruption. Radiology 144:439, 1982.
30. Reich SB: Production of pulmonary edema by aspiration of water-soluble nonabsorbable contrast media. Radiology 92:367, 1969.
31. Gobien RP, Stanley JH, Gobien BS, et al: Percutaneous catheter aspiration and draining of suspected mediastinal abscesses. Radiology 151:69, 1984.
32. Backer CL, LoCicero JD, Hartz RS, et al: Computed tomography in patients with esophageal perforation. Chest 98:1078, 1990.
33. White CS, Templeton PA, Attar S: Esophageal perforation: CT findings. Am J Roentgenol 160:767, 1993.
34. Lee S, Mergo PJ, Ros PR: The leaking esophagus: CT patterns of esophageal rupture, perforation, and fistulization. Crit Rev Diagn Imaging 37:461, 1996.
35. Eriksen KR: Oesophageal fistula diagnosed by microscopic examination of pleural fluid. Acta Chir Scand 128:771, 1964.
36. Wechsler RJ, Steiner RM, Goodman LR, et al: Iatrogenic esophageal-pleural fistula: Subtlety of diagnosis in the absence of mediastinitis. Radiology 144:239, 1982.
37. Craddock DR, Logan A, Mayell M: Traumatic rupture of the oesophagus and stomach. Thorax 23:657, 1968.
38. Lloyd JE, Tillman BF, Atkinson JB, et al: Mediastinal fibrosis complicating histoplasmosis. Medicine 67:295, 1988.
39. Rubin SA, Winer-Muram HT: Thoracic histoplasmosis. J Thorac Imaging 7:39, 1992.
40. Sherrick AD, Brown LR, Harms GF, et al: The radiographic findings of fibrosing mediastinitis. Chest 106:484, 1994.
41. Schowengerdt CG, Suyemoto R, Main FB: Granulomatous and fibrous mediastinitis—a review and analysis of 180 cases. J Thorac Cardiovasc Surg 57:365, 1969.
42. Mole TM, Glober J, Sheppard MN: Sclerosing mediastinitis: A report on 18 cases. Thorax 50:280, 1995.
43. Cohen DM, Goggans EA: Sclerosing mediastinitis and terminal valvular endocarditis caused by fungus suggestive of Aspergillus species. Am J Clin Pathol 56:91, 1971.
44. Ahmad M, Weinstein AJ, Hughes JA, et al: Granulomatous mediastinitis due to Aspergillus flavus in a nonimmunosuppressed patient. Am J Med 70:887, 1981.
45. Leong ASY: Granulomatous mediastinitis due to Rhizopus species. Am J Clin Pathol 70:103, 1978.
46. Lagerstrom CF, Mitchell HG, Graham BS, et al: Chronic fibrosing mediastinitis and superior vena caval obstruction from blastomycosis. Ann Thorac Surg 54:764, 1992.
47. Hoffman-Wellenhof R, Domej W, Schmid C, et al: Mediastinal mass caused by syphilitic aortitis. Thorax 48:568, 1993.
48. Dines DE, Payne WS, Bernatz PE, et al: Mediastinal granuloma and fibrosing mediastinitis. Chest 75:320, 1979.
49. Loyd JE, Tillman BF, Atkinson JB, et al: Mediastinal fibrosis complicating histoplasmosis. Medicine 67:295, 1988.
50. Gurney JW, Conces DJ Jr: Pulmonary histoplasmosis. Radiology 199:297, 1996.
51. Dozois RR, Bernatz PE, Woolner LB, et al: Sclerosing mediastinitis involving major bronchi. Mayo Clin Proc 43:557, 1968.
52. Cameron DD, Ing ST, Boyle M, et al: Idiopathic mediastinal and retroperitoneal fibrosis. Can Med Assoc J 85:227, 1961.
53. Comings DE, Skubi K-B, Eyes JV, et al: Familial multifocal fibrosclerosis. Findings suggesting that retroperitoneal fibrosis, mediastinal fibrosis, sclerosing cholangitis, Riedel's thyroiditis, and pseudotumor of the orbit may be different manifestations of a single disease. Ann Intern Med 66:884, 1967.
54. DuPont HL, Varco RL, Winchell CP: Chronic fibrous mediastinitis simulating pulmonic stenosis, associated with inflammatory pseudotumor of the orbit. Am J Med 44:447, 1968.
55. Graham JR, Suby HI, LeCompte PR, et al: Fibrotic disorders associated with methysergide therapy for headache. N Engl J Med 274:359, 1966.
56. Crotty TB, Colby TV, Gay PC, et al: Desmoplastic malignant mesothelioma masquerading as sclerosing mediastinitis: A diagnostic dilemma. Hum Pathol 23:79, 1992.
57. Flannery MT, Espino M, Altus P, et al: Hodgkin's disease masquerading as sclerosing mediastinitis. South Med J 87:921, 1994.
58. Andrews EC Jr: Five cases of an undescribed form of pulmonary interstitial fibrosis caused by obstruction of the pulmonary veins. Bull Johns Hopkins Hosp 100:28, 1957.
59. Katzenstein ALA, Mazur MT: Pulmonary infarct: An unusual manifestation of fibrosing mediastinitis. Chest 77:521, 1980.
60. Sobrinho-Simões MA, Vaz Saleiro J, Wagenvoort CA: Mediastinal and hilar fibrosis. Histopathology 5:53, 1981.
61. Feigin DS, Eggleston JC, Siegelman SS: The multiple roentgen manifestations of sclerosing mediastinitis. Johns Hopkins Med J 144:1, 1979.
62. Weinstein JB, Aronberg DJ, Sagel SS: CT of fibrosing mediastinitis: Findings and their utility. Am J Roentgenol 141:247, 1983.
63. Kountz PD, Molina PL, Sagel S: Fibrosing mediastinitis in the posterior thorax. Am J Roentgenol 153:489, 1989.
64. Dunn EJ, Ulicny KS Jr, Wright CB, et al: Surgical implication of sclerosing mediastinitis: A report of six cases and review of the literature. Chest 97:338, 1990.
65. Morrison G: Retroperitoneal fibrosis associated with methysergide therapy. J Can Assoc Radiol 19:61, 1968.
66. Wieder S, White TJ III, Salazar J, et al: Pulmonary artery occlusion due to histoplasmosis. Am J Roentgenol 138:243, 1982.
67. Mendelson EB, Mintzer RA, Hidvegi DF: Veno-occlusive pulmonary infarct: An unusual complication of fibrosing mediastinitis. Am J Roentgenol 141:175, 1983.
68. Ramakantan R, Shah P: Dysphagia due to mediastinal fibrosis in advanced pulmonary tuberculosis. Am J Roentgenol 154:61, 1990.
69. Mallin WH, Silberstein EB, Shipley RT, et al: Fibrosing mediastinitis causing nonvisualization of one lung on pulmonary scintigraphy. Clin Nuc Med 18:594, 1993.
70. Farmer DW, Moore E, Amparo E, et al: Calcific fibrosing mediastinitis: Demonstration of pulmonary vascular obstruction by magnetic resonance imaging. Am J Roentgenol 143:1189, 1984.
71. Rholl KS, Levitt RG, Glazer HS: Magnetic resonance imaging of fibrosing mediastinitis. Am J Roentgenol 145:255, 1985.
72. Williams SM, Jones ET: General case of the day. RadioGraphics 17:1324, 1997.
73. Mathisen DJ, Grillo HC: Clinical manifestation of mediastinal fibrosis and histoplasmosis. Ann Thorac Surg 54:1053, 1992.
74. Arnett N, Bacos JM, Macher AM, et al: Fibrosing mediastinitis causing arterial hypertension without pulmonary venous hypertension. Clinical and necropsy observations. Am J Med 63:634, 1977.
75. Dye TE, Saab SB, Almond CH, et al: Sclerosing mediastinitis with occlusion of

pulmonary veins. Manifestations and management. J Thorac Cardiovasc Surg 74:137, 1977.

76. Hicks GL Jr: Fibrosing mediastinitis causing pulmonary artery and vein obstruction with hemoptysis. N Y State J Med 83:242, 1983.
77. Shin MS, Fulmer JD, Ho KJ: Bilateral hilar enlargement and hypoperfusion of the right lower lobe. Chest 90:120, 1986.
78. Wieder S, Rabinowitz JG: Fibrous mediastinitis: A late manifestation of mediastinal histoplasmosis. Radiology 125:305, 1977.
79. Lillard RL, Allen RP: The extrapleural air sign in pneumomediastinum. Radiology 85:1093, 1965.
80. Emery JL: Interstitial emphysema, pneumothorax, and "air-block" in the newborn. Lancet 1:405, 1956.
81. Chasler CN: Pneumothorax and pneumomediastinum in the newborn. Am J Roentgenol 91:550, 1964.
82. Bodey GP: Medical mediastinal emphysema. Ann Intern Med 54:46, 1961.
83. Cyrlak D, Milne EN, Imray TJ: Pneumomediastinum: A diagnostic problem. Crit Rev Diagn Imaging 23(1):75, 1984.
84. Macklin MT, Macklin CC: Malignant interstitial emphysema of the lungs and mediastinum as an important occult complication in many respiratory diseases and other conditions. An interpretation of the clinical literature in the light of laboratory experiment. Medicine 23:281, 1944.
85. Macklin CC: Pneumothorax with massive collapse from experimental local overinflation of the lung substance. Can Med Assoc J 36:414, 1937.
86. Rouby JJ, Lherm T, deLassale EM, et al: Histologic aspects of pulmonary barotrauma in critically ill patients with acute respiratory failure. Intensive Care Med 19:383, 1993.
87. Caldwell EJ, Powell RD Jr, Mullooly JP: Interstitial emphysema: A study of physiologic factors involved in the experimental induction of the lesion. Am Rev Respir Dis 102:516, 1970.
88. Jamadar DA, Kazerooni EA, Hirschl RB: Pneumomediastinum: Elucidation of the anatomic pathway by liquid ventilation. J Comput Assist Tomogr 20:309, 1996.
89. Campbell RE, Boggs TR Jr, Kirkpatrick JA: Early neonatal pneumoperitoneum from progressive massive tension pneumomediastinum. Radiology 114:121, 1975.
90. Kakitsubata Y, Inatsu H, Kakitsubata S, et al: CT manifestations of intraspinal air associated with pneumomediastinum. Acta Radiol 35:305, 1994.
91. Drevelengas A, Kalaitzoglou I, Petridis A: Pneumorrhachis associated with spontaneous pneumomediastinum. Eur J Radiol 18:122, 1994.
92. Millard CE: Pneumomediastinum. Dis Chest 56:297, 1969.
93. Grieve NWT, Bird DRH, Collyer AJ, et al: Pneumomediastinum and diabetic hyperpnoea. BMJ 1:186, 1969.
94. McNicholl B, Murray JP, Egan B: Pneumomediastinum and diabetic hyperpnoea. BMJ 4:493, 1968.
95. Fultz PJ, Melville D, Ekanej A, et al: Nontraumatic rupture of the thoracic aorta: Chest radiographic features of an often unrecognized condition. Am J Roentgenol 171:351, 1998.
96. Gilmartin D: Mediastinal emphysema in Melbourne children: With particular reference to measles and giant-cell pneumonia. Australas Radiol 15:27, 1971.
97. Yalaburgi SB: Subcutaneous and mediastinal emphysema following respiratory tract complications in measles. S Afr Med J 58:521, 1980.
98. Gapany-Gapanavicius M, Yellin A, Almog S, et al: Pneumomediastinum: A complication of chlorine exposure from mixing household cleaning agents. JAMA 248:349, 1982.
99. Hill G, Helenglass G, Powles R, et al: Mediastinal emphysema in marrow transplant recipients. Bone Marrow Transplant 2:315, 1987.
100. Munsell WP: Pneumomediastinum: A report of 28 cases and review of the literature. JAMA 202:689, 1967.
101. Morgan EJ, Henderson DA: Pneumomediastinum as a complication of athletic competition. Thorax 36:155, 1981.
102. Varkey B, Kory RC: Mediastinal and subcutaneous emphysema following pulmonary function tests. Am Rev Respir Dis 108:1393, 1973.
103. Karson EM, Saltzman D, Davis MR: Pneumomediastinum in pregnancy: Two case reports and a review of the literature, pathophysiology, and management. Obstet Gynecol 64(3 Suppl):395, 1984.
104. Dudley DK, Patten DE: Intrapartum pneumomediastinum associated with subcutaneous emphysema. Can Med Assoc J 139:641, 1988.
105. Bejvan SM, Godwin JD: Pneumomediastinum: Old signs and new signs. Am J Roentgenol 166:1041, 1996.
106. Miller WE, Spiekerman RE, Hepper NG: Pneumomediastinum resulting from performing Valsalva maneuvers during marihuana smoking. Chest 62:233, 1972.
107. Shesser R, Davis C, Edelstein S: Pneumomediastinum and pneumothorax after inhaling alkaloid cocaine. Ann Emerg Med 10:213, 1981.
108. Aroesty DJ, Stanley RB, Crockett DM: Pneumomediastinum and cervical emphysema from inhalation of "free based" cocaine: Report of three cases. Laryngol Head Neck Surg 94:372, 1986.
109. Eurman DW, Potash HI, Eyler WR, et al: Chest pain and dyspnea related to "crack" cocaine smoking: Value of chest radiography. Radiology 172:459, 1989.
110. Kirsh MM, Orvald TO: Mediastinal and subcutaneous emphysema complicating acute bronchial asthma. Chest 57:580, 1970.
111. Payne TW, Geppert LJ: Mediastinal and subcutaneous emphysema complicating bronchial asthma in a nine-year-old male. J Allergy 32:135, 1961.
112. Dines DE, Peters GA: Mediastinal emphysema complicating acute asthma—Report of two cases. Minn Med 50:341, 1967.
113. Dattwyler RJ, Goldman MA, Bloch KJ: Pneumomediastinum as a complication of asthma in teenage and young adult patients. J Allergy Clin Immunol 63:412, 1979.

114. Beigelman PM, Miller LV, Martin HE: Mediastinal and subcutaneous emphysema in diabetic coma with vomiting, report of four cases. JAMA 208:2315, 1969.
115. Girard DE, Carlson V, Natelson EA, et al: Pneumomediastinum in diabetic ketoacidosis: Comments on mechanism, incidence, and management. Chest 60:455, 1971.
116. Ruttley M, Mills RA: Subcutaneous emphysema and pneumomediastinum in diabetic ketoacidosis. Br J Radiol 44:672, 1971.
117. Rohlfing BM, Webb WR, Schlobohm RM: Ventilator-related extra-alveolar air in adults. Radiology 121:25, 1976.
118. Altman AR, Johnson TH: Pneumoperitoneum and pneumoretroperitoneum. Consequences of positive end-expiratory pressure therapy. Arch Surg 114:208, 1979.
119. Marcy TW: Barotrauma: Detection, recognition, and management. Chest 104:578, 1993.
120. Tsai SH, Cohen SS, Fenger EPK: Bronchial perforation as a complication of bronchoscopy. Am Rev Tuberc 78:106, 1958.
121. Armen RN, Morrow CS, Sewell S: Mediastinal emphysema: A complication of bronchoscopy. Ann Intern Med 48:1083, 1958.
122. Darch GH: Tracheal neoplasms presenting with mediastinal emphysema. Br J Dis Chest 56:212, 1962.
123. Härmä RA, Koskinen YO, Suukari SO: Spontaneous rupture of the oesophagus. Endoscopic treatment in the primary stage. Thorax 23:210, 1968.
124. Marston EL, Valk HL: Spontaneous perforation of the esophagus: Review of the literature and report of a case. Ann Intern Med 51:590, 1959.
125. Tomsick TA: Dental surgical subcutaneous and mediastinal emphysema: A case report. J Can Assoc Radiol 25:49, 1974.
126. Sandler CM, Libshitz HI, Marks G: Pneumoperitoneum, pneumomediastinum and pneumopericardium following dental extraction. Radiology 115:539, 1975.
127. Thorsøe H: Mediastinal emphysema due to perforation of the intestinal tract. Nord Med 59:286, 1958.
128. Kleinman PK, Brill PW, Whalen JP: Anterior pathway for transdiaphragmatic extension of pneumomediastinum. Am J Roentgenol 131:271, 1978.
129. Halîĉek F, Rosai J: Histioeosinophilic granulomas in the thymuses of 29 myasthenic patients. A complication of pneumomediastinum. Hum Pathol 15:1137, 1984.
130. Landay MJ, Cohen DJ, Deaton CW Jr: Another look at the "ring-around-the-artery" in pneumomediastinum. J Can Assoc Radiol 36:343, 1985.
131. Friedman AC, Lautin EM, Rothenberg L: Mach bands and pneumomediastinum. J Can Assoc Radiol 32:232, 1981.
132. Naclerio E: The "V" sign in the diagnosis of spontaneous rupture of the esophagus (an early roentgen clue). Am J Surg 93:291, 1957.
133. Levin B: The continuous diaphragm sign. A newly recognized sign of pneumomediastinum. Clin Radiol 24:337, 1973.
134. Felson B: The mediastinum. Semin Roentgenol 4:40, 1969.
134a. Tsuji H, Takazakura E, Terade Y, et al: CT demonstration of spinal epidural emphysema complicating bronchial asthma and violent coughing. J Comput Assist Tomogr 13:38, 1989.
134b. Yoshimura T, Takeo G, Souda M, et al: Case report: CT demonstration of spinal epidural emphysema after strenuous exercise. J Comput Assist Tomogr 14:303, 1990.
135. Unger JM, England DM, Bogust GA: Interstitial emphysema in adults: Recognition and prognostic implications. J Thorac Imaging 4:86, 1989.
136. Satoh K, Kobayashi T, Kawase Y, et al: CT appearance of interstitial pulmonary emphysema. J Thorac Imaging 11:153, 1996.
137. Mirvis SE, Bidwell JK, Buddemeyer EU, et al: Value of chest radiography in excluding traumatic aortic rupture. Radiology 163:487, 1987.
138. Creasy JD, Chiles C, Routh WD, et al: Overview of traumatic injury of the thoracic aorta. RadioGraphics 17:27, 1997.
139. Gavant ML, Menke PG, Fabian T, et al: Blunt traumatic aortic rupture: Detection with helical CT of the chest. Radiology 197:125, 1995.
140. Mirvis SE, Shanmuganathan K, Miller BH, et al: Traumatic aortic injury: Diagnosis with contrast-enhanced thoracic CT—five-year experience at a major trauma center. Radiology 200:413, 1996.
141. Posniak HV, Olson MC, Demos TC, et al: CT of thoracic aortic aneurysms. RadioGraphics 10:839, 1990.
142. Gomelsky A, Barry MJ, Wagner RB: Spontaneous mediastinal hemorrhage: A case report with a review of the literature. Md Med J 46:83, 1997.
143. Bethancourt B, Pond GD, Jones SE, et al: Mediastinal hematoma simulating recurrent Hodgkin disease during systemic chemotherapy. Am J Roentgenol 142:1119, 1984.
144. Ellison R, Carrao W, Fox M, et al: Spontaneous mediastinal hemorrhage in patients on chronic hemodialysis. Ann Intern Med 95:704, 1981.
145. MacDonald R, Kelly J: Cervico-mediastinal hematoma following sneezing. Anesthesia 30:50, 1975.
146. Stilwell M, Weisbrod G, Ilves R: Spontaneous mediastinal hematoma. J Assoc Can Radiol 32:60, 1981.
147. Singh S, Ptacin MJ, Bamrah VS: Spontaneous mediastinal hemorrhage. A complication of intracoronary streptokinase infusion for coronary thrombosis. Arch Intern Med 143:562, 1983.
148. Woodring JH, Loh FK, Kryscio RJ: Mediastinal hemorrhage: An evaluation of radiographic manifestations. Radiology 151:15, 1984.
149. Kawashima A, Fishman EK, Kuhlman JE, et al: CT of posterior mediastinal masses. RadioGraphics 11:1045, 1991.
150. Panicek DM, Ewing DK, Markarian B, et al: Interstitial pulmonary hemorrhage from mediastinal hematoma secondary to aortic rupture. Radiology 162(1 Pt 1):165, 1987.

151. Kucich VA, Vogelzang RL, Hartz RS, et al: Ruptured thoracic aneurysm: Unusual manifestation and early diagnosis using CT. Radiology 160:87, 1986.

152. Swensen SJ, McLeod RA, Stephens DH: CT of extracranial hemorrhage and hematomas. Am J Roentgenol 143:907, 1984.

153. Glazer HS, Molina PL, Siegel MJ, et al: High-attenuation mediastinal masses on unenhanced CT. Am J Roentgenol 156:45, 1991.

154. Jivani SKM, Mann JR: Haemomediastinum in a haemophiliac after minor trauma. Thorax 25:372, 1970.

155. Laforet EG: Traumatic hemomediastinum. J Thorac Surg 29:597, 1955.

156. Strax TE, Ryvicker MJ, Elguezabal A: Superior vena caval syndrome due to a mediastinal hematoma secondary to dissecting aortic aneurysm. Dis Chest 55:338, 1969.

CHAPTER 74

Masses Situated Predominantly in the Anterior Mediastinal Compartment

A wide variety of lesions can present as a localized tumor or mass in the mediastinum.[1, 2] Because many of these arise in a specific tissue or structure that is situated in a particular site within the mediastinum, it is logical to classify these lesions on the basis of their anatomic location. One of the most widely used of such classification schemes divides the mediastinum into three compartments: (1) an *anterior* compartment, comprising the tissues in front of the heart, aorta, and brachiocephalic vessels, including the thymus, adipose tissue, and lymph nodes; (2) a *middle* mediastinal compartment, comprising the heart, pericardium, all the major vessels leaving and entering this organ, trachea and main bronchi, paratracheal and tracheobronchial lymph nodes, phrenic nerves, and upper portions of the vagus nerves; and (3) a *posterior* compartment, comprising the descending thoracic aorta, esophagus, thoracic duct, lower portion of the vagus nerves, posterior group of mediastinal lymph nodes, and (usually) the paravertebral tissue between the anterior vertebral bodies and the chest wall.

There are a number of practical and conceptual difficulties with this division, including the following: (1) The tissue adjacent to the vertebral bodies is not actually in the mediastinum; (2) the distinction between the middle and the posterior mediastinal compartments is somewhat artificial because it is often difficult to decide whether a lesion is in one or the other and because many masses actually affect both compartments; (3) the anterior margin of the brachiocephalic vessels and ascending aorta is often difficult to identify on the chest radiograph;[3] and (4) anterior mediastinal masses often project over the heart.[4] For these reasons, we prefer to consider the various masses that affect these anatomic regions in the following three groups: (1) the *anterior mediastinum*, when a mass is situated predominantly in the region in front of a line drawn along the anterior border of the trachea and the posterior border of the heart (Fig. 74–1);[4] (2) the *middle-posterior mediastinum*, when a mass is located predominantly between this line and the anterior aspect of the vertebral bodies; and (3) the *paravertebral region*, when a mass is situated predominantly in the potential space adjacent to a vertebral body.

Overlap is bound to occur; all that this classification implies is that a lesion is present *predominantly* in one or another compartment. For example, aortic aneurysms may be situated in any of the three compartments, as may certain neoplasms, such as leiomyoma and neurofibroma; in addition, lymph node enlargement in lymphoma occurs almost as frequently in the anterior as in the middle-posterior compartment, although it is most likely to be massive at the

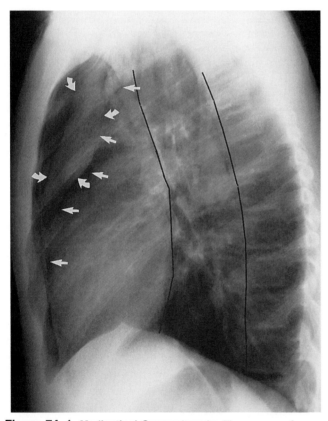

Figure 74–1. Mediastinal Compartments. The presence of a pneumomediastinum in this patient allows identification of the anterior border of the heart, ascending aorta, and brachiocephalic vessels *(straight arrows)*. The anatomic anterior mediastinum is composed of the tissue anterior to these structures and includes the thymus *(curved arrows)*, adipose tissue, and lymph nodes. However, normally the anterior margins of the ascending aorta and brachiocephalic vessels are difficult to visualize. Furthermore, anterior mediastinal masses often project over the heart. Therefore, on the lateral chest radiograph a mass can be considered to probably lie in the anterior mediastinum if it is situated predominantly in the region in front of a line drawn along the anterior border of the trachea and the posterior border of the heart. A mass probably lies in the middle or posterior mediastinum if it is situated between this line and a line drawn along the anterior aspect of the vertebral bodies. Extrapulmonary masses located posterior to this line lie outside of the mediastinum and therefore should be considered paravertebral in location.

former site. Such overlap is inevitable because the anatomic structures in which many masses arise are situated in more than one compartment. Nevertheless, separation into these three groups is helpful in suggesting a diagnosis of many mediastinal and paravertebral tumors, particularly if this information is combined with a knowledge of the patients' clinical manifestations and the CT characteristics of the mass. In fact, a diagnosis can be made with a high degree of confidence in some cases (e.g., an anterior mediastinal mass in a patient who has myasthenia gravis is almost certainly a thymoma, and a bell-shaped tumor in the same location that has fat attenuation on CT and is unassociated with symptoms almost always is a thymolipoma). Despite this relatively high degree of diagnostic accuracy, tissue confirmation is necessary in many cases and is available in the majority after surgical excision of the tumor. Fine-needle aspiration biopsy can be a useful technique in the former circumstance, although results of the procedure must be interpreted carefully: In one investigation of 189 mediastinal abnormalities (including both primary and metastatic neoplasms and inflammatory disorders) from four university centers in the United States, histologic correlation in 78 cases showed a sensitivity and specificity for the detection of neoplasm of 87% and 88%, respectively.[5]

Most mediastinal abnormalities are initially suspected following chest radiography; the need for further investigation and the optimal imaging modality or other test by which it should be conducted are largely dictated by the tentative diagnosis made on this examination. CT and magnetic resonance (MR) imaging allow visualization of the exact location of the lesions and, in some cases, identification of the structures from which they arise; one or both of these techniques are indicated in almost all cases. Because of their anatomic precision, it is preferable to describe the exact location of a lesion in relation to the adjacent mediastinal structures with both of these techniques, rather than limiting the description to a particular mediastinal compartment.

The wide variety of tissues within the mediastinum is reflected in the many forms of neoplastic, developmental, and inflammatory masses that are seen.[6] In a review of the literature before 1971, 34 previous reports of mediastinal tumors, involving 3,364 patients were documented.[7] Excluding metastatic pulmonary carcinoma and inflammatory conditions, the frequency of tumors was as follows: neurogenic neoplasms, 19%; lymphoma, 16%; bronchial and pericardial cysts, 14%; germ cell ("teratodermoid") tumors, 13%; thymoma, 12%; and thyroid tumors, 6%; a variety of miscellaneous tumors composed the remainder. In another 1971 review of 1,064 tumors seen over a 40-year period at the Mayo Clinic, the findings were similar: Neurogenic neoplasms, thymomas, and benign cysts constituted 60% of tumors; lymphomas, teratomas, granulomas, and intrathoracic goiters constituted 30%; and miscellaneous benign or malignant mesenchymal tumors constituted 10%.[8] In nonsurgical series, vascular abnormalities, usually aortic aneurysms, account for 10% of mediastinal masslike lesions.[1] Metastases to the mediastinum are also common, although they are usually not considered in reviews of mediastinal tumors because they are only occasionally the presenting manifestation of cancer. As might be expected, such presentation is most often associated with a primary pulmonary carcinoma; however, other sources occur rarely.[9]

This chapter is concerned with masses that develop in the anterior mediastinum; those that involve the middle-posterior compartment and the paravertebral region are discussed in Chapters 75 and 76. The anterior mediastinum is the site of the majority of clinically important primary mediastinal masses, including thymoma and a variety of other thymic abnormalities, lymphoma, germ cell tumors, and hyperplastic and neoplastic abnormalities of thyroid and ectopic parathyroid tissue. Abnormalities involving the ascending aorta can mimic an anterior mediastinal mass.

TUMORS AND TUMOR-LIKE CONDITIONS OF THE THYMUS

Thymic Hyperplasia

True thymic hyperplasia, as opposed to the lymphoid hyperplasia that is associated with myasthenia gravis (see farther on) can be defined as an increase in the size of the thymus gland associated with a more or less normal gross architecture and histologic appearance.[10, 11] The diagnosis can be made by noting a significant increase in the weight of the thymus compared with that expected for age, by detecting an increase in the size of a histologically normal gland on serial radiographs or CT, or by measuring the gland thickness on CT (see farther on) (Fig. 74–2). The first criterion is somewhat arbitrary because figures for normal thymus weight at different ages are somewhat variable;[13] according to some investigators, a weight greater than 100 gm should be considered to represent true hyperplasia.[13]

The pathogenesis is variable. Most commonly, it appears to be a rebound phenomenon secondary to atrophy caused by chemotherapy for malignancy (usually lymphoma or a germ cell tumor)[14–18] or by hypercortisolism;[19] a similar process has also been reported after treatment of Cushing's syndrome.[21] Such rebound enlargement is not uncommon; in one CT study of 120 patients treated for testicular carcinoma, evidence of thymic enlargement was found in 14 (12%) after therapy.[17] In another investigation in which serial CT scans were performed in 20 patients who were from 2 to 35 years of age and who had various malignancies, the thymic volume decreased an average of 43% after chemotherapy.[23] On further follow-up, rebound hyperplasia occurred in 25% of patients, the volume of the thymus exceeding the baseline volume by 50% (Fig. 74–3).[23] For unexplained reasons, some cases of hyperplasia have been found in association with testicular carcinoma before the induction of chemotherapy.[24]

A second relatively common group of patients with thymic hyperplasia has hyperthyroidism (Graves' disease);[25–28] rare cases of hyperplasia associated with Hodgkin's disease have also been reported.[29] Although the pathogenetic relationship between the thyroid disease and the thymic hyperplasia is not clear, there is evidence that it may be related to the presence of an intrathymic thyrotropin receptor, which may serve as an autoantigen.[30]

A variety of other conditions have been associated with thymic hyperplasia less commonly. Occasionally, there is a history of a "stressful" event,[31] such as sepsis[32] or massive burn.[33] Cases have also been reported in patients who have Beckwith-Wiedemann syndrome (congenital adrenal cortical cytomegaly associated with hyperplasia of various viscera and tissues and postnatal gigantism);[34] sarcoidosis;[35] pure red cell aplasia;[36, 37] and a complex systemic endocrinopathy involving the adrenals, pancreas, ovaries, and kidneys.[38] Analysis of excised hyperplastic tissue has shown no immunochemical, structural, or functional differences from normal thymic tissue.[39]

Thymic hyperplasia is seldom apparent on the chest radiograph in adults.[40] On CT, the most helpful measurement for determining an increase in the size of the thymus is its thickness (Fig. 74–4):[41, 42] The maximal normal thickness in individuals younger than 20 years is 1.8 cm;[41] in those older than 20, it is 1.3 cm. Measurements greater than these are consistent with hyperplasia. In patients who have Hodgkin's disease or non-Hodgkin's lymphoma, rebound thymic hyperplasia must be distinguished from residual or recurrent tumor.[43] Although this cannot be done reliably by CT or MR imaging, it is often possible using gallium scintigraphy,[44–48] gallium uptake being seen in residual tumor but not in fibrotic or necrotic tissue. Although such increased uptake is relatively common in children who have rebound thymic hyperplasia,[47–50] it is rare in adults.[51]

In patients who have no underlying tumor or who have an extrathoracic malignancy, thymic rebound hyperplasia is an incidental finding on CT that seldom causes any diagnostic concern. In fact, there is evidence that it may be a favorable prognostic sign in some patients. In one study of 200 adults who had malignant testicular tumors, 120 who had metastatic disease were treated with chemotherapy, and 80 who had no evidence of metastasis received no treatment.[52] Serial CT scans demonstrated thymic enlargement 3 to 4 months after initiation of treatment in 14 of the 120 patients (12%) who received chemotherapy but in only 1 patient in the control group. Thirteen of the 14 patients (93%) who had thymic enlargement were well and disease-free after a mean follow-up of 45 months compared with 78% of patients in the group who did not have thymic enlargement.

Most patients in whom thymic hyperplasia has been diagnosed are children or young adults.[10, 11] Symptoms are usually absent, although respiratory distress and dysphagia can occur. The diagnosis should be suspected if there is a history of prior chemotherapy; in the absence of such a history, excision of the enlarged thymus is almost certainly required for diagnosis. As might be expected, specimens obtained by transthoracic needle aspiration are unlikely to be diagnostic.[53]

Thymic Follicular Hyperplasia

The term *thymic hyperplasia* also has been used to describe a distinctive histologic reaction in the thymus of patients who have myasthenia gravis. In approximately two thirds of individuals with the latter condition, the thymic cortex is the site of multiple well-defined lymphoid follicles, many containing germinal centers (Fig. 74–5). Because the weight of the thymus gland in these cases is usually within normal limits,[25, 54] the designation *thymic hyperplasia* is, strictly speaking, incorrect; in fact, it has been suggested that the terms *lymphoid* or *follicular* hyperplasia might be more appropriate to describe the abnormality.[25] Such follicular hyperplasia has also been documented in patients who

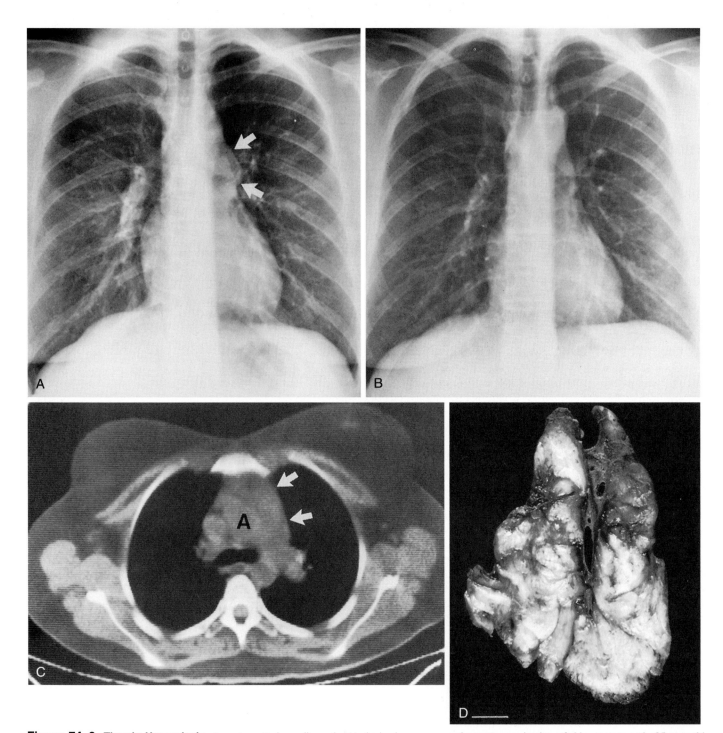

Figure 74–2. Thymic Hyperplasia. A posteroanterior radiograph *(A)* obtained as a pre-employment examination of this asymptomatic 25-year-old nurse reveals a sharply defined opacity protruding to the left at the level of the aortopulmonary window *(arrows)*. Results of a film obtained several years previously *(B)* were normal. A CT scan at the level of the carina *(C)* reveals a homogeneous mass *(arrows)* situated in the anterior mediastinum contiguous with the ascending aorta (A) and main pulmonary artery. The resected specimen *(D)* resembles a normal thymus gland except for size; histologic examination showed normal thymic tissue. The cause of the hyperplasia was not identified. (Bar = 1 cm.)

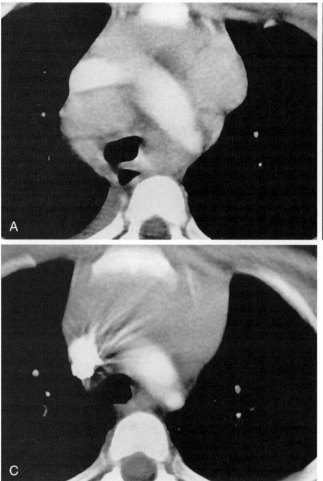

Figure 74–3. Thymic "Rebound": Hyperplasia. A contrast-enhanced CT scan in a 9-year-old child *(A)* demonstrates extensive mediastinal lymphadenopathy (proven to be due to Hodgkin's disease). The patient underwent successful treatment. A CT scan performed 6 months later *(B)* shows a small residual thymus. A scan performed 1 year following the initial scan *(C)* demonstrates a significant increase in thymic size, representing "rebound" hyperplasia. There was no evidence of tumor recurrence. (Courtesy of Dr. Ella Kazerooni, Department of Radiology, University of Michigan Hospital, Ann Arbor, MI.)

have autoimmune connective tissue disease, pure red blood cell hypoplasia,[55] and human immunodeficiency virus (HIV) infection[56] (some of the last-mentioned cases have also been associated with thymic enlargement[57]).

Occasionally, lymphoid follicles can be seen in thymus glands of apparently normal individuals; however, in patients who have myasthenia gravis, they are usually larger and much more numerous. This observation as well as the large

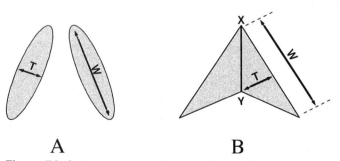

A   B

Figure 74–4. Measurement of Thymic Size on CT. The two thymic lobes are measured separately. The width (W) corresponds to the long axis of the lobe as seen on the transverse CT image and the thickness (T) to the short axis diameter *(A)*. When the two lobes are confluent, the thymus has a triangular or arrowhead shape *(B)*. The thymus is divided in half by a line through the anterior apex of the gland and perpendicular to it (X-Y). The width (W) and thickness (T) of each lobe are then measured. (Measurement described by Baron RL, et al: Radiology 142:121, 1982.)

number of cases of myasthenia gravis associated with thymic lymphoid hyperplasia and the favorable response to thymectomy in many patients who have the abnormality suggests a pathogenetic association between the two conditions;[58] however, the details of this relationship remain unclear.

Thymic lymphoid hyperplasia seldom leads to radiographically apparent abnormalities.[20, 40] Although it may also be associated with a normal-appearing thymus on CT, a diffusely enlarged thymus (Fig. 74–6) or a focal mass is not uncommon.[42] In a retrospective study of 45 patients who had myasthenia gravis, 22 had histologically proven lymphoid hyperplasia.[42] On CT, 10 (45%) of the 22 patients had a normal-appearing thymus, 7 (32%) had a diffusely enlarged thymus, and 5 (23%) had a focal mass. All 7 patients who had a diffusely enlarged thymus had lymphoid hyperplasia; of the 26 patients who had a normal-appearing thymus, 10 (38%) had lymphoid hyperplasia and 16 (62%) had normal histologic findings. Of 12 patients who had a focal mass, 5 (42%) had lymphoid hyperplasia, and 7 (58%) had thymoma.[42] These findings, which have been replicated by other investigators,[59, 60] indicate the limitations of CT in the diagnosis of thymic lymphoid hyperplasia. MR imaging is also of limited value in diagnosis.[59] One case has been reported of a patient who had myasthenia gravis in whom the initial CT scan result was normal, but a repeat scan performed 5 months later, when there was an exacerbation of symptoms,

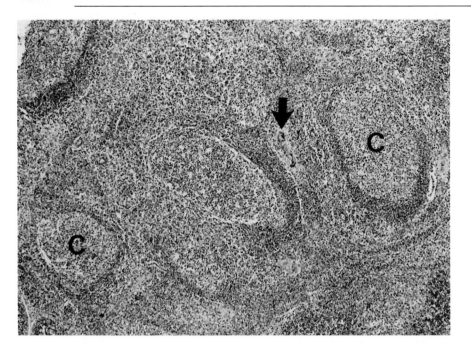

Figure 74–5. Thymic Lymphoid Hyperplasia Associated with Myasthenia Gravis. A section of a grossly normal thymus gland removed from a patient who had myasthenia gravis shows several irregularly shaped germinal centers (C) that cause considerable distortion of normal thymic architecture. Occasional Hassall's corpuscles are evident *(arrow).* (×48.)

showed diffuse thymic enlargement;[61] histologic examination of the resected specimen revealed follicular hyperplasia.

Thymolipoma

Thymolipomas are uncommon anterior mediastinal tumors consisting of an admixture of fat and thymic epithelial and lymphoid tissue. They have been said to constitute 2% to 10% of all thymic tumors;[62] in our experience, the former figure is the more representative. By 1990, approximately 90 cases had been reported;[63] in a review from the Armed Forces Institute of Pathology in 1995, an additional 33 were documented.[64] No sex predilection is evident; although the tumor can occur at any age, young men appear to be more susceptible.[65]

The precise nature of thymolipoma is uncertain.[54, 66] It has been considered to represent no more than a lipoma

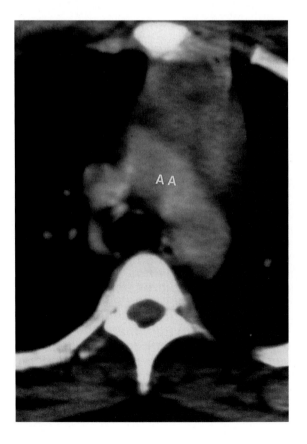

Figure 74–6. Thymic Lymphoid Hyperplasia. A contrast-enhanced CT scan at the level of the aortic arch (AA) in a 29-year-old woman who had myasthenia gravis demonstrates a diffusely enlarged thymus. Diffuse lymphoid follicular hyperplasia was proven surgically. (Courtesy of Dr. Ella Kazerooni, Department of Radiology, University of Michigan Hospital, Ann Arbor, MI.)

occurring within the thymus gland; however, because the thymic tissue itself appears to be increased in amount,[54] this hypothesis appears unlikely. It also has been suggested that the tumor is a mixed lipoma and thymoma, the predominance of fat perhaps reflecting normal involution of the thymus; however, the normal appearance of the thymic tissue makes this interpretation improbable. A final theory proposes that the tumor begins as a true thymic hyperplasia (i.e., an increase in the amount of normal thymic tissue) that subsequently regresses and is replaced by adipose tissue.[54]

Grossly, thymolipomas are typically yellow, soft, and roughly bilobed in shape, somewhat resembling the normal thymus gland. They are often large and can grow to huge proportions; some have been reported to weigh greater than 12,000 gm[62] or measure 36 cm in greatest dimension.[64] Histologically, the tumor consists of mature adipose tissue interspersed with normal thymic lymphoepithelial tissue.[54, 62] Germinal centers are typically absent, even when there is a history of myasthenia gravis. Calcification and cystic degeneration of Hassall's corpuscles are common;[64] striated muscle cells have been noted occasionally.[67] Several unusual histologic variants—one associated with fibrosis (designated *thymofibrolipoma*),[68] one with parathyroid tissue (*lipothymoade-*

noma),[69] and a third with abnormal thymic tissue (*proliferating thymolipoma*)[70]—have been reported.

The characteristic radiographic appearance consists of an anterior mediastinal mass that droops into the lower chest (Fig. 74–7);[1, 62, 71] extension into one or both hemithoraces may be seen. The tumor typically conforms to the adjacent structures and may mimic cardiomegaly or elevation of one or both hemidiaphragms.[22, 62, 71] When small, it is round or oval in shape, mimicking other mediastinal masses.[62] In a review of the radiographic manifestations in 27 patients, 14 masses occupied the entire anteroposterior diameter of the chest;[71] in 14 patients, the low density of the tumor could be appreciated on the radiograph, and in 7, a change of shape or position of the mass was seen when the patient assumed a decubitus position.

CT scans characteristically show predominant fat attenuation or equivalent fat and soft tissue attenuation (Fig. 74–8).[71] The soft tissue may appear as linear whorls intermixed with fat or, less commonly, as small rounded opacities embedded within it.[72, 73] The mass can often be seen to be connected to the thymus. MR imaging demonstrates high signal intensity on T1-weighted spin-echo images as a result of fat and areas of intermediate signal intensity related to

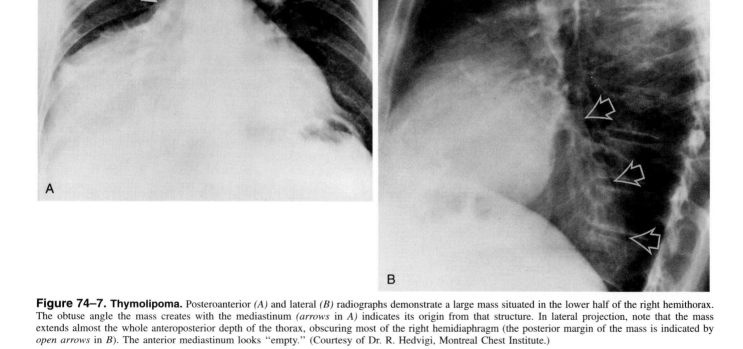

Figure 74–7. Thymolipoma. Posteroanterior *(A)* and lateral *(B)* radiographs demonstrate a large mass situated in the lower half of the right hemithorax. The obtuse angle the mass creates with the mediastinum *(arrows in A)* indicates its origin from that structure. In lateral projection, note that the mass extends almost the whole anteroposterior depth of the thorax, obscuring most of the right hemidiaphragm (the posterior margin of the mass is indicated by *open arrows* in *B*). The anterior mediastinum looks "empty." (Courtesy of Dr. R. Hedvigi, Montreal Chest Institute.)

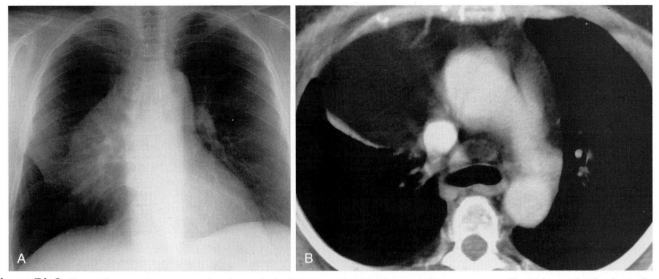

Figure 74–8. Thymolipoma. A posteroanterior chest radiograph *(A)* in a 61-year-old woman demonstrates a mediastinal mass that has lower density than the adjacent soft tissues, consistent with fat. A contrast-enhanced CT scan *(B)* demonstrates that the mass lies in the region of the right lobe of the thymus and that it is made up almost exclusively of fat. The findings are characteristic of thymolipoma. (Courtesy of Dr. Ella Kazerooni, Department of Radiology, University of Michigan Hospital, Ann Arbor, MI.)

soft tissue.[71, 74, 75] The characteristic features of thymolipoma on the radiograph and CT allow distinction from other mediastinal masses in the majority of cases. In one study of 128 patients who had anterior mediastinal masses, three of which were thymolipomas, two independent observers made a correct first-choice diagnosis of thymolipoma based on the chest radiographic findings in two cases and on CT in all three.[76]

Thymolipomas characteristically cause few or no symptoms even when large; thus, the lesion is usually discovered on a screening radiograph. Rare cases have been reported in association with myasthenia gravis,[66, 77] aplastic anemia,[78] Graves' disease, red blood cell hypoplasia, and hypogammaglobulinemia.[77] The behavior is typically benign, no recurrences having been documented after resection; however, an unusual case has been reported of apparent thymic liposarcoma, possibly derived from a thymolipoma.[79]

Thymic Cysts

Thymic cysts are uncommon mediastinal lesions that account for only 1% to 2% of all tumors in the anterior compartment.[80, 81] Although it has been suggested that they represent degeneration and enlargement of Hassall's corpuscles,[82] most are probably derived from remnants of the fetal thymopharyngeal duct. Occasional cysts have been reported after thoracic surgery[83] or chemotherapy for a malignant neoplasm,[84] suggesting a relationship to trauma or drug-related involution. An association with HIV infection has also been documented in some cases.[85, 86]

Pathologically, the cysts are unilocular or multilocular and range in size from microscopic to as large as 18 cm in maximal diameter.[82] They can contain straw-colored fluid or, if hemorrhage has occurred, brown gelatinous or friable material (Fig. 74–9). Histologically, the cyst wall is lined by squamous, transitional, or simple cuboidal or columnar epithelium; ulceration associated with underlying fibrosis and chronic inflammation is fairly common, as is evidence

of remote hemorrhage (hemosiderin-laden macrophages and cholesterol clefts). Considerable epithelial hyperplasia occurs in some cases, possibly reflecting a reparative reaction to such damage.[87] Thymic tissue can be identified focally in the cyst wall (*see* Fig. 74–9) and, in fact, is necessary to make the diagnosis.

An important point in pathologic differential diagnosis is the observation that some malignant tumors, including thymoma, Hodgkin's disease, and germ cell tumors,[88, 89, 89a] can show prominent cystic change, occasionally associated with a relatively small amount of neoplastic tissue; consequently, thorough sampling of every "thymic cyst" must be carried out to exclude the possibility of neoplasia, especially if the cyst wall is focally thickened. In addition to such degenerative changes in a primary neoplasm, it has been suggested that Hodgkin's disease can occasionally develop in the wall of a true thymic cyst.[90] Although rare, carcinoma also has been reported to arise from cyst epithelium.[91–93]

The appearance on the chest radiograph consists of a smoothly marginated anterior mediastinal mass (Fig. 74–10).[1, 80, 81, 94] When large, the cyst may obscure the margins of the adjacent structures and simulate cardiomegaly (Fig. 74–11). On CT, they typically have water density (O H) and thin walls.[94] Occasionally, soft tissue septa or ringlike calcifications are seen within the cyst or foci of linear calcification in the cyst wall, presumably as a result of previous hemorrhage.[6, 94] Bleeding into the cyst also may be manifested by a density measurement greater than water.[94] Thymic cysts have low signal intensity on T1-weighted MR images and high signal intensity on T2-weighted images.[75] Hemorrhage results in increased signal on T1-weighted images as a result of the T1 shortening effect of methemoglobin.[94] Cysts that develop after radiation or chemotherapy usually have a predominant soft tissue component; occasionally, however, they may resemble congenital cysts.[94]

Most patients are asymptomatic. Rare cases have been reported in patients who have myasthenia gravis and Graves' disease[95] and Horner's syndrome.[96] Provided that a neoplastic cyst has been excluded, the prognosis is excellent.

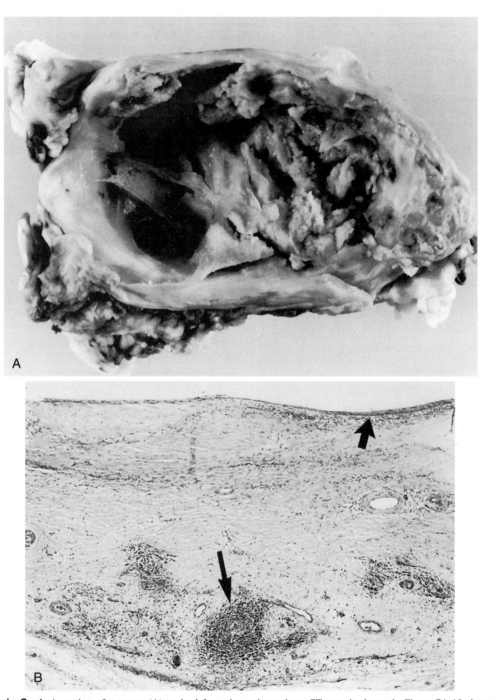

Figure 74–9. Thymic Cyst. A section of a tumor *(A)* excised from the patient whose CT scan is shown in Figure 74–10 shows a thick-walled cyst that contains abundant friable material, reflecting prior hemorrhage. Histologically, the cyst wall *(B)* is composed of fibrous tissue lined by a flattened squamous epithelium *(short arrow)*; a small amount of residual thymic tissue is evident *(long arrow)*. (×60.)

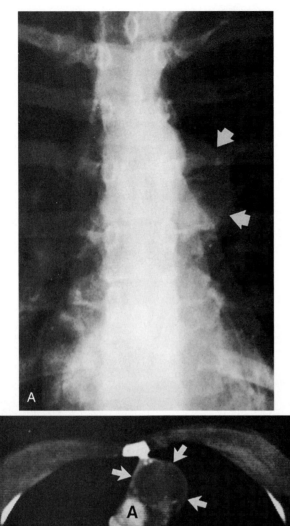

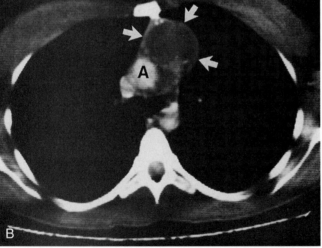

Figure 74–10. Thymic Cyst. A magnified view of the mediastinum from a posteroanterior radiograph *(A)* reveals a sharply defined homogeneous opacity extending to the left at the level of the aortopulmonary window *(arrows)*. A CT scan at the same level *(B)* shows the lesion to be a fluid-filled cyst *(arrows)* relating to the anterior aspect and left side of the ascending aorta (A). The resected specimen is shown in Figure 74–9.

Inflammatory Conditions Causing Thymic Enlargement

Enlargement of the thymus gland is occasionally caused by an inflammatory process. Reported examples include Churg-Strauss syndrome,[97] hydatid disease, tuberculosis,[98, 99] Langerhans' cell histiocytosis,[100] and inflammatory pseudotumor.[101]

Thymoma

Thymomas are neoplasms of thymic epithelium that characteristically consist of rather uniform cells with a variable amount of admixed lymphocytes; although cytologically bland, they can behave in either a benign or a malignant fashion. Thymic epithelial neoplasms composed of cells that have significant cytologic atypia and a high mitotic rate are more appropriately termed *thymic carcinoma* and are discussed separately *(see* page 2897).

Thymoma is the most common primary neoplasm to affect the anterior mediastinum; in a 1993 review, it comprised approximately 20% of all mediastinal tumors.[102] Of a total of 789 cases in five reviews from Sweden,[103] France,[104] Italy,[105] the United States,[106] and Germany,[107] there was a slight female predominance (427 to 362, or 1.2 to 1). Most tumors are discovered in middle-aged adults, the average age at diagnosis in the five series cited being between 45 and 52 years; rarely, they occur in childhood and adolescence.[108, 109]

The cause and pathogenesis are unknown in most cases. The possibility of viral infection has been suggested by the observation of tumor-associated Epstein-Barr virus in some patients;[110, 111] however, the vast majority of tumors show no evidence of the infection. Cases have also been reported in individuals who have HIV[112] or RNA tumor virus infection;[113] however, their rarity is such that a coincidental association cannot be excluded. Although chromosomal abnormalities have been documented in some tumors, no consistent pattern has been found.[114] Rare familial cases have been reported.[115]

Pathologic Characteristics

The vast majority of thymomas arise in the upper portion of the anterior mediastinum, corresponding to the position of the normal thymus gland. Rarely, they are discovered in an unusual location, such as the posterior mediastinum,[116] lower neck,[117] perihilar tissues, pleura,[118] or lung parenchyma.[119]

Grossly the majority of tumors are well encapsulated and round or slightly lobulated. They are usually between 5 and 15 cm in diameter,[54, 106] although they tend to be somewhat smaller in individuals who have myasthenia gravis, presumably because of the presence of symptoms at an earlier stage. Rarely, such tumors are so small that they are identified only microscopically, in which case they may be multifocal.[120, 121] Cut sections of larger tumors often reveal them to be firm, pale gray or tan in color, and subdivided into numerous lobules by variably thick fibrous bands (Fig. 74–12). One or more cysts are not infrequent and are sometimes large, comprising most of the tumor volume;[122] foci of fibrosis, calcification, and hemorrhage also may be seen. Such secondary changes may result in a mistaken impression of an inflammatory or other benign abnormality.[123] Infiltration of the pleura, lung, and (less commonly) the pericardium, chest wall, diaphragm, or mediastinal vessels occurs in 30% to 50% of cases;[114, 124, 125] however, the tumor can be adherent to adjacent structures without actually invading them *(see* Fig. 74–12).[106] Because the natural history of thymoma can be predicted, in part, by the presence or

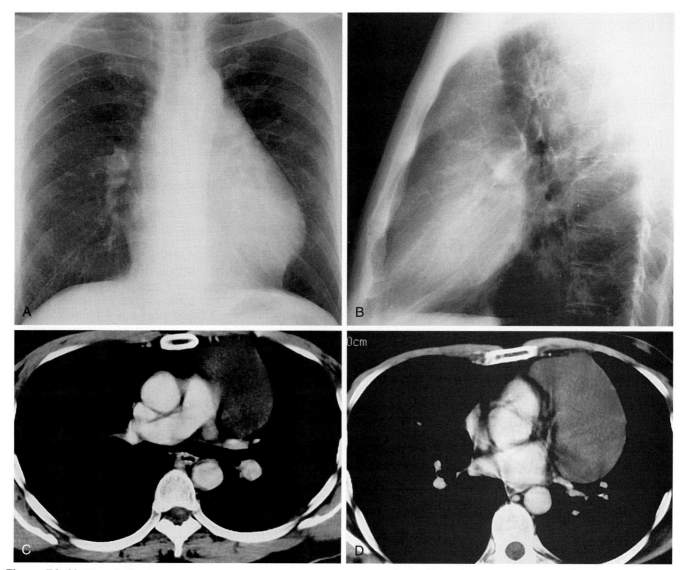

Figure 74–11. Thymic Cyst. A posteroanterior chest radiograph *(A)* in a 53-year-old man shows an unusual contour of the mediastinum and apparent cardiomegaly. A lateral radiograph *(B)* shows poorly defined increased opacity in the anterior mediastinum and normal heart size. Contrast-enhanced CT scans *(C* and *D)* demonstrate a thin-walled, fluid-filled cyst. The presence of a thymic cyst was confirmed surgically.

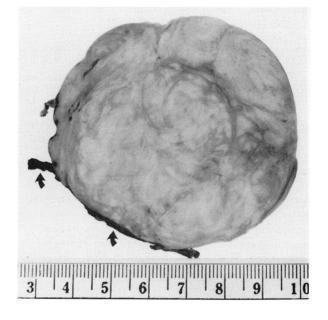

Figure 74–12. Thymoma. A slice of an anterior mediastinal mass shows a well-circumscribed tumor possessing a distinctly lobulated appearance. There is no necrosis or hemorrhage. A small amount of compressed lung is adherent to the tumor *(arrows)*.

absence of local extracapsular invasion (*see* farther on), this must be clearly confirmed histologically.

The cellular composition of thymoma and the appearance of the tumor cells are variable, both within a single tumor and between different tumors. The neoplastic epithelial cells can vary from polygonal to distinctly spindled in shape, and the associated lymphocytic infiltrate can be absent or can be so marked as to obscure almost completely the presence of the epithelial cells. Such histologic variability has given rise to several morphologic classifications of the tumor. One of the earliest and most widely used classification systems divided the tumors into three groups depending on the relative proportions of epithelial cells and lymphocytes:[126] predominantly lymphocytic, mixed lymphoepithelial, and predominantly epithelial (the last-named sometimes being further subdivided into polygonal and spindle cell varieties[127]). Although this classification is useful for descriptive purposes, a consistent association between histologic type and biologic behavior has been difficult to demonstrate.[128–131]

A second classification based on epithelial cell morphology has also been proposed.[132] According to this schema (Müller-Hermelink), tumors are divided into cortical, medullary, and mixed forms, the first-named being, in turn, subdivided into "predominantly" cortical (organoid) and "pure" cortical types. Because there are morphologic, immunohistochemical, and functional differences between the cortical and medullary regions of the normal thymus,[132, 133] such a classification has some theoretical merit; moreover, some investigators have shown a close correspondence between the immunophenotypes of lymphocytes in cortical and medullary thymomas and normal thymic cortical and medullary lymphocytes.[134, 135] Perhaps most important, the histologic types defined in this classification have been shown by a number of workers to be associated with different biologic behaviors and prognosis (*see* farther on).[128, 134, 136–139] Although the reproducibility of diagnoses using this classification scheme has been questioned by some investigators,[140] others have found it to be quite good.[141]

According to the Müller-Hermelink classification, *organoid (predominantly cortical) thymomas* resemble the normal thymus and consist of lobules of lymphocyte-rich tumor separated by a fibrovascular stroma (Fig. 74–13). Although the latter is usually fairly delicate, occasionally, it is markedly thickened and associated with dystrophic calcification (*see* Fig. 74–13), a feature that sometimes can be identified radiographically. The epithelial cells are generally round or polygonal in shape and, because of the tremendous number of admixed lymphocytes, may be inapparent at first glance (Fig. 74–14). (In fact, because the epithelial cells are inconspicuous and the lymphocytes often show some degree of nuclear atypia, a diagnosis of lymphoma may be considered, especially if the amount of tissue examined is small or is obtained from a site other than the anterior mediastinum.[142]) Nuclei are uniform in size and shape and possess small nucleoli. Hassall's corpuscles are relatively common, as are foci of "medullary differentiation," in which the density of lymphocytes is less than that of the surrounding tissue, resulting in distinct areas of relative pallor at low magnification (Fig. 74–15). Another common feature is the presence of perivascular spaces (Fig. 74–16) containing proteinaceous

material and scattered lymphocytes (shown by one group of investigators to have a B-cell phenotype).[143]

Cortical thymomas are composed of single or small clusters of relatively large polygonal epithelial cells separated by a variable number of lymphocytes (Fig. 74–17). Nuclei tend to have prominent nucleoli. Medullary differentiation and Hassall's corpuscles are sparse or absent. One group of investigators has found evidence that the histologic pattern may change from organoid to cortical to well-differentiated carcinoma as the disease progresses (i.e., in recurrent tumor after surgery), suggesting that these patterns may represent a single neoplasm that has different degrees of differentiation.[144]

The *medullary form of thymoma* consists of spindle-shaped epithelial cells with uniform, elongated nuclei and inconspicuous nucleoli (Fig. 74–18). Mitotic activity and Hassall's corpuscles are typically absent, and admixed lymphocytes are few. In one study of 30 thymomas, investigators found abnormal expression of the proto-oncogene *bcl*-2 in medullary tumors;[145] other workers have found it to be present in medullary and mixed tumors but not cortical ones.[146] *Mixed tumors* show a combination of medullary and organoid patterns. The two patterns may be seen as relatively large, more or less separate foci or as more intimately associated nests of spindle cells separated by sheets of lymphocytes and polygonal epithelial cells (Fig. 74–19).

Although the Müller-Hermelink classification of thymoma has been widely adopted, it has not gone without criticism.[147] Some studies relating prognosis to histology have had relatively few examples of some tumor types; moreover, sufficient tumor sampling may not always have been carried out, a problem of particular importance because of the varied histologic appearance of many thymomas.[147] The usefulness of separating predominantly cortical from cortical tumors and in distinguishing them from well-differentiated thymic carcinoma as well as the prognostic independence of histologic features and stage has also been questioned. On the basis of the information available, it seems appropriate to regard the classification as useful; however, additional studies are necessary before it can be considered definitive. Unusual histologic findings in thymoma include a microcystic appearance with signet-ring–like cells[148] and the presence of a prominent plasma cell infiltrate,[149] pseudosarcomatous stroma,[149a] or myoid cell population.[150]

Radiologic Manifestations

Most thymomas are situated near the junction of the heart and great vessels. Radiographically, they are round or oval in shape, and their margins are usually smooth or lobulated (Fig. 74–20).[1, 151] They can protrude to one or both sides of the mediastinum and can displace the heart and great vessels posteriorly. In some cases, calcification is apparent at the periphery of the lesion or throughout its substance (Fig. 74–21).[151] Occasionally, a tumor simulates cardiac enlargement[94, 151] or is located in an unusual site, such as the cardiophrenic angle[151] or posterior mediastinum.[116, 151, 152] The radiographic appearances of invasive and noninvasive tumors are usually indistinguishable.[151] Occasionally, an invasive tumor spreads to the pleural space and leads to focal or diffuse pleural thickening.[151, 153, 154] Such pleural involvement

Text continued on page 2891

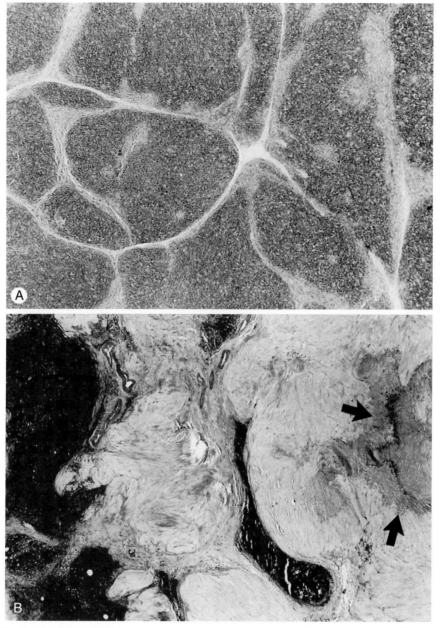

Figure 74–13. Thymoma: Microscopic Lobulation. A low-power view of a predominantly cortical thymoma *(A)* shows the tumor to be divided by thin fibrous bands into numerous lobules of variable size and shape. A section from another tumor *(B)* shows marked thickening of fibrous septa with focal calcification *(arrows)*.

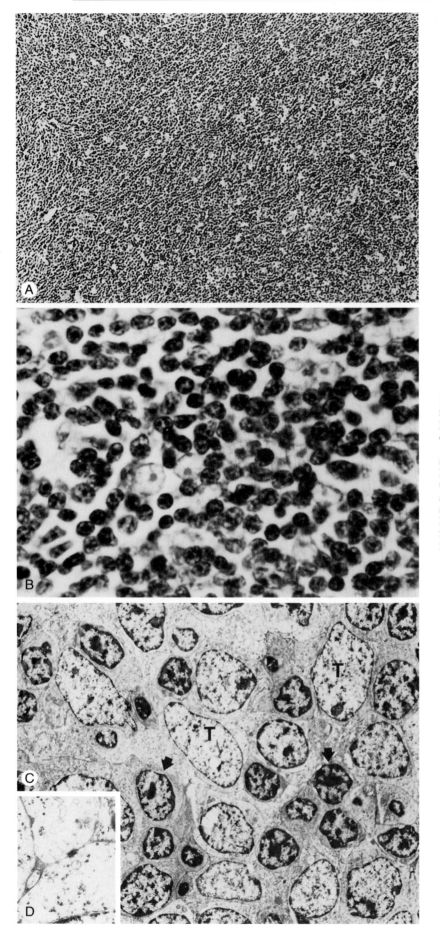

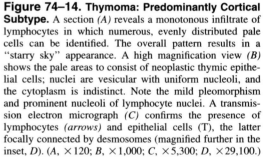

Figure 74–14. Thymoma: Predominantly Cortical Subtype. A section *(A)* reveals a monotonous infiltrate of lymphocytes in which numerous, evenly distributed pale cells can be identified. The overall pattern results in a "starry sky" appearance. A high magnification view *(B)* shows the pale areas to consist of neoplastic thymic epithelial cells; nuclei are vesicular with uniform nucleoli, and the cytoplasm is indistinct. Note the mild pleomorphism and prominent nucleoli of lymphocyte nuclei. A transmission electron micrograph *(C)* confirms the presence of lymphocytes *(arrows)* and epithelial cells (T), the latter focally connected by desmosomes (magnified further in the inset, *D*). (*A*, ×120; *B*, ×1,000; *C*, ×5,300; *D*, ×29,100.)

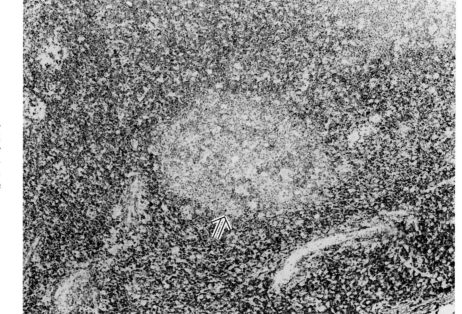

Figure 74–15. Thymoma: Medullary Differentiation. A section of a predominantly cortical thymoma shows a distinct focus of relative pallor *(arrow)* caused by a reduced concentration of lymphocytes. This appearance corresponds to the difference between cortical and medullary regions of the normal thymus. (×70.)

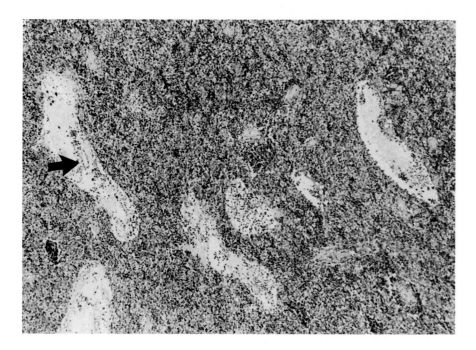

Figure 74–16. Thymoma: Perivascular Spaces. A section of a mixed tumor shows several irregularly shaped clear spaces in which proteinaceous fluid and a few lymphocytes can be identified; a small vessel is present in some *(arrow)*. (×60.)

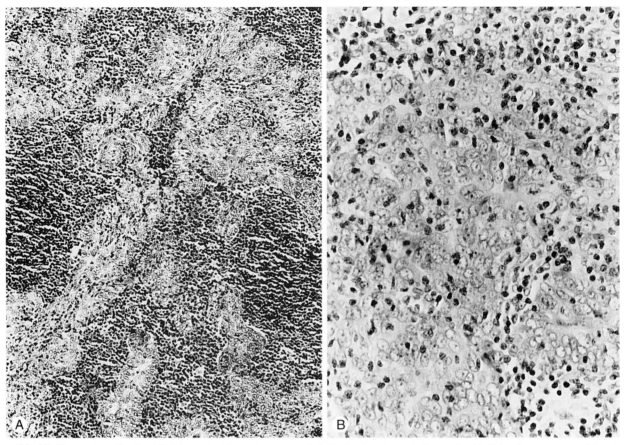

Figure 74–17. Thymoma: Cortical Subtype. In this section *(A)*, well-defined trabeculae and sheets of epithelial cells are separated by clusters of lymphocytes. A magnified view *(B)* shows the epithelial cells to have fairly uniform vesicular nuclei with prominent nucleoli. *(A, ×120, B, ×375.)*

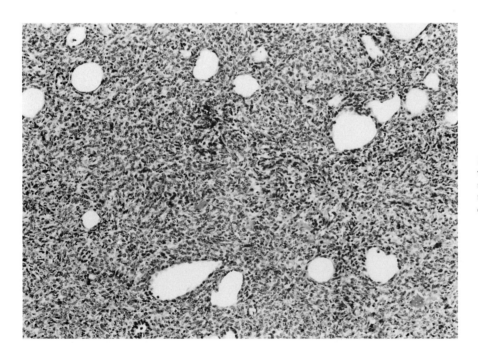

Figure 74–18. Thymoma: Medullary Subtype. This tumor consists almost entirely of uniform polygonal or somewhat spindle-shaped epithelial cells with only occasional admixed lymphocytes. *(×120.)*

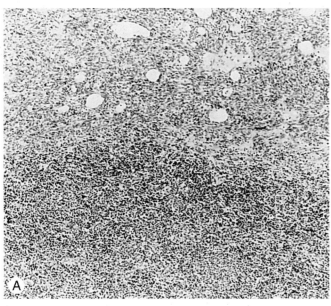
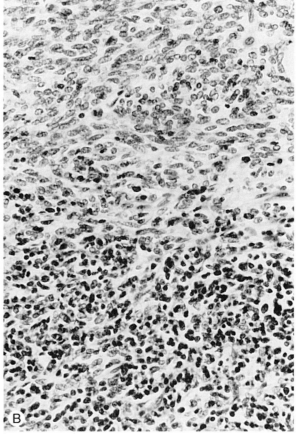

Figure 74–19. Thymoma: Mixed Medullary and Organoid Patterns. The upper half of *A* and *B* shows spindle-shaped cells with sparse lymphocytes, typical of the medullary form of thymoma. The lower half shows numerous lymphocytes separating more rounded cells, characteristic of the organoid (predominantly cortical) pattern.

is usually unilateral; when extensive, it may mimic malignant mesothelioma (Fig. 74–22).[151, 153]

Several investigators have shown that CT is superior to chest radiography in both diagnosis and assessment of tumor extent.[155–158] On CT, the majority of thymomas present as round or oval soft tissue masses that have sharply demarcated margins. Typically, they are located in the region of the thymus anterior to the aortic root and main pulmonary artery and project to one side of the mediastinum (*see* Fig. 74–20).[1, 42, 151, 154] Tumors usually have homogeneous attenuation; less commonly and usually in large tumors, the presence of hemorrhage, necrosis, or cyst formation leads to focal areas of low attenuation.[1, 94, 151] Rarely, such areas are the predominant feature.[76, 151] Foci of calcification may be seen in the capsule or throughout the tumor (*see* Fig. 74–21).[94, 151]

CT does not allow reliable distinction of invasive from noninvasive thymoma. Although preservation of fat planes between the tumor and adjacent structures is most suggestive of a noninvasive tumor, limited invasion cannot be excluded.[1, 151, 159] Similarly, although obliteration of the fat planes is suggestive of invasion (Fig. 74–23), this may be seen with noninvasive tumors.[154, 159, 160] For example, in one investigation of 15 thymomas, partial obliteration of fat planes was present in 8 invasive tumors and 7 noninvasive ones;[159] it was also evident in one thymic cyst (*see* Fig. 74–23). Despite these observations, certain findings on CT are highly suggestive of tumor invasion, including complete obliteration of fat planes,[60] pericardial thickening,[160] encasement of mediastinal vessels,[1, 151] an irregular interface

with the adjacent lung,[151, 161] and focal or diffuse pleural thickening.[151, 160, 162] Pleural implants, when present, are usually unilateral and result in focal or diffuse thickening; associated effusions are uncommon.[1, 163] Because invasive thymomas can extend into the posterior mediastinum, retrocrural space, and retroperitoneum,[151, 161, 164] CT performed for assessment of thymoma should include the upper abdomen.

Thymomas have intermediate signal intensity (equal to that of skeletal muscle) on T1-weighted MR images and increased signal intensity (approaching that of fat) on T2-weighted images (*see* Fig. 74–23).[71, 151, 165] The capsule has low signal intensity. Cystic regions and areas of hemorrhage have low signal intensity on T1-weighted images and high signal intensity on T2-weighted images.[1, 151] Inhomogeneous areas of signal intensity on T2-weighted images are seen more commonly in invasive than in noninvasive tumors. For example, in one investigation of 12 invasive thymomas, 11 showed this feature compared with none of 5 benign tumors;[165] 6 of the invasive thymomas had a lobulated internal architecture on T2-weighted images, internal lobules being separated by low-intensity septations.

Because of the relatively high prevalence of abnormalities in the thymus,[42, 166] CT is also indicated in the investigation of patients who have myasthenia gravis.[42, 167–171] In one study of 57 patients who had this disorder, chest radiographs and CT scans were correlated with pathologic findings after thymectomy;[168] 14 of 16 cases of thymoma were either suspected or definitely diagnosed on CT. In another investigation of 19 patients who had myasthenia gravis and who

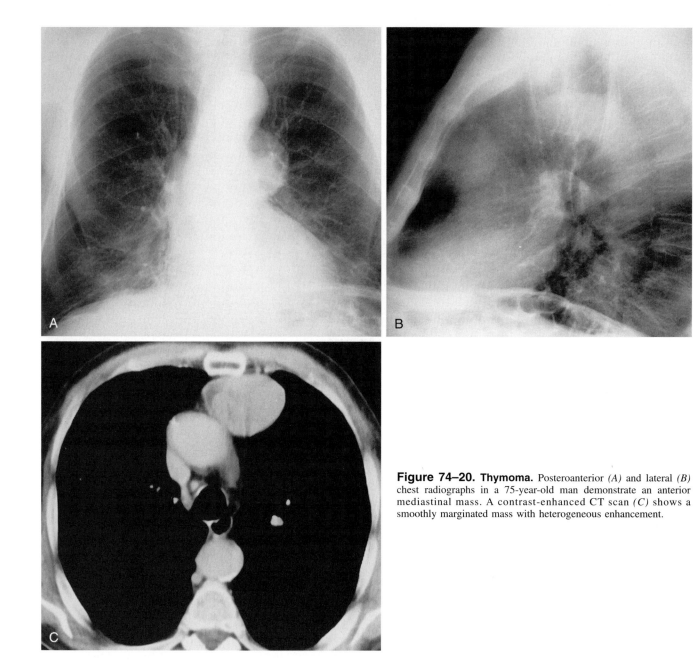

Figure 74–20. Thymoma. Posteroanterior *(A)* and lateral *(B)* chest radiographs in a 75-year-old man demonstrate an anterior mediastinal mass. A contrast-enhanced CT scan *(C)* shows a smoothly marginated mass with heterogeneous enhancement.

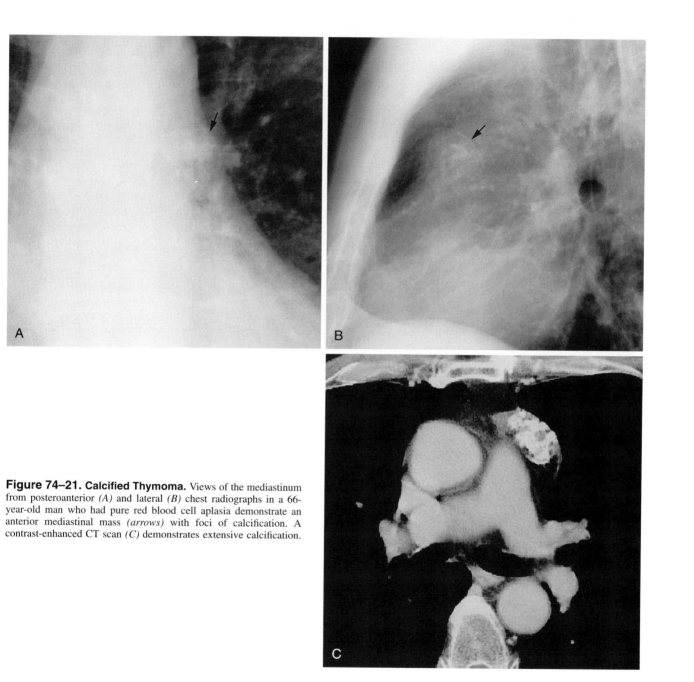

Figure 74–21. Calcified Thymoma. Views of the mediastinum from posteroanterior *(A)* and lateral *(B)* chest radiographs in a 66-year-old man who had pure red blood cell aplasia demonstrate an anterior mediastinal mass *(arrows)* with foci of calcification. A contrast-enhanced CT scan *(C)* demonstrates extensive calcification.

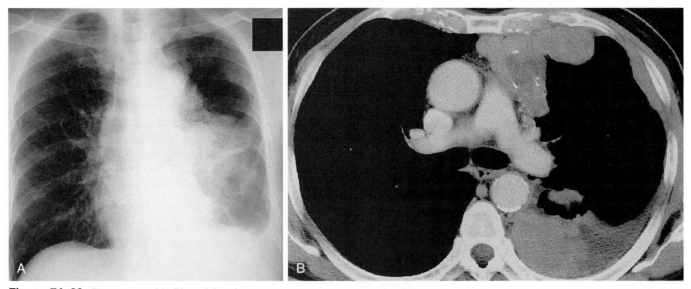

Figure 74–22. Thymoma with Pleural Involvement. A posteroanterior chest radiograph in a 65-year-old man *(A)* shows extensive left pleural thickening and a small left pleural effusion. A contrast-enhanced CT scan *(B)* demonstrates an inhomogeneous anterior mediastinal mass with focal areas of calcification, nodular left pleural thickening, and a small left pleural effusion. The diagnosis of invasive thymoma with left pleural seeding was proven at thoracotomy.

underwent thymectomy, CT was accurate in detecting the nine thymic masses;[170] however, it could not distinguish thymomas from nonthymomatous masses, including cysts.

In an investigation of 45 patients who had myasthenia gravis and who underwent thymectomy, 26 had normal CT findings, 7 had a diffusely enlarged thymus, and 12 had a focal mass.[42] Pathologic assessment demonstrated that 16 of 26 patients who had normal CT findings had normal thymic tissue, and 10 had lymphoid hyperplasia; all 7 patients who had a diffusely enlarged thymus had lymphoid hyperplasia. Five of 12 patients who had a focal mass at CT had lymphoid hyperplasia, and 7 had thymoma. On the basis of these results, one can conclude that the presence of a diffusely enlarged thymus or a focal mass on CT in a patient who has myasthenia gravis indicates the presence of an abnormality, either lymphoid hyperplasia or thymoma; however, CT is of limited value in distinguishing lymphoid hyperplasia from a normal thymus or from thymoma.[42]

Clinical Manifestations

Although some patients who have thymoma are asymptomatic when the tumor is discovered, the majority manifest symptoms related to local compression or invasion of thoracic structures or to systemic paraneoplastic disease. The effects of local compression or invasion are seen in about one third of patients, the most frequent being chest pain, shortness of breath, dysphagia, and cough;[106] hoarseness, evidence of pericarditis (rarely, with cardiac tamponade),[172, 173] and the superior vena cava syndrome[174] (sometimes with intravascular tumor extension[175]) can also be seen. Unusual and uncommon manifestations are spontaneous hemorrhage mimicking aortic dissection[176] and repeated respiratory tract infections associated with immunodeficiency (Good's syndrome).[177] Rare tumors present as a solitary lung metastasis.[178]

Myasthenia gravis is by far the most common para-

neoplastic disease associated with thymoma. Approximately 10% to 15% of patients who have myasthenia have the tumor,[106] and about 35% to 40% of all patients who have thymoma have myasthenia.[106, 137, 138, 179, 180] Although all histologic types can be associated with the complication, it is more common in the cortical form than in mixed or medullary tumors.[134, 136, 137] The tumor is sometimes occult;[120, 121] for example, in one review of 165 patients who had thymoma, 12 were identified who had myasthenia gravis and whose resected thymus was of normal size or was only minimally enlarged.[105] Rarely, patients who have thymoma develop other neurologic abnormalities, such as peripheral neuropathy[181] and limbic encephalitis.[182]

A variety of hematologic abnormalities are also associated with thymoma. Pure red blood cell aplasia (hypoplasia) is probably the most common;[183] of all patients who have this disorder, approximately 10% to 15% have a thymoma, most often of the medullary type.[55] Rarely, the hypoplasia occurs in association with other paraneoplastic disorders, such as myasthenia gravis,[184] polymyositis,[185] or peripheral blood lymphocytosis.[186] Other hematologic conditions associated with thymoma—at least some of which probably represent paraneoplastic phenomena—include aplastic anemia,[187] agranulocytosis,[188] cryoglobulinemia,[189] hypogammaglobulinemia[190] (sometimes associated with persistent candidiasis),[180] hypergammaglobulinemia (in one case associated with a prominent plasma cell infiltrate in the tumor),[184] T-cell lymphocytosis,[191–193] and leukemia.[194]

Many autoimmune diseases have been associated with thymoma. Although some of these may represent true paraneoplastic complications of the tumor, the development of some diseases years after thymectomy suggests that the absence of the thymus itself may be the pathogenetic link.[195, 196] Implicated conditions include systemic lupus erythematosus,[197] rheumatoid disease, polymyositis, Graves' disease, sclerosing cholangitis,[98] inflammatory bowel disease (including Crohn's disease, ulcerative colitis, and, in one

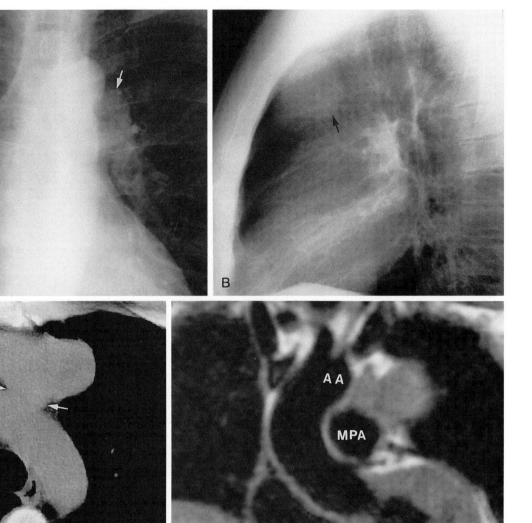

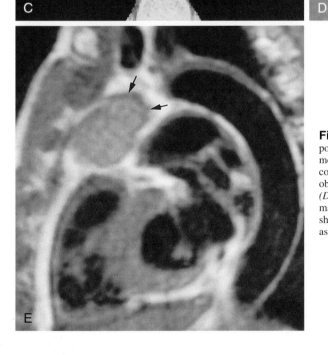

Figure 74–23. Invasive Thymoma. Views of the mediastinum from posteroanterior *(A)* and lateral *(B)* chest radiographs show an anterior mediastinal mass (arrows). A CT scan *(C)* performed without intravenous contrast demonstrates the mass and shows it to be associated with focal obliteration of the fat planes *(arrows)*. A T1-weighted coronal MR image *(D)* shows the close relationship of the mass to the aortic arch (AA) and main pulmonary artery (MPA). A sagittal T1-weighted MR image *(E)* shows low-signal intensity capsule *(arrows)* and high-signal intensity mediastinal fat. The diagnosis was confirmed at surgery.

instance, graft-versus-host–like disease[199]), intestinal pseudo-obstruction,[200] pernicious anemia, Sjögren's syndrome, pemphigus vulgaris, epidermodysplasia verruciformis,[201] and alopecia areata.[104, 106, 107]

Because the neoplastic epithelial cells of thymoma are derived from normal thymic epithelial cells, serologic or clinical manifestations of neuroendocrine disease would not be expected to be associated with the tumor. Nevertheless, cases have been reported in which there was increased urinary excretion of catecholamines[202] and ectopic secretion of parathormone and clinical findings of hyperparathyroidism.[203]

Prognosis and Natural History

The majority of thymomas are slow-growing encapsulated neoplasms whose excision results in cure; however, some are locally aggressive tumors that are unresectable or that recur after apparent complete excision. Recurrence or local invasion at the time of initial diagnosis occurs most commonly in the anterior mediastinal soft tissue, pericardium, or pleura; occasionally, a tumor extends into the lung parenchyma, bronchial lumen,[204] superior vena cava,[175] or right atrium[175, 205] or across the diaphragm (chiefly into the retroperitoneal space).[206] The most common sites of metastasis are the lung; pleura; thoracic skeleton; and mediastinal, supraclavicular, or cervical lymph nodes. Extrathoracic metastases are uncommon; in a review of the literature in 1976, only 29 cases were identified, and it is possible that some of these represented thymic carcinomas.[207] In another review of 283 patients, only 8 (3%) had distant metastases.[106] The diagnosis may be confirmed by fine-needle aspiration cytology.[208]

Numerous investigations have been carried out in an attempt to identify criteria that can accurately assess the likelihood of tumor recurrence or metastasis. Although to some extent correlated, there is evidence that both histologic type and stage are useful in this regard. Several staging schemes have been proposed (Table 74–1),[103, 104, 209, 210] the most widely used being that of Masaoka and colleagues.[211]

There is little question that the best criterion of malignancy or benignancy (apart from metastasis) is the presence or absence of local invasion, a finding that is usually established by the surgeon at the time of thoracotomy. The percentage of thymomas that are reported to show such invasion varies widely in different series, ranging from about 5% to 50% (some of these cases would probably be classified today as thymic carcinoma).[54] Recurrence is not uncommon in individuals who have such grossly invasive tumors because complete resection is usually impossible; however, because they can be slow growing, residual disease may be associated with prolonged survival.[212] Microscopic invasion into fat, pleura, or pericardium adjacent to the thymic tumor is also associated with an increased likelihood of recurrence.[125, 213] Although the presence of invasion is the most important predictor of prognosis, recurrence has sometimes been documented in well-encapsulated tumors that apparently have been completely excised.[106]

As indicated previously, there is evidence that tumor behavior is also associated with the histologic type: Several groups of investigators have shown that the probability of tumor recurrence is relatively high and the prognosis relatively poor with organoid and cortical tumors compared with medullary and mixed forms.[128, 134, 136, 137] Because the likelihood of local invasion is also associated with the presence of the first two patterns, the usefulness of histologic type in predicting behavior can be questioned;[147] nevertheless, multivariate analysis in some studies has shown it to be independent of stage in predicting long-term survival.[214]

Investigations of other parameters that might predict

Table 74–1. STAGING OF THYMOMA

STAGE	BERGH ET AL[103]	MASAOKA ET AL[211]	VERLEY AND HOLLMANN[104]	KORNSTEIN AND DEBLOIS[209]
I	Intact capsule or growth within the capsule	Macroscopically completely encapsulated and microscopically no capsular invasion	Grossly noninvasive a. Without adhesions b. With fibrous adhesions to mediastinal structures	Intact capsule or growth within the capsule
II	Pericapsular growth into the surrounding mediastinal fat tissue	1. Macroscopic invasion into surrounding fatty tissue or mediastinal pleura, *or* 2. Microscopic invasion into capsule	Localized (macroscopic) invasiveness (i.e., pericapsular growth into fat tissue or adjacent pleura or pericardium) a. Complete excision b. Incomplete excision	a. Microscopic invasion through capsule into adjacent mediastinal tissue b. Gross and microscopic invasion through capsule into surrounding fat or adjacent pleura or pericardium
III	Invasive growth into the surrounding organs, intrathoracic metastases, or both	Macroscopic invasion into neighboring organ (i.e., pericardium, great vessels, or lung)	Largely invasive tumor a. Invasion into surrounding organs and/or intrathoracic dissemination b. Lymphogenous or hematogenous metastasis	Invasion into surrounding structures (i.e., great vessels, lung)
IV		a. Pleural or pericardial dissemination b. Lymphogenous or hematogenous metastasis		a. Pleural or pericardial dissemination b. Lymphogenous or hematogenous metastases

Modified from Kornstein MJ, deBlois GG: Tumors of the thymic epithelial cell. *In*: Pathology of the Thymus and Mediastinum. Vol. 33 in Major Problems in Pathology. Philadelphia, WB Saunders, 1995, p 90.

biologic behavior have yielded variable results. The findings of some morphometric studies have suggested that the presence of invasion is more likely in tumors containing cells that have increased nuclear area;[215, 216] however, there is substantial overlap between groups of invasive and noninvasive tumors,[215] and this parameter is not useful in the individual case. Measurement of nuclear DNA content by flow cytometry also has yielded conflicting results, some investigators finding the presence of aneuploidy to have little or no predictive value[215, 217–219] and others finding the presence of aneuploidy to be associated with a worse prognosis.[220, 221] Measurements of cell proliferative activity, as manifested by argyrophilic nucleolar organizer region counts[222, 223] or the degree of proliferation-associated antigen or MIB-1 immunoreactivity,[224] have also been correlated with biologic behavior; although assessment of the last two features has yielded equivocal results, the presence of a high argyrophilic nucleolar organizer region count has been found by several investigators to predict aggressive behavior.[219, 222, 223]

In one immunohistochemical study of P53 expression in 46 noninvasive thymomas, a 10-year survival rate of 100% was found in P53-negative tumors compared with 71% for tumors that were positive.[219] Analysis of another group of 24 tumors, however, showed no evidence of either P53 or bcl-2 activity in neoplastic cells.[225] Other workers have generally found bcl-2 activity to be present in medullary tumors and in the spindle cell component of mixed tumors.[145, 145, 226] In one study, the presence of Fas antigen was associated with the presence of an advanced stage.[146] Some investigators have found evidence that expression of epidermal growth factor or epidermal growth factor receptor is also associated with tumor progression and prognosis.[225, 227]

The response of paraneoplastic syndromes to thymectomy is variable and depends, in part, on the specific syndrome and the underlying thymic pathology. For example, red blood cell aplasia resolves in about 30% to 35% of patients,[228, 229] whereas recovery from hypogammaglobulinemia appears to be uncommon.[229] Remission of myasthenia gravis appears to be more common after thymectomy for nonneoplastic conditions than for thymoma;[230, 231] for example, one group of investigators reported a complete remission rate of 40% at 5 years in the former situation and only 7% in the latter.[232] Recurrent tumor may be associated with recurrence of neurologic symptoms.[230, 231]

For patients who have thymoma, the overall 5-year survival is approximately 60% to 80%;[104, 124, 125, 210] for those who have invasive tumors (stage III or IV), it is about 50% to 60%, and for patients who have apparently completely encapsulated forms, it is about 75% to 90%. Recurrence may be seen many years after thymectomy,[233] and long-term follow-up is necessary before a patient can be considered to be cured.

Thymic Carcinoma

The nosology of malignant thymic epithelial tumors is somewhat confusing. As discussed in the previous section, some thymomas that show histologic features suggestive of a benign neoplasm invade adjacent mediastinal tissues and lung and occasionally metastasize. Although this behavior

indicates that such tumors are malignant and hence might be called carcinomas, the term *carcinoma* is usually reserved for neoplasms that possess the traditional histologic and cytologic features of malignancy, such as nuclear atypia, significant mitotic activity, and necrosis.[233a] Analysis of these latter tumors suggests that they, in turn, can be considered in two groups: (1) those tumors that show no resemblance to any of the histologic variants of thymoma and (2) those tumors that somewhat resemble the cortical form of thymoma (and that may be associated with areas of organoid or cortical thymoma elsewhere in the same tumor) but that show a greater degree of nuclear atypia, relatively few admixed lymphocytes, and an increased number of mitotic figures (so-called well-differentiated thymic carcinoma).[234, 235]

Well-Differentiated Thymic Carcinoma

The neoplastic cells of well-differentiated thymic carcinoma have an epidermoid appearance with little evidence of true squamous differentiation (i.e., keratinization or intercellular bridges).[134, 234] Perivascular spaces similar to those in thymomas are relatively common. As indicated, mitotic activity is greater than that of thymoma, most often between 1 to 5 per 10 high-power fields.[134, 234] It has been speculated that this variant may represent the most aggressive form of a spectrum of thymic tumors showing cortical differentiation;[144] as such, the distinctiveness of the tumor has been questioned and it has been referred to instead as *atypical thymoma*.[147, 233a]

As with thymoma, well-differentiated thymic carcinoma has been found to occur predominantly in adults (average age in one series of 50 years[234]). Many patients have myasthenia gravis (20 of 26 [77%] in one series[234] and 13 of 32 [40%] in another[134]). There are no distinctive radiologic features. The great majority of tumors are found to be locally invasive at the time they are discovered, and a small number eventually metastasize. The prognosis, however, is considerably better than that of most of the histologically more traditional forms of thymic carcinoma.

Other Forms of Thymic Carcinoma

The category of other forms of thymic carcinoma has been reported to include approximately 15% to 35% of all thymic epithelial tumors.[236–239] The cause is unknown in most cases. Some patients who have tumors that show a histologic pattern of lymphoepithelioma have evidence of Epstein-Barr virus infection.[240, 241] Others have a history of prior mediastinal radiotherapy.[239, 264] Rare cases appear to originate in a thymic cyst[242, 243] or a thymoma.[244–246] A particularly aggressive form of disease associated with chromosomal translocation (15;19) has been described.[247]

Pathologically, thymic carcinomas are usually bulky masses that range from 5 to 15 cm in diameter and are often found to invade adjacent structures at the time of diagnosis.[248, 264] A variety of histologic patterns has been reported, the most common being squamous cell carcinoma (some well differentiated and others resembling lymphoepithelioma of the nasopharynx) (Fig. 74–24).[248, 264] Other variants include small cell carcinoma (*see* page 2899); various combinations of adenocarcinoma, small cell carcinoma, and

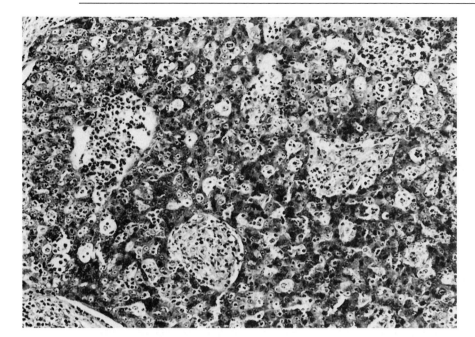

Figure 74–24. Thymic Carcinoma. A section of a well-circumscribed anterior mediastinal mass shows sheets of cytologically atypical cells associated with an extensive infiltrate of polymorphonuclear leukocytes. (×170.)

squamous cell carcinoma;[249] basaloid carcinoma;[243] mucoepidermoid carcinoma;[250] adenoid cystic carcinoma; clear cell carcinoma (resembling renal cell carcinoma);[251] papillary carcinoma;[233a] and spindle cell (sarcomatoid) carcinoma.[248, 252, 253, 264] Exceptional cases have been associated with a neuroblastomatous[254] or neuroendocrine[255] component (the former pattern has also been the sole histologic finding in some tumors[256]).

The distinction between primary thymic and metastatic carcinoma can be difficult, if not impossible, on histologic examination alone and relies more on the lack of a pulmonary neoplasm (the presence of a nonpulmonary origin of metastatic carcinoma being uncommon[257]). Immunohistochemical examination also may be useful in differentiation; in one investigation of nine thymic carcinomas and five pulmonary carcinomas, all thymic tumors and none of the pulmonary tumors reacted with an antibody to cytokeratin 7.[258] Two groups of investigators have found CD5—a molecule associated with T-cell growth—to be present in many thymic carcinomas but not in extrathymic carcinomas.[259, 260]

Differentiation between thymoma and thymic carcinoma is usually straightforward on the basis of cytologic features. However, with small tissue samples and in well-differentiated tumors, it can be difficult; in such cases, strong protein P53 expression,[236] aneuploidy and a high DNA index,[238] strong expression of epithelial membrane antigen,[261] or the absence of MIC2-positive lymphocytes[262] is more likely to be associated with carcinoma; however, none of these features is diagnostic in a specific case. As might be expected, markers of cellular proliferation, such as proliferating-cell nuclear antigen and argyrophilic nuclear organizer regions, are also likely to be more evident in carcinoma.[237] As with the distinction from metastatic carcinoma, immunohistochemical assessment of the presence of CD5 may prove to have greater discriminative power; in one investigation, 16 of 24 thymic carcinomas showed a positive reaction for this substance compared with none of 17 benign thymomas, 15 invasive thymomas, and 6 well-differentiated thymic carcinomas.[260]

Radiologically, thymic carcinomas usually present as large anterior mediastinal masses that have lobulated or poorly defined margins (Fig. 74–25).[1, 76, 162] On CT, they can have homogeneous soft tissue attenuation or heterogeneous attenuation as a result of necrosis; foci of calcification are present in 10% to 40% of cases.[162, 263] Focal or diffuse obliteration of the adjacent fat planes and evidence of extension into the pericardium or pleura is present in the majority.[162, 263] Although local pleural extension and associated effusion are common, distal pleural implants are seldom seen.[162] Mediastinal lymphadenopathy is present in 40% of cases.[162, 263]

Clinically, most patients are symptomatic at the time of diagnosis, the most common complaints being chest pain and cough; systemic findings, such as fever, weight loss, fatigue, and night sweats, are also common.[264] Rarely a radiographically occult tumor produces clinical findings, such as cardiac tamponade.[265] Compared with thymoma, the presence of a paraneoplastic syndrome is uncommon;[252, 266, 267] an association with myasthenia gravis was identified in only four cases in one report published in 1993.[268] Rare cases have been associated with hypercalcemia[269] and hypertrophic osteoarthropathy.[270] Some patients with neuroblastoma have had the syndrome of inappropriate antidiuretic hormone secretion.[256]

The prognosis for thymic carcinoma is poor, with progressive intrathoracic growth and extrathoracic metastases developing in the majority of patients.[252] In one investigation of 20 patients, attempted curative resection was possible in only 7 (35%).[266] The overall survival at 5 years is about 30% to 35%.[252, 264, 266, 267] Factors associated with outcome include stage,[271] grade, and histologic type (well-differentiated squamous cell, mucoepidermoid, and basaloid carcinomas tending to have a better prognosis).[252, 266] There is evidence that the tumors may be more aggressive during pregnancy.[272] In one investigation, the immunocytochemical identification of Mcl-1 (a protein related to *bcl*-2) was more likely to be associated with high-grade (particularly squamous cell) carcinoma;[226] although the investigators suggested

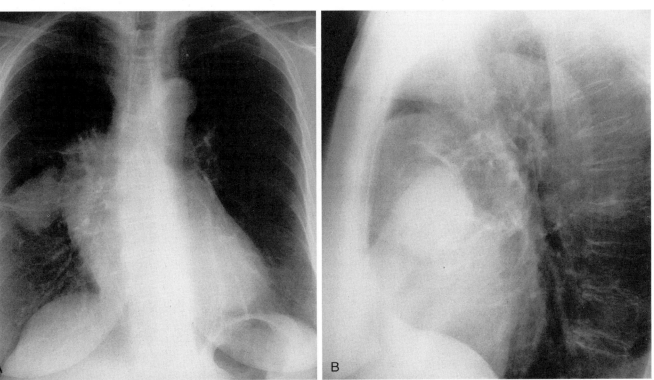

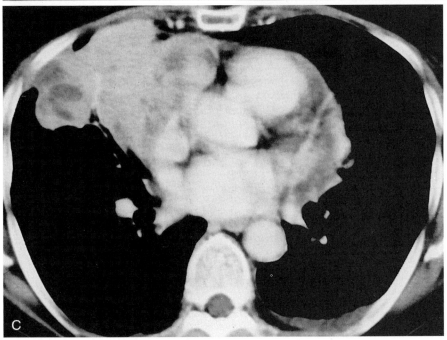

Figure 74–25. Thymic Carcinoma. Posteroanterior (A) and lateral (B) chest radiographs in a 69-year-old woman show a large, lobulated anterior mediastinal mass. Also noted is a soft-tissue component projecting into the right mid lung zone. A contrast-enhanced CT scan (C) also demonstrates a lobulated anterior mediastinal mass with inhomogeneous attenuation and obliteration of the adjacent fat planes. The mass can be seen extending into the right middle lobe. At surgery, this was shown to be a thymic carcinoma with pericardial, pleural, and right middle lobe involvement.

that this might be a useful prognostic marker, its benefit independent of histology or stage has not been shown.

Thymic Neuroendocrine Neoplasms

The term *thymic neuroendocrine neoplasms* encompasses several varieties of thymic neoplasm, all of which have in common histologic, ultrastructural, immunohistochemical, and, occasionally, clinical features of neuroendocrine function.[273] Although specific names have been given to the several histologic varieties, it is possible that they represent a spectrum of differentiation rather than specific entities. The cause and pathogenesis are unknown. The tumors are believed to be derived from neuroendocrine cells analogous to either intestinal Kulchitsky's cells or thyroid C cells (or both) whose presence has been documented in normal thymus.[274] These tumors are uncommon; according to one group of investigators, approximately 100 cases had been reported by 1984.[275] There is a 3 to 1 male-to-female predominance.[275] They may occur at any age,[276] the average at the time of diagnosis being about 45 years.

Pathologic Characteristics

Pathologically, the most common histologic subtype is carcinoid tumor; as with their pulmonary counterparts, these may be well differentiated (typical carcinoid tumor) or may show features suggestive of a more aggressive nature (atypical carcinoid). Grossly the tumors are usually bulky and somewhat lobulated. About half are well circumscribed or clearly encapsulated; the remainder invade the adjacent pleura, pericardium, diaphragm, or mediastinum.[274] The cut surface is usually solid, gray to tan in color, and soft in consistency; foci of necrosis and hemorrhage are frequent and calcification may be evident.[274, 275, 277]

The histologic pattern of typical carcinoid tumor consists most commonly of nests and trabeculae of fairly uniform cells separated by a delicate fibrovascular stroma; small foci of necrosis and mitotic figures are present in many cases. Variants include a spindle cell tumor similar to that of some peripheral pulmonary carcinoid tumors,[278] a tumor resembling thyroid medullary carcinoma (sometimes associated with amyloid),[274] a pigmented (melanocytic) tumor,[279, 280] a sclerotic tumor,[273] a tumor with prominent mucinous stroma,[281] and a tumor with sarcomatoid differentiation.[282, 283] Rare cases have also been reported of carcinoid tumor combined with a thymoma[284] or a thymic carcinoma[285] or after therapy for a mediastinal germ cell tumor.[286] Atypical carcinoid tumors tend to show sheets of cells without a nesting or trabecular appearance; cytologic atypia, necrosis, and mitotic activity are often prominent.[273, 287]

As with carcinoid tumors in other locations, silver stains show intracytoplasmic argyrophilic granules in many cases; ultrastructural examination reveals the presence of neurosecretory granules in virtually all.[274, 277] Immunohistochemical investigation frequently shows a positive reaction to nonspecific neuroendocrine markers, such as chromogranin and synaptophysin, as well as to one or more specific neuropeptides, such as calcitonin, cholecystokinin, neurotensin, gastrin, somatostatin, and adrenocorticotropic hormone.[277, 288, 289] (From a diagnostic point of view, it should be remembered that thymic carcinomas and atypical thymomas may also show a positive reaction for these substances.[289a])

In addition to carcinoid tumor, rare mediastinal tumors are composed predominantly of cells with hyperchromatic nuclei and scanty cytoplasm that resemble small cell carcinoma of the lung.[264, 274, 290] In some cases, an apparent transition between the two histologic patterns can be identified.[264, 290] As with pulmonary carcinoma, occasional tumors have a mixed appearance (usually squamous cell–small cell) by either light[248] or electron microscopy.[248, 264] Rare examples of tumors analogous to large cell neuroendocrine carcinoma of the lung have also been reported.[291] From a practical point of view, metastasis from a pulmonary carcinoma must be carefully excluded before a tumor that has any of these histologic appearances can be considered primary in the anterior mediastinum. Although the diagnosis of mediastinal neuroendocrine tumors is made most often on surgically excised tissue, it can be done on specimens obtained by ultrasound-guided transthoracic needle aspiration.[292–294]

Radiologic Manifestations

The chest radiograph result can be normal, a feature that is particularly likely in patients who have corticotropin-

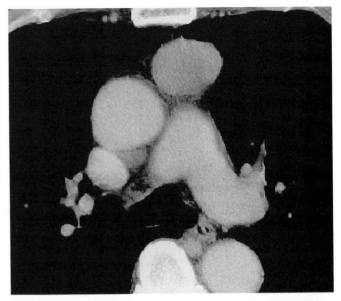

Figure 74–26. Thymic Carcinoid Tumor. A CT scan in a 67-year-old man demonstrates a 3-cm diameter anterior mediastinal mass with homogeneous enhancement. At surgery this was shown to be a "typical" carcinoid tumor.

producing carcinoid tumors;[295, 296] for example, in one investigation of five patients who presented with Cushing's syndrome, four had normal findings on chest radiographs.[295] Nonsecreting tumors or tumors associated with multiple endocrine neoplasia (MEN) syndromes more commonly manifest as large anterior mediastinal masses.[277, 297, 298] On CT, the tumors range from 1 to 25 cm in diameter[296, 298] and have homogeneous attenuation (Fig. 74–26) or heterogeneous attenuation as a result of necrosis or calcification (Fig. 74–27).[1, 295, 296] Evidence of invasion of adjacent structures and metastases to the regional lymph nodes or lungs is not uncommon.[277, 295, 298, 299] Skeletal metastases are typically osteoblastic.[94, 295]

Clinical Manifestations

Many mediastinal carcinoid tumors produce no symptoms and are discovered on screening chest radiography. Signs and symptoms caused by compression or invasion of mediastinal structures may be present, however, and include chest or shoulder pain, dyspnea, cough, superior vena cava syndrome, and pulmonary artery stenosis.[274, 300] Clubbing and hypertrophic osteoarthropathy are seen occasionally.[301] About 5% of patients have an MEN syndrome;[288, 302] almost all affected patients are male, and the majority have MEN type I (pituitary adenoma, parathyroid adenoma, and pancreatic islet cell tumor). Rare patients have neurofibromatosis.[303]

Clinical findings of paraneoplastic disease are present in about one third of patients, reflecting the neuroendocrine nature of these neoplasms.[273] Cushing's syndrome is by far the most common manifestation,[304, 305] having been identified in almost 25% of cases documented in the literature by 1984;[275] other syndromes, including inappropriate secretion of antidiuretic hormone[274] and carcinoid syndrome,[306, 307] are rare. Cushing's syndrome may be related to the production of either adrenocorticotropic hormone or corticotropin-releasing hormone.[308] Tumors associated with ectopic hormone

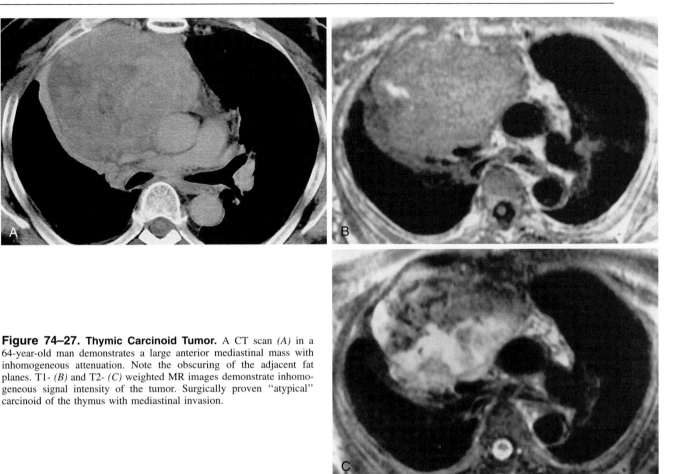

Figure 74–27. Thymic Carcinoid Tumor. A CT scan *(A)* in a 64-year-old man demonstrates a large anterior mediastinal mass with inhomogeneous attenuation. Note the obscuring of the adjacent fat planes. T1- *(B)* and T2- *(C)* weighted MR images demonstrate inhomogeneous signal intensity of the tumor. Surgically proven "atypical" carcinoid of the thymus with mediastinal invasion.

production tend to occur in younger patients and to be smaller than nonfunctioning tumors; in fact, as indicated previously, they are sometimes undetectable on radiographs.

Prognosis

As might be expected, complete excision of well-differentiated (typical), encapsulated carcinoid tumors of the thymus is associated with a good prognosis,[274] even in the few patients in whom regional lymph node metastases are present. The prognosis of patients who have atypical forms is guarded, particularly if there is extension outside the thymus at the time of presentation; in this case, local disease or metastases result in death in most patients.[274, 277, 287] The overall 5-year survival rate is said to be 65%.[275] Small cell carcinomas are so rare that it is difficult to predict behavior on the basis of published reports; however, there is some evidence that they may be somewhat less aggressive than their pulmonary counterparts.[264]

GERM CELL NEOPLASMS

The term *germ cell neoplasms* refers to a group of tumors histologically identical to certain testicular and ovarian neoplasms, all of which are believed to be derived from primitive germ cell elements. They include mature (benign) and malignant teratoma, seminoma, endodermal sinus tumor,

choriocarcinoma, and embryonal carcinoma.[309] The vast majority of these tumors are located in the anterior mediastinum:[310, 311] For example, in a 1971 review of 86 benign and 20 malignant tumors from the Mayo Clinic, 100 (94%) were located at this site;[8] the remaining 6 tumors (4 benign and 2 malignant) were found in the posterior mediastinum. Small foci of thymic tissue can be found at the periphery of some tumors,[312] suggesting an origin in the thymus.

In most cases, tumors become manifest in early adulthood, the mean age at diagnosis being between 20 and 40 years in several studies.[309, 313–315] For unexplained reasons, benign lesions are more common in women, and malignant tumors more frequent in men.[315, 316] For example, of 86 benign neoplasms reported from the Mayo Clinic in 1971, 52 (60%) occurred in women and 34 (40%) in men;[8] by contrast, of 56 malignant tumors reported from the same institution in 1985, 48 cases (86%) involved men.[314] In another investigation of 64 malignant, nonseminomatous mediastinal tumors, all were found to arise in men.[317]

The most common form of mediastinal germ cell tumor is mature teratoma, constituting almost 75% of tumors in two series of 133 cases[8, 310] and 45% in another.[315] The most common malignant tumor is seminoma: in three series that had a total of 103 malignant neoplasms, 29 (28%) were this type;[8, 313, 314] the remaining tumors consisted of 14 embryonal carcinomas, 10 malignant teratomas, 5 choriocarcinomas, and 3 endodermal sinus tumors; 42 tumors had a mixed histologic appearance. In another review of 64 cases of nonseminomatous, nonteratomatous mediastinal neoplasms, the most common pure histologic type was yolk sac tumor (38 cases), followed by choriocarcinoma (8 cases) and embryonal carcinoma (6 cases);[317] 12 tumors had a mixed histologic appearance.

Mediastinal germ cell tumors are generally considered to arise from cells whose journey along the urogenital ridge to the primitive gonad is interrupted in the mediastinum during fetal development. Occasionally, clinical or pathologic examination of a testicle reveals either viable tumor or focal scarring consistent with regressed tumor,[313, 318] indicating that the mediastinal neoplasm represents a metastasis. Although careful clinical examination must be performed in every case of mediastinal germ cell tumor to exclude this possibility, the relatively large number of negative pathologic examinations at autopsy[313] and biopsy[319] and the usual lack of emergence of a gonadal primary tumor during prolonged clinical follow-up indicate that this is a rare event. From a practical point of view, germ cell neoplasms involving the mediastinum that originate in the testis almost always have concomitant retroperitoneal lymph node metastases. Moreover, metastatic tumors in the mediastinum that are associated with a clear-cut gonadal primary are relatively uncommon compared with pulmonary metastases. Although these mediastinal metastases can have the same clinical and radiologic manifestations as primary mediastinal tumors, their clinical course is often different.[320] Such tumors may enlarge after chemotherapy in the absence of histologic evidence of malignancy (the growing teratoma syndrome).[321]

A relationship between mediastinal germ cell neoplasms and Klinefelter's syndrome has been documented by several groups of investigators;[322, 323] in one review of the literature, 21 of 272 tumors (almost 8%) were found to have this association.[322] The reason for the increased risk of germ cell neoplasia in these patients is unclear; possible explanations include the abnormal androgen and gonadotropin secretion that is characteristic of the syndrome or intrinsically abnormal germ cell tissue in patients who have Klinefelter's syndrome. Rare cases have also been reported of Klinefelter's syndrome, mediastinal teratoma, and hematologic neoplasia.[324]

Hematologic malignancies, most commonly nonlymphocytic leukemia and occasionally malignant histiocytosis, have also been associated with mediastinal germ cell neoplasms, particularly teratomas.[325–327] Associations with refractory anemia and excess blasts[328] and thrombocytopenia[329] have also been reported. Some of the leukemias have developed after the institution of chemotherapy or radiotherapy (or both), raising the possibility of therapeutically induced neoplasia. In most, however, the teratoma and hematologic malignancy have been recognized synchronously or within a short time after the induction of therapy, suggesting a common pathogenesis. Three hypotheses have been invoked to explain this association:[327] (1) The hematologic neoplasm represents an intrinsic malignant component of the teratoma, an explanation supported by occasional case reports;[330] (2) the teratoma secretes substances that induce the hematologic malignancy; and (3) the tumors represent independent neoplastic transformation of cells derived from primordial hindgut cells, which form a common source for both germ cells and hematopoietic stem cells.

Although a pathologic diagnosis of a mediastinal germ cell tumor can be made with small tissue samples, such as obtained by transthoracic needle aspiration,[331, 332] because of the tumor's varied histologic appearance, such diagnosis is sometimes difficult. Although this problem is relatively unimportant with respect to specific typing of germ cell tumors, advances in chemotherapy make the distinction from metastatic carcinoma of considerable significance.[333–335] Because such distinction is sometimes difficult, it seems reasonable to suggest that the possibility of a primary germ cell neoplasm be considered in any young patient who has an anterior mediastinal mass in whom a diagnosis of metastatic carcinoma is made in the absence of an extramediastinal primary focus. In this situation, review of pathologic material and testing for the presence of serum and tissue tumor markers, such as α-fetoprotein, β-human chorionic gonadotropin, and CD30, may result in a change in diagnosis.

As a group, nonseminomatous, malignant germ cell tumors are usually seen on radiographs as large anterior mediastinal masses that may have smooth, lobulated, or irregular margins.[76, 336, 337] On CT, these tumors usually have heterogeneous attenuation and contain large areas of low attenuation (Fig. 74–28).[336, 337] Focal areas of calcification may be seen.[337–339] The fat planes between the tumor and the adjacent structures are usually obliterated. Pleural and pericardial effusions are common.[1, 336, 337] CT may also demonstrate pulmonary metastases or irregular interfaces between the tumor and the lung as a result of direct pulmonary extension.[336, 337] Extension into the chest wall, mediastinal lymph node enlargement, and distal metastases can also be seen.[1, 336, 337]

Although the prognosis of malignant nonseminomatous germ cell tumors has improved markedly with the introduction of cisplatin-based chemotherapeutic regimens,[340] it is worse than that associated with their testicular counterparts, and approximately 50% to 70% of patients die from local or metastatic disease.[315, 317, 341, 343] A staging system has

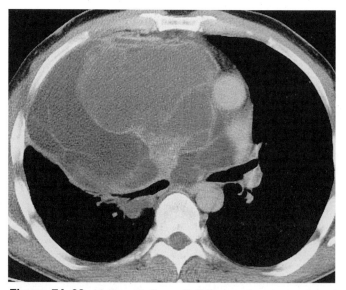

Figure 74–28. Malignant Germ Cell Tumor. A contrast-enhanced CT scan in a 37-year-old man demonstrates a large tumor diffusely infiltrating the mediastinum. The tumor has focal areas of soft tissue attenuation and large areas of low attenuation. Biopsy showed a malignant, nonseminomatous germ cell tumor.

Table 74–2. STAGING OF MEDIASTINAL GERM CELL TUMORS

Stage I	Well-circumscribed tumor with or without focal adhesions to the pleura or pericardium but without microscopic evidence of invasion into adjacent structures
Stage II	Tumor confined to the mediastinum with macroscopic and/or microscopic evidence of infiltration into adjacent structures (such as the pleura, pericardium, and great vessels)
Stage III	Tumor with metastases
IIIA	With metastases to intrathoracic organs (lymph nodes, lung)
IIIB	With extrathoracic metastases

Adapted from Moran CA, Suster S: Primary germ cell tumors of the mediastinum: I. Analysis of 322 cases with special emphasis on teratomatous lesions and a proposal for histopathologic classification and clinical staging. Cancer 80:681, 1997. Copyright © 1997, American Cancer Society. Reprinted by permission of Wiley-Liss, Inc., a subsidiary of John Wiley & Sons, Inc.

been proposed that may aid in predicting prognosis (Table 74–2).[329]

Teratoma

A teratoma can be defined as a neoplasm consisting of one or more types of tissue, usually derived from more than one germ cell layer, at least some of which are not native to the area in which the tumor arises. In the mediastinum, the majority of lesions are cystic and benign; solid neoplasms are usually malignant.[344, 345] The tumor is recognized most often in adolescence or early adulthood, although occasional series consisting of older individuals have been reported.[346] As indicated previously, almost all examples arise in the anterior mediastinum, posterior tumors being rare.[347] An unusual case has been reported of a gastric teratoma that herniated through the diaphragm and manifested as a mediastinal mass.[348]

Pathologic Characteristics

The tumors can be divided into three histologic types: mature teratoma, immature teratoma, and teratoma with malignant transformation. The term *dermoid cyst* is sometimes used to denote a tumor composed solely of ectodermal elements (invariably epidermis and its appendages) that line a keratin-filled cavity. Although not an uncommon variety of teratoma in the ovary, its occurrence in the mediastinum is rare because almost all tumors that grossly resemble a dermoid cyst have foci of endodermal and mesodermal tissue in their walls.[345, 349]

Mature teratomas are by far the most common form. They are usually well delimited from surrounding mediastinal structures and are unicystic or multicystic; solid forms occur occasionally (Fig. 74–29). Most are large when discovered, an average diameter of 8 to 10 cm being reported in several reviews.[298, 349, 350] Histologically, the tumors are composed of irregularly arranged but well-differentiated adult tissues (*see* Fig. 74–29); ectodermal elements, particularly epidermis and skin appendages, predominate.[312, 345, 350] Other relatively common tissues include cartilage, fat, smooth muscle, and respiratory mucosa. Bone, dental tissue, glial tissue, and enteric mucosa are less frequently encountered. A relatively high incidence of pancreatic tissue has

been documented by several investigators[345, 351, 352] and may be associated with a variety of complications (*see* farther on). In fact, anterior mediastinal cysts composed solely of pancreatic tissue have been hypothesized to represent unidirectional differentiation of a teratoma.[353] Mixed tumors composed of mature teratoma and one or more of the other germ cell variants are uncommon.[312]

Immature teratomas consist of the same adult tissues as the mature variety but in addition contain foci of primitive, less well-organized tissue resembling that seen in the developing fetus (Fig. 74–30). Primitive neuroepithelial tissue is most common; embryonic cartilage, bone, and undifferentiated mesenchyme occur in lesser amounts. Chromosomal abnormalities involving 12p have been identified in some cases.[328, 354]

Teratomas with malignant transformation contain a frankly malignant neoplasm in addition to the fetal or well-differentiated adult tissues that are found in the immature and mature varieties. The most common malignancy is sarcoma, usually angiosarcoma or rhabdomyosarcoma;[309, 355, 356] such tumors are probably derived from foci of immature mesenchymal tissue[357] and may become predominant after chemotherapy-induced destruction of the relatively sensitive germ cell portion of the tumor.[355, 356] Among the carcinomas, adenocarcinoma is the most frequent type, followed by squamous cell carcinoma and undifferentiated carcinoma (Fig. 74–31).[358] Neuroendocrine tumors are rare.[359] Teratomas with malignant transformation tend to be larger than their benign counterparts[359, 360] and not infrequently show invasion of contiguous structures at the time of diagnosis.

Radiologic Manifestations

The majority of mediastinal teratomas are seen on radiographs as a localized mass in the anterior compartment close to the origin of the major vessels from the heart (Fig. 74–32).[1, 336, 361] For example, in one investigation of 66 cases, 54 (82%) were found in the anterior mediastinum, 3 (4%) in the middle-posterior mediastinum, and 9 (14%) in multiple compartments;[361] findings included a focal mediastinal mass (in 92% of cases), diffuse mediastinal widening (3%), a mediastinal mass partially obscured by adjacent pulmonary consolidation (3%), and cardiomegaly in 1 (2%). The tumors ranged from 5 to 17 cm in longest dimension (mean, 10 cm). Calcification was evident on the radiograph in 14 mature teratomas (21%) and was classified as amorphous in 6 and as peripheral and curvilinear in 5; in 4 cases, it appeared to represent teeth or bone.

On CT, 59 tumors (89%) had well-defined margins that were smooth or lobulated.[361] Twenty-six mature teratomas (39%) had heterogeneous attenuation with soft tissue, fluid, fat, and calcium attenuation components (Fig. 74–33). Other common combinations included soft tissue, fluid, and fat (in 24% of cases) and soft tissue and fluid (15%). Although soft tissue attenuation was present in all mature cystic teratomas, it was the dominant component (occupying more than 50% of the total volume of the mass) in only two tumors (3%). Fifty-eight teratomas had fluid attenuation on CT, 50 had fat attenuation, and 35 had foci of calcification. MR imaging, performed in eight mature cystic teratomas, demonstrated areas that had soft tissue signal intensity in all cases, signal intensity consistent with fluid in seven (88%), and signal

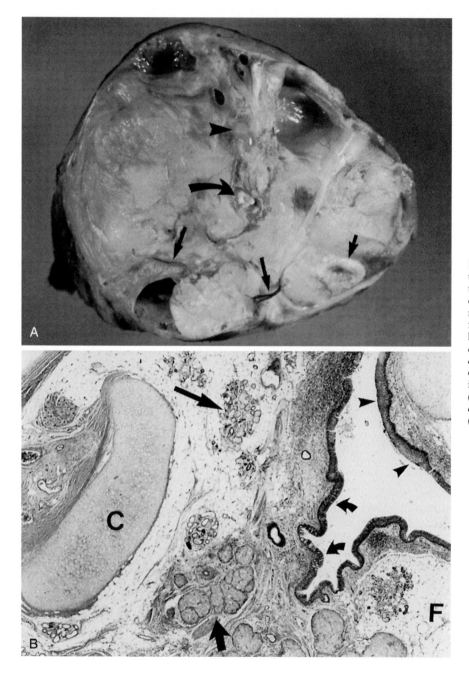

Figure 74–29. Mature Teratoma. A slice through this well-circumscribed anterior mediastinal tumor *(A)* shows mostly solid tissue containing several small cystic spaces. In addition to the relatively nondescript fleshy areas of tumor, there are scattered foci that possess specific differentiation, including hair *(long straight arrows)*, skin *(short straight arrow)*, mucus *(arrowhead)*, and bone *(curved arrow)*. A section *(B)* shows multiple foci of cytologically mature but architecturally disorganized tissue including fat (F), cartilage (C), sebaceous glands *(short arrow)*, salivary or bronchial type glands *(long arrow)*, and squamous *(arrowheads)* and respiratory *(curved arrows)* epithelium. (×25.)

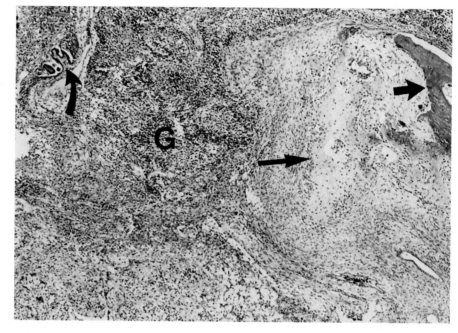

Figure 74–30. Immature Teratoma. The section shows foci of mature bone *(short arrow)*, cartilage *(long arrow)*, and pigmented epithelium *(curved arrow)*. In addition, there is a large focus of disorganized cells with hyperchromatic nuclei (G) that represent immature neuroglial elements. (×48.)

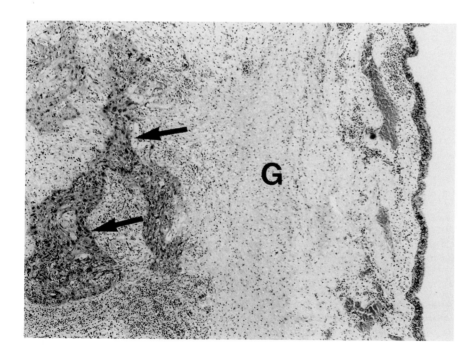

Figure 74–31. Teratoma with Malignant Transformation. A section through a grossly benign, predominantly cystic teratoma shows respiratory type epithelium on the right overlying mature neuroglial tissue (G). On the left are several irregularly shaped sheets of cytologically malignant squamous cells *(arrows).* (×50.)

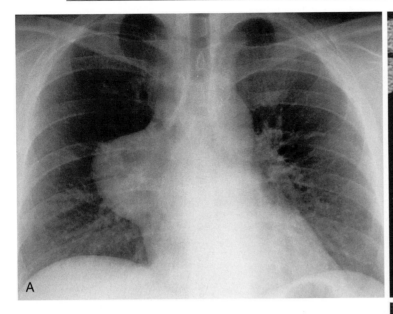

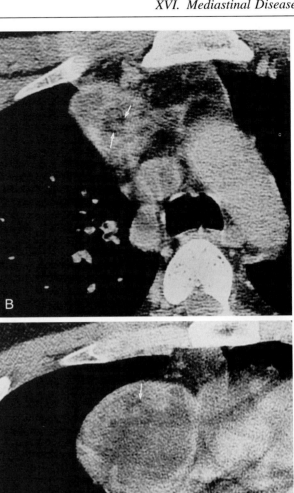

Figure 74–32. Mature Teratoma. A posteroanterior chest radiograph *(A)* in a 36-year-old man shows a smoothly marginated mediastinal mass. Thin-section CT scans *(B* and *C)* show the mass to have inhomogeneous attenuation and small localized areas of fat attenuation *(arrows)*.

intensity consistent with fat in five (63%). Sonography, performed in six cases, demonstrated heterogeneous echogenicity with a predominant fluid component (hypoechoic regions and increased through transmission) *(see* Fig. 74–33).

Occasionally a fat-fluid level is seen on the radiograph and CT (Fig. 74–34).[336, 362] The combination of fat, fluid, and soft tissue allows diagnosis of the majority of mature cystic teratomas on CT. For example, in one study of 128 patients who had anterior mediastinal masses, of whom 16 had teratoma, a confident, correct diagnosis of the tumor was made on the chest radiograph in 2 (13%) and on CT in 10 (63%).[76]

Complications of teratoma that may be evident on either radiographs or CT include atelectasis and obstructive pneumonitis (as a result of airway compression),[336, 361, 363] pneumonitis (after rupture into the lung),[363, 380] and effusion (secondary to rupture into the pleural space or pericardium).[336, 361, 363, 380] Occasionally, an effusion has a fat-fluid level;[364]

rarely, the accumulated fluid is sufficient to cause cardiac tamponade.[336] Perforation of the aorta and superior vena cava are additional rare complications.[363]

Clinical Manifestations

Mature teratomas usually do not produce symptoms and are discovered on a screening chest radiograph. Those that grow to a large size can cause shortness of breath, cough, and a sensation of pressure or pain in the retrosternal area. Large lesions, particularly the malignant forms, also may obstruct the superior vena cava or grow to such a size as to present in the suprasternal notch.[365] Rarely, compression of a bronchus results in recurrent infection;[366] similar compression of the pulmonary artery or right ventricular outflow tract may be associated with signs of pulmonic stenosis.[367]

Occasionally a cystic tumor ruptures and spills its contents into the mediastinum or pleural cavity, with resultant

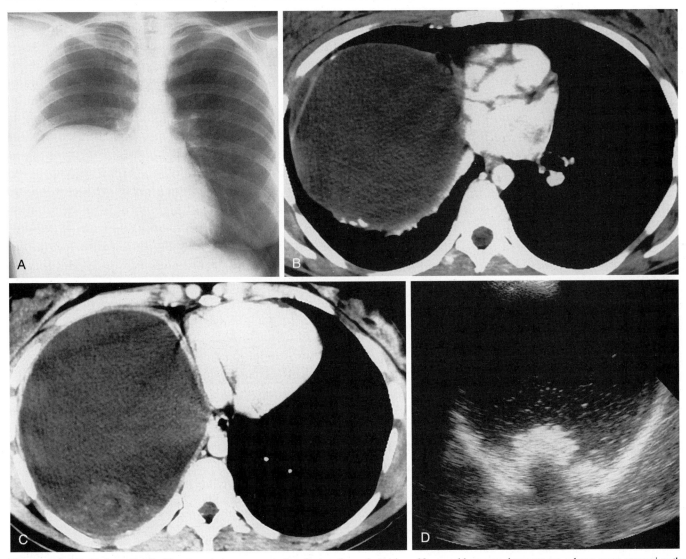

Figure 74–33. Mature Cystic Teratoma. A posteroanterior chest radiograph *(A)* in a 28-year-old woman demonstrates a large mass occupying the lower right hemithorax. A CT scan through the cephalad aspect of the mass *(B)* shows predominantly fluid and fat attenuation and localized areas of calcification. CT at a more caudad level *(C)* shows a nodular soft tissue component. Ultrasound *(D)* demonstrates hypoechoic regions and focal areas of heterogeneous echogenicity. The diagnosis of mature cystic teratoma was confirmed at surgical resection. (Courtesy of Dr. Ella Kazerooni, Department of Radiology, University of Michigan Hospital, Ann Arbor, MI.)

mediastinitis or empyema;[368] similarly, a fistula can develop with adjacent structures, including the pericardium (sometimes causing tamponade),[369] aorta, superior vena cava, esophagus, tracheobronchial tree, or externally through the neck. When communication occurs with the airways, the contents of the cyst may be expectorated; if this material contains hair (trichoptysis), the diagnosis of mature teratoma can be made clinically. The pathogenesis of cyst rupture is not always clear; although it may be caused by infection in some cases, it is also possible that it results from erosion by locally produced pancreatic enzymes.[369, 370] Support for this hypothesis is provided by the relatively common presence of pancreatic tissue in mature teratomas and by the occasional patient in whom a high level of amylase has been found in fluid from a fistulous tract or adjacent lung.[369, 371] Rarely, pancreatic islet tissue has been associated with hypoglycemia and hyperinsulinemia.[372]

Although malignant forms of teratoma can grow rapidly,[373] it is important to recognize that a rapid increase in size does not necessarily indicate malignancy: Hemorrhage into the cyst of a mature teratoma can result in an abrupt increase in size and can cause severe retrosternal pain or discomfort.

Prognosis and Natural History

Mature teratomas are benign tumors; provided that they are completely excised, cure is the rule. Thorough pathologic sampling, however, must be carried out to ensure that small foci of immature tissue, other germ cell tumor, or carcinoma or sarcoma are not present. The behavior of immature teratoma depends somewhat on the age of the patient: Tumors that manifest in infancy or childhood are often treated successfully by surgical excision, whereas those that appear in older individuals frequently follow a highly aggressive course that results in death.[315, 374, 375] As might be expected,

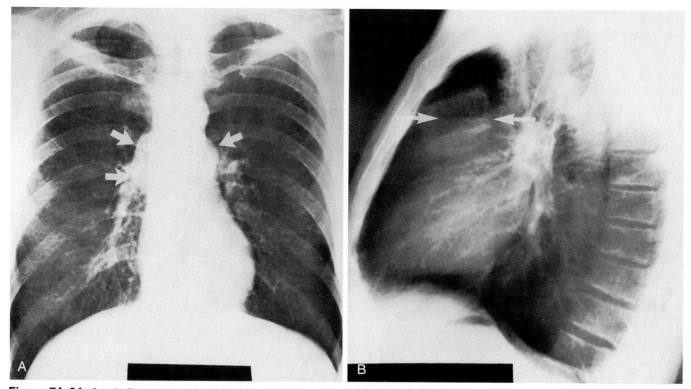

Figure 74–34. Cystic Teratoma of the Anterior Mediastinum Containing a Fat-Fluid Level. Posteroanterior *(A)* and lateral *(B)* radiographs reveal a mass of moderate size situated in the anterior mediastinum. The mass is somewhat lobulated and projects to both sides of the mediastinum *(arrows in A)*. In lateral projection, a fluid level can be seen *(arrows in B)*.

teratomas with malignant transformation are also usually aggressive and cause death within a few months of diagnosis as a result of local spread or metastases, or both.[309] As indicated previously, some teratomas are complicated by synchronous or subsequent leukemia, which may influence the course of disease.

Seminoma

Seminoma (germinoma) is the most frequent mediastinal germ cell neoplasm after teratoma and is the most common form of histologically pure malignant tumor. In one review of the literature reported in 1985, approximately 200 cases were identified.[376] The tumor occurs almost exclusively in men; most patients present in their twenties or thirties.[315, 377, 378]

The majority of mediastinal seminomas are solid, gray-tan tumors greater than 5 cm in diameter; occasionally, there is prominent multilocular cystic change.[379] Histologically, the tumor is composed of nests of cells separated by a variably thick fibrovascular stroma that contains numerous lymphocytes (Fig. 74–35).[378, 381] Tumor cell nuclei are typically round and contain coarsely clumped chromatin and prominent nucleoli; the cytoplasm is usually clear and contains glycogen. In addition to lymphocytes, loosely formed, nonnecrotizing granulomas, germinal centers, or both are found in the stroma of many cases[381] and can be a helpful feature in differentiating the neoplasms from lymphoma, thymoma, and thymic cysts.[25, 382] A positive immunohistochemical reaction to placental alkaline phosphatase is seen in many tumors and is also a helpful finding in differential diagnosis, particularly in small samples.[378, 383] Ultrastructural features are characteristic.[384]

Radiographically, seminomas usually manifest as large masses that may project into one or both sides of the anterior mediastinum.[313, 336, 385, 386] They typically have homogeneous attenuation on CT and enhance only slightly after intravenous administration of contrast material.[336] Occasionally, a few localized areas of low attenuation[337] or ringlike and stippled foci of calcification are seen.[336, 387] Evidence of invasion of adjacent structures is seldom apparent.[1, 337] Metastases may result in regional lymph node enlargement or bone destruction.[1, 386]

Approximately 20% to 30% of patients are asymptomatic at the time of initial diagnosis. When present, symptoms usually derive from pressure or invasion of mediastinal vessels or the major airways and include chest pain and shortness of breath.[378] Superior vena caval obstruction develops in about 10% of patients.[377, 378] Gynecomastia associated with high blood levels of estradiol and β-human chorionic gonadotropin has been reported rarely.[388] Tumors must be distinguished from metastatic testicular seminoma, which occurs in about 5% of patients who have stage III disease.[376] It has been suggested that assessment of the K-ras sequence and P53 immunoreaction profile might aid in distinguishing the two tumors.[360]

Pure seminomas are radiosensitive, and the prognosis is considerably better than that of mixed or nonseminomatous malignant germ cell tumors; the overall 5-year survival rate is in the range of 60% to 80%.[315, 389–391] As might be expected, tumors that have a higher stage (manifested by local

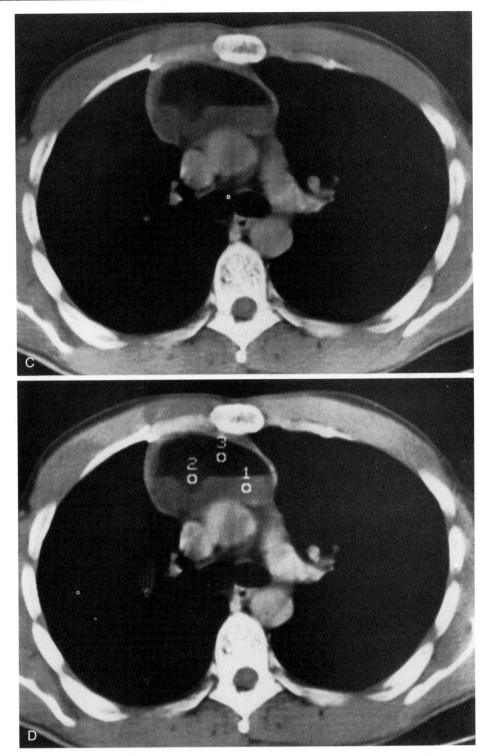

Figure 74–34 *Continued.* A CT scan at the level of the left pulmonary artery *(C)* also shows a fluid level in the center of the mass. A CT scan at the same level *(D)* for measurement of attenuation coefficients revealed the following determinations of Hounsfield units: *1* = 16; *2* = −78; and *3* = −139. The conclusion that can be reached from these measurements is as follows: the material at the bottom of the cyst represents soft tissue detritus of unknown nature; the supernatant represents liquid fat; and the small nubbin (number *2* in *D*) represents material composed of an admixture of fat and soft tissue components. The patient was an asymptomatic middle-aged man. (Reprinted with permission slightly modified from Fulcher AS, Proto AV, and Jolles H: Cystic teratoma of the mediastinum: Demonstration of fat/fluid level. Am J Roentgenol 154:259, 1990.)

mediastinal invasion or regional lymph node metastases) tend to be associated with a worse outcome.[378, 390] Other features that have been found to be associated with a bad prognosis include age older than 35 years, pyrexia, and superior vena cava syndrome.[378, 390]

Endodermal Sinus Tumor

Endodermal sinus tumors are highly malignant germ cell neoplasms believed to show differentiation toward yolk sac endoderm. Origin in the mediastinum is rare; only 38 cases of the pure form had been reported in the English language literature by 1986.[392] The tumor also occurs occasionally in association with other germ cell neoplasms.

Tumors are usually large (often more than 10 cm) with areas of necrosis, hemorrhage, and cystic degeneration; occasionally, the last-named is a prominent feature.[89] The histologic appearance is quite variable; reticular, tubulopapillary, hepatoid,[393] spindle cell,[394] and solid patterns have been described. Perivascular structures resembling the rat endo-

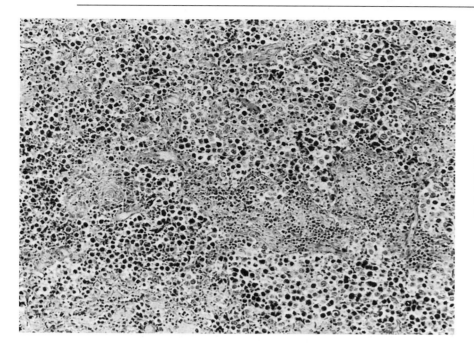

Figure 74–35. Mediastinal Seminoma. A section of an anterior mediastinal tumor from a 23-year-old man shows interconnecting sheets of cells with abundant cytoplasm and fairly uniform, more or less round nuclei; the intervening stroma contains a moderate number of lymphocytes. (× 120.)

dermal sinus (Shiller-Duval bodies) and small intracellular and extracellular globules of periodic acid–Schiff–positive material are characteristic features. Immunohistochemical studies show a positive reaction for α-fetoprotein and alpha₁-antitrypsin in many cases;[383, 392] occasional tumors also show carcinoembryonic antigen and keratin positivity. Extracellular basement membrane–like material is often present on ultrastructural examination.[392, 395]

Most endodermal sinus tumors appear in young adults, the mean age in the 1986 review cited previously being about 23 years;[392] the majority occur in men. Radiographic and CT findings are similar to those of other malignant mediastinal germ cell tumors (Fig. 74–36).[336, 337] Symptoms related to local mediastinal compression or invasion are present in most patients at the time of diagnosis; systemic

symptoms (anorexia, weight loss, and fever) and symptoms related to metastases are also frequent.[392] Serum levels of α-fetoprotein are elevated in virtually all patients and are a useful indicator of tumor recurrence or remission with therapy. Although the prognosis is generally poor, prolonged survival and even cure have been documented in some patients who have been treated aggressively.[396–398] As with other neoplasms, patients who have low-stage tumors tend to have a better survival.[317]

Choriocarcinoma

Choriocarcinoma is a rare variety of mediastinal germ cell neoplasm that is usually seen in combination with other

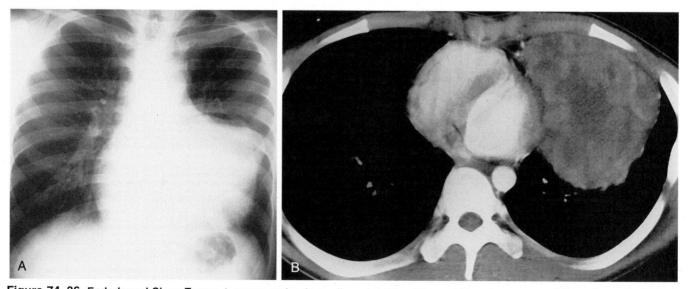

Figure 74–36. Endodermal Sinus Tumor. A posteroanterior chest radiograph *(A)* in a 16-year-old boy demonstrates a left anterior mediastinal mass obscuring the heart border. A contrast-enhanced CT scan *(B)* demonstrates inhomogeneous soft tissue attenuation and focal central areas of decreased attenuation. (Courtesy of Dr. Ella Kazerooni, Department of Radiology, University of Michigan Hospital, Ann Arbor, MI.)

forms, especially embryonal carcinoma.[399–402] As with other malignant germ cell tumors, the peak age incidence is between 20 and 30 years, and most occur in men.[403]

Pathologically, the tumor is typically a bulky lobulated mass associated with prominent necrosis and hemorrhage.[403] Histologically, sheets of cells with vesicular nuclei and abundant eosinophilic cytoplasm (cytotrophoblasts) are located adjacent to large multinucleated giant cells (syncytiotrophoblasts). The latter show a positive immunohistochemical reaction for β-human chorionic gonadotropin;[403] some tumors also express human placental alkaline phosphatase.[383]

The radiographic and CT findings are similar to those of other malignant nonseminomatous germ cell tumors.[1, 336] Most patients are symptomatic at the time of presentation with dyspnea, hemoptysis, hoarseness, stridor, dysphagia, and/or Horner's syndrome.[404] Gynecomastia has been reported in about two thirds of patients[405] and is invariably associated with elevated serum levels of human chorionic gonadotropin. The prognosis is extremely poor, with death occurring in most patients within months of the diagnosis.[403, 406]

PRIMARY MEDIASTINAL LYMPHOMA

Lymphoma is one of the most common cause of mediastinal abnormality: It has been estimated that it constitutes about 20% of all mediastinal neoplasms in adults and 50% in children.[407] A mediastinal mass is also a frequent manifestation of lymphoma; for example, in one series of 650 patients, 121 (approximately 20%) had mediastinal involvement. Most often, such involvement occurs in association with clinical or radiographic evidence of extrathoracic lymphoma; in about 5% of cases the mediastinum is the sole site of abnormality,[408] in which case differentiation from other mediastinal abnormalities can be difficult on the basis of radiologic findings alone. The most common causes of such primary disease are Hodgkin's disease, large cell lymphoma, and lymphoblastic lymphoma; other forms are infrequent.[409–411] Many of these primary mediastinal tumors appear to originate in the thymus. Only a brief summary of the major forms of lymphoma is presented here; further details of the radiologic and clinical features are given in Chapter 35 (see page 1291).

Hodgkin's disease is undoubtedly the most common lymphoma to manifest in the mediastinum, lymph node enlargement being evident on the initial radiograph of approximately 50% of patients.[412, 413] An anterior mediastinal mass involving the thymus is also common.[414, 415] Nodular sclerosis is by far the most frequent histologic subtype (Fig. 74–37); the disease is seen most often in young women.

Lymphoblastic lymphoma constitutes about 60% of cases of primary mediastinal non-Hodgkin's lymphoma,[407] and approximately 50% to 80% of patients with this neoplasm have a prominent mass in the mediastinum at the time of presentation.[416] The majority of patients are children or adolescents, frequently male; immunologic studies show most tumors to have features of thymic T cells. Signs and symptoms related to mediastinal involvement are common and include respiratory distress (as a result of airway com-

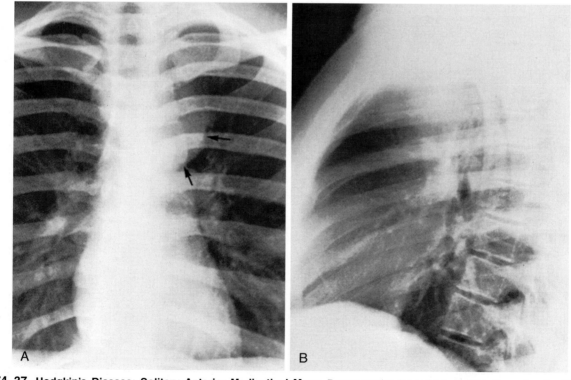

Figure 74–37. Hodgkin's Disease: Solitary Anterior Mediastinal Mass. Posteroanterior *(A)* and lateral *(B)* radiographs of a 15-year-old girl reveal a smooth, homogeneous mass projecting to the left of the upper mediastinum *(arrows)*. Although the mass cannot be outlined clearly in lateral projection, its position in the anterior mediastinum is established by the fact that it fades out superiorly as a result of contiguity with the soft tissues of the neck at the thoracic inlet. (If the mass were posteriorly situated, its superior border would be clearly outlined because of contiguity with air-containing lung.) This mass was the only intrathoracic abnormality visualized. Biopsy revealed Hodgkin's disease of nodular sclerosis type.

pression) and superior vena cava syndrome. Pleural and pericardial effusions are also frequent.[417] The tumor is aggressive, with widespread dissemination (especially to extrathoracic lymph nodes and the central nervous system) occurring in many individuals; a leukemic phase also commonly develops. Despite these features, current therapy results in remission in the majority of patients and a 3-year disease-free survival of approximately 55%.[409]

The remaining 40% of primary mediastinal non-Hodgkin's lymphomas are composed of different histologic subtypes, by far the most common of which is *diffuse large cell lymphoma*.[418–423] Grossly, the tumors are large, averaging almost 12 cm in diameter in one review.[420] Invasion of contiguous mediastinal structures, chest wall, and lung is common at the time of presentation.[420] Immunopathologic examination shows most tumors to be of B-cell origin. Sclerosis, manifested by either a diffuse increase in reticulin or relatively broad bands of fibrous tissue, is a characteristic feature. The majority of tumors occur in young adults; in most series, the sex incidence is about equal, although in some there is a predominance of women.[420, 421] Symptoms referable to the thorax, particularly dyspnea and pain, are present in the majority of patients. Superior vena cava syndrome also occurs in many individuals (in 38 of 93 patients [40%] in three series);[408, 420, 423] compression of the vena cava in the absence of the full-blown clinical syndrome can be identified in some patients.[423] With aggressive chemotherapy and radiation therapy, most investigators have found a complete remission rate of almost 80% and a 50% to 60% 5-year survival.

TUMORS AND TUMOR-LIKE CONDITIONS OF ENDOCRINE ORGANS

Thyroid Tumors

Although extension of thyroid tissue into the thorax is seen in only 1% to 3% of patients subjected to thyroidectomy,[424, 425] such tissue nevertheless constitutes a significant percentage of anterior mediastinal masses. The most frequent pathologic finding is multinodular goiter,[426] a condition that occurs most commonly in women in their forties;[427] occasionally the abnormality is acute[428, 429] or chronic[430] thyroiditis or thyroid carcinoma.[427]

Seventy-five per cent to 80% of mediastinal thyroid tumors arise from a lower pole or the isthmus and extend into the anterior or middle mediastinum. Most of the remainder arise from the posterior aspect of either thyroid lobe and extend into the posterior mediastinum behind the trachea, innominate or brachiocephalic vein, and innominate or subclavian arteries;[431–433] in the last-mentioned location, they are situated almost exclusively on the right.[432] In a small number of cases (probably less than 1%), there is no evident connection between the cervical and intrathoracic thyroid tissue;[427] in these, it is assumed that the intrathoracic tumor arises from ectopic thyroid tissue displaced during fetal development.[434] As might be expected from this discussion, the abnormal thyroid tissue is located in the uppermost portion of the mediastinum in the majority of patients; however, occasionally, growth extends from the neck to the diaphragm.[427]

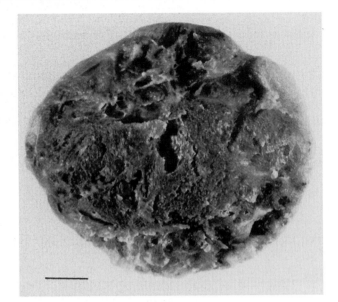

Figure 74–38. Mediastinal Goiter. A cut section of a superior mediastinal tumor shows a well-circumscribed mass that grossly resembles mature thyroid tissue. (Bar = 1 cm.)

Pathologically, most excised mediastinal goiters measure 6 to 10 cm in diameter and have foci of hemorrhage, fibrosis, cyst formation, and calcification (Fig. 74–38). Carcinoma is identified in 2% to 3% of cases.[427] The rare case of intrathoracic oncocytoma may have its origin in ectopic mediastinal thyroid tissue.[435]

Radiologic Manifestations

Radiographically, the appearance of a retrosternal goiter is that of a sharply defined, smooth or lobulated mass that causes displacement and narrowing of the trachea (Fig. 74–39).[94, 436] Anterior and middle mediastinal goiters displace the trachea posteriorly and laterally, whereas those in the posterior mediastinum displace it anteriorly.

Because CT allows accurate assessment of the position of an intrathoracic goiter and its relationship to adjacent structures as well as the diagnosis of other masses that may mimic the abnormality on the chest radiograph, it is currently the imaging modality of choice in the assessment of these tumors. Characteristic features include continuity with the cervical thyroid, focal calcification, a relatively high CT number, an increase in CT number after bolus administration of iodinated contrast material, and prolonged enhancement after contrast administration (Fig. 74–40).[437] The attenuation value of the thyroid is often greater than 100 H before administration of contrast material; because the gland concentrates iodine, it enhances intensely and for a prolonged period (more than 2 minutes) after intravenous injection.[437, 438] The attenuation of the intrathoracic component of a goiter is usually greater than that of muscle but less than that of the cervical thyroid gland. Focal nonenhancing areas of low attenuation as a result of hemorrhage or cyst formation are common.[1, 436] The connection between the intrathoracic thyroid tissue and the thyroid gland is usually readily apparent on CT; rarely, the only connection is a narrow fibrous or vascular pedicle that may not be apparent.[436]

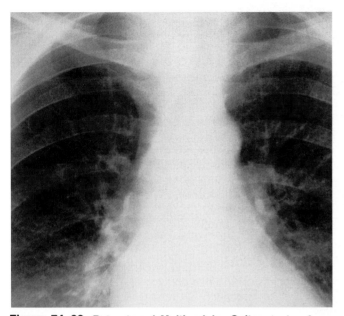

Figure 74–39. Retrosternal Multinodular Goiter. A view from a posteroanterior chest radiograph in a 64-year-old woman demonstrates extrinsic compression and smooth displacement of the trachea by a soft-tissue mass extending from the lower neck into the thoracic inlet.

Thyroid carcinoma usually manifests as a mass of inhomogeneous attenuation in the lower neck, which may extend into the thorax.[439–441] The distinction between carcinoma and a goiter can be made on CT when there is evidence of spread into the adjacent tissue or lymph node enlargement.[438, 441] In many cases, however, the borders of a carcinoma are well defined.[438] Localized areas of low attenuation and foci of calcification can be seen in both benign and malignant masses.[438, 440]

MR imaging, particularly in the coronal and sagittal planes, can demonstrate the extent of intrathoracic thyroid tissue and its relationship to adjacent structures. Multinodular goiters have heterogeneous signal characteristics on both T1- and T2-weighted MR images.[442, 443] Because of its low sensitivity in the detection of calcification and its high cost, MR imaging has a limited, if any, role in the assessment of the intrathoracic thyroid.

The vast majority of intrathoracic goiters show evidence of function on radionuclide imaging.[444–446] Radionuclides used include iodine-123, technetium-99m, and iodine-131,[444] the last-named being the agent of choice.[446] In one investigation of 54 consecutive patients in whom chest radiographs suggested the presence of an upper mediastinal mass, scintigraphy detected 39 of 42 intrathoracic goiters (sensitivity 93%) and correctly excluded goiter in 12 patients (specificity 100%).[444] "False-positive" uptake, however, can be seen in association with hiatal hernia[447, 448] and in the thymus,[449] the latter possibly as a result of binding of iodine to protein in Hassall's corpuscles.

Clinical Manifestations

Many patients who have intrathoracic goiter are asymptomatic,[8, 310, 427] the abnormality being discovered on a screening chest radiograph. When present, symptoms include respiratory distress (which can be worsened by certain move-

ments of the neck) and hoarseness. The latter is usually caused by compression of the recurrent laryngeal nerve;[431] however, its presence should raise the possibility of extracapsular invasion and malignancy. Posterior mediastinal goiters can cause dysphagia, whereas those in the anterior and middle compartment can cause superior vena cava syndrome as a result of obstruction of brachiocephalic vessels.[310, 433, 450, 451] Physical examination usually reveals evidence of a goiter in the neck; inspiratory and expiratory stridor may be apparent. Thyrotoxicosis is present in some patients.[452, 453] An unusual case has been reported in which a huge retrosternal goiter was associated with systemic hypertension (blood pressure 230/130 mm Hg);[454] after removal of the goiter, blood pressure returned to normal and remained so without further medical treatment.

Parathyroid Tumors

Parathyroid tumors constitute a rare cause of an anterior mediastinal mass. Their presence within the mediastinum is best explained on the basis of the normal migration of parathyroid glands with the thymus during embryonic development; although they usually separate and remain in the neck, occasionally they proceed distally, usually in direct continuity with thymic tissue. Most abnormal glands contain an adenoma or are hyperplastic; occasionally, a tumor is malignant (parathyroid carcinoma).[455] Rarely, multiple nodules of hyperplastic parathyroid tissue can be found scattered within mediastinal soft tissue or the thymus ("parathyromatosis") without gross tumor formation.[456] Nonneoplastic parathyroid cysts have also been documented.[457, 458]

Most mediastinal parathyroid lesions are so small as to be invisible radiographically. Occasionally, a tumor is sufficiently large to widen the mediastinal silhouette, usually unilaterally.[459–462] Calcification may also be apparent.[463] On CT, mediastinal parathyroid adenomas usually present as small nodules that show minimal, if any, enhancement after

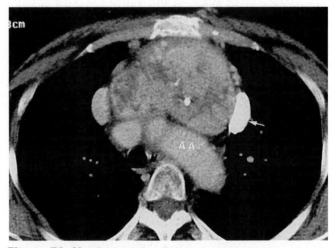

Figure 74–40. Multinodular Goiter. A CT scan performed during intravenous administration of contrast demonstrates a large anterior mediastinal mass that has inhomogeneous attenuation and contains small foci of calcification. The mass lies anterior to the aortic arch (AA) and innominate artery and displaces the left brachiocephalic vein (*arrow*). The patient was a 67-year-old woman with long-standing multinodular goiter.

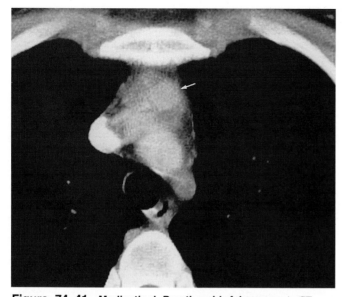

Figure 74–41. Mediastinal Parathyroid Adenoma. A CT scan performed during intravenous administration of contrast demonstrates a poorly defined nodule _(arrow)_ immediately anterior to the lower margin of the left brachiocephalic vein. (Contrast can be seen in the right brachiocephalic vein.) The patient was a 30-year-old woman who had hyperparathyroidism. Surgical excision confirmed the lesion to be a parathyroid adenoma.

intravenous administration of contrast material (Fig. 74–41).[1, 464, 465] The appearance may be similar to that of lymph nodes.[464, 465] Most tumors occur in the upper portion of the anterior mediastinum;[464, 465] they are seen less commonly in the paraesophageal regions[466] and rarely in the aortopulmonary window.[467] Tracheal compression has been seen in association with parathyroid cysts.[468]

On MR imaging, adenomas have signal intensity that is hypointense or isointense relative to muscle on T1-weighted images and high signal intensity on T2-weighted images.[466, 467, 469] Hemorrhage can result in high signal intensity on both T1- and T2-weighted images.[469] The signal intensity also may be altered by the presence of fat or fibrous tissue.[469a] Tumors usually enhance after intravenous administration of gadolinium-based contrast agents.[470] In one investigation of 25 patients, MR imaging had a higher sensitivity (22 of 25 cases, 88%) than did scintigraphy (11 of 19 cases, 58%) or ultrasound (3 of 24 cases, 12%) in detecting tumors.[466]

Radionuclide imaging of mediastinal parathyroid glands can be performed using double-tracer radionuclide imaging (thallium-201 and technetium-99m-pertechnetate),[466] or technetium-99m-sestamibi. Several groups of investigators have shown the last named to be associated with the greatest sensitivity and specificity.[467, 471–473] Optimal assessment is obtained by using technetium-99m-sestamibi combined with single-photon emission computed tomography (SPECT) imaging.[467, 474] In one investigation of nine patients who had ectopic parathyroid tissue (eight adenomas, one hyperplastic gland) in the aortopulmonary window, the abnormal glands were identified on the sestamibi SPECT scans in all six patients in whom the procedure was performed compared to eight of nine patients (89%) on CT and five of eight patients (63%) on MR imaging.[467] Because of the limited spatial resolution of scintigraphy, it has been suggested that the combination of sestamibi SPECT scintigraphy and fast-spin-

echo MR imaging provides the best overall assessment of the presence and anatomic location of hyperfunctioning glands.[469a, 475]

Mediastinal parathyroid glands can also be identified using selective arteriography;[476, 477] however, the technique is invasive and has limited sensitivity for the detection of adenomas. Preliminary results suggest that localization of adenomas can be improved by serial measurement of parathyroid hormone in the superior vena cava during selective arteriography with nonionic contrast media. In one investigation, a 1.4-fold increase in parathyroid hormone level in the superior vena cava within 20 to 120 seconds after arteriography allowed correct prediction of the site of an adenoma in 13 of 20 patients (65%);[477a] eight of nine patients who had positive arteriograms and five of eleven patients who had negative arteriograms had positive results of venous sampling.

In contrast to most other mediastinal masses, parathyroid tumors usually can be diagnosed on the basis of clinical and laboratory findings. Because most are functioning, patients present with signs and symptoms of hyperparathyroidism, including anorexia, weakness, fatigue, nausea, vomiting, constipation, and hypotonicity of muscles. Skeletal abnormalities typical of hyperparathyroidism may be seen on radiographs. Laboratory studies reveal hypercalcemia, hypophosphatemia, elevation of serum alkaline phosphatase, and hypercalciuria. Adenomas or hyperplastic glands are seldom large enough to cause symptoms or signs of local compression, although this has been documented in patients who have parathyroid cysts.[478]

SOFT TISSUE TUMORS AND TUMOR-LIKE CONDITIONS

Soft tissue tumors account for about 5% of all mediastinal masses[479] and include benign and malignant neoplasms of fat, fibrous tissue, smooth and striated muscle, blood and lymphatic vessels, bone, and neural tissue.[480] In addition, several developmental and acquired abnormalities composed predominantly of mesenchymal tissue (such as hemangioma and lipomatosis) can present as mediastinal masses. Each of these can occur in any mediastinal compartment; however, tumors of neural tissue are most common in the paravertebral region (_see_ page 2974), whereas most of the others are more frequently located anteriorly.

Tumors of Adipose Tissue

Lipoma

Although uncommon compared with other neoplasms, extrathymic lipoma is probably the most common nonneurogenic mesenchymal tumor to occur in the mediastinum; in one series of 396 mediastinal neoplasms, it constituted 2.3% of the total.[481] Pathologically, most are encapsulated tumors composed of cytologically bland adipocytes. Spindle cell, pleomorphic, and vascular (angiolipoma) variants have also been reported.[482–484]

Certain radiographic features of mediastinal lipomas aid in diagnosis. Because the density of fat is lower than that of other soft tissues, the radiographic density of lipomas is often—albeit not always—less than that of other mediastinal masses. This is particularly true if the mass happens to be surrounded by mediastinal tissue of unit density (Fig. 74–42).[485] In some patients, the mass has an hourglass configuration, part of the lesion being in either the neck or the chest wall.[486, 487] Most tumors project from only one side of the mediastinum.[459] CT is usually diagnostic, the characteristic finding consisting of a mass that has homogeneous fat attenuation.[488] The presence of heterogeneous attenuation with soft tissue components should raise the possibility of a liposarcoma. Perhaps because of their pliability, mediastinal lipomas usually do not cause symptoms, even when massive.[481] Surgical excision is curative in virtually all cases.

Lipomatosis

Lipomatosis is an unusual nonneoplastic abnormality of mediastinal adipose tissue characterized by the excessive accumulation of fat in its normal locations. (The condition should not be confused with lipoblastomatosis, an abnormality of young children characterized by a proliferation of immature but fundamentally benign lipoblastic tissue.[489, 490]) Lipomatosis is most commonly seen in conditions associated with hypercortisolism, such as Cushing's syndrome,[491, 492] ectopic adrenocorticotropic hormone syndrome,[493] and long-term corticosteroid therapy.[478, 492, 494–497] In all these situations, there is a redistribution of normal adipose tissue with excessive deposition in the upper mediastinum and in the pleuro-pericardial angles (Fig. 74–43). The abnormality has also been described in obese individuals not receiving corticosteroid therapy (Fig. 74–44).[498] Typically, patients do not have symptoms from the fat deposits. One case has been reported of an asthmatic patient who developed cough that was attributed to compression of the trachea and main bronchi.[478]

Radiologically, mediastinal widening tends to be smooth and symmetric, although the margins can be lobulated if the accumulation is large (Fig. 74–45). The widening usually extends from the thoracic inlet to the hila bilaterally (*see* Fig. 74–44); occasionally, the accumulation is predominantly paraspinal and symmetric (Fig. 74–46).[499] Increasing size of the pleuropericardial fat pads may be evident on serial radiographs.[494, 495, 497] In cases in which doubt exists on conventional radiographs, CT is invariably diagnostic.[499, 500]

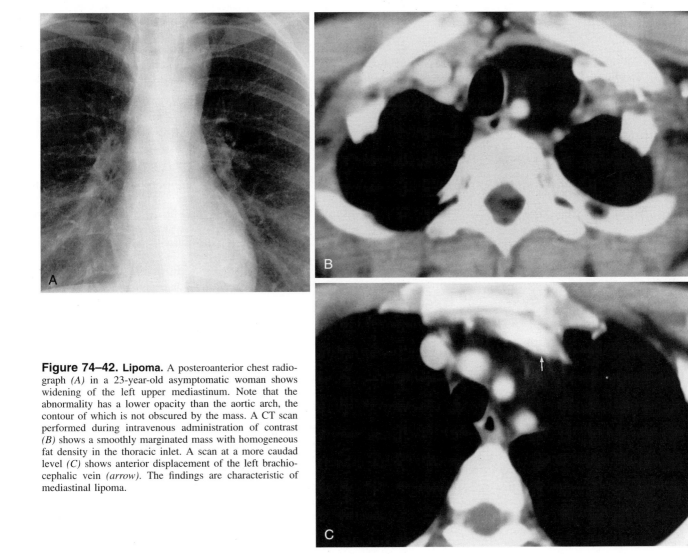

Figure 74–42. Lipoma. A posteroanterior chest radiograph *(A)* in a 23-year-old asymptomatic woman shows widening of the left upper mediastinum. Note that the abnormality has a lower opacity than the aortic arch, the contour of which is not obscured by the mass. A CT scan performed during intravenous administration of contrast *(B)* shows a smoothly marginated mass with homogeneous fat density in the thoracic inlet. A scan at a more caudad level *(C)* shows anterior displacement of the left brachiocephalic vein *(arrow)*. The findings are characteristic of mediastinal lipoma.

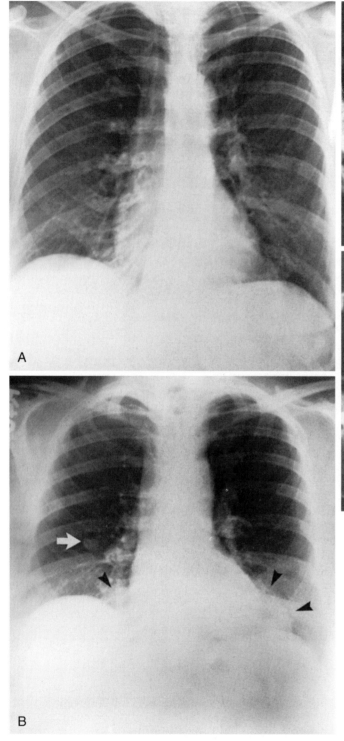

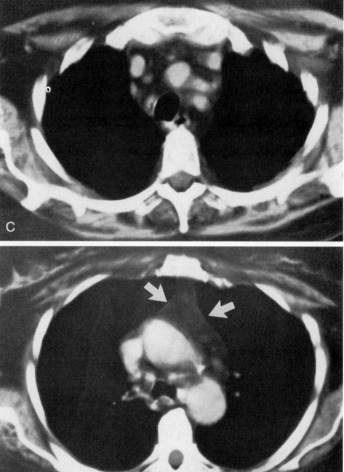

Figure 74–43. Mediastinal Lipomatosis Secondary to Paraneoplastic Cushing's Syndrome. A posteroanterior radiograph *(A)* of this 68-year-old woman is normal. Two years later, during which time the patient had gained a great deal of weight, a repeat posteroanterior radiograph *(B)* reveals considerable widening of the upper half of the mediastinum and appreciable enlargement of the pleuropericardial fat pads bilaterally *(arrowheads).* In addition, a solitary nodule measuring 12 mm in diameter had appeared in the lower portion of the right lung *(arrow).* CT scans through the upper half of the mediastinum *(C and D)* reveal the presence of a large amount of fat separating the vessels in the upper mediastinum *(C)* and anterior to the aorta *(arrows in D).* The solitary pulmonary nodule proved to be a carcinoid tumor. (Courtesy of Dr. Anthony Proto, Virginia Commonwealth University, Medical College of Virginia, Richmond, Virginia.)

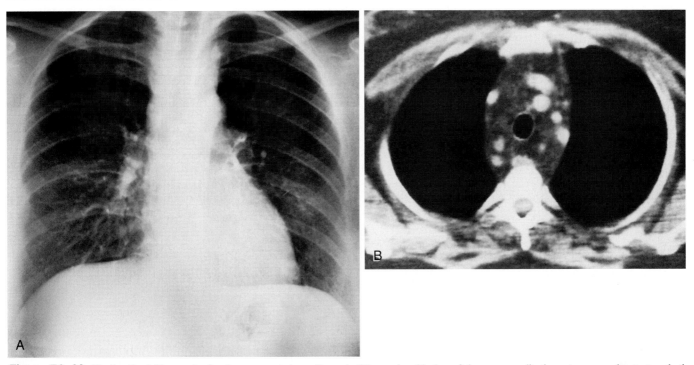

Figure 74–44. Mediastinal Lipomatosis. A posteroanterior radiograph *(A)* reveals widening of the upper mediastinum to an equal extent on both sides. The contour is smooth. No other abnormalities are apparent other than thickening of bronchial walls consistent with chronic bronchitis. A CT scan at the level of the left brachiocephalic vein *(B)* demonstrates wide separation of vessels as a result of an accumulation of a large amount of fat. This 58-year-old woman was receiving no therapy nor did she have any underlying condition to which the lipomatosis could be attributed: she was simply obese. The widened mediastinum returned to normal following a 40-pound weight loss.

Liposarcoma

Liposarcomas of the mediastinum are rare, only about 60 cases having been reported by 1993;[500–503] an additional 28 cases were documented in a report from the Memorial Sloan-Kettering Cancer Center in 1995.[504] An origin in the thymus has been noted in some cases.[504] Pathologically, most tumors can be classified as lipoma-like or myxoid types;[504, 505] pleomorphic and round cell patterns are uncommon. A single case composed of a mixture of liposarcoma and leiomyosarcoma has been reported.[505a] The diagnosis was made by transthoracic needle aspiration.[506]

The radiographic findings consist of a mediastinal mass, which is usually large and has well-defined margins.[507–509] On CT, well-differentiated tumors have areas of fat and areas of soft tissue attenuation, whereas poorly differentiated ones have homogeneous soft tissue attenuation.[509]

Most tumors are discovered in adults (mean age of 43 years in the Memorial Sloan-Kettering series).[504] Many are locally invasive at the time of diagnosis and are associated with dyspnea, wheezing, chest pain, or cough;[501, 510] superior vena cava syndrome is a rare manifestation.[510] The behavior of these tumors depends on the grade and extent of local invasion: In low-grade encapsulated forms, cure can be expected;[503] by contrast, locally invasive forms often recur and may result in death, particularly if high grade. Extrathoracic metastases are seldom observed.[481, 504]

Tumors of Vascular Tissue

Hemangioma

Hemangiomas have been estimated to constitute about 0.5% of all mediastinal tumors;[511] approximately 100 cases

had been reported by 1987.[512] Many are located in the superior portion of the mediastinum; some appear to arise in the thymus.[512] The majority, if not all, probably represent developmental malformations rather than true neoplasms. They can be an isolated abnormality or can occur as part of a multifocal hemangiomatous malformation affecting several organs (Osler-Weber-Rendu syndrome [*see* page 655]).[511, 513] Their occasional association with teratoma has also suggested that they might represent unidirectional development in this neoplasm;[514] however, such an event must be rare.

Hemangiomas are often encapsulated or well-circumscribed, red-brown tumors with a spongy appearance on cut section;[511, 514, 515] occasionally, they extend into adjacent tissues.[512, 514] Histologically, the tumors are composed of thin-walled or thick-walled vessels of large, small, or mixed size, corresponding to cavernous, capillary, or mixed hemangiomas. Regressive changes, including cyst formation, fibrosis, and ossification, are seen in some cases.[515] Significant cytologic atypia and mitotic activity are absent.

Radiographically, hemangiomas tend to be smooth in outline but are sometimes lobulated. Most are located in the upper portion of the anterior mediastinum;[511, 512, 516, 517] they are seen less commonly in the posterior mediastinum[516, 517] and rarely in the middle mediastinum.[517] Phleboliths, a virtually diagnostic sign, can be identified in approximately 10% of cases.[459, 516] Rarely, adjacent ribs are hypertrophied[518] or eroded.[519] On CT, the tumors usually have sharply defined smooth margins and heterogeneous attenuation and show heterogeneous enhancement after intravenous administration of contrast material.[517] In one investigation of 14 patients, 10 (71%) had sharply defined margins, 3 (21%) had focal obliteration of adjacent fat planes, and 1 had diffuse infiltra-

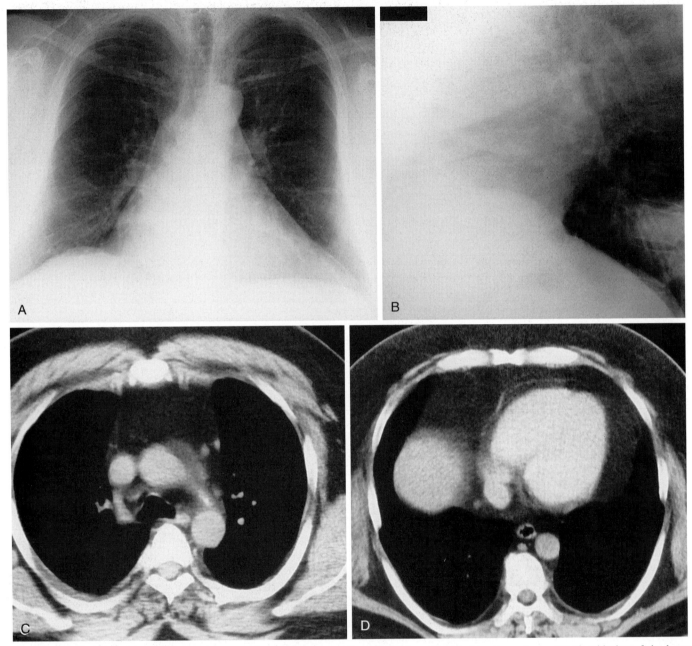

Figure 74–45. Mediastinal Lipomatosis. A posteroanterior chest radiograph *(A)* in a 42-year-old woman shows smooth widening of the lower mediastinum and prominent pericardial fat pads. A lateral radiograph *(B)* shows filling of the retrosternal airspace. CT scans performed without intravenous contrast *(C and D)* demonstrate mediastinal lipomatosis.

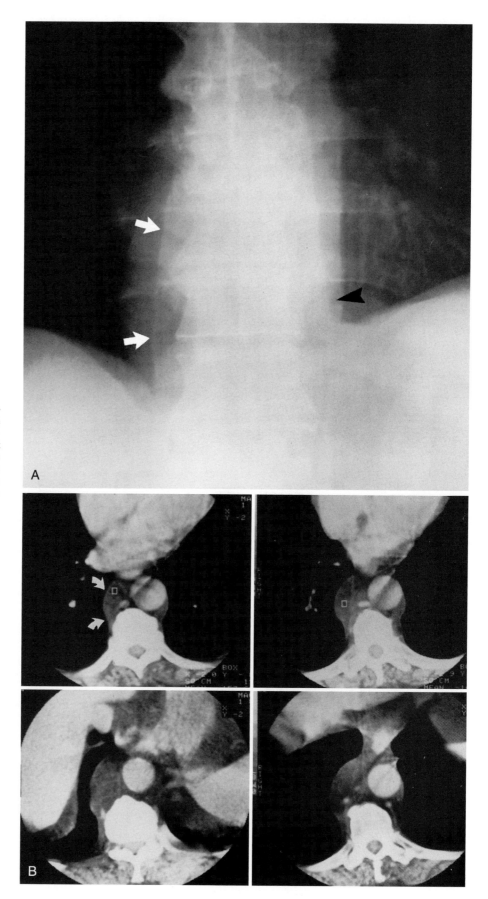

Figure 74–46. Posterior Mediastinal Lipomatosis. An overexposed radiograph of the lower thoracic spine in anteroposterior projection *(A)* reveals widening of the paraspinal soft tissues, more marked on the right *(arrows)*. The left paraspinal line is wider than normal in its lower portion *(arrowhead)*. Serial CT scans through the lower mediastinum *(B)* demonstrate paraspinal lipomatosis.

tion of the mediastinum.[517] Six (60%) showed predominantly central enhancement after intravenous administration of contrast material, a finding considered highly suggestive of the diagnosis.[517] Three of 14 tumors had punctate calcifications and 1 had phleboliths.[517]

The majority of tumors are discovered in young individuals.[511, 514] Many patients are symptomatic at the time of presentation,[514] the chief complaints being chest pain and dyspnea. Superior vena cava and Horner's syndromes have been reported occasionally.[514] Rarely, a tumor projects superiorly from the upper portion of the mediastinum and can be appreciated as a fullness in the neck.[514] The prognosis is almost invariably good, even in tumors that are incompletely excised.[512, 515]

Epithelioid Hemangioendothelioma

Epithelioid hemangioendothelioma (hemangioendothelioma, histiocytoid hemangioma) has been reported rarely in the mediastinum.[520–522] Most are large (5 to 15 cm in diameter);[522] they may be encapsulated or locally infiltrative. Histologically the tumor consists of round-to-oval epithelioid cells, either isolated or arranged in small nests within a fibrous stroma. Intracytoplasmic lumens believed to represent primitive vascular differentiation can be identified in some cells; the endothelial nature of the cells is best demonstrated by ultrastructural examination, the presence of a

positive immunohistochemical reaction for factor VIII– related antigen, or the binding of *Ulex* lectin. Metaplastic bone formation and a prominent osteoclast-like giant cell reaction have been identified in many tumors (Fig. 74–47).[522–524]

The radiologic manifestations consist of a smoothly marginated or lobulated mass, which can contain foci of calcification (Fig. 74–48). In one review of 12 cases, the mean age at the time of diagnosis was 49 years (range, 19 to 62 years);[522] 7 patients presented with symptoms related to compression of mediastinal structures, and the remainder were asymptomatic. The tumor is best regarded as a low-grade sarcoma because both local recurrence after attempted surgical excision and metastases can occur. In the study of 12 patients previously cited, however, follow-up of 9 indicated that 7 were alive and without evidence of disease 2 to 21 years (mean, 8 years) after diagnosis;[522] 1 died of surgical complications related to excision of a recurrence 1 year after initial diagnosis, and another died of undetermined causes.

Angiosarcoma

Angiosarcoma is a rare mediastinal tumor: In a 1963 review of the literature, only eight well-documented cases were identified,[514] and few have been reported since that time.[479, 525] Most occur in the anterior mediastinum and have no obvious source; a single case has been reported that

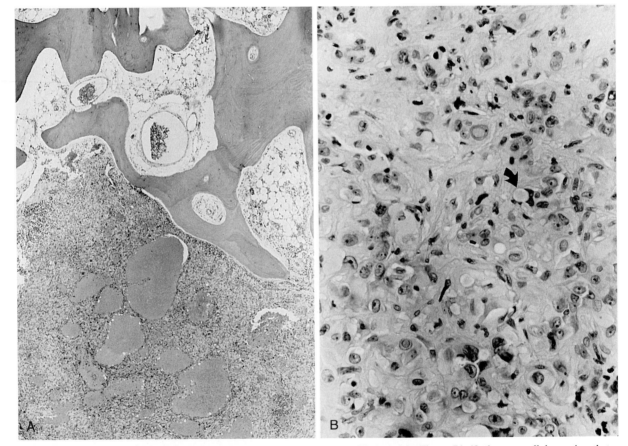

Figure 74–47. Epithelioid Hemangioendothelioma. A section of the tumor illustrated in Figure 74–48 shows a cellular region that contains a number of variably sized cystic spaces filled with blood. Abundant mature bone with interspersed bone marrow is also evident. A magnified view *(B)* shows the neoplastic cells to have abundant lightly staining cytoplasm, in some cells associated with prominent intracellular lumina *(arrow).*

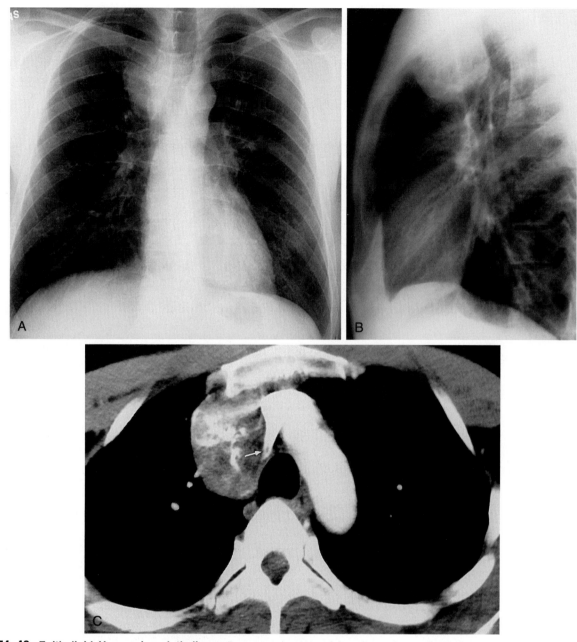

Figure 74–48. Epithelioid Hemangioendothelioma. Posteroanterior *(A)* and lateral *(B)* chest radiographs in a 36-year-old man demonstrate a lobulated mediastinal mass that contains foci of calcification. A CT scan performed during intravenous administration of contrast *(C)* better demonstrates the foci of calcification within the tumor. Note medial and posterior displacement of the superior vena cava *(arrow)*. Sections of the resected specimen are shown in Figure 74–47.

apparently arose in the superior vena cava.[525] The tumors are aggressive and are usually associated with chest pain at the time of diagnosis. Most patients die within 3 years of diagnosis.

Hemangiopericytoma

Similar to its pulmonary counterpart (*see* page 1336), hemangiopericytoma of the mediastinum is believed to be derived from the vascular pericyte. Few well-documented cases have been reported.[514] The tumor can be locally infiltrative and aggressive or can be encapsulated and apparently benign; histologic features of the two varieties are virtually

identical. Radiologic and clinical manifestations are nonspecific.

Lymphangioma

Mediastinal lymphangiomas have two clinicopathologic forms: (1) a variety that extends from the neck into the mediastinum and usually occurs in infants (cystic hygroma) (Fig. 74–49)[526–528] and (2) a more or less well-circumscribed variety that usually is discovered in adults and is located in the lower anterior (occasionally middle posterior [Fig. 74–50]) mediastinum remote from the neck.[529–532] As with hemangiomas, lymphangiomas probably represent developmental

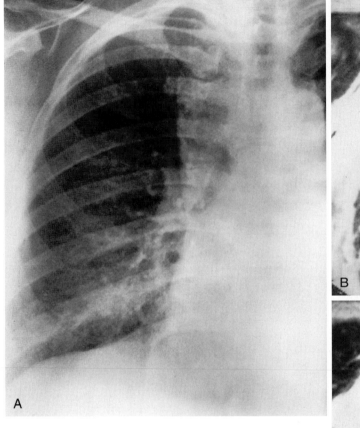

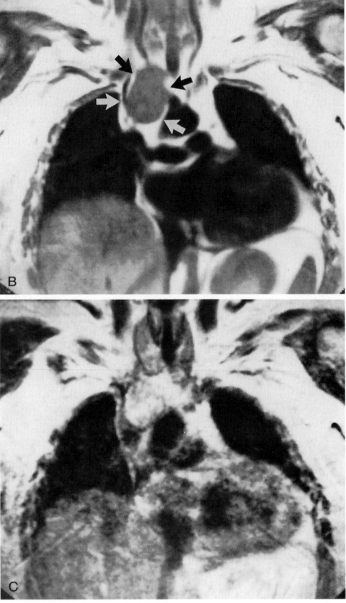

Figure 74–49. Lymphangioma of the Anterior Mediastinum.
A view of the right lung and mediastinum *(A)* of this asymptomatic
48-year-old woman reveals an opacity in the paramediastinal region,
extending superiorly from the upper portion of the right hilum. A T1-
weighted MR scan *(B)* reveals a sharply defined, homogeneous mass
extending from just above the thoracic inlet downward into the right
side of the mediastinum *(arrows)*. A T2-weighted image *(C)* shows
increased signal intensity consistent with the presence of fluid.

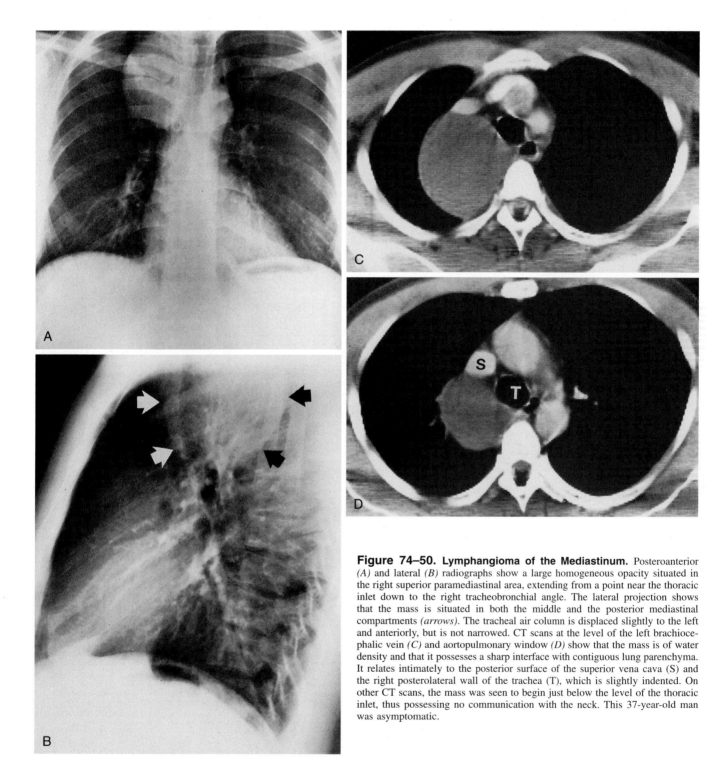

Figure 74–50. Lymphangioma of the Mediastinum. Posteroanterior
(A) and lateral *(B)* radiographs show a large homogeneous opacity situated in
the right superior paramediastinal area, extending from a point near the thoracic
inlet down to the right tracheobronchial angle. The lateral projection shows
that the mass is situated in both the middle and the posterior mediastinal
compartments *(arrows)*. The tracheal air column is displaced slightly to the left
and anteriorly, but is not narrowed. CT scans at the level of the left brachiocephalic vein *(C)* and aortopulmonary window *(D)* show that the mass is of water
density and that it possesses a sharp interface with contiguous lung parenchyma.
It relates intimately to the posterior surface of the superior vena cava (S) and
the right posterolateral wall of the trachea (T), which is slightly indented. On
other CT scans, the mass was seen to begin just below the level of the thoracic
inlet, thus possessing no communication with the neck. This 37-year-old man
was asymptomatic.

anomalies rather than true neoplasms. Pathologically, the tumor consists of thin-walled, usually multilocular cysts containing numerous thin-walled vascular spaces lined by endothelial cells. The wall is composed of connective tissue with a variable amount of lymphoid tissue.[8]

The radiographic findings are nonspecific and consist of a sharply defined, smoothly marginated mediastinal mass, which frequently displaces adjacent mediastinal structures.[533] One case was associated with adjacent rib and clavicle erosion.[534] In one investigation of 19 adult patients, 7 tumors (37%) were located in the anterior mediastinum, 5 (26%) in the middle mediastinum, 3 (16%) in the posterior mediastinum, 3 (16%) in the thoracic inlet, and 1 in the lung.[535]

The most common CT appearance, seen in about 60% of cases, consists of a smoothly marginated cystic mass with homogeneous water density (Fig. 74–51).[533–536] Multiple loculations can be seen within the mass in approximately one third.[535, 536] The mass can displace or surround adjacent vessels.[535, 536] Less common findings include foci of calcification, homogeneous soft tissue density, and spiculated margins.[535] Hemorrhage results in an increase in the size of the mass and an increase in the attenuation values on CT.[536] The

findings on MR imaging in three patients were variable and nonspecific.[535]

Because of their soft consistency, lymphangiomas seldom cause symptoms, even when large;[537] occasionally, however, they cause symptoms by compressing the tracheobronchial tree,[8] or the superior vena cava or its major tributaries.[538] In younger patients particularly, a soft tissue mass may be visible in the neck. Chylothorax develops in some cases.[529, 539]

Lymphangiomatosis

Lymphangiomatosis is a rare abnormality characterized by a poorly delimited proliferation of lymphatic vessels at several sites throughout the body (*see* page 663). Mediastinal involvement may be complicated by chylothorax as well as by vascular infiltration of adjacent soft tissue, lung, and pleura.[540–542] Most affected patients are children. The radiologic findings include mediastinal widening, bilateral pleural effusions, and pulmonary interstitial opacities characterized mainly by interlobular septal thickening.[543, 544] In one investigation of eight patients, all had diffuse increased density of

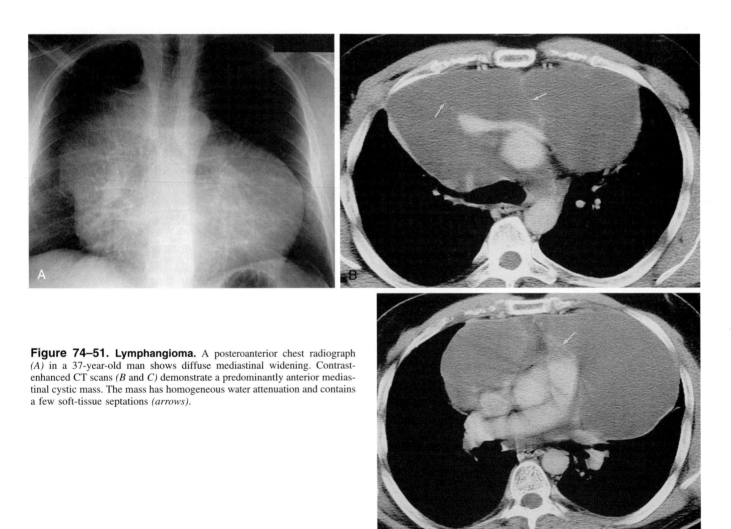

Figure 74–51. Lymphangioma. A posteroanterior chest radiograph *(A)* in a 37-year-old man shows diffuse mediastinal widening. Contrast-enhanced CT scans *(B* and *C)* demonstrate a predominantly anterior mediastinal cystic mass. The mass has homogeneous water attenuation and contains a few soft-tissue septations *(arrows).*

the mediastinal fat with attenuation values approximating that of water on CT.[544]

Tumors of Muscle

Leiomyoma and Leiomyosarcoma

Smooth muscle neoplasms are rare in the mediastinum;[545] in one review of the literature published in 1988, only 13 examples were identified.[546] Because some reported tumors have been located in the paravertebral region and because smooth muscle differentiation has not been confirmed immunohistochemically or ultrastructurally in all cases,[547] it is possible that some are, in fact, neurogenic neoplasms.

Apart from the esophagus, the origin of mediastinal smooth muscle tumors is often not clear. Although it has been suggested that they represent unidirectional differentiation in a teratoma,[481, 548] it seems more likely that the majority are derived from the walls of small mediastinal blood vessels; apparent origin in the superior vena cava,[549] pulmonary artery, trachea,[550] and the wall of a mediastinal bronchial cyst[548] also has been reported. A possible association between leiomyosarcoma and prior radiotherapy was documented in one case.[551] Pathologic findings are those of a spindle cell neoplasm with varying degrees of nuclear atypia and mitotic activity.[545]

Radiologic features are nonspecific. In one review of 10 well-documented cases, the average age at the time of presentation was about 55 years;[545] patients who had tumors in the paraspinal region were usually asymptomatic, whereas those who had anterior tumors had signs and symptoms related to compression of adjacent structures. The prognosis is related to histologic grade and the extent of local extension of tumor in mediastinal soft tissue.

Rhabdomyoma and Rhabdomyosarcoma

Primary mediastinal rhabdomyosarcoma is rare.[481, 552, 553] As with smooth muscle tumors, its origin is usually unclear, although the well-documented occurrence of rhabdomyosarcoma in association with immature teratoma[355–357] suggests that some may be derived from this neoplasm. Various histologic types of tumor have been reported, including alveolar, embryonal, and pleomorphic.[553] The majority of tumors develop in children and pursue an aggressive course.[552] A single case has been reported of a rhabdomyoma that arose in the superior portion of the medastinum unattached to the heart.[554]

Fibrous and Fibrohistiocytic Tumors

Fibroma and Fibrosarcoma

Because it is likely that some neoplasms reported as fibroma or fibrosarcoma are better classified as other forms of soft tissue tumor (e.g., a neurogenic neoplasm), the precise incidence of primary mediastinal fibrous tumors is difficult to determine; however, it is certainly low.[481] Some tumors are histologically identical to fibrous tumor of the pleura (see page 2828).[555, 556] There are no distinctive radiologic or clinical features.

Benign and Malignant Fibrous Histiocytoma

Benign fibrous histiocytoma (xanthogranuloma) of the mediastinum is a rare tumor.[481] As with their pulmonary counterparts (see page 1371), the precise nature of these tumors is uncertain, particularly with respect to their inflammatory or neoplastic character. Pathologically the tumors are usually well encapsulated and are composed of a variable number of intermingled fibroblasts, histiocytes, and multinucleated giant cells.[481] Nuclear atypia, mitotic activity, and necrosis are absent or minimal.

Malignant fibrous histiocytoma of the mediastinum is also rare, only 10 cases having been documented by 1991.[480, 557] Most are aggressive tumors associated with signs and symptoms at the time of presentation and relatively rapid progression to death.

Tumors of Bone and Cartilage

The origin of cartilaginous and osteogenic tumors in the mediastinum is uncertain; although some are presumably derived from soft tissue unrelated to bone,[559] the observation that many develop in the paravertebral region suggests that others may originate in the vertebral bone.[559, 560] All histologic forms of tumor are rare; examples include chondroma,[561] chondrosarcoma,[562] and osteosarcoma. Only six cases of the last-mentioned neoplasm were identified in one literature review in 1995;[563] one was possibly related to previous radiotherapy.[564] As might be expected, the prognosis of the malignant tumors is usually poor.

TUMORS SITUATED IN THE ANTERIOR CARDIOPHRENIC ANGLE

Although masses in the vicinity of the cardiophrenic angle on either side originate in the middle mediastinum, they project into the anterior compartment and are thus discussed at this point. The differential diagnosis of such masses is extensive and includes lesions arising in the lung parenchyma, in the visceral or parietal pleura or pleural space, in the pericardium or contiguous myocardium, and in or beneath the diaphragm. Although lesions arising in any of these anatomic regions can produce similar radiographic findings, specific diagnoses can usually be made on CT.[76, 438, 565, 566] Only three are considered in any detail at this point—pleuropericardial fat, mesothelial cysts, and enlargement of diaphragmatic lymph nodes. Although hernia through the foramina of Morgagni appears radiographically as a homogeneous shadow usually indistinguishable from a large pleuropericardial fat pad (Fig. 74–52), for convenience these lesions are discussed in Chapter 77 (see page 3001).

Pleuropericardial Fat

Accumulations of fat that normally occupy the cardiophrenic angles can attain a considerable size. Although such pleuropericardial fat pads are always bilateral, they

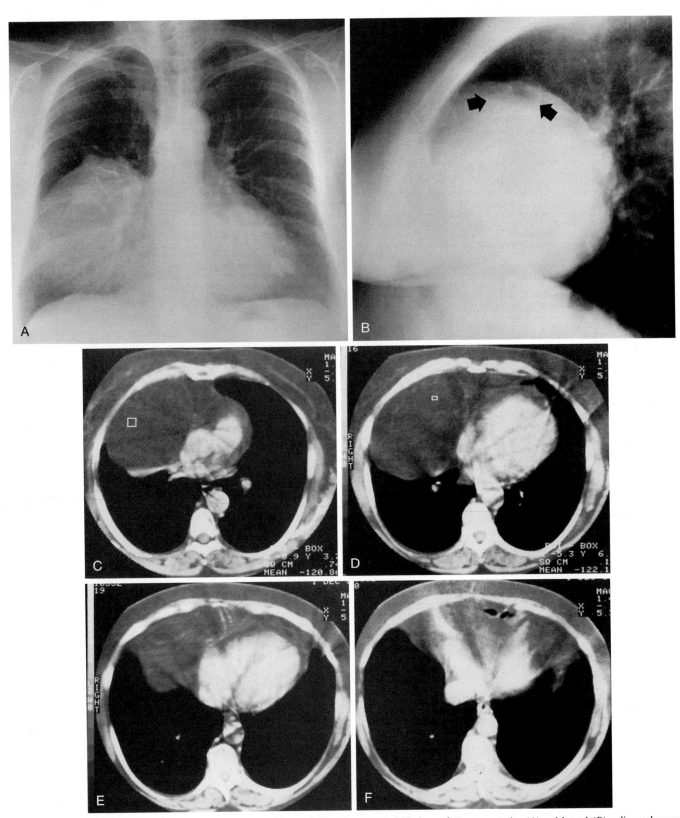

Figure 74–52. Herniation of Omentum and Bowel Through the Foramen of Morgagni. Posteroanterior *(A)* and lateral *(B)* radiographs reveal a large mass situated in the inferior portion of the right hemithorax, lying chiefly anteriorly and obliterating the right border of the heart. Its density is homogeneous except for a small radiolucency situated in its most superior portion *(arrows in B)*. Serial CT scans through the lower mediastinum *(C–F)* reveal a large mass of fat density (mean attenuation, −120 Hounsfield units) situated in the region of the right cardiophrenic angle and extending around the anterior aspect of the heart. In the lower left scan, two small loops of bowel can be readily identified. The patient was an asymptomatic 67-year-old man.

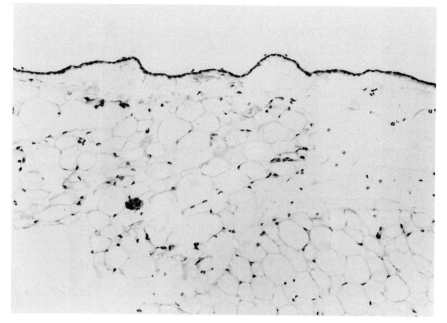

Figure 74–53. Mesothelial Cyst. A section through the wall of a smooth-walled cyst that was situated contiguous with the pericardium shows adipose tissue lined by a layer of flattened mesothelial cells. This appearance is characteristic of a pericardial mesothelial cyst. (×150.)

may be asymmetric. They can increase substantially in size over time, as a result of either obesity or hyperadrenocorticism (e.g., Cushing's syndrome); as such, they can cause a potentially confusing radiographic opacity (*see* Fig. 74–43). The diagnosis can be readily made on CT (*see* Fig. 74–45)[76, 566, 567] or MR imaging.[568] Rarely, the fat pads undergo necrosis, an event associated with the abrupt onset of retrosternal pain, sometimes resembling that caused by pulmonary thromboembolism or myocardial infarction.[569] Affected patients are typically obese; the only radiographic sign of note is a large pleuropericardial fat pad.

Mesothelial (Pericardial) Cysts

The vast majority of mesothelial (pericardial, pleuropericardial) cysts are congenital and result from aberrations in the formation of the coelomic cavities. Rarely an otherwise typical "congenital" cyst has developed years after an episode of acute pericarditis,[570] suggesting that some may be acquired. The cysts are spherical or oval in shape, thin walled, and often translucent; the vast majority are unilocular and contain clear or straw-colored fluid.[8] Histologically, the cyst wall is composed of a thin layer of fibrous tissue lined by a single layer of flattened or cuboidal cells resembling mesothelial cells (Fig. 74–53);[570a] other tissues, such as cartilage, smooth muscle, and glandular tissue, are absent.

Radiographically, the majority of mesothelial cysts are located in the cardiophrenic angles (Fig. 74–54). For example, in one study of 72 cases, 54 were identified at this site and 18 at a higher level;[8] 11 of the latter extended into the superior aspect of the mediastinum (Fig. 74–55). Most—almost 75% of cases in the study cited[8]—are located

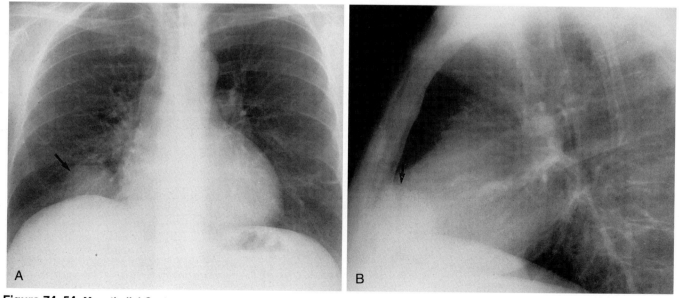

Figure 74–54. Mesothelial Cyst. Posteroanterior *(A)* and lateral *(B)* chest radiographs in an asymptomatic 47-year-old woman demonstrate a smoothly marginated mass in the right anterior cardiophrenic angle *(arrows).*

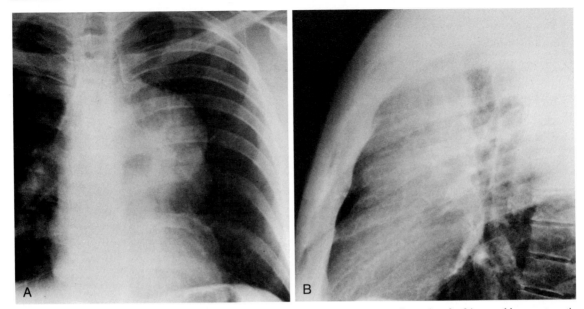

Figure 74–55. Anterior Mediastinal Mesothelial Cyst. Posteroanterior *(A)* and lateral *(B)* radiographs of a 34-year-old asymptomatic man reveal a large lobulated mass of homogeneous density projecting to the left of the mediastinum and situated anteriorly in the crotch between the heart and the ascending aorta. At thoracotomy, the mass was found to be a multiloculated cyst containing clear watery fluid.

on the right side.[571] Typically, the cysts are smooth in contour and round or oval in shape. Most are between 3 and 8 cm in diameter; rare examples have been reported to be as small as 1 cm or as large as 28 cm.[572–574]

The benign cystic nature of these masses can usually be confirmed by CT (Fig. 74–56),[438, 575, 576] MR imaging,[577] or ultrasonography,[570, 574, 578, 579] even when their location is atypical, such as the superior portion of the mediastinum.[576, 580, 581] The characteristic CT appearance consists of a water density smooth, round, or oval cystic lesion abutting the pericardium. Occasional cysts have soft tissue attenuation, presumably as a result of the presence of viscous mater-

ial;[571, 582] such lesions cannot be reliably distinguished from a neoplasm.[76] A case has been reported in which the wall of a pericardial cyst was calcified.[583] Cysts typically have low echogenicity and increased through transmission on ultrasound.

Symptoms are almost invariably absent, most cysts being discovered on a screening chest radiograph. Occasionally, a large cyst gives rise to a sensation of retrosternal pressure or to dyspnea.[584] Rare complications include infection,[487] erosion of the superior vena cava,[585] cardiac tamponade,[586] development of mesothelioma,[587] and atrial fibrillation.[588]

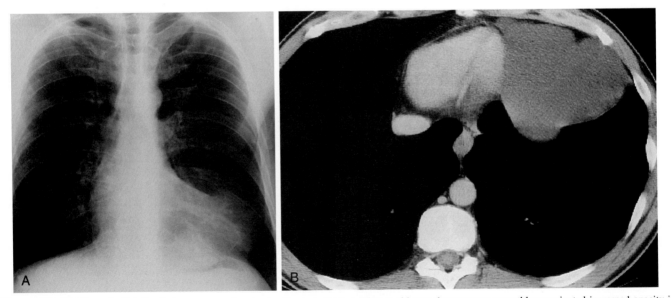

Figure 74–56. Mesothelial Cyst. A posteroanterior chest radiograph *(A)* in a 46-year-old man demonstrates smoothly marginated increased opacity in the left cardiophrenic angle. A contrast-enhanced CT scan *(B)* demonstrates a water density cyst. The diagnosis was confirmed at thoracotomy.

Enlargement of Diaphragmatic Lymph Nodes

The superior diaphragmatic lymph nodes are distributed in three clusters: anterior (prepericardiac), middle (lateral pericardiac), and posterior.[589, 590] They can be affected by tumors arising above the diaphragm—most commonly lymphoma and Hodgkin's disease and less commonly carcinoma of the breast and lung—or by tumors arising below the diaphragm, particularly carcinoma of the colon and ovary.[589–592]

The nodes are normally not visible on chest radiographs because of their small size and their investment with fat and other connective tissue adjacent to the pleura. When enlarged, they displace the pleura laterally and produce a smooth or lobulated mass projecting out of the cardiophrenic angle, an appearance that can simulate pleuropericardial fat pads. Although such enlargement may be apparent on conventional radiographs, CT is a superior method of assessment.[589–593] In one investigation of 274 CT scans obtained on 209 patients who had lymphoma (153 Hodgkin's disease and 56 non-Hodgkin's lymphoma), evidence of enlargement of cardiophrenic angle lymph nodes was found in 14 (7%);[593] in only 3 of these was node enlargement clearly evident on conventional radiographs. Although node enlargement can occur as the initial presentation in patients who have Hodgkin's disease,[594, 595] it is more common during a relapse of the disease.[594] Thus, it is important to compare the cardiophrenic angles on serial chest radiographs.

MISCELLANEOUS ANTERIOR MEDIASTINAL TUMORS

Benign[596, 597] and malignant[481] mediastinal mesenchymomas are rare tumors composed of a mixture of two or more mesodermal tissues. Their precise nature is debated, some authors considering them to represent hamartomas (at least the benign forms) and others true neoplasms. It is possible that some represent predominant mesodermal differentiation in a teratoma. Other rare neoplasms that have been reported to occur in the mediastinum include myxoma,[598] granulocytic sarcoma,[599, 600] alveolar soft-part sarcoma,[558] synovial sarcoma,[601] and pleomorphic adenoma (possibly derived from ectopic tracheobronchial gland tissue within a mediastinal lymph node).[602]

REFERENCES

1. Strollo DC, Rosado-de-Christenson ML, Jett JR: Primary mediastinal tumors: Part 1. Tumors of the anterior mediastinum. Chest 112:511, 1997.
2. Strollo DC, Rosado-de-Christenson ML, Jett JR: Primary mediastinal tumors: Part II. Tumors of the middle and posterior mediastinum. Chest 112:1344, 1997.
3. Landay MJ: Anterior clear space: How clear? How often? How come? Radiology 192:165, 1994.
4. Felson B: Chest Roentgenology. Philadelphia, WB Saunders, 1973.
5. Powers CN, Silverman JF, Geisinger KR, et al: Fine-needle aspiration biopsy of the mediastinum: A multi-institutional analysis. Am J Clin Pathol 105:168, 1996.
6. Marchevsky A: The mediastinum. Pathology 3:339, 1996.
7. Ingels GW, Campbell DC, Giampetro AM, et al: Malignant schwannomas of the mediastinum: Report of two cases and review of the literature. Cancer 27:1190, 1971.
8. Wychulis AR, Payne WS, Clagett OT, et al: Surgical treatment of mediastinal tumors: A 40-year experience. J Thorac Cardiovasc Surg 62:379, 1971.
9. Mattana J, Kurtz B, Miah A, et al: Renal cell carcinoma presenting as a solitary anterior superior mediastinal mass. J Med 27:205, 1996.
10. Linegar AG, Odell JA, Fennell WM, et al: Massive thymic hyperplasia. Ann Thorac Surg 55:1197, 1993.
11. Langer CJ, Keller SM, Erner SM: Thymic hyperplasia with hemorrhage simulating recurrent Hodgkin disease after chemotherapy-induced complete remission. Cancer 70:2082, 1992.
12. Kendall MD, Johnson HRM, Singh J: The weight of the human thymus gland at necropsy. J Anat 131:485, 1980.
13. Arliss J, Scholes J, Dickson PR, et al: Massive thymic hyperplasia in an adolescent. Ann Thorac Surg 45:220, 1988.
14. Carmosino L, DiBenedetto A, Feffer S: Thymic hyperplasia following successful chemotherapy. Cancer 56:1526, 1985.
15. Düe W, Dieckmann K-P, Stein H: Thymic hyperplasia following chemotherapy of a testicular germ cell tumor: Immunohistological evidence for a simple rebound phenomenon. Cancer 63:446, 1989.
16. Choyke PL, Zeman RK, Gootenberg JE, et al: Thymic atrophy and regrowth in response to chemotherapy: CT evaluation. Am J Roentgenol 149:269, 1987.
17. Kissin CM, Husband JE, Nicholas D, et al: Benign thymic enlargement in adults after chemotherapy: CT demonstration. Radiology 163:67, 1987.
18. Simmonds P, Silberstein M, McKendrick J: Thymic hyperplasia in adults following chemotherapy for malignancy. Aust N Z J Med 23:264, 1993.
19. Tabarin A, Catargi B, Chanson P, et al: Pseudo-tumors of the thymus after correction of hypercortisolism in patients with ectopic ACTH syndrome: A report of five cases. Clin Endocrinol 42:207, 1995.
20. Mizuno T, Hashimoto T, Masaoka A, et al: Thymic follicular hyperplasia manifested as an anterior mediastinal mass. Surg Today 27:275, 1997.
21. Doppman JL, Oldfield EH, Chrousos GP, et al: Rebound thymic hyperplasia after treatment of Cushing's syndrome. Am J Roentgenol 147:1145, 1986.
22. Sidhu US, Malhotra V, Chhina GS: Roentgenogram of the month: An unusual case of pseudocardiomegaly. Chest 113:1711, 1998.
23. Choyke PL, Zeman RK, Gootenberg JE, et al: Thymic atrophy and regrowth in response to chemotherapy: CT evaluation. Am J Roentgenol 149:269, 1987.
24. Moul JW, Fernandez EB, Bryan MG, et al: Thymic hyperplasia in newly diagnosed testicular germ cell tumors. J Urol 152:1480, 1994.
25. Levine GD, Rosai J: Thymic hyperplasia and neoplasia: A review of current concepts. Hum Pathol 9:495, 1978.
26. Fyfe B, Dominguez F, Poppiti RJ: Thymic hyperplasia: A clue to the diagnosis of hyperthyroidism. Am J Forensic Med Pathol 11:257, 1990.
27. Bergman TA, Mariash CN, Oppenheimer JH: Anterior mediastinal mass in a patient with Graves' disease. J Clin Endocrinol Metab 55:587, 1982.
28. Beddingfield GW, Campbell DC Jr, Hood RH Jr, et al: Simultaneous disorders of thyroid and thymus: Report of two cases. Ann Thorac Surg 4:445, 1967.
29. Pendlebury SC, Boyages S, Koutts J, et al: Thymic hyperplasia associated with Hodgkin disease and thyrotoxicosis. Cancer 70:1985, 1992.
30. Murakami M, Hosoi Y, Negishi T, et al: Thymic hyperplasia in patients with Graves' disease: Identification of thyrotropin receptors in human thymus. J Clin Invest 98:2228, 1996.
31. Judd RL: Massive thymic hyperplasia with myoid cell differentiation. Hum Pathol 18:1180, 1987.
32. Williams DJ: True thymic hyperplasia: An unrecognized cause of cardiac murmur? Thymus 12:135, 1988.
33. Gelfand DW, Goldman AS, Law EJ, et al: Thymic hyperplasia in children recovering from thermal burns. J Trauma 12:813, 1972.
34. Balcom RJ, Hakanson DO, Werner A, et al: Massive thymic hyperplasia in an infant with Beckwith-Wiedemann syndrome. Arch Pathol Lab Med 109:153, 1985.
35. Pardo-Mindan FJ: Immunological aspects of sarcoidosis associated with true thymic hyperplasia. Allerg Immunopathol (Paris) 8:91, 1980.
36. Konstantopoulos K, Androulaki A, Aessopos A, et al: Pure red cell aplasia associated with true thymic hyperplasia. Hum Pathol 26:1160, 1995.
37. Wong KF, Chau KF, Chan JK, et al: Pure red cell aplasia associated with thymic lymphoid hyperplasia and secondary erythropoietin resistance. Am J Clin Pathol 103:346, 1995.
38. Declich P, Sironi M, Isimbaldi G, et al: Atrio-ventricular nodal tumor associated with polyendocrine anomalies. Pathol Res Pract 192:54, 1996.
39. Rice HE, Flake AW, Hori T, et al: Massive thymic hyperplasia: Characterization of a rare mediastinal mass. J Pediatr Surg 29:1561, 1994.
40. Freundlich IM, McGavran MH: Abnormalities of the thymus. J Thorac Imaging 11:58, 1996.
41. Baron RL, Lee JKT, Sagel SS, et al: Computed tomography of the normal thymus. Radiology 142:121, 1982.
42. Nicolaou S, Müller NL, Li DKB, et al: Thymus in myasthenia gravis: Comparison of CT and pathologic findings and clinical outcome after thymectomy. Radiology 201:471, 1996.
43. Suzuki K, Kurokawa K, Suzuki T, et al: Anterior mediastinal metastasis of testicular germ cell tumor: Relation to benign thymic hyperplasia. Eur Urol 32:371, 1997.
44. Iosilevsky G, Front D, Bettman L, et al: Uptake of ^{67}Ga citrate and (2 H-3)deoxyglucose in the tumor model, following chemotherapy and radiotherapy. J Nucl Med 26:278, 1985.
45. Canellos G: Residual mass in lymphoma may not be residual disease. J Clin Oncol 6:931, 1988.
46. Israel O, Front D, Lam M, et al: Gallium-67 imaging in monitoring lymphoma response to treatment. Cancer 61:2439, 1988.
47. Front D, Ben-Haim S, Israel O, et al: Lymphoma: Predictive value of Ga-67 scintigraphy after treatment. Radiology 182:359, 1992.
48. Israel O: Benign mediastinal and parahilar uptake of Gallium-67 in treated lymphoma: Do we have all the answers? J Nucl Med 34:1330, 1993.
49. Harris EW, Rakow JI, Weiner M, et al: Thallium-201 scintigraphy for assessment of a gallium-67 avid mediastinal mass following therapy for Hodgkin's disease. J Nucl Med 34:1326, 1993.
50. Rettenbacher L, Galvan G: Differentiation between residual cancer and thymic hyperplasia in malignant non-Hodgkin's lymphoma with somatostatin receptor scintigraphy. Clin Nucl Med 19:64, 1994.
51. Small EJ, Venook AP, Damon LE: Gallium-avid thymic hyperplasia in an adult after chemotherapy for Hodgkin disease. Cancer 72:905, 1993.
52. Kissin CM, Husband JE, Nicholas D, et al: Benign thymic enlargement in adults after chemotherapy: CT demonstration. Radiology 163:67, 1987.
53. Riazmontazer N, Bedayat G: Aspiration cytology of an enlarged thymus presenting as a mediastinal mass: A case report. Acta Cytol 37:427, 1993.
54. Rosai J, Levine GD: Atlas of Tumor Pathology: Tumors of the Thymus. Second Series, Fascicle 13. Washington, DC, Armed Forces Institute of Pathology, 1976.
55. Wong KF, Chau KF, Chan JK, et al: Pure red cell aplasia associated with thymic lymphoid hyperplasia and secondary erythropoietin resistance. Am J Clin Pathol 103:346, 1995.
56. Burke AP, Anderson D, Benson W, et al: Localization of human immunodeficiency virus 1 RNA in thymic tissues from asymptomatic drug addicts. Arch Pathol Lab Med 119:36, 1995.
57. Prevot S, Audouin J, Andre-Bougaran J, et al: Thymic pseudotumorous enlargement due to follicular hyperplasia in a human immunodeficiency virus seropositive patient: Immunohistochemical and molecular biological study of viral infected cells. Am J Clin Pathol 97:420, 1992.
58. Clark RE, Marbarger JP, West PN, et al: Thymectomy for myasthenia gravis in the young adult: Long-term results. J Thorac Cardiovasc Surg 80:696, 1980.
59. Batra P, Herrmann C Jr, Mulder D: Mediastinal imaging in myasthenia gravis: Correlation of chest radiography, CT, MR and surgical findings. Am J Roentgenol 148:515, 1987.
60. Chen J, Weisbrod GL, Herman SJ: Computed tomography and pathologic correlations of thymic lesions. J Thorac Imaging 3:61, 1988.
61. Goldberg RE, Haaga JR, Yulish BS: Serial CT scans in thymic hyperplasia. J Comput Assist Tomogr 11:539, 1987.
62. Teplick JG, Nedwich A, Haskin ME: Roentgenographic features of thymolipoma. Am J Roentgenol 117:873, 1973.
63. Nishimura O, Naito Y, Noguchi Y, et al: Thymolipoma: A report of three cases. Jpn J Surg 20:234, 1990.
64. Moran CA, Rosado-de-Christenson M, Suster S: Thymolipoma: Clinicopathologic review of 33 cases. Mod Pathol 8:741, 1995.
65. Levine S, Labiche H, Chandor S: Thymolipoma. Am Rev Respir Dis 98:875, 1968.
66. Le Marc'hadour F, Pinel N, Pasquier B, et al: Thymolipoma in association with myasthenia gravis. Am J Surg Pathol 15:802, 1991.
67. Iseki M, Tsuda N, Kishikawa M, et al: Thymolipoma with striated myoid cells: Histological, immunohistochemical, and ultrastructural study. Am J Surg Pathol 14:395, 1990.
68. Moran CA, Zeren H, Koss MN: Thymofibrolipoma: A histologic variant of thymolipoma. Arch Pathol Lab Med 118:281, 1994.
69. van Hoeven KH, Brennan MF: Lipothymoadenoma of the parathyroid. Arch Pathol Lab Med 117:312, 1993.
70. Hull MT, Warfel KA, Kotylo P, et al: Proliferating thymolipoma: Ultrastructural, immunohistochemical, and flow cytometric study. Ultrastruct Pathol 19:75, 1995.
71. Rosado-de-Christenson M, Pugatch RD, Moran CA, et al: Thymolipoma: Analysis of 27 cases. Radiology 193:121, 1994.
72. Yeh H-C, Gordon A, Kirschner PA, et al: Computed tomography and sonography of thymolipoma. Am J Roentgenol 140:1131, 1983.
73. Faerber EN, Balsara RK, Schidlow DV, et al: Thymolipoma: Computed tomographic appearances. Pediatr Radiol 20:196, 1990.

74. Shirkhoda A, Chasen MH, Eftekhari F, et al: MR imaging of mediastinal thymolipoma. J Comput Assist Tomogr 11:364, 1987.

75. Molina PL, Siegel MJ, Glazer HS: Thymic masses on MR imaging. Am J Roentgenol 155:495, 1990.

76. Ahn JM, Lee KS, Goo JM, et al: Predicting the histology of anterior mediastinal masses: Comparison of chest radiography and CT. J Thorac Imaging 11:265, 1996.

77. Otto HF, Löning T, Lachenmayer L, et al: Thymolipoma in association with myasthenia gravis. Cancer 50:1623, 1982.

78. Barnes RDS, O'Gorman P: Two cases of aplastic anaemia associated with tumours of the thymus. J Clin Pathol 15:264, 1962.

79. Havlicek F, Rosai J: A sarcoma of thymic stroma with features of liposarcoma. Am J Clin Pathol 82:217, 1984.

80. McCafferty MH, Bahnson HT: Thymic cyst extending into the pericardium: A case report and review of thymic cysts. Ann Thorac Surg 33:503, 1982.

81. Indeglia RA, Shea MA, Grage TB: Congenital cysts of the thymus gland. Arch Surg 94:149, 1967.

82. Bieger RC, McAdams AJ: Thymic cysts. Arch Pathol 82:535, 1966.

83. Jaramillo D, Perez-Atayde A, Griscom NT: Apparent association between thymic cysts and prior thoracotomy. Radiology 172:207, 1989.

84. Borgna-Pignatti C, Andreis IB, Rugolotto S, et al: Thymic cyst appearing after treatment of mediastinal non-Hodgkin lymphoma. Med Pediatr Oncol 22:70, 1994.

85. Mishalani SH, Lones MA, Said JW: Multilocular thymic cyst: A novel thymic lesion associated with human immunodeficiency virus infection. Arch Pathol Lab Med 119:467, 1995.

86. Avila NA, Mueller BU, Carrasquillo JA, et al: Multilocular thymic cysts: Imaging features in children with human immunodeficiency virus infection. Radiology 201:130, 1996.

87. Suster S, Barbuto D, Carlson G, et al: Multilocular thymic cysts with pseudoepitheliomatous hyperplasia. Hum Pathol 22:455, 1991.

88. Suster S, Rosai J: Cystic thymomas: A clinicopathologic study of ten cases. Cancer 69:92, 1992.

89. Moran CA, Suster S: Mediastinal yolk sac tumors associated with prominent multilocular cystic changes of thymic epithelium: A clinicopathologic and immunohistochemical study of five cases. Mod Pathol 10:800, 1997.

89a. Moran CA, Suster S: Mediastinal seminomas with prominent cystic changes. A clinicopathologic study of 10 cases. Am J Surg Pathol 19:1047, 1995.

90. Smith PLC, Jobling C, Rees A: Hodgkin's disease in a large thymic cyst in a child. Thorax 38:392, 1983.

91. Leong AS-Y, Brown JH: Malignant transformation in a thymic cyst. Am J Surg Pathol 8:471, 1984.

92. Yamashita S, Yamazaki H, Kato T, et al: Thymic carcinoma which developed in a thymic cyst. Intern Med 35:215, 1996.

93. Babu MK, Nirmala V: Thymic carcinoma with glandular differentiation arising in a congenital thymic cyst. J Surg Oncol 57:277, 1994.

94. Brown LR, Aughenbaugh GL: Masses of the anterior mediastinum: CT and MR imaging. Am J Roentgenol 157:1171, 1991.

95. Peacey SR, Belchetz PE: Graves' disease: Associated ocular myasthenia gravis and a thymic cyst. J R Soc Med 86:297, 1993.

96. Fraile G, Rodriguez-Garcia JL, Monroy C, et al: Thymic cyst presenting as Horner's syndrome. Chest 101:1170, 1992.

97. Jessurun J, Azevedo M, Saldana M: Allergic angiitis and granulomatosis (Churg-Strauss syndrome): Report of a case with massive thymic involvement in a nonasthmatic patient. Hum Pathol 17:637, 1986.

98. Duprez A, Cordier R, Schmitz P: Tuberculoma of the thymus: First case of surgical excision. J Thorac Cardiovasc Surg 44:445, 1962.

99. FitzGerald JM, Mayo JR, Miller RR, et al: Tuberculosis of the thymus. Chest 102:1604, 1992.

100. Siegal GP, Dehner LP, Rosai J: Histiocytosis X (Langerhans' cell granulomatosis) of the thymus: A clinicopathologic study of four childhood cases. Am J Surg Pathol 9:117, 1985.

101. Harpaz N, Gribetz AR, Krellenstein DJ, et al: Inflammatory pseudotumor of the thymus. Ann Thorac Surg 42:331, 1986.

102. Hoffman OA, Gillespie DJ, Aughenbaugh GL, et al: Primary mediastinal neoplasms (other than thymoma). Mayo Clin Proc 68:880, 1993.

103. Bergh NP, Gatzinsky P, Larsson S, et al: Tumors of the thymus and thymic region: I. Clinicopathological studies on thymomas. Ann Thorac Surg 25:91, 1978.

104. Verley JM, Hollmann KH: Thymoma: A comparative study of clinical stages, histologic features, and survival in 200 cases. Cancer 55:1074, 1985.

105. Maggi G, Giaccone G, Donadio M, et al: Thymomas: A review of 169 cases, with particular reference to results of surgical treatment. Cancer 58:765, 1986.

106. Lewis JE, Wick MR, Scheithauer BW, et al: Thymoma: A clinicopathologic review. Cancer 60:2727, 1987.

107. Hofmann W, Möller P, Manke H-G, et al: Thymoma: A clinicopathologic study of 98 cases with special reference to three unusual cases. Pathol Res Pract 179:337, 1985.

108. Pescarmona E, Giardini R, Brisigotti M, et al: Thymoma in childhood: A clinicopathological study of five cases. Histopathology 21:65, 1992.

109. Cajal SR, Suster S: Primary thymic epithelial neoplasms in children. Am J Surg Pathol 15:466, 1991.

110. McGuire LJ, Huang DP, Teoh R, et al: Epstein-Barr virus genome in thymoma and thymic lymphoid hyperplasia. Am J Pathol 131:385, 1988.

111. Teoh R, McGuire L, Wong K, et al: Increased incidence of thymoma in Chinese myasthenia gravis: Possible relationship with Epstein-Barr virus. Acta Neurol Scand 80:221, 1989.

112. Buff DD, Greenberg SD, Leong P, et al: Thymoma, *Pneumocystis carinii* pneumonia, and AIDS. N Y State J Med 88:276, 1988.

113. Ono A, Saito H, Kondo S, et al: RNA tumor virus in human thymomas and thymus hyperplasia. Semin Surg Oncol 1:139, 1985.

114. Dal Cin P, De Wolf-Peeters C, Deneffe G, et al: Thymoma with a t(15;22)(p11;q11). Cancer Genet Cytogenet 89:181, 1996.

115. Lam WW, Chan FL, Lau YL, et al: Paediatric thymoma: Unusual occurrence in two siblings. Pediatr Radiol 23:124, 1993.

116. Cooper GN Jr, Narodick BG: Posterior mediastinal thymoma: Case report. J Thorac Cardiovasc Surg 63:561, 1972.

117. Miller WT Jr, Gefter WB, Miller WT: Thymoma mimicking a thyroid mass. Radiology 184:75, 1992.

118. Moran CA, Travis WD, Rosado-de-Christenson M, et al: Thymomas presenting as pleural tumors: Report of eight cases. Am J Surg Pathol 16:138, 1992.

119. Moran CA, Suster S, Fishback NF, et al: Primary intrapulmonary thymoma: A clinicopathologic and immunohistochemical study of eight cases. Am J Surg Pathol 19:304, 1995.

120. Puglisi F, Finato N, Mariuzzi L, et al: Microscopic thymoma and myasthenia gravis. J Clin Pathol 48:682, 1995.

121. Pescarmona E, Rosati S, Pisacane A, et al: Microscopic thymoma: Histological evidence of multifocal cortical and medullary origin. Histopathology 20:263, 1992.

122. Suster S, Rosai J: Cystic thymomas: A clinicopathologic study of ten cases. Cancer 69:92, 1992.

123. Suster S, Moran CA: Malignant thymic neoplasms that may mimic benign conditions. Semin Diagn Pathol 12:98, 1995.

124. Maggi G, Casadio C, Cavallo A, et al: Thymoma: Results of 241 operated cases. Ann Thorac Surg 51:152, 1991.

125. Kornstein MJ, Curran WJ Jr, Turrisi AT, et al: Cortical versus medullary thymomas: A useful morphologic distinction? Hum Pathol 19:1335, 1988.

126. Salyer WR, Eggleston JC: Thymoma: A clinical and pathological study of 65 cases. Cancer 37:229, 1976.

127. Lewis JE, Wick MR, Scheithauer BW, et al: Thymoma: A clinicopathologic review. Cancer 60:2727, 1987.

128. Pescarmona E, Rendina EA, Venuta F, et al: The prognostic implication of thymoma histologic subtyping: A study of 80 consecutive cases. Am J Clin Pathol 93:190, 1990.

129. Ricci C, Rendina EA, Pescarmona EO, et al: Correlations between histological type, clinical behaviour, and prognosis in thymoma. Thorax 44:455, 1989.

130. Verley JM, Hollmann KH: Thymoma: A comparative study of clinical stages, histologic features and survival in 200 cases. Cancer 55:1074, 1985.

131. Gray GF, Gutowski WT: Thymoma: A clinicopathologic study of 54 cases. Am J Surg Pathol 3:235, 1979.

132. Marino M, Müller-Hermelink HK: Thymoma and thymic carcinoma: Relation of thymoma epithelial cells to the cortical and medullary differentiation of thymus. Virchows Arch (Pathol Anat) 407:119, 1985.

133. Lee D, Wright DH: Immunohistochemical study of 22 cases of thymoma. J Clin Pathol 41:1297, 1988.

134. Quintanilla-Martinez L, Wilkins EW Jr, Ferry JA, et al: Thymoma—morphologic subclassification correlates with invasiveness and immunohistologic features: A study of 122 cases. Hum Pathol 24:958, 1993.

135. Chan JK, Tsang WY, Seneviratne S, et al: The MIC2 antibody 013: Practical application for the study of thymic epithelial tumors. Am J Surg Pathol 19:1115, 1995.

136. Ho FCS, Fu KH, Lam SY, et al: Evaluation of a histogenetic classification for thymic epithelial tumours. Histopathology 25:21, 1994.

137. Pan C-C, Wu H-P, Yang C-F, et al: The clinicopathological correlation of epithelial subtyping in thymoma: A study of 112 consecutive cases. Hum Pathol 25:893, 1994.

138. Quintanilla-Martinez L, Wilkins EW Jr, Choi N, et al: Histologic subclassification is an independent prognostic factor. Cancer 74:606, 1994.

139. Moreno EA, Aguayo AJL, Parrilla PP, et al: Prognostic factors of thymomas. Eur J Surg Oncol 21:482, 1995.

140. Dawson A, Ibrahim NBN, Gibbs AR: Observer variation in the histopathological classification of thymoma: Correlation with prognosis. J Clin Pathol 47:519, 1994.

141. Close PM, Kirchner T, Uys CJ, et al: Reproducibility of a histogenetic classification of thymic epithelial tumours. Histopathology 26:339, 1995.

142. Salter DM, Krajewski AS: Metastatic thymoma: A case report and immunohistological analysis. J Clin Pathol 39:275, 1986.

143. Fend F, Kirchner T, Marx A, et al: B-cells in thymic epithelial tumours: An immunohistochemical analysis of intra- and extraepithelial B-cell compartments. Virchows Arch (B) 63:241, 1993.

144. Pescarmona E, Rendina EA, Venuta F, et al: Recurrent thymoma: Evidence for histological progression. Histopathology 27:445, 1995.

145. Brocheriou I, Carnot F, Briere J: Immunohistochemical detection of bcl-2 protein n thymoma. Histopathology 27:251, 1995.

146. Tateyama H, Eimoto T, Tada T, et al: Apoptosis, bcl-2 protein, and fas antigen in thymic epithelial tumors. Mod Pathol 10:983, 1997.

147. Moran CA, Suster S: Current status of the histologic classification of thymoma. Int J Surg Pathol 3:67, 1995.

148. Fukuda T, Ohnishi Y, Emura I, et al: Microcystic variant of thymoma: Histological and immunohistochemical findings in two cases. Virchows Arch (A) 420:185, 1992.

149. Moran CA, Suster S, Koss MN: Plasma cell-rich thymoma. Am J Clin Pathol 102:199, 1994.

149a. Suster S, Moran CA, Chan JKC: Thymoma with pseudosarcomatous stroma: Report of an unusual histologic variant of thymic epithelial neoplasm that may simulate carcinosarcoma. Am J Surg Pathol 21:1316, 1997.

150. Moran CA, Koss MN: Rhabdomyomatous thymoma. Am J Surg Pathol 17:633, 1993.

151. Rosado-de-Christenson ML, Galobardes J, Moran CA. Thymoma: Radiologic-pathologic correlation. Radiographics 12:151, 1992.

152. Tan A, Holdener GP, Hecht A, et al: Malignant thymoma in an ectopic thymus: CT appearance. J Comput Assist Tomogr 15:842, 1991.

153. Hofmann W, Möller P, Manke HG, et al: Thymoma: A clinicopathologic study of 98 cases with special reference to three unusual cases. Pathol Res Pract 179:337, 1985.

154. Morgenthaler TI, Brown LR, Colby TV, et al: Thymoma. Mayo Clin Proc 68:1110, 1993.

155. Brown LR, Muhm JR, Gray JE: Radiographic detection of thymoma. Am J Roentgenol 134:1181, 1980.

156. Dixon AK, Hilton CJ, Williams GT: Computed tomography and histological correlation of the thymic remnant. Clin Radiol 32:255, 1981.

157. Machida K, Tasaka A, Yoshitake T: Computed tomography in the evaluation of benign and malignant thymoma. Nippon J Tomogr 9:56, 1982.

158. Baron RL, Lee JKT, Sagel SS, et al: Computed tomography of the abnormal thymus. Radiology 142:127, 1982.

159. Chen J, Weisbrod GL, Herman SJ: Computed tomography and pathologic correlations of thymic lesions. J Thorac Imaging 3:61, 1988.

160. Keen SJ, Libshitz HI: Thymic lesions: Experience with computed tomography in 24 patients. Cancer 59:1520, 1987.

161. Zerhouni EA, Scott WW Jr, Baker RR, et al: Invasive thymomas: Diagnosis and evaluation by computed tomography. J Comput Assist Tomogr 6:92, 1982.

162. Do YS, Im J-G, Lee BH, et al: CT findings in malignant tumors of thymic epithelium. J Comput Assist Tomogr 19:192, 1995.

163. Verstandig AG, Epstein DM, Miller WT, et al: Thymoma: Report of 71 cases and a review. Crit Rev Diagn Imaging 33:201, 1992.

164. Scatarige JC, Fishman EK, Zerhouni EA, et al: Transdiaphragmatic extension of invasive thymoma. Am J Roentgenol 144:31, 1985.

165. Sakai F, Sone S, Kiyono K, et al: MR imaging of thymoma: Radiologic-pathologic correlation. Am J Roentgenol 158:751, 1992.

166. Hale DA, Cohen AJ, Schaefer P, et al: Computed tomography in the evaluation of myasthenia gravis. South Med J 83:414, 1990.

167. Mink JH, Bein ME, Sukov R, et al: Computed tomography of the anterior mediastinum in patients with myasthenia gravis and suspected thymoma. Am J Roentgenol 130:239, 1978.

168. Fon GT, Bein ME, Mancuso AA, et al: Computed tomography of the anterior mediastinum in myasthenia gravis: A radiologic-pathologic correlative study. Radiology 142:135, 1982.

169. Moore AV, Korobkin M, Powers B, et al: Thymoma detection by mediastinal CT: Patients with myasthenia gravis. Am J Roentgenol 138:217, 1982.

170. Brown LR, Muhm JR, Sheedy PF II, et al: The value of computed tomography in myasthenia gravis. Am J Roentgenol 140:31, 1983.

171. Ellis K, Austin JHM, Ill AJ: Radiologic detection of thymoma in patients with myasthenia gravis. Am J Roentgenol 151:873, 1988.

172. Venegas RJ, Sun NCJ: Cardiac tamponade as a presentation of malignant thymoma. Acta Cytol 32:257, 1988.

173. Shishido M, Yano K, Ichiki H, et al: Pericarditis as the initial manifestation of malignant thymoma: Disappearance of pericardial effusion with corticosteroid therapy. Chest 106:313, 1994.

174. Dib HR, Friedman B, Khouli HI, et al: Malignant thymoma: A complicated triad of SVC syndrome, cardiac tamponade, and DIC. Chest 105:941, 1994.

175. Futami S, Yamasaki T, Minami R, et al: Intracaval and intracardiac extension of malignant thymoma. Intern Med 32:257, 1993.

176. Templeton PA, Vainright JR, Rodriguez A, et al: Mediastinal tumors presenting as spontaneous hemothorax, simulating aortic dissection. Chest 93:828, 1988.

177. Jeandel C, Gastin I, Blain H, et al: Thymoma with immunodeficiency (Good's syndrome) associated with selective cobalamin malabsorption and benign IgM-kappa gammopathy. J Intern Med 235:179, 1994.

178. Rosen VJ, Christiansen TW, Hughes RK: Metastatic thymoma presenting as a solitary pulmonary nodule. Cancer 19:527, 1966.

179. Bertelsen S, Malmstrøm J, Heerfordt J, et al: Tumours of the thymic region. Thorax 30:19, 1975.

180. Rosenthal T, Hertz M, Samra Y, et al: Thymoma: Clinical and additional radiologic signs. Chest 65:428, 1974.

181. Perini M, Ghezzi A, Basso PF, et al: Association of neuromyotonia with peripheral neuropathy, myasthenia gravis and thymoma: A case report. Ital J Neurol Sci 15:307, 1994.

182. Cunningham JD, Burt ME: Limbic encephalitis secondary to malignant thymoma. Ann Thorac Surg 58:250, 1994.

183. Masaoka A, Hashimoto T, Shibata K, et al: Thymomas associated with pure red cell aplasia: Histologic and follow-up studies. Cancer 64:1872, 1989.

184. Bailey RO, Dunn HG, Rubin AM, et al: Myasthenia gravis with thymoma and pure red blood cell aplasia. Am J Clin Pathol 89:687, 1988.

185. Katabami S, Sugiyama T, Kodama T, et al: Polymyositis associated with thymoma and the subsequent development of pure red cell aplasia. Intern Med 34:569, 1995.

186. Handa SI, Schofield KP, Sivakumaran M, et al: Pure red cell aplasia associated with malignant thymoma, myasthenia gravis, polyclonal large granular lymphocytosis and clonal thymic T cell expansion. J Clin Pathol 47:676, 1994.

187. De Giacomo T, Rendina EA, Venuta F, et al: Pancytopenia associated with thymoma resolving after thymectomy and immunosuppressive therapy: Case report. Scand J Thorac Cardiovasc Surg 29:149, 1995.

188. Postiglione K, Ferris R, Jaffe JP, et al: Immune mediated agranulocytosis and anemia associated with thymoma. Am J Hematol 49:336, 1995.

189. Athanassiou P, Ioakimidis D, Weston J, et al: Type 1 cryoglobulinaemia associated with a thymic tumour: Successful treatment with plasma exchange. Br J Rheumatol 34:285, 1995.

190. Honda T, Hayasaka M, Hachiya T, et al: Invasive thymoma with hypogammaglobulinemia spreading within the bronchial lumen. Respiration 62:294, 1995.

191. Lishner M, Ravid M, Shapira J, et al: Delta-T-lymphocytosis in a patient with thymoma. Cancer 74:2924, 1994.

192. Smith GP, Perkins SL, Segal GH, et al: T-cell lymphocytosis associated with invasive thymomas. Am J Clin Pathol 102:447, 1994.

193. Medeiros LJ, Bhagat SK, Naylor P, et al: Malignant thymoma associated with T-cell lymphocytosis: A case report with immunophenotypic and gene rearrangement analysis. Arch Pathol Lab Med 117:279, 1993.

194. Friedman HD, Inman DA, Hutchison RE, et al: Concurrent invasive thymoma and T-cell lymphoblastic leukemia and lymphoma: A case report with necropsy findings and literature review of thymoma and associated hematologic neoplasm. Am J Clin Pathol 101:432, 1994.

195. Rosman A, Atsumi T, Khamashta MA, et al: Development of systemic lupus erythematosus after chemotherapy and radiotherapy for malignant thymoma. Br J Rheumatol 34:1175, 1995.

196. Mevorach D, Perrot S, Buchanan NM, et al: Appearance of systemic lupus erythematosus after thymectomy: Four case reports and review of the literature. Lupus 4:33, 1995.

197. Zandman-Goddard G, Lorber M, Schoenfeld Y: Systemic lupus erythematosus and thymoma—a double-edged sword. Int Arch Allergy Immunol 108:99, 1995.

198. Yoshioka R, Sato Y, Kogure A, et al: Association of primary sclerosing cholangitis, thymoma and hypogammaglobulinemia. Liver 15:53, 1995.

199. Kornacki S, Hansen FC 3rd, Lazenby A: Graft-versus-host–like colitis associated with malignant thymoma. Am J Surg Pathol 19:224, 1995.

200. Tan CK, Ng HS, Ho JS, et al: Acute intestinal pseudo-obstruction due to malignant thymoma. Singapore Med J 34:175, 1993.

201. Jacyk WK, Hazelhurst JA, Dreyer L, et al: Epidermodysplasia verruciformis and malignant thymoma. Clin Exp Dermatol 18:89, 1993.

202. Ho WK, Wilson JD: Hypothermia, hyperhidrosis, myokymia and increased urinary excretion of catecholamines associated with a thymoma. Med J Aust 158:787, 1993.

203. Rizzoli R, Pache JC, Didierjean L, et al: A thymoma as a cause of true ectopic hyperparathyroidism. J Clin Endocrinol Metab 79:912, 1994.

204. Asamura H, Morinaga S, Shimosato Y, et al: Thymoma displaying endobronchial polypoid growth. Chest 94:647, 1988.

205. Missault L, Duprez D, De Buyzere M, et al: Right atrial invasive thymoma with protrusion through the tricuspid valve. Eur Heart J 13:1726, 1992.

206. Scatarige JC, Fishman EK, Zerhouni EA, et al: Transdiaphragmatic extension of invasive thymoma. Am J Roentgenol 144:31, 1985.

207. Nickels J, Franssila K: Thymoma metastasizing to extrathoracic sites. Acta Pathol Microbiol Scand Sect A 84:331, 1976.

208. Reddy VB, Reyes C, Wang H, et al: Cytologic patterns of metastatic thymoma: Diagnosis by fine-needle aspiration biopsy. Diagn Cytopathol 11:182, 1994.

209. Kornstein MJ, deBlois GG: Pathology of the thymus and mediastinum. In: Major Problems in Pathology. Vol. 33. Philadelphia, WB Saunders, 1995.

210. Regnard JF, Magdeleinat P, Dromer C, et al: Prognostic factors and long-term results after thymoma resection: A series of 307 patients. J Thorac Cardiovasc Surg 112:376, 1996.

211. Masaoka A, Monden Y, Nakahara K, et al: Follow-up study of thymomas with special reference to their clinical stages. Cancer 48:2485, 1981.

212. Park HS, Shin DM, Lee JS, et al: Thymoma: A retrospective study of 87 cases. Cancer 73:2491, 1994.

213. Wilkins EW Jr, Grillo HC, Scannell G, et al: Role of staging in prognosis and management of thymoma. Ann Thorac Surg 51:888, 1991.

214. Blumberg D, Port JL, Weksler B, et al: Thymoma: A multivariate analysis of factors predicting survival. Ann Thorac Surg 60:908, 1995.

215. Asamura H, Nakajima T, Mukai K, et al: Degree of malignancy of thymic epithelial tumors in terms of nuclear DNA content and nuclear area: An analysis of 39 cases. Am J Pathol 133:615, 1988.

216. Nomori H, Horinouchi H, Kaseda S, et al: Evaluation of the malignant grade of thymoma by morphometric analysis. Cancer 61:982, 1988.

217. Sauter ER, Sardi A, Hollier LH, et al: Prognostic value of DNA flow cytometry in thymomas and thymic carcinomas. South Med J 83:656, 1990.

218. Kuo T-T, Lo S-K: DNA flow cytometric study of thymic epithelial tumors with evaluation of its usefulness in the pathologic classification. Hum Pathol 24:746, 1993.

219. Pich A, Chiarle R, Chiusa L, et al: P53 expression and proliferative activity predict survival in noninvasive thymomas. Int J Cancer 69:180, 1996.

220. Davies SE, Macartney JC, Camplejohn RS, et al: DNA flow cytometry of thymomas. Histopathology 15:77, 1989.

221. Pollack A, El-Naggar AK, Cox JD, et al: Thymoma: The prognostic significance of flow cytometric DNA analysis. Cancer 69:1702, 1992.

222. Pich A, Chiarle R, Chiusa L, et al: Argyrophilic nucleolar organizer region counts predict survival in thymoma. Cancer 74:1568, 1994.

223. Pich A, Chiarle R, Chiusa L, et al: Long-term survival of thymoma patients by histologic pattern and proliferative activity. Am J Surg Pathol 19:918, 1995.

224. Yang W-I, Efird JT, Quintanilla-Martinez L, et al: Cell kinetic study of thymic epithelial tumors using PCNA (PC10) and Ki-67 (MIB-1) antibodies. Hum Pathol 27:70, 1996.

225. Gilhus NE, Jones M, Turley H, et al: Oncogene proteins and proliferation antigens in thymomas: Increased expression of epidermal growth factor receptor and Ki67 antigen. J Clin Pathol 48:447, 1995.

226. Chen FF, Yan JJ, Chang KC, et al: Immunohistochemical localization of Mcl-1 and bcl-2 proteins in thymic epithelial tumours. Histopathology 29:541, 1996.

227. Hayashi Y, Ishii N, Obayashi C, et al: Thymoma: Tumour type related to expression of epidermal growth factor (EGF), EGF-receptor, P53, v-erb B and ras p21. Virchows Arch 426:43, 1995.

228. Zeok JV, Todd EP, Dillon M, et al: The role of thymectomy in red cell aplasia. Ann Thorac Surg 28:257, 1979.

229. Masaoka A, Hashimoto T, Shibata K, et al: Thymomas associated with pure red cell aplasia: Histologic and follow-up studies. Cancer 64:1872, 1989.

230. Ohmi M, Ohuchi M: Recurrent thymoma in patients with myasthenia gravis. Ann Thorac Surg 50:243, 1990.

231. Rivner MH, Swift TR: Thymoma: Diagnosis and management. Semin Neurol 10:83, 1990.

232. Slater G, Papatestas A, Genkins G, et al: Thymomas in patients with myasthenia gravis. Ann Surg 188:171, 1978.

233. Gotti G, Paladini P, Haid MM, et al: Late recurrence of thymoma and myasthenia gravis. Scand J Thorac Cardiovasc Surg 29:37, 1995.

233a. Suster S, Moran CA: Thymic carcinoma: Spectrum of differentiation and histologic types. Pathology 30:111, 1998.

234. Kirchner T, Schalke B, Buchwald J, et al: Well-differentiated thymic carcinoma: An organotypical low-grade carcinoma with relationship to cortical thymoma. Am J Surg Pathol 16:1153, 1992.

235. Pescarmona E, Rosati S, Rendina EA, et al: Well-differentiated thymic carcinoma: A clinico-pathological study. Virchows Arch A 420:179, 1992.

236. Tateyama H, Eimoto T, Tada T, et al: P53 protein expression and P53 gene mutation in thymic epithelial tumors: An immunohistochemical and DNA sequencing study. Am J Clin Pathol 104:375, 1995.

237. Tateyama H, Mizuno T, Tada T, et al: Thymic epithelial tumours: Evaluation of malignant grade by quantification of proliferating cell nuclear antigen and nucleolar organizer regions. Virchows Arch (A) 422:265, 1993.

238. Kuo TT, Lo SK: DNA flow cytometric study of thymic epithelial tumors with evaluation of its usefulness in the pathologic classification. Hum Pathol 24:746, 1993.

239. Jensen MO, Antonenko D: Thyroid and thymic malignancy following childhood irradiation. J Surg Oncol 50:206, 1992.

240. Iezzoni JC, Gaffey MJ, Weiss LM: The role of Epstein-Barr virus in lymphoepithelioma-like carcinomas. Am J Clin Pathol 103:308, 1995.

241. Fujii T, Kawai T, Saito K, et al: EBER-1 expression in thymic carcinoma. Acta Pathol Jpn 43:107, 1993.

242. Yamashita S, Yamazaki H, Kato T, et al: Thymic carcinoma which developed in a thymic cyst. Intern Med 35:215, 1996,

243. Iezzoni JC, Nass LB: Thymic basaloid carcinoma: A case report and review of the literature. Mod Pathol 9:21, 1996.

244. Herezeg E, Kahn LB: Primary thymic carcinoma: An unusual case originating in a lymphocytic rich thymoma. Virchows Arch (Pathol Anat) 409:163, 1986.

245. Suarez Vilela D, Salas Valien JS, Gonzalez Moran MA, et al: Thymic carcinosarcoma associated with a spindle cell thymoma: An immunohistochemical study. Histopathology 21:263, 1992.

246. Suster S, Moran CA: Primary thymic epithelial neoplasms showing combined features of thymoma and thymic carcinoma: A clinicopathologic study of 22 cases. Am J Surg Pathol 20:1469, 1996.

247. Lee AC, Kwong YI, Fu KH, et al: Disseminated mediastinal carcinoma with chromosomal translocation (15;19): A distinctive clinicopathologic syndrome. Cancer 72:2273, 1993.

248. Snover DC, Levine GD, Rosai J: Thymic carcinoma: Five distinctive histological variants. Am J Surg Pathol 6:451, 1982.

249. Matsuno Y, Mukai K, Noguchi M, et al: Histochemical and immunohistochemical evidence of glandular differentiation in thymic carcinoma. Acta Pathol Jpn 39:433, 1989.

250. Moran CA, Suster S: Mucoepidermoid carcinomas of the thymus: A clinicopathologic study of six cases. Am J Surg Pathol 19:826, 1995.

251. Hasserjian RP, Klimstra DS, Rosai J: Carcinoma of the thymus with clear-cell features: Report of eight cases and review of the literature. Am J Surg Pathol 19:835, 1995.

252. Suster S, Rosai J: Thymic carcinoma: A clinicopathologic study of 60 cases. Cancer 67:1025, 1991.

253. Nishimura M, Kodama T, Nishiyama H, et al: A case of sarcomatoid carcinoma of the thymus. Pathol Int 47:260, 1992.

254. Alguacil-Garcia A, Halliday WC: Thymic carcinoma with focal neuroblastoma differentiation. Am J Surg Pathol 11:474, 1987.

255. Sensaki K, Aida S, Takagi K, et al: Coexisting undifferentiated thymic carcinoma and thymic carcinoid tumor. Respiration 60:247, 1993.

256. Argani P, Erlandson RA, Rosai J: Thymic neuroblastoma in adults: Report of three cases with special emphasis on its association with the syndrome of inappropriate secretion of antidiuretic hormone. Am J Clin Pathol 108:537, 1997.

257. Hayashi S, Hamanaka Y, Sueda T, et al: Thymic metastasis from prostatic carcinoma: Report of a case. Surg Today 23:632, 1993.

258. Fukai I, Masaoka A, Hashimoto T, et al: Differential diagnosis of thymic carcinoma and lung carcinoma with the use of antibodies to cytokeratins. J Thorac Cardiovasc Surg 110:1670, 1995.

259. Hishima T, Fukayama M, Fujisawa M, et al: CD5 expression in thymic carcinoma. Am J Pathol 145:268, 1994.

260. Dorfman DM, Shahsafaei A, Chan JK: Thymic carcinomas, but not thymomas and carcinomas of other sites, show CD5 immunoreactivity. Am J Surg Pathol 21:936, 1997.

261. Fukai I, Masaoka A, Hashimoto T, et al: The distribution of epithelial membrane antigen in thymic epithelial neoplasms. Cancer 70:2077, 1992.

262. Chan JK, Tsang WY, Seneviratne S, et al: The MIC2 antibody 013: Practical application for the study of thymic epithelial tumors. Am J Surg Pathol 19:1115, 1995.

263. Lee JD, Choe KO, Kim SJ, et al: CT findings in primary thymic carcinoma. J Comput Assist Tomogr 15:429, 1991.

264. Wick MR, Weiland LH, Scheithauer BW, et al: Primary thymic carcinomas. Am J Surg Pathol 6:613, 1982.

265. Ando Y, Hirabayashi N, Minami H, et al: Occult thymic carcinoma presenting as malignant cardiac tamponade. Intern Med 34:393, 1995.

266. Hsu CP, Chen CY, Chen CL, et al: Thymic carcinoma: Ten years' experience in twenty patients. J Thorac Cardiovasc Surg 107:615, 1994.

267. Chang HK, Wang CH, Liaw CC, et al: Prognosis of thymic carcinoma: Analysis of 16 cases. J Formos Med Assoc 91:764, 1992.

268. Sungur A, Ruacan S, Gungen Y, et al: Myasthenia gravis and primary squamous cell carcinoma of the thymus. Arch Pathol Lab Med 117:937, 1993.

269. Negron-Soto JM, Cascade PN: Squamous cell carcinoma of the thymus with paraneoplastic hypercalcemia. Clin Imaging 19:122, 1995.

270. Ilhan I, Kutluk T, Gogus S, et al: Hypertrophic pulmonary osteoarthropathy in a child with thymic carcinoma: An unusual presentation in childhood. Med Pediatr Oncol 23:140, 1994.

271. Tsuchiya R, Koga K, Matsuno Y, et al: Thymic carcinoma: Proposal for pathological TNM and staging. Pathol Int 44:505, 1994.

272. Peleg D, Zabari A, Shalev E: Relapsing thymic carcinoma during pregnancy. Acta Obstet Gynecol Scand 71:398, 1992.

273. Wick MR, Rosai J: Neuroendocrine neoplasms of the mediastinum. Semin Diagn Pathol 8:35, 1991.

274. Rosai J, Levine G, Weber WR, et al: Carcinoid tumors and oat cell carcinomas of the thymus. Pathol Ann 11:201, 1976.

275. Viebahn R, Hiddemann W, Klinke F, et al: Thymus carcinoid. Pathol Res Pract 180:445, 1985.

276. Gartner LA, Voorhess ML: Adrenocorticotropic hormone–producing thymic carcinoid in a teenager. Cancer 71:106, 1993.

277. Wick MR, Bernatz PE, Carney JA, et al: Primary mediastinal carcinoid tumors. Am J Surg Pathol 6:195, 1982.

278. Levine GD, Rosai J: A spindle cell variant of thymic carcinoid tumor. Arch Pathol Lab Med 100:293, 1976.

279. Ho FCS, Ho JCI: Pigmented carcinoid tumor of the thymus. Histopathology 1:363, 1977.

280. Lagrange W, Dahm H-H, Karstens J, et al: Melanocytic neuroendocrine carcinoma of the thymus. Cancer 59:484, 1987.

281. Suster S, Moran CA: Thymic carcinoid with prominent mucinous stroma: Report of a distinctive morphologic variant of thymic neuroendocrine neoplasm. Am J Surg Pathol 19:1277, 1995.

282. Paties C, Zangrandi A, Vassallo G, et al: Multidirectional carcinoma of the thymus with neuroendocrine and sarcomatoid components and carcinoid syndrome. Pathol Res Pract 187:170, 1991.

283. Kuo TT: Carcinoid tumor of the thymus with divergent sarcomatoid differentiation: Report of a case with histogenetic consideration. Hum Pathol 25:319, 1994.

284. Cho KJ, Ha CW, Koh JS, et al: Thymic carcinoid tumor combined with thymoma-neuroendocrine differentiation in thymoma? J Korean Med Sci 8:458, 1993.

285. de Montpreville VT, Macchiarini P, Dulmet E: Thymic neuroendocrine carcinoma (carcinoid): A clinicopathologic study of fourteen cases. J Thorac Cardiovasc Surg 111:134, 1996.

286. Warren JS, Yum MN: Carcinoid tumor arising in a treated primary germ cell tumor of the mediastinum. South Med J 80:259, 1987.

287. Valli M, Fabris GA, Dewar A, et al: Atypical carcinoid tumour of the thymus: A study of eight cases. Histopathology 24:371, 1994.

288. Herbst WM, Kummer W, Hofmann W, et al: Carcinoid tumors of the thymus: An immunohistochemical study. Cancer 60:2465, 1987.

289. Wick MR, Scheithauer BW: Thymic carcinoid: A histologic, immunohistochemical, and ultrastructural study of 12 cases. Cancer 53:475, 1984.

289a. Hishima T, Fukayama M, Hayashi Y, et al: Neuroendocrine differentiation in thymic epithelial tumors with special reference to thymic carcinoma and atypical thymoma. Hum Pathol 29:330, 1998.

290. Wick MR, Scheithauer BW: Oat-cell carcinoma of the thymus. Cancer 49:1652, 1982.

291. Chetty R, Batitang S, Govender D: Large cell neuroendocrine carcinoma of the thymus. Histopathology 31:274, 1997.

292. Wang DY, Kuo SH, Chang DB, et al: Fine needle aspiration cytology of thymic carcinoid tumor. Acta Cytol 39:423, 1995.

293. Wang DY, Chang DB, Kuo SH, et al: Carcinoid tumours of the thymus. Thorax 49:357, 1994.

294. Gherardi G, Marveggio C, Placidi A: Neuroendocrine carcinoma of the thymus: Aspiration biopsy, immunocytochemistry, and clinicopathologic correlates. Diagn Cytopathol 12:158, 1995.

295. Brown LR, Aughenbaugh GL, Wick MR, et al: Roentgenologic diagnosis of primary corticotropin-producing carcinoid tumors of the mediastinum. Radiology 142:143, 1982.
296. Felson B, Castleman B, Levinsohn EM, et al: Cushing syndrome associated with mediastinal mass. Am J Roentgenol 138:815, 1982.
297. Birnberg FA, Webb WR, Selch MT, et al: Thymic carcinoid tumors with hyperparathyroidism. Am J Roentgenol 139:1001, 1982.
298. Wang DY, Chang DB, Kuo SH, et al: Carcinoid tumours of the thymus. Thorax 49:357, 1994.
299. Economopoulos GC, Lewis JW Jr, Lee MW, et al: Carcinoid tumors of the thymus. Ann Thorac Surg 50:58, 1990.
300. Lynch M, Blevins LS, Martin RP: Acquired supravalvular pulmonary stenosis due to extrinsic compression by a metastatic thymic carcinoid tumor. Int J Card Imaging 12:61, 1996.
301. Lowenthal RM, Gumpel JM, Kreel L, et al: Carcinoid tumor of the thymus with systemic manifestations: A radiologic and pathological study. Thorax 29:553, 1974.
302. Zeiger MA, Swartz SE, MacGillivray DC, et al: Thymic carcinoid in association with MEN syndromes. Am Surg 58:430, 1992.
303. de Montpreville VT, Macchiarini P, Dulmet E: Thymic neuroendocrine carcinoma (carcinoid): A clinicopathologic study of fourteen cases. J Thorac Cardiovasc Surg 111:134, 1996.
304. Felson B, Castleman B, Levinsohn EM, et al: Cushing syndrome associated with mediastinal mass: Radiologic-pathologic correlation conference. SUNY Upstate Medical Center. Am J Roentgenol 138:815, 1982.
305. Brown LR, Aughenbaugh GL, Wick MR, et al: Roentgenologic diagnosis of primary corticotropin-producing carcinoid tumors of the mediastinum. Radiology 142:143, 1982.
306. Hughes JP, Ancalmo N, Leonard GL, et al: Carcinoid tumour of the thymus gland: Report of a case. Thorax 30:470, 1975.
307. Lowenthal RM, Gumpel JM, Kreel L, et al: Carcinoid tumour of the thymus with systemic manifestations: A radiological and pathological study. Thorax 29:553, 1974.
308. Kimura N, Ishikawa T, Sasaki Y, et al: Expression of prohormone convertase, PC2, in adrenocorticotropin-producing thymic carcinoid with elevated plasma corticotropin-releasing hormone. J Clin Endocrinol Metab 81:390, 1996.
309. Moran CA, Suster S: Primary germ cell tumors of the mediastinum: I. Analysis of 322 cases with special emphasis on teratomatous lesions and a proposal for histopathologic classification and clinical staging. Cancer 80:681, 1997.
310. Benjamin SP, McCormack LJ, Effler DB, et al: Critical review—"Primary tumours of the mediastinum." Chest 62:297, 1972.
311. Nichols CR: Mediastinal germ cell tumors. Semin Thorac Cardiovasc Surg 4:45, 1992.
312. Dehner LP: Germ cell tumors of the mediastinum. Semin Diagn Pathol 7:266, 1990.
313. Luna MA, Valenzuela-Tamariz J: Germ-cell tumors of the mediastinum, postmortem findings. Am J Clin Pathol 65:450, 1976.
314. Knapp RH, Hurt RD, Payne WS, et al: Malignant germ cell tumors of the mediastinum. J Thorac Cardiovasc Surg 89:82, 1985.
315. Dulmet EM, Macchiarini P, Suc B, et al: Germ cell tumors of the mediastinum: A 30-year experience. Cancer 72:1894, 1993.
316. Albuquerque KV, Mistry RC, Deshpande RK, et al: Primary germ cell tumours of the mediastinum. Indian J Cancer 31:250, 1994.
317. Moran CA, Suster S, Koss MN: Primary germ cell tumors of the mediastinum: III. Yolk sac tumor, embryonal carcinoma, choriocarcinoma, and combined non-teratomatous germ cell tumors of the mediastinum—a clinicopathologic and immunohistochemical study of 64 cases. Cancer 80:699, 1997.
318. Aliotta PJ, Castillo J, Englander LS, et al: Primary mediastinal germ cell tumors: Histologic patterns of treatment failures at autopsy. Cancer 62:982, 1988.
319. Daugaard G, Rorth M, von der Maase H, et al: Management of extragonadal germ-cell tumors and the significance of bilateral testicular biopsies. Ann Oncol 3:283, 1992.
320. Hejase MJ, Donohue JP, Foster RS, et al: Post-chemotherapy resection of non-seminomatous germ cell testicular tumors metastatic to the mediastinum. J Urol 156:1345, 1996.
321. Afifi HY, Bosl GJ, Burt ME: Mediastinal growing teratoma syndrome. Ann Thorac Surg 64:359, 1997.
322. Lachman MF, Kim K, Koo B-C: Mediastinal teratoma associated with Klinefelter's syndrome. Arch Pathol Lab Med 110:1067, 1986.
323. McNeil MM, Leong A S-Y, Sage RE: Primary mediastinal embryonal carcinoma in association with Klinefelter's syndrome. Cancer 47:343, 1981.
324. Zon R, Orazi A, Neiman RS, et al: Benign hematologic neoplasm associated with mediastinal mature teratoma in a patient with Klinefelter's syndrome: A case report. Med Pediatr Oncol 23:376, 1994.
325. Landanyi M, Roy I: Mediastinal germ cell tumors and histiocytosis. Hum Pathol 19:586, 1988.
326. DeMent SH, Eggleston JC, Spivak JL: Association between mediastinal germ cell tumors and hematologic malignancies: Report of two cases and review of the literature. Am J Surg Pathol 9:23, 1985.
327. deMent SH: Association between mediastinal germ cell tumors and hematologic malignancies: An update. Hum Pathol 21:699, 1990.
328. Sole F, Bosch F, Woessner S, et al: Refractory anemia with excess of blasts and isochromosome 12p in a patient with primary mediastinal germ-cell tumor. Cancer Genet Cytogenet 77:111, 1994.
329. Garnick MB, Griffin JD: Idiopathic thrombocytopenia in association with extragonadal germ cell cancer. Ann Intern Med 98:926, 1983.
330. Larsen M, Evans WK, Shepherd FA, et al: Acute lymphoblastic leukemia: Possible origin from a mediastinal germ cell tumor. Cancer 53:441, 1984.
331. Motoyama T, Yamamoto O, Iwamoto H, et al: Fine needle aspiration cytology of primary mediastinal germ cell tumors. Acta Cytol 39:725, 1995.
332. Collins KA, Geisinger KR, Wakely PE Jr, et al: Extragonadal germ cell tumors: A fine-needle aspiration biopsy study. Diagn Cytopathol 12:223, 1995.
333. Richardson RL, Schoumacher RA, Mehmet F, et al: The unrecognized extragonadal germ cell cancer syndrome. Ann Intern Med 94:181, 1981.
334. Fox RM, Woods RL, Tattersall MH, et al: Undifferentiated carcinoma in young men: The atypical teratoma syndrome. Lancet 1:1316, 1979.
335. Greco FA, Vaughn WK, Hainsworth JD: Advanced poorly differentiated carcinoma of unknown primary site: Recognition of a treatable syndrome. Ann Intern Med 104:547, 1986.
336. Rosado-de-Christenson ML, Templeton PA, Moran CA: Mediastinal germ cell tumors: Radiologic and pathologic correlation. Radiographics 12:1013, 1992.
337. Lee KS, Im J-G, Han CH, et al: Malignant primary germ cell tumors of the mediastinum: CT features. Am J Roentgenol 153:947, 1989.
338. Levitt RG, Husband JE, Glazer HS: CT of primary germ-cell tumors of the mediastinum. Am J Roentgenol 142:73, 1984.
339. Blomlie V, Lien HH, Fosså SD, et al: Computed tomography in primary nonseminomatous germ cell tumors of the mediastinum. Acta Radiol 29:289, 1988.
340. Childs WJ, Goldstraw P, Nicholls JE, et al: Primary malignant mediastinal germ cell tumours: Improved prognosis with platinum-based chemotherapy and surgery. Br J Cancer 67:1098, 1993.
341. Nichols CR, Saxman S, Williams SD, et al: Primary mediastinal nonseminomatous germ cell tumors: A modern single institution experience. Cancer 65:1641, 1990.
342. Wright CD, Kesler KA, Nichols CR, et al: Primary mediastinal nonseminomatous germ cell tumors: Results of a multimodality approach. J Thorac Cardiovasc Surg 99:210, 1990.
343. Gerl A, Clemm C, Lamerz R, et al: Cisplatin-based chemotherapy of primary extragonadal germ cell tumors: A single institution experience. Cancer 77:526, 1996.
344. Templeton AW: Malignant mediastinal teratoma with bone metastases: A case report. Radiology 76:245, 1961.
345. Schlumberger HG: Teratoma of the anterior mediastinum in the group of military age. Arch Pathol 41:398, 1946.
346. Le Roux BT: Mediastinal teratomata. Thorax 15:333, 1960.
347. Karl SR, Dunn J: Posterior mediastinal teratomas. J Pediatr Surg 20:508, 1985.
348. Chiba T, Suzuki H, Hebiguchi T, et al: Gastric teratoma extending into the mediastinum. J Pediatr Surg 15:191, 1980.
349. Inada K, Nakano A: Structure and genesis of the mediastinal teratoma. AMA Arch Pathol 66:183, 1958.
350. Pachter MR, Lattes R: "Germinal" tumors of the mediastinum: A clinicopathologic study of adult teratomas, teratocarcinomas, choriocarcinomas and seminomas. Dis Chest 45:301, 1964.
351. Bordi C, De Viia O, Pollice L: Full pancreatic endocrine differentiation in a mediastinal teratoma. Hum Pathol 16:961, 1985.
352. Dunn PJS: Pancreatic endocrine tissue in benign mediastinal teratoma. J Clin Pathol 37:1105, 1984.
353. Perez-Ordonez B, Wesson DE, Smith CR, et al: A pancreatic cyst of the anterior mediastinum. Mod Pathol 9:210, 1996.
354. van Echten J, de Jong B, Sinke RJ, et al: Definition of a new entity of malignant extragonadal germ cell tumors. Genes Chromosomes Cancer 12:8, 1995.
355. Manivel C, Wick MR, Abenoza P, et al: The occurrence of sarcomatous components in primary mediastinal germ cell tumors. Am J Surg Pathol 10:711, 1986.
356. Caballero C, Gomez S, Matias-Guiu X, et al: Rhabdomyosarcomas developing in association with mediastinal germ cell tumours. Virchows Arch (A) 420:539, 1992.
357. Ulbright TM, Loehrer PJ, Roth LM, et al: The development of nongerm cell malignancies within germ cell tumors. Cancer 54:1824, 1984.
358. Morinaga S, Nomori H, Kobayashi R, et al: Well-differentiated adenocarcinoma arising from mature cystic teratoma of the mediastinum (teratoma with malignant transformation): Report of a surgical case. Am J Clin Pathol 101:531, 1994.
359. Lancaster KJ, Liang CY, Myers JC, et al: Goblet cell carcinoid arising in a mature teratoma of the mediastinum. Am J Surg Pathol 21:109, 1997.
360. Przygodzki RM, Moran CA, Suster S, et al: Primary mediastinal and testicular seminomas: A comparison of K-ras-2 gene sequence and P53 immunoperoxidase analysis of 26 cases. Hum Pathol 27:975, 1996.
361. Moeller KH, Rosado-de-Christenson ML, Templeton PA: Mediastinal mature teratoma: Imaging features. Am J Roentgenol 169:985, 1997.
362. Fulcher AS, Proto AV, Jolles H: Cystic teratoma of the mediastinum: Demonstration of fat/fluid level. Am J Roentgenol 154:259, 1990.
363. Sasaka K, Kurihara Y, Nakajima Y, et al: Spontaneous rupture: A complication of benign mature teratomas of the mediastinum. Am J Roentgenol 170:323, 1998.
364. Yeoman LJ, Dalton HR, Adam EJ: Fat-fluid level in pleural effusion as a complication of a mediastinal dermoid: CT characteristics. J Comput Assist Tomogr 14:305, 1990.
365. Rusby NL: Dermoid cysts and teratomata of the mediastinum: A review. J Thorac Surg 13:169, 1944.
366. Clagett OT, Woolner LB: Clinicopathologic Conference—recurrent chest infection in a teen-ager. Mayo Clin Proc 43:134, 1968.
367. Marshall ME, Trump DL: Acquired extrinsic pulmonic stenosis caused by mediastinal tumors. Cancer 49:1496, 1982.
368. Cobb CJ, Wynn J, Cobb SR, et al: Cytologic findings in an effusion caused by

rupture of a benign cystic teratoma of the mediastinum into a serous cavity. Acta Cytol 29:1015, 1985.

369. Southgate J, Slade PR: Teratodermoid cyst of the mediastinum with pancreatic enzyme secretion. Thorax 37:476, 1982.

370. Sommerlad BC, Cleland WP, Yong NK: Physiological activity in mediastinal teratomata. Thorax 30:510, 1975.

371. Suda K, Mizuguchi K, Hebisawa A, et al: Pancreatic tissue in teratoma. Arch Pathol Lab Med 108:835, 1984.

372. Honicky RE, dePapp EW: Mediastinal teratoma with endocrine function. Am J Dis Child 126:650, 1973.

373. Taniyama K, Ohta S, Suzuki H, et al: Alpha-fetoprotein–producing immature mediastinal teratoma showing rapid and massive recurrent growth in an adult. Acta Pathol Jpn 42:911, 1992.

374. Carter D, Bibro M, Touloukian RJ: Benign clinical behavior of immature mediastinal teratoma in infancy and childhood: Report of two cases and review of the literature. Cancer 49:398, 1982.

375. Harms D, Jänig U: Immature teratomas of childhood: Report of 21 cases. Pathol Res Pract 179:388, 1985.

376. Moriconi WJ, Taylor S, Huntrakoon M, et al: Primary mediastinal germinomas in females: A case report and review of the literature. J Surg Oncol 29:176, 1985.

377. Polansky SM, Barwick KW, Ravin CE: Primary mediastinal seminoma. Am J Roentgenol 132:17, 1979.

378. Moran CA, Suster S, Przygodzki RM, et al: Primary germ cell tumors of the mediastinum: II. Mediastinal seminomas—a clinicopathologic and immunohistochemical study of 120 cases. Cancer 80:691, 1997.

379. Moran CA, Suster S: Mediastinal seminomas with prominent cystic changes: A clinicopathologic study of 10 cases. Am J Surg Pathol 19:1047, 1995.

380. Choi S-J, Lee JS, Song KS, et al: Mediastinal teratoma: CT differentiation of ruptured and unruptured tumors. Am J Roentgenol 171:591, 1998.

381. Schantz A, Sewall W, Castleman B: Mediastinal germinoma: A study of 21 cases with excellent prognosis. Cancer 30:1189, 1981.

382. Burns BF, McCaughey WTE: Unusual thymic seminomas. Arch Pathol Lab Med 110:539, 1986.

383. Niehans GA, Manivel JC, Copland GT, et al: Immunohistochemistry of germ cell and trophoblastic neoplasms. Cancer 62:1113, 1988.

384. Levine GD: Primary thymic seminoma—a neoplasm ultrastructurally similar to testicular seminoma and distinct from epithelial thymoma. Cancer 31:729, 1973.

385. Hochholzer L, Theros EG, Rosen SH: Some unusual lesions of the mediastinum: Roentgenologic and pathologic features. Semin Roentgenol 4:74, 1969.

386. Aygun C, Slawson RG, Bajaj K, et al: Primary mediastinal seminoma. Urology 23:109, 1984.

387. Shin MS, Ho KJ: Computed tomography of primary mediastinal seminomas. J Comput Assist Tomogr 7:990, 1983.

388. Nagi DK, Jones WG, Belchetz PE: Gynaecomastia caused by a primary mediastinal seminoma. Clin Endocrinol 40:545, 1994.

389. Economou JS, Trump DL, Holmes EC, et al: Management of primary germ cell tumors of the mediastinum. J Thorac Cardiovasc Surg 83:643, 1982.

390. Hurt RD, Bruckman JE, Farrow GM, et al: Primary anterior mediastinal seminoma. Cancer 49:1658, 1982.

391. Raghavan D, Barrett A: Mediastinal seminomas. Cancer 46:1187, 1980.

392. Truong LD, Harris L, Mattioli C, et al: Endodermal sinus tumor of the mediastinum: A report of seven cases and review of the literature. Cancer 58:730, 1986.

393. Moran CA, Suster S: Hepatoid yolk sac tumors of the mediastinum: A clinicopathologic and immunohistochemical study of four cases. Am J Surg Pathol 21:1210, 1997.

394. Moran CA, Suster S: Yolk sac tumors of the mediastinum with prominent spindle cell features: A clinicopathologic study of three cases. Am J Surg Pathol 21:1173, 1997.

395. Mukai K, Adams WR: Yolk sac tumor of the anterior mediastinum: Case report with light- and electron-microscopic examination and immunohistochemical study of alpha-fetoprotein. Am J Surg Pathol 3:77, 1979.

396. Kuzur ME, Cobleigh MA, Greco A, et al: Endodermal sinus tumor of the mediastinum. Cancer 50:766, 1982.

397. Rusch VW, Logothetis C, Samuels M: Endodermal sinus tumor of the mediastinum: Report of apparent cure in two patients with extensive disease. Chest 86:745, 1984.

398. Sham JST, Fu KH, Chiu CSW, et al: Experience with the management of primary endodermal sinus tumor of the mediastinum. Cancer 64:756, 1989.

399. Sandhaus L, Strom RL, Mukai K: Primary embryonal-choriocarcinoma of the mediastinum in a woman: A case report with immunohistochemical study. Am J Clin Pathol 75:573, 1981.

400. Knapp RH, Fritz SR, Reiman HM: Primary embryonal carcinoma and choriocarcinoma of the mediastinum. Arch Pathol Lab Med 106:507, 1982.

401. Fine G, Smith RW Jr, Pachter MR: Primary extragenital choriocarcinoma in the male subject: Case report and review of the literature. Am J Med 32:776, 1962.

402. Cohen BA, Needle MA: Primary mediastinal choriocarcinoma in a man. Chest 67:106, 1975.

403. Moran CA, Suster S: Primary mediastinal choriocarcinomas: A clinicopathologic and immunohistochemical study of eight cases. Am J Surg Pathol 21:1007, 1997.

404. Wenger ME, Dines DE, Ahmann DL, et al: Primary mediastinal choriocarcinoma. Mayo Clin Proc 43:570, 1968.

405. Leading article: Primary mediastinal choriocarcinoma. BMJ 2:135, 1969.

406. Yurick BS, Ottoman RE: Primary mediastinal choriocarcinoma. Radiology 75:901, 1960.

407. Waldron JA Jr, Dohring EJ, Farber LR: Primary large cell lymphomas of the mediastinum: An analysis of 20 cases. Semin Diagn Pathol 2:281, 1985.

408. Levitt LJ, Aisenberg AC, Harris NL, et al: Primary non-Hodgkin's lymphoma of the mediastinum. Cancer 50:2486, 1982.

409. Yokose T, Kodama T, Matsuno Y, et al: Low-grade B cell lymphoma of mucosa-associated lymphoid tissue in the thymus of a patient with rheumatoid arthritis. Pathol Int 48:74, 1998.

410. Suematsu N, Watanabe S, Shimosato Y: A case of large "thymic granuloma": Neoplasm of T-zone histiocyte. Cancer 54:2480, 1984.

411. Szporn AH, Dikman S, Jagirdar J: True histiocytic lymphoma of the thymus: Report of a case and a study of the distribution of histiocytic cells in the fetal and adult thymus. Am J Clin Pathol 82:734, 1984.

412. Martin JJ: The Nisbet Symposium: Hodgkin's disease: Radiological aspects of the disease. Australas Radiol 11:206, 1967.

413. Fisher AMH, Kendall R, Van Leuven BD: Hodgkin's disease: A radiological survey. Clin Radiol 13:115, 1962.

414. Keller AR, Castleman B: Hodgkin's disease of the thymus gland. Cancer 33:1615, 1974.

415. Wernecke K, Vassallo P, Rutsch F, et al: Thymic involvement in Hodgkin's disease: CT and sonographic findings. Radiology 181:375, 1991.

416. Trump DL, Mann RB: Diffuse large cell and undifferentiated lymphomas with prominent mediastinal involvement: A poor prognostic subset of patients with non-Hodgkin's lymphoma. Cancer 50:277, 1982.

417. Picozzi VJ, Coleman CN: Lymphoblastic lymphoma. Semin Oncol 17:96, 1990.

418. Yousem SA, Weiss LM, Warnke RA: Primary mediastinal non-Hodgkin's lymphomas: A morphologic and immunologic study of 19 cases. Am J Clin Pathol 83:676, 1985.

419. Lamarre L, Jacobson JO, Aisenberg AC, et al: Primary large cell lymphoma of the mediastinum: A histologic and immunophenotypic study of 29 cases. Am J Surg Pathol 13:730, 1989.

420. Perrone T, Frizzera G, Rosai J: Mediastinal diffuse large-cell lymphoma with sclerosis: A clinicopathologic study of 60 cases. Am J Surg Pathol 10:176, 1986.

421. Möller P, Lämmler B, Eberlein-Gonska M, et al: Primary mediastinal clear cell lymphoma of B-cell type. Virchows Arch Pathol Anat 409:79, 1986.

422. Menestrina F, Chilosi M, Bonetti F, et al: Mediastinal large-cell lymphoma of B-type, with sclerosis: Histopathological and immunohistochemical study of eight cases. Histopathology 10:589, 1986.

423. Lazzarino M, Orlandi E, Paulli M, et al: Primary mediastinal B-cell lymphoma with sclerosis: an aggressive tumor with distinctive clinical and pathologic features. J Clin Oncol 11:2306, 1993.

424. Crile G Jr: Intrathoracic goiter. Cleve Clin Q 6:313, 1939.

425. Lahey FH: Intrathoracic goiters. Surg Clin North Am 25:609, 1945.

426. Nielsen VM, Løvgreen NA, Elbrønd O: Intrathoracic goitre: Surgical treatment in an ENT department. J Laryngol Otol 97:1039, 1983.

427. Katlic MR, Wang C, Grillo HC: Substernal goiter. Ann Thorac Surg 39:391, 1985.

428. Karadeniz A, Hacihanefioglu U: Abscess formation in an intrathoracic goitre. Thorax 37:556, 1982.

429. Irwin RS, Pratter MR, Hamolsky MW: Chronic persistent cough: An uncommon presenting complaint of thyroiditis. Chest 81:386, 1982.

430. Ward MJ, Davies D: Riedel's thyroiditis with invasion of the lungs. Thorax 36:956, 1981.

431. Dontas NS: Intrathoracic goitre. Br J Tuberc 52:154, 1958.

432. Rietz K-A, Werner B: Intrathoracic goiter. Acta Chir Scand 119:379, 1960.

433. Fragomeni LS, Ceratti de Zambuja P: Intrathoracic goitre in the posterior mediastinum. Thorax 35:638, 1980.

434. Spinner RJ, Moore KL, Gottfried MR, et al: Thoracic intrathymic thyroid. Ann Surg 220:91, 1994.

435. Meijer S, Hoitsma FW: Malignant intrathoracic oncocytoma. Cancer 49:97, 1982.

436. Bashist B, Ellis K, Gold RP: Computed tomography of intrathoracic goiters. Am J Roentgenol 140:455, 1983.

437. Glazer GM, Axel L, Moss AA: CT diagnosis of mediastinal thyroid. Am J Roentgenol 138:495, 1982.

438. Tecce PM, Fishman EK, Kuhlman JE: CT evaluation of the anterior mediastinum: Spectrum of disease. Radiographics 14:973, 1994.

439. Glazer HS, Molina PL, Siegel MJ, et al: High-attenuation mediastinal masses on unenhanced CT. Am J Roentgenol 156:45, 1991.

440. Mori K, Eguchi K, Moriyama H, et al: Computed tomography of anterior mediastinal tumors. Acta Radiol 28:395, 1987.

441. Takashima S, Morimoto S, Ikezoe J, et al: CT evaluation of anaplastic thyroid carcinoma. Am J Roentgenol 154:1079, 1990.

442. Gefter WB, Spritzer CE, Eisenberg B, et al: Thyroid imaging with high-field-strength surface-coil MR. Radiology 164:483, 1987.

443. Noma S, Nishimura K, Togashi K, et al: Thyroid gland: MR imaging. Radiology 164:495, 1987.

444. Park H-M, Tarver RD, Siddiqui AR, et al: Efficacy of thyroid scintigraphy in the diagnosis of intrathoracic goiter. Am J Roentgenol 148:527, 1987.

445. Irwin RS, Braman SS, Arvanitidis AN, et al: 131I thyroid scanning in preoperative diagnosis of mediastinal goiter. Ann Intern Med 89:73, 1978.

446. Irwin RS: Two asymptomatic patients with mediastinal disease. Chest 112:1677, 1997.

447. Schneider JA, Divgi CR, Scott AM, et al: Hiatal hernia on whole-body radioiodine survey mimicking metastatic thyroid cancer. Clin Nucl Med 18:751, 1993.

448. Willis LL, Cowan RJ: Mediastinal uptake of I-131 in a hiatal hernia mimicking recurrence of papillary thyroid carcinoma. Clin Nucl Med 18:961, 1993.

449. Vermiglio F, Baudin E, Travagli JP, et al: Iodine concentration by the thymus in thyroid carcinoma. J Nucl Med 37:1830, 1996.

450. Silverstein GE, Burke G, Goldberg D, et al: Superior vena caval system obstruction caused by benign endothoracic goiter. Dis Chest 56:519, 1969.

451. Hershey CO, McVeigh RC, Miller RP: Transient superior vena cava syndrome due to propylthiouracil therapy in intrathoracic goiter. Chest 79:356, 1981.

452. Owen WJ, Gleeson MJ, McColl I: Thyroid crisis and tracheal compression in patient with retrosternal goitre. BMJ 2:997, 1978.

453. Samanta A, Jones GR, Burden AC, et al: Thoracic inlet compression due to amiodarone induced goitre. Postgrad Med J 61:249, 1985.

454. Holden MP, Wooler GH, Ionescu MI: Massive retrosternal goitre presenting with hypertension. Thorax 27:772, 1972.

455. Murphy MN, Glennon PG, Diocee MS, et al: Nonsecretory parathyroid carcinoma of the mediastinum: Light microscopic, immunocytochemical, and ultrastructural features of a case, and review of the literature. Cancer 58:2468, 1986.

456. Kollmorgen CF, Aust MR, Ferreiro JA, et al: Parathyromatosis: A rare yet important cause of persistent or recurrent hyperparathyroidism. Surgery 116:111, 1994.

457. Landau O, Chamberlain DW, Kennedy RS, et al: Mediastinal parathyroid cysts. Ann Thorac Surg 63:951, 1997.

458. Gurbuz AT, Peetz ME: Giant mediastinal parathyroid cyst: An unusual cause of hypercalcemic crisis—case report and review of the literature. Surgery 120:795, 1996.

459. Leigh TF, Weens HS: Roentgen aspects of mediastinal lesions. Semin Roentgenol 4:59, 1969.

460. Lee YT, Hutcheson JK: Mediastinal parathyroid carcinoma detected on routine chest film. Chest 65:354, 1974.

461. Becker FO, Tausk K: Radiologically evident functioning mediastinal parathyroid adenoma. Chest 58:79, 1970.

462. Braxel C, Haemers S, van der Straeten M: Mediastinal parathyroid adenoma detected on a routine chest X-ray. Scand J Respir Dis 60:367, 1979.

463. Hanson DJ Jr: Unusual radiographic manifestations of parathyroid adenoma: Report of a case. N Engl J Med 267:1080, 1962.

464. Stark DD, Gooding GAW, Moss AA, et al: Parathyroid imaging: Comparison of high-resolution CT and high-resolution sonography. Am J Roentgenol 141:633, 1983.

465. Yousem DM, Scheff AM: Thyroid and parathyroid gland pathology. Otolaryngol Clin North Am 28:621, 1995.

466. Kang YS, Rosen K, Clark OH, et al: Localization of abnormal parathyroid glands of the mediastinum with MR imaging. Radiology 189:137, 1993.

467. Doppman JL, Skarulis MC, Chen CC, et al: Parathyroid adenomas in the aortopulmonary window. Radiology 201:456, 1996.

468. Hauet EJ, Paul MA, Salu MK: Compression of the trachea by a mediastinal parathyroid cyst. Ann Thorac Surg 64:851, 1997.

469. Auffermann W, Gooding GA, Okerlung MD, et al: Diagnosis of recurrent hyperparathyroidism: Comparison of MR imaging and other imaging techniques. Am J Roentgenol 150:1027, 1988.

469a. Lee VS, Spritzer CE: MR imaging of abnormal parathyroid glands. Am J Roentgenol 170:1097, 1998.

470. Seelos KC, DeMarco R, Clark OH, et al: Persistent and recurrent hyperparathyroidism: Assessment with gadopentetate dimeglumine-enhanced MR imaging. Radiology 177:373, 1990.

471. O'Doherty M, Kettle A, Wells P, et al: Parathyroid imaging with Tc-99m-sestamibi: Preoperative localization and tissue uptake studies. J Nucl Med 33:313, 1992.

472. Wei J, Burke GJ, Mansberger AR: Preoperative imaging of abnormal parathyroid glands in patients with hyperparathyroid disease using combination Tc-99m-pertechnetate and Tc-99m-sestamibi radionuclide scans. Ann Surg 219:568, 1994.

473. Gordon BM, Gordon L, Hoang K, et al: Parathyroid imaging with 99mTc-sestamibi. Am J Roentgenol 167:1563, 1996.

474. Udelsman R: Parathyroid imaging: The myth and the reality. Radiology 201:317, 1996.

475. Lee VS, Spritzer CE, Coleman RE, et al: The complementary roles of fast spin-echo MR imaging and double-phase 99mTc-sestamibi scintigraphy for localization of hyperfunctioning parathyroid glands. Am J Roentgenol 167:1555, 1996.

476. Krudy AG, Doppman JL, Brennan MF, et al: The detection of mediastinal parathyroid glands by computed tomography, selective arteriography and venous sampling: An analysis of 17 cases. Radiology 140:739, 1981.

477. Krudy AG, Doppman JL, Miller DL, et al: Detection of mediastinal parathyroid glands by nonselective digital arteriography. Am J Roentgenol 142:693, 1984.

477a. Doppman JL, Skarulis MC, Chang R, et al: Hypocalcemic stimulation and nonselective venous sampling for localizing parathyroid adenomas: Work in progress. Radiology 208:145, 1998.

478. Sorhage F, Stover DE, Mortazavi A: Unusual etiology of cough in a woman with asthma. Chest 110:852, 1996.

479. Gibbs AR, Johnson NF, Giddings JC, et al: Primary angiosarcoma of the mediastinum: Light and electron microscopic demonstration of factor VIII–related antigen in neoplastic cells. Hum Pathol 15:687, 1984.

480. Swanson PE: Soft tissue neoplasms of the mediastinum. Semin Diagn Pathol 8:14, 1991.

481. Pachter MR, Lattes R: Mesenchymal tumors of the mediastinum: I. Tumors of fibrous tissue, adipose tissue, smooth muscle, and striated muscle. Cancer 16:74, 1963.

482. Politis J, Funahasi A, Gehlsen JA, et al: Intrathoracic lipomas: Report of three cases and review of the literature with emphasis on endobronchial lipoma. J Thorac Cardiovasc Surg 77:550, 1979.

483. Sarama RF, DiGiacomo WA, Safirstein BH: Primary mediastinal lipoma. J Med Soc N J 78:901, 1981.

484. Tangthangtham A, Wongsangiem M, Supakul V, et al: Pleomorphic lipoma in the middle mediastinum. J Med Assoc Thai 78:437, 1995.

485. Wilson ES: Radiolucent mediastinal lipoma. Radiology 118:44, 1976.

486. Hodge J, Aponte G, McLaughlin E: Primary mediastinal tumors. J Thorac Surg 37:730, 1959.

487. Lyons HA, Calvy GL, Sammons BP: The diagnosis and classification of mediastinal masses: I. A study of 782 cases. Ann Intern Med 51:897, 1959.

488. Mendez G Jr, Isikoff MB, Isikoff SK, et al: Fatty tumors of the thorax demonstrated by CT. Am J Roentgenol 133:207, 1979.

489. Tabrisky J, Rowe JH, Cristie SG, et al: Benign mediastinal lipoblastomatosis. J Pediatr Surg 9:399, 1974.

490. Dudgeon DL, Haller JA Jr: Pediatric lipoblastomatosis: Two unusual cases. Surgery 95:371, 1984.

491. Santini LC, Williams JL: Mediastinal widening (presumably lipomatosis) in Cushing's syndrome. N Engl J Med 284:1357, 1971.

492. Price JE, Rigler LG: Widening of the mediastinum resulting from fat accumulation. Radiology 96:497, 1970.

493. Drasin GF, Lynch T, Temes GP: Ectopic ACTH production and mediastinal lipomatosis. Radiology 127:610, 1978.

494. Koerner HJ, Sun DI-C: Mediastinal lipomatosis secondary to steroid therapy. Am J Roentgenol 98:461, 1966.

495. Bodman SF, Condemi JJ: Mediastinal widening in iatrogenic Cushing's syndrome. Ann Intern Med 67:399, 1967.

496. Teates CD: Steroid-induced mediastinal lipomatosis. Radiology 96:501, 1970.

497. van de Putte LBA, Wagenaar JPM, San KH: Paracardiac lipomatosis in exogenous Cushing's syndrome. Thorax 28:653, 1973.

498. Lee WJ, Fattal G: Mediastinal lipomatosis in simple obesity. Chest 70:308, 1976.

499. Streiter ML, Schneider HJ, Proto AV: Steroid-induced thoracic lipomatosis: Paraspinal involvement. Am J Roentgenol 139:679, 1982.

500. Chalaoui J, Sylvestre J, Dussault RG, et al: Thoracic fatty lesions: Some usual and unusual appearances. J Can Assoc Radiol 32:197, 1981.

501. Standerfer RJ, Armistead SH, Paneth M: Liposarcoma of the mediastinum: Report of two cases and review of the literature. Thorax 36:693, 1981.

502. Dogan R, Ayrancioglu K, Aksu O: Primary mediastinal liposarcoma. A report of a case and review of the literature. Eur J Cardiothorac Surg 3:367, 1989.

503. Grewal RG, Prager K, Austin JHM, et al: Long term survival in nonencapsulated primary liposarcoma of the mediastinum. Thorax 48:1276, 1993.

504. Klimstra DS, Moran CA, Perino G, et al: Liposarcoma of the anterior mediastinum and thymus: A clinicopathologic study of 28 cases. Am J Surg Pathol 19:782, 1995.

505. Sekine Y, Hamaguchi K, Miyahara Y, et al: Thymus-related liposarcoma: Report of a case and review of the literature. Surg Today 26:203, 1996.

505a. Gómez-Román JJ, Val-Bernal JF: Lipoleiomyosarcoma of the mediastinum. Pathology 29:428, 1997.

506. Attal H, Jensen J, Reyes CV: Myxoid liposarcoma of the anterior mediastinum: Diagnosis by fine needle aspiration biopsy. Acta Cytol 39:511, 1995.

507. Dogan R, Ayrancioglu K, Aksu Ö: Primary mediastinal liposarcoma: A report of a case and review of the literature. Eur J Cardiothorac Surg 3:367, 1989.

508. Grewal RG, Prager K, Austin JHM, et al: Long term survival in nonencapsulated primary liposarcoma of the mediastinum. Thorax 48:1276, 1993.

509. Santamaria G, Serres X, Pruna X: Primary mediastinal liposarcoma with moderately high CT attenuation. Am J Roentgenol 167:1064, 1996.

510. Schweitzer DL, Aguam AS: Primary liposarcoma of the mediastinum. J Thorac Cardiovasc Surg 74:83, 1977.

511. Gindhart TD, Tucker WY, Choy SH: Cavernous hemangioma of the superior mediastinum: Report of a case with electron microscopy and computerized tomography. Am J Surg Pathol 3:353, 1979.

512. Cohen AJ, Sbaschnig RJ, Hochholzer L, et al: Mediastinal hemangiomas. Ann Thorac Surg 43:656, 1987.

513. Kings GLM: Multifocal haemangiomatous malformation: A case report. Thorax 30:485, 1975.

514. Pachter MR, Lattes R: Mesenchymal tumors of the mediastinum: II. Tumors of blood vascular origin. Cancer 16:95, 1963.

515. Moran CA, Suster S: Mediastinal hemangiomas: A study of 18 cases with emphasis on the spectrum of morphological features. Hum Pathol 26:416, 1995.

516. Davis JM, Mark GJ, Greene R: Benign blood vascular tumors of the mediastinum. Radiology 126:581, 1978.

517. McAdams HP, Rosado-de-Christenson ML, Moran CA: Mediastinal hemangioma: Radiographic and CT features in 14 patients. Radiology 193:399, 1994.

518. Leigh TF: Mass lesions of the mediastinum. Radiol Clin North Am 1:377, 1963.

519. Leibovici D, Oner V: Hemangioma of the posterior mediastinum: Review of the literature and report of a case. Am Rev Respir Dis 86:415, 1962.

520. Yousem SA, Hochholzer L: Unusual thoracic manifestations of epithelioid hemangioendothelioma. Arch Pathol Lab Med 111:459, 1987.

521. Moreno A, Canadas MA, Minguella J, et al: Histiocytoid hemangioma of the innominate vein. Pathol Res Pract 183:785, 1988.

522. Suster S, Moran CA, Koss MN: Epithelioid hemangioendothelioma of the anterior mediastinum: Clinicopathologic, immunohistochemical, and ultrastructural analysis of 12 cases. Am J Surg Pathol 18:871, 1994.

523. Lamovec J, Sobel HJ, Zidar A, et al: Epithelioid hemangioendothelioma of the anterior mediastinum with osteoclast-like giant cells: Light microscopic, immunohistochemical and electron microscopic study. Am J Clin Pathol 93:813, 1990.

524. Weidner N: Atypical tumor of the mediastinum: Epithelioid hemangioendothelioma containing metaplastic bone and osteoclastlike giant cells. Ultrastruct Pathol 15:481, 1991.

525. Abratt RP, Williams M, Raff M, et al: Angiosarcoma of the superior vena cava. Cancer 52:740, 1983.
526. Ochsner JL, Ochsner SF: Congenital cysts of the mediastinum: 20-year experience with 42 cases. Ann Surg 163:909, 1966.
527. Summer TE, Volberg FM, Kiser PE, et al: Mediastinal cystic hygroma in children. Pediatr Radiol 11:160, 1981.
528. Bratu M, Brown M, Carter M, et al: Cystic hygroma of the mediastinum in children. Am J Dis Child 119:348, 1970.
529. Pachter MR, Lattes R: Mesenchymal tumors of the mediastinum: III. Tumors of lymph vascular origin. Cancer 16:108, 1963.
530. Feng Y-F, Masterson JB, Riddell RH: Lymphangioma of the middle mediastinum as an incidental finding on a chest radiograph. Thorax 35:955, 1980.
531. Brown LR, Reiman HM, Rosenow EC III, et al: Intrathoracic lymphangioma. Mayo Clin Proc 61:882, 1986.
532. Topcu S, Soysal O, Balkan E, et al: Mediastinal cystic lymphangioma: Report of two cases. Thorac Cardiovasc Surg 45:209, 1997.
533. Pannell TL, Jolles H: Adult cystic mediastinal lymphangioma simulating a thymic cyst. J Thorac Imaging 7:86, 1991.
534. Pilla TJ, Wolverson MK, Sundaram M, et al: CT evaluation of cystic lymphangiomas of the mediastinum. Radiology 144:841, 1982.
535. Shaffer K, Rosado-de-Christenson ML, Patz EF Jr, et al: Thoracic lymphangioma in adults: CT and MR imaging features. Am J Roentgenol 162:283, 1994.
536. Miyake H, Shiga M, Takaki H, et al: Mediastinal lymphangiomas in adults: CT findings. J Thorac Imaging 11:83, 1996.
537. Khoury GH, Demong CV: Mediastinal cystic hygroma in childhood. J Pediatr 62:432, 1963.
538. Daniel TM, Staub EW, Clark DE: Symptomatic venous compression from a mediastinal cystic lymphangioma. Chest 63:834, 1973.
539. Matsuzoe D, Iwasaki A, Hideshima T, et al: Postoperative chylothorax following partial resection of mediastinal lymphangioma: Report of a case. Surg Today 25:827, 1995.
540. Gilsanz V, Yeh HC, Baron MG: Multiple lymphangiomas of the neck, axilla, mediastinum and bones in an adult. Radiology 120:161, 1976.
541. Watts MA, Gibbons JA, Aaron BL: Mediastinal and osseous lymphangiomatosis, case report and review. Ann Thorac Surg 34:324, 1982.
542. Ramani P, Shah A: Lymphangiomatosis: Histologic and immunohistochemical analysis of four cases. Am J Surg Pathol 17:329, 1993.
543. Fan LL, Mullen ALW, Brugman SM, et al: Clinical spectrum of chronic interstitial lung disease in children. J Pediatr 121:867, 1992.
544. Swensen SJ, Hartman TE, Mayo JR, et al: Diffuse pulmonary lymphangiomatosis: CT findings. J Comput Assist Tomogr 19:348, 1995.
545. Moran CA, Suster S, Perino G, et al: Malignant smooth muscle tumors presenting as mediastinal soft tissue masses: A clinicopathologic study of 10 cases. Cancer 74:2251, 1994.
546. Uno A, Sakurai M, Onuma K, et al: A case of giant mediastinal leiomyoma with long-term survival. Tohoku J Exp Med 156:1, 1988.
547. Rasaretnam R, Panabokke RG: Leiomyosarcoma of the mediastinum. Br J Dis Chest 69:63, 1975.
548. Bernheim J, Griffel B, Versano S, et al: Mediastinal leiomyosarcoma in the wall of a bronchial cyst (letter to the editor). Arch Pathol Lab Med 104:221, 1980.
549. Sunderrajan EV, Luger AM, Rosenholtz MJ, et al: Leiomyosarcoma in the mediastinum presenting as superior vena cava syndrome. Cancer 53:2553, 1984.
550. Rodriguez E, Pombo F, Aguilera C, et al: Recurring tracheal leiomyoma presenting as a calcified mediastinal mass. Eur J Radiol 23:82, 1996.
551. Weiss KS, Zidar BL, Wang S, et al: Radiation-induced leiomyosarcoma of the great vessels presenting as superior vena cava syndrome. Cancer 60:1238, 1987.
552. Crist WM, Raney RB, Newton W, et al: Intrathoracic soft tissue sarcomas in children. Cancer 50:598, 1982.
553. Suster S, Moran CA, Koss MN: Rhabdomyosarcomas of the anterior mediastinum: Report of four cases unassociated with germ cell, teratomatous, or thymic carcinomatous components. Hum Pathol 25:349, 1994.
554. Miller R, Kurtz SM, Powers MJ: Mediastinal rhabdomyoma. Cancer 42:1983, 1978.
555. Witkin GB, Rosai J: Solitary fibrous tumor of the mediastinum: A report of 14 cases. Am J Surg Pathol 13:547, 1989.
556. Hanau CA, Miettinen M: Solitary fibrous tumor: Histological and immunohistochemical spectrum of benign and malignant variants presenting at different sites. Hum Pathol 26:440, 1995.
557. Chen W, Chan CW, Mok CK: Malignant fibrous histiocytoma of the mediastinum. Cancer 50:797, 1982.
558. Flieder DB, Moran CA, Suster S: Primary alveolar soft-part sarcoma of the mediastinum: a clinicopathological and immunohistochemical study of two cases. Histopathology 31:469, 1997.
559. Venuta F, Pescarmona EO, Rendina EA, et al: Primary osteogenic sarcoma of the posterior mediastinum: Case report. Scand J Thorac Cardiovasc Surg 27:169, 1993.
560. Suster S, Moran CA: Malignant cartilaginous tumors of the mediastinum: Clinicopathological study of six cases presenting as extraskeletal soft tissue masses. Hum Pathol 28:588, 1997.
561. Widdowson DJ, Lewis-Jones HG: A large soft-tissue chondroma arising from the posterior mediastinum. Clin Radiol 39:333, 1988.
562. Chelty R: Extraskeletal mesenchymal chondrosarcoma of the mediastinum. Histopathology 17:261, 1990.
563. Lin J, Ho J, Chan A, et al: Extraosseous osteogenic sarcoma of the mediastinum occurring in a Chinese patient. Clin Oncol 7:200, 1995.
564. Catanese J, Dutcher JP, Dorfman HD, et al: Mediastinal osteosarcoma with extension to lungs in a patient treated for Hodgkin's disease. Cancer 62:2252, 1988.
565. Modic MT, Janicki PC: Computed tomography of mass lesions of the right cardiophrenic angle. J Comput Assist Tomogr 4:521, 1980.
566. Glazer HS, Wick MR, Anderson DJ, et al: CT of fatty thoracic masses. Am J Roentgenol 159:1181, 1992.
567. Paling MR, Williamson BRJ: Epipericardial fat pad: CT findings. Radiology 165:335, 1987.
568. Rodríguez, Soler R, Gayol A, et al: Massive mediastinal and cardiac fatty infiltration in a young patient. J Thorac Imaging 10:225, 1995.
569. Behrendt DM, Scannell JG: Pericardial fat necrosis: An unusual cause of severe chest pain and thoracic "tumor." N Engl J Med 279:473, 1968.
570. Peterson DT, Katz LM, Popp RL: Pericardial cyst 10 years after acute pericarditis. Chest 67:719, 1975.
570a. Salyer DC, Salyer WR, Eggleston JC: Benign developmental cysts of the mediastinum. Arch Pathol Lab Med 101:136, 1977.
571. Stoller JK, Shaw C, Matthay RA: Enlarging, atypically located pericardial cyst: Recent experience and literature review. Chest 89:402, 1986.
572. Ochsner JL, Ochsner SF: Congenital cysts of the mediastinum: 20-year experience with 42 cases. Ann Surg 163:909, 1966.
573. Pader E, Kirschner PA: Pericardial diverticulum. Dis Chest 55:344, 1969.
574. Snyder SN: Massive pericardial coelomic cyst: Diagnostic features and unusual presentation. Chest 71:100, 1977.
575. Pugatch RD, Braver JH, Robbins AH, et al: CT diagnosis of pericardial cysts. Am J Roentgenol 131:515, 1978.
576. Ikezoe J, Sone S, Morimoto S, et al: Computed tomography reveals atypical localization of benign mediastinal tumors. Acta Radiol 30:175, 1989.
577. Vinee P, Stover B, Sigmund G, et al: MR imaging of the pericardial cyst. J Magn Reson Imaging 2:593, 1992.
578. Felner JM, Fleming WH, Franch RH: Echocardiographic identification of a pericardial cyst. Chest 68:386, 1975.
579. Padder FA, Conrad AR, Manzar KJ, et al: Echocardiographic diagnosis of pericardial cyst. Am J Med Sci 313:191, 1997.
580. Rogers CI, Seymour EQ, Brock JG: Atypical pericardial cyst location: The value of computed tomography. Case report. J Comput Assist Tomogr 4:683, 1980.
581. Stoller JK, Shaw C, Matthay RA: Enlarging, atypically located pericardial cyst: Recent experience and literature review. Chest 89:402, 1986.
582. Brunner DR, Whitley NO: A pericardial cyst with high CT numbers. Am J Roentgenol 142:279, 1984.
583. Zhao F, Wang C, Song XL: Calcified pericardial cyst—a case report and the roentgenologic and pathologic differentiation from other calcified mediastinal cysts. J Thorac Cardiovasc Surg 32:193, 1984.
584. Daniel RA Jr, Diveley WL, Edwards WH, et al: Mediastinal tumors. Ann Surg 151:783, 1960.
585. Mastroroberto P, Chello M, Bevacqua E, et al: Pericardial cyst with partial erosion of the superior vena cava. An unusual case. J Cardiovasc Surg 37:323, 1996.
586. Bandeira FC, de Sa VP, Moriguti JC, et al: Cardiac tamponade: an unusual complication of pericardial cyst. J Am Soc Echocardiogr 9:108, 1996.
587. Bierhoff E, Pfeifer U: Malignant mesothelioma arising from a benign mediastinal mesothelial cyst. Gen Diagn Pathol 142:59, 1996.
588. Vlay SC, Hartman AR: Mechanical treatment of atrial fibrillation: removal of pericardial cyst by thoracoscopy. Am Heart J 129:616, 1995.
589. Aronberg DJ, Peterson RP, Glazer HS, et al: Superior diaphragmatic lymph nodes: CT assessment. J Comput Assist Tomogr 10:937, 1986.
590. Schwartz EE, Wechsler RJ: Diaphragmatic and paradiaphragmatic tumors and pseudotumors. J Thorac Imaging 4:19, 1989.
591. Vock P, Hodler J: Cardiophrenic angle adenopathy: Update on causes and significance. Radiology 159:395, 1986.
592. Sussman SK, Halvorsen RA Jr, Silverman PM, et al: Paracardiac adenopathy: CT evaluation. Am J Roentgenol 149:29, 1987.
593. Cho CS, Blank N, Castellino RA: CT evaluation of cardiophrenic angle lymph nodes in patients with malignant lymphoma. Am J Roentgenol 143:719, 1984.
594. Castellino RA, Blank N: Adenopathy of the cardiophrenic angle (diaphragmatic) lymph nodes. Am J Roentgenol 114:509, 1972.
595. Fayos JV, Lampe I: Cardiac apical mass in Hodgkin's disease. Radiology 99:15, 1971.
596. Majeski JA, Paxton ES, Wirman JA, et al: A thoracic benign mesenchymoma in association with hemihypertrophy. Am J Clin Pathol 76:827, 1981.
597. Pachter MR: Benign mesenchymoma of the mediastinum: A case with extramedullary hematopoiesis within the tumor and vascular malformations in the lungs. Arch Pathol 74:179, 1962.
598. Jaituni S, Arkee MSK, Caterine JM: Mediastinal myxoma: A case report. J Iowa Med Soc 64:107, 1974.
599. McCluggage WG, Boyd HK, Jones FGC, et al: Mediastinal granulocytic sarcoma. A report of two cases. Arch Pathol Lab Med 122:545, 1998.
600. Chubachi A, Miura I, Takahashi N, et al: Acute myelogenous leukemia associated with a mediastinal tumor. Leuk Lymphoma 12:143, 1993.
601. Witkin GB, Miettinen M, Rosai J: A biphasic tumor of the mediastinum with features of synovial sarcoma: A report of four cases. Am J Surg Pathol 13:490, 1989.
602. Feigin GA, Robinson B, Marchevsky A: Mixed tumor of the mediastinum. Arch Pathol Lab Med 110:80, 1986.

CHAPTER 75

Masses Situated Predominantly in the Middle-Posterior Mediastinal Compartment

As discussed in Chapter 74 (*see* page 2875), we prefer to consider the middle and posterior mediastinal compartments together in a discussion of mediastinal masses. For practical purposes, a tumor can be considered to lie in this region when, on the lateral chest radiograph, it is situated between a line drawn along the anterior border of the trachea and the posterior border of the heart and one drawn along the anterior aspect of the vertebral bodies (*see* Fig. 74–1, page 2876). The most common abnormalities of this region are lymph node enlargement and aortic aneurysms;[1] esophageal lesions and congenital cysts are less frequent, and most other lesions are rare.

LYMPH NODE ENLARGEMENT

Lymph node enlargement is the most common abnormality of the middle-posterior mediastinum. It is caused most often by lymphoma, metastatic carcinoma (Fig. 75–1), sarcoidosis, and infection (either directly by organisms such as *Histoplasma capsulatum* and *Mycobacterium tuberculosis* or as a hyperplastic reaction to the presence of organisms within the lungs). Most of these and other less common conditions are discussed elsewhere in this book; only giant lymph node hyperplasia (Castleman's disease) and granulomatous mediastinitis are considered in any detail here.

Clinicopathologic effects of enlarged lymph nodes in the middle-posterior mediastinum are usually minimal or absent altogether. However, because of their intimate association with the airways and vessels that course through this region, stenosis or obstruction may ensue and result in signs and symptoms, sometimes associated with life-threatening consequences.[2]

Giant Lymph Node Hyperplasia (Castleman's Disease)

Giant lymph node hyperplasia (Castleman's disease, angiofollicular lymph node hyperplasia) is an unusual condition of unknown etiology and pathogenesis originally described by Castleman in 1954[3] and elaborated upon in greater detail by Keller and colleagues in 1972.[4] In the latter report, the authors described two distinct histologic variants. The *hyaline vascular type* is the more common (74 of 81 cases in Keller and colleagues' study) and is characterized by the presence of numerous germinal centers interspersed in a population of mononuclear cells (predominantly lymphocytes) and numerous capillaries (Fig. 75–2); some of the capillaries, often with thickened hyalinized walls, extend into the germinal centers themselves. The lymphocytes surrounding the germinal centers may be arranged in a concentric ("onionskin") pattern (*see* Fig. 75–2). This form of disease is usually unassociated with symptoms and is discovered as a mass in the mediastinum or hilum on a screening chest radiograph.

The second variant, termed the *plasma cell type*, is characterized histologically by the presence of numerous plasma cells between the germinal centers, which are often larger than those in the hyaline vascular type; relatively few capillaries are present. In contrast to those who have the hyaline vascular type, patients who have this variant tend to have systemic manifestations of disease, most often nonspe-

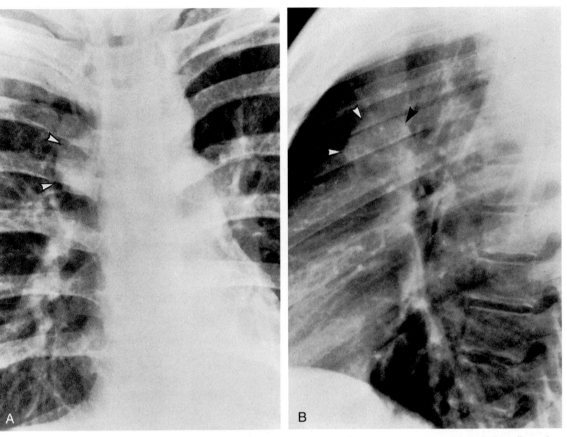

Figure 75–1. Enlarged Azygos Lymph Node Caused by Metastatic Carcinoma. Posteroanterior *(A)* and lateral *(B)* radiographs reveal a well-defined homogeneous mass *(arrowheads)* situated just anterior to the right tracheobronchial angle. This is the anatomic location of both the azygos vein and the azygos lymph node, and an opacity such as is visualized in this patient can be the result of distention of the vein or enlargement of the node. In this case, it was caused by metastatic carcinoma of the adrenal gland.

cific findings such as fever, anemia, weight loss, and hypergammaglobulinemia.[4] A variety of other clinical manifestations have also been reported occasionally,[5] including a syndrome of growth failure and anemia in children,[6, 7] nephrotic syndrome, myelofibrosis,[8] peripheral neuropathy,[9] and thrombotic thrombocytopenic purpura.[10]

The lesions described by Castleman and by Keller and colleagues were usually solitary, in the majority of patients (70 of 81) involving only the mediastinum or hilum.[3, 4] Both histologic types of this localized form of the disease tend to occur in young adults and are associated with a good prognosis following surgical excision;[7] systemic manifestations associated with the plasma cell variant usually resolve, and there is typically no tendency to recurrence or the development of new disease.

Patients have also been identified who have multifocal disease that tends to affect superficial lymph node groups with or without involvement of the mediastinum. Such "multicentric Castleman's disease" (multicentric lymph node hyperplasia) often affects persons older than those who have isolated Castleman's disease and is frequently associated with evidence of systemic disease such as hepatosplenomegaly, anemia, hypergammaglobulinemia, alterations in measurements of liver function, skin rash, and renal and central nervous system abnormalities.[5, 11–13] The condition appears to represent an unusual histologic reaction to a number of agents, rather than a specific entity; for example,

some patients are seropositive on testing for human immunodeficiency virus (HIV) or have Kaposi's sarcoma, in which case evidence of infection by herpesvirus 8 is not uncommon.[14, 15] An association with the POEMS syndrome (*p*olyneuropathy, *o*rganomegaly, *e*ndocrinopathy, *m*onoclonal gammopathy, and *s*kin changes) also has been reported.[16] The prognosis associated with the multicentric variant of giant lymph node hyperplasia is distinctly poorer than that associated with the solitary form; in many patients, there is progression of the lymphoid proliferation, the development of serious infectious complications, or evolution to frank lymphoma.

The fundamental nature of giant lymph node hyperplasia and the relationship between the solitary and multicentric forms are uncertain.[5] It has been suggested that the solitary form may represent a hamartoma of lymphoid tissue, a focus of lymphoid hyperplasia, or an infectious lymphadenitis.[5] The diffuse nature of the multicentric form, its association with conditions known to be accompanied by an abnormal immune reaction such as HIV infection, the relatively frequent progression to lymphoma, and the occasional documentation of altered helper-suppressor T-cell ratios[17] suggest an underlying abnormality of the immune system.

The radiographic appearance of the localized form of giant lymph node hyperplasia is that of a solitary, smooth or lobulated mass situated most commonly in the left or right hilum or middle-posterior mediastinum; less commonly, an-

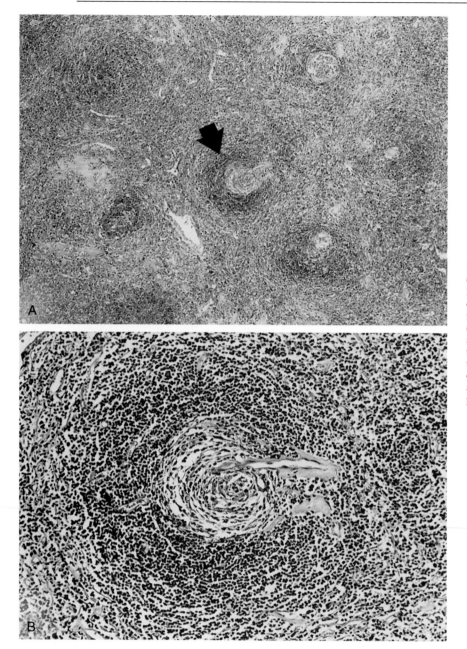

Figure 75–2. Giant Lymph Node Hyperplasia (Castleman's Disease). A section from a large lobulated anterior mediastinal mass *(A)* reveals an extensive infiltrate of lymphoid cells admixed with numerous vessels and several germinal centers *(arrow)*. Although this appearance superficially resembles a lymph node, the absence of sinusoids and the configuration of the germinal centers indicate that this is not a normal nodal structure. A magnified view of one germinal center *(B)* shows a small vessel with a thickened, hyalinized wall extending into its mid portion. *(A, ×40; B, ×150.)*

terior mediastinum is affected. (Fig. 75–3).[18–22a] In multicentric disease, the lymphadenopathy often involves multiple mediastinal compartments (Fig. 75–4).[11, 12, 22] The latter form can be associated with pulmonary parenchymal involvement, consisting on CT scans of areas of ground-glass attenuation, poorly defined centrilobular nodules, thickening of the bronchoarterial bundles, and interlobular septal thickening (Fig. 75–5).[12, 23] The enlarged nodes typically show marked homogeneous enhancement following intravenous administration of contrast;[11, 22, 22a] such enhancement is less marked in the plasma cell type than in the hyaline vascular type of disease.[12] Focal calcification can be seen.[11, 21, 22, 24] Magnetic resonance (MR) studies show a signal that is hypointense compared with that characteristic for mediastinal fat but hyperintense compared with that of skeletal muscle on T1-weighted images and high signal intensity on T2-weighted images.[25, 26] The lesions enhance following administration of

gadolinium-based contrast medium.[22a] Foci of calcification result in localized areas of low signal intensity.[25] Because of the highly vascular nature of the mass, it has been suggested that arteriography may be helpful in planning the surgical approach.[27]

Granulomatous Lymphadenitis

The term *granulomatous lymphadenitis* refers mainly to chronic disease attributable to infection, such as tuberculosis or histoplasmosis, or to sarcoidosis. In both forms, paratracheal and tracheobronchial lymph node enlargement may be the predominant finding. In the infectious granulomas ("mediastinal granuloma"), node enlargement tends to be predominantly unilateral; in sarcoidosis, it tends to be bilateral and symmetric and, in contrast with the lymphoma, is

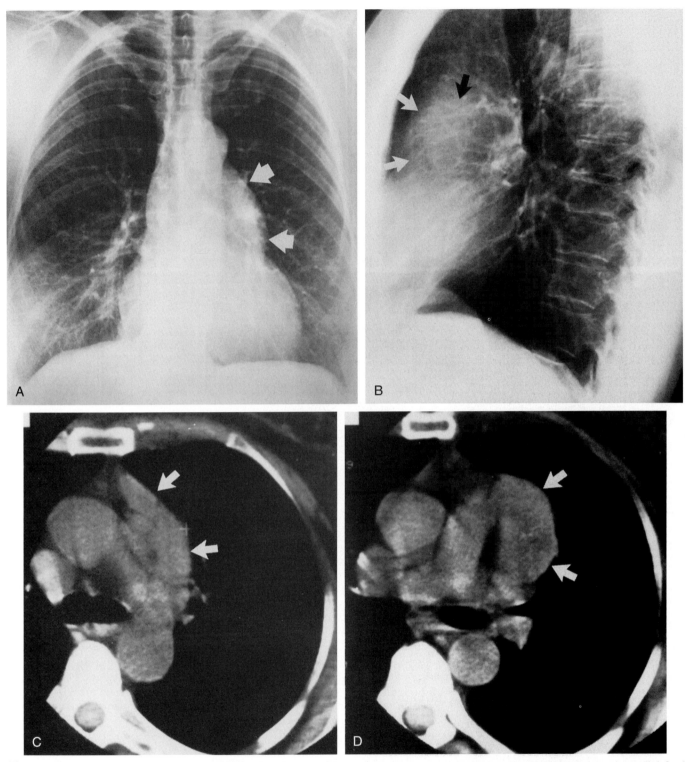

Figure 75–3. Giant Lymph Node Hyperplasia (Castleman's Disease). Posteroanterior *(A)* and lateral *(B)* radiographs reveal a well-defined opacity protruding to the left from the region of the main pulmonary artery *(arrows in A)*. In the lateral projection, an ill-defined opacity can be identified in the anterior mediastinum *(arrows)*. CT scans at the level of the aortopulmonary window *(C)* and main pulmonary artery *(D)* reveal a well-defined, homogeneous mass *(arrows)* contiguous with the left side of the mediastinum and protruding into the left hemithorax. The patient was a 63-year-old woman who had no symptoms referable to her chest.

almost invariably associated with bronchopulmonary node enlargement.

The presence of granulomatous inflammation of middle-posterior mediastinal lymph nodes does not, by itself, result in untoward effects in most cases. Occasionally, infection spreads outside of the nodal capsule into adjacent tissue; in some cases, this results in localized or diffuse acute mediastinitis or in fibrosing mediastinitis *(see* page 2856). Fibrosis

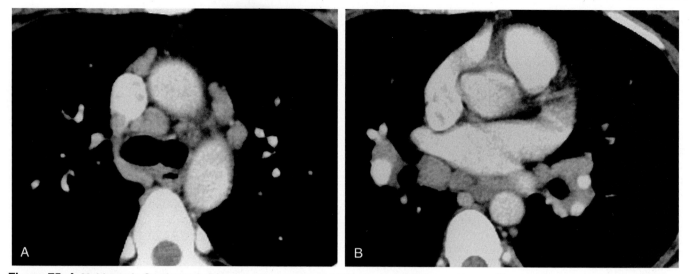

Figure 75–4. Multicentric Castleman's Disease. Contrast-enhanced CT scans (*A* and *B*) from a 44-year-old woman demonstrate enlarged mediastinal and bilateral hilar lymph nodes. The diagnosis of Castleman's disease was proved by lymph node biopsy. (Courtesy of Dr. Takeshi Johkoh, Department of Radiology, Osaka University Medical School, Osaka, Japan.)

of posterior mediastinal lymph nodes can exert local effects on the esophagus, including traction diverticula and esophagobronchial fistula.

TUMORS AND TUMOR-LIKE CONDITIONS

Primary Tracheal Neoplasms

Although pulmonary carcinoma is usually manifested in the mediastinum in the form of metastases to lymph nodes from a primary lesion in the lung, rarely the carcinoma arises in the trachea or main bronchi just distal to the carina and thus is situated within the middle mediastinum. If the neoplasm extends outward into the paratracheal space, it may widen the mediastinum to either side. An irregular,

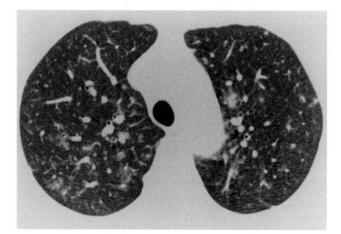

Figure 75–5. Multicentric Castleman's Disease. An HRCT scan from a 43-year-old woman with multicentric Castleman's disease shows mild bilateral peribronchial and perivascular interstitial thickening and poorly defined centrilobular nodular opacities. Open lung biopsy showed an extensive infiltrate of plasma cells localized predominantly in the peribronchovascular interstitial tissue. A scalene lymph node excised 2 years previously had demonstrated plasma cell–type giant lymph node hyperplasia.

shaggy mass is usually evident within the tracheal air column on standard radiographs or CT scans. A similar appearance can be caused by other primary tracheal neoplasms and by endotracheal metastases. Symptoms include cough, hemoptysis, and (sometimes) severe dyspnea and wheezing; stridor may be apparent.

Aorticopulmonary Paraganglioma

Paragangliomas (chemodectomas) arise from small macroscopic or microscopic collections of neuroendocrine cells (paraganglia) in intimate association with the autonomic nervous system. In the thorax, they generally occur in one of two locations:[28] (1) the perivascular adventitial tissue bounded by the aorta superiorly, the pulmonary artery inferiorly, and the ligamentum arteriosum and right pulmonary artery on either side (aorticopulmonary paragangliomas); and (2) in association with the segmental ganglia of the sympathetic chain in the paravertebral region adjacent to the posterior aspects of the ribs (paravertebral paragangliomas; *see* page 2977). Tumors in the former site are relatively uncommon, only about 100 cases having been reported by 1994.[29] The mean age at the time of diagnosis is about 45 to 50 years, and there is a slight female preponderance.[30] Tumors are occasionally multiple, both within and outside the thorax.

The lesions can be manifested grossly as discrete, encapsulated nodules or as poorly circumscribed growths that encompass adjacent vascular structures.[31–33] Histologic features consist of fairly uniform cell nests ("Zellballen") separated by a prominent fibrovascular stroma. Individual tumor cells usually have a moderate amount of clear or granular eosinophilic cytoplasm and more or less round, regular nuclei; mitotic figures are typically sparse. Evidence of neuroendocrine differentiation can be demonstrated by several techniques: argyrophilic intracytoplasmic granules can be seen with appropriate silver stains, electron microscopic examination reveals dense core intracytoplasmic granules,[30] and immunohistochemical studies show a positive reaction for chromogranin, synaptophysin, and (occasionally) specific hormones such as glucagon, adrenocorticotropic hormone (ACTH), and calcitonin.[34, 35] Rare tumors are associated with melanin production.[36]

Radiographic features of aorticopulmonary paragangliomas are those of a mass in the mediastinum in close relation to the base of the heart and aortic arch.[30] Occasional tumors are located in the subcarinal region[37, 38] or extend into the paratracheal soft tissue (Fig. 75–6). CT demonstrates a soft tissue mass that can have homogeneous attenuation or can contain large central areas of low attenuation as a result of necrosis.[37–40] Tumors usually show marked enhancement following intravenous administration of contrast.[38–40] In fact, use of contrast is essential in the identification of paragangliomas, particularly when they are located within the pericardium; in one investigation of eight such tumors, six were missed on unenhanced CT scans, whereas all eight were evident following intravenous administration of contrast.[38]

On MR studies, paragangliomas have signal intensity that is hypointense or isointense to muscle on T1-weighted images and hyperintense on T2-weighted images.[38] Areas of signal void may be seen on T1-weighted images owing to flowing blood.[37] Angiography demonstrates multiple feeding vessels, hypervascularity, and homogeneous capillary blush.[40] Scintigraphy is the imaging modality of choice to confirm the presence of a paraganglioma.[38, 41] Approximately 90% of tumors show abnormal uptake on [131]I- or ^{123}I-metaiodobenzylguanidine (MIBG) scintigraphy.[38, 41, 42] Preliminary reports suggest that the use of ^{111}In-octreotide may yield superior results.[43, 44] The main role of contrast-enhanced CT or MR imaging is in providing detailed assessment of the extent of tumor and its relationship to adjacent structures prior to surgical resection.[38]

Clinically, most aorticopulmonary paragangliomas do not induce symptoms and are discovered on a screening chest radiograph; sometimes, they compress or invade local structures and cause cough, chest pain, hoarseness, dysphagia, or (occasionally) the superior vena cava syndrome. Some patients, invariably young women, also have a gastric

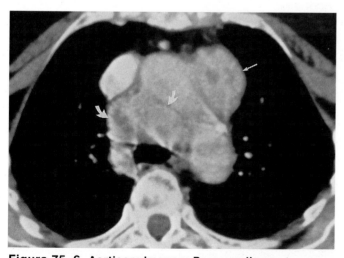

Figure 75–6. Aorticopulmonary Paraganglioma. A contrast-enhanced CT scan demonstrates an inhomogeneous soft tissue mass involving the aortopulmonary window *(straight arrow)* and paratracheal region *(curved arrows)*. The patient was a 68-year-old woman with surgically proven middle mediastinal paraganglioma.

stromal neoplasm and pulmonary chondromas, either synchronously or metachronously (Carney's triad; *see* page 1343). Rare tumors secrete catecholamines in sufficient amounts to cause a paraneoplastic syndrome.

The prognosis for patients who have aorticopulmonary paragangliomas is guarded. Because of their location and vascularity, the operative mortality is high (almost 10% of patients in one review[30]). In addition, complete excision frequently cannot be achieved;[30] in one review of the literature published in 1994, the overall local recurrence rate was about 55%.[29] Despite this, the growth rate may be slow, and survival for a number of years following partial excision is possible. Metastases have been documented in about 25% of patients;[29] no reliable morphologic criteria are available that permit the distinction between tumors that do and do not metastasize.

Localized Infectious Mediastinitis

Apart from tuberculous and histoplasma lymphadenitis, localized infection of the middle mediastinum is very uncommon. The most common cause is probably an abscess, as may occur following esophageal rupture or thoracic surgery (*see* page 2851). Echinococcal (hydatid) cysts have been reported rarely and may be associated with erosion of the great vessels.[45] One case of an inflammatory mass located adjacent to the aorta and extending from its "knuckle" to the tracheal bifurcation has been interpreted as an unusual manifestation of syphilitic aortitis.[46]

CYSTS

Bronchogenic Cyst

Congenital bronchogenic cysts of the mediastinum are described in detail in Chapter 22 (*see* page 612) and are reviewed only briefly here. Although these cysts can occur anywhere in the mediastinum, the majority are located in the paratracheal or subcarinal region.[1, 47–49] They are usually discovered in childhood or early adult life but can be seen as an incidental finding at autopsy in elderly persons. Although they may grow very large without inducing symptoms, even small ones can cause airway obstruction in infants and children,[51] particularly if they undergo an abrupt increase in size as a result of hemorrhage or infection. Rarely, a cyst appears to undergo spontaneous resolution.[52]

Esophageal Cyst

Esophageal cysts (esophageal duplication cysts) have been hypothesized to result from either abnormal budding of the foregut or a failure of complete vacuolation of the originally solid esophagus to produce a hollow tube.[49] Some cases have been associated with developmental cystic abnormalities of the lung.[54] The cysts are lined by nonkeratinizing squamous or ciliated columnar epithelium. A double layer of smooth muscle in their walls and a lack of cartilage are necessary findings to exclude a diagnosis of bronchogenic cyst; however, as indicated previously (*see* page 609), the distinction between the two may be difficult, and the relatively noncommittal term "simple cyst" is sometimes the best designation.

The cysts are usually located within or adjacent to the wall of the esophagus. The CT findings consist of a round mass of homogeneous water density or soft tissue density that does not enhance following intravenous administration of contrast (Fig. 75–7).[1, 53, 55–59] On MR studies, the cysts can have low or high signal intensity on T1-weighted images but characteristically have very high signal intensity on T2-weighted images.[1, 50, 60] The CT findings and MR signal characteristics are indistinguishable from those of bronchogenic cysts (Fig. 75–8). Transesophageal ultrasonography has been utilized successfully in diagnosis.[61]

Many patients are asymptomatic, the abnormality sometimes being discovered incidentally at an advanced age.[61] Occasionally, esophageal compression is manifested by dysphagia;[49] chronic cough, misinterpreted as a symptom of asthma or bronchitis, has also been attributed to airway impingement by a cyst.[62] Rare cases have been complicated by the development of carcinoma.[63, 64]

Pancreatic Pseudocyst

Pancreatic pseudocysts are encapsulated collections of pancreatic secretions often containing blood and necrotic

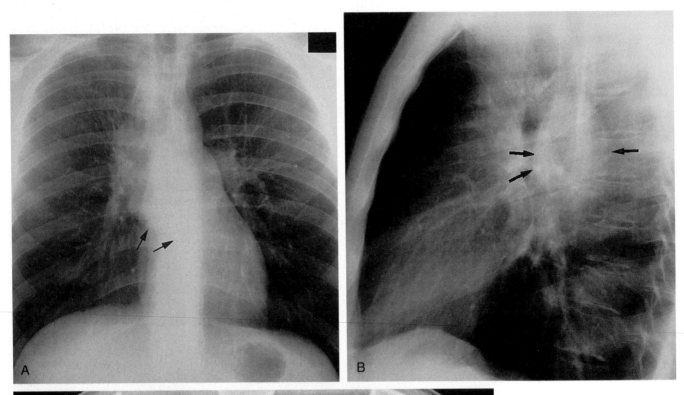

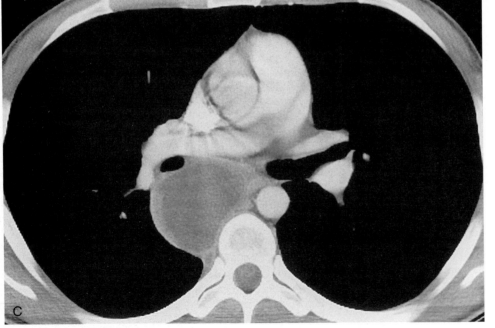

Figure 75–7. Esophageal Cyst. A posteroanterior chest radiograph *(A)* from a 22-year-old man shows a subcarinal mass displacing the azygoesophageal recess interface *(arrows)*. A lateral radiograph *(B)* shows the mass posterior to the bronchus intermedius *(arrows)*. A CT scan obtained following intravenous administration of contrast *(C)* demonstrates a nonenhancing cystic mass adjacent to the esophagus. The lesion was surgically proved to be an esophageal duplication cyst.

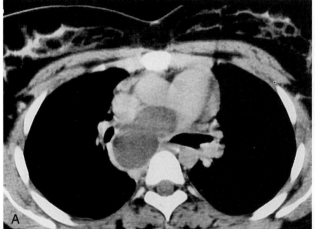

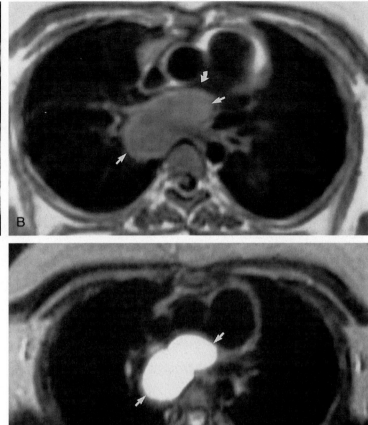

Figure 75–8. Middle and Posterior Mediastinal Broncho-genic Cyst. A contrast-enhanced CT scan from a 26-year-old woman *(A)* demonstrates a dumbbell-shaped mass with inhomogeneous low attenuation in the subcarinal region. The lesion has both middle and posterior mediastinal components and compresses the proximal right pulmonary artery. The attenuation values within the mass were greater than 20 HU. A transverse T1-weighted (TR 645, TE 20) MR image *(B)* demonstrates a slightly inhomogeneous mass *(straight arrows)* with a signal intensity similar to that of chest wall muscle. Note marked narrowing of the right pulmonary artery *(curved arrow)*. A transverse T2-weighted (TR 2581, TE 90) spin-echo MR image *(C)* demonstrates homogeneous high signal intensity *(arrows)* characteristic of fluid. At surgery this was shown to be a mediastinal bronchogenic cyst associated with a partial pericardial defect.

material.[59] The vast majority occur in patients who have acute or chronic pancreatitis and are located in the peripancreatic tissue. Occasionally, a lesion extends into the posterior mediastinum through the esophageal or aortic hiatus.[59, 65, 66] Usually, the cysts are of water density on CT scans (Fig. 75–9); however, hemorrhage or infection can result in areas of soft tissue attenuation.[59] The diagnosis can usually be readily made by CT by showing continuity with pancreatic or peripancreatic fluid collections.[59]

Thoracic Duct Cyst

Thoracic duct cyst is a rare type of middle-posterior mediastinal mass that can occur anywhere from the thoracic inlet to the diaphragm and can communicate with the thoracic duct either superiorly or inferiorly.[67–69] (Rare cases have also been described in the supraclavicular region.[70]) Nineteen cases were documented in a review of the literature published in 1992.[71] The abnormality should be distinguished from trauma-associated "lymphocele" ("chyloma"; *see* page 2636).

The cysts can be large enough to displace the mediastinum to the opposite side. Patients may be asymptomatic or complain of dysphagia or back pain;[67–69] rarely, tracheal compression results in acute respiratory insufficiency.[71, 72] The diagnosis can be suggested by appearance on

lymphangiography[73, 74] and by analysis of fluid obtained by fluoroscopically or CT-guided needle aspiration.[75, 77]

VASCULAR ABNORMALITIES

Dilation of the Main Pulmonary Artery

Dilation of the main pulmonary artery may be of sufficient degree to suggest a mediastinal mass.[76] The great majority of cases are associated with either pulmonary arterial hypertension or left-to-right shunt; some are related to pulmonary valve stenosis,[76] pulmonary artery banding,[78, 79] infection, or vasculitis (typically Behçet's disease) (*see* page 1518).

On the posteroanterior chest radiograph, dilation of the main pulmonary artery results in a focal convexity caudal to the aortic arch and cephalic to the left main bronchus (Fig. 75–10). It is usually accompanied by dilation of the pulmonary trunk and enlargement of the right ventricle, findings that are most readily apparent on the lateral radiograph.

Idiopathic dilation invariably does not give rise to symptoms and is unassociated with evidence of hemodynamic abnormality on radiologic examination or during cardiac catheterization.[76, 77, 80] Physical examination of a patient who has a severe degree of dilation may reveal a widely

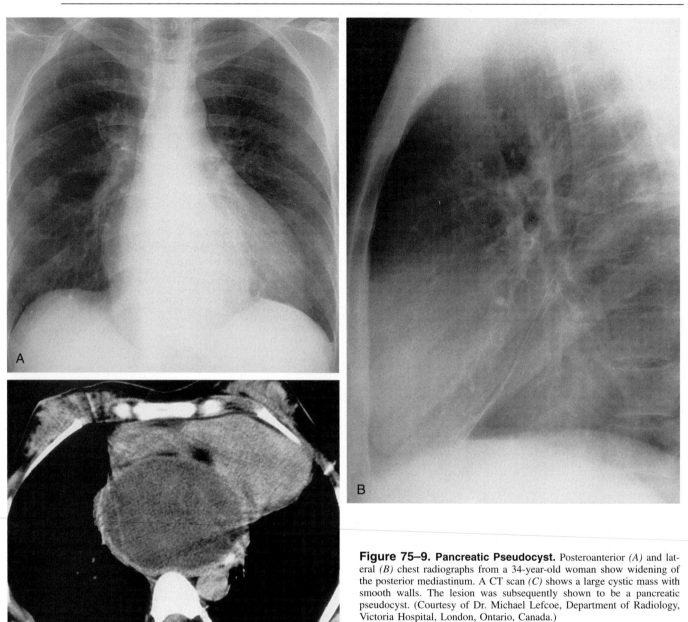

Figure 75–9. Pancreatic Pseudocyst. Posteroanterior *(A)* and lateral *(B)* chest radiographs from a 34-year-old woman show widening of the posterior mediastinum. A CT scan *(C)* shows a large cystic mass with smooth walls. The lesion was subsequently shown to be a pancreatic pseudocyst. (Courtesy of Dr. Michael Lefcoe, Department of Radiology, Victoria Hospital, London, Ontario, Canada.)

split second heart sound, varying little with respiration. The ostensible reason for this sign is a delay in impulse rebound caused by loss of compliance of the dilated pulmonary trunk.[81] When there is significant dilation, an echocardiogram may reveal increased distance of the pulmonic valve from the chest wall and a fine fluttering of the valve, presumably caused by turbulence.[82]

Dilation of the Mediastinal Veins

Superior and Inferior Vena Cava

The great majority of cases of dilation of the superior vena cava (SVC) are the result of raised central venous pressure, most commonly from cardiac decompensation; rare causes include tricuspid valvular stenosis and cardiac tamponade secondary to pericardial effusion or constrictive pericarditis. The radiographic appearance is distinctive, consisting of a smooth, well-defined widening of the right side of the mediastinum (Fig. 75–11). The width of the vena cava (and therefore of the mediastinum itself) varies considerably with the phase of respiration. The azygos vein is almost always dilated as well; in fact, this is a more dependable sign of systemic venous hypertension because the diameter of the vein in the right tracheobronchial angle can be precisely measured. (The azygos vein can be considered to be dilated if its diameter is greater than 10 mm when the patient is in the erect position or 15 mm when the patient is recumbent.)

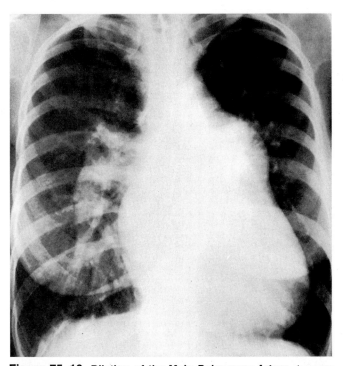

Figure 75–10. Dilation of the Main Pulmonary Artery. A poster-oanterior chest radiograph shows dilation of the hilar and peripheral pulmonary arteries, indicating pulmonary pleonemia. The main pulmonary artery is greatly dilated, creating a smooth protuberance of the left border of the cardiovascular silhouette. The patient was known to have a patent ductus arteriosus.

Occasionally, a right superior mediastinal opacity is caused by a nondilated but laterally displaced SVC.[83] Rarely, the SVC has an aneurysmal dilation, presumably congenital in origin;[84–86] the aneurysm may be fusiform or saccular in type[87, 88] and typically changes in appearance on radiographs obtained with the patient in the erect and supine positions.[89] The diagnosis is readily apparent on CT scans (Fig. 75–12). A case has been described of a patient who developed progressive right superior mediastinal widening on the radiograph as a result of an intravascular lipoma of the right brachiocephalic vein and SVC;[90] CT demonstrated the characteristic fatty attenuation of the tumor. Occasionally, the inferior vena cava (IVC) undergoes localized aneurysmal dilation and is visible as a smooth, sharply circumscribed opacity in the right cardiophrenic angle.[91] All other anomalies of the IVC occur within the abdomen and possess no intrathoracic manifestations other than those associated with azygos continuation (*see* farther on).[92–94]

Persistence of a left SVC is an uncommon anomaly that occurs in 0.3% of normal persons and in 4.4% of patients who have congenital heart disease. The right SVC develops partly from the right anterior cardinal vein, while the left anterior cardinal vein normally regresses; persistence of the latter results in a left SVC. In such circumstances, a straight-edged shadow is present on the left side of the mediastinum that overlies the aortic arch and proximal descending aorta;[95] drainage is usually via the coronary sinus. Rarely, the left SVC drains into the left atrium, thus creating a right-to-left shunt.[96] The diagnosis of a left SVC can be

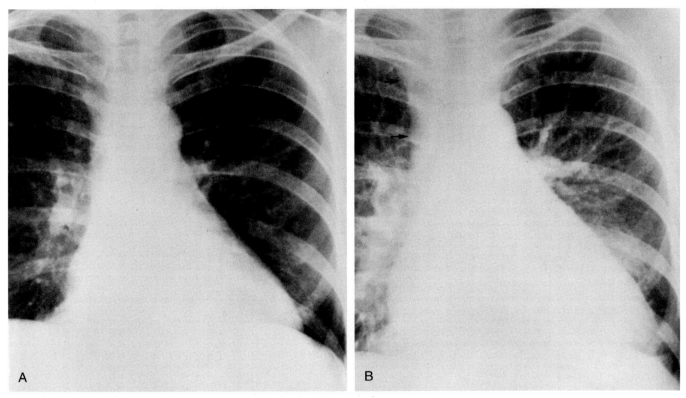

Figure 75–11. Dilation of the Superior Vena Cava. During a remission, the chest radiograph *(A)* of a 35-year-old woman with systemic lupus erythematosus revealed no significant abnormalities. On the occasion of an exacerbation several months later (at which time she had clinical evidence of cardiac decompensation), a chest radiograph *(B)* demonstrated moderate cardiac enlargement (due predominantly to pericardial effusion) and generalized interstitial pulmonary edema. Note the widening of the superior mediastinum caused by dilation of the superior vena cava *(arrows)*.

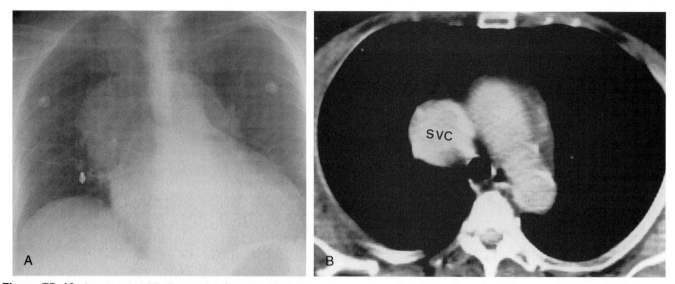

Figure 75–12. Aneurysmal Dilation of the Superior Vena Cava. An anteroposterior chest radiograph *(A)* shows a soft tissue opacity in the right paratracheal region. A contrast-enhanced CT scan *(B)* demonstrates aneurysmal dilation of the superior vena cava (SVC). The patient was an 83-year-old woman. The abnormality had been present on the radiograph for many years.

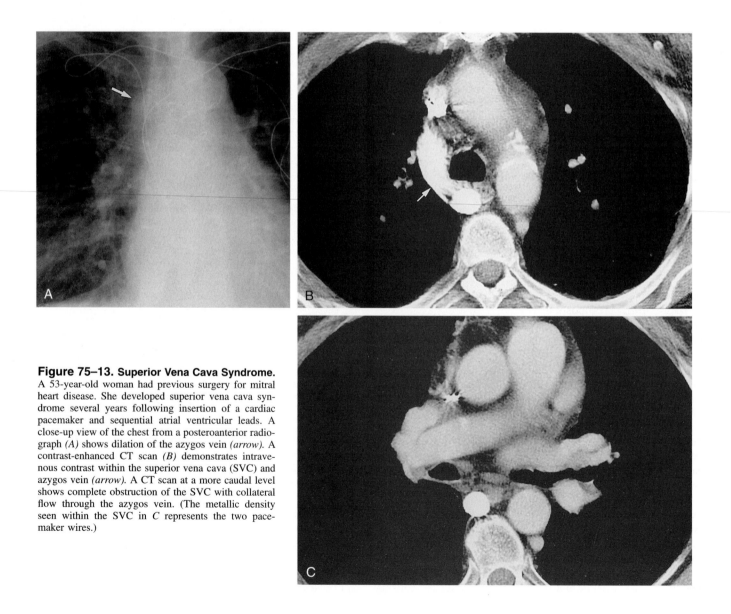

Figure 75–13. Superior Vena Cava Syndrome. A 53-year-old woman had previous surgery for mitral heart disease. She developed superior vena cava syndrome several years following insertion of a cardiac pacemaker and sequential atrial ventricular leads. A close-up view of the chest from a posteroanterior radiograph *(A)* shows dilation of the azygos vein *(arrow)*. A contrast-enhanced CT scan *(B)* demonstrates intravenous contrast within the superior vena cava (SVC) and azygos vein *(arrow)*. A CT scan at a more caudal level shows complete obstruction of the SVC with collateral flow through the azygos vein. (The metallic density seen within the SVC in *C* represents the two pacemaker wires.)

Table 75–1. ETIOLOGY OF SUPERIOR VENA CAVA SYNDROME

CAUSATIVE DISORDER/FACTOR	COMMENT	SELECTED REFERENCE(S)
Infection		
Histoplasmosis	In association with fibrosing mediastinitis	*See* page 2856
Syphilis	Secondary to aortic aneurysm	281
Tuberculosis		282
Filariasis	Secondary to mediastinal lymph node involvement	283
Traumatic		
Intravenous catheter		111, 112, 304
Cardiac surgery	Related to pericardial hematoma	284
Neoplasms		
Metastatic carcinoma		285, 286
Mediastinal thymic or germ cell tumors		287, 288
Soft tissue neoplasms		289, 291
Lymphoma, leukemia		290, 292, 293
Thyroid enlargement	Multinodular goiter	294, 295
	Graves' disease	296
Primary sarcoma of the superior vena cava		297, 298
Drugs		
Megestrol acetate		299
Vascular Abnormalities		
Innominate artery aneurysm		300
Right subclavian artery aneurysm		301
Aortic dissection		302, 303
Syphilitic aortic aneurysm		281
Post-traumatic aortic pseudoaneurysm		305
Miscellaneous		
Radiation		306
Pulmonary bulla		307
Sarcoidosis		308
Langerhans' cell histiocytosis		309
Behçet's disease		310

readily confirmed by CT,[97–99] MR imaging,[96] or transesophageal echocardiography.[100] The right SVC is often decreased in size;[96, 101] in approximately 15% of cases, it is absent.[96, 97]

Superior Vena Cava Syndrome

The SVC syndrome is characterized by edema of the face, neck, upper extremities, and thorax, often associated with prominent, dilated chest wall veins. It is caused by obstruction of the vena cava, by either external compression or intraluminal thrombosis or neoplastic infiltration; not infrequently, a combination of all three processes is involved.[102] In most published series, the causative disorder is malignancy in 95% or more of cases;[103–105] pulmonary carcinoma is the cause in 80% to 85%, and lymphoma and metastatic carcinoma of nonpulmonary origin in 5% to 10%. Of the pulmonary carcinomas, small cell is the most common histologic type.[106, 107] SVC syndrome is also a common feature of pulmonary carcinoma; in one review of approximately 6,500 patients who had this tumor, 249 (almost 4%) developed the complication;[108] in two other series of 1,090 cases of small cell carcinoma, approximately 10% had the syndrome at the time of diagnosis.[109, 110]

Although precise figures are not available, it is possible that the most common benign abnormality causing the SVC syndrome today is the insertion of intravenous devices such as cardiac pacemakers[111, 112] and Hickman catheters.[113] The pathogenesis of the obstruction in these cases is presumably thrombosis and (following thrombus organization) fibrosis. The most common noniatrogenic benign disorder causing

the SVC syndrome is probably fibrosing mediastinitis;[104, 114] reports of a great variety of other diseases have also been published (Table 75–1).

In most cases, the chest radiograph shows a mass widening the mediastinum on the right; a prominent azygos vein may also be evident (Fig. 75–13). In patients who develop SVC thrombosis related to indwelling central venous catheters, radiographs commonly show lateral displacement of the catheter.[115] The diagnosis can be confirmed by CT,[115–118] MR imaging,[119] or venography.[105] With CT, it is based on decreased or absent opacification of the SVC and the presence of opacification of collateral veins following the intravenous administration of contrast (Fig. 75–14).[116, 117] Both findings need to be present in order to make a definitive diagnosis, because opacification of collateral vessels is seen in about 5% of patients who do not have SVC obstruction.[117] Either CT or ultrasound-guided transthoracic needle aspiration constitutes a reliable and rapid means of diagnosis in cases caused by a malignant neoplasm.[120–123]

The most common symptoms are dyspnea and a feeling of fullness in the head. Physical findings include facial swelling and dilation of the veins of the neck and upper chest; proptosis and conjunctival suffusion can be seen in some patients.[124] Although vascular dilation is usually bilateral, in the rare case in which obstruction is limited to one or the other brachiocephalic vein it may be unilateral.[125] In one investigation of approximately 250 patients in whom the syndrome was caused by metastatic pulmonary carcinoma, symptoms were present in about 30% for 1 week or less prior to diagnosis and in 50% for over 2 weeks.[108]

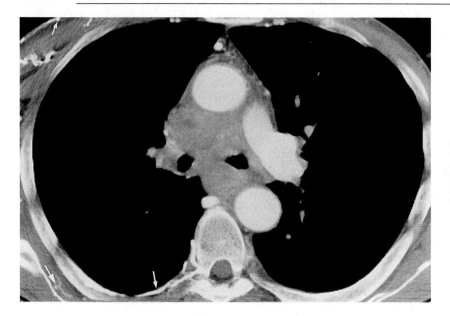

Figure 75–14. Superior Vena Cava Syndrome. A contrast-enhanced CT scan demonstrates extensive mediastinal lymphadenopathy, lack of opacification of the superior vena cava (SVC), and extensive collateral venous circulation in the chest wall *(arrows)* and mediastinum. The patient was a 61-year-old man who had extensive mediastinal metastases from pulmonary carcinoma.

The concept that the SVC syndrome represents a medical emergency is no longer generally accepted.[104, 126] As might be expected, the prognosis is usually poor in patients in whom the syndrome is caused by a malignant neoplasm.[103, 105, 108] Nevertheless, some (albeit not all[110]) investigators have found a better prognosis in patients who have pulmonary small cell carcinoma associated with SVC syndrome than in those who do not have the complication.[127]

Azygos and Hemiazygos Veins

Dilation of the azygos and hemiazygos veins has many causes (Table 75–2). Elevated central venous pressure secondary to cardiac decompensation is by far the most common; other causes of elevated right-sided pressure, such as tricuspid stenosis, acute pericardial tamponade, or constrictive pericarditis, are less frequent. Rarely, dilation of either venous system is present without discernible cause.[128–130] The dilated region of the azygos vein can measure up to 12 cm in diameter[129] and tends to decrease markedly in size when the patient is in the erect position.[130]

Table 75–2. ETIOLOGY OF AZYGOS AND HEMIAZYGOS VEIN DILATION

CAUSATIVE DISORDER/FACTOR	SELECTED REFERENCE(S)
Elevated central venous pressure secondary to cardiac disease	
Intrahepatic and extrahepatic portal vein obstruction	311, 312
Anomalous pulmonary venous drainage	
Acquired occlusion of the inferior or superior vena cava	313
Azygos continuation (infrahepatic interruption) of the inferior vena cava	314, 315
Persistence of the left superior vena cava	
Hepatic vein obstruction (Budd-Chiari syndrome or veno-occlusive disease)	
Idiopathic	129, 130

Radiographically, dilation of the azygos vein is manifested by a round or oval shadow in the right tracheobronchial angle more than 10 mm in diameter on radiographs exposed with the patient in the erect position.[131] In one study of 54 patients from 23 to 77 years of age, a vein diameter greater than 15 mm as measured on an anteroposterior chest radiograph obtained with the patient in the supine position corresponded to a central venous pressure greater than 10 cm of water.[132] In another investigation in 48 patients, none of whom had any lesion known to cause azygos vein enlargement, the mean diameter of the vein was shown to be 14 mm when the patient was in the supine position.[133] Measurements exceeding 10 mm on radiographs obtained when the patient was in the erect position or exceeding 15 mm when the patient was in the supine position indicated increase in either pressure or flow.

A dilated azygos vein can be differentiated from an enlarged azygos lymph node fairly easily by comparing the diameters of the shadow on radiographs exposed in the erect and supine positions: when the shadow is the vein, there is a noticeable difference in size. This technique was employed to advantage in a patient in whom a dilated azygos vein was situated in an anomalous azygos fissure; the dilation was subsequently shown to be caused by azygos continuation of the IVC (Fig. 75–15).[134]

Dilation of the posterior portions of the azygos or hemiazygos vein may result in widening and irregularity of the paraspinal line, on the right or on the left side, respectively (Fig. 75–16).[135–137] Extreme tortuosity of a dilated azygos arch may simulate a pulmonary mass on a lateral chest radiograph.[138] The normal anatomy of the azygos and hemiazygos veins and their abnormalities are well visualized by both CT[118, 139, 140] and MR imaging.[96, 119]

The symptoms and signs of azygos and hemiazygos vein dilation depend entirely on the cause. Azygos continuation of the IVC is often associated with a congenital cardiac malformation (Fig. 75–17),[141, 142] with errors in abdominal situs,[143] or with asplenia or polysplenia.[144] Most patients are asymptomatic; however, some have symptoms or signs attributable to the associated heart disease. Rarely, marked

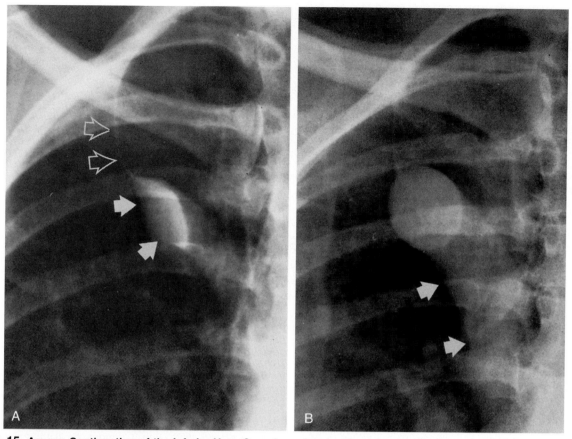

Figure 75–15. Azygos Continuation of the Inferior Vena Cava Associated with an Azygos Fissure. A close-up view of the upper portion of the right hemithorax from a posteroanterior radiograph *(A)* reveals a large oval opacity *(solid arrows)* situated at the lower end of a curvilinear opacity representing an azygos fissure *(open arrows)*. To prove that this actually represented a dilated azygos vein, the patient was placed in a supine position and the radiograph repeated *(B)*. By this procedure, the vein has undergone a remarkable degree of dilation and now can be seen to extend inferiorly to the right side of the mediastinum *(arrows)*. (Courtesy of Dr. Anthony Proto, Virginia Commonwealth University, Medical College of Virginia, Richmond.)

azygos vein dilation causes obstruction of the SVC[129] or compression of the right main bronchus.[130]

Left Superior Intercostal Vein

Dilation of the left superior intercostal vein has the same causes as those associated with dilation of the azygos vein, although visibility of this vein radiographically is not nearly so frequent as that of the azygos. The normal left superior intercostal vein originates from a confluence of the second, third, and fourth left intercostal veins. As it passes anteriorly from the spine it relates intimately to some portion of the aortic arch and in this location is seen end-on as the "aortic nipple," a local protuberance in the contour of the arch that is identifiable in about 10% of normal persons.[145] On posteroanterior chest radiographs taken with the patient in an erect position, the maximum normal diameter of the aortic nipple is 4.5 mm.[146] A diameter greater than this is a useful sign of circulatory abnormalities, the most common of which are azygos continuation of the IVC, hypoplasia of the left innominate vein, cardiac decompensation, portal hypertension, Budd-Chiari syndrome, obstruction of the superior or IVC (Fig. 75–18),[146] and congenital absence of the azygos vein.[147]

Abnormalities of the Aorta and Its Branches

Aneurysms of the Thoracic Aorta

The normal vessel diameter is 3.7 ± 0.3 cm at the level of the aortic root, 3.3 ± 0.6 cm at the level of the ascending aorta, and 2.4 ± 0.3 cm at the level of the descending thoracic aorta.[148] An aneurysm is considered to be present when the diameter is 5 cm or greater. They can be classified according to the composition of their wall, their location, or their shape. The wall of a true aneurysm is composed of intima, media, and adventitia, whereas that of a false aneurysm (pseudoaneurysm) is composed of fibrous tissue or compressed blood clot, or both.

The majority of true thoracic aortic aneurysms are the result of atherosclerosis and occur in the descending portion.[149–152] They are usually fusiform, start immediately distal to the takeoff of the left subclavian artery, and often extend into the abdomen.[151, 152] Such aneurysms are typically seen in elderly persons and are more common in men.[152–154] Aneurysms of the ascending aorta are less common and can be the result of atherosclerosis, cystic medial degeneration ("cystic medial necrosis"), or, rarely, infection (mycotic aneurysm).[150–152] Cystic medial degeneration is the most common pathologic finding associated with aneurysms of the ascending aorta.[152, 155, 156] The abnormality can be idio-

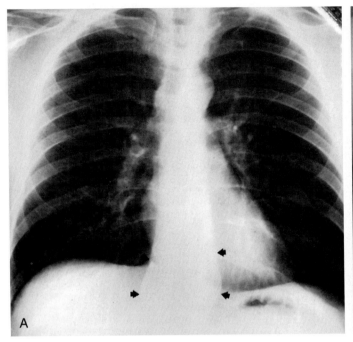

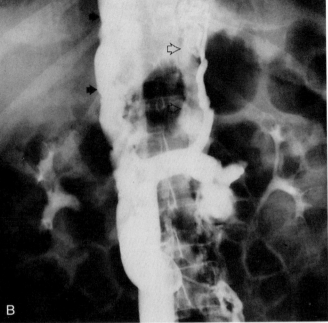

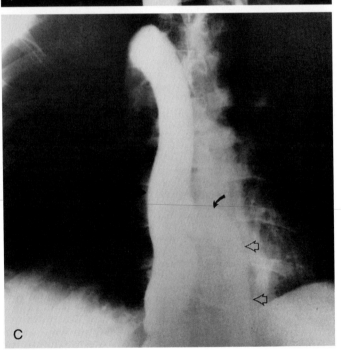

Figure 75–16. Proximal Interruption (Azygos and Hemiazygos Continuation) of the Inferior Vena Cava. A chest radiograph *(A)* from a 31-year-old asymptomatic man reveals an increased width of the paraspinal soft tissues in the lower thoracic region bilaterally *(arrows).* The shadow of the azygos vein in the right tracheobronchial angle measures 10 mm, the upper limit of normal. Following insertion of a catheter into the inferior vena cava, contrast medium was injected *(B).* Excellent opacification of the inferior vena cava was observed up to the level of the renal veins, but flow proximal to that point was by way of markedly dilated azygos *(solid arrows)* and hemiazygos *(open arrows)* veins. Within the thorax *(C),* the hemiazygos vein *(open arrows)* passed across the midline to join the azygos *(solid arrows)* at the level of T8 *(curved arrow).* The markedly dilated azygos then continued cephalad to terminate in the superior vena cava at its normal location in the right tracheobronchial angle.

pathic or associated with a connective tissue disorder such as Marfan's syndrome or Ehlers-Danlos syndrome.[152, 155] The majority of mycotic aneurysms of the aorta are true aneurysms;[152] predisposing conditions include bacterial endocarditis, drug abuse, atherosclerosis, and immunosuppression.[152, 157] Syphilis is now a relatively rare cause.

False aneurysms are most often the result of blunt trauma and are usually eccentric or saccular in shape.[151, 152, 158–160] Such aneurysms are typically located in the proximal descending thoracic aorta just beyond the origin of the left subclavian artery *(see* page 2626). Occasionally, a false aneurysm follows penetrating trauma or iatrogenic injury; rarely, it is associated with tuberculosis.[151, 152, 161]

On the chest radiograph, aneurysms of the ascending

aorta and proximal aortic arch usually project anteriorly and to the right (Fig. 75–19), while those of the distal arch and descending aorta project posteriorly and to the left (Fig. 75–20). In fact, aortic aneurysms should be considered in the differential diagnosis for any abnormal opacity that is contiguous with any part of the aorta. Calcification of the aneurysm wall is relatively common *(see* Fig. 75–19).

The diagnosis can be confirmed using CT (Fig. 75–21),[150, 152, 162, 163] MR imaging (Fig. 75–22),[164, 165, 165a, 165b] transesophageal echocardiography,[166] or angiography (Fig. 75–23). Contrast-enhanced CT is currently the most commonly used technique. It allows accurate assessment of the presence and extent of the aneurysm, its relationship to adjacent structures, and the presence of complications such

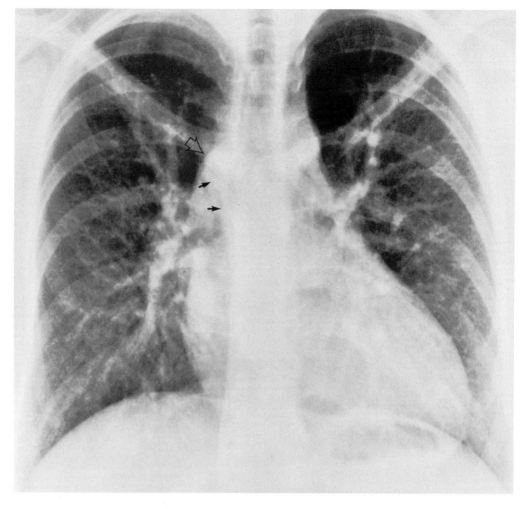

Figure 75–17. Azygos Continuation (Proximal Interruption) of the Inferior Vena Cava Associated with Ventricular Septal Defect. A radiograph of the chest in posteroanterior projection from a 20-year-old asymptomatic woman reveals a smooth, well-defined opacity in the right tracheobronchial angle *(open arrow)*. This represents a moderately dilated azygos vein (width 20 mm). In its course superiorly, the dilated vein has displaced the right mediastinal pleura laterally, thus creating a right paraspinal interface *(solid arrows)* analogous to the left paraspinal interface caused by the aorta. The radiograph also shows moderate pulmonary pleonemia and mild ventricular enlargement attributable to a ventricular septal defect.

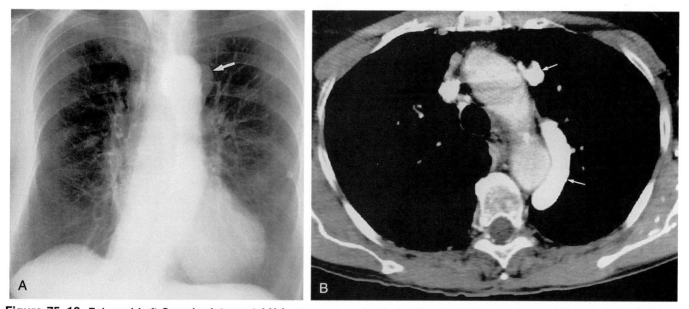

Figure 75–18. Enlarged Left Superior Intercostal Vein. A posteroanterior chest radiograph *(A)* demonstrates a prominent aortic nipple *(arrow)*. (Incidental note is made of a calcified granuloma in the left lung.) A contrast-enhanced CT scan *(B)* demonstrates a dilated left superior intercostal vein *(arrows)* due to collateral blood flow from the left brachiocephalic vein into the hemiazygos and azygos veins. Also note collateral blood flow in the left axilla. The patient was a 77-year-old woman who had long-standing superior vena cava obstruction related to fibrosing mediastinitis (presumed to be due to histoplasmosis). Note calcified paratracheal lymph nodes.

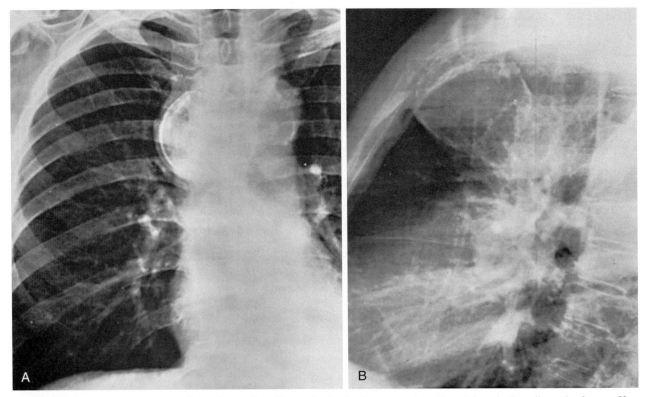

Figure 75–19. Saccular Aneurysm of the Ascending Thoracic Aorta. Posteroanterior *(A)* and lateral *(B)* radiographs from a 52-year-old asymptomatic man reveal a well-circumscribed mass projecting anteriorly and to the right. Its wall is densely calcified. The etiology of the aneurysm was not established.

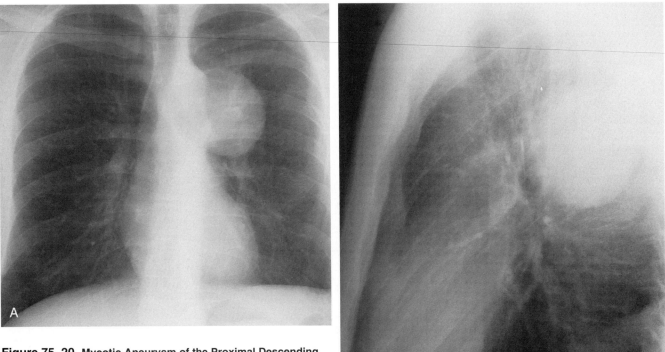

Figure 75–20. Mycotic Aneurysm of the Proximal Descending Thoracic Aorta. Posteroanterior *(A)* and lateral *(B)* radiographs from a 22-year-old man demonstrate a well-circumscribed mass abutting the aorta and projecting posteriorly and to the left. The lesion was surgically proved to be mycotic aneurysm.

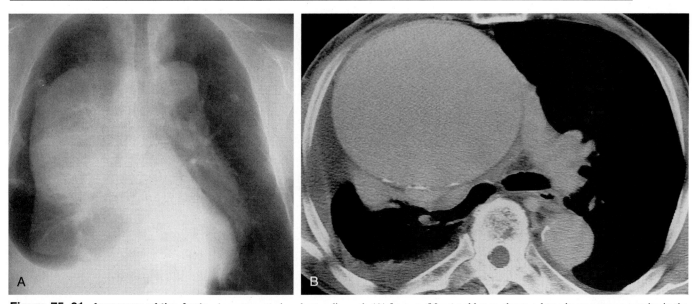

Figure 75–21. Aneurysm of the Aorta. A posteroanterior chest radiograph *(A)* from an 86-year-old man shows a large homogeneous opacity in the right upper mediastinum. A CT scan performed without intravenous contrast *(B)* demonstrates an aneurysm of the ascending thoracic aorta measuring 11 cm in diameter. Note focal intimal calcification in the ascending and descending thoracic aorta and the presence of small bilateral pleural effusions. The cause of the aneurysm was not established.

as compression of the trachea, bronchi, or pulmonary arteries or veins and SVC.[152, 167, 168] Foci of intimal calcification are seen on CT scans in approximately 75% of cases. Mural thrombus is also frequently evident, particularly in patients who have large aneurysms (Fig. 75–24).[152, 169] Because of its ability to demonstrate mural thrombus, CT allows better assessment of the true diameter of the aorta than is possible with angiography.[152] Optimal anatomic assessment of the aorta is obtained by using spin-echo MR imaging with T1-weighting and electrocardiographic gating.[165b] However, spin-echo sequences are prone to artifacts secondary to slow blood flow, and alternative techniques, such as cine gradient-echo and cine phase-contrast MR imaging, may be required to distinguish such artifacts from mural thrombus.[165b]

Many patients are asymptomatic. Clinical manifestations vary according to the size and location of the aneurysm.

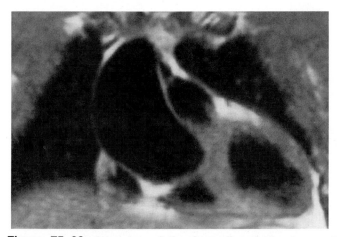

Figure 75–22. Aneurysm of the Ascending Aorta. A coronal cardiac-gated MR image demonstrates a 5-cm-diameter ascending aortic aneurysm that showed cystic medial "necrosis" on histologic examination. The patient was a 28-year-old man.

Symptoms caused by aneurysms of the transverse arch are particularly notable and result from compression of the SVC, recurrent laryngeal nerve, or tracheobronchial tree. They include a brassy cough, hemoptysis, and hoarseness. Aneurysms of the descending aorta may cause bone erosion leading to severe pain; they can also cause dysphagia as a result of esophageal compression.[170] Respiratory insufficiency has been reported to result from tracheobronchial compression by a large calcified aneurysm of the descending aorta,[171] and an anterior spinal artery syndrome has been described as a result of compression from an aneurysm of the descending aorta years after trauma.[172]

Aortic Dissection

Aortic dissection occurs when blood collects in the media and divides it into two distinct layers. In the majority of patients, the primary event is an intimal tear.[173–175] Because it is under high pressure, the blood cleaves a channel in the media, resulting in the formation of a false lumen for blood flow, in addition to the true aortic lumen.[176] Such dissection can proceed both proximal and distal to the entry site. As it progresses, it may be associated with multiple tears in the intima, leading to additional entry and exit sites. Occasionally, dissection occurs as a result of bleeding from the vasa vasorum into the media and is followed by a tear of the intima.[175, 177] In a small number of cases, rupture of the vasa vasorum results in thickening of the aortic wall without intimal rupture.[178]

The most widely accepted classification of aortic dissection is the Stanford Classification System, which designates dissections involving the ascending aorta as type A, regardless of the distal extension of the dissection, and all other types of dissection as type B. Depending on the series, about 55% to 90% of dissections are type A.[179–181] They can extend into the perivalvular region and result in aortic insufficiency,[182] extend to and occlude the branches of the aortic

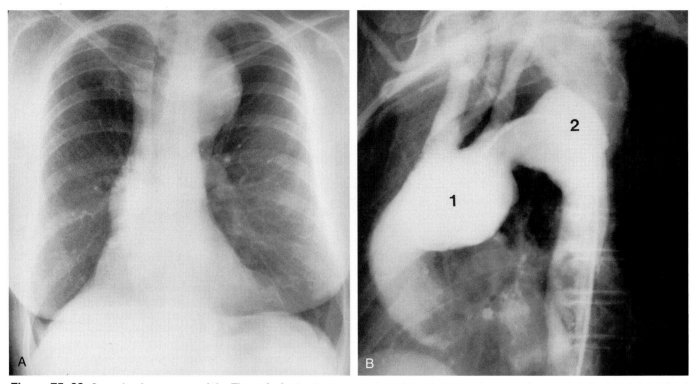

Figure 75–23. Saccular Aneurysms of the Thoracic Aorta. A posteroanterior radiograph *(A)* reveals a rather large, well-defined, slightly lobulated opacity projecting to the left of the superior mediastinum, suggestive of a large aortic aneurysm. No other abnormalities are apparent. An aortogram in left anterior oblique projection *(B)* reveals a double aneurysm of the aortic arch, one situated at the level of the origin of the brachiocephalic artery (number 1) and the other in the distal transverse portion of the arch distal to the takeoff of the left subclavian artery (number 2).

arch,[182] or rupture into the pericardial sac and cause tamponade.[183]

Aortic dissection is seen most commonly in patients who have systemic arterial hypertension or Marfan's syndrome; less common causes include Ehlers-Danlos syndrome, aortitis, and vascular catheterization.[174, 176, 182, 184] In many cases, cystic medial degeneration is evident in the aortic wall. Because most patients are older, atherosclerosis is often present; however, it is more likely to be a coincidental finding than a significant contributing factor in the dissection. Dissection most commonly involves the ascending aorta, in which atherosclerosis tends to be relatively mild, and dissections rarely begin in the lower abdominal aorta, where arteriosclerosis is very common and often severe.[185]

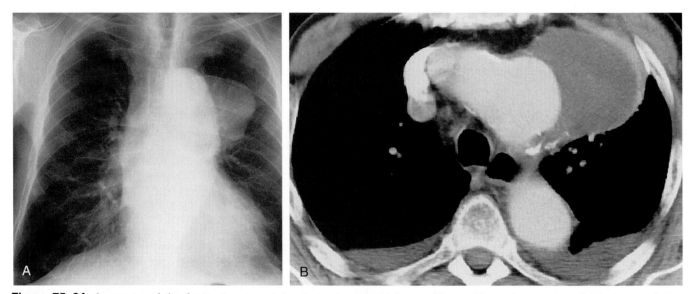

Figure 75–24. Aneurysm of the Aorta. A posteroanterior chest radiograph *(A)* from an 87-year-old man demonstrates a homogeneous soft tissue opacity abutting the proximal descending thoracic aorta. A contrast-enhanced CT scan *(B)* shows a focal saccular aneurysm involving the proximal descending thoracic aorta and containing a large mural thrombus. Small bilateral pleural effusions are also evident. The aneurysm was proved to be secondary to atherosclerosis.

The most common radiographic manifestations of aortic dissection are widening of the superior mediastinum and aorta, a double contour of the aortic arch, increase in size of the aorta or change in configuration on serial chest radiographs, and displacement of a calcified plaque by 10 mm or more (Fig. 75–25).[151, 175, 183, 186, 187] Enlargement of the aorta is a nonspecific finding seen in many patients who have systemic arterial hypertension or atherosclerosis. However, acute enlargement on serial chest radiographs should raise the possibility of dissection.[175] A normal configuration of the aorta does not exclude the diagnosis, as it is seen in approximately 25% of patients who have acute dissection.[175, 188] Displacement of intimal calcification is also not a reliable diagnostic finding:[175, 183] the lateral border of the visualized aorta may not be at the same level as that of the calcified plaque, thus mimicking displacement of the calcification;[175, 183] in addition, other processes such as accumulation of fat or a neoplasm can simulate the appearance of aortic wall thickening.[183] Because of the equivocal significance of these features, the plain chest radiograph is of limited value in the diagnosis of aortic dissection. For example, in one investigation in 75 patients, the diagnosis of aortic dissection or thoracic aortic aneurysm was suggested prospectively based on the findings on the chest radiograph in only 19 (25%);[189] retrospective analysis of the chest radiographs showed that only 36 patients (48%) had abnormalities suggestive of aortic dissection.

CT is a rapid and relatively noninvasive method for diagnosing acute aortic dissection. The diagnostic accuracy using dynamic or spiral CT technique following intravenous administration of contrast in various studies has ranged from 88% to 100%.[181, 190–193] In one investigation of 110 patients who had clinically suspected dissection and in whom the final diagnosis was proved by either contrast angiography, intraoperative inspection, or autopsy, CT had a sensitivity of 94% and a specificity of 87% in the detection of aortic dissection.[181] In another investigation of 49 patients, spiral CT had an accuracy of 100%.[193]

The characteristic CT findings consist of a linear filling defect (intimal flap) and the presence of a false lumen (Fig. 75–26). The true and false lumens former have differential enhancement on CT scans, the former showing greater enhancement than the latter. Another sign of dissection is increased attenuation of the thrombosed false lumen or of the aortic wall.[175, 183, 194] Such increased attenuation is present in the acute phase and decreases gradually as the hematoma resolves.[183] Although acute dissection is characteristically associated with central displacement of intimal calcification, this finding is not diagnostic. For example, in one study of 136 patients, it was seen in 33 (24%) who had an aortic aneurysm unassociated with dissection;[195] the abnormality in such cases is the result of calcification of thrombus within the aneurysm. False-negative or false-positive diagnoses based on CT appearance can result from insufficient contrast enhancement or from motion artifacts.[175, 177, 183, 196]

MR imaging is comparable to CT in the evaluation of patients who have suspected aortic dissection (Fig. 75–27).[181, 183, 193, 196] The diagnosois can usually be made using conventional spin-echo MR technique with electrocardiographic gating and T1-weighting; however, slow flow of blood within the false lumen may mimic intramural thrombus on spin-echo MR imaging.[165b] The distinction can be readily made using gradient-echo MR imaging, cine phase-contrast imaging, or gadolinium-enhanced MR angiography.[165b]

Transthoracic echocardiography is a rapid and noninvasive method for assessment of the ascending aorta but does not provide adequate visualization of the aortic arch and descending aorta. Better assessment of these portions of the vessel can be obtained using transesophageal echocardiography. In one study of 110 patients who had clinically suspected dissection of the thoracic aorta, the sensitivities for detecting dissection were similar for CT, MR imaging, and transesophageal echocardiography (98%, 98%, and 94%, respectively) but was considerably lower for transthoracic echocardiography (59%).[181] The specificity for both transthoracic (83%) and transesophageal echocardiography (77%) was lower than that for either contrast-enhanced CT (87%) or MR imaging (98%). Echocardiography should therefore be limited to the assessment of patients who are too unstable to be moved.

For many years, angiography was considered the imaging modality of choice in the diagnosis of aortic dissection.[197, 198] However, the procedure has several limitations, including the time required to assemble the angiography team, its invasiveness, and its relatively low sensitivity (about 80% to 90%).[198–200] False-negative angiograms can result from lack of visualization of the intimal flap, poor opacification of the false lumen, or thrombosis of the false lumen.[183, 187, 198, 199]

The diagnosis of aortic dissection is usually suggested by the clinical history.[201] Typically, the onset is sudden and associated with severe pain, which may be described as tearing or ripping in nature and often radiates to the throat, jaw, back, or abdomen as the dissection extends from its point of origin. Nausea and vomiting, sweating, and faintness are other manifestations in some individuals. Most patients have a history of hypertension. Physical examination may reveal evidence of acute peripheral arterial occlusion, aortic insufficiency, or bruits over the affected portion of aorta.[202]

As might be expected, untreated aortic dissection is often rapidly fatal, particularly if it involves the ascending aorta.[183, 203, 204] The death rate in patients who have untreated dissection is 1% per hour for the first 48 hours.[203] With appropriate medical and surgical treatment, survival rates are about 80% to 90% at 30 days and 60% to 70% at 5 years.[182, 183, 205]

Buckling and Aneurysm of the Innominate Artery

Buckling and aneurysm of the innominate artery are both manifested radiographically as a smooth, well-defined opacity in the right superior paramediastinal area, extending upward from the aortic arch. Buckling is a relatively common condition that occurs in about 15% of patients who have hypertension or atherosclerosis, or both (Fig. 75–28).[206] Aneurysms are much less common.

The innominate artery is about 5 cm long and is firmly fixed proximally at its origin from the aorta and distally by the subclavian and carotid arteries. When the thoracic aorta elongates and dilates as a result of atherosclerosis, the arch moves cephalad, carrying with it the origin of the innominate artery. Because of its fixation superiorly, the latter buckles to the right.[207] Occasionally, the buckling occurs posteriorly

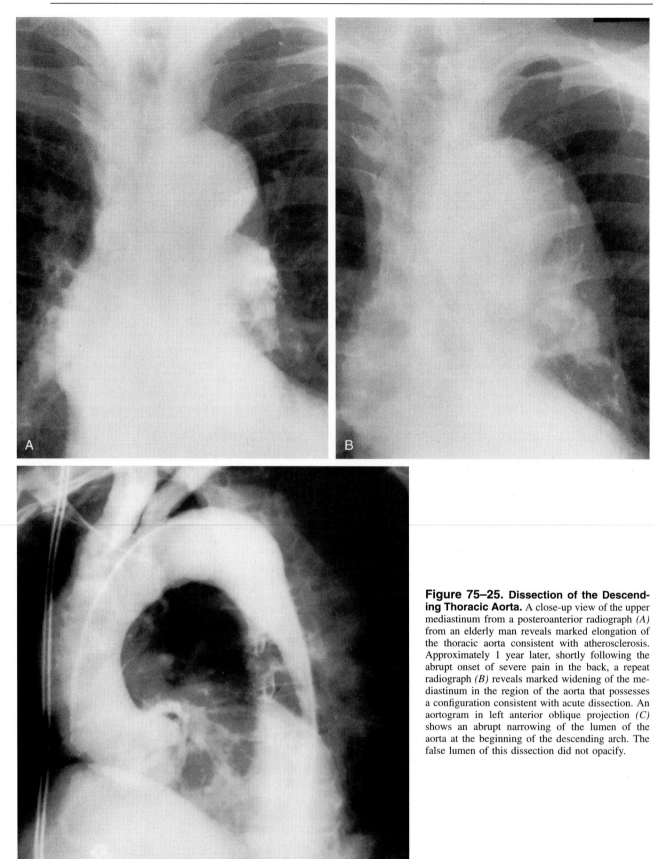

Figure 75–25. Dissection of the Descending Thoracic Aorta. A close-up view of the upper mediastinum from a posteroanterior radiograph *(A)* from an elderly man reveals marked elongation of the thoracic aorta consistent with atherosclerosis. Approximately 1 year later, shortly following the abrupt onset of severe pain in the back, a repeat radiograph *(B)* reveals marked widening of the mediastinum in the region of the aorta that possesses a configuration consistent with acute dissection. An aortogram in left anterior oblique projection *(C)* shows an abrupt narrowing of the lumen of the aorta at the beginning of the descending arch. The false lumen of this dissection did not opacify.

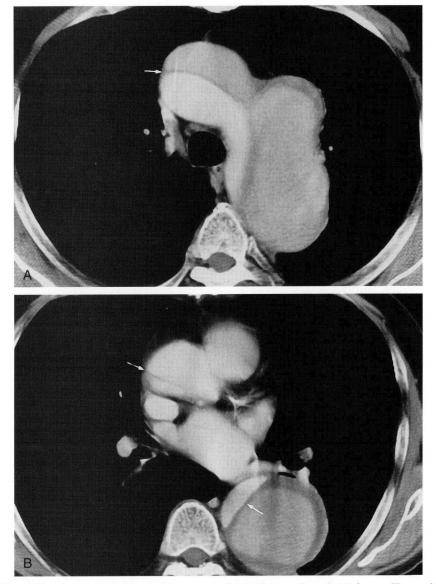

Figure 75–26. Aortic Dissection. A contrast-enhanced CT scan at the level of the aortic arch *(A)* from a 57-year-old man demonstrates marked enhancement of the true aortic lumen and poor enhancement of the false lumen of the dissection. Note the presence of a linear filling defect (intimal flap) *(arrows)* separating the true from the false lumen. A CT scan at a more caudal level *(B)* shows that the dissection involves the ascending aorta (type A), which is of normal caliber; the descending thoracic aorta shows aneurysmal dilation. The patient had systemic arterial hypertension.

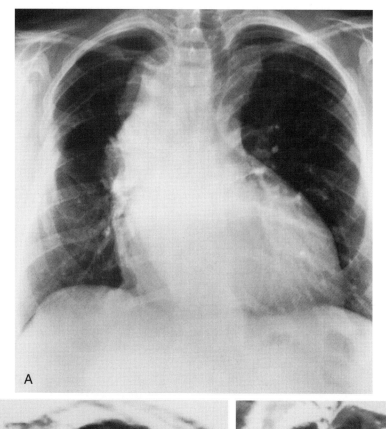

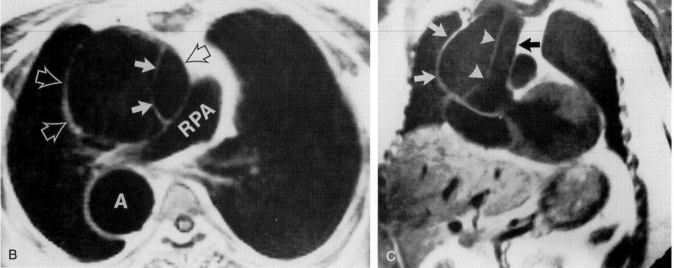

Figure 75–27. Dissection of the Ascending Aorta in a Patient with a Right Aortic Arch. A posteroanterior radiograph *(A)* reveals evidence of a former right thoracotomy that had been performed many years previously for repair of a coarctation and aortic valvotomy. The trachea is deviated markedly to the left by a right-sided aortic arch. The width of the aorta at the point of maximal tracheal displacement is obviously greater than normal. A T1-weighted magnetic resonance scan in transverse section *(B)* at the level of the right pulmonary artery (RPA) shows a markedly dilated ascending aorta *(open arrows)*. Situated within it is a curvilinear shadow *(arrows)* representing the intimal flap; the smaller area to the left of the flap represents the true lumen, and the larger area to the right, the false lumen. Note that the descending aorta *(A)* at this level is still on the right side. A coronal reconstruction *(C)* again reveals the markedly dilated ascending aorta *(arrows)* containing the intimal flap *(arrowheads)*; again, the true lumen is on the left and the false lumen on the right. The patient was a 27-year-old woman who had Turner's syndrome.

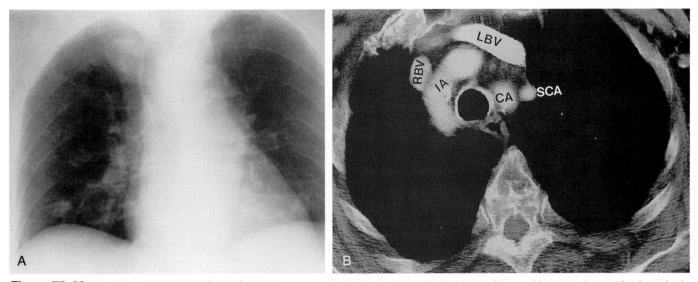

Figure 75–28. Buckling of the Innominate Artery. An anteroposterior chest radiograph *(A)* from an 86-year-old woman shows a focal opacity in the right superior paramediastinal area. A contrast-enhanced CT scan *(B)* shows that the opacity is the result of buckling of the innominate artery (IA). Contrast is also present in the left brachiocephalic vein (LBV), right brachiocephalic vein (RBV), left carotid artery (CA), and left subclavian artery (SCA).

and laterally, in which case the vessel becomes almost completely surrounded by lung parenchyma and simulates a nodule.[208–210] Sometimes, a similar appearance is caused by an aneurysm or pseudoaneurysm of the right carotid artery; in one case, this resulted in a resemblance to a Pancoast tumor.[211] Buckling of the left common carotid artery can also simulate a mediastinal neoplasm.[212]

Aneurysms of the innominate artery can cause pain, cough, dyspnea, hoarseness, dysphagia, Horner's syndrome, and clubbing of the fingers of the right hand. A pulsatile mass may be evident at the base of the neck.[206] Although buckling seldom causes symptoms, it may give rise to a small, palpable, pulsatile mass in the right supraclavicular fossa, indicating that the common carotid artery also is affected.[206, 207] Buckling occurs most often in middle-aged or older obese women who have clinical evidence of atherosclerosis and hypertension. Its presence in patients under the age of 30 years should suggest the possibility of coarctation of the aorta.[207]

Congenital Anomalies of the Aorta

Although most congenital malformations of the aortic arch become evident during the first year of life,[213] occasional examples are not recognized until adulthood.[214, 215] A congenital aortic vascular ring results from persistence of the two aortic arches or of the right aortic arch and left ductus arteriosus; in a minority of patients, the right subclavian artery, also of anomalous origin, arises from the descending aorta.[216] The radiographic diagnosis can be made by the demonstration of a double aortic arch and of a vessel posterior to the esophagus. On the frontal view, the trachea is midline; on the lateral radiograph, the trachea is displaced posteriorly by the larger anterior arch. A specific diagnosis can be made using CT or MR imaging.[163, 165b, 217, 218] Symptoms result from compression of the trachea or esophagus and include those due to recurrent respiratory infections, shortness of breath, and dysphagia.

Other congenital anomalies of the aorta that result in

abnormalities of mediastinal contour include (1) pseudocoarctation of the aorta (Fig. 75–29), in which a left paramediastinal "mass" is visible just above the aortic arch as a result of elongation and buckling of the aorta;[219, 220] (2) a cervical aortic arch, in which the aortic arch extends into the soft tissues of the neck before turning downward on itself to become the descending aorta;[221, 222] (3) aortic diverticula;[223] and (4) by far the most common, a right aortic arch (Fig. 75–30).[224] The last-named is present in about 0.1% to 0.2% of the population.[225] In approximately 70% of cases, there is also an aberrant left subclavian artery.[225] Occasionally, the abnormal arch compresses the trachea sufficiently to result in a clinical picture that can be confused with asthma.[226]

In approximately 0.5% of the population, a normal left aortic arch is associated with an aberrant right subclavian artery.[225] Occasionally, this vessel can be visualized as a soft tissue opacity, typically having an oblique course from left to right and extending cephalad from the aortic arch (Fig. 75–31).[227] The proximal portion of the aberrant artery is frequently dilated, a finding known as a diverticulum of Kommerell (Fig. 75–32).[225, 228] The diagnosis can be readily confirmed using contrast-enhanced CT (Fig. 75–33), MR imaging, or angiography (Fig. 75–32).[218, 225]

DISEASES OF THE ESOPHAGUS

Esophageal lesions that may present radiographically as mediastinal masses or as diffuse mediastinal widening include neoplasms, diverticula, hiatal hernia (*see* page 2996), and megaesophagus.

Neoplasms

Carcinoma. Although barium examination and esophagoscopy are the two definitive procedures in the diagnosis of primary carcinoma of the esophagus, conventional radiographs of the chest can provide clues to its presence (Fig.

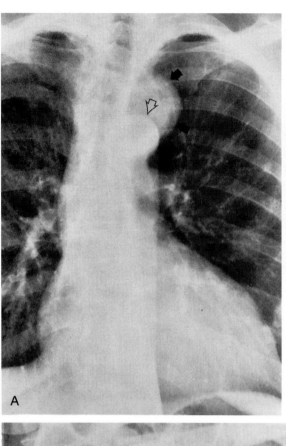

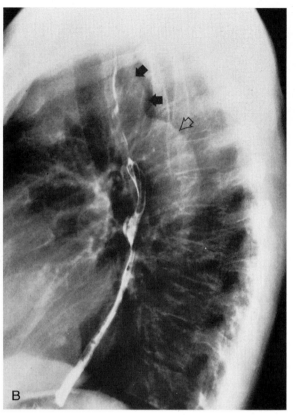

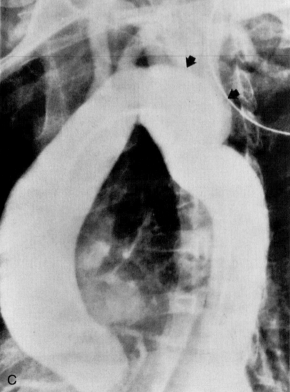

Figure 75–29. Pseudocoarctation of the Aorta. A posteroanterior view *(A)* of the chest of a 63-year-old asymptomatic woman reveals a homogeneous soft tissue opacity *(solid arrows)* that projects above the shadow of the aortic arch *(open arrow).* In lateral projection *(B),* the posterior aspect of the "mass" is again identified by *solid arrows* and the posterior portion of the aortic arch by an *open arrow.* On the basis of this plain film evidence the findings were thought to be compatible with pseudocoarctation of the aorta; however, an aortogram was performed for confirmation. In oblique projection *(C),* this study confirms the fact that the abnormal opacity observed on the plain radiograph is due to an unusually high aortic arch *(solid arrows)* that buckled in its descending portion so as to produce a prominent notch on its posterior and left lateral aspects.

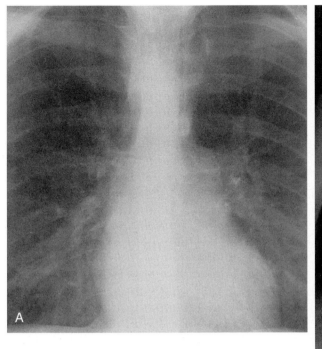

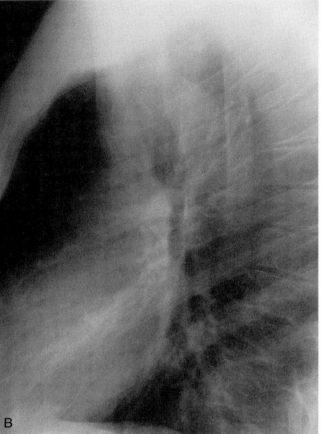

Figure 75–30. Right Aortic Arch. Close-up views from posteroanterior *(A)* and lateral *(B)* chest radiographs from a 33-year-old man demonstrate a right aortic arch causing smooth deviation of the trachea anteriorly and to the left. The patient was asymptomatic.

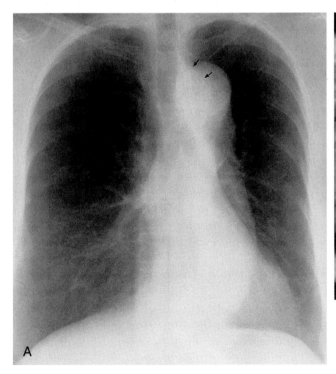

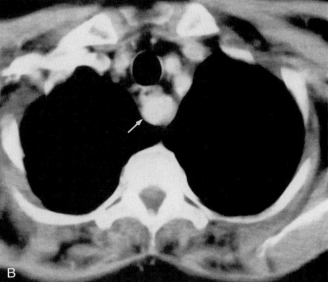

Figure 75–31. Aberrant Right Subclavian Artery. A posteroanterior chest radiograph *(A)* demonstrates an oblique opacity extending cephalad from the aortic arch to the right *(arrows)*. A CT scan *(B)* demonstrates an aberrant right subclavian artery *(arrow)* coursing to the right, posterior to the esophagus.

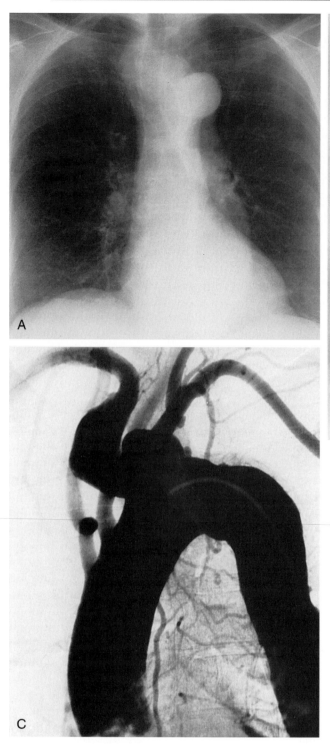

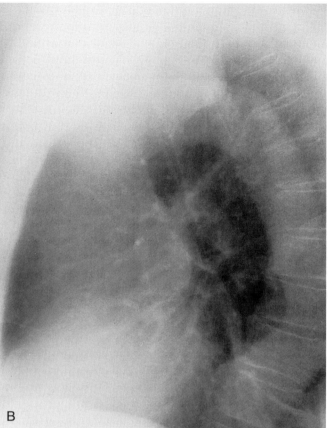

Figure 75–32. Diverticulum of Kommerell. Posteroanterior *(A)* and lateral *(B)* chest radiographs from an 80-year-old woman demonstrate a soft tissue opacity coursing obliquely from the level of the aortic arch cephalad from left to right. On the lateral radiograph, the opacity causes a smooth indentation of the posterior wall of the trachea. An aortogram *(C)* demonstrates dilation of the proximal portion of the aberrant right subclavian artery (diverticulum of Kommerell).

75–34).[229–233] In a review of 103 patients, significant abnormalities were found in 49.[229] The most frequent abnormalities included an abnormal azygoesophageal recess interface (27%), a widened mediastinum (18%), a posterior tracheal indentation or mass (16%), a widened retrotracheal stripe (11%), and tracheal deviation (10%). Less common abnormalities included deformity of the gastric air bubble, a retrocardiac mass, an esophageal fluid level, and a retrohilar mass. In another plain film study of 102 patients who had carcinoma of the middle third of the esophagus, 63 (62%)

had thickening of the retrotracheal stripe, anterior bowing of the posterior wall of the trachea, or a combination of these findings.[230] Progressive thickening of the retrotracheal stripe also has been shown to be a useful marker for recurrent esophageal carcinoma following surgery or radiation therapy.[231]

CT manifestations of esophageal carcinoma include esophageal wall thickening, proximal dilation, obscuration of the periesophageal fat planes, and periesophageal lymph node enlargement.[232, 234–236] Although esophageal wall thick-

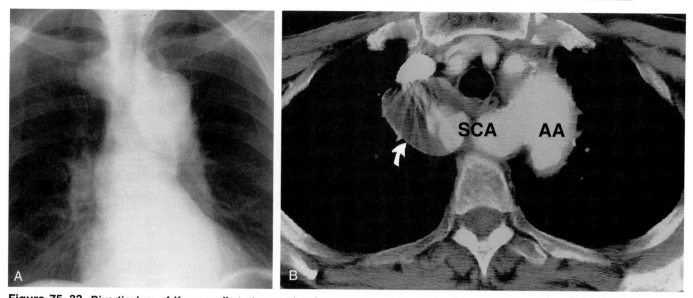

Figure 75–33. Diverticulum of Kommerell. A close-up view from a posteroanterior chest radiograph *(A)* from a 74-year-old woman shows a soft tissue opacity in the superior mediastinum. A contrast-enhanced CT scan *(B)* demonstrates the upper aspect of the aortic arch (AA) and the aberrant right subclavian artery (SCA). The latter is ectatic (diverticulum of Kommerell) and contains thrombus *(curved arrow).*

ening is the earliest manifestation of carcinoma, it is by no means diagnostic. In one study of 200 consecutive CT examinations in which thickened esophageal walls (over 3 mm) were found in 35%, esophageal carcinoma was identified as the cause in only half;[235] other causes included reflux and monilial esophagitis, varices, and post-irradiation scarring.

CT is also helpful in the staging of esophageal carcinoma.[59, 237–240] The tumor may invade the adjacent mediastinal soft tissue, aorta, trachea, or bronchi and metastasize to mediastinal and upper abdominal lymph nodes, the lungs, and extrathoracic organs, most commonly the liver. Extension into mediastinal fat can be detected by the presence of increased periesophageal soft tissue density, often ill defined.[232] The assessment of aortic invasion using CT is based on the evaluation of the arc of contact between the esophageal mass and the aorta (in turn based on a 360-degree aortic circumference).[232] Some authors have considered an interface arc of less than 45 degrees as reliably excluding aortic invasion, an arc between 45 and 90 degrees as indeterminate, and an arc greater than 90 degrees as highly suggestive of invasion;[237] however, use of these criteria is associated with a large number of indeterminate cases.[232] As a result, other investigators have considered arcs less than 90 degrees as excluding invasion and those greater than 90 degrees as suggestive of invasion.[241, 242] Although several workers have shown CT to have a high degree of accuracy in the assessment of aortic invasion,[237, 238, 243] others have found it to be considerably less;[205, 244] in fact, the reported sensitivity of CT in the detection of aortic invasion has ranged from 6% to 100%, the specificity from 52% to 96%, and the accuracy from 55% to 96%.[232]

Findings suggestive of tracheobronchial invasion include posterior indentation of the airway and focal thickening of the airway wall. The reported sensitivity of CT in the detection of tracheobronchial involvement in various studies has ranged from 31% to 100%, the specificity from 86% to 98%, and the accuracy from 74% to 97%.[232] Similarly, there has been considerable variation in the reported

efficacy of CT in the detection of metastases to regional lymph nodes, its sensitivity ranging from 34% to 61%, specificity from 88% to 97%, and accuracy from 51% to 70%.[232]

The results of these studies indicate that CT is helpful in identifying advanced local disease and the presence of metastases to the lungs, liver, and intra-abdominal lymph nodes.[232, 244] However, it has limited value in the detection of early periesophageal tumor extension or involvement of mediastinal lymph nodes.[244] Several investigators have shown that endoscopic ultrasound examination is superior to CT in the detection of local tumor spread.[241, 242, 245] It has also been shown that the combination of CT and endoscopic ultrasound examination provides greater diagnostic accuracy than either modality alone.[242, 246] MR imaging has not been found to have any significant advantages over CT and plays a limited role in the assessment of these patients.[247, 248] Preliminary results suggest that positron emission tomography using 2-[^{18}F]-fluoro-2-deoxy-D-glucose (FDG) is comparable to CT in the demonstration of the extent of esophageal carcinoma and involvement of periesophageal nodes and is superior to it in the detection of distant metastases.[248a]

Mesenchymal Neoplasms. Leiomyosarcomas constitute fewer than 1% of malignant esophageal tumors.[249, 250] In one series of 10 patients, 9 presented with dysphagia and 5 had a mediastinal mass evident on the chest radiograph.[251] Barium swallow showed an intramural esophageal lesion in 6 patients, an intraluminal mass in 2, and infiltrative lesions in 2. In 3 patients, CT demonstrated a large exophytic component containing gas or contrast material.

Benign neoplasms of the esophagus consist mostly of leiomyomas, fibromas, and lipomas. Although the majority are too small to result in radiographic abnormalities or clinical manifestations, they can grow to a large size. In this situation, the tumor presents radiographically as a rounded mass projecting to one or both sides of the posterior mediastinum.[252] In one series of 81 primary neoplasms of the mediastinum in adults, 4 were leiomyomas of the esophagus,

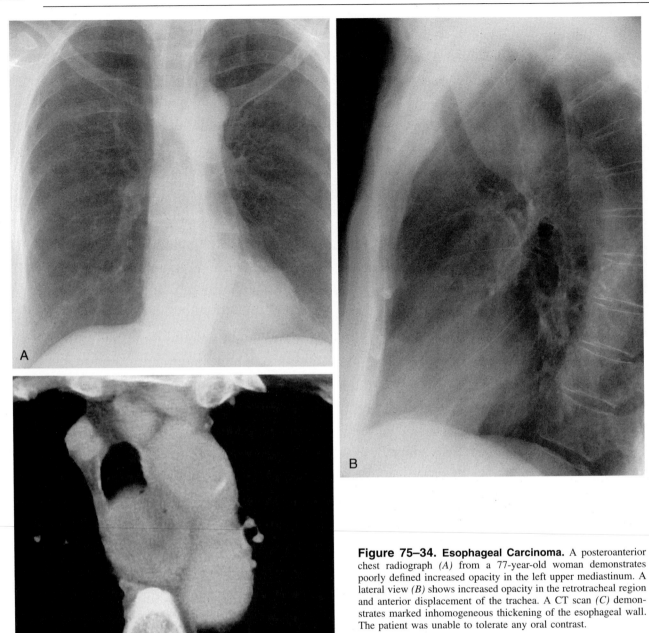

Figure 75–34. Esophageal Carcinoma. A posteroanterior chest radiograph *(A)* from a 77-year-old woman demonstrates poorly defined increased opacity in the left upper mediastinum. A lateral view *(B)* shows increased opacity in the retrotracheal region and anterior displacement of the trachea. A CT scan *(C)* demonstrates marked inhomogeneous thickening of the esophageal wall. The patient was unable to tolerate any oral contrast.

all originating in the lower third.[253] Although such tumors are usually solitary, multiple tumors occur in about 4% of cases.[254] The appearance of leiomyomas and fibromas is that of a nonspecific intramural soft tissue mass. Lipomas have a characteristic appearance on CT scans consisting of homogeneous fat attenuation.[255]

Diverticula

Diverticula occur in the pharyngeal region (Zenker's diverticulum), in the mid-thoracic region as a result of cicatricial contraction from healed infected lymph nodes (traction diverticula), and in the lower esophagus as a result of

outpouching of the mucosa through defects in the muscular wall at the point of entry of blood vessels (pulsion diverticula). Unlike the other two varieties, traction diverticula are seldom, if ever, visible on plain radiographs.

Zenker's diverticulum originates between the transverse and oblique fibers of the inferior pharyngeal constrictor muscle. It may become large enough to be identified in the superior mediastinum on plain radiographs, in which case it frequently contains an air-fluid level. If large, it can compress the esophagus or, rarely, cause tracheal narrowing.[256] Barium studies not only clearly outline the sac but also reveal the degree of anterior displacement of the proximal esophagus. The diagnosis can also be readily made using

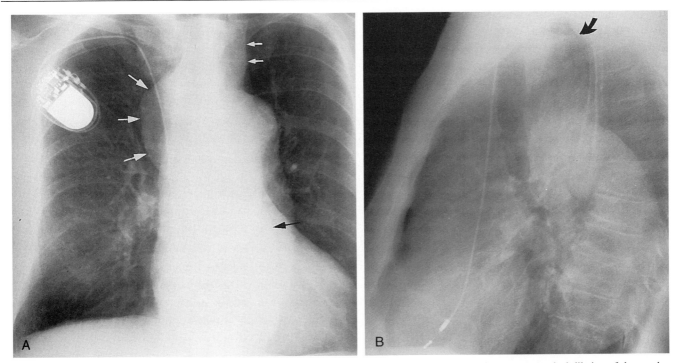

Figure 75–35. Achalasia. Posteroanterior *(A)* and lateral *(B)* chest radiographs from a 74-year-old man demonstrate marked dilation of the esophagus *(straight arrows),* which contains an air-fluid level *(curved arrow)* and displaces the trachea anteriorly. The patient had long-standing achalasia.

CT. Symptoms include dysphagia, chronic cough due to aspiration, and recurrent pneumonia.

Diverticula arising from the lower third of the esophagus are almost always congenital in origin and present as round, cystlike structures to the right of the midline just above the diaphragm. An air-fluid level is usually present. Barium studies are again diagnostic.[257] A rare form of multiple pulsion diverticula has also been described that closely resembles that seen in the colon.[258]

Megaesophagus

Esophageal dilation has many causes, including stenosis secondary to reflux esophagitis or fibrosing mediastinitis, progressive systemic sclerosis (PSS), carcinoma, and achalasia. Among these, achalasia causes the most severe generalized dilation. The dilated esophagus is usually apparent radiographically as a shadow projecting entirely to the right side of the mediastinum. Because it is behind the heart, it does not cause a silhoutte sign with that structure. The trachea may be displaced anteriorly (Fig. 75–35). Depending on the underlying cause, an air-fluid level may be observed in the dilated esophagus, most frequently in achalasia and seldom in PSS. Although a barium study is the diagnostic procedure of choice, CT also allows the diagnosis, even in patients in whom the condition is not suspected.[259, 260] On conventional chest radiographs, an air-containing esophagus may be identified in some patients who have PSS and, in the appropriate clinical context, is suggestive of the diagnosis. Air in the esophagus can also be seen postoperatively[261] and in patients who employ esophageal speech after laryngectomy.[262]

Symptoms of achalasia include dysphagia, pain on swallowing, and chronic cough; recurrent pneumonia may result from aspiration. Stridor is observed occasionally.[263, 264]

Acute trapping of air within the esophagus distal to the cricopharyngeal sphincter has been described as a cause of tracheal obstruction and vena caval compression.[263]

Tracheoesophageal and Bronchoesophageal Fistulas

Fistulas between the esophagus and the airways can be congenital or acquired. Although congenital fistula is usually identified in neonates, it may not be recognized until adolescence or adulthood. In most cases of delayed recognition, there is a long history of cough, often with expectoration of food; occasionally, there is associated bronchiectasis.[265, 266] Such congenital communication is considered in greater detail in Chapter 22 (*see* page 627).

The most common cause of acquired fistula between the esophagus and the respiratory tract is carcinoma of the esophagus; in some instances, fistula formation is the result of radiation therapy.[267–269] This complication is not rare; in one series of 474 patients who had received radiotherapy for carcinoma of the esophagus, it occurred in 25 (approximately 5%).[267] As might be expected, once a fistula has developed, the prognosis is extremely poor, most patients dying within weeks to months. Acquired nonmalignant tracheoesophageal fistulas can be caused by cuffed tracheal tubes, surgical trauma, blunt injuries, and foreign bodies.[270–272] Although generally diagnosed by endoscopic or barium examination, they have also been detected by CT.[273]

Esophageal Varices

Paraesophageal varices occasionally result in abnormalities on the chest radiograph (Fig. 75–36).[274, 275] In one review of 352 patients who had portal hypertension, these were evident in 17 (5%);[275] they included middle-posterior

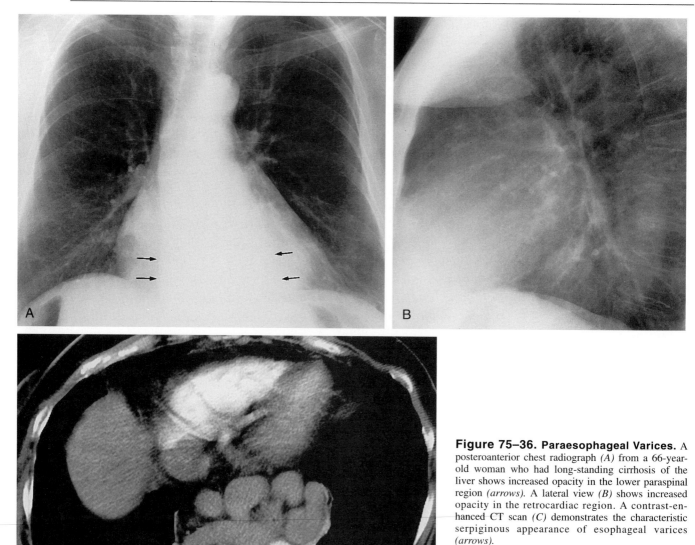

Figure 75–36. Paraesophageal Varices. A posteroanterior chest radiograph *(A)* from a 66-year-old woman who had long-standing cirrhosis of the liver shows increased opacity in the lower paraspinal region *(arrows)*. A lateral view *(B)* shows increased opacity in the retrocardiac region. A contrast-enhanced CT scan *(C)* demonstrates the characteristic serpiginous appearance of esophageal varices *(arrows)*.

mediastinal or paravertebral opacities, a soft tissue opacity adjacent to the descending thoracic aorta, and obscuration of the aorta.[275] In a second investigation of 100 patients, abnormalities consistent with esophageal varices were seen on chest radiographs in 20 and on CT in 38;[275a] most of the varices detected on the radiographs were greater than 2.5 cm in diameter. Rarely, blood flows from the abdomen through the diaphragm into the thorax and drains into the pericardiophrenic vein;[276, 277] such a portosystemic shunt can result in an abnormal soft tissue shadow at the level of the left cardiophrenic angle.[277] The diagnosis of esophageal varices and transdiaphragmatic portosystemic shunt can be readily made by CT.[275, 277, 278]

Although esophageal varices do not in themselves occasion respiratory symptoms, complicating hematemesis may be confused with hemoptysis. In addition, transient pleural effusions and mediastinal opacities have been identified on radiographs following endoscopic injection sclerotherapy;[279] in one patient, this form of treatment was associated with formation of an esophageal-pleural fistula.[280]

REFERENCES

1. Strollo DC, Rosado-de-Christenson ML, Jett JR: Primary mediastinal tumors: Part II. Tumors of the middle and posterior mediastinum. Chest 112:1344, 1997.
2. Azizkhan RG, Dudgeon DL, Buck JR, et al: Life-threatening airway obstruction as a complication to the management of mediastinal masses in children. J Pediatr Surg 20:816, 1985.
3. Castleman B (ed): Case Records of the Massachusetts General Hospital, Case 40011. N Engl J Med 250:26, 1954.
4. Keller AR, Hochholzer L, Castleman B: Hyaline-vascular and plasma-cell types of giant lymph node hyperplasia of the mediastinum and other locations. Cancer 29:670, 1972.
5. Frizzera G: Castleman's disease: More questions than answers. Hum Pathol 16:202, 1985.
6. Neerhout RC, Larson W, Mansur P: Mesenteric lymphoid hamartoma associated with chronic hypoferremia, anemia, growth failure and hyperglobulinemia. N Engl J Med 280:922, 1969.
7. Maier HC, Sommers SC: Mediastinal lymph node hyperplasia, hypergammaglobulinemia, and anemia. J Thorac Cardiovasc Surg 79:860, 1980.
8. Karcher DS, Pearson CE, Butler WM, et al: Giant lymph node hyperplasia involving the thymus with associated nephrotic syndrome and myelofibrosis. Am J Clin Pathol 77:100, 1982.
9. Yu GSM, Carson JW: Giant lymph-node hyperplasia, plasma-cell type, of the mediastinum, with peripheral neuropathy. Am J Clin Pathol 66:46, 1976.
10. Couch WD: Giant lymph node hyperplasia associated with thrombotic thrombocytopenic purpura. Am J Clin Pathol 74:340, 1980.
11. Kirsch CFE, Webb EM, Webb WR: Multicentric Castleman's disease and POEMS syndrome: CT findings. J Thorac Imaging 12:75, 1997.
12. Johkoh T, Müller NL, Ichikado K, et al: Intrathoracic multicentric Castleman's disease: CT findings in 12 patients. Radiology 209:477, 1998.
13. Weisenburger DD, Nathwani BN, Winberg CD, et al: Multicentric angiofollicular lymph node hyperplasia. Hum Pathol 16:162, 1985.
14. Cesarman E, Knowles DM: Kaposi's sarcoma–associated herpesvirus: A lymphotropic human herpesvirus associated with Kaposi's sarcoma, primary effusion lymphoma, and multicentric Castleman's disease. Semin Diagn Pathol 14:54, 1997.
15. Oksenhendler E, Duarte M, Soulier J, et al: Multicentric Castleman's disease in HIV infection: A clinical and pathological study of 20 patients. AIDS 10:61, 1996.
16. Bitter MA, Komaiko W, Franklin WA: Giant lymph node hyperplasia with osteoblastic bone lesions and the POEMS (Takatsuki's) syndrome. Cancer 56:188, 1985.
17. Carbone A, Manconi R, Volpe R, et al: Immunohistochemical, enzyme histochemical, and immunologic features of giant lymph node hyperplasia of the hyaline-vascular type. Cancer 58:908, 1986.
18. Wychulis AR, Payne WS, Clagett OT, et al: Surgical treatment of mediastinal tumors. A 40-year experience. J Thorac Cardiovasc Surg 62:379, 1971.
19. Culver GJ, Choi BK: Benign lymphoid hyperplasia (Castleman's tumor) mimicking a posterior mediastinal neurogenic tumor. Chest 62:516, 1972.
20. Gibbons JA, Rosencrantz H, Posey DJ, et al: Angiofollicular lymphoid hyperplasia (Castleman's tumor) resembling a pericardial cyst: Differentiation by computerized tomography. Ann Thorac Surg 32:193, 1981.
21. Kim JH, Jun TG, Sung SW, et al: Giant lymph node hyperplasia (Castleman's disease) in the chest. Ann Thorac Surg 59:1162, 1995.
22. Moon WK, Im J-G, Kim JS, et al: Mediastinal Castleman disease: CT findings. J Comput Assist Tomogr 18:43, 1994.
22a. McAdams HP, Rosado-de-Christenson M, Fishback NF, Templeton PA: Castleman disease of the thorax: Radiologic features with clinical and histopathologic correlation. Radiology 209:221, 1998.
23. Barrie JR, English JC, Müller NL: Castleman's disease of the lung: Radiographic, high-resolution CT, and pathologic findings. Am J Roentgenol 166:1055, 1996.
24. Breatnach E, Myers JD, McElvein RB, et al: Unusual cause of a calcified anterior mediastinal mass. Chest 89:113, 1986.
25. Moon WK, Im J-G, Han MC: Castleman's disease of the mediastinum: MR imaging features. Clin Radiol 49:466, 1994.
26. Khan J, von Sinner W, Akhtar M, et al: Castleman's disease of the chest: Magnetic resonance imaging features. Chest 105:1608, 1994.
27. Samuels TH, Hamilton PA, Ngan B: Mediastinal Castleman's disease: Demonstration with computed tomography and angiography. Can Assoc Radiol J 41:380, 1990.
28. Glenner GG, Grimley PM: Atlas of Tumor Pathology: Second Series, Fascicle 9. Tumors of the extra-adrenal paraganglion system (including chemoreceptors). Washington, DC, Armed Forces Institute of Pathology, 1974.
29. Lamy AL, Fradet GJ, Luoma A, et al: Anterior and middle mediastinum paraganglioma: Complete resection is the treatment of choice. Ann Thorac Surg 57:249, 1994.
30. Lack EE, Stillinger RA, Colvin DB, et al: Aorticopulmonary paraganglioma. Report of a case with ultrastructural study and review of the literature. Cancer 43:269, 1979.
31. Odze R, Bégin LR: Malignant paraganglioma of the posterior mediastinum. Cancer 65:564, 1990.
32. Olson JL, Salyer WR: Mediastinal paraganglioma (aortic body tumor): A report of four cases and a review of the literature. Cancer 41:2405, 1978.
33. Moran CA, Suster S, Fishback N, et al: Mediastinal paragangliomas. A clinicopathologic and immunohistochemical study of 16 cases. Cancer 72:2358, 1993.
34. Wick MR, Simpson RW, Nichans GA, et al: Anterior mediastinal tumors: A clinicopathologic study of 100 cases, with emphasis on immunohistochemical analysis. Prog Surg Pathol 11:79, 1990.
35. Assaf HM, Al-Momen AA, Martin JG: Aorticopulmonary paraganglioma: A case report with immunohistochemical studies and literature review. Arch Pathol Lab Med 116:1085, 1992.
36. Moran CA, Albores-Saavedra J, Wenig BM, et al: Pigmented extraadrenal paragangliomas. A clinicopathologic and immunohistochemical study of five cases. Cancer 79:398, 1997.
37. Ros PR, Rosado-de-Christenson ML, Buetow PC, et al: The Radiological Society of North America 83rd Scientific Assembly and Annual Meeting. Image interpretation session: 1997. Radiographics 18:195, 1998.
38. Hamilton BH, Francis IR, Gross BH, et al: Intrapericardial paragangliomas (pheochromocytomas): Imaging features. Am J Roentgenol 168:109, 1997.
39. Ogawa J, Inoue H, Koide S, et al: Functioning paraganglioma in the posterior mediastinum. Ann Thorac Surg 33:507, 1982.
40. Drucker EA, McLoud TC, Dedrick CG, et al: Mediastinal paraganglioma: Radiologic evaluation of an unusual vascular tumor. Am J Roentgenol 148:521, 1987.
41. Bomanji J, Conry BG, Britton KE, et al: Imaging neural crest tumors with ^{123}I-meta-iodobenzylguanidine and x-ray computed tomography: A comparative study. Clin Radiol 39:502, 1988.
42. van Gils AP, Falke TA, van Erkel AR, et al: MR imaging and MIBG scintigraphy of pheochromocytomas and extra-adrenal functioning paragangliomas. RadioGraphics 11:37, 1991.
43. Kwekkeboom DJ, van Urk H, Pauw BK, et al: Octreotide scintigraphy for the detection of paragangliomas. J Nucl Med 34:873, 1993.
44. van Gelder T, Verhoeven GT, de Jong P, et al: Dopamine-producing paraganglioma not visualized by iodine-123-MIBG scintigraphy. J Nucl Med 36:620, 1995.
45. Rakower J, Milwidsky H: Primary mediastinal echinococcosis. Am J Med 29:73, 1960.
46. Hofmann-Wellenhof R, Domej W, Schmid C, et al: Mediastinal mass caused by syphilitic aortitis. Thorax 48:568, 1993.
47. Salyer DC, Salyer WR, Eggleston JC: Benign developmental cysts of the mediastinum. Arch Pathol Lab Med 101:136, 1977.
48. Reed JC, Sobonya RE: Morphologic analysis of foregut cysts in the thorax. Am J Roentgenol 120:851, 1974.
49. Snyder ME, Luck SR, Hernandez R, et al: Diagnostic dilemmas of mediastinal cysts. J Pediatr Surg 20:810, 1985.
50. Naidich DP, Rumancik WM, Ettenger NA, et al: Congenital anomalies of the lungs in adults: MR diagnosis. Am J Roentgenol 151:13, 1988.
51. Leigh TF: Mass lesions of the mediastinum. Radiol Clin North Am 1:377, 1963.
52. Sanders DE: Asymptomatic resorption of mediastinal cysts: A further report of two cases. J Can Assoc Radiol 20:239, 1969.
53. Rappaport DC, Herman SJ, Weisbrod GL: Congenital bronchopulmonary diseases in adults: CT findings. Am J Roentgenol 162:1295, 1994.
54. Kitano Y, Iwanaka T, Tsuchida Y, et al: Esophageal duplication cyst associated with pulmonary cystic malformations. J Pediatr Surg 30:1724, 1995.
55. Weiss LM, Fagelman D, Warhit JM: CT demonstration of an esophageal duplication cyst. J Comput Assist Tomogr 7:716, 1983.
56. Nakata H, Nakayama C, Kimoto T, et al: Computed tomography of mediastinal bronchogenic cysts. J Comput Assist Tomogr 6:733, 1982.
57. Mendelson DS, Rose JS, Efremidis SC, et al: Bronchogenic cysts with high CT numbers. Am J Roentgenol 140:463, 1983.
58. Kuhlman JE, Fishman EK, Wang KP, et al: Mediastinal cysts: Diagnosis by CT and needle aspiration. Am J Roentgenol 150:75, 1988.
59. Kawashima A, Fishman EK, Kuhlman JE, et al: CT of posterior mediastinal masses. RadioGraphics 11:1045, 1991.
60. Murayama S, Murakami J, Watanabe H, et al: Signal intensity characteristics of mediastinal cystic masses on T1-weighted MRI. J Comput Assist Tomogr 19:188, 1995.
61. Endo S, Sohara Y, Yamaguchi T, et al: The effectiveness of transesophageal ultrasonography in preoperatively diagnosing an esophageal cyst in a 75-year-old woman: Report of a case. Surg Today 24:356, 1994.
62. Bowton DL, Katz PO: Esophageal cyst as a cause of chronic cough. Chest 86:150, 1984.
63. Olsen JB, Clemmensen O, Andersen K: Adenocarcinoma arising in a foregut cyst of the mediastinum. Ann Thorac Surg 51:497, 1991.
64. Tapia RH, White VA: Squamous cell carcinoma arising in duplication cyst of the esophagus. Am J Gastroenterol 80:325, 1985.
65. Kirchner SG, Heller RM, Smith CN: Pancreatic pseudocyst of the mediastinum. Radiology 123:37, 1977.
66. Zeilender S, Turner MA, Glauser FL: Mediastinal pseudocyst associated with chronic pleural effusion. Chest 97:1014, 1990.
67. Sambrook Gowar FJ: Mediastinal thoracic duct cyst. Thorax 33:800, 1978.
68. Hori S, Harada K, Morimoto S, et al: Lymphangiographic demonstration of thoracic duct cyst. Chest 789:652, 1980.
69. Tsuchiya R, Sugiura Y, Ogata T, et al: Thoracic duct cyst of the mediastinum. J Thorac Cardiovasc Surg 79:856, 1980.
70. Wax MK, Treloar Me: Thoracic duct cyst: An unusual supraclavicular mass. Head Neck 14:502, 1992.

71. Mori M, Kidogawa H, Isoshima K: Thoracic duct cyst in the mediastinum. Thorax 47:325, 1992.

72. Fromang DR, Seltzer MB, Tobias JA: Thoracic duct cyst causing mediastinal compression and acute respiratory insufficiency. Chest 67:725, 1975.

73. Tsuchiya R, Sugiura Y, Ogata T, et al: Thoracic duct cyst of the mediastinum. J Thorac Cardiovasc Surg 79:856, 1980.

74. Hori S, Harada K, Morimoto S, et al: Lymphangiographic demonstration of thoracic duct cyst. Chest 78:652, 1980.

75. Morettin LB, Allen TE: Thoracic duct cyst: Diagnosis with needle aspiration. Radiology 161:437, 1986.

76. Buckingham WB, Sutton GC, Meszaros WT: Abnormalities of the pulmonary artery resembling intrathoracic neoplasms. Dis Chest 40:698, 1961.

77. Hom M, Jolles H: Traumatic mediastinal lymphocele mimicking other thoracic injuries: Case report. J Thorac Imaging 7:78, 1992.

78. Hoeffel JC, Pernot C, Worms AM, et al: Calcified aneurysm of the main pulmonary artery: A complication of banding. Radiology 113:167, 1974.

79. Shin MS, Ceballos R, Bini RM, et al: CT diagnosis of false aneurysm of the pulmonary artery not demonstrated by angiography. Case report. J Comput Assist Tomogr 7:524, 1983.

80. Befeler, MacLeod CA, Baum GL, et al: Idiopathic dilatation of the pulmonary artery. Am J Med Sci 254:667, 1967.

81. Kumar S, Murthy KV, Brandfonbrener M: Possible mechanism of wide splitting of second sound in idiopathic dilatation of the pulmonary artery. Chest 68:739, 1975.

82. Asayama J, Matsunra T, Endo N, et al: Echocardiographic findings of idiopathic dilatation of pulmonary artery. Chest 71:671, 1977.

83. Drasin E, Sayre RW, Castellino RA: Non-dilated superior vena cava presenting as a superior mediastinal mass. J Can Assoc Radiol 23:273, 1972.

84. Leigh TF, Weens HS: Roentgen aspects of mediastinal lesions. Semin Roentgenol 4:59, 1969.

85. Farr JE, Anderson WT, Brundage BH: Congenital aneurysm of the superior vena cava. Chest 65:566, 1974.

86. Okay NH, Bryk D, Kroop IG, et al: Phlebectasia of the jugular and great mediastinal veins. Radiology 95:6291, 1970.

87. Hidvegi RS, Modry DL, LaFléche L: Congenital saccular aneurysm of the superior vena cava: Radiographic features. Am J Roentgenol 133:924, 1979.

88. Mok CK, Chan CW, Clarke RT, et al: Coexisting congenital primary superior vena cava aneurysm and rheumatic mitral stenosis. Thorax 36:638, 1981.

89. Picou MA, Antonovic R, Holden WE: Position-dependent mediastinal mass: Aneurysm of the superior vena cava (letter). Am J Roentgenol 161:1110, 1993.

90. Vinnicombe S, Wilson AG, Morgan R, et al: Intravascular lipoma of the superior vena cava: CT features. J Comput Assist Tomogr 18:824, 1994.

91. Oh KS, Dorst JP, Haroutunian LM: Inferior vena caval varix. Radiology 109:161, 1973.

92. Mayo J, Gray R, St Louis E, et al: Anomalies of the inferior vena cava. Am J Roentgenol 140:339, 1983.

93. Jasinski RW, Yang C-F, Rubin JM: Vena cava anomalies simulating adenopathy on computed tomography. Case report. J Comput Assist Tomogr 5:921, 1981.

94. Alexander ES, Clark RA, Gross BH, et al: CT of congenital anomalies of the inferior vena cava. Comput Radiol 6:219, 1982.

95. Fleming JS, Gibson RV: Absent right superior vena cava as an isolated anomaly. Br J Radiol 37:696, 1964.

96. White CS, Baffa JM, Haney PJ, et al: MR imaging of congenital anomalies of the thoracic veins. RadioGraphics 17:595, 1997.

97. Webb WR, Gamsu G, Speckman JM, et al: Computed tomographic demonstration of mediastinal venous anomalies. Am J Roentgenol 139:157, 1982.

98. Kellman GM, Alpern MB, Sandler MA, et al: Computed tomography of vena caval anomalies with embryologic correlation. RadioGraphics 8:533, 1988.

99. Cormier MG, Yedlicka JW, Gray RJ, et al: Congenital anomalies of the superior vena cava: A CT study. Semin Roentgenol 24:77, 1989.

100. Voci P, Luzi G, Agati L: Diagnosis of persistent left superior vena cava by multiplane transesophageal echocardiography. Cardiologia 40:273, 1995.

101. Dillon EH, Camputaro C: Partial anomalous pulmonary venous drainage of the left upper lobe vs duplication of the superior vena cava: Distinction based on CT findings. Am J Roentgenol 160:375, 1993.

102. Escalante CP: Causes and management of superior vena cava syndrome. Oncology 7:61, 1993.

103. Lochridge SK, Knibbe WP, Doty DB: Obstruction of the superior vena cava. Surgery 85:14, 1979.

104. Schraufnagel DE, Hill R, Leech JA, et al: Superior vena caval obstruction: Is it a medical emergency? Am J Med 70:1169, 1981.

105. Davies PF, Shevland JE: Superior vena caval obstruction: An analysis of seventy-six cases, with comments on the safety of venography. Angiology 36:354, 1985.

106. Shimm DS, Logue GL, Rigsby LC: Evaluating the superior vena cava syndrome. JAMA 245:951, 1981.

107. Chan RH, Dar AR, Yu E, et al: Superior vena cava obstruction in small-cell lung cancer. Int J Radiat Oncol 38:513, 1997.

108. Gauden SJ: Superior vena cava syndrome induced by bronchogenic carcinoma: Is this an oncological emergency? Australas Radiol 37:363, 1993.

109. Spiro SG, Shah S, Harper PG, et al: Treatment of obstruction of the superior vena cava by combination chemotherapy with and without irradiation in small-cell carcinoma of the bronchus. Thorax 38:501, 1983.

110. Urban T, Lebeau B, Chastang C, et al: Superior vena cava syndrome in small-cell lung cancer. Arch Intern Med 153:384, 1993.

111. Kastner RJ, Fisher WG, Blacky AR, et al: Pacemaker-induced superior vena

cava syndrome with successful treatment by balloon venoplasty. Am J Cardiol 77:789, 1996.

112. Dhondt E, Hutse W, Vanmeerhaeghe X, et al: Superior vena cava syndrome after implantation of a transvenous cardioverter defibrillator. Eur Heart J 16:716, 1995.

113. Richmond G, Handwerger S, Schoenfeld N, et al: Superior vena cava syndrome: A complication of Hickman catheter insertion in patients with the acquired immunodeficiency syndrome. N Y State J Med 92:65, 1992.

114. Doty DB: Bypass of superior vena cava: 6 years' experience with spiral vein graft for obstruction of superior vena cava due to benign and malignant disease. J Thorac Cardiovasc Surg 83:326, 1982.

115. Brown G, Husband JE: Mediastinal widening: A valuable radiographic sign of superior vena cava thrombosis. Clin Radiol 47:415, 1993.

116. Engel IA, Auh YH, Rubenstein WA, et al: CT diagnosis of mediastinal and thoracic inlet venous obstruction. Am J Roentgenol 141:521, 1983.

117. Kim H-J, Kim HS, Chung SH: CT diagnosis of superior vena cava syndrome: Importance of collateral vessels. Am J Roentgenol 161:539, 1993.

118. Gosselin MV, Rubin GD: Altered intravascular contrast material flow dynamics: Clues for refining thoracic CT diagnosis. Am J Roentgenol 169:1597, 1997.

119. Weinreb JC, Mootz A, Cohen JM: MRI evaluation of mediastinal and thoracic inlet venous obstruction. Am J Roentgenol 146:679, 1986.

120. Morrissey B, Adams H, Gibbs AR, et al: Percutaneous needle biopsy of the mediastinum: Review of 94 procedures. Thorax 48:632, 1993.

121. Bressler EL, Kirkham JA: Mediastinal masses: Alternative approaches to CT-guided needle biopsy. Radiology 191:391, 1994.

122. Belfiore G, Camera L, Moggio G, et al: Middle mediastinum lesions: Preliminary experience with CT-guided fine-needle aspiration biopsy with a suprasternal approach. Radiology 202:870, 1997.

123. Ko JC, Yang PC, Yuan A, et al: Superior vena cava syndrome. Rapid histologic diagnosis by ultrasound-guided transthoracic needle aspiration biopsy. Am J Respir Crit Care Med 149:783, 1994.

124. Hirschmann JV, Raugi GJ: Dermatologic features of the superior vena cava syndrome. Arch Dermatol 128:953, 1992.

125. Forman JW, Unger KM: Unilateral superior vena caval syndrome. Thorax 35:314, 1980.

126. Bell DR, Woods RL, Levi JA: Superior vena caval obstruction: A 10-year experience. Med J Aust 145:566, 1986.

127. Wurschmidt F, Bunemann H, Heilmann HP: Small cell lung cancer with and without superior vena cava syndrome: A multivariate analysis of prognostic factors in 408 cases. Int J Radiat Oncol Biol Phys 33:77, 1995.

128. Stern WZ, Bloomberg AE: Idiopathic azygos phlebectasia simulating mediastinal tumor. Radiology 77:622, 1961.

129. Seebauer L, Prauer HW, Gmeinwieser J, et al: A mediastinal tumour simulated by a sacculated aneurysm of the azygos vein. Thorac Cardiovasc Surg 37:112, 1989.

130. Mehta M, Towers M: Computed tomography appearance of idiopathic aneurysm of the azygos vein. Can Assoc Radiol J 47:288, 1996.

131. Felson B: Chest Roentgenology. Philadelphia, WB Saunders, 1973.

132. Preger L, Hooper TI, Steinbach HL, et al: Width of azygos vein related to central venous pressures. Radiology 93:521, 1969.

133. Doyle FH, Read AE, Evans KT: The mediastinum in portal hypertension. Clin Radiol 12:114, 1961.

134. Pomeranz SJ, Proto AV: Tubular shadow in the lung. Chest 89:447, 1986.

135. Campbell HE, Baruch RJ: Aneurysm of hemiazygos vein associated with portal hypertension. Am J Roentgenol 83:1024, 1960.

136. Steinberg I: Dilatation of the hemiazygos veins in superior vena caval occlusion simulating mediastinal tumor. Am J Roentgenol 87:248, 1962.

137. Floyd GD, Nelson WP: Developmental interruption of the inferior vena cava with azygos and hemiazygos substitution. Unusual radiographic features. Radiology 119:55, 1976.

138. Rockoff SD, Druy EM: Tortuous azygos arch simulating a pulmonary lesion. Am J Roentgenol 138:577, 1982.

139. Allen HA, Haney PJ: Left-sided inferior vena cava with hemiazygos continuation. Case report. J Comput Assist Tomogr 5:917, 1981.

140. Breckenridge JW, Kinlaw WB: Azygos continuation of inferior vena cava: CT appearance. J Comput Assist Tomogr 4:392, 1980.

141. Petersen RW: Infrahepatic interruption of the inferior vena cava with azygos continuation (persistent right cardinal vein). Radiology 84:304, 1965.

142. Milledge RD: Absence of the inferior vena cava. Radiology 85:860, 1965.

143. Pacofsky KB, Wolfel DA: Azygos continuation of the inferior vena cava. Am J Roentgenol 113:362, 1971.

144. Berdon WE, Baker DH: Plain film findings in azygos continuation of the inferior vena cava. Am J Roentgenol 104:452, 1968.

145. Ball JB Jr, Proto AV: The variable appearance of the left superior intercostal vein. Radiology 144:445, 1982.

146. Friedman AC, Chambers E, Sprayregen S: The normal and abnormal left superior intercostal vein. Am J Roentgenol 131:599, 1978.

147. Hatfield MK, Vyborny CJ, MacMahon H, et al: Congenital absence of the azygos vein: A cause for "aortic nipple" enlargement. Am J Roentgenol 149:273, 1987.

148. Guthaner DF, Wexler L, Harell G: CT demonstration of cardiac structures. Am J Roentgenol 133:75, 1979.

149. Hirose Y, Hamade S, Takamiya M, et al: Aortic aneurysms: Growth rates measured with CT. Radiology 185:249, 1992.

150. Godwin JD: Conventional CT of the aorta. J Thorac Imaging 5:18, 1990.

151. Chen JTT: Plain radiographic evaluation of the aorta. J Thorac Imaging 5:1, 1990.

152. Posniak HV, Olson MC, Demos TC, et al: CT of thoracic aortic aneurysms. RadioGraphics 10:839, 1990.

153. McNamara JJ, Pressler VM: Natural history of arteriosclerotic thoracic aortic aneurysms. Ann Thorac Surg 26:468, 1978.
154. Pressler V, McNamara JJ: Thoracic aortic aneurysm: Natural history and treatment. J Thorac Cardiovasc Surg 79:489, 1980.
155. Moreno-Cabral CE, Miller DC, Mitchell RS, et al: Degenerative and atherosclerotic aneurysms of the thoracic aorta: Determinants of early and late surgical outcome. J Thorac Cardiovasc Surg 88:1020, 1984.
156. Frist WH, Miller DC: Aneurysms of ascending thoracic aorta and transverse aortic arch. Cardiovasc Clin 17:263, 1987.
157. Johansen K, Devin J: Mycotic aortic aneurysms: A reappraisal. Arch Surg 118:583, 1983.
158. Heystraten FM, Rosenbusch G, Kingma LM, et al: Chronic posttraumatic aneurysm of the thoracic aorta: Surgically correctable occult threat. Am J Roentgenol 146:303, 1986.
159. Mirvis SE, Shanmuganathan K, Miller BH, et al: Traumatic aortic injury: Diagnosis with contrast-enhanced thoracic CT—five-year experience at a major trauma center. Radiology 200:413, 1996.
160. Gavant ML, Flick P, Menke P, et al: CT aortography of thoracic aortic rupture. Am J Roentgenol 166:955, 1996.
161. Felson B, Akers PV, Hall GS, et al: Mycotic tuberculous aneurysm of the thoracic aorta. JAMA 237:1104, 1977.
162. Adachi H, Ino T, Mizuhara A, et al: Assessment of aortic disease using three-dimensional CT angiography. J Card Surg 9:673, 1994.
163. Chung JW, Park JH, Im J-G, et al: Spiral CT angiography of the thoracic aorta. RadioGraphics 16:811, 1996.
164. Dinsmore RE, Liberthson RR, Wismer GL, et al: Magnetic resonance imaging of thoracic aortic aneurysms: comparison with other imaging methods. Am J Roentgenol 146:309, 1986.
165. Link KM, Lesko NM: The role of MR imaging in the evaluation of acquired diseases of the thoracic aorta. Am J Roentgenol 158:1115, 1992.
165a. Alley MT, Shifrin RY, Pelc NJ, Herfkens RJ: Ultrafast contrast-enhanced three-dimensional MR angiography: State-of-the-art. Radiographics 18:273, 1998.
165b. Ho VB, Prince MR: Thoracic MR aortography: Imaging techniques and strategies. Radiographics 18:287, 1998.
166. Kamp O, van Rossum AC, Torenbeek R: Transesophageal echocardiography and magnetic resonance imaging for the assessment of saccular aneurysm of the transverse thoracic aorta. Int J Cardiol 33:330, 1991.
167. Cramer M, Foley WD, Palmer TE, et al: Compression of the right pulmonary artery by aortic aneurysms: CT demonstration. J Comput Assist Tomogr 9:310, 1985.
168. Duke RA, Barrett MR, Payne SD, et al: Compression of left main bronchus and left pulmonary artery by thoracic aortic aneurysm. Am J Roentgenol 149:261, 1987.
169. Heiberg E, Wolverson MK, Sundaram M, et al: CT characteristics of aortic atherosclerotic aneurysm versus aortic dissection. J Comput Assist Tomogr 9:78, 1985.
170. Birnholz JC, Ferrucci JT, Wyman SM: Roentgen features of dysphagia aortica. Radiology 111:93, 1974.
171. Charrette EJ, Winton TL, Salerno TA: Acute respiratory insufficiency from an aneurysm of the descending thoracic aorta. J Thorac Cardiovasc Surg 85:467, 1983.
172. Conti VR, Calverley J, Safley WL, et al: Anterior spinal artery syndrome with chronic traumatic thoracic aortic aneurysm. Ann Thorac Surg 33:81, 1982.
173. Schlatmann TJ, Becker AE: Pathogenesis of dissection aneurysm of aorta. Am J Cardiol 39:21, 1977.
174. Wilson SK, Hutchins GM: Aortic dissecting aneurysms: causative factors in 204 subjects. Arch Pathol Lab Med 106:175, 1982.
175. Fisher ER, Stern EJ, Godwin JD: Acute aortic dissection: Typical and atypical imaging features. RadioGraphics 14:1263, 1994.
176. Roberts WC: Aortic dissection: Anatomy, consequences, and causes. Am Heart J 101:195, 1981.
177. Godwin JD, Breiman RS, Speckman JM: Problems and pitfalls in the evaluation of thoracic aortic dissection by computed tomography. J Comput Assist Tomogr 6:750, 1982.
178. Yamada T, Tada S, Harada J: Aortic dissection without intimal rupture: Diagnosis with MR imaging and CT. Radiology 168:347, 1988.
179. Hirst AE Jr, Johns VJ Jr, Kime SW Jr: Dissecting aneurysm of the aorta: A review of 505 cases. Medicine 37:217, 1958.
180. Wolff KA, Herold CJ, Tempany CM, et al: Aortic dissection: Atypical patterns seen at MR imaging. Radiology 181:489, 1991.
181. Nienaber CA, von Kodolitsch Y, Nicolas V, et al: The diagnosis of thoracic aortic dissection by noninvasive imaging procedures. N Engl J Med 328:1, 1993.
182. DeBakey ME, McCollum H, Crawford ES, et al: Dissection and dissecting aneurysms of the aorta: Twenty-year follow-up of five hundred twenty-seven patients treated surgically. Surgery 92:1118, 1982.
183. Petasnick JP: Radiologic evaluation of aortic dissection. Radiology 180:297, 1991.
184. Sakamoto I, Hayashi K, Matsunaga N, et al: Aortic dissection caused by angiographic procedures. Radiology 191:467, 1994.
185. Beachley MC, Ranniger K, Roth FJ: Roentgenographic evaluation of dissecting aneurysms of the aorta. Am J Roentgenol 121:617, 1974.
186. Beachley MC, Ranniger K, Roth FJ: Roentgenographic evaluation of dissecting aneurysms of the aorta. Am J Roentgenol 121:617, 1974.
187. Earnest FIV, Muhm JR, Sheedy PF II: Roentgenographic findings in thoracic aortic dissection. Mayo Clin Proc 54:43, 1979.
188. Demos TC, Posniak HV, Marsan RE: CT of aortic dissection. Semin Roentgenol 24:22, 1989.
189. Luker GD, Glazer HS, Eagar G, et al: Aortic dissection: Effect of prospective chest radiographic diagnosis on delay to definitive diagnosis. Radiology 193:813, 1994.
190. Vasile N, Mathieu D, Keita K, et al: Computed tomography of thoracic aortic dissection: Accuracy and pitfalls. J Comput Assist Tomogr 10:211, 1986.
191. Thorsen MK, San Dretto MA, Lawson TL, et al: Dissecting aortic aneurysms: Accuracy of computed tomographic diagnosis. Radiology 148:773, 1983.
192. White RD, Lipton MJ, Higgins CB, et al: Noninvasive evaluation of suspected thoracic aortic disease by contrast-enhanced computed tomography. Am J Cardiol 57:282, 1986.
193. Sommer T, Fehske W, Holzknecht N, et al: Aortic dissection: A comparative study of diagnosis with spiral CT, multiplanar transesophageal echocardiography, and MR imaging. Radiology 199:347, 1996.
194. Heiberg E, Wolverson MK, Sundaram M, et al: CT characteristics of aortic atherosclerotic aneurysm versus aortic dissection. J Comput Assist Tomogr 9:78, 1985.
195. Torres WE, Maurer DE, Steinberg HV, et al: CT of aortic aneurysms: The distinction between mural and thrombus calcification. Am J Roentgenol 150:1317, 1988.
196. Heiberg E, Wolverson M, Sundaram M, et al: CT findings in aortic dissection. Am J Roentgenol 136:13, 1981.
197. DeSanctis RW, Doroghazi RM, Austen WG, et al: Aortic dissection. N Engl J Med 317:1060, 1987.
198. Cigarroa JE, Isselbacher EM, DeSanctis RW, et al: Medical progress. Diagnostic imaging in the evaluation of suspected aortic dissection: Old standards and new directions. Am J Roentgenol 161:485, 1993.
199. Shuford WH, Sybers RG, Weens HS: Problems in the aortographic diagnosis of dissecting aneurysm of the aorta. N Engl J Med 280:225, 1969.
200. Wilbers CRH, Carrol CL, Hnilica MA: Optimal diagnostic imaging of aortic dissection. Tex Heart Inst J 17:271, 1990.
201. Eagle KA, DeSanctis RW: Aortic dissection. Current Prob Cardiol 14:225, 1989.
202. O'Donovan TPB, Osmundson PJ, Payne WS: Painless dissecting aneurysm of the aorta. Report of a case. Circulation 29:782, 1964.
203. Wheat MW: Treatment of dissecting aneurysms of the aorta: Current status. Prog Cardiovasc Dis 16:87, 1973.
204. Williams DM, LePage MA, Lee DY: The dissected aorta: Part I. Early anatomic changes in an in vitro model. Radiology 203:23, 1997.
205. Crawford ES, Svensson LG, Coselli JS, et al: Aortic dissection and dissecting aortic aneurysms. Ann Surg 208:254, 1988.
206. Green RA: Enlargement of the innominate and subclavian arteries simulating mediastinal neoplasm. Am Rev Tuberc 79:790, 1959.
207. Schneider HJ, Felson B: Buckling of the innominate artery simulating aneurysm and tumor. Am J Roentgenol 85:1106, 1961.
208. Christensen EE, Landay MJ, Dietz GW, et al: Buckling of the innominate artery simulating a right apical lung mass. Am J Roentgenol 131:119, 1978.
209. Tamaki M, Tanabe H, Kamiuchi H, et al: Buckling of the distal innominate artery simulating a nodular lung mass. Chest 83:829, 1983.
210. Christensen EE, Landay MJ, Dietz GW, et al: Buckling of the innominate artery simulating a right apical lung mass. Am J Roentgenol 131:119, 1978.
211. Rong SH: Carotid pseudoaneurysm simulating Pancoast's tumor. Am J Roentgenol 142:495, 1984.
212. Sandler CM, Toombs BD, Lester RG: Buckling of the left common carotid artery simulating mediastinal neoplasm. Am J Roentgenol 133:312, 1979.
213. Hallman GL, Cooley DA: Congenital aortic vascular ring. Surgical considerations. Arch Surg 88:666, 1964.
214. Lam CR, Kabbani S, Arciniegas E: Symptomatic anomalies of the aortic arch. Surg Gynecol Obstet 147:673, 1978.
215. Idbeis B, Levinsky L, Srinivasan V, et al: Vascular rings: Management and a proposed nomenclature. Ann Thorac Surg 31:255, 1981.
216. Engelman RM, Madayag M: Aberrant right subclavian artery aneurysm: A rare cause of a superior mediastinal tumor. Chest 62:45, 1972.
217. Van Son JA, Julsrud PR, Hagler DJ, et al: Imaging strategies for vascular rings. Ann Thorac Surg 57:604, 1994.
218. VanDyke CW, White RD: Congenital abnormalities of the thoracic aorta presenting in the adult. J Thorac Imaging 9:230, 1994.
219. Soto B, Shin MS, Papapietro SE: Nonobstructive coarctation. Cardiovasc Radiol 2:231, 1979.
220. Gaupp RJ, Fagan CJ, Davis M, et al: Pseudocoarctation of the aorta. Case report. J Comput Assist Tomogr 5:571, 1981.
221. Moncada R, Shannon R, Miller R, et al: The cervical aortic arch. Am J Roentgenol 125:591, 1975.
222. Kennard DR, Spigos DG, Tan WS: Cervical aortic arch: CT correlation with conventional radiologic studies. Am J Roentgenol 141:295, 1983.
223. Salomonowitz E, Edwards JE, Hunter DW, et al: The three types of aortic diverticula. Am J Roentgenol 142:673, 1984.
224. Shuford WH, Sybers RG, Edwards FK: The three types of right aortic arch. Am J Roentgenol 109:67, 1970.
225. Raymond GS, Miller RM, Müller NL, Logan PM. Congenital thoracic lesions that mimic neoplastic disease on chest radiographs of adults. Am J Roentgenol 168:763, 1997.
226. Bevelaqua F, Schicchi JS, Haas F, et al: Aortic arch anomaly presenting as exercise-induced asthma. Am Rev Respir Dis 140:805, 1989.
227. Branscom JJ, Austin JHM: Aberrant right subclavian artery: Findings seen on plain chest roentgenograms. Am J Roentgenol 119:539, 1973.

228. Kommerell B: Verlagerung des Oesophagus durch eine abnorm verlaufende Arteria subclavia dextra (Arteria lusoria). Fortschr Geb Rontgenstr Nuklearmed 54:590, 1936.

229. Lindell MM Jr, Hill CA, Libshitz HI: Esophageal cancer: Radiographic chest findings and their prognostic significance. Am J Roentgenol 133:461, 1979.

230. Daffner RH, Postlethwait RW, Putman CE: Retrotracheal abnormalities in esophageal carcinoma: Prognostic implications. Am J Roentgenol 130:719, 1978.

231. Yrjana J: The posterior tracheal band and recurrent esophageal carcinoma. Radiology 146:433, 1983.

232. Wolfman NT, Scharling ES, Chen MYM: Esophageal squamous carcinoma. Radiol Clin North Am 32:1183, 1994.

233. Levine MS: Esophageal cancer: Radiologic diagnosis. Radiol Clin North Am 35:265, 1997.

234. Quint LE, Glazer GM, Orringer MB, et al: Esophageal carcinoma: CT findings. Radiology 155:171, 1985.

235. Reinig JW, Stanley JH, Schabel SI: CT evaluation of thickened esophageal walls. Am J Roentgenol 140:931, 1983.

236. Rankin S, Mason R: Staging of oesophageal carcinoma. Clin Radiol 46:373, 1992.

237. Picus D Balfe DM, Koehler RE, et al: Computed tomography in the staging of esophageal carcinoma. Radiology 146:433, 1983.

238. Thompson WM, Halvorsen RA, Foster WL Jr, et al: Computed tomography for staging esophageal and gastroesophageal cancer: Reevaluation. Am J Roentgenol 141:951, 1983.

239. Botet JF, Lightdale CJ, Zauber AG, et al: Preoperative staging of esophageal cancer: Comparison of endoscopic US and dynamic CT. Radiology 181:419, 1991.

240. Noh HM, Fishman EK, Forastiere AA, et al: CT of the esophagus: Spectrum of disease with emphasis on esophageal carcinoma. RadioGraphics 15:1113, 1995.

241. Vilgrain V, Mompoint D, Palazzo L, et al: Staging of esophageal carcinoma: Comparison of results with endoscopic sonography and CT. Am J Roentgenol 155:277, 1990.

242. Botet JF, Lightdale CJ, Zauber AG, et al: Preoperative staging of esophageal cancer: Comparison of endoscopic US and dynamic CT. Radiology 181:419, 1991.

243. Sharma OP, Chandermohan M, Mashankar AS, et al: Role of computed tomography in preoperative evaluation of esophageal carcinoma. Indian J Cancer 31:12, 1994.

244. Maerz LL, Deveney CW, Lopez RR, et al: Role of computed tomographic scans in the staging of esophageal and proximal gastric malignancies. Am J Surg 165:558, 1993.

245. Heintz A, Höhne U, Schweden F, et al: Preoperative detection of intrathoracic tumor spread of esophageal cancer. Endosonography versus computed tomography. Surg Endosc 5:75, 1991.

246. Armengol Miro JR, Benjamin S, Binmoeller K, et al: Clinical applications of endoscopic ultrasonography in gastroenterology: State of the art 1993. Results of a Consensus Conference, Orlando, Florida, 19 January 1993. Endoscopy 25:358, 1993.

247. Takashima S, Takeuchi N, Shiozaki H, et al: Carcinoma of the esophagus: CT vs MR imaging in determining resectability. Am J Roentgenol 156:297, 1991.

248. Thompson WM, Halvorsen RA Jr: Staging esophageal carcinoma II: CT and MRI. Semin Oncol 21:447, 1994.

248a. Rankin SC, Taylor H, Cook GJR, Mason R: Computed tomography and positron emission tomography in the pre-operative staging of oesophageal carcinoma. Clin Radiol 53:659, 1998.

249. Rainer WG, Brus R: Leiomyosarcoma of the esophagus. Surgery 58:343, 1965.

250. Choh JH, Khazei AH, Ihm HJ: Leiomyosarcoma of the esophagus: Report of a case and review of the literature. J Surg Oncol 32:223, 1986.

251. Levine MS, Buck JL, Pantongrag-Brown L, et al: Leiomyosarcoma of the esophagus: Radiographic findings in 10 patients. Am J Roentgenol 167:27, 1996.

252. Cohen AM, Cunat JS: Giant esophageal leiomyoma as a mediastinal mass. J Can Assoc Radiol 32:129, 1981.

253. Daniel RA Jr, Diveley WL, Edwards WH, et al: Mediastinal tumors. Ann Surg 151:783, 1960.

254. Godard JE, McCranie D: Multiple leiomyomas of the esophagus. Am J Roentgenol 117:259, 1973.

255. Glazer HS, Wick MR, Anderson DJ, et al: CT of fatty thoracic masses. Am J Roentgenol 159:1181, 1992.

256. Stemermen DH, Mercader V, Kramer G, et al: An unusual presentation of Zenker's diverticulum. Clin Imaging 20:112, 1996.

257. Jalundhwala JM, Shah RC: Epiphrenic esophageal diverticulum. Chest 57:97, 1970.

258. Montgomery RD, Mendl K, Stephenson SF: Intramural diverticulosis of the oesophagus. Thorax 30:278, 1975.

259. Tishler JM, Shin MS, Stanley RJ, et al: CT of the thorax in patients with achalasia. Dig Dis Sci 28:692, 1983.

260. Rabushka LS, Fishman EK, Kuhlman JE: CT evaluation of achalasia. J Comput Assist Tomogr 15:434, 1991.

261. Blomquist G, Mahoney PS: Noncollapsing air-filled esophagus in diseased and postoperative chests. Acta Radiol 55:32, 1961.

262. Schabel SI, Stanley JH: Air esophagram after laryngectomy. Am J Roentgenol 136:19, 1981.

263. McLean RDW, Stewart CJ, Whyte DGC: Acute thoracic inlet obstruction in achalasia of the oesophagus. Thorax 31:456, 1976.

264. Giustra PE, Killoran PJ, Wasgatt WN: Acute stridor in achalasia of the esophagus (cardiospasm). Am J Gastroenterol 60:160, 1973.

265. Grant DM, Thompson GE: Diagnosis of congenital tracheoesophageal fistula in the adolescent and adult. Anesthesiology 49:139, 1978.

266. Osinowo O, Harley HR, Janigan D: Congenital broncho-oesophageal fistula in the adult. Thorax 38:138, 1983.

267. Fitzgerald RH, Bartles DM, Parker EF: Tracheoesophageal fistulas secondary to carcinoma of the esophagus. J Thorac Cardiovasc Surg 82:194, 1981.

268. Little AG, Ferguson MK, DeMeester TR, et al: Esophageal carcinoma with respiratory tract fistula. Cancer 53:1322, 1984.

269. Symbas PN, McKeown PP, Hatcher CR Jr, et al: Tracheoesophageal fistula from carcinoma of the esophagus. Ann Thorac Surg 38:382, 1984.

270. Keszler P, Buzna E: Surgical and conservative management of esophageal perforation. Chest 80:158, 1981.

271. Hjelms E, Jensen H, Lindewald H: Nonmalignant oesophagobronchial fistula. Eur J Respir Dis 63:351, 1982.

272. Hilgenberg AD, Grillo MC: Acquired nonmalignant tracheoesophageal fistula. J Thorac Cardiovasc Surg 85:492, 1983.

273. Leeds WM, Morley TF, Zappasodi SJ, et al: Computed tomography for diagnosis of tracheoesophageal fistula. Crit Care Med 14:591, 1986.

274. Moult PJA, Waite DW, Dick W: Posterior mediastinal venous masses in patients with portal hypertension. Gut 16:57, 1975.

275. Ishikawa T, Saeki M, Tsukune Y, et al: Detection of paraesophageal varices by plain films. Am J Roentgenol 144:701, 1985.

275a. Lee SJ, Lee KS, Kim SA, et al: Computed radiography of the chest in patients with paraesophageal varices: Diagnostic accuracy and characteristic findings. Am J Roentgenol 170:1527, 1998.

276. Arakawa A, Nagata Y, Miyagi S, et al: Case report: Interruption of inferior vena cava with anomalous continuations. J Comput Tomogr 11:341, 1987.

277. Minami M, Kawauchi N, Itai Y, et al: Transdiaphragmatic portosystemic shunt to the pericardiacophrenic vein. Am J Roentgenol 161:569, 1993.

278. Wachsberg RH, Yaghmai V, Javors BR, et al: Cardiophrenic varices in portal hypertension: Evaluation with CT. Radiology 195:553, 1995.

278a. Ibukuro K, Tsukiyama T, Mori K, Inoue Y: Preaortic esophageal veins: CT appearance. Am J Roentgenol 170:1535, 1998.

279. Saks BJ, Kilbey AE, Dietrich PA, et al: Pleural and mediastinal changes following endoscopic injection sclerotherapy of esophageal varices. Radiology 149:639, 1983.

280. Reddy SC: Esophagopleural fistula. J Comput Assist Tomogr 7:376, 1983.

281. Phillips PL, Amberson JB, Libby DM: Syphilitic aortic aneurysm presenting with the superior vena cava syndrome. Am J Med 71:171, 1981.

282. Harbecke RG, Schlueter DP, Rosenzweig DY: Reversible superior vena caval syndrome due to tuberculosis. Thorax 34:410, 1979.

283. Seetharaman ML, Bahadur P, Shrinivas V, et al: Filarial mediastinal lymphadenitis. Another cause of superior vena caval syndrome. Chest 94:871, 1988.

284. Maggiano HJ, Higgins TL, Lobo W, et al: Superior vena cava syndrome after open heart surgery. Cleve Clin J Med 59:93, 1992.

285. Biswal BM, Sandhu MS, Mohanti BK, et al: Carcinoma of the uterine cervix presenting as superior vena cava syndrome: Report of three cases and a review of literature. J Obstet Gynecol 21:437, 1995.

286. Montalban C, Moreno MA, Molina JP, et al: Metastatic carcinoma of the prostate presenting as a superior vena cava syndrome. Chest 104:1278, 1993.

287. Venegas RJ, Sun NCJ: Cardiac tamponade as a presentation of malignant thymoma. Acta Cytol 32:257, 1988.

288. Shishido M, Yano K, Ichiki H, et al: Pericarditis as the initial manifestation of malignant thymoma. Disappearance of pericardial effusion with corticosteroid therapy. Chest 106:313, 1994.

289. Attal H, Jensen J, Reyes CV: Myxoid liposarcoma of the anterior mediastinum. Diagnosis by fine needle aspiration biopsy. Acta Cytol 39:511, 1995.

290. Dingerkus H, Voller H, Albrecht A, et al: Mediastinal chloroma affecting the right heart with superior vena cava syndrome. Am Heart J 127:465, 1994.

291. Rutegard J, Granstrand M, Aberg T: Intracaval paraganglioma causing superior vena cava syndrome. Eur J Cardiothorac Surg 6:337, 1992.

292. Lazzarino M, Orlandi E, Paulli M, et al: Primary mediastinal B-cell lymphoma with sclerosis: An aggressive tumor with distinctive clinical and pathologic features. J Clin Oncol 11:2306, 1993.

293. Varma S, Varma N, Dhar S, et al: Cytodiagnosis of granulocytic sarcoma presenting as superior vena cava syndrome in acute myeloblastic leukemia. A case report. Acta Cytol 36:371, 1992.

294. McKellar DP, Verazin GT, Lim KM, et al: Superior vena cava syndrome and tracheal obstruction due to multinodular goiter. Head Neck 16:72, 1994.

295. Hershey CO, McVeigh RC, Miller RP: Transient superior vena cava syndrome due to propylthiouracil therapy in intrathoracic goiter. Chest 79:356, 1981.

296. Ishihara T, Kurahachi H, Hattori N, et al: Superior vena cava syndrome due to Graves' disease. Intern Med 32:80, 1993.

297. Sumiyoshi Y, Kikuchi M: Leiomyosarcoma of the superior vena cava producing superior vena cava syndrome and heart tamponade. Pathol Int 45:691, 1995.

298. Downes AJ, Jones TJ, Wilson RS: Intimal sarcoma of the superior vena cava. Postgrad Med J 69:155, 1993.

299. Abulafia O, Sherer DM: Recurrent transient superior vena cava–like syndrome possibly associated with megestrol acetate. Obstet Gynecol 85:899, 1995.

300. McFarland JJ, Kahn MB, Bellows CF, et al: Superior vena cava syndrome caused by aneurysm of the innominate artery. Ann Thorac Surg 59:227, 1995.

301. Cave EM, Virdi IS, Ruttley MS: Case report: An unusual case of the superior vena cava syndrome—aneurysm of an aberrant right subclavian artery. Clin Radiol 49:834, 1994.

302. Rosenzweig BP, Kronzon I: Transesophageal echocardiographic diagnosis of the

superior vena cava syndrome resulting from aortic dissection: A multiplane study. J Am Soc Echocardiogr 7:414, 1994.

303. Link MS, Pietrzak MP: Aortic dissection presenting as superior vena cava syndrome. Am J Emerg Med 12:326, 1994.

304. Seelig MH, Oldenburg WA, Klingler PJ, et al: Superior vena cava syndrome caused by chronic hemodialysis catheters: Autologous reconstruction with a pericardial tube graft. J Vasc Surg 28:556, 1998.

305. Razzouk A, Gundry S, Wang N, et al: Pseudoaneurysms of the aorta after cardiac surgery or chest trauma. Am Surg 59:818, 1993.

306. Lee Y, Doering R, Jihayel A: Radiation-induced superior vena cava syndrome. Tex Heart Inst J 22:103, 1995.

307. Nemoto T, Terada Y, Matsunobe S, et al: Superior vena cava syndrome caused by a right apical tense bulla. Chest 105:611, 1994.

308. McPherson JG III, Yeoh CB: Rare manifestations of sarcoidosis. J Natl Med Assoc 85:869, 1993.

309. Mogul M, Hartman G, Donaldson S, et al: Langerhans' cell histiocytosis presenting with the superior vena cava syndrome: A case report. Med Pediatr Oncol 21:456, 1993.

310. Thomas I, Helmold ME, Nychay S: Behçet's disease presenting as superior vena cava syndrome. J Am Acad Dermatol 26:863, 1992.

311. Blendis LM, Laws JW, Williams R, et al: Calcified collateral veins and gross dilatation of the azygos vein in cirrhosis. Br J Radiol 41:909, 1968.

312. Wu M-T, Pan H-B, Chen C, et al: Azygos blood flow in cirrhosis: Measurement with MR imaging and correlation with variceal hemorrhage. Radiology 198:457, 1996.

313. Milner LB, Marchan R: Complete absence of the inferior vena cava presenting as a paraspinous mass. Thorax 35:798, 1980.

314. Schneeweiss A, Bleiden LC, Deutsch V, et al: Uninterrupted inferior vena cava with azygos continuation. Chest 80:114, 1981.

315. Van der Horst RL, Hastreiter AR: Congenital interruption of the inferior vena cava. Chest 80:638, 1981.

CHAPTER 76

Masses Situated Predominantly in the Paravertebral Region

As discussed in Chapter 74, the paravertebral region is bounded in the front by the anterior surface of the vertebral column and in the back by the chest wall. It is in a sense almost a potential space, because it normally contains only a small amount of connective tissue, blood vessels, the sympathetic nerve chains, and peripheral nerves. However, neoplasms that originate in the last two structures as well as abnormalities related to the spinal canal can expand to present as masses in this region. Although herniation of abdominal contents through a posterior diaphragmatic defect and infectious, traumatic, or neoplastic diseases of the thoracic spine also can be manifested by a paravertebral mass, for convenience these are discussed elsewhere (*see* pages 2997 and 3020).

TUMORS AND TUMOR-LIKE CONDITIONS OF NEURAL TISSUE

Neoplasms of neural tissue account for about 20% of all primary "mediastinal" neoplasms in adults[1-3] and as many as 35% in children;[3] they are by far the most common type in the paravertebral compartment.[2, 4] From a histogenetic point of view, there are two basic types: those arising from the peripheral nerves and those originating from sympathetic ganglia.

Tumors Arising from Peripheral Nerves

The vast majority of neural tumors that arise in the thorax originate in an intercostal nerve in the paravertebral region. Neoplasms arising from other nerves, including the vagus and phrenic nerves and small unnamed branches, are rare.[5, 6] The etiology of most tumors is unknown; however, some have been associated with a history of irradiation[7] and others with neurofibromatosis. Malignant tumors are particularly likely to be seen in patients who have the latter condition.[8]

Several histologic forms can be seen, including neurilemoma (schwannoma), neurofibroma (both plexiform and non-plexiform types), neurogenic sarcoma (malignant schwannoma), and peripheral primitive neuroectodermal tumor; neurilemoma is the most common. The majority of neurilemomas and neurofibromas are encapsulated, more or less spherical masses that expand into the paravertebral space; some tumors extend through a spinal foramen and grow in a dumbbell fashion in both spinal canal and paravertebral region—a feature that has been noted in as many as 10% of cases in some series.[9] Although malignant tumors can show invasion of contiguous structures at the time of diagnosis, they also can be encapsulated.

Histologically, neurofibromas are somewhat variable in appearance and consist of a mixture of spindle cells, myxoid stroma, and mature collagen. Neurilemomas are composed of spindle cells arranged in either a relatively compact and orderly architecture (so-called Antoni A pattern) or more haphazardly in a loose myxomatous stroma (Antoni B pattern). As might be expected, neurogenic sarcomas tend to show features that are usually associated with malignancy, such as nuclear atypia, necrosis, and mitotic activity; nevertheless, histologic distinction between benign and malignant forms can be difficult in some cases. Sarcomas should not be confused with the cellular form of benign schwannoma, which can show considerable nuclear atypia and has been reported to have a predilection for the posterior mediastinum.[10] Peripheral primitive neuroectodermal tumor (Askin's tumor) is composed of small cells with scanty cytoplasm similar to those of Ewing's sarcoma (*see* page 3028).[11]

In most cases, neurilemomas and neurofibromas are manifested radiographically as sharply defined round, smooth or lobulated paraspinal masses.[12, 13] They typically span only one or two posterior rib interspaces but can become quite large.[12, 13] In approximately 50% of cases, they are associated with bony abnormalities such as expansion of the neural foramina, erosion of the vertebral bodies, and erosion or deformity of the ribs.[13] On computed tomography

(CT) scans, both forms of tumor can have homogeneous or heterogeneous attenuation; in the majority of cases, attenuation is slightly lower than that of chest wall muscle (Fig. 76–1).[13-15] Tumors usually show heterogeneous enhancement following intravenous administration of contrast medium (Fig. 76–2),[13-16] a feature related to the presence of lipid within myelin and to areas of hypocellularity, cystic degeneration, or hemorrhage.[13-15] Punctate foci of calcification are seen in 10% of cases.[15] A plexiform neurofibroma may be manifested on CT scans as a mass that has poorly defined margins and diffusely infiltrates the mediastinum along the distribution of the sympathetic chains and various large nerves (including the phrenic, recurrent laryngeal, and vagus nerves).[17] On magnetic resonance (MR) imaging scans, schwannomas and neurofibromas have low to intermediate signal intensity on T1-weighted images and focal areas with intermediate to high signal intensity on T2-weighted images (Fig. 76–3).[18] The procedure is particularly helpful in determining the nerve of origin for tumors in the thoracic inlet.[18a]

Neurogenic sarcomas usually present radiographically as round masses greater than 5 cm in diameter.[13, 19] CT typically demonstrates areas of low attenuation related to hemorrhage and necrosis.[13, 20] The tumors may have either well-defined smooth margins[13, 20] or poorly defined margins due to infiltration of the chest wall or adjacent mediastinal structures.[13-15] Calcification is evident in some cases.[13]

Most tumors are discovered in young adults. Many do not cause symptoms and are discovered on a screening chest radiograph; for example, in one series of 49 patients, 32 (65%) were asymptomatic.[21] In some patients, compression of intercostal nerves, proximal airways, or superior vena cava gives rise to pain or dyspnea;[2, 4, 22] associated neurologic signs are not uncommon in such circumstances.[2, 4] As might be expected, signs and symptoms are more frequent in patients who have malignant tumors.[3]

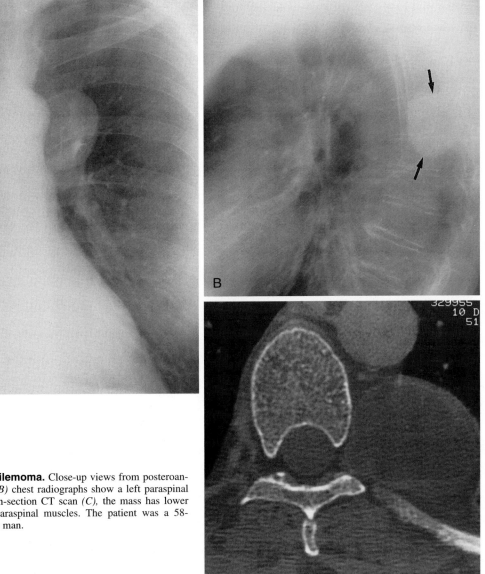

Figure 76–1. Neurilemoma. Close-up views from posteroanterior *(A)* and lateral *(B)* chest radiographs show a left paraspinal mass *(arrows)*. On thin-section CT scan *(C)*, the mass has lower attenuation than the paraspinal muscles. The patient was a 58-year-old asymptomatic man.

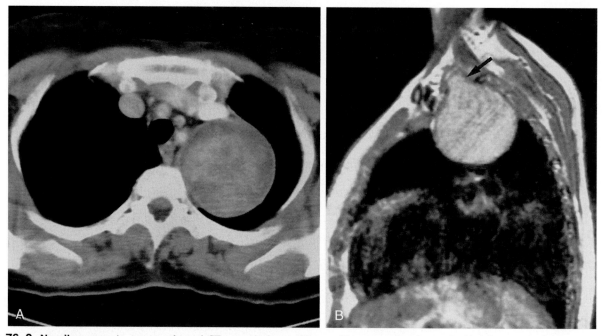

Figure 76–2. Neurilemoma. A contrast-enhanced CT scan *(A)* from a 39-year-old woman who presented with left arm pain demonstrates a sharply marginated mass in the left upper chest. The mass has inhomogeneous attenuation, a finding commonly seen in neurogenic tumors. A sagittal MR image (TR 1700, TE 30) *(B)* demonstrates that the mass has a pedicle *(arrow)* extending to the brachial plexus. At surgery, a neurilemoma was found to arise from the left T1 nerve root.

The majority of tumors are benign, only about 5% to 25% having pathologic or clinical features of malignancy.[1, 2, 8, 23, 24] Provided complete surgical excision can be achieved, the prognosis associated with the former group is excellent. By contrast, malignant neoplasms are typically aggressive and not uncommonly associated with hematogenous metastases, usually to the lungs.[13, 14] In one review of 40 patients who had malignant schwannoma, 29 (almost 75%) died, the average survival from the time of diagnosis being only 2 years.[1]

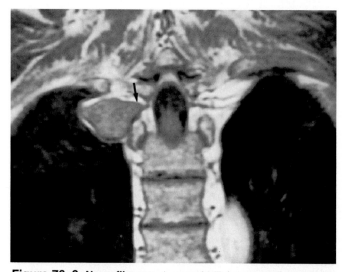

Figure 76–3. Neurofibroma. A coronal MR image obtained using T1-weighted spin-echo technique (TR 800, TE 15) demonstrates a paraspinal tumor. The mass has heterogeneous signal intensity and can be seen to originate from a nerve root *(arrow).*

Tumors Arising from Sympathetic Ganglia

The principal tumors in this group are ganglioneuroma, ganglioneuroblastoma, neuroblastoma, and paraganglioma; because of their similarity to each other and their differences from paraganglioma, the first three are conveniently discussed together. Melanocytic schwannoma, a rare tumor believed to originate in sympathetic ganglia, has also been reported.[25, 26] Almost all of these tumors arise in the paravertebral region; however, rare examples have also been reported to originate in the anterior mediastinum.[27]

Ganglioneuroma, Ganglioneuroblastoma, and Neuroblastoma

Ganglioneuroma, ganglioneuroblastoma, and neuroblastoma are a group of tumors representing a continuum whose histologic appearance varies from mature, fully differentiated tissue in the first-named to immature tissue in the last. Because of this, distinction between the neoplasms is to some extent arbitrary and sometimes difficult.[28] Ganglioneuromas are composed of an admixture of mature Schwann cells, collagen, and ganglion cells, whereas neuroblastomas consist of primitive-appearing cells, usually with scanty cytoplasm and pleomorphic, hyperchromatic nuclei; rosette formation is common in the latter neoplasm. Ganglioneuroblastomas show features of both tumors in varying degrees.[28]

The radiographic appearance consists of sharply defined oblong masses located along the anterolateral surface of the thoracic spine (Fig. 76–4).[12, 13, 29] These tumors can usually be distinguished from neurogenic tumors by their vertical orientation and elongated, tapering appearance. Calcification occurs in approximately 25% of cases (Fig. 76–5).[30] The ribs or vertebrae are eroded in some cases, just as often by

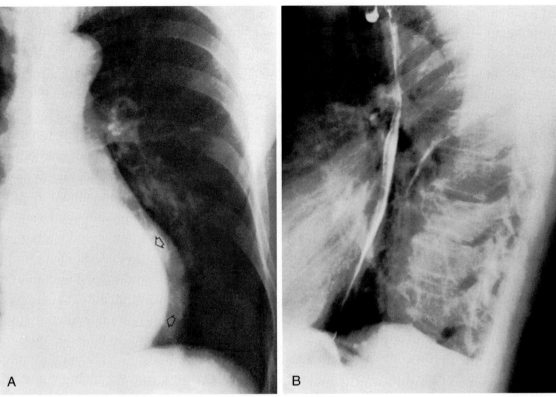

Figure 76–4. Ganglioneuroma. Close-up views of the left hemithorax from posteroanterior *(A)* and lateral *(B)* radiographs from a 42-year-old asymptomatic man show a smooth, well-defined, homogeneous mass in the paravertebral region *(arrows)*. It contains no visible calcium. The thoracic spine showed no abnormality.

benign as by malignant forms; such erosion can be striking in neuroblastoma but tends to be more subtle in ganglioneuroma.[29] The tumors can exhibit homogeneous or heterogeneous attenuation on CT.[13] MR imaging usually demonstrates homogeneous, intermediate signal intensity on both T1- and T2-weighted images.[13, 31] Occasionally, curvilinear bands of low signal intensity are seen on both T1- and T2-weighted images, causing a whorled appearance.[18]

Neuroblastomas and ganglioneuroblastomas occur most commonly in infants and children, whereas ganglioneuromas tend to occur in adolescents and young adults.[28] Many patients are asymptomatic; some have chest wall pain. Uncommon clinical manifestations include paraplegia, Horner's syndrome, diarrhea (related to the secretion of vasoactive intestinal peptide), and hemothorax (secondary to erosion of an intercostal artery).[28, 32] Urinary catecholamines are elevated in some patients.[28]

Ganglioneuromas are benign neoplasms that may grow very slowly over a period of many years;[33] complete excision typically results in cure. By contrast, neuroblastomas are aggressive tumors; although there is evidence that the course may be more prolonged in adults than in children, recurrence and metastases are common even in these patients, in whom the 5-year survival rate may be no more than 30%.[34] The prognosis with ganglioneuroblastoma is less predictable and depends to some extent on the age at diagnosis (a younger age being associated with a better outcome), stage, and the histologic pattern; in one review of 55 patients followed for 2 to 23 years, the 5-year actuarial survival rate was approximately 90%.[28]

Paraganglioma

As discussed in Chapter 75 (*see* page 2942), intrathoracic paragangliomas usually occur either in the middle mediastinum in relation to the aortopulmonary paraganglia or in the paravertebral region in relation to the aorticosympathetic paraganglia. As with tumors arising in the former location, those in the paravertebral region are uncommon; one group of investigators documented only 47 reported cases by 1990.[35] The average age at the time of diagnosis is about 30 to 40 years, and there is a male-to-female predominance of about 2 to 1.[35, 36] Histologic and immunohistochemical features are similar to those of aorticopulmonary tumors (*see* page 2942);[36] melanin pigmentation has been noted occasionally.[37]

Radiographically, most tumors are sharply defined, round or oval masses indistinguishable from other neurogenic neoplasms. Most are located in the mid-thoracic region adjacent to the fifth, sixth, or seventh rib; there is a right-sided predominance of 2 to 1.[38] CT demonstrates a soft tissue mass that can have homogeneous attenuation or can contain large central areas of low attenuation as a result of necrosis; marked enhancement following intravenous administration of contrast is typical.[39, 40] Approximately 90% of tumors show abnormal uptake on [131]I- or ^{123}I-metaiodobenzylguanidine (MIBG) scintigraphy.[41, 42] Preliminary results suggest that ^{111}In-octreotide scintigraphy may be superior to MIBG scintigraphy.[43, 44]

About 50% of patients are asymptomatic or complain of chest pain.[38] The remainder have signs and symptoms related to excess catecholamine production, including head-

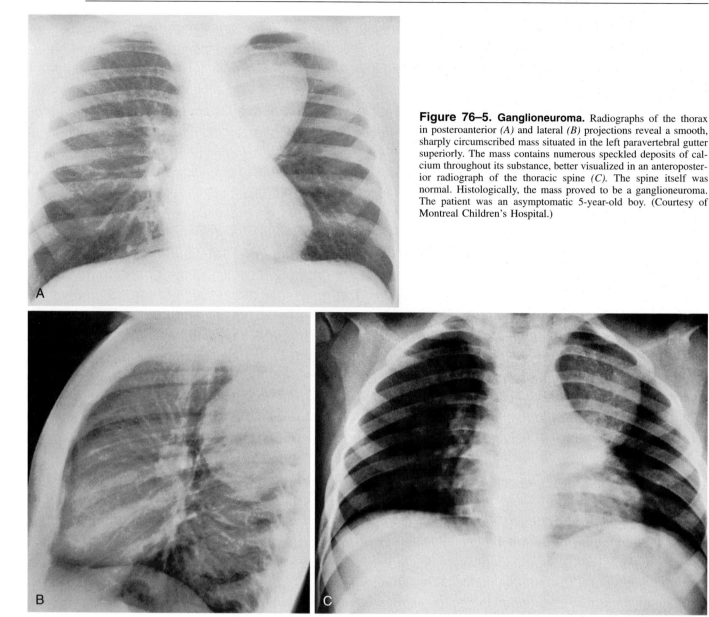

Figure 76–5. Ganglioneuroma. Radiographs of the thorax in posteroanterior *(A)* and lateral *(B)* projections reveal a smooth, sharply circumscribed mass situated in the left paravertebral gutter superiorly. The mass contains numerous speckled deposits of calcium throughout its substance, better visualized in an anteroposterior radiograph of the thoracic spine *(C)*. The spine itself was normal. Histologically, the mass proved to be a ganglioneuroma. The patient was an asymptomatic 5-year-old boy. (Courtesy of Montreal Children's Hospital.)

ache, sweating, tachycardia, palpitations, dyspnea, and nausea. Hypertension is present in most patients, as are increased levels of plasma and urinary catecholamines.[45, 46] Rare clinical manifestations include Horner's syndrome and neurologic findings secondary to spinal cord compression.[47]

The prognosis in patients who have aorticosympathetic paragangliomas is better than that in those who have aorticopulmonary tumors, complete surgical excision and cure being possible in many cases.[36, 38] In a few patients, local invasion or extensive hemorrhage during surgery precludes complete excision; in these situations, the neoplasm usually recurs, although sometimes after a prolonged interval. Metastases were documented in only 7% of patients in one review.[38] Many patients have adrenal or other extrathoracic paraganglionic tumors that can present either synchronously or metachronously.[38]

Meningocele and Meningomyelocele

Meningocele and meningomyelocele are rare anomalies that consist of herniation of the leptomeninges through an intervertebral foramen; a meningocele contains cerebrospinal fluid only, whereas a meningomyelocele also contains neural tissue. The abnormalities occur slightly more often on the right side than on the left and can be situated anywhere between the thoracic inlet and the diaphragm. Approximately 75% of patients present between the ages of 30 and 60 years;[48] many have neurofibromatosis.[49]

On conventional radiographs, the lesions show no specific features that distinguish them from neurogenic neoplasms. However, the diagnosis can usually be readily made on CT or MR imaging scans, both of which demonstrate continuity between the cerebrospinal fluid in the thecal sac and the meningocele (Fig. 76–6).[13, 49] Kyphoscoliosis is frequent, being observed in 47 of 70 patients in one series;[48] the meningocele was usually situated at the apex of the curvature on its convex side. Enlargement of the intervertebral foramen is present in the vast majority of cases.[48] An association with vertebral and rib anomalies is fairly frequent and should suggest the diagnosis.[50, 51]

An unusual lesion has been described in a 19-year-old

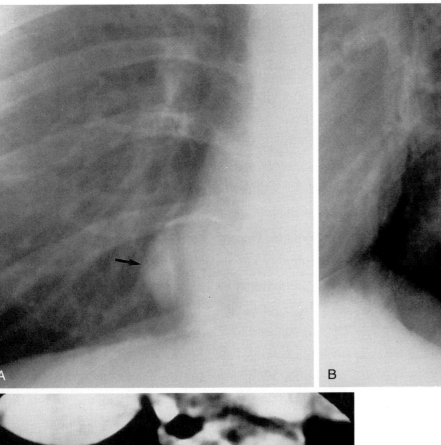

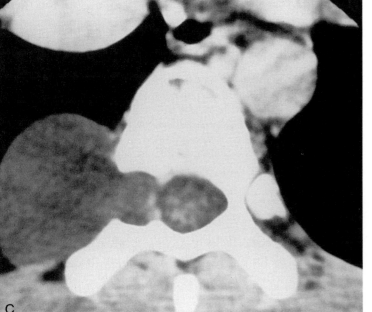

Figure 76–6. Meningocele. Close-up views from postero-anterior *(A)* and lateral *(B)* chest radiographs show a paraspinal opacity *(arrows)* at the level of T10. A CT scan *(C)* demonstrates characteristic fluid attenuation of the meningocele, which communicates with the thecal sac. The patient was a 29-year-old man.

man following trauma that resulted in a fracture of the right first rib, separation of the lateral aspect of the C7–T1 intervertebral disk, and a dural tear at that level.[52] Termed "pseudomeningocele" by the authors, the lesion consisted of a collection of cerebrospinal fluid in the extrapleural space overlying the lung apex; contrast medium entered and exited the cavity freely.

Miscellaneous Neural Tumors

Rare forms of paravertebral neural tumors include *chordoma* (a malignant neoplasm believed to be derived from fetal notochord rests and usually located in the upper paravertebral region),[53, 54] *ependymoma*,[55, 56] and *meningioma*.[57]

CYSTS

Several forms of cyst can occur in the paravertebral region, the most common being gastroenteric.

Gastroenteric (Neurenteric) Cyst

Gastroenteric cysts are lined in whole or in part by gastric and/or small intestinal epithelium; when such a cyst is associated with anomalies of the spinal column (such as spina bifida and hemivertebrae), the designation *neurenteric* is usually applied. It has been hypothesized that the cysts result from incomplete separation of endoderm from the notochord during early fetal life[58] or that they are the result of herniation of a portion of the gut anlage into a gap in the notochord ("split notochord" syndrome).[59]

Histologically, the cysts are lined by a variety of epithelial types, including gastric, small intestinal, duodenal, and bronchial.[58] Gastric epithelium can be functional and associated with peptic ulceration and perforation.[60] The cyst wall is composed of a variably thick muscle layer that may contain salivary gland, duodenal gland, pancreatic, or adrenal tissue.[58, 61, 62] (Rare cysts whose wall has been composed entirely of pancreatic tissue have also been reported.[63])

The radiographic appearance is that of a sharply defined, round or lobulated opacity of homogeneous density.[13, 64] Because of their fluid content, the cysts tend to mold themselves to surrounding structures. They are often connected by a stalk to the meninges and commonly also to a portion of the gastrointestinal tract.[64, 65] If attachment is to the esophagus, communication is rare; however, if it is to the gastrointestinal tract, there is usually communication, permitting gas to enter the cyst. In fact, the cyst may opacify with barium during examination of the upper gastrointestinal tract. Approximately 50% of cases are associated with incomplete closure of the neural tube (spinal dysraphism) or with butterfly vertebrae or hemivertebrae.[13, 49, 66] Very large cysts may be associated with scoliosis.[67] MR imaging is required to exclude intraspinal extension.[13]

Neurenteric cysts typically produce symptoms and therefore manifest themselves early in life;[68] in fact, the vast majority are diagnosed in the first year of life.[13, 69] They can grow very large and cause compression atelectasis, thereby leading to respiratory distress. Peptic ulceration can cause pain.[67] The development of carcinoma is a rare complication.[70]

Hydatid Cyst

Mediastinal echinococcosis is relatively rare compared with the pulmonary form of the disease. It appears to be most common in the paravertebral region; in one review of 80 cases, 74 of which were derived from the literature and 6 were new, cysts were identified at this site in 65%, in the anterior mediastinum in 36%, and in the posterior or middle mediastinum in only 9%.[71] Cysts situated in the paravertebral region tend to erode ribs and vertebrae and compress the spinal cord; those in the middle or posterior mediastinum can compress the trachea and great vessels. CT is helpful in determining the presence of the cysts and in demonstrating their relationship to adjacent structures (Fig. 76–7).[72]

EXTRAMEDULLARY HEMATOPOIESIS

Extramedullary hematopoiesis occurs as a compensatory phenomenon in various diseases in which there is inadequate production or excessive destruction of blood cells. The most common sites of extramedullary hematopoiesis are the liver and spleen; however, foci can occur in many other organs and tissues including the paravertebral areas of the thorax, the pleura,[73] the pulmonary parenchyma,[74, 75] and the bronchial wall.[76] Of all these intrathoracic sites, the paravertebral region is by far the most commonly affected; by 1980, 56 cases had been reported.[77]

The pathogenesis and fundamental nature of extramedullary hematopoiesis are not entirely clear in all cases. Although some of the lesions appear to be true foci of compensatory hyperplasia of bone marrow elements secondary to myelofibrosis, it is possible that others represent an abnormal (dysplastic) cellular proliferation. The latter hypothesis is supported by the extent and degree of cytologic immaturity as well as the apparent invasion of normal tissue in some cases.[75] It has been postulated that extramedullary hematopoiesis in the paravertebral regions occurs either by exten-

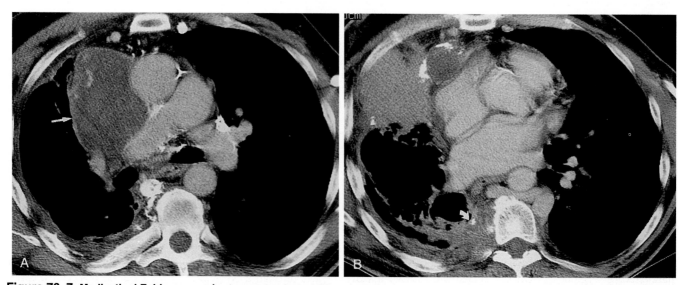

Figure 76–7. Mediastinal Echinococcosis. A contrast-enhanced CT scan *(A)* demonstrates a cystic lesion *(straight arrow)* in the middle mediastinum causing superior vena cava (SVC) obstruction. Note marked collateral venous circulation in the chest wall and mediastinum. A scan at a more caudad level *(B)* shows extensive paravertebral *(curved arrow)* and pleural involvement. The patient was a 52-year-old man who had long-standing *Echinococcus granulosus* infection involving the mediastinum, pleura, right lung, and liver.

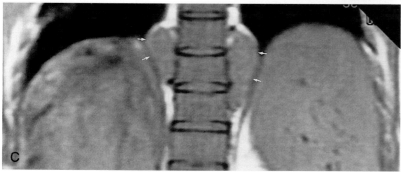

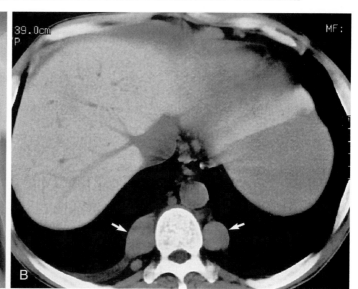

Figure 76–8. Extramedullary Hematopoiesis. A posteroanterior chest radiograph *(A)* from a 39-year-old man shows displacement of the paraspinal interfaces *(arrows)*. A CT scan obtained without intravenous contrast *(B)* shows paraspinal soft tissue masses *(arrows)*. Note the increased attenuation of the liver as a result of hemosiderosis. A coronal T1-weighted MR image *(C)* better demonstrates the extent of the extramedullary hematopoiesis *(arrows)*. The patient had thalassemia intermedia.

sion of hyperplastic marrow from adjacent bone or lymph nodes or by "primary" development in embryonic nests of primitive hematopoietic tissue.[78] In one study, CT showed that the bone in the region in which the mass had developed was usually wider and thinner than elsewhere,[79] supporting the hypothesis that extrusion of marrow occurs through thinned rib trabeculae.[80] It has been speculated that negative intrathoracic pressure may facilitate such extrusion,[79] perhaps explaining the observation that the proliferation of paravertebral marrow is usually intrathoracic rather than extrathoracic.

Foci of extramedullary hematopoiesis can be solitary or multiple and appear pathologically as soft, reddish nodules that can resemble hematomas.[77] Histologically, all marrow elements can be identified, usually associated with erythroid hyperplasia;[81] lymphocytes and a variable amount of adipose tissue are also present. Fibrosis is prominent in some cases, particularly when the foci of hematopoiesis are located in the pulmonary interstitium and pleura;[82] it has been hypothesized that this reaction may be related to the release of fibroblast growth factor from the hematopoietic cells.[82]

The characteristic radiographic finding is one or several smooth but often lobulated masses situated in the paravertebral regions in the lower chest (Fig. 76–8).[83–85] Less commonly, masses occur at multiple levels or involve the entire paravertebral region.[83, 84] On CT scans, the masses usually have homogeneous soft tissue density;[83, 85–87] occasionally, there is a large fatty component.[88, 89] In some tumors, fatty replacement appears to be the result of adipocytic metaplasia

following resolution of the underlying hemolytic disorder.[90, 91] Other features include widening of the ribs as a result of expansion of the medullary cavity, a lacy appearance of the vertebrae, and absence of bony erosion.[85] Radionuclide bone marrow scans may[85, 92, 93] or may not[94] show uptake within the mass.

The majority of cases of extramedullary hematopoiesis are associated with congenital hemolytic anemia (usually hereditary spherocytosis) or thalassemia (most often thalassemia major or intermedia);[77, 95] occasional cases have been reported in association with sickle cell disease,[96] hemoglobin C disease,[97] primary or vitamin deficiency–related macrocytosis,[98] and myelofibrosis (agnogenic myeloid metaplasia). Rarely, no cause is evident.[99] The masses seldom induce symptoms; however, hemothorax has been documented,[100] and paraplegia has been reported to develop as a result of spinal cord compression.[77] Rarely, pulmonary interstitial involvement has been complicated by rapidly fatal respiratory failure.[101]

MISCELLANEOUS MASSES

Rare paravertebral tumors include plasmacytoma,[102] chondrosarcoma,[103] thymoma,[104] and soft tissue tumors, such as lipoma and leiomyoma. Omental fat occasionally herniates through a congenital or an acquired posterior diaphragmatic defect and causes a paravertebral mass (*see* page 2997). Another unusual non-neoplastic cause of a paravertebral mass is ectopic kidney.[105]

REFERENCES

1. Ingels GW, Campbell DC, Giampetro AM, et al: Malignant schwannomas of the mediastinum. Cancer 27:1190, 1971.
2. Hoffman OA, Gillespie DJ, Aughenbaugh GL, et al: Primary mediastinal neoplasms (other than thymoma). Mayo Clin Proc 68:880, 1993.
3. Azarow KS, Pearl RH, Zurcher R, et al: Primary mediastinal masses. A comparison of adult and pediatric populations. J Thorac Cardiovasc Surg 106:67, 1993.
4. Saenz NC, Schnitzer JJ, Eraklis AE, et al: Posterior mediastinal masses. J Pediatr Surg 28:172, 1993.
5. Dabir RR, Piccione W Jr, Kittle CF: Intrathoracic tumors of the vagus nerve. Ann Thorac Surg 50:494, 1990.
6. Sugio K, Inoue T, Inoue K, et al: Neurogenic tumors of the mediastinum originating from the vagus nerve. Eur J Surg Oncol 21:214, 1995.
7. Ducatman BS, Scheithauer BW: Postirradiation neurofibrosarcoma. Cancer 51:1028, 1983.
8. Gale AW, Jelihovsky T, Grant AF, et al: Neurogenic tumors of the mediastinum. Ann Thorac Surg 17:434, 1974.
9. Heltzer JM, Krasna MJ, Aldrich F, et al: Thoracoscopic excision of a posterior mediastinal "dumbbell" tumor using a combined approach. Ann Thorac Surg 60:431, 1995.
10. Lodding P, Kindblom L-G, Angervall L, et al: Cellular schwannoma: A clinicopathologic study of 29 cases. Virchows Arch 416:237, 1990.
11. Askin FA, Rosai J, Sibley RK, et al: Malignant small cell tumor of the thoracopulmonary region in childhood: A distinctive clinicopathologic entity of uncertain histogenesis. Cancer 43:2438, 1979.
12. Reed JC, Kagan-Hallett K, Feigin DS: Neural tumors of the thorax: Subject review from the AFIP. Radiology 126:9, 1978.
13. Strollo DC, Rosado-de-Christenson ML, Jett JR. Primary mediastinal tumors. Part II. Tumors of the middle and posterior mediastinum. Chest 112:1344, 1997.
14. Kumar AJ, Kuhajda FP, Martinez CR, et al: Computed tomography of the extracranial nerve sheath tumors with pathological correlation. J Comput Assist Tomogr 7:857, 1983.
15. Ko S-F, Lee T-Y, Lin J-W, et al: Thoracic neurilemomas: An analysis of computed tomography findings in 36 patients. J Thorac Imaging 13:21, 1998.
16. Cohen LM, Schwartz AM, Rockoff SD: Benign schwannomas: Pathologic basis for CT inhomogeneities. Am J Roentgenol 147:141, 1986.
17. Bourgouin PM, Shepard JO, Moore EH, et al: Plexiform neurofibromatosis of the mediastinum: CT appearance. Am J Roentgenol 151:461, 1988.
18. Sakai F, Sone S, Kiyono K, et al: Intrathoracic neurogenic tumors: MR-pathologic correlation. Am J Roentgenol 159:279, 1992.
18a. Sakai F, Sone S, Kiyono K, et al: Magnetic resonance imaging of neurogenic tumors of the thoracic inlet: Determination of the parent nerve. J Thorac Imaging 11:272, 1996.
19. Ducatman BS, Scheithauer BW, Piepgras DG, et al: Malignant peripheral nerve sheath tumors: A clinicopathologic study of 120 cases. Cancer 57:2006, 1986.
20. Coleman BG, Arger PH, Dalinka MK, et al: CT of sarcomatous degeneration in neurofibromatosis. Am J Roentgenol 140:383, 1983.
21. Benjamin SP, McCormack LJ, Effler DB, et al: Critical review—"primary tumours of the mediastinum." Chest 62:297, 1972.
22. El Oakley R, Grotte GJ: Progressive tracheal and superior vena caval compression caused by benign neurofibromatosis. Thorax 49:380, 1994.
23. Cohen AJ, Thompson L, Edwards FH, et al: Primary cysts and tumors of the mediastinum. Ann Thorac Surg 51:378, 1991.
24. Harjula A, Mattila S, Luosto R, et al: Mediastinal neurogenic tumours: Early and late results of surgical treatment. Scand J Thorac Cardiovasc Surg 20:115, 1986.
25. Krausz T, Azzopardi JG, Pearse E: Malignant melanoma of the sympathetic chain: With a consideration of pigmented nerve sheath tumours. Histopathology 8:881, 1984.
26. Kayano H, Katayama I: Melanotic schwannoma arising in the sympathetic ganglion. Hum Pathol 19:1355, 1988.
27. Asada Y, Marutsuka K, Mitsukawa T, et al: Ganglioneuroblastoma of the thymus: An adult case with the syndrome of inappropriate secretion of antidiuretic hormone. Hum Pathol 27:506, 1996.
28. Adam A, Hochholzer L: Ganglioneuroblastoma of the posterior mediastinum. A clinicopathologic review of 80 cases. Cancer 47:373, 1981.
29. Bar-Ziv J, Nogrady MB: Mediastinal neuroblastoma and ganglioneuroma. The differentiation between primary and secondary involvement on the chest roentgenogram. Am J Roentgenol 125:380, 1975.
30. Schweisguth O, Mathey J, Renault P, et al: Intrathoracic neurogenic tumors in infants and children: A study of forty cases. Ann Surg 150:29, 1959.
31. Wang YM, Li YW, Sheih CP, et al: Magnetic resonance imaging of neuroblastoma, ganglioneuroblastoma and ganglioneuroma. Acta Paediatr Sin 36:420, 1995.
32. Baydur A, Cabula OS, Krishnareddy N, et al: Fatal intrathoracic hemorrhage in a patient with von Recklinghausen's disease. Respiration 62:104, 1995.
33. Viskens D, Deneffe G, Ryckaert R, et al: Intrathoracic ganglioneuroma: Case report. Acta Chir Belg 93:215, 1993.
34. Franks LM, Bollen A, Seeger RC, et al: Neuroblastoma in adults and adolescents: An indolent course with poor survival. Cancer 79:2028, 1997.
35. Odze R, Bégin LR: Malignant paraganglioma of the posterior mediastinum. A case report and review of the literature. Cancer 65:564, 1990.
36. Moran CA, Suster S, Fishback N, et al: Mediastinal paragangliomas. A clinicopathologic and immunohistochemical study of 16 cases. Cancer 72:2358, 1993.
37. Hofman WJ, Wockel W, Thetter O, et al: Melanotic paraganglioma of the posterior mediastinum. Virchows Arch 425:641, 1995.
38. Gallivan MVE, Chun B, Rowden G, et al: Intrathoracic paravertebral malignant paraganglioma. Arch Pathol Lab Med 104:46, 1980.
39. Ogawa J, Inoue H, Koide S, et al: Functioning paraganglioma in the posterior mediastinum. Ann Thorac Surg 33:507, 1982.
40. Drucker EA, McLoud TC, Dedrick CG, et al: Mediastinal paraganglioma: Radiologic evaluation of an unusual vascular tumor. Am J Roentgenol 148:521, 1987.
41. Bomanji J, Conry BG, Britton KE, et al: Imaging neural crest tumors with ^{123}I-meta-iodobenzylguanidine and x-ray computed tomography: A comparative study. Clin Radiol 39:502, 1988.
42. van Gils AP, Falke TA, van Erkel AR, et al: MR imaging and MIBG scintigraphy of pheochromocytomas and extra-adrenal functioning paragangliomas. RadioGraphics 11:37, 1991.
43. Kwekkeboom DJ, van Urk H, Pauw BK, et al: Octreotide scintigraphy for the detection of paragangliomas. J Nucl Med 34:873, 1993.
44. Van Gelder T, Verhoeven GT, de Jong P, et al: Dopamine-producing paraganglioma not visualized by iodine-123-MIBG scintigraphy. J Nucl Med 36:620, 1995.
45. Nigam BK, Hyer SL, Taylor EJ, et al: Intrathoracic chemodectoma with noradrenaline secretion. Thorax 36:66, 1981.
46. Ogawa J, Inoue H, Koide S, et al: Functioning paraganglioma in the posterior mediastinum. Ann Thorac Surg 33:507, 1982.
47. Noorda RJ, Wuisman PI, Kummer AJ, et al: Nonfunctioning malignant paraganglioma of the posterior mediastinum with spinal cord compression. A case report. Spine 21:1703, 1996.
48. Miles J, Pennybacker J, Sheldon P: Intrathoracic meningocele. Its development and association with neurofibromatosis. J Neurol Neurosurg Psychiatry 32:99, 1969.
49. Glazer HS, Siegel MJ, Sagel SS: Low-attenuation mediastinal masses on CT. Am J Roentgenol 152:1173, 1989.
50. Wychulis AR, Payne WS, Clagett OT, et al: Surgical treatment of mediastinal tumors. A 40-year experience. J Thorac Cardiovasc Surg 62:379, 1971.
51. Cabooter M, Bogaerts Y, Javaheri S, et al: Intrathoracic meningocele. Eur J Respir Dis 63:347, 1982.
52. Epstein BS, Epstein JA: Extrapleural intrathoracic apical traumatic pseudomeningocele. Am J Roentgenol 120:887, 1974.
53. Maesen F, Baur C, Lamers J, et al: Chordoma of the thorax. Eur J Respir Dis 68:68, 1986.
54. Clemons RL, Blank RH, Hutcheson JB, et al: Chordoma presenting as a posterior mediastinal mass. A choristoma. J Thorac Cardiovasc Surg 63:922, 1972.
55. Doglioni C, Bontempini L, Iuzzolino P, et al: Ependymoma of the mediastinum. Arch Pathol Lab Med 112:194, 1988.
56. Nobles E, Russell L, Kircher T: Mediastinal ependymoma. Hum Pathol 22:94, 1991.
57. Wilson AJ, Ratliff JL, Lagios MD, et al: Mediastinal meningioma. Am J Surg Pathol 3:557, 1979.
58. Salyer DC, Salyer WR, Eggleston JC: Benign developmental cysts of the mediastinum. Arch Pathol Lab Med 101:136, 1977.
59. Bajpai M, Mathur M: Duplications of the alimentary tract: Clues to the missing links. J Pediatr Surg 29:1361, 1994.
60. Kirwan WO, Walbaum PR, McCormack RJM: Cystic intrathoracic derivatives of the foregut and their complications. Thorax 28:424, 1973.
61. Spock A, Schneider S, Baylin GJ: Mediastinal gastric cysts: A case report and review of English literature. Am Rev Respir Dis 94:97, 1966.
62. Wright JR Jr, Gillis DA: Mediastinal foregut cyst containing an intramural adrenal cortical rest: A case report and review of supradiaphragmatic adrenal rests. Pediatr Pathol 13:401, 1993.
63. Carr MJT, Deiraniya AK, Judd PA: Mediastinal cyst containing mural pancreatic tissue. Thorax 32:512, 1977.
64. Ochsner JL, Ochsner SF: Congenital cysts of the mediastinum: 20-year experience with 42 cases. Ann Surg 163:909, 1966.
65. Leigh TF: Mass lesions of the mediastinum. Radiol Clin North Am 1:377, 1963.
66. Kirwan WO, Walbaum PR, McCormack RJM: Cystic intrathoracic derivatives of the foregut and their complications. Thorax 28:424, 1973.
67. Lyons HA, Calvy GL, Sammons BP: The diagnosis and classification of mediastinal masses. I. A study of 782 cases. Ann Intern Med 51:897, 1959.
68. Benton C, Silverman FN: Some mediastinal lesions in children. Semin Roentgenol 4:91, 1969.
69. Snyder ME, Luck SR, Hernandez R, et al: Diagnostic dilemmas of mediastinal cysts. J Pediatr Surg 20:810, 1985.
70. Chuang MT, Barba FA, Kaneko M, et al: Adenocarcinoma arising in an intrathoracic duplication cyst of foregut origin: A case report with review of the literature. Cancer 47:1887, 1981.
71. Rakower J, Milwidsky H: Primary mediastinal echinococcosis. Am J Med 29:73, 1960.
72. Von Sinner WN, Linjawi T, Al Watban J: Mediastinal hydatid disease: Report of three cases. J Can Assoc Radiol 41:79, 1990.
73. Yazdi HM: Cytopathology of extramedullary hematopoiesis in effusions and peritoneal washings. Diagn Cytopathol 2:326, 1986.
74. Wood DJ, Krishnan K, Stocks P, et al: Catamenial haemoptysis: A rare cause. Thorax 48:1048, 1993.

75. Glew RH, Haese WH, McIntyre PA: Myeloid metaplasia with myelofibrosis: The clinical spectrum of extramedullary hematopoiesis and tumor formation. Johns Hopkins Med J 132:253, 1973.

76. Gowitt GT, Zaatari GS: Bronchial extramedullary hematopoiesis preceding chronic myelogenous leukemia. Hum Pathol 16:1069, 1985.

77. Verani R, Olson J, Moake JL: Intrathoracic extramedullary hematopoiesis. Report of a case in a patient with sickle cell disease–β-thalassemia. Am J Clin Pathol 73:133, 1980.

78. Da Costa JL, Loh YS, Hanam E: Extramedullary hemopoiesis with multiple tumor-simulating mediastinal masses in hemoglobin E–thalassemia disease. Chest 65:210, 1974.

79. Long JA Jr, Doppman JL, Nienhuis AW: Computed tomographic studies of thoracic extramedullary hematopoiesis. J Comput Assist Tomogr 4:67, 1980.

80. Ross P, Logan W: Roentgen findings in extramedullary hematopoiesis. Am J Roentgenol 106:604, 1969.

81. Moran CA, Suster S, Fishback N, et al: Extramedullary hematopoiesis presenting as posterior mediastinal mass: A study of four cases. Mod Pathol 8:249, 1995.

82. Asakura S, Colby TV: Two cases of agnogenic myeloid metaplasia with extramedullary hematopoiesis and fibrosis in the lung. Chest 105:1866, 1994.

83. Gumbs R, Ford EAH, Tea JS, et al: Intrathoracic extramedullary hematopoiesis in sickle cell disease. Am J Roentgenol 149:889, 1987.

84. Papavasiliou C, Gouliamos A, Andreou J: The marrow heterotopia in thalassemia. Eur J Radiol 6:92, 1986.

85. Alam R, Padmanabhan K, Rao H: Paravertebral mass in a patient with thalassemia intermedia. Chest 112:265, 1997.

86. Long JA Jr, Doppman JL, Nienhuis AW: Computed tomographic studies of thoracic extramedullary hematopoiesis. J Comput Assist Tomogr 4:67, 1980.

87. Fielding JR, Owens M, Naimark A: Intrathoracic extramedullary hematopoiesis secondary to B₁₂ and folate deficiency: CT appearance. J Comput Assist Tomogr 15:308, 1991.

88. Yamato M, Fuhrman CR: Computed tomography of fatty replacement in extramedullary hematopoiesis. J Comput Assist Tomogr 11:541, 1987.

89. Joy G, Logan PM: Intrathoracic extramedullary hematopoiesis secondary to idiopathic myelofibrosis. Can Assoc Radiol J 49:200, 1998.

90. Martin J, Palacio A, Petit J, et al: Fatty transformation of thoracic extramedullary hematopoiesis following splenectomy: CT features. J Comput Assist Tomogr 14:477, 1990.

91. Glazer HS, Wick MR, Anderson DJ, et al: CT of fatty thoracic masses. Am J Roentgenol 159:1181, 1992.

92. Stebner FC, Bishop CR: Bone marrow scan and radioiron uptake of an intrathoracic mass. Clin Nucl Med 7:86, 1982.

93. Coates GG, Eisenberg B, Dail DH: Tc-99m sulfur colloid demonstration of diffuse pulmonary interstitial extramedullary hematopoiesis in a patient with myelofibrosis. A case report and review of the literature. Clin Nucl Med 19:1079, 1994.

94. Harnsberger HR, Datz FL, Knockel JQ, et al: Failure to detect extramedullary hematopoiesis during bone marrow imaging with indium-111 to technetium-99m sulphur colloid. J Nucl Med 23:589, 1982.

95. Papavasiliou CG: Tumor simulating intrathoracic extramedullary hemopoiesis. Clinical and roentgenologic considerations. Am J Roentgenol 93:695, 1965.

96. Gumbs RV, Higginbotham-Ford EA, Teal JS, et al: Thoracic extramedullary hematopoiesis in sickle cell disease. Am J Roentgenol 149:889, 1987.

97. Koudieh MS, Afzal M, Rasul K, et al: Intrathoracic extramedullary hematopoietic tumor in hemoglobin C disease. Arch Pathol Lab Med 120:504, 1996.

98. De Montpréville VT, Dulmet EM, Chapelier AR, et al: Extramedullary hematopoietic tumors of the posterior mediastinum related to asymptomatic refractory anemia. Chest 104:1623, 1993.

99. Elbers H, Stadt JVD, Wagenaar SSC: Tumor-simulating thoracic extramedullary hematopoiesis. Ann Thorac Surg 30:584, 1980.

100. Smith PR, Manjoney DL, Teitcher JB, et al: Massive hemothorax due to intrathoracic extramedullary hematopoiesis in a patient with thalassemia intermedia. Chest 94:658, 1988.

101. Yusen RD, Kollef MH: Acute respiratory failure due to extramedullary hematopoiesis. Chest 108:1170, 1995.

102. Miyazaki T, Kohno S, Sakamoto A, et al: A rare case of extramedullary plasmacytoma in the mediastinum. Intern Med 31:1363, 1992.

103. Suster S, Moran CA: Malignant cartilaginous tumors of the mediastinum: Clinicopathological study of six cases presenting as extraskeletal soft tissue masses. Hum Pathol 28:588, 1997.

104. Cooper GN Jr, Narodick BG: Posterior mediastinal thymoma. Case report. J Thorac Cardiovasc Surg 63:561, 1972.

105. Leite de Noronha L, Freitas E, Costa M, Magalhães Godinho MT: Thoracic kidney. Am Rev Respir Dis 109:678, 1974.

PART XVII

DISEASE OF THE DIAPHRAGM AND CHEST WALL

CHAPTER 77

The Diaphragm

The thoracic cage, including the chest wall and diaphragm, serves the dual purpose of enclosing and protecting the contents of the thorax and of producing the movements that result in the changes in pleural pressure necessary for respiration. A multitude of abnormalities involve these structures that can affect either or both of these two major functions. This chapter deals with disorders of the diaphragm and Chapter 78 is concerned with disorders involving the other components of the thoracic cage. The material is primarily related to acquired and congenital diseases; the effects of trauma are discussed in Chapter 66.

The normal embryology, anatomy, physiology, and radiology of the diaphragm are described in detail in Chapter 10. The topography of the diaphragm has been reviewed in detail,[1] as have methods for imaging the chest wall and diaphragm.[2] Briefly, the diaphragm consists of a musculotendinous sheet that separates the thoracic and abdominal contents into two compartments (Fig. 77–1). It can be divided into three anatomic components: (1) a *sternal* portion that originates from the xiphoid process of the sternum; (2) a *costal* portion that arises from the lower six ribs; and (3) a *crural* portion that originates from the anterolateral aspects of the first three lumbar vertebrae on the right and the first two lumbar vertebrae on the left. A portion of the crural (or lumbar) diaphragm arises from the medial and lateral arcuate ligaments and the thickening of the thoracolumbar fascia overlying the anterior surfaces of the psoas and quadratus lumborum muscles. The muscle fibers from all three components insert into the boomerang-shaped central tendon.

Three diaphragmatic discontinuities normally allow communication of a variety of structures between the thorax and abdomen (see Fig. 77–1). The *aortic aperture* is located posterior to the left median arcuate ligament at the level of the twelfth thoracic vertebra; in addition to the aorta, it contains the thoracic duct and other smaller lymphatic vessels and the azygos and hemiazygos veins. The *esophageal aperture* consists of a splitting of the medial fibers of the right crus of the crural diaphragm; in addition to the esophagus, this aperture allows passage of the vagal nerves and the gastric vessels. The *inferior vena cava aperture* is the most anterior discontinuity, located at the level of T-8 between the costal portion of the right hemidiaphragm and the central tendon. In addition to these normal openings, the diaphragm has two symmetric "weak areas" known eponymously as the foramina of Morgagni and Bochdalek, the former located anteriorly and the latter posterolaterally; each may be the site of herniation of abdominal contents into the thorax.

On the chest radiograph, the superior surface of the diaphragm forms a dome-shaped interface with the lungs. The inferior surface is obscured by the organs and soft tissues of the abdomen. In one investigation of 500 healthy subjects, posteroanterior radiographs showed the cupola or dome of the right hemidiaphragm to project into a plane ranging from the anterior end of the fifth rib to the sixth anterior interspace in about 95% of individuals;[3] it projected at the level of the sixth rib anteriorly in about 40% and at or below the level of the seventh rib in only 4%. In most people, the right hemidiaphragm projects half an interspace higher than the left, being at the same level as or lower than the left hemidiaphragm in only about 10%.[4] The discrepancy in position of the two hemidiaphragms is the result of the position of the ventricular mass of the heart rather than that of the liver, as is commonly believed: in patients who have dextrocardia without dextroversion of the abdominal viscera, the right hemidiaphragm is on a plane lower than the left, despite the right-sided position of the liver.[5, 6] Variations in diaphragmatic contour, such as scalloping[4] and prominence of the costophrenic muscle slips, are fairly common and should not be interpreted as evidence of disease.

Excursion of the diaphragm is estimated to account for 60% to 75% of vital capacity,[7] with the remainder being the result of intercostal and accessory muscle contraction. There is a wide range of diaphragmatic excursion in healthy people. In one study of inspiratory-expiratory radiographs of 350 subjects aged 30 to 80 years who had no evidence of respiratory disease, the mean excursions of the right and left hemidiaphragms were 3.3 cm and 3.5 cm, respectively.[8] In another investigation of 114 healthy young men, the range of

FORAMINA OF MORGAGNI

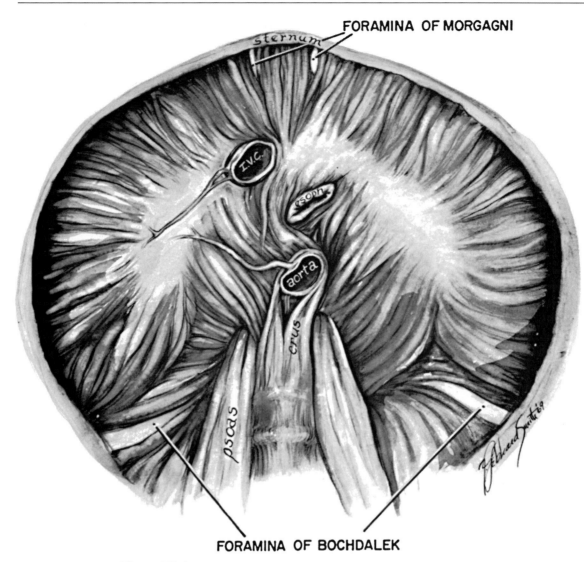

FORAMINA OF BOCHDALEK

Figure 77–1. Anatomy of the Normal Diaphragm Viewed from Below.

excursion was 0.8 to 8.1 cm overall, 5 to 7 cm in 57 individuals (50%), and less than 3 cm in 16 (14%);[9] there was no relationship between diaphragmatic movement and vital capacity. Unequal movement of the two hemidiaphragmatic domes was common; movements were equal in only 10 individuals, greater on the right in 73 (never by more than 1.9 cm), and greater on the left in 31 (exceeding 1.4 cm in only one instance). These observations are in agreement with the results of two other studies.[10, 11] In a more recent investigation of 55 normal adults in whom measurements were obtained by ultrasound, the mean right and left hemidiaphragmatic excursions were 53 ± 16 mm (mean ± SD) and 46 ± 12 mm, respectively, and the ratio of right to left diaphragmatic excursion was about 1.2.[12] There is evidence that the mean diaphragmatic excursion of older people is less than that of younger ones.[13]

Radiologic assessment of diaphragmatic motion is best accomplished fluoroscopically[14-16] or using real-time ultrasound.[17-19] Although major asymmetry of excursion may be seen on radiographs exposed at total-lung capacity (TLC) and residual volume (RV) (e.g., in the assessment of air-trapping from obstructing endobronchial lesions or in unilat-

eral emphysema), minor degrees of asymmetry may become evident only when the motion of both hemidiaphragms is observed simultaneously. Fluoroscopic examination should be carried out not only in posteroanterior projection but also in various degrees of obliquity to reveal any localized regional disturbance in motion. Movement should be observed during tidal breathing, while the patient breathes deeply and preferably rapidly, and while he or she sniffs ("sniff test"). The latter test is accomplished by having the subject produce a rapid inspiration, usually through the nostrils because this is an easily accomplished respiratory maneuver for untrained subjects. In many cases, sniffing reveals restriction or paradoxical motion not clearly apparent during either tidal or deep breathing. Of some importance is the observation that sniffing by normal people may produce paradoxical excursion of one hemidiaphragm;[14] according to one observer, such a finding can be regarded as pathologic only if paradoxical excursion exceeds 2 cm and if it involves the whole hemidiaphragm as seen in oblique or lateral projection.

It has been suggested that ultrasonography may be superior to fluoroscopy in the assessment of abnormalities of diaphragmatic movement.[17] In one investigation of 30 patients referred for evaluation of suspected abnormalities of diaphragmatic movement, fluoroscopic examination was not possible in 4 because of obscuration of a hemidiaphragm by pleural effusion or thoracoplasty.[17] In 21 of the remaining 26 patients, the fluoroscopic and ultrasound evaluations of the diaphragmatic motion were concordant; in 5, they were discordant. All patients who had an abnormal sniff test or paradoxical movement on fluoroscopy showed similar findings on ultrasound; however, ultrasound showed abnormalities of diaphragmatic motion in 5 patients who had normal fluoroscopy. The main advantages of ultrasound are the lack of radiation, direct visualization of the diaphragm, and portability.

In addition to excursion, ultrasound has been employed to measure diaphragmatic thickness, configuration, and the extent of the zone of apposition with the rib cage.[12, 19–21] The technique has also been used to measure the change in diaphragmatic thickness during maximal contraction in the area of apposition. In one study of 13 healthy men, the mean value for thickness was 1.7 ± 0.2 mm at functional residual capacity (FRC) and 4.5 ± 0.9 mm at TLC.[22] The thickness shows a strong positive correlation with the maximal inspiratory pressure that can be generated voluntarily and appears to represent an indicator of diaphragmatic strength.[23] The shape, motion, and thickness of the diaphragm can also be measured by CT and magnetic resonance (MR) imaging.[24–27] For example, in one MR imaging investigation of 10 supine normal subjects, the mean maximal excursions of the right and left hemidiaphragms were 4.4 and 4.2 cm, respectively;[26] regional motion was greater anteriorly and laterally. Using CT, a large range of maximal crural diaphragmatic thickness has been reported in both men (1.8 to 18.8 mm) and women (1.8 to 21.1 mm).[24] Spiral CT and MR imaging also allow three-dimensional reconstruction of the diaphragm and assessment of changes in muscle length, surface area, and shape.[28]

ABNORMALITIES OF DIAPHRAGMATIC POSITION OR MOTION

Unilateral Diaphragmatic Paralysis

Paralysis of a hemidiaphragm usually results from interruption of transmission of the nerve impulses through the phrenic nerve and is associated with many causes (Table 77–1). The most common is invasion of the nerve by a neoplasm, usually of pulmonary origin. The second most frequent category is paralysis of unknown etiology; in these idiopathic cases, the paralysis is almost invariably right sided and usually occurs in males. It has been suggested that this variety may result from an episode of infectious neuritis or may be caused by viral neurotoxin.[29] In support of this hypothesis is the observation that unilateral diaphragmatic paralysis can be a manifestation of herpes zoster infection, presumably as a result of extension of disease from the dorsal root to adjacent posterior and lateral portions of the spinal cord and anterior horn cells.[30]

Unilateral diaphragmatic paralysis can also occur as a complication of neck[31] or thoracic[32, 33] surgery, especially coronary artery bypass surgery.[34–37] The mechanism by which the hemidiaphragm is paralyzed has not been definitively

Table 77–1. UNILATERAL DIAPHRAGMATIC PARALYSIS

ETIOLOGY	SELECTED REFERENCE
Neoplasms	
Phrenic nerve injury	
Surgical section or stretch	46
Cooling	37
Cervical manipulation	46
Cervical venipuncture	50
Birth injury	208
Neuritis	
Brachial neuritis (Parsonage-Turner syndrome)	190
Herpes zoster virus infection	192
Vasculitis (mononeuritis multiplex)	
CNS or spinal cord abnormalities	
Neuralgic amyotrophy	191
Stroke	
Multiple sclerosis	55
Rhizotomy	53
Neural compression	
Cervical spondylosis	82
Mediastinal lymph node enlargement	193
Substernal goiter	
Miscellaneous	
Diabetes mellitus	
Carbon monoxide poisoning	194
Upper abdominal surgery	58
Liver transplantation	116a

established in the latter circumstance; however, there is evidence that it may be the result of cold topical cardioplegia. During cardiopulmonary bypass and aortocoronary bypass grafting, ice slush cooled to subfreezing temperatures by the addition of salt is sometimes packed into the pericardial cavity around the heart. Because the left phrenic nerve runs within the posterior pericardium on the left side, temporary cold-induced injury can theoretically occur.[38, 39] In support of this hypothesis is the observation that cooling of the phrenic nerves in experimental animals causes reversible diaphragmatic paralysis.[40] It has also been suggested that left lower lobe atelectasis may be attributable to left phrenic nerve palsy and that it can be alleviated to some extent by the use of a pericardial insulation technique.[41, 42] Despite the foregoing, one group of investigators who studied 57 patients undergoing coronary artery bypass grafting in which cold topical cardioplegia was employed found that only 10% of the patients demonstrated unequivocal evidence of phrenic nerve damage, whereas most had significant atelectasis of the left lower lobe.[37] Cold topical cardioplegia has also been associated rarely with bilateral phrenic nerve damage.[43–45]

Phrenic nerve damage can also result from chiropractic manipulation of the cervical spine[46, 47] and from catheterization of the large cervical veins.[48–50] Abnormalities of the nerve roots from C-3 to C-5 can also cause diaphragmatic paralysis in cases of severe cervical spondylosis[51, 52] or as a consequence of rhizotomy.[53] Occasionally, unilateral diaphragmatic paralysis is a localized expression of a more diffuse neuropathy.[54] Both unilateral and bilateral upper motor neuron phrenic palsy have been reported in patients who have multiple sclerosis,[55, 56] and transient hemidiaphragmatic elevation can occur on the side contralateral to a supratentorial stroke.[57] Unilateral diaphragmatic paralysis has been reported as a complication of carbon monoxide poisoning.[194] A form of transient unilateral diaphragmatic dysfunction frequently occurs after upper abdominal surgery as a result of stimulation of inhibitory afferent endings in the diaphragm.[58]

Radiologically, an elevated, paralyzed hemidiaphragm presents an accentuated dome configuration in both posteroanterior and lateral projections (Fig. 77–2). Because the peripheral points of attachment of the diaphragm are fixed, costophrenic and costovertebral sulci tend to be deepened, narrowed, and sharpened (Fig. 77–3). If the paralysis is left sided, the stomach and splenic flexure of the colon relate to the inferior surface of the elevated hemidiaphragm and usually contain more gas than normal (Fig. 77–4). In many cases, the stomach undergoes mesenteroaxial volvulus, so that its greater curvature faces upward; in such circumstances, two fluid levels are apparent within the stomach, one in the inverted fundus and the other in the body or

antrum. This broad relationship of distended stomach and colon to the inferior surface is a valuable sign in the differentiation of eventration or diaphragmatic paralysis from traumatic diaphragmatic hernia.[4] Rarely, paralysis or eventration of the right hemidiaphragm is associated with inversion of the liver and a suprahepatic position of the gallbladder.[59] Invasion or compression of the phrenic nerve by such abnormalities as pulmonary carcinoma or calcified lymph nodes can be clarified by CT should the nature of the abnormalities be unclear from conventional radiographic studies.[60]

In a review of the radiographic manifestations of unilateral diaphragmatic paralysis, four cardinal signs were described:[10] (1) elevation of a hemidiaphragm above the normal range; (2) diminished, absent, or paradoxical motion during respiration; (3) paradoxical motion under conditions of augmented load, such as sniffing; and (4) mediastinal swing during respiration. There are several potential pitfalls in the assessment of these signs:[61] (1) the judgment that there is

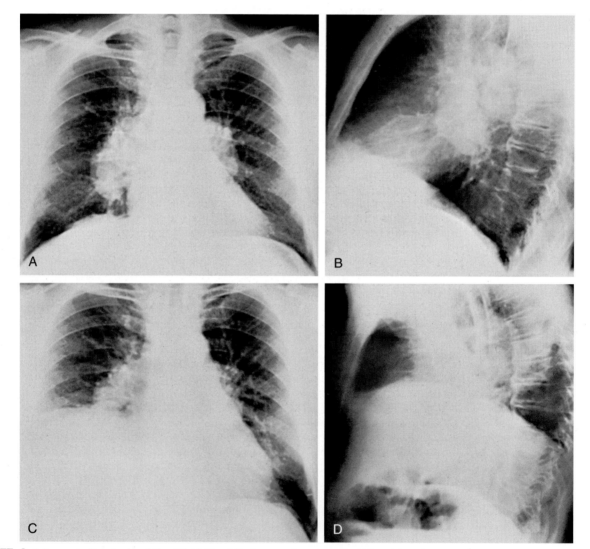

Figure 77–2. Iatrogenic Paralysis of the Right Hemidiaphragm. Posteroanterior *(A)* and lateral *(B)* radiographs of a 49-year-old patient reveal marked enlargement of the hilar lymph nodes bilaterally. No other intrathoracic abnormality is evident. Note the normal position of both hemidiaphragms. As part of the investigation, a right scalene node biopsy was performed, during which the right phrenic nerve was accidentally severed. Ten days later, radiograph of the chest in posteroanterior *(C)* and lateral *(D)* projections demonstrate marked elevation of the right hemidiaphragm. The contour of the hemidiaphragm is smooth and arcuate but does not present the sharp costophrenic angles that usually characterize diaphragmatic paralysis. The scalene node biopsy revealed organisms compatible with *Histoplasma capsulatum.* It was assumed that the hilar lymph node enlargement was the result of histoplasmosis.

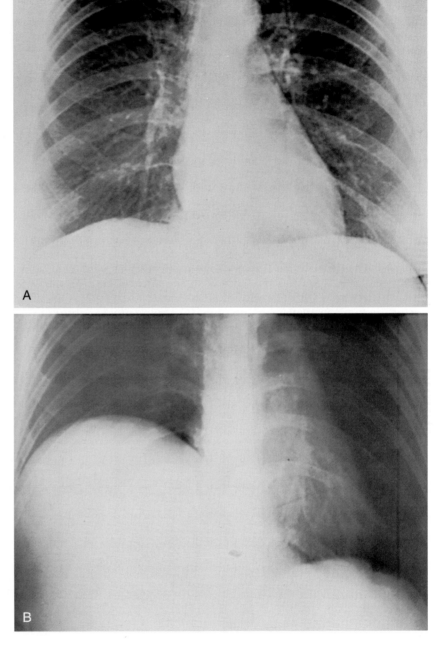

Figure 77–3. Iatrogenic Paralysis of the Right Hemidiaphragm. This 33-year-old woman was admitted to the hospital for repair of a lacerated finger tendon. A view of the lower half of the thorax from a preoperative radiograph *(A)* revealed a normal position of both hemidiaphragms. Anesthesia was established by brachial plexus block, 45 mL of 1% Carbocaine with Adrenalin being injected by way of a supraclavicular approach. One hour after the anesthesia, the patient complained of mild dyspnea, and a radiograph of the chest *(B)* revealed marked elevation of the right hemidiaphragm in a contour typical of diaphragmatic paralysis.

Illustration continued on following page

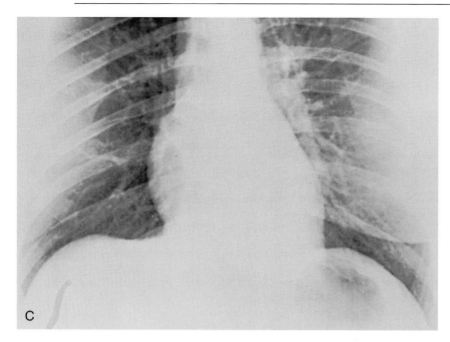

Figure 77–3 *Continued.* The patient received supportive therapy only, and a radiograph exposed 12 hours after anesthesia *(C)* demonstrated return of the right hemidiaphragm to its normal level. The dyspnea had disappeared.

an abnormal elevation may be erroneous because of the considerable variation in the normal height of the hemidiaphragms; (2) mediastinal swing during respiration is a totally unreliable sign in the presence of bronchial obstruction or atelectasis; (3) motion may be absent or paradoxical during respiration in various pulmonary, pleural, and subphrenic diseases, which makes this sign unreliable unless such diseases can be excluded; and (4) sniffing can cause paradoxical motion of one hemidiaphragm in some healthy people, and in order for it to be considered pathologic, it should consist of a reverse excursion of at least 2 cm. Despite these observations, with reasonable care, the diagnosis of unilateral diaphragmatic paralysis can be made radiologically in most cases.

The most reliable radiologic maneuver to detect hemidiaphragmatic paralysis is the sniff test. Normally, both hemidiaphragms descend sharply during a sniff; with unilateral diaphragmatic paralysis, there is paradoxical upward motion of the affected side. Although significant paradoxical motion provides strong evidence for diaphragmatic paralysis or eventration, the incidence of false-positive results is about 5%; in addition, false-negative results can be recorded if the subject uses the abdominal musculature to elevate the diaphragm during the expiratory phase of breathing.[14]

As discussed previously, preliminary results suggest that ultrasound is superior to fluoroscopy in the demonstration of abnormalities of hemidiaphragmatic motion.[17] One investigation of the diaphragm in 30 subjects included 5 who

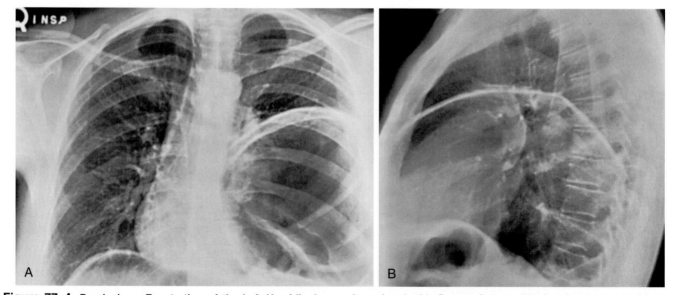

Figure 77–4. Paralysis or Eventration of the Left Hemidiaphragm Associated with Severe Colonic Dilation Secondary to Sigmoid Volvulus. Posteroanterior *(A)* and lateral *(B)* radiographs reveal a remarkable degree of elevation of the left hemidiaphragm. Severely dilated loops of colon are situated beneath this hemidiaphragm and to a lesser extent beneath the right one. The mediastinum is displaced considerably into the right hemithorax.

had bilateral diaphragmatic paralysis, 7 who had unilateral paralysis, 3 who had inspiratory weakness but normally functioning diaphragm, and 5 healthy control subjects.[19] In this study, the thickness of the diaphragm at FRC was significantly less in patients who had bilateral diaphragmatic paralysis (1.8 ± 0.2 mm) than in normal subjects (2.8 ± 0.4 mm, $P < 0.001$); paralyzed diaphragms showed no change in thickness during inspiration in the patients, compared with a change in thickness from FRC to TLC of 37% ± 9% in the normal subjects. In patients who had unilateral paralysis, the thickness of the paralyzed hemidiaphragm at FRC (1.7 ± 0.2 mm) was significantly less than that of the normally functioning hemidiaphragm (2.7 ± 0.5 mm, $P < 0.01$), and the change in thickness with inspiration significantly lower (-8.5% ± 13%, compared with +65% ± 26%).

Patients who have a paralyzed hemidiaphragm usually do not have symptoms; however, some complain of dyspnea on effort or (rarely) orthopnea,[30] the severity of either symptom relating to the rapidity of development of the paralysis and to the presence or absence of underlying pulmonary disease. Physical examination may reveal an elevated hemidiaphragm and decreased breath sounds over the affected side, although distinction from a pleural effusion may be impossible. Diaphragmatic excursion as assessed by percussion is decreased. Examination of the anterior abdominal wall of some patients in the supine position may reveal paradoxical inward movement of the ipsilateral abdominal wall.

Pulmonary function tests typically show a mild restrictive pattern. TLC is about 85% of predicted, whereas vital capacity is reduced to about 75% of predicted; FRC and the ratio of FEV_1 to forced vital capacity (FVC) are usually normal.[61–63] Maximal inspiratory pressures, measured either at the mouth (PI Max) or across the diaphragm (Pdi Max), are only mildly reduced, and values are similar whether the paralysis is right or left sided.[64, 65] Lower values for vital capacity, PI Max, and Pdi Max are observed in patients who have concomitant cardiopulmonary disease.[64] The decrease in lung volumes is greater when measured in the supine, rather than in the upright, position.[66, 67] The average decrease in vital capacity when normal subjects move from the erect to the supine posture is 7.5% ± 6%; a decrease of 20% or greater indicates the need for a study of diaphragmatic function[68] (see pages 419 and 3059). Hypoxemia is usually absent or mild, although it may develop when patients assume a supine position[66, 69] as well as during sleep.[70] Regional ventilation is decreased, particularly of the lung base on the side of the paralyzed hemidiaphragm.[30] Plication of the paralyzed hemidiaphragm can improve lung volumes and arterial blood gases, presumably by stiffening the paralyzed side and preventing paradoxical motion.[71, 72]

Patients who have unilateral hemidiaphragmatic paralysis can manifest an abnormal pattern of gastric pressure swings in relation to pleural or esophageal pressure swings. Normally, gastric pressure becomes more positive as esophageal pressure becomes more negative during inspiration. In one investigation of 15 patients who had unilateral diaphragmatic paralysis, 12 showed an abnormal pattern of gastric pressure swings during quiet tidal breathing;[64] gastric pressure became more *negative* during inspiration, although to a lesser extent than the negative swing in esophageal pressure.

In patients who have bilateral diaphragmatic paralysis (see farther on), gastric pressure decreases to the same extent as esophageal pressure during tidal breathing, so that no active transdiaphragmatic pressure is generated.[67] This pattern of pressure swings could be caused by either an upward movement of the paralyzed hemidiaphragm that was greater than the downward movement of the functioning hemidiaphragm, or by recruitment of expiratory muscles and a sudden relaxation of these muscles at the onset of inspiration.

A definitive diagnosis of phrenic nerve dysfunction as the cause of hemidiaphragmatic paralysis can be obtained by employing the technique of phrenic nerve stimulation in the neck and the measurement of phrenic nerve latency.[37, 73] One method to do this involves the placement of felt-tipped electrodes over the phrenic nerve in the neck; the stimulation voltage is increased in a step-wise fashion while the compound action potential of the ipsilateral hemidiaphragm is recorded using surface electrodes placed on the anterolateral aspect of the chest in the eighth and ninth intercostal spaces or by placing intraesophageal or intradiaphragmatic electrodes.[74–76] A recent modification of this technique uses stimulation with a magnet, a process that circumvents the use of inaccurate surface electrodes and painful needle electrodes.[77–79]

Phrenic nerve latency is the time from stimulation of the nerve to the first detection of the compound action potential; in normal individuals, it ranges from 7 to 9 milliseconds, with an upper limit of 9.75 milliseconds.[80] When the phrenic nerve is completely interrupted or is significantly demyelinated, the compound action potential of the hemidiaphragm is absent or shows prolonged latency. Although this technique can be useful in detecting complete phrenic nerve interruption, it may not be sensitive in identifying partial axonal degeneration because latency may be normal when only a portion of the phrenic nerve axons are conducting. Unfortunately, measurements of the magnitude of the compound action potential from surface electrodes do not accurately reflect the extent of activation of the underlying diaphragm. A useful maneuver may be to combine phrenic nerve stimulation with fluoroscopic or ultrasound examination of diaphragmatic motion.

Bilateral Diaphragmatic Paralysis

In contrast to patients who have unilateral diaphragmatic paralysis, those who have bilateral paralysis have profound respiratory symptoms and functional derangement.[81] Bilateral diaphragmatic weakness causes less severe symptoms than paralysis but can be recognized when dyspnea is exaggerated in the supine position.[82] The causes of bilateral diaphragmatic paralysis are similar to those of unilateral paralysis (Table 77–2). Severe diaphragmatic weakness may be the principal manifestation of a generalized disorder such as myopathy[81, 83] or muscular dystrophy.[84] A rare hereditary form of bilateral diaphragmatic paralysis has been described in monozygotic twins.[85]

The radiographic appearance of bilateral diaphragmatic paralysis consists of elevated hemidiaphragms in both posteroanterior and lateral projections.[14] Linear atelectasis may be present at the lung bases. Paradoxical upward motion of both hemidiaphragms during an inspiratory effort or sniff

Table 77–2. BILATERAL DIAPHRAGMATIC PARALYSIS

ETIOLOGY	SELECTED REFERENCE(S)
Phrenic nerve injury	
Birth injury	195
Topical cardiac hypothermia	44, 45
Cervical disk surgery	
Chiropractic manipulation of the cervical spine	47
Blunt chest trauma	196
Neuritis	
Brachial neuritis (Parsonage-Turner syndrome)	197, 198
Paraneoplastic neuritis	199
CNS or spinal cord abnormalities	
Infantile spinomuscular atrophy	91, 200
Neuralgic amyotrophy	191
Arnold-Chiari malformation	201
Syringomyelia	202
Peripheral neuropathy	203
Multiple sclerosis	56, 204
Miscellaneous	
Diabetes mellitus	205
Mediastinal irradiation	207
Myopathies	
Idiopathic	206

is usually observed on fluoroscopic examination, although recruitment of abdominal expiratory muscles can cause a false-negative sniff test result.[81, 86] Some patients actively expire to a lung volume below the true FRC and then use the elastic recoil forces of the abdominothoracic structures to assist the next inspiration passively; the sudden downward motion of the diaphragm coincident with abdominal muscle relaxation may be misinterpreted as diaphragmatic contraction when viewed fluoroscopically. Despite these potential pitfalls, fluoroscopy can be effectively used to evaluate the condition.[87] The characteristic findings consist of cephalad movement of the paralyzed diaphragm during inspiration accompanied by outward chest wall and inward abdominal wall motion, a phenomenon known as *thoracoabdominal paradox*.[87] Diaphragmatic motion can also be monitored by ultrasonography.[17–19, 88, 89] Because ultrasound also permits assessment of diaphragmatic thickness and changing thickness with respiration,[18, 19] it may be superior to fluoroscopy.

Most patients who have bilateral diaphragmatic paralysis or significant weakness eventually develop ventilatory respiratory failure and hypercapnia; some present with evidence of cor pulmonale and right ventricular failure. Dyspnea on exertion and on assuming the supine position is a characteristic complaint. Dyspnea during recumbency is particularly distressing and can interfere with adequate sleep and result in daytime hypersomnolence. We have seen patients who were able to sleep only when on their hands and knees. The inadequate inspiratory effort also predisposes to atelectasis and respiratory infection.

On physical examination, percussion reveals dullness at both bases and decreased or absent diaphragmatic excursion as a result of the elevated resting position of the diaphragm. Patients are usually tachypneic and clearly using accessory inspiratory muscles. The characteristic physical finding, readily detectable in the supine position, is a paradoxical

inward motion of the anterior abdominal wall on inspiration (Fig. 77–5). This motion is caused by an upward movement of the flaccid diaphragm during inspiration as a result of the negative intrathoracic pressure generated by the normally contracting external intercostal and accessory muscles. Just as activation of abdominal expiratory muscles can cause a false-negative fluoroscopic sniff test result, it can mask the physical finding of paradoxical motion. However, abdominal muscle activation during expiration can be detected by gentle palpation of the abdominal wall during the breathing cycle. In addition, a biphasic abdominal motion may be appreciated—an outward motion at the beginning of inspiration as a result of the sudden relaxation of the abdominal muscles and a later inward motion as the relaxed abdominal wall follows the paradoxical upward movement of the paralyzed diaphragm. Paradoxical abdominal motion can be quantified by magnetometry.[90]

The presence of bilateral diaphragmatic paralysis can be confirmed by measuring transdiaphragmatic pressure swings during tidal breathing and maximal inspiratory efforts.[81, 86, 90] The former is measured by recording gastric and esophageal pressures. During inspiration, gastric pressure normally becomes positive and esophageal pressure negative; in the presence of diaphragmatic paralysis, weakness, or fatigue, the diaphragm acts as a flaccid membrane with the result that the negative intrathoracic pressure is transmitted to the abdominal cavity so that transdiaphragmatic pressure does not change. Even with maximal inspiratory effort, no transdiaphragmatic pressure develops, although maximal expiration may be associated with some transdiaphragmatic pressure as the diaphragm is passively stretched near residual volume.[90]

Bilateral diaphragmatic paralysis causes severe lung restriction. TLC and FRC are between 55% and 65% predicted, and vital capacity is in the range of 45% to 50% predicted.[85, 90a] The FEV_1 is usually decreased in proportion to the FVC so that the ratio of FEV_1 to FVC is normal. Maximal inspiratory mouth pressure is reduced to well below the normal range; maximal transdiaphragmatic pressure is characteristically zero in the presence of complete paralysis. Blood gas measurements show arterial hypoxemia and, in some cases, hypercarbia. The former is related to ventilation-perfusion mismatching at the lung bases and is exacerbated in the supine position.[92]

Eventration

Eventration is a congenital anomaly consisting of failure of muscular development of part or all of one or both hemidiaphragms.[93–95] In some cases, it may be difficult or impossible to distinguish it from diaphragmatic paralysis.[96, 97] When marked diaphragmatic elevation can be attributed to a specific cause (e.g., interruption of the phrenic nerve by an invasive neoplasm or surgical section), it is clearly possible to employ specific terminology in describing the condition. In some cases, however, there is no way of knowing whether elevation is caused by congenital absence of muscle or by phrenic paralysis. In an extensive radiographic survey of individuals older than nursery school age, a group of Japanese investigators showed that the incidence of partial eventration of the right hemidiaphragm increased with age, particularly among women over the age of 60 years;[98] the authors concluded that most right-sided eventrations are acquired and may be attributable to dietary and dressing habits!

Pathologically, a totally eventrated hemidiaphragm consists of a thin membrane attached to normal muscle at points of origin from the rib cage. Sometimes referred to as *Petit's eventration*, this variant occurs almost exclusively on the left side, a point that may be of value in its differentiation from diaphragmatic paralysis. The latter has an approximately equal incidence on the two sides, except in idiopathic cases, in which it occurs almost invariably on the right.[29] Bilateral total eventration is extremely rare.[99] Partial eventration is more common than the total form and is usually present at the anteromedial portion of the right hemidiaphragm;[93, 100, 101] it occurs with equal frequency in men and women,[102] rarely on the left, and occasionally in the central portion of either cupola.

A confident diagnosis of partial eventration can be established by CT[15, 16, 103, 104] or ultrasonography.[15, 105] The main value of these procedures is in distinguishing partial eventration from a focal bulge on the diaphragmatic contour caused by a diaphragmatic tumor or hernia. In eventration, the diaphragm, although thin, can be seen as a continuous layer above the elevated abdominal viscera and retroperitoneal or omental fat. On fluoroscopy and real-time ultrasound, the abnormal region can be seen to move downward with the normal portions of the hemidiaphragm, although it may have a slight lag in its inspiratory excursion.[15, 106] The radiologic signs of complete eventration are identical to those described for diaphragmatic paralysis. In patients who have partial eventration, the affected hemidiaphragm shows a smaller than normal inspiratory excursion. On fluoroscopy or real-time ultrasound, it may have an initial inspiratory lag or small paradoxical motion; however, later in inspiration, it has downward motion.[15]

Characteristically, eventration is unassociated with symptoms and is discovered on a screening chest radiograph. However, symptoms may be present in obese patients as a result of raised intra-abdominal pressure. Although these symptoms are usually related to the gastrointestinal tract, respiratory embarrassment and, rarely, cardiac dysfunction have been attributed to the anomaly.[93, 107]

Restriction of Diaphragmatic Motion

A great variety of diseases of the lungs, pleura, intra-abdominal organs, and diaphragm can lead to restriction of diaphragmatic motion. In some, the limitation is imposed by the character of the disease itself—for example, the severe pulmonary overinflation and air-trapping that categorize diffuse emphysema or acute severe asthma prevent normal ascent of the diaphragm during expiration. In other diseases, local irritation causes "splinting" of a hemidiaphragm that is manifested not only by reduced excursion but also by elevation; such splinting can be caused by acute lower lobe pneumonia or infarction, acute pleuritis, rib fractures, and acute intra-abdominal processes, such as subphrenic abscess, cholecystitis, and peritonitis.

Although other skeletal muscle groups react to irritation or injury by spasm, the diaphragm appears to react by relaxation; this is the only way to explain the elevation that characteristically accompanies local inflammation. The

mechanism by which the diaphragm is splinted in the postoperative period is thought to be neural inhibition of diaphragmatic activation,[108–110] possibly as a result of stimulation of diaphragmatic or splanchnic afferents. A localized decrease in neural activation electromyographically and reduced transdiaphragmatic pressure have been demonstrated following upper abdominal surgery in dogs.[109] Similar diaphragmatic dysfunction was found following laparotomy by one group of investigators who measured diaphragmatic muscle shortening with sonomicrometry crystals;[111] general anesthesia alone and lower abdominal surgery did not produce similar results. Diaphragmatic dysfunction is maximal in patients 8 hours after upper abdominal surgery, with function improving over the subsequent 2 to 7 days.[108] The decreased diaphragmatic activation is not directly related to pain because narcotic analgesia does not improve the deficit in transdiaphragmatic pressure generation.[110] Similarly, postoperative diaphragmatic dysfunction is not caused by a decrease in diaphragmatic contractility because direct stimulation of the phrenic nerve can result in a normal transdiaphragmatic pressure.[112]

Miscellaneous Causes of Disturbance in Diaphragmatic Motion

Several conditions other than restriction or paradox may be associated with abnormal movements of the diaphragm. *Tonic contraction* may occur in tetany, tetanus, rabies, strychnine poisoning, and the pleurodynia that accompanies Coxsackie B virus infection. *Diaphragmatic "flutter"* (respiratory myoclonus) was originally described in 1723 by van Leeuwenhoek when he recognized that he was having abnormal contractions of his diaphragm.[113] Some cases appear to develop as a result of abnormalities of the phrenic nerve or the diaphragm itself and may be precipitated by emotional tension or excitement.[114, 115] Other patients appear to suffer from a central epileptic focus, with involvement of all muscles of respiration, including the accessory muscles.[113] This disorder may present as part of a symptom complex that includes palatal, oropharyngeal, eye, and facial muscle myoclonus. The rapid diaphragmatic contractions may result in pain and dyspnea. In one patient, diaphragmatic flutter was documented and followed by respiratory inductive plethysmography.[116] In *persistent hiccups,* a form of chronic contraction of the diaphragm that occurs at a much lower frequency than flutter, an inspiratory sound is created as air is drawn into the thorax through a partially closed glottis. We have seen one patient who manifested periodic irregular, sudden diaphragmatic contractions late in the expiratory phase of respiration that seemed analogous to a premature heart beat but caused the patient considerably more discomfort.

DIAPHRAGMATIC HERNIAS

Herniation of abdominal or retroperitoneal organs or tissues into the thorax may occur through congenital or acquired weak areas in the diaphragm or through rents resulting from trauma (the latter are discussed in Chapter 66, page 2636). The most common nontraumatic diaphragmatic

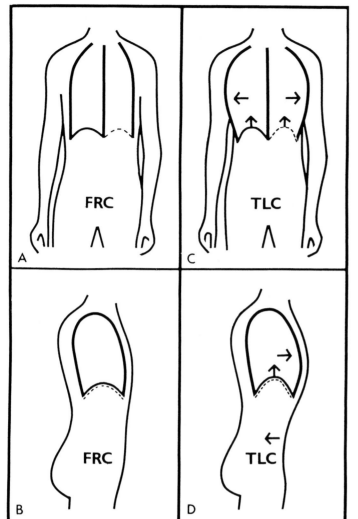

Figure 77–5. Schematic Depiction of Chest Cage and Diaphragmatic Movements Throughout the Respiratory Cycle: Bilateral Diaphragmatic Paralysis. On inspiration to TLC from FRC *(A to D)*, the increased negative intrapleural pressure "sucks" the diaphragm up and draws the abdominal wall in.

hernia occurs through the esophageal hiatus; less common forms include those through the pleuroperitoneal hiatus (Bochdalek's hernias) and through the parasternal hiatus (Morgagni's hernias).

Hernia Through the Esophageal Hiatus

Although a congenital weakness of the esophageal hiatus may be partly responsible for the development of hiatus hernia, there is little doubt that acquired factors play a significant role, the most important being obesity and pregnancy. The prevalence increases with age; in one investigation of 120 patients, the hernias were seen in 2 of 40 (5%) patients under the age of 40 years, 12 of 40 (30%) between the ages of 40 and 59 years, and 26 of 40 (65%) between the ages of 60 and 79 years (Fig. 77–6).[117]

Because the hernia is related to the esophageal hiatus, the stomach is by far the most common herniated structure. Plain radiographs of the chest often show a retrocardiac mass, usually containing air or an air-fluid level (Fig. 77–7). Definitive diagnosis, however, sometimes requires barium study of the esophagogastric junction or the use of CT.[117, 118]

Occasionally, large hernias are located predominantly on one side of the hemithorax and mimic a lung abscess on the radiograph (Fig. 77–8). In cases in which most of the stomach has herniated through the hiatus, the stomach may undergo volvulus within the mediastinum and present as a large mass, sometimes containing a double air-filled level (Fig. 77–9); incarceration of such hernial contents is common, and strangulation may occur.[119, 120] (A number of cases also have been reported of strangulation of contents that have herniated through the diaphragmatic incision made for *repair* of hiatus hernia.[121]) The development of acute upper gastrointestinal tract symptoms in a patient who has a herniated stomach should immediately raise the suspicion of strangulation;[122] the complication is life-threatening and necessitates immediate surgical intervention.

Although the stomach is the most common hernial content, other structures are seen occasionally, including a portion of the transverse colon, a pancreatic pseudocyst,[123] omentum, or liver.[124] In addition, ascitic fluid can extend from the peritoneal cavity into the posterior mediastinum through the esophageal hiatus, an occurrence that can be demonstrated to excellent advantage on CT.[125] In one patient, a large calcified leiomyoma arose from the herniated portion

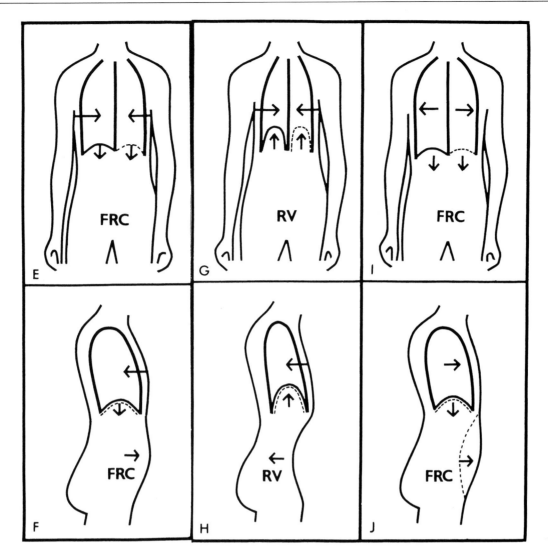

Figure 77–5 *Continued.* On expiration to FRC *(E* and *F)*, the diaphragm descends, and the abdomen protrudes. With a deeper expiration to RV accompanied by active contraction of the abdominal muscles *(G* and *H)*, the diaphragm rises. Subsequently, during the first part of inspiration to FRC *(I* and *J)*, abdominal muscle recoil is associated with descent of the flaccid diaphragm, creating the false impression of active contraction.

of stomach in a large hiatus hernia and presented as a mediastinal mass.[126]

Most patients who have esophageal hiatus hernias do not have symptoms, and the abnormality is discovered on a screening chest radiograph or examination of the upper gastrointestinal tract for unrelated complaints. When present, symptoms consist of retrosternal "burning" and pain, typically occurring after meals and accentuated when the patient lies down; they are relieved by the ingestion of antacid. Symptoms of anemia caused by blood loss may be predominant. In one investigation of 267 patients, 61 (23%) had evidence of blood loss attributable to the hernia;[127] 27 (10%) of the patients presented with hematemesis, 19 (7%) with melena or a history thereof, and 16 (6%) with established iron-deficiency anemia and only a trace of blood or none in the stool.

Hernia Through the Foramen of Bochdalek

In infants, herniation through a persistent embryonic pleuroperitoneal hiatus is not only the most common form

of diaphragmatic hernia but also by far the most serious. Its incidence is 1 in 2,200 live births.[15, 128] Seventy-five to 90% occur on the left side.[129–131] When large, the hernias are associated with a high death rate unless surgically corrected. Even with surgery, the mortality rate is about 30% as a result of hypoplasia of the underlying lung and pulmonary arterial hypertension.[131]

The size of the defect ranges widely. When large, as with complete or almost complete absence of a hemidiaphragm, almost the entire abdominal contents may be in the left hemithorax, thereby interfering with normal lung development and resulting in hypoplasia [132, 133] (*see* page 598). Rarely, there is bilateral agenesis.[134] In most large hernias, there is no peritoneal sac, and communication between the pleural and peritoneal cavities is wide open. When the defect is small, a sac lined by pleura and containing retroperitoneal fat, a portion of the spleen or kidney,[135] or omentum may be the only discernible abnormality.[136, 137]

In adults, small Bochdalek's hernias are much more common than in infants and are almost always unassociated with symptoms. Their incidence increases with age, sug-

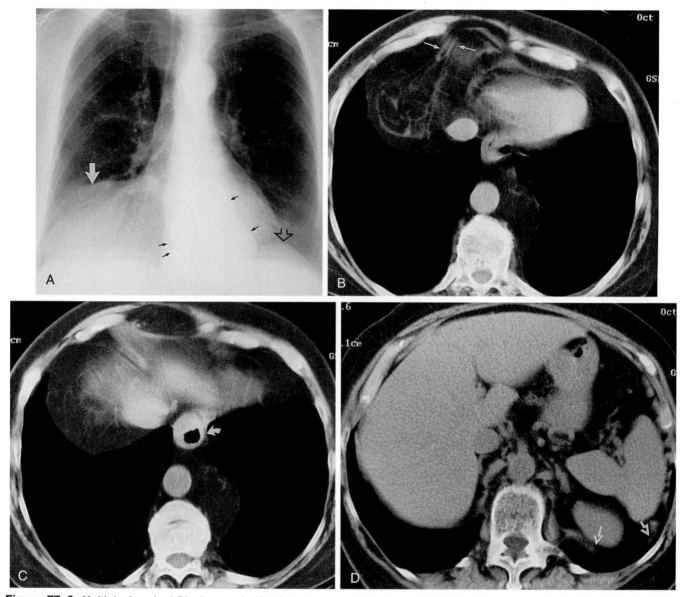

Figure 77–6. Multiple Acquired Diaphragmatic Hernias. A posteroanterior chest radiograph *(A)* in a 69-year-old woman demonstrates a large mass with fat density in the right costophrenic sulcus *(white arrow),* a mass displacing the azygoesophageal recess and left paraspinal interface *(black arrows),* and a mass adjacent to the left hemidiaphragm *(open arrow).* A CT scan *(B)* demonstrates vessels *(arrows)* extending from a defect in the right parasternal region into the mass in the right costophrenic sulcus, a finding diagnostic of Morgagni's hernia. A scan at a more caudad level *(C)* demonstrates a hiatus hernia *(curved arrow)* with associated herniation of omental fat. A scan at a more caudad level *(D)* demonstrates a defect in the left hemidiaphragm *(open arrows)* with herniation of retroperitoneal fat (Bochdalek's hernia).

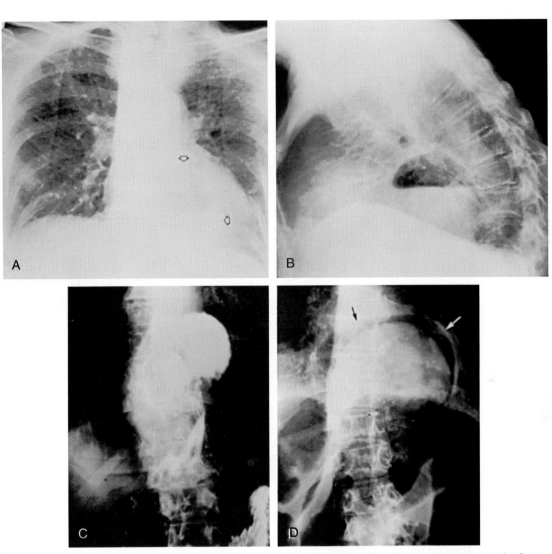

Figure 77–7. Hiatus Hernia. Posteroanterior *(A)* and lateral *(B)* radiographs of the chest of an 87-year-old woman reveal a large soft tissue mass containing a prominent air-fluid level occupying the posteroinferior portion of the mediastinum *(arrows in A)*. An anteroposterior radiograph of the lower mediastinum and upper abdomen following the ingestion of barium *(C)* confirms the presence of herniation of a large portion of stomach into the posterior mediastinum. The patient had no symptoms referable to this hernia. Somewhat later, the patient developed an acute abdomen, with severe abdominal distention and signs of peritonitis. An anteroposterior radiograph *(D)* revealed a double density in the posterior mediastinum, the hernial sac being outlined by gas *(arrows)* and the central portion of the sac containing a homogeneous mass representing a fluid-filled gastric fundus. A hollow abdominal viscus had perforated, releasing gas into the peritoneal space; some of the gas had passed through the esophageal hiatus, outlining the sac.

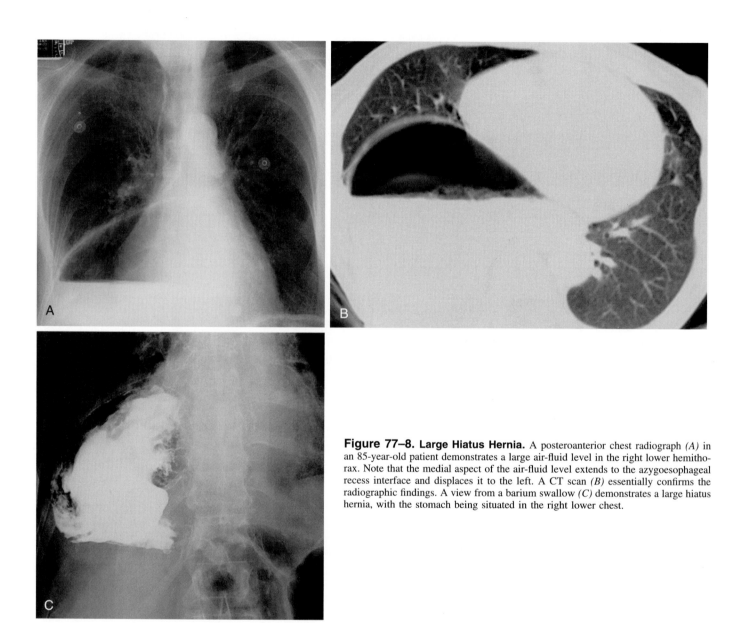

Figure 77–8. Large Hiatus Hernia. A posteroanterior chest radiograph *(A)* in an 85-year-old patient demonstrates a large air-fluid level in the right lower hemithorax. Note that the medial aspect of the air-fluid level extends to the azygoesophageal recess interface and displaces it to the left. A CT scan *(B)* essentially confirms the radiographic findings. A view from a barium swallow *(C)* demonstrates a large hiatus hernia, with the stomach being situated in the right lower chest.

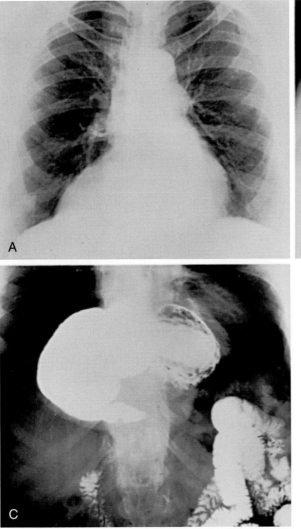

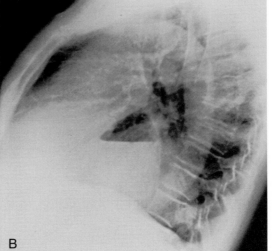

Figure 77–9. Hiatus Hernia. Posteroanterior *(A)* and lateral *(B)* radiograph reveal a large soft tissue mass in the posterior mediastinum, projecting to the right as a smooth, well-defined shadow in the plane of the cardiophrenic angle. A prominent air-fluid level is present within it. Note the downward displacement of the right hemidiaphragm. A radiograph following ingestion of barium *(C)* shows herniation of the whole stomach through the esophageal hiatus into the posterior mediastinum; in the process, the stomach has undergone complete organoaxial volvulus. The shadow projected in the plane of the right cardiophrenic angle on the posteroanterior radiograph is caused by the rotated greater curvature of the stomach. The patient was a 65-year-old woman who had no definite symptoms referable to the hernia.

gesting that they are acquired. In one review of CT scans of the chest and abdomen performed in 940 adult patients, 60 Bochdalek's hernias were found in 52 patients, a prevalence of 6%.[138] Thirty-nine hernias (65%) were left sided and 21 (35%) right sided. In all cases, the hernias contained only fat and were unassociated with symptoms. Another group of investigators correlated the frequency of diaphragmatic defects seen on CT with age in 120 patients ranging from 20 to 79 years of age.[116a] Bochdalek's hernias were seen in 14 patients (12%). They were present in one of 20 (5%) patients between 40 and 49 years of age, 3 of 20 (15%) between 50 and 59 years, 3 of 20 (15%) between 60 and 69 years of age, and 7 of 20 (35%) between 70 and 79 years old; none were present in patients less than 40 years of age. Sixty-five percent of the defects involved the left hemidiaphragm; 60% involved the posterior diaphragm, 27% were at the junction of the lateral arm of the crus and the posterior diaphragm, and 13% were located in the crus or laterally near the costal region of the diaphragm. The frequency of diaphragmatic defects did not correlate with the amount of skeletal muscle or with obesity but was greater in patients who had emphysema.

On the chest radiograph, Bochdalek's hernias can present as a focal bulge in the hemidiaphragm or as a mass adjacent to the posteromedial aspect of either hemidiaphragm (Fig. 77–10). Although the diagnosis can often be suspected by the typical location and by the lower than soft tissue density of the mass as a result of its fat content, the appearance can mimic that of pulmonary, mediastinal, or paravertebral masses.[139–141] The diagnosis is readily made on CT.[117, 138, 141] Occasionally, spiral CT with coronal or sagittal reformations may be required to demonstrate the defects.[142, 143]

Hernia Through the Foramen of Morgagni

Morgagni's (retrosternal or parasternal) hernia is an uncommon form of diaphragmatic hernia. Because the left foramen relates to the heart, most herniations occur on the right; in one series of 50 cases, 4 were bilateral and only 1 was solely left sided.[144] Although the defects are developmental in origin, hernias are more commonly seen in adults than in children and are often associated with obesity, severe effort, or other causes of increased intra-abdominal pressure or trauma;[15, 145, 146] in fact, affected patients are usually overweight, middle-aged women. In contrast to Bochdalek's hernias, a peritoneal sac is present in most cases. The content

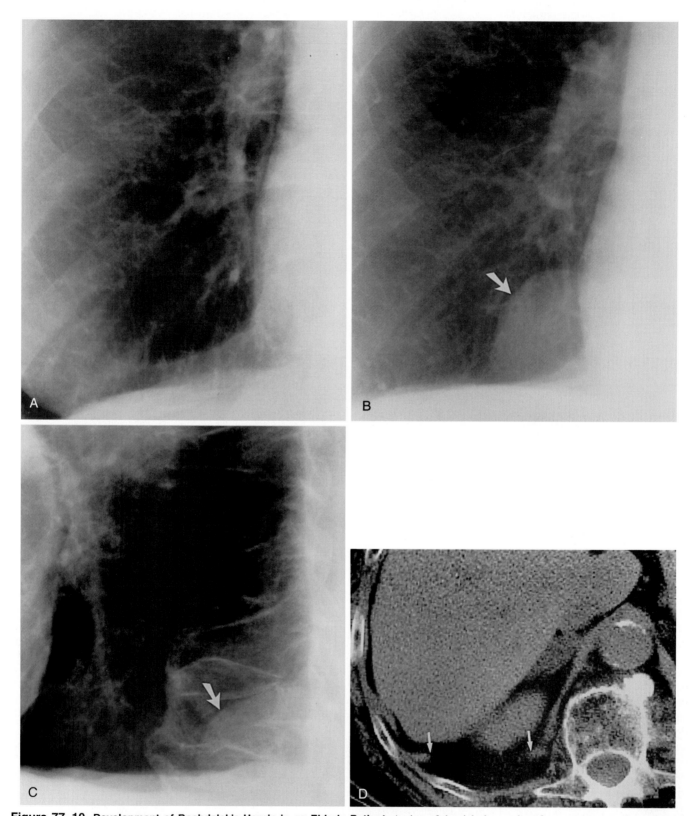

Figure 77–10. Development of Bochdalek's Hernia in an Elderly Patient. A view of the right lower chest from a posteroanterior radiograph *(A)* in a 78-year-old woman is unremarkable. Views from posteroanterior *(B)* and lateral *(C)* radiographs performed 5 years later demonstrate a large mass adjacent to the posteromedial aspect of the right hemidiaphragm *(arrows)*. The mass has lower opacity than the heart and soft tissues of the abdomen, consistent with fat. A view of the right hemidiaphragm from a CT scan *(D)* demonstrates a focal defect *(arrows)* in the posterior aspect of the right hemidiaphragm with herniation of retroperitoneal fat. The patient had no symptoms related to the hernia.

of the hernial sac is usually omentum[147] and sometimes liver or bowel; rarely, other structures, such as a stone-filled gallbladder,[148] stomach,[149] or a congenital hepatic cyst,[150] have been identified. Cases have been reported in which the defect has extended into the pericardial sac, allowing displacement of abdominal contents into this site.[151, 152]

Radiologically, the typical appearance is that of a smooth, well-defined opacity in the right cardiophrenic angle (Fig. 77–11). In most patients, the shadow is of homogeneous density. Occasionally, it is inhomogeneous as a result of either an air-containing loop of bowel or the predominantly fatty nature of the hernial contents (Fig. 77–12). In the latter situation, the hernia is likely to contain omentum, and CT or barium enema reveals the transverse colon to be situated high in the abdomen with a peak situated anteriorly and superiorly, a finding that is virtually diagnostic. Bilateral anteromedial defects in the diaphragm produce a characteristic radiographic pattern when abdominal organs herniate through a single midline opening.[153] In the rare case in which the hernia penetrates into the pericardial sac, loops of air-containing bowel may be identified anterior to the cardiac shadow.[151, 152] The diagnosis of Morgagni's hernia can be readily made on CT [16, 141, 154] or MR imaging.[15]

Most hernias through the foramen of Morgagni do not give rise to symptoms. The minority of adults who have symptoms complain of epigastric or lower sternal pressure and discomfort[147] and (sometimes) cardiorespiratory and gastrointestinal symptoms.[155] In one highly selected series of nine patients, four had gastrointestinal symptoms, two had respiratory symptoms, and one had retrosternal pain.[156] When the sac contains portions of the gastrointestinal tract, strangulation and obstruction may occur, and complications have been reported in 10% to 15% of cases.[147] Extension of the defect into the pericardial sac may produce severe cardiorespiratory symptoms and necessitate prompt corrective surgery, particularly in infants. Abrupt enlargement of a

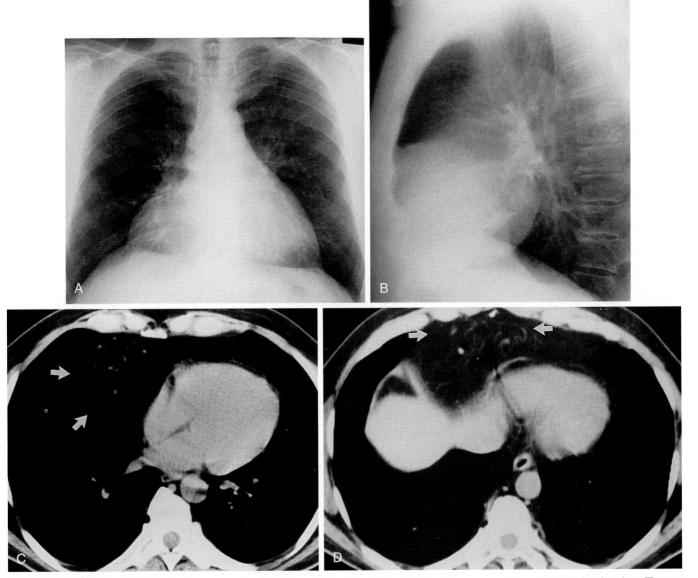

Figure 77–11. Morgagni's Hernia. Posteroanterior *(A)* and lateral *(B)* chest radiographs demonstrate a mass in the right costophrenic sulcus. The mass has a lower than soft tissue density consistent with fat. CT scans *(C* and *D)* demonstrate herniation of omental fat *(arrows)* through the right lower parasternal region diagnostic of Morgagni's hernia. The patient was a 49-year-old man.

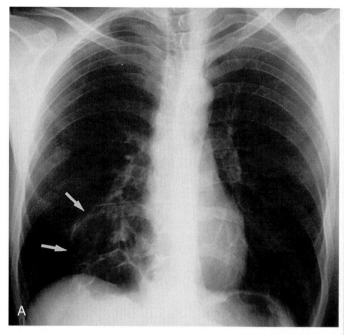

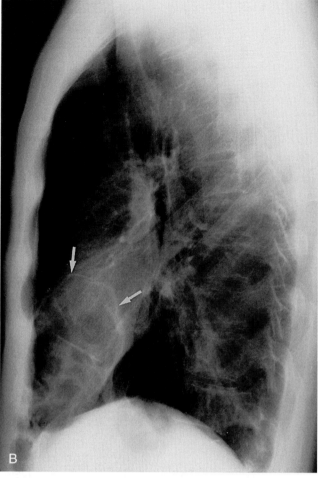

Figure 77–12. Morgagni's Hernia. Posteroanterior *(A)* and lateral *(B)* chest radiographs demonstrate Morgagni's hernia with herniation of colon *(arrows)*. The patient was a 39-year-old man. (Courtesy of Dr. Jim Barrie, University of Alberta Hospital, Edmonton, Alberta.)

previously existing diaphragmatic hernia with subsequent strangulation has been reported as a complication of pregnancy and labor.[157]

NEOPLASMS OF THE DIAPHRAGM

Primary Neoplasms

Primary neoplasms of the diaphragm are rare.[158, 159] In a review of the literature from 1868 to 1968, one group of investigators identified only 84 cases.[159] Most develop from the tendinous or anterior muscular portion. Benign and malignant forms occur with relatively equal frequency.[160] The former include lipoma (the most common),[162–164] angiofibroma, neurofibroma, neurilemoma,[165] leiomyoma, teratoma (Fig. 77–13),[166, 167] desmoid tumor,[168] and tumors with various mesenchymal admixtures.[160] Because fat pads and herniations of omental fat are common in the region of the diaphragm, the radiologic diagnosis of lipoma requires demonstration of a true capsule.[164] Malignant neoplasms include fibrosarcoma (the most common),[164, 169] malignant fibrous histiocytoma,[170] hemangiopericytoma,[171] germ cell tumors,[172] pheochromocytoma,[173] epithelioid hemangioendothelioma,[174] leiomyosarcoma,[161, 175] and chondrosarcoma.[164, 176, 177] Various non-neoplastic abnormalities that form localized tumors, such as lymphangioma and endometrioma,[158] are also occasionally found.

Radiologically, most diaphragmatic tumors present as smooth or lobulated soft tissue masses protruding into the inferior portion of the lung (Fig. 77–14). Benign neoplasms may calcify. In many cases, malignant tumors involve much of one hemidiaphragm and thus simulate diaphragmatic elevation; associated pleural effusion is common. The presence of an intradiaphragmatic mass can be established most easily by CT.[15, 163, 164, 166] When the tumor is large, it may not be possible to determine whether it arose from the diaphragm, pleura, lungs, or liver.[164] Variations in diaphragmatic thickness on CT occasionally mimic an intradiaphragmatic mass or a tumor in an adjacent organ.[178] The distinction can be readily made by careful analysis of sequential images. Rarely, muscular hypertrophy of a diaphragmatic crus simulates a paraspinal mass on the radiograph.[179]

Characteristically, benign neoplasms are unassociated with symptoms; by contrast, most patients who have primary malignant neoplasms complain of epigastric or lower chest pain, cough, dyspnea, and gastrointestinal discomfort.[158, 159]

Secondary Neoplasms

Secondary neoplastic involvement of the diaphragm occurs most frequently by direct extension of neoplasm from the basal pleura in cases of pulmonary carcinoma or mesothelioma; however, any neoplasm that metastasizes to

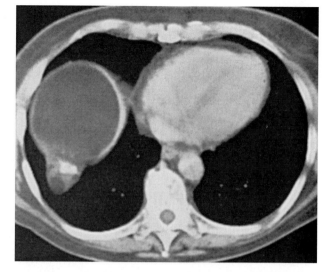

Figure 77–13. Cystic Teratoma of the Right Hemidiaphragm. A CT scan at the level of the right hemidiaphragm shows a mass containing fat (CT attenuation, −70 HU), a small amount of soft tissue posteriorly, and two small areas of calcification. The mass was resected and proved to be a cystic teratoma on pathologic examination; it was shown to contain a tooth. This 65-year-old woman presented with a 1-year history of right upper quadrant pain and nausea. (From Müller NL: J Comput Assist Tomogr 10:325, 1986.)

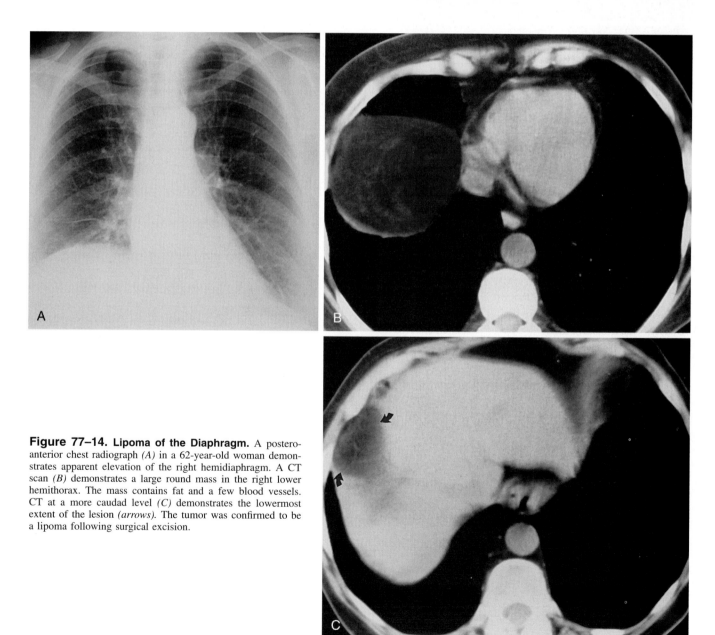

Figure 77–14. Lipoma of the Diaphragm. A postero-anterior chest radiograph *(A)* in a 62-year-old woman demonstrates apparent elevation of the right hemidiaphragm. A CT scan *(B)* demonstrates a large round mass in the right lower hemithorax. The mass contains fat and a few blood vessels. CT at a more caudad level *(C)* demonstrates the lowermost extent of the lesion *(arrows)*. The tumor was confirmed to be a lipoma following surgical excision.

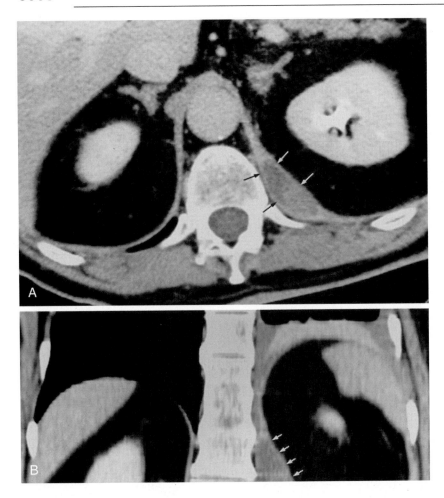

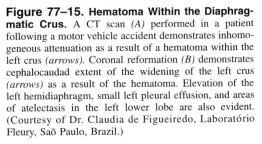

Figure 77–15. Hematoma Within the Diaphragmatic Crus. A CT scan *(A)* performed in a patient following a motor vehicle accident demonstrates inhomogeneous attenuation as a result of a hematoma within the left crus *(arrows)*. Coronal reformation *(B)* demonstrates cephalocaudad extent of the widening of the left crus *(arrows)* as a result of the hematoma. Elevation of the left hemidiaphragm, small left pleural effusion, and areas of atelectasis in the left lower lobe are also evident. (Courtesy of Dr. Claudia de Figueiredo, Laboratório Fleury, Saõ Paulo, Brazil.)

the pleura or that involves the basal lung, liver, or subphrenic peritoneum can spread into the diaphragm. Ovarian carcinoma is particularly likely to be the cause when the initial site of involvement is the peritoneum.[180] Discrete diaphragmatic metastases, derived from either lymphatic or hematogenous spread, are rare. Radiographic features and clinical manifestations are usually related to the presence of neoplasm in contiguous structures or elsewhere, rather than in the diaphragm itself.

MISCELLANEOUS DIAPHRAGMATIC ABNORMALITIES

Accessory diaphragm is a rare anomaly in which the right hemithorax is partitioned into two compartments by a musculotendinous membrane resembling a diaphragm.[181–183] About 30 cases had been reported by 1995.[184] The accessory leaf usually is situated within the oblique fissure, separating the lower lobe from the remainder of the right lung. It is attached medially to the pericardium, inferiorly and anteriorly to the diaphragm, and laterally and posteriorly to the chest wall. Radiologically, it may be mistaken for a somewhat thickened major fissure. The anomaly has been associ

ated with pulmonary hypoplasia and can cause neonatal respiratory distress,[184] but usually does not give rise to symptoms.

Diaphragmatic defects, too small to allow passage of a hernial sac, may explain in part the pleural effusions that develop in patients with conditions such as Meigs' syndrome or cirrhosis and ascites.[185, 186] Such defects may be congenital or acquired and can be demonstrated either directly at autopsy or indirectly by the development of pneumothorax following intraperitoneal administration of gas.[186] Similar small defects have been postulated as the entry sites for tissue or air in some cases of pleural endometriosis and catamenial pneumothorax[187] (*see* page 2767).

Intradiaphragmatic cysts are rare and usually represent extralobar sequestration. The abnormality is presumably caused by entrapment of an accessory lung bud within the diaphragm during its development. In most cases, the cyst receives its blood supply from the abdominal aorta or one of its branches and characteristically drains by way of the systemic veins.[188] The anomaly relates to the left hemidiaphragm in 90% of cases and is usually associated with diaphragmatic eventration.[189] Occasionally, intradiaphragmatic cysts are the result of a degenerated traumatic hematomas[15] (Fig. 77–15). Rarely, cystic lesions of the liver, such as amebic or hydatid cysts, simulate a diaphragmatic cyst (Fig. 77–16).

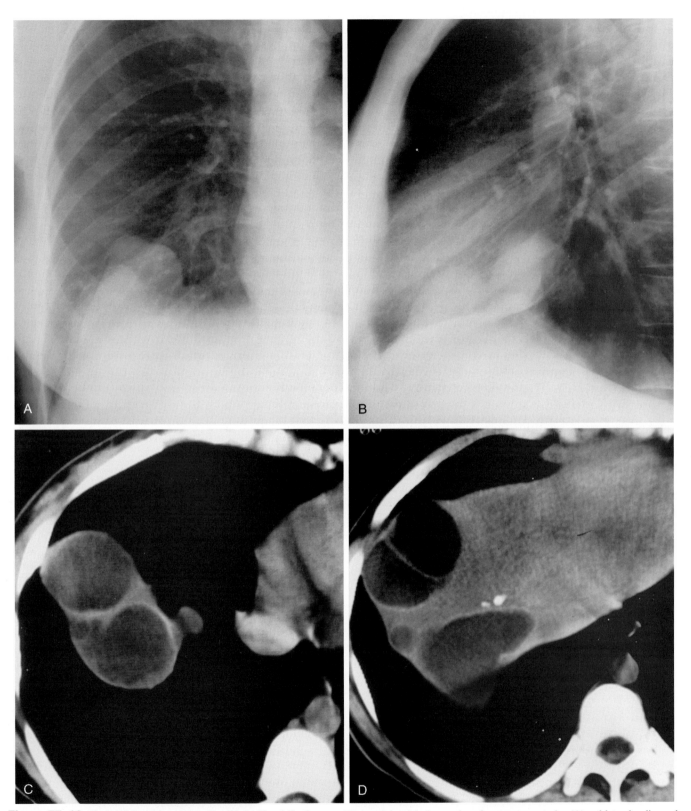

Figure 77–16. Hydatid Cyst Involving the Right Hemidiaphragm. Views of the right lower chest from posteroanterior *(A)* and lateral radiographs *(B)* reveal a lobulated mass extending from the right hemidiaphragm into the inferior aspect of the right middle lobe. CT scans *(C and D)* demonstrate several cystic lesions in the right lower chest and in the liver. Also noted are foci of calcification in the liver. At surgery, the patient was found to have hydatid disease of the liver that extended through the diaphragm and into the lung. This 30-year-old woman presented with right upper quadrant pain.

REFERENCES

1. Whitelaw WA: Topography of the diaphragm. *In* Lengant C (ed): The Thorax. Part A: Physiology: Lung Biology in Health and Disease. New York, Marcel Dekker, 1995, pp 587.
2. Malagari K, Fraser RG: Imaging of the chest wall and diaphragm. *In* Lenfant C (ed): The Thorax. Part A: Physiology: Lung Biology in Health and Disease. New York, Marcel Dekker, 1995, pp 1763.
3. Lennon EA, Simon G: The height of the diaphragm in the chest radiograph of normal adults. Br J Radiol 38:937, 1965.
4. Felson B: Chest Roentgenology. Philadelphia, WB Saunders, 1973.
5. Wittenborg MH, Aviad I: Organ influence on the normal posture of the diaphragm: A radiological study of inversions and heterotaxias. Br J Radiol 36:280, 1963.
6. Reddy V, Sharma S, Cobanoglu A: What dictates the position of the diaphragm: The heart or the liver? A review of sixty-five cases. J Thoracic Cardiovasc Surg 108:687, 1994.
7. Lasser EC: Some aspects of pulmonary dynamics revealed by concurrent roentgen kymography of spirometric movements and diaphragmatic excursions. Radiology 77:434, 1961.
8. Fraser RG: Unpublished observations.
9. Young DA, Simon G: Certain movements measured on inspiration-expiration chest radiographs correlated with pulmonary function studies. Clin Radiol 23:37, 1972.
10. Alexander C: Diaphragm movements and the diagnosis of diaphragmatic paralysis. Clin Radiol 17:79, 1966.
11. Schmidt S: Anatomic and physiologic aspects of respiratory kymography. Acta Radiol (Diagn) 8:409, 1969.
12. Houston JG, Morris AD, Howie CA, et al: Technical report: Quantitative assessment of diaphragmatic movement: A reproducible method using ultrasound. Clin Radiol 46:705, 1992.
13. Simon G, Bonnell J, Kazantzis G, et al: Some radiological observations on the range of movement of the diaphragm. Clin Radiol 20:213, 1969.
14. Alexander C: Diaphragm movements and the diagnosis of diaphragmatic paralysis. Clin Radiol 17:79, 1966.
15. Tarver RD, Conces DJ Jr, Cory DA, et al: Imaging the diaphragm and its disorders. J Thorac Imaging 4:1, 1989.
16. Graham NJ, Müller NL: The diaphragm. Can Assoc Radiol J 43:250, 1992.
17. Houston JG, Fleet M, Cowan MD, et al: Comparison of ultrasound with fluoroscopy in the assessment of suspected hemidiaphragmatic movement abnormality. Clin Radiol 50:95, 1995.
18. Ueki J, De Bruin PF, Pride NB: *In vivo* assessment of diaphragm contraction by ultrasound in normal subjects. Thorax 50:1157, 1995.
19. Gottesman E, McCool FD: Ultrasound evaluation of the paralyzed diaphragm. Am J Respir Crit Care Med 155:1570, 1997.
20. Jousela I, Tahvanainen J, Makelainen A, et al: Diaphragmatic movement studied with ultrasound during spontaneous breathing and mechanical ventilation with intermittent positive pressure ventilation (IPPV) and airway pressure release ventilation (APRV) in man. Anaesthesiologie und Reanimation 19:43, 1994.
21. McCool FD, Hoppin FG: Ultrasonography of the diaphragm. *In* Lenfant C (ed): The Thorax. Part B: Applied Physiology: Lung Biology in Health and Disease. New York, Marcel Dekker, 1995, pp 1295.
22. Ueki J, De Bruin PF, Pride NB: In vivo assessment of diaphragm contraction by ultrasound in normal subjects. Thorax 50:1157, 1995.
23. Cohn DB, Benditt JO, Sherman CB, et al: Diaphragm thickness: An index of respiratory muscle strength. Am Rev Respir Dis 147:A694, 1993.
24. Dovgan DJ, Lenchik L, Kaye AD: Computed tomographic evaluation of maximal diaphragmatic crural thickness. Conn Med 58:203, 1994.
25. Kanematsu M, Imaeda T, Mochizuki R, et al: Dynamic MRI of the diaphragm. J Comput Assist Tomogr 19:67, 1995.
26. Gierada DS, Curtin JJ, Erickson SJ, et al: Diaphragmatic motion: Fast gradient recalled-echo MR imaging in healthy subjects. Radiology 194:879, 1995.
27. Gauthier AP, Verbanck S, Estenne M, et al: Three-dimensional reconstruction of the *in vivo* human diaphragm shape at different lung volumes. J Appl Physiol 76:495, 1994.
28. Pettiaux N, Cassart M, Paiva M, et al: Three-dimensional reconstruction of human diaphragm with the use of spiral computed tomography. J Appl Physiol 82:998, 1997.
29. Riley EA: Idiopathic diaphragmatic paralysis: A report of eight cases. Am J Med 32:404, 1962.
30. Ridyard JB, Stewart RM: Regional lung function in unilateral diaphragmatic paralysis. Thorax 31:438, 1976.
31. Moorthy SS, Gibbs PS, Losasso AM, et al: Transient paralysis of the diaphragm following radical neck surgery. Laryngoscope 93:642, 1983.
32. Smith CD, Sade RM, Crawford FA, et al: Diaphragmatic paralysis and eventration in infants. J Thorac Cardiovasc Surg 91:490, 1986.
33. Heine MF, Asher EF, Roy TM, et al: Phrenic nerve injury following scalenectomy in a patient with thoracic outlet obstruction. J Clin Anesth 7:75, 1995.
34. Markand ON, Moorthy S, Mahomed J, et al: Postoperative phrenic nerve palsy in patients with open heart surgery. Ann Thorac Surg 39:68, 1985.
35. Large FR, Heywood LJ, Flower CD, et al: Incidence and aetiology of a raised hemidiaphragm after cardiopulmonary bypass. Thorax 40:444, 1985.
36. Estenne N, Yernault JC, De Smett JN, et al: Phrenic and diaphragm function after coronary artery bypass grafting. Thorax 40:293, 1985.
37. Wilcox P, Baile EM, Hards J, et al: Phrenic nerve function and its relationship to atelectasis after coronary artery bypass surgery. Chest 93:693, 1988.
38. Benjamin JJ, Cascade PN, Reubenfire N, et al: Left lower atelectasis and consolidation following cardiac surgery: The effect of topical cooling on the phrenic nerve. Radiology 142:11, 1982.
39. Rousou JA, Parker T, Angelman RM, et al: Phrenic nerve paresis associated with the use of iced slush and the cooling jacket for topical hypothermia. J Thorac Cardiovasc Surg 89:921, 1985.
40. Nochomovitz ML, Goldman M, Mitra J, et al: Respiratory responses in reversible diaphragm paralysis. J Appl Physiol 51:1150, 1981.
41. Esposito RA, Spencer FC: The effect of pericardial insulation on hypothermic phrenic nerve injury during open heart surgery. Ann Thorac Surg 43:303, 1987.
42. Wheeler WE, Rubis LJ, Jones CW, et al: Etiology and prevention of topical cardiac hypothermia-induced phrenic nerve injury and left lower lobe atelectasis during cardiac surgery. Chest 88:680, 1985.
43. Kohorst WR, Schonfeld SA, Altman M: Bilateral diaphragmatic paralysis following topical cardiac hypothermia. Chest 85:65, 1984.
44. Cabrera MR, Edsall JR: Bilateral diaphragm paralysis associated with topical cardiac hypothermia. N Y State J Med 87:514, 1987.
45. Olopade CO, Staats BA: Time course of recovery from frostbitten phrenics after coronary artery bypass graft surgery. Chest 99:1112, 1991.
46. Heffner JE: Diaphragmatic paralysis following chiropractic manipulation of the cervical spine. Arch Intern Med 145:562, 1985.
47. Pandit A, Kalra S, Woodcock A: An unusual cause of bilateral diaphragmatic paralysis. Thorax 47:201, 1992.
48. Drachler DH, Koepke GW, Weg G: Phrenic nerve injury from subclavian vein catheterization: Diagnosis by electromyography. JAMA 236:2280, 1976.
49. Best JB, Pereira M, Senior RM: Phrenic nerve injury associated with the venipuncture of the internal jugular vein. Chest 28:777, 1980.
50. Hadeed HA, Braun TW: Paralysis of the hemidiaphragm as a complication of internal jugular vein cannulation: Report of a case. J Oral Maxillofac Surg 46:409, 1988.
51. Buszek MC, Szymke TE, Honet JC, et al: Hemidiaphragmatic paralysis: An unusual complication of cervical spondylosis. Arch Phys Med Rehab 64:601, 1983.
52. Mellem H, Johansen B, Nakstad P, et al: Unilateral phrenic nerve paralysis caused by osteoarthritis of the cervical spine. Eur J Respir Dis 71:56, 1987.
53. Lenz H, Rohr H: Zur radikulären Genese der sogenannten Relaxatio diaphragmatis. (Radicular genesis of so-called relaxatio diaphragmatis.) Fortschr Roentgenstr 103:540, 1965.
54. Lagueny A, Ellie E, Saintarailles J, et al: Unilateral diaphragmatic paralysis: An electrophysiological study. J Neurol Neurosurg Psychiatr 55:316, 1992.
55. Balbierz JM, Ellenberg M, Honet JC: Complete hemidiaphragmatic paralysis in a patient with multiple sclerosis. Am J Phys Med Rehabil 67:161, 1988.
56. Aisen M, Arlt G, Foster S: Diaphragmatic paralysis without bulbar or limb paralysis in multiple sclerosis. Chest 98:499, 1990.
57. Santamaria J, Ruiz C: Diaphragmatic elevation in stroke. Eur Neurol 28:81, 1988.
58. Ford GT, Whitelaw WA, Rosenal TW, et al: Diaphragm function after upper abdominal surgery in humans. Am Rev Respir Dis 127:431, 1983.
59. Anderson RD, Connell TH, Lowman RM: Inversion of the liver and suprahepatic gallbladder associated with eventration of the diaphragm. Radiology 97:87, 1970.
60. Shin MS, Ho K-J: Computed tomographic evaluation of the pathologic lesion for the idiopathic diaphragmatic paralysis. J Comput Tomogr 6:257, 1982.
61. Arborelius M, Lilja B, Senyk J: Regional and total lung function studies in patients with hemidiaphragmatic paralysis. Respiration 32:253, 1975.
62. Ridyard JB, Stewart RM: Regional lung function in unilateral diaphragmatic paralysis. Thorax 31:438, 1976.
63. Easton PA, Fleetham JA, de la Rocha A, et al: Respiratory function after paralysis of the right hemidiaphragm. Am Rev Respir Dis 127:1125, 1983.
64. Lisboa C, Paré PD, Pertuze J, et al: Inspiratory muscle function in unilateral diaphragmatic paralysis. Am Rev Respir Dis 134:488, 1986.
65. LaRoche CM, Mier AK, Mixham J, et al: Diaphragm strength in patients with recent hemidiaphragm paralysis. Thorax 43:170, 1988.
66. Clague HW, Hall DR: Effect of posture on lung volume, airway closure and gas exchange in hemidiaphragmatic paralysis. Thorax 34:523, 1979.
67. Newsom Davis J, Goldman M, Loh L, et al: Diaphragm function and alveolar hypoventilation. Q J Med 45:87, 1976.
68. Allen SM, Hunt B, Green M: Fall in vital capacity with posture. Br J Dis Chest 79:267, 1985.
69. Cordero PJ, Morales P, Mora V, et al: Transient right-to-left shunting through a patent foramen ovale secondary to unilateral diaphragmatic paralysis. Thorax 49:933, 1994.
70. Patakas D, Tsara V, Zoglopitis F, et al: Nocturnal hypoxia in unilateral diaphragmatic paralysis. Respiration 58:95, 1991.
71. Wright CD, Williams JG, Ogilvie CM, et al: Results of diaphragmatic plication for unilateral diaphragmatic paralysis. J Thorac Cardiovasc Surg 90:195, 1985.
72. Schonfeld T, O'Neal MH, Platzker ACG, et al: Function of the diaphragm before and after plication. Thorax 35:631, 1980.
73. Shochina M, Ferber I, Wolf E: Evaluation of the phrenic nerve in patients with neuromuscular disorders. Int J Rehabil Res 6:455, 1983.
74. Silverman JL, Rodriquez AA: Needle electromyographic evaluation of the diaphragm. Electromyog Clin Neurophysiol 34:509, 1994.

75. Saadeh PB, Crisafulli CF, Sosner J, Wolf E: Needle electromyography of the diaphragm: A new technique. Muscle Nerve 16:15, 1993.
76. Gea J, Espadaler JM, Guiu R, et al: Diaphragmatic activity induced by cortical stimulation: Surface versus esophageal electrodes. J Appl Physiol 74:655, 1993.
77. Machetanz J, Bischoff C, Pilchlmeier R, et al: Magnetically induced muscle contraction caused by motor nerve stimulation and not by direct muscle activation. Muscle Nerve 17:1170, 1994.
78. Similowski T, Fleury B, Launois S, et al: Cervical magnetic stimulations: A new painless method for bilateral phrenic nerve stimulation in conscious humans. J Appl Physiol 67:1311, 1989.
79. Mills GH, Kyroussis D, Hamnegard CH, et al: Unilateral magnetic stimulation of the phrenic nerve. Thorax 50:1162, 1995.
80. Newsom Davis J: Phrenic nerve conduction in man. J Neurol Neurosurg Psychiatry 30:420, 1967.
81. Newsom Davis J, Goldman M, Loh L, et al: Diaphragm function and alveolar hypoventilation. Q J Med 45:87, 1976.
82. Mier A, Brophy C, Green M: Diaphragm weakness. J R Soc Med 80:315, 1987.
83. Schiani EA, Roncoroni AJ, Duy RJM: Isolated bilateral diaphragmatic paralysis with interstitial lung disease. Am Rev Respir Dis 129:337, 1984.
84. Skatrud J, Iber C, McHugh W, et al: Determinants of hypoventilation during wakefulness and sleep in diaphragmatic paralysis. Am Rev Respir Dis 121:580, 1980.
85. Molho M, Katz I, Schwartz E, et al: Familial bilateral paralysis of the diaphragm. Chest 91:464, 1987.
86. Loh L, Goldman M, Newsom Davis J: The assessment of diaphragm function. Medicine 56:165, 1977.
87. Ch'en IY, Armstrong JD II. Value of fluoroscopy in patients with suspected bilateral hemidiaphragmatic paralysis. Am J Roentgenol 160:29, 1993.
88. Ambler R, Gruenewald SJ: Ultrasound monitoring of diaphragm activity in bilateral diaphragmatic paralysis. Arch Dis Child 60:170, 1985.
89. Diament MJ, Boechat MI, Kangarloo H: Real-time sector ultrasound in the evaluation of suspected abnormalities of diaphragmatic motion. J Clin Ultrasound 13:539, 1985.
90. Kreitzer SM, Feldman NT, Saunders NA, et al: Bilateral diaphragmatic paralysis with hypercapnic respiratory failure. Am J Med 65:89, 1978.
90a. Chan CK, Loke J, Virgulto JA, et al: Bilateral diaphragmatic paralysis: Clinical spectrum, prognosis, and diagnostic approach. Arch Phys Med Rehabil 69:976, 1988.
91. Bove KE, Iannaccone ST: Atypical infantile spinomuscular atrophy presenting as acute diaphragmatic paralysis. Pediatr Pathol 8:95, 1988.
92. Loh L, Hughes JBM, Newsom Davis J: Gas exchange problems in bilateral diaphragm paralysis. Bull Eur Physiopathol Respir 15:137, 1979.
93. Chin EF, Lynn RB: Surgery of eventration of the diaphragm. J Thorac Surg 32:6, 1956.
94. Prasad R, Nath J, Mukerji PK: Eventration of diaphragm. J Indian Med 84:187, 1986.
95. Bhattacharya SK, Singh NK, Lahiri TK: Eventration of diaphragm. J Indian Med 84:15, 1986.
96. Tamas A, Dunbar JS: Eventration of the diaphragm. J Can Assoc Radiol 8:1, 1957.
97. Paris F, Blasco E, Canto A, et al: Diaphragmatic eventration in infants. Thorax 28:66, 1973.
98. Okuda K, Nomura F, Kawai M, et al: Age-related gross changes of the liver and right diaphragm, with special reference to partial eventration. Br J Radiol 52:870, 1979.
99. Avnet NL: Roentgenologic features of congenital bilateral anterior diaphragmatic eventration. Am J Roentgenol 88:743, 1962.
100. Laustela E: Partial eventration of the left diaphragm: An unusual case. Ann Chir Gynaecol Fenn 48:218, 1959.
101. Vogl A, Small A: Partial eventration of the right diaphragm (congenital diaphragmatic herniation of the liver). Ann Intern Med 43:61, 1955.
102. Tarver RD, Godwin JD, Putman CE: The diaphragm. Radiol Clin North Am 22:615, 1984.
103. Rubinstein ZJ, Solomon A: CT findings in partial eventration of the right diaphragm. J Comput Assist Tomogr 5:719, 1981.
104. Brink JA, Heiken JP, Semenkovich J, et al: Abnormalities of the diaphragm and adjacent structures: Findings on multiplanar spiral CT scans. Am J Roentgenol 163:307, 1994.
105. Yeh H-C, Halton KP, Gray CE: Anatomic variations and abnormalities in the diaphragm seen with US. Radiographics 10:1019, 1990.
106. Larson RK, Evans BH: Eventration of the diaphragm. Am Rev Respir Dis 87:753, 1963.
107. Symbas PN, Hatcher CR, Waldon W: Diaphragmatic eventration in infancy and childhood. Ann Thorac Surg 4:113, 1977.
108. Ford GT, Whitelaw WA, Rosenal TW, et al: Diaphragm function after upper abdominal surgery in humans. Am Rev Respir Dis 127:431, 1983.
109. Road JD, Burgess KR, Whitelaw WA, et al: Diaphragm function and respiratory response after upper abdominal surgery in dogs. J Appl Physiol 57:576, 1984.
110. Simonneau G, Vivien A, Sartene R, et al: Diaphragm dysfunction induced by upper abdominal surgery: Role of postoperative pain. Am Rev Respir Dis 128:899, 1983.
111. Easton PA, Fitting JW, Arnoux R, et al: Recovery of diaphragm function after laparotomy and chronic sonomicrometer implantation. J Appl Physiol 66:613, 1989.
112. Bertrand D, Viires N, Cantineau J-P, et al: Diaphragmatic contractility after upper abdominal surgery. J Appl Physiol 61:1775,1986.
113. Phillips JR, Eldridge FL: Respiratory myoclonus (Leeuwenhoek's disease). N Engl J Med 289:1390, 1973.
114. Ting EY, Karliner JS, Williams MH Jr: Diaphragmatic flutter associated with apneustic respiration: A case report with pulmonary function studies. Am Rev Respir Dis 88:833, 1963.
115. Rigatto M, De Medieros NP: Diaphragmatic flutter: Report of a case and review of literature. Am J Med 32:103, 1962.
116. Barrio JL, Feinerman D, Hesla PE, et al: Diaphragmatic flutter in a patient with lymphoma. Mt Sinai J Med 54:188, 1987.
116a. Smyrniotis V, Andreani P, Muiesan P, et al: Diaphragmatic nerve palsy in young children following liver transplantation. Trans Internat 11:281, 1998.
117. Caskey CI, Zerhouni EA, Fishman EK, Rahmouni AD: Aging of the diaphragm: A CT study. Radiology 171:385, 1989.
118. Bogaert J, Weemaes K, Verschakelen JA, et al: Spiral CT findings in a postoperative intrathoracic gastric herniation: A case report. Eur Radiol 5:192, 1995.
119. Carter BN, Giuseffi J: Strangulated diaphragmatic hernia. Ann Surg 128:210, 1948.
120. Pearson S: Strangulated diaphragmatic hernia: Report of four cases. Arch Surg 66:155, 1953.
121. Hoffman E: Strangulated diaphragmatic hernia. Thorax 23:541, 1968.
122. Menuck L: Plain film findings of gastric volvulus herniating into the chest. Am J Roentgenol 126:1169, 1976.
123. Johnston RH Jr, Owensby LC, Vargas GM, et al: Pancreatic pseudocyst of the mediastinum. Ann Thorac Surg 41:210, 1986.
124. Poe RG, Schowengerdt CG: Two cases of atraumatic herniation of the liver. Am Rev Respir Dis 105:959, 1972.
125. Godwin JD, MacGregor JM: Extension of ascites into the chest with hiatal hernia: Visualization on CT. Am J Roentgenol 148:31, 1987.
126. Graham JC Jr, Blanchard IT, Scatliff JH: Calcified gastric leiomyoma presenting as a mediastinal mass. Am J Roentgenol 1114:529, 1972.
127. Felder SL, Masley PM, Wolff WI: Anemia as a presenting symptom of esophageal hiatal hernia of the diaphragm. Arch Intern Med 105:873, 1960.
128. Naeye RL, Shochat SJ, Whitman V, et al: Unsuspected pulmonary abnormalities associated with diaphragmatic hernia. Pediatrics 58:902, 1976.
129. Reed JO, Lang EF: Diaphragmatic hernia in infancy. Am J Roentgenol 82:437, 1959.
130. Young DG: Contralateral pneumothorax with congenital diaphragmatic hernia. BMJ 4:433, 1968.
131. Mallik K, Rodgers BM, McGahren ED: Congenital diaphragmatic hernia: Experience in a single institution from 1978 through 1994. Ann Thorac Surg 60:1331, 1995.
132. Vanamo K: A 45-year perspective of congenital diaphragmatic hernia. Br J Surg 83:1758, 1996.
133. Muraskas JK, Husain A, Myers TF, et al: An association of pulmonary hypoplasia with unilateral agenesis of the diaphragm. J Pediat Surg 28:999, 1993.
134. Jasnosz KM, Hermansen MC, Snider C, et al: Congenital complete absence (bilateral agenesis) of the diaphragm: A rare variant of congenital diaphragmatic hernia. Am J Perinatol 11:340, 1994.
135. Lundius B: Intrathoracic kidney. Am J Roentgenol 125:678, 1975.
136. Le Roux BT: Supraphrenic herniation of perinephric fat. Thorax 20:376, 1965.
137. Israël-Asselain R, Uzzan D, Dérrida J: Image pseudo-tumorale par hernie diaphragmatique de graisse supra-rénale. (Transdiaphragmatic herniation of suprarenal fat simulating a tumor mass.) J Franc Med Chir Thorac 20:567, 1966.
138. Gale ME: Bochdalek hernia: Prevalence and CT characteristics. Radiology 156:449, 1985.
139. De Martini WJ, House AJS: Partial Bochdalek's herniation: Computerized tomographic evaluation. Chest 77:702, 1980.
140. Curley FJ, Hubmayr RD, Raptopoulos V: Bilateral diaphragmatic densities in a 72-year-old woman. Chest 86:915, 1984.
141. Raymond GS, Miller RM, Müller NL, Logan PM: Congenital thoracic lesions that mimic neoplastic disease on chest radiographs of adults. Am J Roentgenol 168:763, 1997.
142. Yamana D, Ohba S: Three-dimensional image of Bochdalek diaphragmatic hernia: A case report. Radiat Med 12:39, 1994.
143. Van Hise ML, Primack SL, Israel RS, Müller NL: CT in blunt chest trauma: Indications and limitations. Radiographics 18:1071, 1998.
144. Comer TP, Clagett OT: Surgical treatment of hernia of the foramen of Morgagni. J Thorac Cardiovasc Surg 52:461, 1966.
145. Paris F, Tarazona V, Casillas M, et al: Hernia of Morgagni. Thorax 28:631, 1973.
146. Thomas GG, Clitherow NR: Herniation through the foramen of Morgagni in children. Br J Surg 64:215, 1977.
147. Betts RA: Subcostosternal diaphragmatic hernia, with report of five cases. Am J Roentgenol 75:269, 1956.
148. Fischel RE, Joel EM: Herniation of a stone-filled gallbladder through the diaphragm. Acta Radiol (Diagn) 2:172, 1964.
149. Vaughan BF: Diaphragmatic hernia as a finding in the chest radiograph. Proc Coll Radiol Aust 3:42, 1959.
150. Chu DY, Olson AL, Mishaalany HG: Congenital liver cyst presenting as congenital diaphragmatic hernia. J Pediatr Surg 21:897, 1986.
151. Smith L, Lippert KM: Peritoneopericardial diaphragmatic hernia. Ann Surg 148:798, 1958.
152. Wallace DB: Intrapericardial diaphragmatic hernia. Radiology 122:596, 1977.
153. Robinson AE, Gooneratne NS, Blackburn WR, et al: Bilateral anteromedial defect of the diaphragm in children. Am J Roentgenol 135:301, 1980.
154. Panicek DM, Benson CB, Gottlieb RH, et al: The diaphragm: Anatomic, pathologic, and radiologic considerations. Radiographics 8:385, 1988.

155. Boyd DP, Wooldridge BF: Diaphragmatic hernia through the foramen of Morgagni. Surg Gynecol Obstet 104:727, 1957.
156. Paris F, Tarazona V, Casillas M, et al: Hernia of Morgagni. Thorax 28:631, 1973.
157. Reed MWR, de Silva PHP, Mostafa SM, et al: Diaphragmatic hernia in pregnancy. Br J Surg 74:435, 1987.
158. Anderson LS, Forrest JV: Tumors of the diaphragm. Am J Roentgenol 119:259, 1973.
159. Olafsson G, Rausing A, Holen O: Primary tumors of the diaphragm. Chest 59:568, 1971.
160. Ochsner A, Ochsner A Jr: Tumors of the diaphragm. In Spain D (ed): Diagnosis and Treatment of Tumors of the Chest. New York, Grune & Stratton, 1960, p 240.
161. Blondeel PN, Christiaens MR, Thomas J, et al: Primary leiomyosarcoma of the diaphragm. Eur J Surg Oncol 21:429, 1995.
162. Ferguson DD, Westcott JL: Lipoma of the diaphragm: Report of a case. Radiology 118:527, 1976.
163. Tihansky DP, Lopez G: Bilateral lipomas of the diaphragm. N Y State J Med 88:151, 1988.
164. Schwartz EE, Wechsler RJ: Diaphragmatic and paradiaphragmatic tumors and pseudotumors. J Thorac Imaging 4:19, 1989.
165. McHenry CR, Pickleman J, Winters G, et al: Diaphragmatic neurilemoma. J Surg Oncol 37:198, 1988.
166. Müller NL: CT features of cystic teratoma of the diaphragm. J Comput Assist Tomogr 10:325, 1986.
167. Dubost C, Hugues FC, Gossot D, et al: Cystic teratoma of the diaphragm. Apropos of a case, review of the literature. J Chir (Paris) 121:273, 1984.
168. Soysal O, Libshitz HI: Diaphragmatic desmoid tumor. Am J Roentgenol 166:1496, 1996.
169. Sbokos CG, Salama FD, Powell V, et al: Primary fibrosarcoma of the diaphragm. Br J Dis Chest 71:49, 1977.
170. Yamamoto H, Watanabe K, Takayama W, et al: Primary malignant fibrous histiocytoma of the diaphragm: Report of a case. Surg Today 24:744, 1994.
171. Seaton D: Primary diaphragmatic haemangiopericytoma. Thorax 29:595, 1974.
172. Kekomaki M, Ekfors TO, Nikkanen V, et al: Intrapleural endodermal sinus tumor arising from the diaphragm. J Pediatr Surg 19:312, 1984.
173. Buckley KM, Whitman GJ, Chew FS: Radiologic-pathologic conferences of the Massachusetts General Hospital: Diaphragmatic pheochromocytoma. Am J Roentgenol 165:260, 1995.
174. Bevelaqua FA, Valensi Q, Hulnick D: Epithelioid hemangioendothelioma: A rare tumor with variable prognosis presenting as a pleural effusion. Chest 93:665, 1988.
175. Parker MC: Leiomyosarcoma of the diaphragm: A case report. Eur J Surg Oncol 11:171, 1985.
176. Ujiki GT, Method HL, Putong PB, et al: Primary chondrosarcoma of the diaphragm. Am J Surg 122:132, 1971.
177. Gordon LF, Ramchandani P, Goldenberg NC, et al: Thoraco-abdominal mass: Roentgenologic CPC. Invest Radiol 16:451, 1981.
178. Federle MP, Mark AS, Guillaumin ES: CT of subpulmonic pleural effusions and atelectasis: Criteria for differentiation from subphrenic fluid. Am J Roentgenol 146:685, 1986.
179. Woodring JH, Bognar B: Muscular hypertrophy of the left diaphragmatic crus: An unusual cause of a paraspinal "mass." J Thorac Imaging 13:144, 1998.
180. Kapnick SJ, Griffiths CT, Finkler NJ: Occult pleural involvement in stage III ovarian carcinoma: Role of diaphragm resection. Gynecol Oncol 39:135, 1990.
181. Campbell JA: The diaphragm in roentgenology of the chest. Radiol Clin North Am 1:395, 1963.
182. Nigogosyan G, Ozarda A: Accessory diaphragm: A case report. Am J Roentgenol 85:309, 1961.
183. Hashida Y, Sherman FE: Accessory diaphragm associated with neonatal respiratory distress. J Pediatr 59:529, 1961.
184. Becmeur F, Horta P, Donato L, et al: Accessory diaphragm: Review of 31 cases in the literature. Eur J Pediatr Surg 5:43, 1995.
185. Lieberman FL, Hidemura R, Peters RL, et al: Pathogenesis and treatment of hydrothorax complicating cirrhosis with ascites. Ann Intern Med 64:341, 1966.
186. Lieberman FL, Peters RL: Cirrhotic hydrothorax: Further evidence that an acquired diaphragmatic defect is at fault. Arch Intern Med 125:114, 1970.
187. Slasky BS, Siewers RD, Lecky JW, et al: Catamenial pneumothorax: The roles of diaphragmatic defects and endometriosis. Am J Roentgenol 138:639, 1982.
188. Ranniger K, Valvassori GE: Angiographic diagnosis of intralobar pulmonary sequestration. Am J Roentgenol 92:540, 1964.
189. Wier JA: Congenital anomalies of the lung. Ann Intern Med 52:330, 1960.
190. Biberstein MP, Eisenberg H: Unilateral diaphragmatic paralysis in association with Erb's palsy. Chest 75:209, 1979.
191. Graham AN, Martin PD, Haas LF: Neuralgic amyotrophy with bilateral diaphragmatic palsy. Thorax 40:635, 1985.
192. Dervaux L, Lacquet LM: Hemidiaphragmatic paralysis after cervical herpes zoster. Thorax 37:870, 1982.
193. Shin MS, Ho K-J: Computed tomographic evaluation of the pathologic lesion for the idiopathic diaphragmatic paralysis. J Comput Assist Tomogr 6:257, 1982.
194. Joiner TA, Sumner JR, Catchings TT: Unilateral diaphragmatic paralysis secondary to carbon monoxide poisoning. Chest 97:498, 1990.
195. Bowman ED, Murton LJ: A case of neonatal bilateral diaphragmatic paralysis requiring surgery. Aust Paediatr J 20:331, 1984.
196. Sandham JD, Shaw DT, Guenter CA: Acute supine respiratory failure due to bilateral diaphragmatic paralysis. Chest 72:97, 1977.
197. Patterson DL, DeRemee RA, Hunt LW: Severe asthma complicated by bilateral diaphragmatic paralysis attributed to Parsonage-Turner syndrome. Mayo Clin Proceed 69:774, 1994.
198. Walsh NE, Dumitru D, Kalantri A, et al: Brachial neuritis involving the bilateral phrenic nerves. Arch Phys Med Rehabil 68:46, 1987.
199. Thomas NE, Passamonte PM, Sunderrajan EV, et al: Bilateral diaphragmatic paralysis as a possible paraneoplastic syndrome from renal cell carcinoma. Am Rev Respir Dis 129:507, 1984.
200. McWilliam RC, Gardner-Medwyn D, Doyle D, et al: Diaphragmatic paralysis due to spinal muscular atrophy. Arch Dis Child 60:145, 1985.
201. Montserrat JM, Picado CF, Agusti-Vidal A: Arnold-Chiari malformation and paralysis of the diaphragm. Respiration 53:128, 1988.
202. Mier A, Brophy C, Green M: Diaphragm weakness and syringomyelia. J R Soc Med 81:59, 1988.
203. Goldstein RL, Hyde RW, Lapham LW, et al: Peripheral neuropathy presenting with respiratory insufficiency as the primary complaint. Am J Med 56:443, 1974.
204. Cooper CB, Trend PJ, Wiles CM: Severe diaphragm weakness in multiple sclerosis. Thorax 40:633, 1985.
205. White JE, Bullock RE, Hudgson P, et al: Phrenic neuropathy in association with diabetes. Diabetic Med 9:954, 1992.
206. Morales P, Cases E, Gudin J: Nontraumatic bilateral diaphragmatic myopathy: An unusual disturbance. Lung 175:363, 1997.
207. De Vito EL, Quadrelli SA, Montiel GC, et al: Bilateral diaphragmatic paralysis after mediastinal radiotherapy. Respiration 63:187, 1996.
208. Smith CD, Sade RM, Crawford FA, et al: Diaphragmatic paralysis and eventration in infants. J Thorac Cardiovasc Surg 91:490, 1986.

CHAPTER 78

The Chest Wall

ABNORMALITIES OF THE PECTORAL GIRDLE AND ADJACENT STRUCTURES

Congenital Anomalies

Several congenital anomalies affect the pectoral girdle. Although the majority do not result in serious disability, their recognition is important, particularly for the radiologist. The precise cause of these anomalies is uncertain; however, it has been postulated that Sprengel's deformity, Klippel-Feil deformity, and Poland's syndrome may be the result of an interruption of the early embryonic blood supply provided by the subclavian or vertebral arteries or their branches.[1]

Cleidocranial Dysostosis

The most common congenital anomaly of the clavicle is cleidocranial dysostosis, a syndrome characterized by incomplete ossification associated with defective development of the pubic bones, vertebral column, and long bones. A case has also been described of bilateral retrosternal subluxation of the medial ends of the clavicles that was considered by the author to be congenital in origin;[2] the posterior position of the medial ends of the clavicles suggested a retrosternal mass on a lateral radiograph.

Sprengel's and Klippel-Feil Deformities

Sprengel's deformity is characterized by a failure of the scapula to descend normally so that its superior angle lies on a plane higher than the neck of the first rib (Fig. 78–1). It is frequently associated with fusion of two or more cervical vertebrae, resulting in a short, wide neck with considerably limited movement, that is, the Klippel-Feil deformity.[3] The latter has in turn been associated with an increased prevalence of scoliosis[4, 5] and with agenesis of the right upper and middle lung lobes.[6] The extent and nature of the cervical abnormalities can be appreciated using computed tomography (CT) and magnetic resonance (MR) imaging.[7] Other anomalies of the scapula include ununited apophyses, an abnormality that is frequently bilateral and symmetric and that may simulate fracture, and pseudoforamen, in which the supraspinatous and infraspinatous fossae are formed by fibrous tissue rather than by bone, creating the radiographic appearance of lytic lesions. A similar "foramen" may be formed at the superior border of the scapula by calcification of the superior transverse ligament.

Poland's Syndrome

Poland's syndrome is a congenital anomaly consisting of hypoplasia or aplasia of the pectoralis major muscle and ipsilateral syndactyly;[8] rarely, the hypoplasia-aplasia is bilateral.[9] Other anomalies that may be associated include absence of the pectoralis minor muscle, absence or atrophy of ipsilateral ribs two to five, aplasia of the ipsilateral breast or nipple, dextrocardia,[10] and simian crease in the affected extremity.[8] Mild cases may consist only of asymmetry of breast size.[11] Unilateral absence of the pectoralis muscles results in unilateral hyperlucency on the chest radiograph, not to be confused with the Swyer-James syndrome (Fig. 78–2). Poland's syndrome has also been reported to be

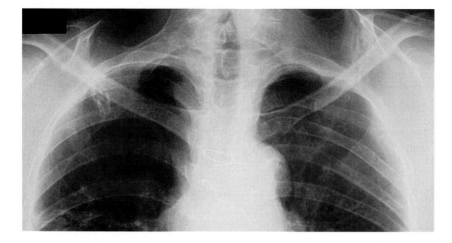

Figure 78–1. Sprengel's Deformity. A view of the upper chest in a 37-year-old woman demonstrates elevation of both scapulae (Sprengel's deformity). Also note bone union of left sixth and seventh cervical ribs, which are articulating with the elevated left scapula (omovertebral bones). A single right C7 omovertebral bone is present. Incidental note is made of mild right upper lobe scarring related to previous tuberculosis and of postoperative findings related to previous sternotomy.

associated with an increased incidence of lung hernia,[12] leukemia, and (possibly) non-Hodgkin's lymphoma, neuroblastoma, leiomyosarcoma, and Wilms' tumor.[13–17] The extent of the muscle abnormalities in the shoulder girdle can be described and quantified using CT, MR imaging, or both.[18, 19]

Acquired Abnormalities

Radical Neck Dissection

The radiologic appearance of the chest following radical neck dissection is characterized by a number of abnormalities. In one review of 30 cases, the authors found the following, in decreasing order of frequency: hyperlucent supraclavicular fossa (28 cases), absent sternocleidomastoid muscle

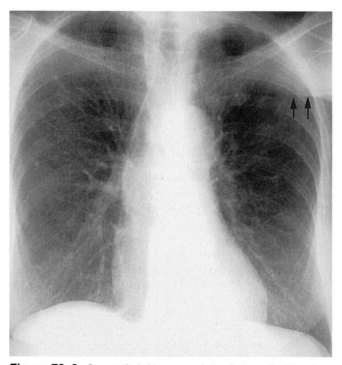

Figure 78–2. Congenital Absence of the Pectoralis Muscle. A posteroanterior chest radiograph demonstrates increased radiolucency of the left hemithorax. The course of the left anterior axillary fold *(arrows)* is horizontal as a result of absence of the left pectoralis muscle. Note that the breast shadows are symmetric. The patient was a 67-year-old woman.

(23 cases), drooping shoulder (20 cases), medial continuation of the ipsilateral companion shadow (19 cases), and sternoclavicular subluxation (8 cases).[20] The last-named appears to occur as a later complication of the drooping pectoral girdle, which in turn is a result of muscle resection and interruption of the spinal accessory nerve.

Pulmonary Hernia

A pulmonary hernia can be defined as a protrusion of the lung beyond the confines of the rib cage. It is an uncommon abnormality, only approximately 300 cases having been reported by 1996.[12] Approximately 20% are congenital and 80% acquired.[12] The hernias can be classified as cervical (approximately one third), intercostal (two thirds), or diaphragmatic (about 1%).[12, 21, 22] The majority of acquired hernias develop following penetrating injury, blunt trauma associated with multiple rib fractures, thoracotomy, or insertion of multiple chest tubes.[12, 21] Rarely, they occur secondary to rib destruction by tuberculosis or fungal infection or chest wall invasion by pulmonary carcinoma.[12, 21] Herniation through a chest wall defect is more likely to occur in patients who have emphysema or who are receiving positive-pressure ventilation. "Spontaneous" lung hernias can also occur following vigorous, prolonged episodes of cough in patients who have chronic obstructive pulmonary disease (COPD).[12]

The radiographic manifestations include a well-circumscribed lucency extending beyond the rib cage or an air collection in the tissues overlying the chest wall.[12, 21] Unless the hernia is tangential to the x-ray beam, it may not be apparent on the radiograph. The diagnosis can be readily made using CT (Fig. 78–3).[12, 21] The majority of patients are asymptomatic. Occasionally, the patient may feel a painless, local bulge during cough. On palpation, the swelling is compressible and may demonstrate crepitus.[12] Rarely, there is localized pain.[12, 23] Isolated cases have been reported of incarceration of the herniated lung complicated by ischemic injury and perforation.[12, 24]

ABNORMALITIES OF THE RIBS

Congenital Anomalies

Cervical Rib

An anomalous accessory rib in the cervical region is a relatively common finding, being seen in about 0.5% of the

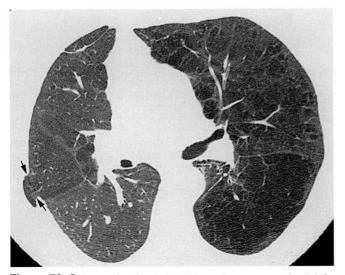

Figure 78–3. Lung Hernia. An HRCT scan demonstrates a focal defect in the right chest wall *(arrows)* with associated lung hernia. The patient was a 64-year-old woman who had undergone right lung transplantation for emphysema.

general population.[25] It usually arises from the seventh cervical vertebra. Both the anomaly and the symptoms that derive therefrom are said to be more common in women, occurring in a ratio of approximately 2.5 to 1.[25] In about 90% of cases, the rib does not cause symptoms; however, when it compresses the cervical spinal cord,[26] the subclavian vessels, or the brachial plexus (thoracic outlet syndrome), symptoms may be present and are sometimes disabling.[27, 28]

The diagnosis of thoracic outlet syndrome secondary to a cervical rib can be made when there is radiographic evidence of a cervical rib associated with the typical symptoms and signs of pain and weakness of the arm, swelling of the hand, and variation in the intensity of the pulses in the two arms when the affected extremity is in certain positions. The syndrome can also occur after trauma or in association with narrowing of the scalene triangle by spasm of the scalene muscle, an abnormally long or drooping transverse process

of the seventh cervical rib, or exostosis of the clavicle or first thoracic rib.[29–33] A brachiocephalic vascular syndrome has been described in which pressure exerted by a cervical rib results in subclavian artery thrombosis that extends to the ipsilateral carotid artery, producing symptoms of cerebrovascular insufficiency.[34] Bilateral thoracic outlet obstruction caused by bone deformity and compression of the main arterial vessels has been described in one patient who experienced episodes of tetany of the hands that were relieved by resection of the first ribs.[35]

In patients who have symptoms or signs indicative of vascular compression, arteriography, contrast-enhanced spiral CT, and MR imaging can be of considerable assistance in evaluation and are occasionally essential for diagnosis and preoperative evaluation.[36–39] Spiral CT allows assessment of the entire course of the cervical rib in multiple planes and its relationship to adjacent vessels and nerves, as well as the presence of associated skeletal abnormalities (Fig. 78–4). When performing angiography or spiral CT, it is important to keep in mind that venous and, to a lesser extent, arterial compression occurs normally in the thoracic outlet during abduction of the upper extremity.[40] In one investigation of 10 healthy individuals in which spiral CT was performed when the arm was in the neutral position and when it was abducted 90 degrees or more, the distances between the anterior scalene muscle and the clavicle, and between the clavicle and the first rib, were found to be decreased with abduction.[40] Compression of the subclavian vein occurred at both locations in all subjects during upper arm abduction, with a mean decrease in diameter of approximately 50%; arterial compression was less common and milder in degree, with a mean decrease in diameter of approximately 15%.

When considering the diagnosis of thoracic outlet syndrome, it should be remembered that causes other than cervical rib can also be seen (e.g., tumor of the first rib[41] or of the lung apex).

Intrathoracic Rib

Intrathoracic rib is a rare congenital anomaly, only 17 cases having been reported by 1979.[42] The rib arises from

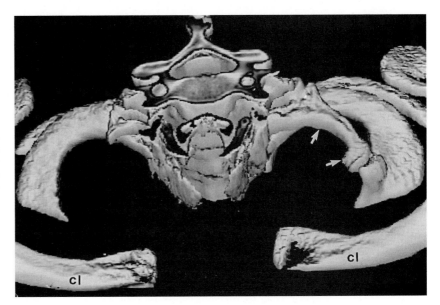

Figure 78–4. Cervical Rib. A three-dimensional reconstruction image from a spiral CT demonstrates a left cervical rib *(arrows)* articulating with the left first thoracic rib. Also seen are the right and left clavicles (cl). The patient presented with left thoracic outlet syndrome.

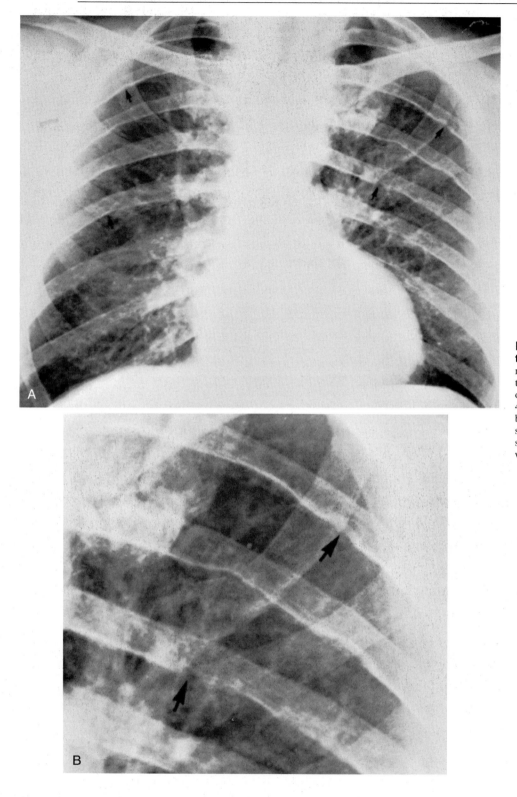

Figure 78–5. Rib Notching: Coarctation of the Aorta. A posteroanterior radiograph *(A)* and a magnified view of the left upper ribs *(B)* demonstrate numerous defects of the inferior surfaces of ribs 4 to 8 bilaterally (several are indicated by *arrows*). The configuration of vascular shadows in the region of the aortic arch is strongly suggestive of coarctation. This was a proven case in a 58-year-old man.

the anterior or posterior surface of a normal rib or from a vertebral body, more commonly on the right; it usually extends downward and slightly laterally to end at or near the diaphragm.[42, 42a] In one patient, the supernumerary rib originated from the posterior portion of the left third rib and extended through lung substance to join the anterior portion of the left second rib.[43] Typically, these accessory structures are unassociated with symptoms. The diagnosis may be apparent on the radiograph or may require the use of CT.[44]

Miscellaneous Abnormalities

Fusion of two or more ribs and various types of bifid ribs are relatively common and are of little or no significance. Rarely, an anomalous rib arises from the right side of the last sacral vertebra, forming a pelvic rib.[45] Asphyxiating thoracic dystrophy of the newborn is characterized by very short and stubby ribs that extend no farther than the mid-axilla.[46] The anomaly results in poor respiratory mobility, frequent respiratory infections, and, frequently, death.

Fibrodysplasia ossificans progressiva is a rare hereditary condition that can cause severe chest wall restriction. This inherited disorder is characterized by progressive ossification of voluntary muscles and ligaments associated with a characteristic skeletal malformation consisting of short big toes containing only a single phalanx.[47] Affected patients are usually infertile and die of pneumonia in their third or fourth decade. Because ventilatory capacity is maintained by relatively preserved diaphragmatic function, respiratory failure is unusual except in the terminal stages.

Acquired Abnormalities

Rib Notching and Erosion

Notching of ribs may occur on the inferior or superior aspect; it is most frequent in the former location and has many causes (Table 78–1).[48] By far the most common—coarctation of the aorta—typically produces notching several centimeters lateral to the costovertebral junction on the inferior aspect of ribs three to nine (Fig. 78–5). The notches result from erosion by pulsating, dilated intercostal arteries taking part in collateral arterial flow. These arteries may become extremely tortuous and may even extend to and erode the superior aspects of contiguous ribs. Rib notching secondary to coarctation of the aorta seldom is seen in

Table 78–1. CAUSES OF INFERIOR RIB NOTCHING

ARTERIAL

Aortic obstruction
  1. Coarctation of the aortic arch
  2. Thrombosis of the abdominal aorta
Subclavian artery obstruction
  1. Blalock-Taussig operation
  2. Takayasu's arteritis
Widened arterial pulse pressure
Decreased pulmonary blood flow
  1. Tetralogy of Fallot
  2. Pulmonary atresia (pseudotruncus)
  3. Ebstein's malformation
  4. Pulmonary valve stenosis
  5. Unilateral absence of the pulmonary artery
  6. Pulmonary emphysema

VENOUS

Superior vena cava obstruction

ARTERIOVENOUS

Pulmonary arteriovenous fistula
Intercostal arteriovenous fistula

NEUROGENIC

Intercostal neurogenic tumor

OSSEOUS

Hyperparathyroidism

IDIOPATHIC

Table 78–2. CAUSES OF SUPERIOR RIB NOTCHING

DISTURBANCE OF OSTEOBLASTIC ACTIVITY (DECREASED OR DEFICIENT BONE FORMATION)

1. Paralytic poliomyelitis (bulbar or spinal)
2. Connective tissue diseases (rheumatoid arthritis, progressive systemic sclerosis, lupus erythematosus, Sjögren's syndrome)
3. Localized pressure (rib retractors, chest tubes, multiple hereditary exostoses, neurofibromatosis, thoracic neuroblastoma, coarctation of the aorta)
4. Osteogenesis imperfecta
5. Marfan's syndrome
6. Radiation damage

DISTURBANCE OF OSTEOCLASTIC ACTIVITY (INCREASED BONE RESORPTION)

1. Hyperparathyroidism
2. Hypervitaminosis D

IDIOPATHIC

patients before the age of 6 or 7 years and usually is not well developed until the early teens.[49]

Rib notching occasionally occurs in association with other causes of aortic obstruction; for example, Takayasu's arteritis has been reported to be associated with notching of ribs 9 and 10 bilaterally.[50] Inferior notching may also occur in a variety of other cardiovascular disorders, particularly the tetralogy of Fallot. In one study of 245 patients who had this condition, 19 showed rib notching;[51] it was unilateral on the left side in most cases and occurred after both Blalock-Taussig anastomosis (Fig. 78–6) and after thoracotomy without vascular anastomosis.

Notching or erosion of the superior aspects of the ribs is considerably less common than that of the inferior aspects; however, we suspect that it may be present more often than is generally recognized because of its more subtle radiographic appearance. Superior marginal rib defects can be classified into three major groups (Table 78–2):[52] (1) abnormalities associated with a disturbance of osteoblastic activity (decreased or deficient bone formation), (2) abnormalities associated with a disturbance of osteoclastic activity (increased bone resorption), and (3) idiopathic.

Formerly, the most common cause of notching or erosion of the superior aspects of the ribs was undoubtedly chronic paralytic poliomyelitis.[52–54] However, the rarity with which this disease is now seen places it far down on the list in the differential diagnosis; because the same mechanism is in effect in patients who are quadriplegic as a result of cervical cord injury, this condition has replaced poliomyelitis as the most common cause.[55] The radiographic appearance typically consists of shallow indentations ranging from 1 to 4 cm in length on the superior margins of ribs 3 to 9 posterolaterally. The erosions were considered at one time to result from continued pressure of the medial margins of the scapulae; however, for a variety of reasons, this mechanism appears to be most unlikely.[52] A more reasonable explanation is the absence of the "stress stimulus" provided by repetitive contraction of the intercostal muscles as a result of atrophy of accessory inspiratory muscles.[52] The cause of superior rib erosions in the connective tissue diseases such as rheumatoid arthritis and progressive systemic sclerosis is unknown; however, it may be related to intercostal muscle

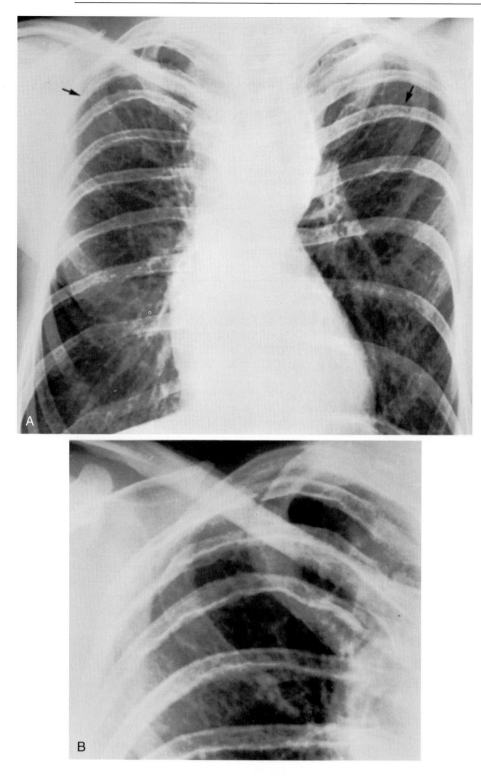

Figure 78–6. Rib Notching: Postoperative Bilateral Blalock-Taussig Anastomosis for Tetralogy of Fallot. A posteroanterior radiograph *(A)* reveals extensive notching of ribs 3 to 7 bilaterally, affecting both the inferior surface (as in Figure 78–5) and, in some areas, the superior surface *(arrows).* The erosions are seen to advantage on a magnified view of the right upper ribs *(B).* Such notching is the result of hypertrophy of intercostal arteries to provide anastomotic circulation to the upper extremities. The patient was a 25-year-old man.

hypertrophy associated with restrictive lung disease.[56] However, we have not seen similar erosions in patients who have idiopathic interstitial pulmonary fibrosis and suspect that it is not the restrictive lung disease *per se* that leads to the osseous abnormality.

Osteomyelitis

Primary infection of the ribs is rare and may be difficult to appreciate radiologically until bone destruction is ad-

vanced. More commonly, osteomyelitis is secondary to infectious processes in the lung (usually due to *Mycobacterium tuberculosis, Actinomyces israelii,* or *Nocardia asteroides*) or to empyema (empyema necessitatis). In one series of 16 patients who had pyogenic osteomyelitis of the ribs, 9 had pre-existing empyema and 14 presented with discharging chest wall sinuses;[57] *Staphylococcus aureus* was the causative organism in 8 of the 16 cases.

Rib involvement is occasionally the first manifestation

of tuberculosis.[58] It may begin as a chondritis or osteitis.[58] The radiographic manifestations of these two forms evolve somewhat differently but eventually are characterized by destructive lesions often associated with a periosteal reaction and a soft tissue mass;[58–60] the appearance may suggest malignancy.[61] These abnormalities are often difficult to visualize on the radiograph but can be detected readily on CT.[59, 60, 62] The most common finding consists of a juxtacostal soft tissue mass that has central low attenuation and shows peripheral enhancement following intravenous administration of contrast; this was seen in all 10 patients in two series (Fig. 78–7).[59, 60] Rib destruction is evident in approximately 50% of cases and is manifested by cortical irregularities or expansile osteolytic lesions.[59, 60] Only half of the patients have evidence of underlying pleural or parenchymal disease on CT. Rarely, rib involvement or pleural tuberculosis leads to the development of retromammary or intramammary tuberculous abscesses.[63, 64] Rib lesions of this and other types often can be detected by bone scanning before they are apparent on chest radiography.[65] It should be remembered that unilateral enlargement of the ribs can occur in association with chronic pleural disease (in one series, most often the result of tuberculosis);[66] such enlargement reflects a reaction of the ribs to adjacent pleural inflammation rather than to direct bone infection.

Primary costal echinococcosis is rare, only 38 cases having been reported by 1973.[67] In its early form, it manifests as a solitary expanding osteolytic lesion within a rib and is unassociated with layering of periosteal new bone. In more advanced disease, the posterior portions of the ribs and the vertebrae tend to be affected, usually in association with soft tissue masses. Sometimes, extraosseous lesions, such as pleural hydatid cysts, cause pressure atrophy of the ribs.[67]

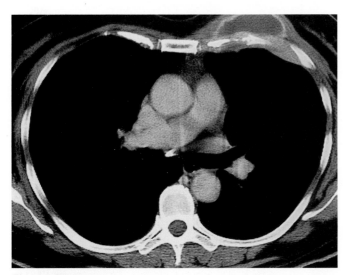

Figure 78–7. Tuberculous Osteitis and Chondritis. A CT scan performed following intravenous administration of contrast demonstrates irregularity of the left anterior third rib and costal cartilage. A soft tissue mass that has a low attenuation center and rim enhancement is present anterior to the rib, consistent with an abscess. Note the presence of a calcified subcarinal lymph node consistent with previous pulmonary tuberculosis. The patient was a 53-year-old woman who had no evidence of active pulmonary tuberculosis at the time of the chest wall disease. Biopsy of the mass confirmed the diagnosis.

Costochondral Osteochondritis

Costochondral osteochondritis (Tietze's syndrome) is characterized by painful, nonsuppurative swelling of one or more costochondral or sternochondral joints.[68] By 1983, reports of 316 cases had appeared in the world literature.[69] In the majority of these, sternocostal joint involvement was an isolated finding; in some, it was associated with a systemic arthritic disorder, psoriasis, or relapsing polychondritis.[70] The condition shows no gender predominance.[71] It becomes manifest almost invariably in the second to fourth decades of life, with the very young and the very old rarely being affected.[72]

The etiology and pathogenesis are unknown. It has been suggested that the underlying abnormality may be chronic postural stress that is exacerbated by coughing or trauma.[73] An outbreak of the disease has been described in six employees of a copper mine, leading to speculation that it might be caused by a virus;[74] however, affected cartilage is said to be histologically normal.[75, 76] The association with arthritis or polychondritis suggests an immunologic component in some cases.

Although the majority of affected patients undoubtedly manifest no radiologic changes, hypertrophy and excess calcification of the costal cartilages can be identified in some.[71] The second ribs are the most commonly involved. The affected ribs may show evidence of periosteal reaction and increased size and density anteriorly. When subperiosteal new bone formation develops, it tends to occur along the superior aspects. Enlargement and alteration of the trabecular pattern of the anterior portion of the first ribs may also occur and may lead to an extremely dense appearance of the bone. CT can sometimes help to distinguish the swelling of Tietze's syndrome from that of more serious disease:[77, 78] for example, in six patients who had Tietze's syndrome in one series, CT showed no abnormality in two, ventral angulation of the involved costal cartilage in two, and enlargement of the costal cartilage at the site of the complaint in two.[78]

Ultrasonography has also been shown to be useful in demonstrating and following the costal cartilage abnormalities.[79, 80] Pinhole skeletal scintigraphy has been suggested as an accurate method of differential diagnosis in patients who have anterior chest wall swelling and pain;[81, 82] however, in one study of 20 patients and 10 controls in which scintigraphic imaging was performed using technetium Tc 99m methylene diphosphonate, there was high sensitivity but poor specificity in detecting the presence and location of costochondritis.[83]

The clinical picture consists of painful swelling of one or more upper rib cartilages, without apparent cause; some patients experience episodes of remission and exacerbation. The pain and tenderness may antedate or coincide with the swelling and is accentuated by movement, deep respiration, and cough. Multiple sites are involved in approximately one third of cases.[71] Weeks or months may elapse before the swelling and pain disappear, and slight chest deformity may remain. Symptomatic improvement has been reported following treatment with anti-inflammatory agents and calcitonin.[84] A variant of Tietze's syndrome, termed *costosternal chondrodynia*, is characterized by local pain and tenderness in the upper or middle costal cartilages without associated swelling.[85]

ABNORMALITIES OF THE STERNUM

Pectus Excavatum

This common deformity, also known as "funnel chest," consists of depression of the sternum so that the ribs on each side protrude anteriorly more than the sternum itself. It is generally believed to result from a genetically determined abnormality of the sternum and portions of the diaphragm; the condition can occur either sporadically or with a dominant pattern of inheritance.[86, 87] The prevalence in the general population has been estimated to range from 0.13% to 0.4%.[86]

Several mechanisms have been proposed for its development: (1) an overstimulation of the anterior fibers of the diaphragm; (2) an anomalous position of the heart to the left of the midline, leaving the retrosternal area "empty" and permitting the sternum and costal cartilages to be "sucked in" to fill the empty space;[88] and (3) an inherent defect in connective tissue of the skeleton itself. The last possibility is supported by the frequent association of the deformity with congenital connective tissue disorders, such as Marfan's syndrome, Poland's syndrome, scoliosis, and Pierre Robin syndrome.[72, 86] Occasionally, the deformity is associated with multiple congenital defects.[89]

The radiographic manifestations are easily recognized (Fig. 78–8). In posteroanterior projection, the heart is displaced to the left and rotated in a way suggestive of a "mitral configuration."[90] The parasternal soft tissues of the anterior chest wall, which are seen in profile rather than *en face*, are apparent as increased density over the inferomedial portion of the right hemithorax and should not be mistaken for disease of the right middle lobe, even though the right heart border is obscured (*see* Fig. 78–8). The degree of sternal depression is easily seen on lateral radiographs. Pectus excavatum is associated with exaggerated respiratory movements of the diaphragm.[91] Possibly as a result of upward compression deformity of the heart and great vessels, the abnormality occasionally is associated with an unusual mediastinal configuration that can simulate a mediastinal mass;[92] in such cases, the true nature of the configuration can usually be readily clarified by CT. By altering the normal anatomic position of the adjacent structures, pectus excavatum can also be associated with false-positive results on scintigraphic studies by mimicking a mass in the liver or lungs.[93, 94]

The severity of the defect is best quantified by CT or MR imaging. The "pectus index" can be derived by dividing the transverse diameter of the chest by the anteroposterior diameter. In one series, the normal value of this index was found to be 2.56 ($\pm$ 0.35 SD);[95] the investigators suggested that patients who have a ratio of 3.25 or greater require surgical correction. Similar indices derived from CT have been employed to assess the results of surgical repair.[96]

The vast majority of patients are symptom free, except

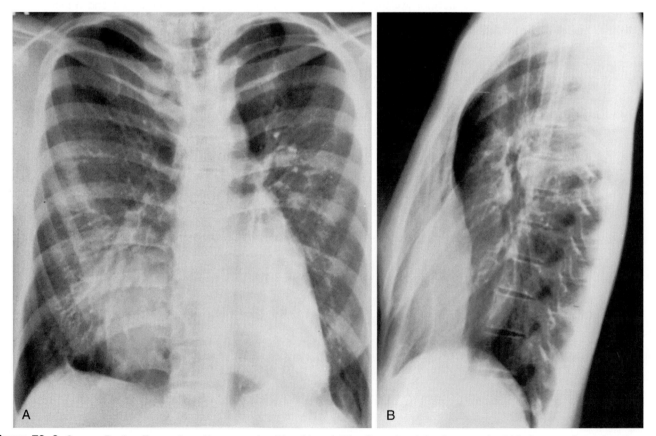

Figure 78–8. Severe Pectus Excavatum. Posteroanterior *(A)* and lateral *(B)* radiographs of the chest reveal a fairly large opacity projected over the lower portion of the right hemithorax contiguous with the shadow of the thoracic spine. The pulmonary arteries to the right lower lobe are displaced laterally and the heart is displaced to the left. The severe deformity of the sternum can be readily identified in lateral projection and is of sufficient degree to displace the heart posteriorly such that the contour of the left ventricle is projected over the thoracic vertebral bodies. The patient was a young woman who had no symptoms.

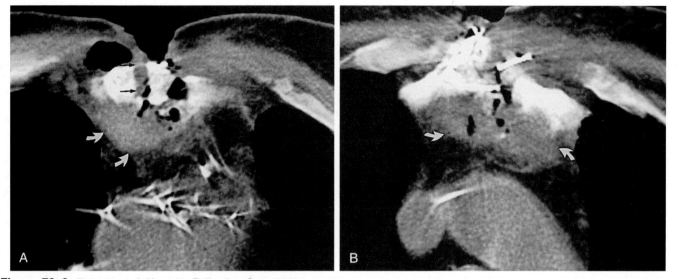

Figure 78–9. Retrosternal Abscess Following Sternotomy. A CT scan at the level of the main pulmonary artery *(A)* demonstrates a draining sinus *(straight arrows)* that communicates with a retrosternal collection *(curved arrows)*. The collection extends cephalad to the level of the aortic arch *(B)*. Note sternal dehiscence and broken sternal wires. The presence of a retrosternal abscess was confirmed at surgery; cultures grew *Staphylococcus aureus*. The patient was a 64-year-old man who had persistent wound infection 5 weeks after coronary artery bypass surgery.

perhaps for the anxiety occasioned by the physical deformity.[86, 97] However, cardiac[98, 99] or respiratory[100] symptoms are occasionally attributed to the abnormality. A heart murmur is also fairly common; for example, in one study of 54 children who had pectus excavatum, a murmur was identified in 24 (44%), the most common simulating pulmonic stenosis and probably resulting from kinking of the pulmonary artery.[86] Increased splitting of the second heart sound also was frequently observed and, in association with the pulmonic murmur, suggested an atrial septal defect. The electrocardiogram usually showed increased left-sided potentials, presumably as a result of leftward displacement of the heart. Although auscultatory, electrocardiographic, and radiographic abnormalities suggestive of significant heart disease were frequent in this series, the researchers considered that all 54 children had normal hearts. Only two children were symptomatic, both experiencing infrequent episodes of mild syncope. In some individuals, a murmur is caused by mitral valve prolapse.[101] The incidence of Wolff-Parkinson-White syndrome also is increased in children who have pectus excavatum.[102] Results of pulmonary function tests are usually normal or reveal only slight decreases in vital capacity (VC); however, occasional patients manifest severe restriction.

Pectus Carinatum

The reverse of pectus excavatum is pectus carinatum ("pigeon breast"), a congenital or acquired deformity in which the sternum protrudes anteriorly more than normal. It occurs more often in males than in females and is associated with a family history of chest wall deformity in about 25% of patients and of scoliosis in about 10%.[103] The most common variety of congenital disease consists of simple anterior protrusion of the sternum and costal cartilages that develops with growth.[104] A rare variety is associated with premature ossification of the sternal suture lines that results in forward angulation of the body of the sternum.[105]

The most common abnormalities associated with acquired pectus carinatum are atrial and ventricular septal defects.[106] The character of the deformity is slightly different in these two anomalies; in the former, the forward bulging tends to be predominantly unilateral and directly over the right ventricle, whereas in the latter, the protuberance is symmetric and affects chiefly the upper portion of the sternum. Approximately 50% of patients who have atrial and ventricular septal defects have a pigeon breast deformity.[106] Another condition associated with acquired pectus carinatum is prolonged and severe asthma dating from early childhood.[107]

The great majority of patients who have congenital pectus carinatum are asymptomatic; however, it has been suggested that children who have the deformity are more subject to respiratory infections.[104] Pulmonary hypertension develops in most patients in whom ventricular septal defect is associated with pigeon breast deformity, but it is undoubtedly caused by the heart disease rather than by the sternal abnormality.[106]

Infection of the Sternum and Its Articulations

Inflammatory diseases affecting the sternum and sternal articulations are uncommon and occur most frequently as a complication of median sternotomy for open heart surgery. Local infection occurs in 0.5% to 5% of patients undergoing sternotomy.[108, 109] Occasionally, evidence of sternal osteomyelitis or retrosternal abscess is apparent on the lateral radiograph;[110, 111] however, CT is the imaging method of choice in the assessment of patients suspected of having poststernotomy complications.[109, 111] CT findings include irregularity of the bony sternotomy margins, periosteal new bone formation, bony sclerosis, and peristernal soft tissue masses, which may contain areas of low attenuation owing to abscess formation (Fig. 78–9).[109, 111, 112] Early sternal osteomyelitis is difficult to distinguish from normal sternal irregularities following the surgical procedure.[109] Bone scintigraphy or sequential use of bone scintigraphy and gallium 67 scintigraphy also can be helpful in evaluating these patients.[109, 111]

Heroin addicts are unusually prone to develop septic arthritis of the sternoclavicular and sternochondral joints, the most common causative organisms being *Pseudomonas aeruginosa* and *S. aureus*;[113] occasionally, *Candida albicans* is the cause.[114] Hydatid disease rarely affects the sternum.[111]

Sternocostoclavicular Hyperostosis

This is a disease of unknown etiology consisting of clublike, symmetric enlargement of the clavicles associated with venous congestion of the upper half of the body as a result of bilateral subclavian vein occlusion. Radiographically, there is symmetric hyperostosis of the sternal ends and midportions of the clavicles; synostosis of the sternoclavicular joints; a widened, thickened sternum; and varying degrees of similar disease of the upper ribs.[115, 116] The abnormalities are seen particularly well on CT.[116] Bone scintigraphy shows increased uptake.[116]

ABNORMALITIES OF THE THORACIC SPINE

Kyphoscoliosis

Abnormalities of curvature of the thoracic spine may be predominantly lateral (scoliosis), predominantly posterior (kyphosis), or a combination of the two (kyphoscoliosis). Although such abnormalities are common, particularly scoliosis, deformity of sufficient degree to cause symptoms and signs of cardiac or pulmonary disease is rare. In the United States, the incidence of scoliosis in which the Cobb angle (*see* farther on) is less than 35 degrees is 1 in 1,000; the incidence of the deformity with an angle greater than 70 degrees is 1 in 10,000.[117]

Abnormalities of curvature of the spine can be considered in three groups according to etiology: (1) congenital, including anomalies of the thoracic spine such as hemivertebrae, and various hereditary disorders in which spinal deformity constitutes only a part of the clinical picture (e.g., neurofibromatosis, Friedreich's ataxia, muscular dystrophy, Morquio's syndrome, Ehlers-Danlos syndrome, and Marfan's syndrome);[107, 118–122] (2) paralytic, including poliomyelitis (Fig. 78–10), muscular dystrophy, or cerebral palsy; and (3) idiopathic. Patients in the last group constitute approximately 80% of individuals who have severe kyphoscoliosis; this variety shows a female predominance of 4 to 1.

Pathologic examination in severe cases reveals small lungs that show alveolar dilation in some regions and collapse in others.[123, 124] Muscular hypertrophy of pulmonary arteries is common and is associated with a reduction in the cross-sectional area of the pulmonary vascular bed.[125] The major influence in the development of these vascular changes is probably chronic hypoxic vasoconstriction, although mechanical factors such as compression of small intraparenchymal vessels may also contribute. In addition, pulmonary vessels may fail to develop fully when the deformity occurs during the growth period of childhood.[123, 126]

In the great majority of cases, the scoliosis is convex

to the right. The severity is best determined by the Cobb method:[127] lines are drawn parallel to the upper border of the highest and the lower border of the lowest vertebral bodies of the curvature as seen on an anteroposterior radiograph of the spine, and the angle is measured at the intersection point of lines drawn perpendicular to these. The angle also can be measured simply by drawing lines parallel to the upper and lower borders of the vertebral bodies encompassing the curvature and calculating the angle at the intersection. Assessment of cardiac size and of the state of the pulmonary parenchyma and vasculature can be exceedingly difficult because of the severe deformity of the thoracic cage. Occasionally, regional areas of oligemia may be detected; they suggest a local reduction in perfusion, presumably resulting from hypoxic vasoconstriction secondary to hypoventilation.

Disability from kyphoscoliosis is related to the angle of scoliosis and to age.[128] It has been suggested that it is the combination of the kyphotic and scoliotic defects that determines the severity of symptoms and the likelihood of developing ventilatory failure,[123] lesser degrees of scoliosis causing more severe impairment in the presence of severe kyphosis and vice versa. In general, adults whose scoliotic angle is 100 degrees or more will develop ventilatory failure.

The major pathophysiologic effect of severe kyphoscoliosis is restrictive lung disease that results in alveolar hypoventilation, hypoxic vasoconstriction, and, eventually, pulmonary arterial hypertension and cor pulmonale. Symptoms and signs of cardiopulmonary disease usually do not appear until the fourth or fifth decade, at which time the course is usually rapidly downhill and is characterized by repeated episodes of ventilatory and right heart failure, often precipitated by pulmonary infection. Despite the foregoing, even adults who have severe kyphoscoliosis can remain asymptomatic; in one study of 500 patients, cardiorespiratory failure did not develop if the VC remained more than 40% of predicted.[129]

Tests of pulmonary function characteristically reveal a decrease in VC and total lung capacity (TLC) and normal or increased values of residual volume.[130, 131] In patients who have cor pulmonale, TLC may be as low as 2 liters.[132, 133] (Because predicted values for lung volumes are based at least partly on height, it has been suggested that it is more accurate to use arm span in predicting values in patients who have kyphoscoliosis.[134]) Restriction is the result of decreased compliance of both the lung and the chest wall.[135, 136] Expiratory flow rates are usually reduced only in proportion to the reduction in VC, and direct measurement of airway resistance reveals normal values in the majority.[132] However, some patients have airway obstruction in addition to lung restriction; this has been shown to be related to bronchial torsion and compression of central airways[137] or, in one patient who had tracheal obstruction, to a combination of thoracic deformity and a tortuous aorta.[138] Measurement of steady-state diffusing capacity reveals relatively normal values for gas transfer corrected for the reduction in alveolar volume in patients who have mild or moderate restriction;[139] however, in patients who are hypercapnic and in heart failure, the values are decreased out of proportion to the reduced lung volumes. Mixing efficiency may[140] or may not[130] be impaired, perhaps depending on the degree of scoliosis.

Arterial blood gas values are almost invariably abnor-

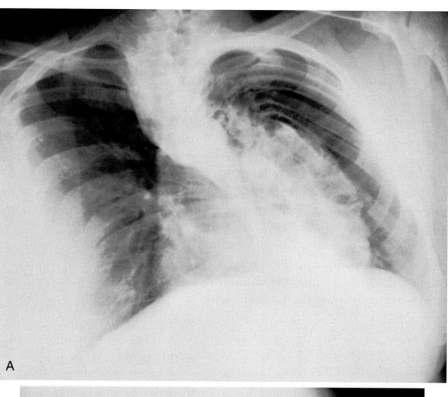

Figure 78–10. Kyphoscoliosis. Posteroanterior *(A)* and lateral *(B)* radiographs reveal severe deformity of the thoracic skeleton, the spine possessing a marked scoliosis to the left in the midthoracic region and severe kyphosis in the mid and lower regions. Deformity of the rib cage is as might be anticipated from the thoracic curvature. The 48-year-old woman had no significant complaints referable to her respiratory tract; her thoracic deformity was the result of remote poliomyelitis. Pulmonary function tests revealed remarkably normal values, there being only a slight reduction in vital capacity and functional residual capacity.

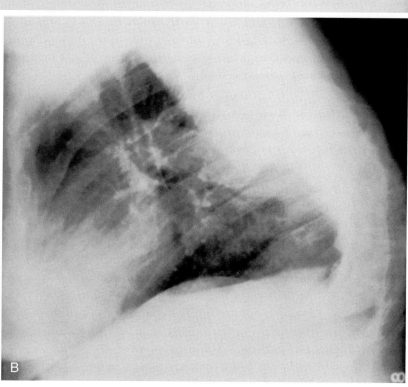

mal in adults and occasionally in adolescents.[123, 130, 133, 140] In the more advanced cases, it is common to find both hypoxemia and hypercapnia, findings that can be attributed to alveolar hypoventilation secondary to shallow respiration[123, 133] and to a ventilation-perfusion ($\dot{V}/\dot{Q}$) imbalance.[131, 140] Studies in which radioactive xenon has been used have shown defects in both ventilation and perfusion.[142, 143] In one series in which a bolus method of xenon injection was employed, no consistent difference in perfusion of the lungs on the convex and concave sides of the curvature was identified;[143] although the lung bases were more severely affected than the apices, perfusion and ventilation were reduced equally and progressively with increasing spinal deformity. In this study, the defect in gas exchange was thought to result from regional inhomogeneity of ventilation and perfusion, a finding that is seen more often in older patients. In one series of 40 patients who had idiopathic scoliosis, 17 showed evidence of airway closure at lung volumes greater than functional residual capacity (FRC),[128] whereas in another study of 19 patients whose average age was younger, closing volumes were all below FRC.[130] This discrepancy almost certainly can be explained by the age of the patients and the degree of scoliosis.

Although the arterial hypoxemia associated with severe kyphoscoliosis can be ascribed to both gas exchange impairment and hypoventilation, the relative contribution of gas exchange abnormalities is much less than that in patients who have similar degrees of alveolar hypoventilation secondary to COPD.[139] In patients who have mild or moderate kyphoscoliosis, the alveolar-arterial oxygen tension gradient may be in the normal range. In fact, even in the presence of advanced disease associated with pulmonary arterial hypertension and cor pulmonale, the majority of the arterial hypoxemia is caused by alveolar hypoxia rather than by $\dot{V}/\dot{Q}$ mismatch or shunt. The relative preservation of the lung's ability to function as a gas-exchanging organ, if adequately ventilated, is also evidenced by the normal or low values for dead space.[144] In contrast to patients who have COPD—in whom hypoventilation develops because of increased dead space despite normal or increased levels of minute ventilation—patients who have kyphoscoliosis develop alveolar hypoventilation primarily as a result of a decrease in minute ventilation secondary to small tidal volumes. Patients who have kyphoscoliosis can be particularly susceptible to ventilatory depression and oxygen desaturation during sleep;[145–148] desaturation is especially profound during rapid eye movement sleep.[146, 149]

Compliance of both the chest wall and the lung is decreased in kyphoscoliosis. The decrease in chest wall compliance may be profound and correlates significantly with the angle of scoliosis.[150] The mechanism by which lung compliance is reduced is unclear but could be related to microatelectasis or to an increase in the surface tension resulting from failure of the lung to inflate because of the chest wall restriction (or both). In a study of six kyphoscoliotic patients who had combined cardiorespiratory failure, a highly significant increase in compliance was found after 5 minutes of positive-pressure breathing;[151] the investigators attributed the improvement to a decrease in alveolar surface forces, although they could not exclude expansion of collapsed air spaces as a contributory factor.

The abnormalities of pulmonary function in patients who have paralytic scoliosis are somewhat different from those in patients who have the idiopathic variety, probably because of the additional component of respiratory muscle dysfunction.[131] However, a decrease in respiratory muscle and diaphragmatic function also has been reported in patients who have advanced idiopathic kyphoscoliosis; it is probably attributable to altered muscle length and inefficiency related to the deformed thorax.[152] Respiratory muscle performance can be improved in patients who have kyphoscoliosis by specific muscle training programs and can be accompanied by an increase in lung volumes and a reduction in dyspnea.[153]

A reasonable pathophysiologic mechanism for the development of ventilatory respiratory failure in patients who have kyphoscoliosis is the increased work of breathing caused by stiffness of the respiratory system. In the presence of increased work of breathing and decreased respiratory muscle performance, the normal ventilatory depression that occurs during sleep results in progressive alveolar hypoventi-

lation. Although the development of such respiratory failure was formerly associated with a relatively rapid downhill course, the results of more recent studies suggest that the prognosis may be considerably improved by the use of domiciliary oxygen and intermittent mechanical ventilation.[141, 148, 154–156] Either cuirass-type or positive-pressure ventilation applied during the nocturnal hours can result in a prolonged interim improvement in pulmonary gas exchange and lung mechanics and a reduction in pulmonary artery pressures and the severity of symptoms. It is unclear whether these benefits are the consequence of a simple improvement in respiratory system mechanics resulting from the maintenance of larger tidal volumes, or if they are related to an improvement in respiratory drive or alleviation of chronic respiratory muscle fatigue.

Ankylosing Spondylitis

Ankylosing spondylitis is an immunologic disorder that develops in approximately 1 in 2,000 persons in the general population. It is strongly associated with the histocompatibility antigen HLA-B27.[157, 158] Twenty per cent of HLA-B27–positive subjects will develop the disease,[159] and approximately 88% of patients who have ankylosing spondylitis have the antigen.[158] Although the disease has been reported to occur four to eight times more frequently in males than in females, the distribution of HLA-B27–positive individuals is equal in the two sexes.[160] The discrepancy in sex incidence is related to the fact that the disease in women tends to be milder and therefore is diagnosed less often.[160] In any event, the typical patient who has ankylosing spondylitis is a young man who has a history of onset of symptoms early in the third decade of life. Although peripheral joint involvement develops eventually in about 20% to 25% of patients, there is little question that ankylosing spondylitis is distinct from rheumatoid arthritis.[161]

The abnormality is characterized pathologically by synovitis, chondritis, and juxta-articular osteitis of the sacroiliac, apophyseal, and costovertebral articulations. Progression of the disease is marked by erosion of subchondral bone, destruction of cartilage, and bony ankylosis. Calcification and ossification deep to the paraspinal ligaments are late changes. Aortic valvulitis develops in approximately 5% of patients,[161, 162] an incidence that increases to 10% in patients who have had the disease for 30 years.[162]

In addition to the characteristic changes in the thoracic skeleton, approximately 1% to 2% of patients develop pleuropulmonary manifestations,[163, 164] most commonly in the form of upper lobe fibrobullous disease (*see* page 1438).[165–167] The bullae can be secondarily infected and associated with significant hemoptysis;[168] usually, this is related to the formation of a fungus ball and, occasionally, to nontuberculous mycobacterial infection. Approximately 100 cases of upper lobe fibrobullous disease associated with ankylosing spondylitis were identified in a review of the literature published in 1977;[163] 8 of the patients developed spontaneous pneumothorax, an incidence well above that expected in the population at large. Bronchocentric granulomatosis confined to the upper lobes also has been described as a complication.[169] CT, particularly HRCT, is useful in characterizing the extent and nature of the upper lobe changes as well as in detecting or excluding an intracavitary fungus ball.[170, 171] In one review of 26 patients who had ankylosing spondylitis, 19 (70%) showed an abnormality on HRCT compared with only 4 (15%) on chest radiography.[172] The most frequently detected abnormalities were bronchial wall thickening and bronchiectasis (in 6 patients), nonapical interstitial disease (4), paraseptal emphysema (4), mediastinal lymph node enlargement (3), tracheal dilation (2), apical fibrosis (2), fungus ball (1), and interstitial lung disease (in 12). In another series of 2,080 patients, an unexpected number manifested evidence of pleuritis with effusion.[163] Bilateral pleural effusions have also been reported in a patient who had clinically inactive joint disease.[173]

The clinical picture is characterized by intermittent or continuous low back pain, sometimes associated with constitutional symptoms such as fatigue, weight loss, anorexia, and low-grade fever. The back pain can be distinguished from that of a mechanical or nonspecific type by its insidious onset, its duration (usually more than 3 months before the patient seeks medical help), its association with morning stiffness, and its improvement with exercise.[159] As the disease progresses upward and affects the thoracic spine, the patient may complain of chest pain that is sometimes accentuated during respiration.[174] Involvement of the costovertebral articulations results in a limitation of chest expansion, which correlates with a decrease in VC.[175] As the spine fuses, the kyphotic curvature gradually increases and chest expansion progressively diminishes. Few patients complain of dyspnea.

Involvement of the thoracic spine by ankylosing spondylitis results in fixation of the chest cage in an inspiratory position and leads to the paradoxical combination of hyperinflation (increased FRC) and lung restriction (decreased TLC and VC) on pulmonary function testing. VC is reduced, often to 70% or less of predicted values; residual volume and FRC are usually, but not always, increased.[177, 178] Mild interstitial lung disease, which cannot be appreciated radiographically, may contribute to lung restriction in some cases.[172, 179] Airway resistance is usually normal.[180] In one study of six patients who had moderate disease (TLC 85% ± 5% predicted), maximal exercise capacity was only mildly reduced;[181] ventilatory impairment was not the factor that limited exercise. Mixing efficiency and flow resistance are normal. Maximal static inspiratory transpulmonary pressure is diminished.

Although ventilation-perfusion relationships are usually normal,[182] one group of investigators found evidence in some patients of inequality that gave rise to mild arterial hypoxemia and an increase in the physiologic dead space;[183] this was attributed to underventilation of upper lobes in contrast to relative hyperventilation of lower lobes as a consequence of maintenance of diaphragmatic movement. Employing xenon 133, one group of investigators also showed an overall diminution in lung volume and a reduced proportion of inhaled xenon reaching the lung apices;[184] however, distribution of injected xenon was normal.

In an investigation of age-specific death rates of 836 patients who had ankylosing spondylitis,[176] a high mortality was found in men for those diseases known to be associated with spondylitis, including ulcerative colitis, nephritis, and tuberculosis or other respiratory disease.

Infectious Spondylitis

Pyogenic or tuberculous spondylitis can result in destruction of the vertebral body and intervertebral disk and development of a paraspinal mass evident on the chest radiograph. The mass is often fusiform and has its maximal diameter at the point of major bone destruction (Fig. 78–11). Tuberculous spondylitis shows a predilection for the lower thoracic and upper lumbar spine.[185, 186] CT demonstrates bony destruction and associated soft tissue masses that usually contain areas of low attenuation and show rim enhancement following intravenous administration of contrast.[186] Foci of calcification are frequently present within the soft tissue masses.[186] The extent of bony destruction and paraspinal abscess formation are particularly well seen on MR imaging (Fig. 78–12).[187] Early vertebral osteomyelitis and disk space infection are more readily apparent on MR imaging than on plain radiographs or CT.[187–189] The MR findings consist of decreased signal intensity in the disk space and adjacent vertebra on T1-weighted images and increased signal intensity on T2-weighted images.[187–190] With disease progression, there is gradual loss in disk space and increasing bone destruction. Gadolinium enhancement is helpful in assessing extraosseous extension of the inflammatory process, including extension into the epidural space.[190, 191]

Miscellaneous Abnormalities

Occasional individuals have deep paraspinal gutters associated with a position of the thoracic spine that is much more anterior than normal.[192] Because the distance between the sternum and the spine is reduced, the heart may be displaced into the left hemithorax, as in pectus excavatum. The "abnormality" seldom, if ever, results in disturbed cardiorespiratory function or in symptoms and signs. Another spinal "deformity" is the absence of physiologic thoracic kyphosis known as the "straight back syndrome"; extensive pulmonary function assessment, both at rest and during exercise, has shown that despite some decrease in TLC, affected individuals manifest no significant impairment of pulmonary function.[193]

Fractures of thoracic vertebral bodies can result in extraosseous hemorrhage and the development of unilateral or bilateral paraspinal hematomas. Although the fracture is usually visible radiographically, the major evidence of its presence may be deformity of the contiguous paraspinal soft tissues.

NEOPLASMS AND NON-NEOPLASTIC TUMORS OF THE CHEST WALL

The etiology of most primary chest wall neoplasms is unknown. An exception is those in individuals who have received prior chest wall radiation, in whom the risk of developing sarcoma is clearly increased (Fig. 78–13).[194–197] A history of breast carcinoma or, less commonly, Hodgkin's disease is present in most of these patients; rarely, the complication has been related to previous pulmonary carcinoma.[198] In one series, the latency between irradiation and the appearance of the sarcoma ranged from 5 to 28 years

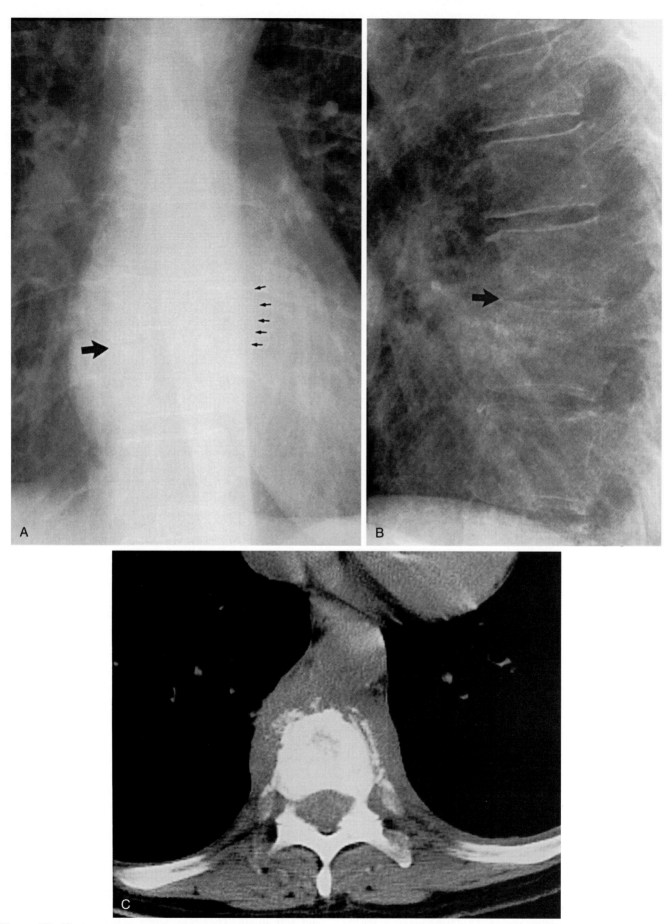

Figure 78–11. Staphylococcal Diskitis and Osteomyelitis. Posteroanterior *(A)* and lateral *(B)* chest radiographs in a 54-year-old intravenous drug abuser show narrowing of the T9–10 intervertebral disk space *(large arrows),* mild anterior wedging of the T9 vertebral body, and focal displacement of the left paraspinal interface *(small arrows).* A CT scan *(C)* demonstrates erosion of the T9 vertebral body, paravertebral inflammatory tissue, and a small left pleural effusion. Biopsy and blood cultures grew *Staphylococcus aureus.*

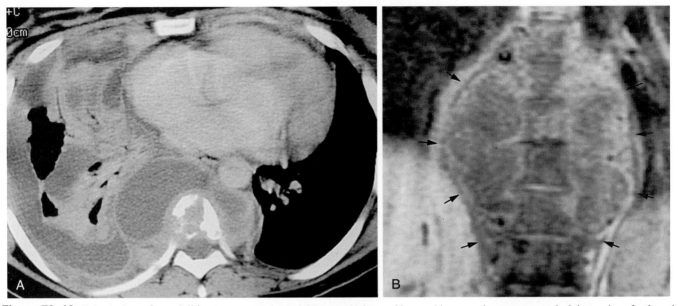

Figure 78–12. Tuberculous Spondylitis. A contrast-enhanced CT scan *(A)* from a 22-year-old woman demonstrates marked destruction of a thoracic vertebral body and extensive paraspinal soft tissue infiltration with low attenuation center and rim enhancement characteristic of abscess formation. Also note right empyema and consolidation and atelectasis of the right middle and lower lobes. A T1-weighted coronal MR image *(B)* shows cephalocaudal extent of the paraspinal abscesses *(arrows)*. (Courtesy of Dr. Sandy Rubin, University of Texas Medical Branch, Galveston, TX.)

(mean, 13 years).[194] The most common neoplasms that develop in these circumstances are malignant fibrohistiocytoma, fibrosarcoma, and osteogenic sarcoma; other histologic types are rare.[199] A possible pathogenetic association between repeated trauma and the development of a rib chondrosarcoma has been reported in one patient[200] and between prior surgery and the formation of a periosteal chondroma in several others.[201]

Although the following discussion divides tumors of the chest wall into soft tissue and skeletal groups, it should be remembered that confident determination of the origin of a neoplasm is not always possible, particularly if it is large.

Neoplasms of Soft Tissue

Primary neoplasms of the soft tissues of the chest wall are rare. In adults, the most common benign lesion is lipoma; other benign tumors include neurogenic neoplasms of the intercostal nerves (neurofibroma and schwannoma), and fibromas and angiofibromas of the intercostal muscles.[202] Desmoid tumors arise most commonly from the aponeurosis of the abdominal wall musculature in multiparous females; however, several examples have been reported to arise in the chest wall, usually after trauma.[203-205] The most common primary malignant neoplasms are fibrosarcoma and malignant fibrohistiocytoma; however, virtually any form of mesenchymal tumor may be seen.[207] Lymphoma and plasmacytomas are almost always secondary to adjacent skeletal disease; however, chest wall involvement is rarely the presenting manifestation of Hodgkin's disease, in which it probably represents direct spread from internal mammary lymph nodes.[208] Non-neoplastic tumors, such as elastofibromas (particularly in the subscapular region),[209, 210] abscesses, granulomas, and echinococcal cysts, also must be considered in the differential diagnosis of a chest wall mass.[202, 211, 212]

CT scanning has been shown to be a sensitive method of evaluating possible chest wall involvement by lymphoma[213, 214] and of assessing the extent of primary neoplasms of the chest wall.[215] However, its accuracy in the evaluation of chest wall invasion by intrapulmonary lesions is open to question.[216, 217] In one investigation of 20 patients who underwent CT, chest wall involvement was suggested by apparent extension of the mass into fat or muscle of the chest wall or around ribs or on the definite presence of bone destruction;[217] chest wall invasion was proved in 11 of the 20 cases at surgery or autopsy, but in 6 of the 9 remaining cases it was shown to be not present.

A soft tissue neoplasm of the chest wall may be identified radiographically in asymptomatic subjects or may become evident clinically as a soft tissue mass outside the chest wall. The tumor is likely to be malignant if it occasions pain. Rare neoplasms have been associated with hypertrophic osteoarthropathy.[218]

Lipoma

The point of origin of a lipoma in the chest wall establishes its mode of presentation: When it originates adjacent to the parietal pleura, it causes a soft tissue mass that indents the lung and possesses a contour characteristic of its extrapulmonary origin; when it arises outside the rib cage, it manifests as a palpable soft tissue mass that may be visualized radiographically if viewed in profile or, if of sufficient size, even *en face*. Most lipomas that arise between the ribs have a dumbbell or an hourglass configuration, part projecting inside and part outside the thoracic cage (Fig. 78–14). The density of lipomas is intermediate between that of air and soft tissue. Therefore, when a lipoma relates to lung parenchyma it may not be readily distinguishable from other soft tissue masses on the chest radiograph, whereas when it

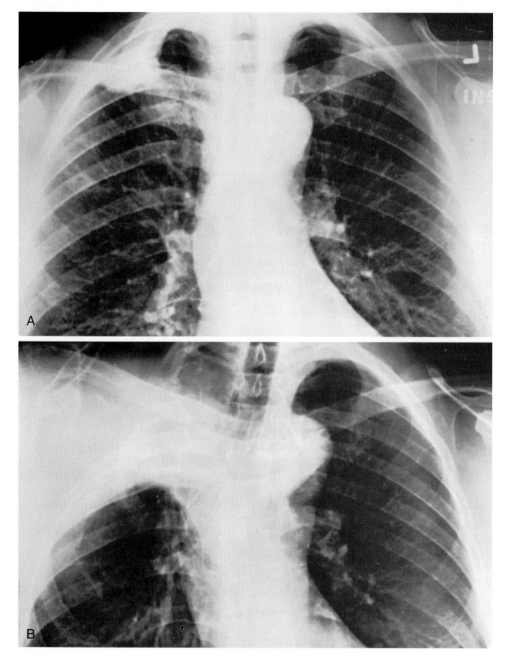

Figure 78–13. Fibrosarcoma of the Chest Wall Following Radiation Therapy. A posteroanterior radiograph of the upper half of the chest *(A)* from a 52-year-old man reveals a homogeneous mass at the apex of the right lung. Biopsy revealed squamous cell carcinoma, and a right upper lobectomy was performed. At thoracotomy, there was evidence of chest wall invasion, and postoperative radiation therapy was administered. Seven years later *(B)*, there had developed a large opacity in the right apical region associated with extensive destruction of ribs.

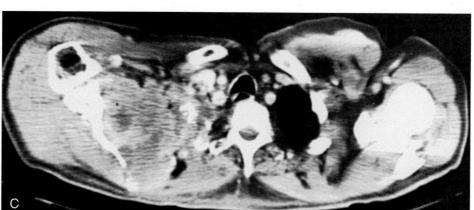

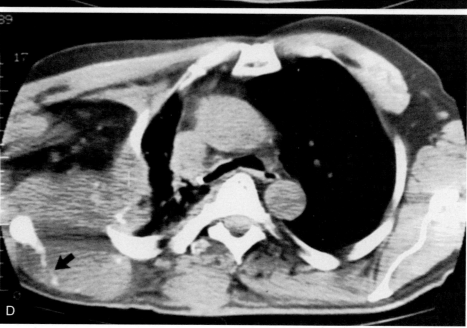

Figure 78–13 *Continued.* CT scans just below the thoracic inlet *(C)* and at the level of the main bronchi *(D)* reveal an almost complete absence of ribs in the apical region and extensive invasion of the soft tissues of the chest wall. The scapula has been partly destroyed, seen to best advantage in *D (arrow)*. Biopsy showed a high-grade sarcoma, with features consistent with those of fibrosarcoma.

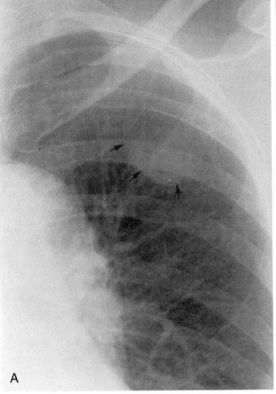

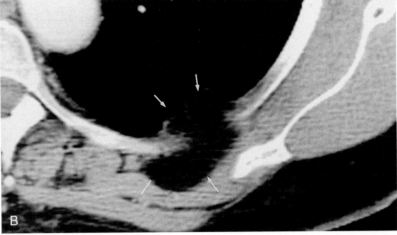

Figure 78–14. Lipoma. A view of the left upper chest from a posteroanterior chest radiograph *(A)* shows a soft tissue opacity *(arrows)* projecting over the left posterior fifth rib. The opacity has well-defined lower margins and poorly defined upper margins suggesting that it abuts the lung and the chest wall. A CT scan *(B)* demonstrates that the mass *(arrows)* has homogeneous fat attenuation and an hourglass configuration. The findings are diagnostic of a lipoma, presumably originating from the extrapleural fat. The patient was a 22-year-old woman who presented with chest wall pain. Because of this symptom, the tumor was resected and was confirmed to be a lipoma.

relates to the chest wall the contrast with contiguous soft tissues usually permits its identification as of fat origin.[219–221]

As a result of the specificity of CT in identifying fat-containing structures, this technique is especially valuable in the diagnosis of chest wall lipomas.[222, 223] The characteristic CT appearance consists of a well-defined mass that has homogeneous fat attenuation. The presence of any soft tissue strands should suggest the possibility of liposarcoma (Fig. 78–15).[223] Foci of calcification may be present in areas of fat necrosis.[223, 224] The diagnosis can also be made on MR imaging, which shows signal intensities characteristic of fat on all pulse sequences (high signal intensity on T1-weighted images, lower signal intensity on T2-weighted images, and low signal intensity on fat-saturation images).[224, 225]

Neurogenic Tumors

Neurogenic tumors may affect the thoracic spine roots, the paraspinal ganglia of the sympathetic chain, the intercostal nerves along the thoracic cage, or the peripheral nerves on the chest wall. Plexiform neurofibromas, seen in patients who have neurofibromatosis, can involve the chest wall extensively.[223] Tumors arising from the intercostal nerves can result in rib erosion, notching, and sclerosis (Fig. 78–16).[223] On CT, neurogenic tumors usually manifest as well-circumscribed cylindrical masses. They may have homogeneous or heterogeneous attenuation that may be lower or equal to that of chest wall muscle (Fig. 78–17).[226, 227] They usually show inhomogeneous enhancement following intravenous administration of contrast and often contain single or multiple areas of low attenuation.[223]

On MR imaging, neurogenic tumors usually have low to intermediate signal intensity on T1-weighted images and

inhomogeneously high signal intensity on T2-weighted images.[223, 225, 228] Neurilemomas often have peripheral high signal intensity on T2-weighted images and contain central areas with low signal intensity. Ganglioneuromas typically have a whorled appearance on both T1- and T2-weighted images caused by the presence of curvilinear or nodular bands of low signal intensity.[228]

Peripheral Primitive Neuroectodermal Tumor

Peripheral primitive neuroectodermal tumors (PPNETs) are a group of clinically aggressive neoplasms characterized histologically by the presence of small round cells arranged in a lobular pattern and associated with rosettes or pseudorosettes and immunohistochemical and ultrastructural evidence of neural differentiation.[229–231] Although the tumors may arise in many sites, they most often affect the periosteum and soft tissue of the thoracic wall (hence the synonym "malignant small cell tumor of the thoracopulmonary region"). (The tumor was first described in 1979 by Askin and his colleagues and has also been referred to eponymously as "Askin tumor."[232]) The neoplasm is believed to be derived from cells originating in the neural crest and has a number of features in common with Ewing's sarcoma.[231, 233, 234] An abnormality of chromosome 22 (e.g., reciprocal translocation of the long arms of chromosomes 11 and 22, or deletion of the long arm of 22) is characteristically present.[233] The pathogenesis is unknown; however, a number of tumors have developed following thoracic irradiation, usually for Hodgkin's disease.[197, 235]

Although PPNET may arise at any age, most tumors are seen in children, adolescents, or young adults.[229, 230] Chest wall pain is the usual presenting symptom;[230] some patients

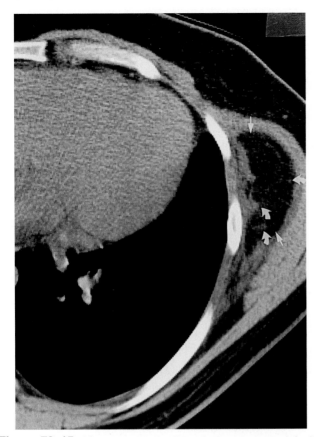

Figure 78–15. Liposarcoma. A CT scan demonstrates a left chest wall tumor displacing the adjacent muscles. The tumor contains large areas of fat attenuation *(straight arrows)* and focal areas of soft tissue attenuation *(curved arrows).* The appearance is characteristic of low-grade liposarcoma. The patient was a 32-year-old man.

have complicating pleural effusion extensive enough to result in dyspnea.[236] Radiologic findings include a unilateral chest wall mass, rib destruction, pleural thickening or effusion, soft tissue extension into the adjacent lung, pulmonary nodules, and, occasionally, mediastinal lymph node enlargement.[237, 238] The tumor has inhomogeneous attenuation on CT and inhomogeneous signal intensity on T2-weighted MR imaging.[237, 238]

The prognosis is poor. The overall 2-year survival rate in one series of 30 patients was 38%.[230] In another review of 54 patients, the 2-year progression-free survival of the 43 patients who had localized disease at the time of presentation was only 25%;[229] all of the patients who had disseminated disease at the time of diagnosis died within 5 years (approximately 80% in less than 2 years).

PPNET may be confused histologically with other forms of malignant small cell tumor in the chest wall. The most common of such tumors are undoubtedly metastatic pulmonary small cell carcinoma and lymphoma; rare varieties include small cell mesothelioma,[239] Ewing's sarcoma, neuroblastoma, rhabdomyosarcoma, and desmoplastic small round-cell tumor (an aggressive neoplasm that usually arises in the abdomen of young men).[240, 241] Despite the difficulty in diagnosis in some cases, the diagnosis has been made on samples derived by fine needle aspiration.[242]

Neoplasms and Non-neoplastic Tumors of Bone

Neoplasms of the thoracic skeleton are uncommon, accounting for only 5% of all neoplasms of bones and joints in one series.[243] Of the 134 cases of thoracic bone tumors in this review, 84 (63%) were primary (48 benign and 36

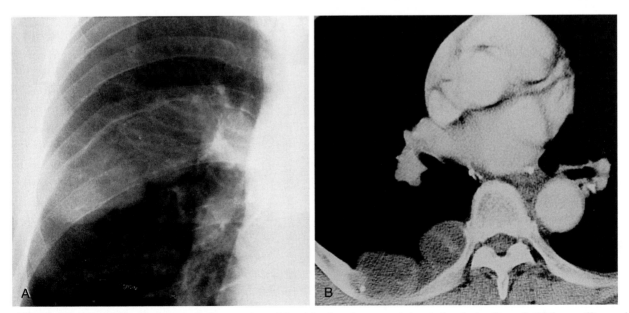

Figure 78–16. Intercostal Neurilemoma. A close-up view of the right chest from an anteroposterior chest radiograph *(A)* from a 69-year-old man demonstrates a soft tissue tumor adjacent to and parallel to the right seventh rib. Also note notching and sclerosis of the undersurface of the rib and widening of the interspace between the seventh and eighth ribs. A contrast-enhanced CT scan *(B)* shows the tumor to have inhomogeneous attenuation and to contain cystic areas. Note erosion of the posterior seventh rib. (Courtesy of Dr. Eun-Young Kang, Department of Radiology, Korea University Guro Hospital, Seoul, Korea.)

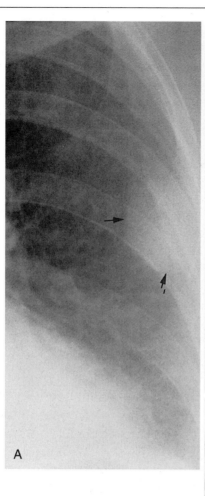

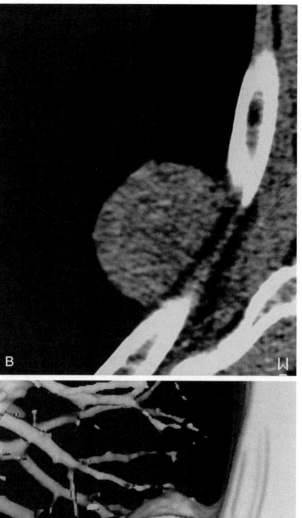

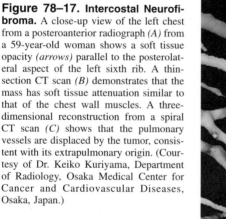

Figure 78–17. Intercostal Neurofibroma. A close-up view of the left chest from a posteroanterior radiograph *(A)* from a 59-year-old woman shows a soft tissue opacity *(arrows)* parallel to the posterolateral aspect of the left sixth rib. A thin-section CT scan *(B)* demonstrates that the mass has soft tissue attenuation similar to that of the chest wall muscles. A three-dimensional reconstruction from a spiral CT scan *(C)* shows that the pulmonary vessels are displaced by the tumor, consistent with its extrapulmonary origin. (Courtesy of Dr. Keiko Kuriyama, Department of Radiology, Osaka Medical Center for Cancer and Cardiovascular Diseases, Osaka, Japan.)

malignant) and the remainder metastatic.[243] The majority of the latter were from primary tumors in the lung and breast. The average age of the patients with malignant neoplasms was 48 years and of those with benign neoplasms, 26 years.

Most osseous neoplasms occur in the ribs. For example, in one series of 100 patients, tumor was localized to the ribs in 78 and to the sternum in 22;[244] in the review of 134 patients cited previously, 72 involved the ribs, 26 the scapulae, 15 the thoracic vertebrae, 14 the clavicles, and 7 the

sternum.[243] In the latter study, the following characteristics were noted: (1) rib lesions were most commonly metastatic; (2) the majority of lesions arising in the sternum were malignant, most often chondrosarcoma; (3) involvement of the clavicles was most often by metastatic neoplasm, with benign neoplasms the next most common; (4) primary neoplasms in the scapulae were more numerous than metastatic ones, with the majority benign; and (5) involvement of the thoracic vertebrae was almost invariably metastatic in origin.

Benign Tumors and Tumor-like Lesions

Osteochondroma is the most common benign neoplasm of the thoracic skeleton. Complications include compression of nerves, blood vessels, and the spinal cord and (rarely) hemothorax or diaphragmatic perforation.[245a, 245b, 248] Approximately 0.5% to 2% of the tumors undergo malignant transformation.[248] Additional rare osteocartilaginous abnormalities of the chest wall include enchondroma, osteoblastoma,[245] and endostoma ("bone islands").

The most common non-neoplastic tumor of the thoracic skeleton is fibrous dysplasia (Fig. 78–18). The lesion is usually monostotic and asymptomatic; rarely, multiple lesions are sufficient to result in progressive restrictive lung disease, pulmonary hypertension, and cor pulmonale.[206] Langerhans' cell histiocytosis, hemangioma, and aneurysmal bone cyst occur occasionally.[243, 246, 247] Involvement of the rib cage by Paget's disease represents a typical radiographic appearance similar to that in any other bone (Fig. 78–19).

Gorham's syndrome is an unusual disorder consisting of an intraosseous proliferation of vascular or lymphatic channels that can cause progressive osteolysis, affect the chest wall diffusely, and prove fatal.[249] In a review of 97 patients who had this abnormality, the ages of affected individuals ranged from 1 to 75 years (mean age 27). Sixty-four per cent were males, 57% had a history of previous thoracic trauma, and 16 (16%) died of the disorder;[249] in 10 patients, death was attributed to chest wall disease, and in 3, it was caused by spinal cord involvement by the proliferating tissue. The chest wall involvement in Gorham's syndrome can be imaged using a combined CT and nuclear medicine approach.[250] Chylothorax is seen in some patients.[251]

The SAPHO syndrome (synovitis, acne, pustulosis, hyperostosis, and osteitis) is an uncommon disorder in which the bone lesions most often affect the anterior chest wall (frequently the clavicle).[252] The radiographic features of the osseous lesions often suggest a neoplasm; however, pathologic examination shows the lesions to consist of acute inflammation, edema, and periosteal bone formation in the early stage and sclerotic bone trabeculae in long-standing disease.[252] The most common clinical presentation is pain related to the sites of osseous involvement.

The majority of benign neoplasms of the thoracic skeleton cause no symptoms and usually are detected in asymptomatic subjects on a screening chest radiograph. Rarely, thoracic outlet syndrome has been caused by a benign tumor of the first rib.[41]

Malignant Neoplasms

Sternal metastases most frequently originate in the breast, thyroid, or lung and may be associated with pathologic fractures.[253] Hodgkin's disease can also affect the sternum and parasternal chest wall as a result of contiguous spread from retrosternal lymph nodes.[254] A wide variety of primary neoplasms can involve the thoracic spine; however, metastatic carcinoma is much more common. In a few cases, the major radiographic finding is an extraosseous soft tissue mass, and identification of the primary bone lesion requires careful radiographic study. Lymphoma, particularly Hodgkin's disease, may be manifested radiologically as a fusiform

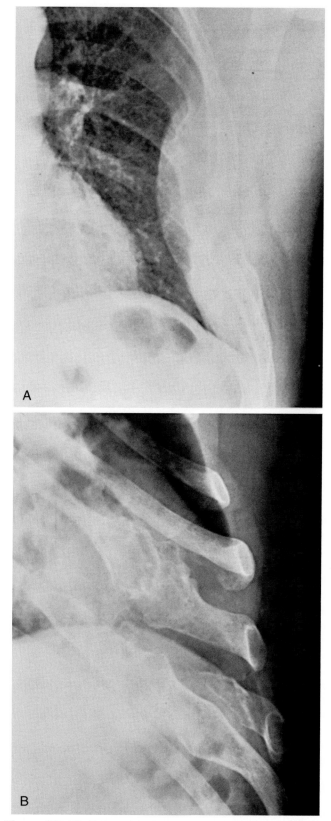

Figure 78–18. Polyostotic Fibrous Dysplasia of the Left Rib Cage. Posteroanterior *(A)* and oblique *(B)* views of the left rib cage reveal considerable expansion and distortion of ribs along the lower axillary lung zone (one rib has been removed). The left innominate bone and left tibia were affected in a similar manner. Bone involvement is thus unilateral, representing the osseous manifestation of Albright's syndrome.

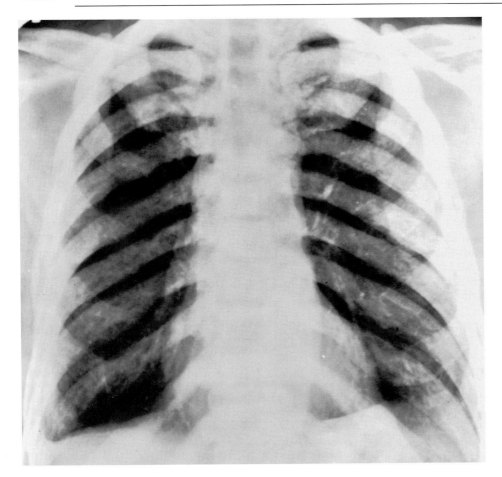

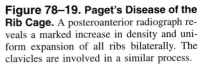

Figure 78–19. Paget's Disease of the Rib Cage. A posteroanterior radiograph reveals a marked increase in density and uniform expansion of all ribs bilaterally. The clavicles are involved in a similar process.

paraspinal soft tissue mass produced by enlargement of the posterior parietal group of lymph nodes; in such cases, contiguous vertebrae may be eroded by extranodal invasion.

The most common malignant mesenchymal neoplasm of the rib is chondrosarcoma;[245] osteogenic sarcoma, chondroblastoma, malignant fibrohistiocytoma, hemangiopericytoma, angiosarcoma, and giant cell tumor fibrosarcoma occur occasionally (Fig. 78–20).[243, 255-262] Radiographically, these tumors usually appear as a mass on the lateral chest wall; sometimes, they arise in the posterior aspect of a rib, in which case they may appear as a paravertebral mass.[261] Chondrosarcomas are usually large masses with indistinct margins, cortical breakthrough and soft tissue involvement.[245c] Foci of calcification may be seen within the cartilaginous matrix. The foci of calcification and soft tissue extension are better seen on CT than on radiographs. The MR imaging signal characteristics are nonspecific, with intermediate signal intensity on T1-weighted images and inhomogeneous areas of high signal intensity on T2-weighted images.[245c]

Myeloma and (occasionally) solitary plasmacytoma are the most frequent malignant lymphoid neoplasms, followed by Hodgkin's disease and non-Hodgkin's lymphoma.[243, 263] In older patients, particularly men, the association of a destructive lesion of one or more ribs with a soft tissue mass

that protrudes into the thorax and indents the lung is highly suggestive of myeloma (Fig. 78–21).[264] However, a similar appearance can be seen in association with a primary pulmonary carcinoma that invades the chest wall and with other primary or metastatic chest wall neoplasms (Fig. 78–22). Advanced myelomatosis of the rib cage may be associated with expansion of bone (Fig. 78–23). Pathologic fractures, particularly of the sternum (Fig. 78–24), may result in severe deformity of the chest wall.

Clinical manifestations of these neoplasms are varied. A pathologic fracture occasionally causes a patient to seek medical advice. Malignant neoplasms may cause pain and, if extensive, respiratory insufficiency (Fig. 78–25); hemothorax occurs occasionally.[265] Tumors of the vertebrae may compress the cord and result in neurologic signs and symptoms.[201] Radiologic assessment may be useful in suggesting the diagnosis; however, definitive diagnosis requires correlation between the histologic and radiologic appearances of the neoplasm. CT and MR imaging are helpful in characterizing the tumor and in assessing its extent. CT is superior to MR imaging in the demonstration of foci of calcification in chondrosarcomas and osteosarcomas.[111, 223, 225] However, because of its greater ability to distinguish tumor from normal soft tissue, MR imaging is the modality of choice in the assessment of the extent of chest wall tumors and their relationship to adjacent structures.[111, 223, 225]

Text continued on page 3039

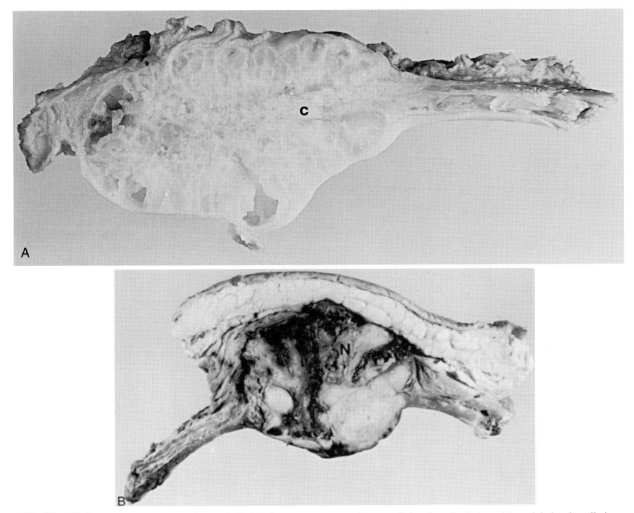

Figure 78–20. Rib Sarcoma. A gross specimen of rib *(A)* shows a segment to be expanded and partly destroyed by a lobulated, well-circumscribed mass composed of gelatinous, somewhat translucent tissue and more solid white areas resembling mature cartilage (c). Histologic examination showed a low-grade chondrosarcoma. A segment of rib from another patient *(B)* is similarly expanded and destroyed by a well-defined mass, in this case with focal necrosis (N) and hemorrhage. Fat and skin of the chest wall are present above the mass. Histologic examination showed a malignant fibrous histiocytoma.

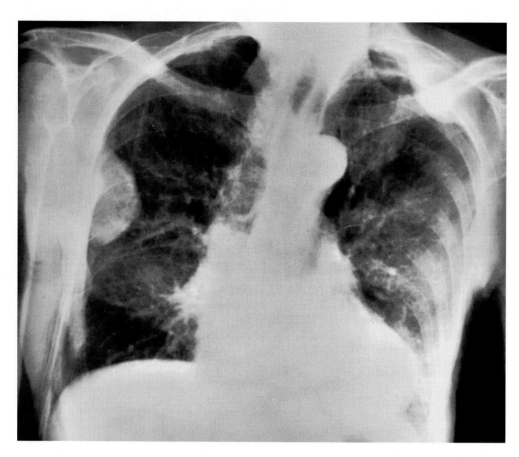

Figure 78–21. Multiple Myeloma of the Rib Cage. A posteroanterior radiograph reveals large homogeneous masses protruding into the thorax along the right axillary lung zone and left apex. The obtuse angle that these masses create with the pleura indicates their origin from either the pleura or the chest wall. Such an appearance is highly suggestive of multiple myeloma affecting the rib cage but also can be produced by metastatic carcinoma.

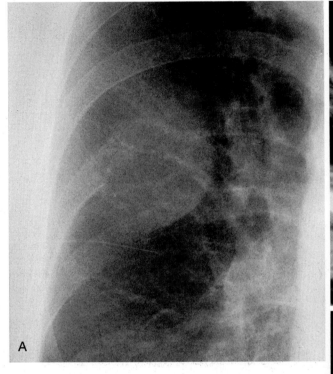

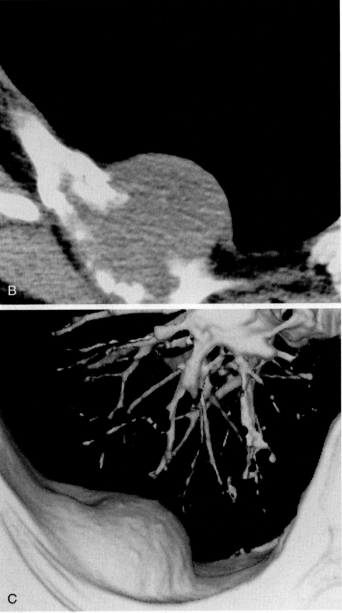

Figure 78–22. Metastatic Thyroid Carcinoma. A view of the right chest from a posteroanterior radiograph *(A)* from a 62-year-old woman demonstrates a soft tissue mass adjacent to the posterior right seventh rib. Note destruction of the inferior cortical margin of the rib. A CT scan *(B)* demonstrates rib destruction by an expansile lesion. A three-dimensional reconstruction from a spiral CT scan *(C)* demonstrates the characteristic appearance of an extrapulmonary mass. (Courtesy of Dr. Keiko Kuriyama, Department of Radiology, Osaka Medical Center for Cancer and Cardiovascular Diseases, Osaka, Japan.)

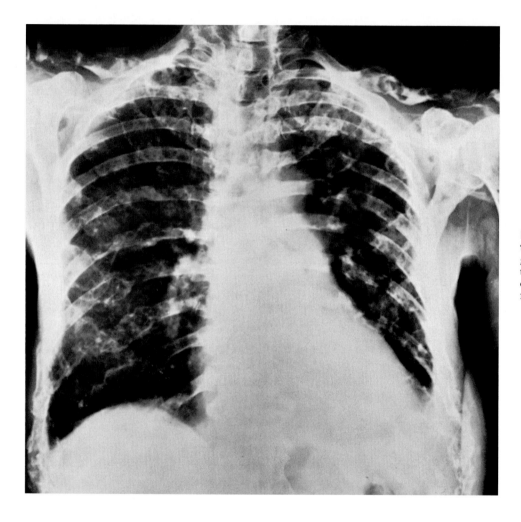

Figure 78–23. Multiple Myeloma of the Rib Cage. A posteroanterior radiograph reveals extensive destruction of virtually all ribs bilaterally. Note that several of the ribs have been expanded, a common feature in multiple myeloma of ribs.

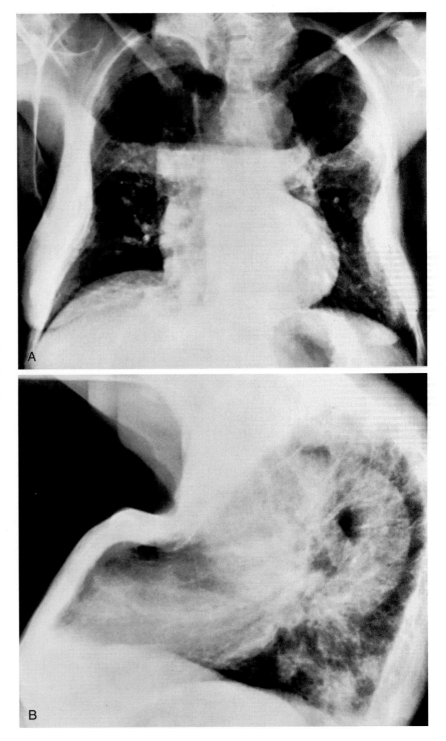

Figure 78–24. Collapse of the Anterior Chest Wall Caused by Involvement of the Sternum in Multiple Myeloma. In posteroanterior projection *(A)*, a rather unusual broad opacity can be identified passing across the whole of the chest from side to side. This opacity obviously cannot arise from *within* the thorax. In lateral projection *(B)*, it is evident that the upper portion of the anterior chest wall has collapsed inward, thus creating a horizontal ''shelf'' that casts the unusual shadow in posteroanterior projection. The patient was a 63-year-old woman who had widespread multiple myeloma. Note the extensive involvement of the rib cage.

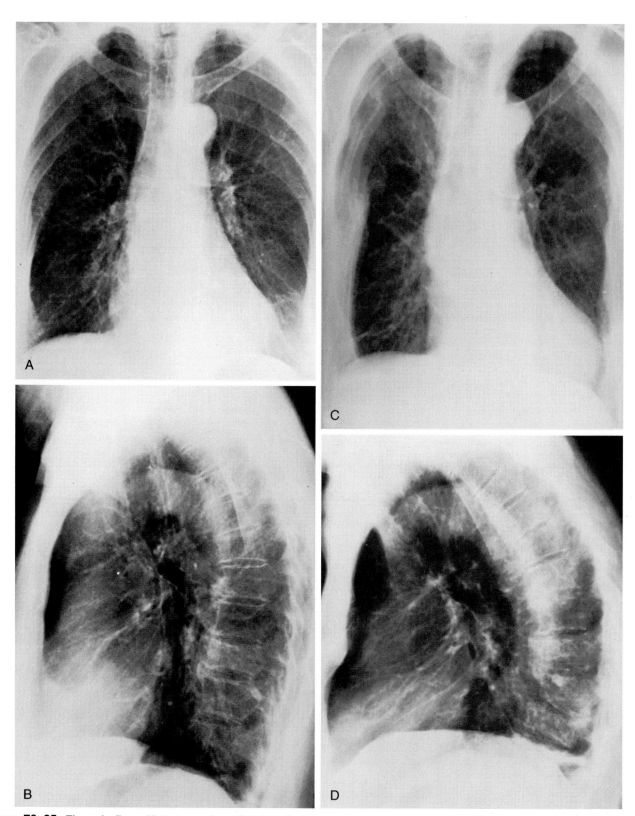

Figure 78–25. Thoracic Bony Metastases from Cervical Carcinoma. Posteroanterior *(A)* and lateral *(B)* chest radiographs show a normal skeleton except for several vertebral osteophytes. Five months later, similar examinations *(C* and *D)* reveal fractures of the ribs bilaterally and of the sternum; these were associated clinically with a flail sternum and collapse of virtually the entire chest wall that resulted in respiratory failure. The patient was an elderly woman who had squamous cell carcinoma of cervix and biopsy-proven skeletal metastases. (Courtesy of Dr. Jim Gruber, Montreal General Hospital.)

REFERENCES

1. Bavinck JNB, Weaver DD: Subclavian artery supply disruption sequence: Hypothesis of a vascular etiology for Poland, Klippel-Feil, and Möbius anomalies. Am J Med Genet 23:903, 1986.
2. Newlin NS: Congenital retrosternal subluxation of the clavicle simulating an intrathoracic mass. Am J Roentgenol 130:1184, 1978.
3. Greenspan A, Cohen J, Szabo RM: Klippel-Feil syndrome. An unusual association with Sprengel deformity, omovertebral bone, and other skeletal, hematologic, and respiratory disorders. A case report. Bull Hosp Joint Dis Orthop Inst 51:54, 1991.
4. Theiss SM, Smith MD, Winter RB: The long-term follow-up of patients with Klippel-Feil syndrome and congenital scoliosis. Spine 22:1219, 1997.
5. Tomsen MN, Schneider U, Weber M, et al: Scoliosis and congenital anomalies associated with Klippel-Feil syndrome types I–III. Spine 22:396, 1997.
6. Bhagat R, Pant K, Singh VK, et al: Pulmonary developmental anomaly associated with Klippel-Feil syndrome and anomalous atrioventricular conduction. Chest 101:1157, 1992.
7. Ulmer JL, Elster AD, Ginsberg LE, et al: Klippel-Feil syndrome: CT and MR of acquired and congenital abnormalities of cervical spine and cord. J Comput Assist Tomogr 17:215, 1993.
8. Pearl M, Chow TF, Friedman E: Poland's syndrome. Radiology 101:619, 1976.
9. Karnak I, Tanyel C, Tuncbilek E, et al: Bilateral Poland anomaly. Am J Med Genet 75:505, 1998.
10. Fraser FC, Teebi AS, Walsh S, et al: Poland sequence with dextrocardia: Which comes first? Am J Med Genet 73:194, 1997.
11. Perez Aznar JM, Urbano J, Garcia Laborda E, et al: Breast and pectoralis muscle hypoplasia. A mild degree of Poland's syndrome. Acta Radiol 37:759, 1996.
12. Moncada R, Vade A, Gimenez C, et al: Congenital and acquired lung hernias. J Thorac Imaging 11:75, 1996.
13. Esquembre C, Ferris J, Verdeguer A, et al: Poland syndrome and leukaemia. Eur J Pediatr 146:444, 1987.
14. Sackey K, Odone V, Geroge S, et al: Poland's syndrome associated with childhood non-Hodgkin's lymphoma. Am J Dis Child 138:600, 1984.
15. Caksen H, Patiroglu T, Ozdemir MA, et al: Neuroblastoma and Poland syndrome in a 15-year-old boy. Acta Paediatr Jpn 39:701, 1997.
16. Athale UH, Warrier R: Poland's syndrome and Wilms' tumor: An unusual association. Med Pediatr Oncol 30:67, 1998.
17. Shaham D, Ramu N, Bar-Ziv J: Leiomyosarcoma in Poland's syndrome. A case report. Acta Radiol 33:444, 1992.
18. Wright AR, Milner RH, Bainbridge LC, et al: MR and CT in the assessment of Poland syndrome. J Comput Assist Tomogr 16:442, 1992.
19. Bainbridge LC, Wright AR, Kanthan R: Computed tomography in the preoperative assessment of Poland's syndrome. Br J Plast Surg 44:604, 1991.
20. Mueller CF, Moseley RD Jr: Roentgenologic appearance of the chest following radical neck dissection. Am J Roentgenol 117:840, 1973.
21. Bhalla M, Leitman BS, Forcade C, et al: Lung hernia: Radiographic features. Am J Roentgenol 154:51, 1990.
22. Munnell ER: Herniation of the lung. Ann Thorac Surg 5:204, 1968.
23. Meek JC, Bollen E, Koudstaal J, et al: Pain in scar as an early symptom of acquired thoracic hernia. Eur Respir J 4:505, 1991.
24. Sloth-Nielsen J, Jurik AG: Spontaneous intercostal pulmonary hernia with subsegmental incarceration. Eur J Cardiothorac Surg 3:562, 1989.
25. Fisher MS: Eve's rib (letters to the editor). Radiology 140:841, 1981.
26. Rock JP, Spickler EM: Anomalous rib presenting as cervical myelopathy: A previously unreported variant of Klippel-Feil syndrome. Case report. J Neurosurg 75:465, 1991.
27. Novak CB, Mackinnon SE: Thoracic outlet syndrome. Orthop Clin North Am 27:747, 1996.
28. Mackinnon SE, Patterson GA, Novak CB: Thoracic outlet syndrome: A current overview. Semin Thorac Cardiovasc Surg 8:176, 1996.
29. Siegel RS, Steichen FM: Cervicothoracic outlet syndrome. Vascular compression caused by congenital abnormality of thoracic ribs: A case report. J Bone Joint Surg 49A:1187, 1967.
30. Capistrant TD: Thoracic outlet syndrome in whiplash injury. Ann Surg 185:175, 1977.
31. Machleder HI, Moll F, Verity MA: The anterior scalene muscle in thoracic outlet compression syndrome. Arch Surg 131:1141, 1986.
32. Bilbey JH, Müller NL, Connell DG, et al: Thoracic outlet syndrome: Evaluation with CT. Radiology 171:381, 1989.
33. Nguyen TT, Baumgartner F, Nelems B: Bilateral rudimentary first ribs as a cause of thoracic outlet syndrome. J Natl Med Assoc 89:69, 1997.
34. De Villiers JC: A brachiocephalic vascular syndrome associated with cervical rib. BMJ 2:140, 1966.
35. Lagerquist LG, Tyler FH: Thoracic outlet syndrome with tetany of the hands. Am J Med 59:281, 1975.
36. Dick R: Arteriography in neurovascular compression at the thoracic outlet, with special reference to embolic patterns. Am J Roentgenol 110:141, 1970.
37. Remy-Jardin M, Doyen J, Remy J, et al: Functional anatomy of the thoracic outlet: Evaluation with spiral CT. Radiology 205:843, 1997.
38. Matsumura JS, Rilling WS, Pearce WH, et al: Helical computed tomography of the normal thoracic outlet. J Vasc Surg 26:776, 1997.
39. Esposito MD, Arrington JA, Blackshear MN, et al: Thoracic outlet syndrome in a throwing athlete diagnosed with MRI and MRA. J Magn Reson Imaging 7:598, 1997.
40. Matsumura JS, Rilling WS, Pearce WH, et al: Helical computed tomography of the normal thoracic outlet. J Vasc Surg 26:776, 1997.
41. Melliere D, Ben Yahia NE, Etienne G, et al: Thoracic outlet syndrome caused by tumor of the first rib. J Vasc Surg 14:235, 1991.
42. Kelleher J, O'Connell DJ, MacMahon H: Intrathoracic rib: Radiographic features of two cases. Br J Radiol 52:181, 1979.
42a. Kinane TB, Cleveland RH: Spare rib. Am J Roentgenol 171:118, 1998.
43. Shoop JD: Transthoracic rib. Radiology 93:1335, 1969.
44. Peterson MS, Plunkett MB: CT demonstration of an intrathoracic rib (letter). Am J Roentgenol 160:895, 1993.
45. Sullivan D, Cornwell WS: Pelvic rib: Report of a case. Radiology 110:355, 1974.
46. Pirnar T, Neuhauser EBD: Asphyxiating thoracic dystrophy of the newborn. Am J Roentgenol 98:358, 1966.
47. Connor JM, Evans CC, Evans DAP: Cardiopulmonary function in fibrodysplasia ossificans progressiva. Thorax 36:419, 1981.
48. Boone ML, Swenson BE, Felson B: Rib notching: Its many causes. Am J Roentgenol 91:1075, 1964.
49. Ferris RA, LoPresti JM: Rib notching due to coarctation of the aorta: Report of a case initially observed at less than one year of age. Br J Radiol 47:357, 1974.
50. Chinitz LA, Kronzon I, Trehan N, et al: Total occlusion of the abdominal aorta in a patient with Takayasu's arteritis: The importance of lower rib notching in the differential diagnosis. Cath Cardiovasc Diagn 12:405, 1986.
51. Sturm A Jr, Loogen F: Rippenusuren ohne Aortenisthrusstenose, unter besonderer Berücksichtigung der Fallotschen Tetralogie und Pentalogie. (Notching of the ribs in the absence of coarctation of the aorta, with particular consideration to Fallot's tetralogy and pentalogy.) Fortschr Roentgenstr 97:464, 1962.
52. Sargent EN, Turner AF, Jacobson G: Superior marginal rib defects. An etiologic classification. Am J Roentgenol 106:491, 1969.
53. Gilmartin D: Cartilage calcification and rib erosion in chronic respiratory poliomyelitis. Clin Radiol 17:115, 1966.
54. Bernstein C, Loeser WD, Manning LG: Erosive rib lesions in paralytic poliomyelitis. Radiology 70:368, 1958.
55. Wignall BK, Williamson BRJ: The chest x-ray in quadriplegia: A review of 119 patients. Clin Radiol 31:81, 1980.
56. Keats TE: Superior marginal rib defects in restrictive lung disease. Am J Roentgenol 124:449, 1975.
57. Osinowo O, Adebo OA, Okubanjo AO: Osteomyelitis of the ribs in Ibadan. Thorax 41:58, 1986.
58. Wolstein D, Rabinowitz JG, Twersky J: Tuberculosis of the rib. J Can Assoc Radiol 25:307, 1974.
59. Adler BD, Padley SPG, Müller NL: Tuberculosis of the chest wall: CT findings. J Comput Assist Tomogr 17:271, 1993.
60. Lee G, Im J-G, Kim JS, et al: Tuberculosis of the ribs: CT appearance. J Comput Assist Tomogr 17:363, 1993.
61. Ip M, Chen NK, So SY, et al: Unusual rib destruction in pleuropulmonary tuberculosis. Chest 95:242, 1989.
62. Fitzgerald R, Hutchinson CE: Tuberculosis of the ribs: Computed tomographic findings. Br J Radiol 65:822, 1992.
63. Chung SY, Yang I, Bae SH, et al: Tuberculous abscess in retromammary region: CT findings. J Comput Assist Tomogr 20:766, 1996.
64. Frouge C, Miquel A, Cochan-Priollet B, et al: Breast mass due to rib tuberculosis. Eur J Radiol 19:118, 1995.
65. Fogelman I: Lesions in the ribs detected by bone scanning. Clin Radiol 31:317, 1980.
66. Eyler WR, Monsein LH, Beute GH, et al: Rib enlargement in patients with chronic pleural disease. Am J Roentgenol 167:921, 1996.
67. Bonakdarpour A, Zadeh YFA, Maghssoudi H, et al: Costal echinococcosis. Report of six cases and review of the literature. Am J Roentgenol 118:371, 1973.
68. Aeschlimann A, Kahn MF: Tietze's syndrome: A critical review. Clin Exp Rheumatol 8:407, 1990.
69. Jurik AG, Graudal H: Sternocostal joint swelling—clinical Tietze's syndrome. Scand J Rheumatol 17:33, 1988.
70. Lim MC, Chan HL: Relapsing polychondritis—a report on two Chinese patients with severe costal chondritis. Ann Acad Med Singapore 19:396, 1990.
71. Skorneck AB: Roentgen aspects of Tietze's syndrome. Painful hypertrophy of costal cartilage and bone—osteochondritis? Am J Roentgenol 83:748, 1960.
72. Calabro JJ, Marchesano JM: Tietze's syndrome: Report of a case with juvenile onset. J Pediatr 68:985, 1966.
73. Dunlop RF: Tietze revisited (letter to the editor). Clin Orthop 62:223, 1969.
74. Gill GV: Epidemic of Tietze's syndrome. BMJ 2:499, 1977.
75. Pohl R: Zur Aetiologie des Tietze-Syndrome. (Etiology of Tietze's syndrome.) Wien Klin Wochenschr 69:370, 1957.
76. Ausubel H, Cohen BD, LaDue JS: Tietze's disease of eight years' duration. N Engl J Med 261:190, 1959.
77. Edelstein G, Levitt RG, Slaker DP, et al: CT observation of rib abnormalities: Spectrum of findings. J Comput Assist Tomogr 9:65, 1985.
78. Edelstein G, Levitt RG, Slaker DP, et al: Computed tomography of Tietze syndrome. J Comput Assist Tomogr 8:20, 1984.
79. Choi YW, Im JG, Song CS, et al: Sonography of the costal cartilage: Normal anatomy and preliminary clinical application. J Clin Ultrasound 23:243, 1995.

80. Antico A, Ghidotti I, Allegri M, et al: Tietze's syndrome: A case report and topical methods in diagnostic imaging. Monaldi Arch Chest Dis 49:208, 1994.
81. Yang W, Bahk YW, Chung SK, et al: Pinhole skeletal scintigraphic manifestations of Tietze's disease. Eur J Nucl Med 21:947, 1994.
82. Massie JD, Sebes, Cowles SJ: Bone scintigraphy and costochondritis. J Thorac Imaging 8:137, 1993.
83. Mendelson G, Mendelson H, Horowitz SF, et al: Can (99m)technetium methylene diphosphonate bone scans objectively document costochondritis? Chest 111:1600, 1997.
84. Ricevuti G: Effects of human calcitonin on pain in the treatment of Tietze's syndrome. Clin Ther 7:669, 1985.
85. Carabasi RK, Christian JJ, Brindley HH: Costosternal chondrodynia: A variant of Tietze's syndrome? Dis Chest 41:559, 1962.
86. Guller B, Hable K: Cardiac findings in pectus excavatum in children: Review and differential diagnosis. Chest 66:165, 1974.
87. Leung AKC, Hoo JJ: Familial congenital funnel chest. Am J Med Genet 26:887, 1987.
88. Wooler GH, Mashhour YAS, Garcia JB, et al: Pectus excavatum. Thorax 24:557, 1969.
89. Ravitch MM, Matzen RN: Pulmonary insufficiency in pectus excavatum associated with left pulmonary agenesis, congenital clubbed feet and extromelia. Dis Chest 54:58, 1968.
90. Backer Ole G, Brünner S, Larsen V: Radiologic evaluation of funnel chest. Acta Radiol 55:249, 1961.
91. Mosetitsch W: Pectus excavatum. Fortschr Roentgenstr 100:31, 1964.
92. Soteropoulos GC, Cigtay OS, Schellinger D: Pectus excavatum deformities simulating mediastinal masses. J Comput Assist Tomogr 3:596, 1979.
93. Moreno AJ, Parker AL, Fredericks P, et al: Pectus excavatum defect on liver-spleen scintigraphy. Eur J Nucl Med 12:309, 1986.
94. Muherji S, Zeissman HA, Earll JM, et al: False-positive iodine-131 whole body scan due to pectus excavatum. Clin Nucl Med 13:207, 1988.
95. Haller JA, Kramer SS, Lietman SA: Use of CT scans in selection of patients for pectus excavatum surgery: A preliminary report. J Pediatr Surg 22:904, 1987.
96. Nakahara K, Ohno K, Shinichiro M, et al: An evaluation of operative outcome in patients with funnel chest diagnosed by means of the computed tomogram. J Thorac Cardiovasc Surg 93:577, 1987.
97. Clark JB, Grenville-Mathers R: Pectus excavatum. Br J Dis Chest 56:202, 1962.
98. Wachtel FW, Ravitch MM, Grishman A: The relation of pectus excavatum to heart disease. Am Heart J 52:121, 1956.
99. Skinner EF: Xiphoid horn in pectus excavatum. Thorax 24:750, 1969.
100. Fink A, Rivin A, Murray JF: Pectus excavatum. An analysis of twenty-seven cases. Arch Intern Med 108:427, 1961.
101. Shamberger RC, Welch K, Sanders SP: Mitral valve prolapse associated with pectus excavatum. J Pediatr 111:404, 1987.
102. Park JM, Farmer AR: Wolff-Parkinson-White syndrome in children with pectus excavatum. J Pediatr 112:926, 1988.
103. Schamberger RC, Welch KJ: Surgical correction of pectus carinatum. J Pediatr Surg 22:48, 1987.
104. Lester CW: Pectus carinatum, pigeon breast and related deformities of the sternum and costal cartilages. Arch Paediatr 77:399, 1960.
105. Currarino G, Silverman FN: Premature obliteration of the sternal sutures and pigeon-breast deformity. Radiology 70:532, 1958.
106. Davies H: Chest deformities in congenital heart disease. Br J Dis Chest 53:151, 1959.
107. Zorab PA: Chest deformities. BMJ 1:1155, 1966.
108. Goodman LR, Kay HR, Teplick SK, et al: Complications of median sternotomy: Computed tomographic evaluation. Am J Roentgenol 141:225, 1983.
109. Templeton PA, Fishman EK: CT evaluation of poststernotomy complications. Am J Roentgenol 159:45, 1992.
110. Biesecker GL, Aaron BL, Mullen JT: Primary sternal osteomyelitis. Chest 63:236, 1973.
111. Franquet T, Giménez A, Alegret X, et al: Imaging findings of sternal abnormalities. Eur Radiol 7:492, 1997.
112. Kay HR, Goodman LR, Teplick SK, et al: Use of computed tomography to assess mediastinal complications after median sternotomy. Ann Thorac Surg 36:706, 1983.
113. Goldin RH, Chow AW, Edwards JE Jr, et al: Sternoarticular septic arthritis in heroin users. N Engl J Med 289:616, 1973.
114. Gimferrer J-M, Callejas M-A, Sánchez-Lloret J, et al: *Candida albicans* costochondritis in heroin addicts. Ann Thorac Surg 41:89, 1986.
115. Kohler H, Uehlinger E, Kutzner J, et al: Sternocostoclavicular hyperostosis: Painful swelling of the sternum, clavicles, and upper ribs. Ann Intern Med 87:192, 1977.
116. Sartoris DJ, Schreiman JS, Kerr R, et al: Sternocostoclavicular hyperostosis: A review and report of 11 cases. Radiology 158:125, 1986.
117. Kane WJ: Prevalence of scoliosis. Clin Orthop 126:43, 1977.
118. Loop JW, Akeson WH, Clawson DK: Acquired thoracic abnormalities in neurofibromatosis. Am J Roentgenol 93:416, 1965.
119. Murray JF: Pulmonary disability in the Hurler syndrome (lipochondrodystrophy). A study of two cases. N Engl J Med 261:378, 1959.
120. Buhain WJ, Rammohan G, Berger HW: Pulmonary function in Morquio's disease—a study of two siblings. Chest 68:41, 1975.
121. Joseph KN, Bowen JR, MacEwen GD: Unusual orthopedic manifestations of neurofibromatosis. Clin Orthop 278:17, 1992.
122. Pope FM, Nicholls AC, Palan A, et al: Clinical features of an affected father and daughter with Ehlers-Danlos syndrome type VIIB. Br J Dermatol 126:77, 1992.

123. Bergofsky EH, Turino GM, Fishman AP: Cardiorespiratory failure in kyphoscoliosis. Medicine 38:263, 1959.
124. Reid L: Pathological changes in the lungs in scoliosis. *In* Zorab PA (ed): Symposium on Scoliosis. 2nd ed. New York, Longman, 1969.
125. Naeye RL: Kyphoscoliosis and cor pulmonale. A study of the pulmonary vascular bed. Am J Pathol 38:561, 1961.
126. Reid L: Autopsy studies of the lungs in kyphoscoliosis. *In* Zorab PA (ed): Proceedings of a Symposium on Scoliosis. London, National Fund for Research in Poliomyelitis and Other Crippling Diseases, 1966, p 71.
127. James JIP: Scoliosis. Baltimore, Williams & Wilkins, 1968.
128. Bjure J, Grimby G, Kasalicky J, et al: Respiratory impairment and airway closure in patients with untreated idiopathic scoliosis. Thorax 25:451, 1970.
129. Godfrey S: Respiratory and cardiovascular consequences of scoliosis. Respiration 27(suppl):67, 1970.
130. Weber B, Smith JP, Briscoe WA, et al: Pulmonary function in asymptomatic adolescents with idiopathic scoliosis. Am Rev Respir Dis 111:389, 1975.
131. Kafer ER: Respiratory function in paralytic scoliosis. Am Rev Respir Dis 110:450, 1974.
132. Bates DV, Macklem PT, Christie RV: Respiratory Function in Disease: An Introduction to the Integrated Study of the Lung. 2nd ed. Philadelphia, WB Saunders, 1971.
133. Bruderman I, Stein M: Physiologic evaluation and treatment of kyphoscoliotic patients. Ann Intern Med 55:94, 1961.
134. Hepper NGG, Black LF, Fowler WS: Relationships of lung volume to height and arm span in normal subjects and in patients with spinal deformity. Am Rev Respir Dis 91:356, 1965.
135. Conti G, Rocco M, Antonelli M, et al: Respiratory system mechanics in the early phase of acute respiratory failure due to severe kyphoscoliosis. Intensive Care Med 23:539, 1997.
136. Baydur A, Swank SM, Stiles C, et al: Respiratory mechanics in anesthetized young patients with kyphoscoliosis. Immediate and delayed effects of corrective spinal surgery. Chest 97:1157, 1990.
137. Al-Kattan K, Simonds A, Chung KF, et al: Kyphoscoliosis and bronchial torsion. Chest 111:1134, 1997.
138. Wright PM, Alexander JP: Acute airway obstruction, hypertension and kyphoscoliosis. Anaesthesia 46:119, 1991.
139. Bergofsky EH: Respiratory failure in disorders of the thoracic cage. Am Rev Respir Dis 119:643, 1979.
140. Shaw DB, Read J: Hypoxia and thoracic scoliosis. BMJ 2:1486, 1960.
141. Chailleux E, Fauroux B, Binet F, et al: Predictors of survival in patients receiving domiciliary oxygen therapy or mechanical ventilation. A 10-year analysis of ANTADIR Observatory. Chest 109:41, 1996.
142. Dollery CT, Gillam PMS, Hugh-Jones P, et al: Regional lung function in kyphoscoliosis. Thorax 20:175, 1965.
143. Bake B, Bjure J, Kasalichy J, et al: Regional pulmonary ventilation and perfusion distribution in patients with untreated idiopathic scoliosis. Thorax 27:703, 1972.
144. Kafer E: Idiopathic scoliosis. Gas exchange and the age dependence of arterial blood gases. J Clin Invest 58:825, 1976.
145. Kryger MH: Sleep in restrictive lung disorders. Clin Chest Med 6:675, 1985.
146. Sawicka EH, Branthwaite MA: Respiration during sleep in kyphoscoliosis. Thorax 42:801, 1987.
147. George CF, Kryger MH: Sleep in restrictive lung disease. Sleep 10:409, 1987.
148. McNicholas WT: Impact of sleep in respiratory failure. Eur Respir J 10:920, 1997.
149. Cirignotta F, Gerardi R, Mondini S, et al: Breathing disorders during sleep in chest wall diseases. Monaldi Arch Chest Dis 48:315, 1993.
150. Kafer E: Idiopathic scoliosis. Mechanical properties of the respiratory system and the ventilatory response to carbon dioxide. J Clin Invest 55:1153, 1975.
151. Sinha R, Bergofsky EH: Prolonged alteration of lung mechanics in kyphoscoliosis by positive pressure hyperinflation. Am Rev Respir Dis 106:47, 1972.
152. Lisboa C, Moreno R, Fava M, et al: Inspiratory muscle function in patients with severe kyphoscoliosis. Am Rev Respir Dis 132:48, 1985.
153. Hornstein S, Inman S, Ledsome JR: Ventilatory muscle training in kyphoscoliosis. Spine 12:859, 1987.
154. Garay S, Turino G, Goldring R: Sustained reversal of chronic hypercapnia in patients with alveolar hypoventilation syndromes. Am J Med 70:269, 1981.
155. Hoeppner V, Cockcroft D, Dosman J, et al: Nighttime ventilation improves respiratory failure in secondary kyphoscoliosis. Am Rev Respir Dis 129:240, 1984.
156. Wiers W, LeCoulture R, Dallinga O, et al: Cuirass respiratory treatment of chronic respiratory failure in scoliotic patients. Thorax 32:221, 1977.
157. Brewerton DA, Caffrey M, Hart FD, et al: Ankylosing spondylitis and HLA 27. Lancet 1:904, 1973.
158. Schlosstein L, Terasaki PI, Bluestone R, et al: High association of an HLA antigen, W27, with ankylosing spondylitis. N Engl J Med 288:704, 1973.
159. Calin A, Porta J, Fried JF, et al: Clinical history as a screening test for ankylosing spondylitis. JAMA 237:2613, 1977.
160. Calin A, Fries JF: Striking prevalence of ankylosing spondylitis in "healthy" W27 positive males and females. A controlled study. N Engl J Med 293:835, 1975.
161. Boland EW: Ankylosing spondylitis. *In* Hollander JL (ed): Arthritis and Allied Conditions. 7th ed. Philadelphia, Lea & Febiger, 1966, pp 633–655.
162. Graham DC, Smythe HA: The carditis and aortitis of ankylosing spondylitis. Bull Rheum 9:171, 1958.
163. Rosenow EC III, Strimlan CV, Muhm JR, et al: Pleuropulmonary manifestations of ankylosing spondylitis. Mayo Clin Proc 52:641, 1977.

164. Luthra HS: Extra-articular manifestations of ankylosing spondylitis. Mayo Clin Proc 52:655, 1977.
165. Jessamine AG: Upper lobe fibrosis in ankylosing spondylitis. Can Med Assoc J 98:25, 1968.
166. Campbell AH, MacDonald CB: Upper lobe fibrosis associated with ankylosing spondylitis. Br J Dis Chest 59:90, 1965.
167. Ferdoutsis M, Bouros D, Meletis G, et al: Diffuse interstitial lung disease as an early manifestation of ankylosing spondylitis. Respiration 62:286, 1995.
168. Strobel ES, Fritschka E: Case report and review of the literature. Fatal pulmonary complication in ankylosing spondylitis. Clin Rheumatol 16:617, 1997.
169. Rohatgi PK, Turrisi BC: Bronchocentric granulomatosis and ankylosing spondylitis. Thorax 39:317, 1984.
170. Rumancik WM, Firooznia H, Davis MS, et al: Fibrobullous disease of the upper lobes: An extraskeletal manifestation of ankylosing spondylitis. J Comput Tomogr 8:225, 1984.
171. Fenlon HM, Casserly I, Sant SM, et al: Plain radiographic and thoracic high-resolution CT in patients with ankylosing spondylitis. Am J Roentgenol 168:1067, 1997.
172. Casserly IP, Fenlon HM, Breatnach E, et al: Lung findings on high-resolution computed tomography in idiopathic ankylosing spondylitis—correlation with clinical findings, pulmonary function testing and plain radiography. Br J Rheumatol 36:677, 1997.
173. Kinnear WJ, Shneerson JM: Acute pleural effusions in inactive ankylosing spondylitis. Thorax 40:150, 1985.
174. Good AE: The chest pain of ankylosing spondylitis. Its place in the differential diagnosis of heart pain. Ann Intern Med 58:926, 1963.
175. Fisher LR, Cawley MI, Holgate ST: Relation between chest expansion, pulmonary function, and exercise tolerance in patients with ankylosing spondylitis. Ann Rheum Dis 49:921, 1990.
176. Radford EP, Doll R, Smith PG: Mortality among patients with ankylosing spondylitis not given x-ray therapy. N Engl J Med 297:572, 1977.
177. Miller JM, Sproule BJ: Pulmonary function in ankylosing spondylitis. Am Rev Respir Dis 90:376, 1964.
178. Franssen MJ, van Herwaarden CL, van de Putte LB: Lung function in patients with ankylosing spondylitis. A study of the influence of disease activity and treatment with nonsteroidal anti-inflammatory drugs. J Rheumatol 13:936, 1986.
179. Kchir MM, Mtimet S, Kochbati S, et al: Bronchoalveolar lavage and transbronchial biopsy in spondyloarthropathies. J Rheumatol 19:913, 1992.
180. van Noord JA, Cauberghs M, Van de Woestijne KP, et al: Total respiratory resistance and reactance in ankylosing spondylitis and kyphoscoliosis. Eur Respir J 4:945, 1991.
181. Elliott CG, Hill TE, Crapo RO, et al: Exercise performance of subjects with ankylosing spondylitis and limited chest expansion. Bull Eur Physiopathol Respir 21:363, 1985.
182. Travis DM, Cook CD, Julian DG, et al: The lungs in rheumatoid spondylitis. Gas exchange and lung mechanics in a form of restrictive pulmonary disease. Am J Med 29:623, 1960.
183. Renzetti AD Jr, Nicholas W, Dutton RE Jr, et al: Some effects of ankylosing spondylitis on pulmonary gas exchange. N Engl J Med 262:215, 1960.
184. Stewart RM, Ridyard JB, Pearson JD: Regional lung function in ankylosing spondylitis. Thorax 31:433, 1976.
185. Weaver P, Lifeso RM: The radiological diagnosis of tuberculosis of the adult spine. Skeletal Radiol 12:178, 1984.
186. Coppola J, Müller NL, Connell DG: Computed tomography of musculoskeletal tuberculosis. J Can Assoc Radiol 38:199, 1987.
187. de Roos A, van Persijn van Meerten EL, Bloem JL, et al: MRI of tuberculous spondylitis. Am J Roentgenol 146:79, 1986.
188. Modic MT, Feiglin DH, Paraino DW, et al: Vertebral osteomyelitis: Assessment using MR. Radiology 157:157, 1985.
189. Smith AS, Weinstein MA, Mizushima A, et al: MR imaging characteristics of tuberculous osteomyelitis vs vertebral osteomyelitis. AJNR Am J Neuroradiol 153:399, 1989.
190. Post MJD, Sze G, Quencer RM, et al: Gadolinium enhanced MR in spinal infection. J Comput Assist Tomogr 14:721, 1990.
191. Hlavin ML, Kaminski HY, Ross JS, et al: Spinal epidural abscess: A ten-year perspective. Neurosurgery 27:177, 1990.
192. Cimmino CV: The paraspinal-thoracic ratio in chest teleroentgenograms. Radiology 69:251, 1957.
193. Gould KG, Cooper KH, Harkleroad LE: Pulmonary function and work capacity in the absence of physiologic dorsal kyphosis of the spine. Dis Chest 55:405, 1969.
194. Souba WW, McKenna RJ Jr, Meis J, et al: Radiation-induced sarcomas of the chest wall. Cancer 57:610, 1986.
195. Huvos AG, Woodard HQ, Cahan WG, et al: Postradiation osteogenic sarcoma of bone and soft tissues. A clinicopathologic study of 66 patients. Cancer 55:1244, 1985.
196. Chapelier AR, Bacha EA, de Montpreville VT, et al: Radical resection of radiation-induced sarcoma of the chest wall: Report of 15 cases. Ann Thorac Surg 63:214, 1997.
197. Delgado-Chavez R, Sobrevilla-Calvo P, Green-Schneeweiss L, et al: Peripheral neuroectodermal tumor of the chest wall in a patient treated for Hodgkin's disease. Leuk Lymphoma 17:509, 1995.
198. Sauter ER, Keller SM, Curran WJ, et al: Radiation-induced chest-wall chondrosarcoma following surgical resection and radiotherapy for non–small-cell lung cancer. J Natl Cancer Inst 85:162, 1993.
199. Lo TCM, Silverman ML, Edelstein A: Postirradiation hemangiosarcoma of the chest wall. Report of a case. Acta Radiol Oncol 24:237, 1985.
200. Ron IG, Amir G, Inbar MJ, et al: Clear cell chondrosarcoma of rib following repetitive low-impact trauma. Am J Clin Oncol 18:87, 1995.
201. Morisaki Y, Takagi K, Ishii Y, et al: Periosteal chondroma developing in a rib at the side of a chest wall wound from a previous thoracotomy: Report of a case. Surg Today 26:57, 1996.
202. Rami-Porta R, Bravo-Bravo JL, Aroca-Gonzalez MJ, et al: Tumours and pseudotumours of the chest wall. Scand J Thorac Cardiovasc Surg 19:97, 1985.
203. Jones ER, Golebiowski A: Desmoid tumour of chest wall. BMJ 2:1134, 1960.
204. Nickell WK, Kittle CF, Boley JO: Desmoid tumour of the chest. Thorax 13:218, 1958.
205. Klein DL, Gamsu G, Gant TD: Intrathoracic desmoid tumor of the chest wall. Am J Roentgenol 129:524, 1977.
206. King RM, Payne WS, Olafsson S, et al: Surgical palliation of respiratory insufficiency secondary to massive exuberant polyostotic fibrous dysplasia of the ribs. Ann Thorac Surg 39:185, 1985.
207. Jain, SK, Afzal M, Mathew M, et al: Malignant mesenchymoma of the chest wall in an adult. Thorax 48:407, 1993.
208. Meis JM, Butler JJ, Osborne BM: Hodgkin's disease involving the breast and chest wall. Cancer 57:1859, 1986.
209. Nielsen T, Sneppen O, Myhre-Jensen O, et al: Subscapular elastofibroma: A reactive pseudotumor. J Shoulder Elbow Surg 5:209, 1996.
210. Berthoty DP, Shulman NS, Miller HAB: Elastofibroma: Chest wall pseudotumor. Radiology 160:341, 1986.
211. Sabanathan S, Salama FD, Morgan WE, et al: Primary chest wall tumors. Ann Thorac Surg 39:4, 1985.
212. Alvarez-Sala R, Gomez de Terreros FJ, Caballero P: Echinococcus cyst as a cause of chest wall tumor. Ann Thorac Surg 43:689, 1987.
213. Cho CS, Blank N, Castellino RA: Computerized tomography evaluation of chest wall involvement in lymphoma. Cancer 55:1892, 1985.
214. Frija J, Bellin M-F, Laval-Jeantet M, et al: Role of CT in the study of recurrences of Hodgkin's disease on the chest wall. Eur J Radiol 7:229, 1987.
215. Gouliamos AD, Carter BL, Emami B: Computed tomography of the chest wall. Radiology 134:433, 1980.
216. Shin MS, Anderson SD, Myers J, et al: Pitfalls in CT evaluation of chest wall invasion by lung cancer. Case report. J Comput Assist Tomogr 10:136, 1986.
217. Pearlberg JL, Sandler MA, Beute GH, et al: Limitations of CT in evaluation of neoplasms involving chest wall. J Comput Assist Tomogr 11:290, 1987.
218. Trivedi SA: Neurilemmoma of the diaphragm causing severe hypertrophic pulmonary osteoarthropathy. Br J Tuberc 52:214,1958.
219. Seltzer RA: Subpleural lipoma. Lancet 84:100, 1964.
220. Doubleday LC, Durham ME Jr, Durham ME Sr: Lipoma of a chest wall. Report of a case. Texas State J Med 59:24, 1963.
221. Rosenberg RF, Rubinstein BM, Messinger NH: Intrathoracic lipomas. Chest 60:507, 1971.
222. Castillo M, Shirkhoda A: Computed tomography of diaphragmatic lipoma. J Comput Assist Tomogr 9:167, 1985.
223. Kuhlman JE, Bouchardy L, Fishman EK, et al: CT and MR imaging evaluation of chest wall disorders. Radiographics 14:571, 1994.
224. Sulzer MA, Goei R, Bollen EC, et al: Lipoma of the external thoracic wall. Eur Respir J 7:207, 1994.
225. Fortier M, Mayo JR, Swensen SJ, et al: MR imaging of chest wall lesions. Radiographics 14:597, 1994.
226. Cohen LM, Schwartz AM, Rockoff SD: Benign schwannomas: Pathologic basis for CT inhomogeneities. Am J Roentgenol 147:141, 1986.
227. Ko S-F, Lee T-Y, Lin J-W, et al: Thoracic neurilemomas: An analysis of computed tomography findings in 36 patients. J Thorac Imaging 13:21, 1998.
228. Sakai F, Sone S, Kiyono K, et al: Intrathoracic neurogenic tumors: MR-pathologic correlation. Am J Roentgenol 159:279, 1992.
229. Kushner BH, Hajdu SI, Gulati SC, et al: Extracranial primitive neuroectodermal tumors. The Memorial Sloan-Kettering Cancer Center experience. Cancer 67:1825, 1991.
230. Contesso G, Llombart-Bosch A, Terrier P, et al: Does malignant small round cell tumor of the thoracopulmonary region (Askin tumor) constitute a clinicopathologic entity? Cancer 69:1012, 1992.
231. Cavazzana AO, Ninfo V, Roberts J, et al: Peripheral neuroepithelioma: A light microscopic, immunocytochemical, and ultrastructural study. Mod Pathol 5:71, 1992.
232. Askin FB, Rosai J, Sibley RK, et al: Malignant small cell tumor of the thoracopulmonary region in childhood. A distinctive clinicopathologic entity of uncertain histogenesis. Cancer 43:2438, 1979.
233. Ambros IM, Ambros PF, Strehl S, et al: MIC2 is a specific marker for Ewing's sarcoma and peripheral primitive neuroectodermal tumors. Evidence for a common histogenesis of Ewing's sarcoma and peripheral primitive neuroectodermal tumors from MIC2 expression and specific chromosome aberration. Cancer 67:1886, 1991.
234. Scotlandi K, Serra M, Manara MC, et al: Immunostaining of the p30/32MIC2 antigen and molecular detection of EWS rearrangements for the diagnosis of Ewing's sarcoma and peripheral neuroectodermal tumor. Hum Pathol 27:408, 1996.
235. Anselmo AP, Cartoni C, Pacchiarotti A, et al: Peripheral neuroectodermal tumor of the chest (Askin tumor) as secondary neoplasm after Hodgkin's disease: A case report. Ann Hematol 68:311, 1994.
236. Takahashi K, Dambara T, Uekusa T, et al: Massive chest wall tumor diagnosed

as Askin tumor. Successful treatment by intensive combined modality therapy in an adult. Chest 104:287, 1993.

237. Winer-Muram HT, Kauffman WM, Gronemeyer SA, et al: Primitive neuroectodermal tumors of the chest wall (Askin tumors): CT and MR findings. Am J Roentgenol 161:265, 1993.

238. Saifuddin A, Robertson RJH, Smith SEW: The radiology of Askin tumors. Clin Radiol 43:19, 1991.

239. Mayall FG, Gibbs AR: The histology and immunohistochemistry of small cell mesothelioma. Histopathology 20:47, 1992.

240. Venkateswaran L, Jenkins JJ, Kaste SC, et al: Disseminated intrathoracic desmoplastic small round-cell tumor: A case report. J Pediatr Hematol Oncol 19:172, 1997.

241. Parkash V, Gerald WL, Parma A, et al: Desmoplastic small round cell tumor of the pleura. Am J Surg Pathol 19:659, 1995.

242. Kumar PV: Fine needle aspiration cytologic findings in malignant small cell tumor of the thoracopulmonary region (Askin tumor). Acta Cytol 38:702, 1994.

243. Ochsner A Jr, Lucas GL, McFarland GB Jr: Tumors of the thoracic skeleton. Review of 134 cases. J Thorac Cardiovasc Surg 52:311, 1966.

244. Pairolero PC, Arnold PG: Chest wall tumors: Experience with 100 consecutive patients. J Thorac Cardiovasc Surg 90:367, 1985.

245. Marcove RC, Huvos AG: Cartilaginous tumors of the ribs. Cancer 27:794, 1971.

245a. Labram EK, Mohan J: Diaphyseal aclasis with spinal cord compression. J Neurosurg 84:518, 1996.

245b. Teijeira FJ, Baril C, Younge D: Spontaneous hemothorax in a patient with hereditary multiple exostoses. Ann Thorac Surg 48:717, 1989.

246. Robinson AE, Thomas RL, Monson DM: Aneurysmal bone cyst of the rib. A report of two unusual cases. Am J Roentgenol 100:526, 1967.

247. Mendl K, Evans CJ: Cyst-like and cystic lesions of the rib with special reference to their radiological differential diagnosis based on the discussion of five cases. Br J Radiol 31:146, 1958.

248. Meyer CA, White CS: Cartilaginous disorders of the chest. Radiographics 18:1109, 1998.

249. Choma ND, Biscotti CV, Bauer TW, et al: Gorham's syndrome: A case report and review of the literature. Am J Med 83: 1151, 1987.

250. Igel BJ, Shah H, Williamson MR, et al: Gorham's syndrome. Correlative imaging using nuclear medicine, plain film, and 3-D CT. Clin Nucl Med 19:1017, 1994.

251. Riantawan P, Tansupasawasdikul S, Subhannachart P: Bilateral chylothorax complicating massive osteolysis (Gorham's syndrome). Thorax 51:1277, 1996.

252. Reith JD, Bauer TW, Schils JP: Osseous manifestations of SAPHO (synovitis, acne, pustulosis, hyperostosis, osteitis) syndrome. Am J Surg Pathol 20:1368, 1996.

253. Urovitz EPM, Fornasier VL, Czitrom AA: Sternal metastases and associated pathological fractures. Thorax 32:444, 1977.

254. Goldman JM: Parasternal chest wall involvement in Hodgkin's disease. Chest 59:133, 1971.

255. Graeber GM, Snyder RJ, Fleming AW, et al: Initial and long-term results in the management of primary chest wall neoplasms. Ann Thorac Surg 34:664, 1982.

256. King RM, Pairolero PC, Trastek VF, et al: Primary chest wall tumors: Factors affecting survival. Ann Thorac Surg 41:597, 1986.

257. Laverdiere JT, Abrahams TG, Jones MA: Primary osseous malignant fibrous histiocytoma involving a rib. Skeletal Radiol 24:152, 1995.

258. Batt H, Sasken H: Primary angiosarcoma of the rib. South Med J 90:454, 1997.

259. Tanaka F, Wada H, Mizuno H, et al: A case of giant cell tumor of the rib with magnetic resonance imaging. Eur J Cardiothorac Surg 10:214, 1996.

260. Ascoli V, Facciolo F, Muda AO, et al: Chondroblastoma of the rib presenting as an intrathoracic mass. Report of a case with fine needle aspiration biopsy, immunocytochemistry and electron microscopy. Acta Cytol 36:423, 1992.

261. Ishida T, Kuwada Y, Motoi N, et al: Dedifferentiated chondrosarcoma of the rib with a malignant mesenchymomatous component: An autopsy case report. Pathol Int 47:397, 1997.

262. Ogose A, Motoyama T, Hotta T, et al: Clear cell chondrosarcomas arising from rare sites. Pathol Int 45:684, 1995.

263. Eygelaar A, Homan Van Der Heide JN: Diagnosis and treatment of primary malignant costal and sternal tumors. Dis Chest 52:683, 1967.

264. Wolfel DA, Dennis JM: Multiple myeloma of the chest wall. Am J Roentgenol 89:1241, 1963.

265. Karlawish JH, Smith GW, Gabrielson EW, et al: Spontaneous hemothorax caused by a chest wall chondrosarcoma. Ann Thorac Surg 59:231, 1995.

PART XVIII

PULMONARY DISEASE ASSOCIATED WITH A NORMAL CHEST RADIOGRAPH

CHAPTER 79

Respiratory Disease Associated with a Normal Chest Radiograph

Considerable experimental and clinical evidence indicates that significant pulmonary and pleural disease, sometimes of life-threatening severity, can be present despite a normal appearance on the chest radiograph. This limitation exists both in the early and healing stages of various inflammatory air-space and interstitial diseases and in a variety of noninflammatory disorders. In many cases, the lack of radiographic abnormality constitutes a significant diagnostic feature and excludes those diseases in which respiratory symptoms and signs are commonly associated with radiographic abnormalities.

In addition to cases in which the radiograph is undoubtedly normal, from time to time a radiographic pattern is encountered that can be judged to be at the outer range of normal but is not unequivocally abnormal. An example of such a radiographic finding is elevation of one or both hemidiaphragms beyond the normal range; although a high diaphragm is often a reflection of suboptimal inspiration (not necessarily the result of poor patient effort, as is sometimes implied), it can be an important indication of small lung volume. Both the equivocal and unequivocal cases are most easily discussed in terms of whether disease is localized or generalized. In each instance, a subsequent radiograph may resolve the problem by showing progression or regression, or comparison with previous radiographs may establish whether there has been a change in the radiographic pattern.

In this chapter the local and diffuse diseases of the lung parenchyma, airways, vasculature, and pleura that may be associated with a normal chest radiograph are discussed. Conditions that can cause alveolar hypoventilation and hyperventilation (usually associated with a normal chest radiograph) are also described. Finally, the anatomic and biochemical abnormalities that can cause decreased oxygen-carrying capacity of the blood and the development of pulmonary symptoms, despite a normal chest radiograph and normal values on conventional pulmonary function tests, are reviewed.

PULMONARY PARENCHYMAL, AIRWAY, VASCULAR, AND PLEURAL DISEASE ASSOCIATED WITH A NORMAL RADIOGRAPH

Diseases of the Pulmonary Parenchyma

The limitations of radiographic visibility in alveolar and interstitial pulmonary disease are discussed in Chapter 11 (*see* page 278). Even in ideal circumstances, with technically perfect radiographs interpreted carefully by experienced observers, abnormalities may be so small as to be imperceptible, or they may be hidden behind or juxtaposed against skeletal or vascular shadows. A solitary uncalcified lesion less than 6 mm in diameter is rarely appreciated and then usually only in retrospect when the lesion has grown and is detected on subsequent radiographs. A solitary nodule 8 to 10 mm in diameter has an approximately 50% chance of being detected.[1, 2] Larger nodules—sometimes as big as 3 to 4 cm in diameter—also may be overlooked, particularly if they are situated over the convexity of the lung or in the paramediastinal area, where the rib cage, large vessels, and mediastinal contents tend to obscure them. This problem was illustrated in one investigation of 27 patients who had resectable pulmonary carcinomas that were initially overlooked by the radiologist;[2] the missed tumors ranged from 0.6 to 3.4 cm in diameter (mean, 1.6 cm). Six consultant radiologists who were aware that the cases involved missed carcinomas were also individually shown the radiographs of 22 of the patients; the consultants missed a mean of 26% of the lesions. In contrast to solitary nodules, multiple micronodular opacities measuring no more than 1 or 2 mm in diameter are usually appreciated, presumably because of the effect of superimposition. Reference is made throughout this book to those diseases that at some point in their clinical course have no detectable radiographic manifestations; this chapter is concerned primarily with those in which a normal chest radiograph is more than an occasional finding.

Localized Disease

Localized acute air-space disease such as that caused by bacterial infection or alveolar hemorrhage characteristically produces radiographic shadows at a very early stage. By contrast, acute local disease confined largely to the pulmonary interstitium (e.g., viral or mycoplasmal pneumonia) can cause symptoms that precede radiographic signs by 48 hours or longer.[3] Localized abnormalities of the pulmonary vascular system, particularly acute thromboembolism, also may show no radiographic signs on the chest film. For example, in one investigation of 1,063 patients suspected of having pulmonary thromboembolism, the chest radiograph was interpreted as normal in 45 of 363 patients (12%) who had angiographically proven disease.[4] Even in patients in whom thromboembolism results in an infarct, an opacity may not be visible until 12 to 24 hours following the embolic episode. This clinical observation is supported by experimental investigations showing a delay of 1 to 7 days until the radiologic appearance of pulmonary hemorrhage after the occlusion of a pulmonary artery.[5]

Chronic pulmonary disease also may be present and active for months or even years before it becomes radiographically visible. It has been estimated, for example, that a focus of active tuberculosis does not become radiologically detectable until 2 or 3 months after initial infection.[3] Similarly, most pulmonary carcinomas are present for years before they become visible; studies of the growth rate of primary lung neoplasms and back-extrapolation of the doubling time indicate that these tumors are invisible during two thirds to three quarters of their existence (*see* page 1142).[6] Although the majority of such tumors do not occa-

sion symptoms during this time, occasionally there are signs and symptoms related to intra- or extrathoracic metastases or to the secretion of a variety of biologically active substances (paraneoplastic syndromes).[7]

Generalized Disease

Diffuse granulomatous and fibrotic pulmonary disease may be present in association with a normal chest radiograph. In contrast to localized pulmonary tuberculosis, in which symptoms and signs may not appear for many weeks *after* the chest radiograph has become abnormal, clinical manifestations such as fever, general malaise, and headaches may develop some weeks *before* the detection of radiologic abnormality in miliary tuberculosis; in some instances the pulmonary lesions are not recognized before death. In one investigation of 71 patients who had miliary tuberculosis, three independent chest radiologists were able to identify the presence of parenchymal abnormalities on the chest radiograph in 42, 44, and 49 individuals (sensitivity, 59% to 69%);[8] nodules could not be seen on the radiograph at the time of diagnosis, even in retrospect, in 30% of patients.

A variety of conditions are associated with radiographically invisible interstitial disease, even in the presence of symptoms and disturbances of pulmonary function. For example, cases of sarcoidosis have been reported in which chest radiographs were normal despite abnormal findings in biopsy specimens[9-11] or reduced compliance,[12] vital capacity, and diffusing capacity.[11, 13, 14] Some patients who have idiopathic pulmonary fibrosis[10, 15] or extrinsic allergic alveolitis[10, 16] also have been shown to have interstitial fibrosis histologically despite normal chest radiographs. Among the connective tissue diseases, progressive systemic sclerosis is frequently associated with a lowered diffusing capacity and arterial blood oxygen tension (PaO_2) despite a normal chest radiograph.[13, 17, 18] By contrast, pulmonary involvement in rheumatoid disease is often detectable radiologically before pulmonary function becomes impaired,[19] although subclinical interstitial involvement can also be detected by HRCT in a significant percentage of patients.[20]

In systemic lupus erythematosus, the presence and extent of parenchymal abnormalities are frequently underestimated on the chest radiograph[21] (*see* page 1426). The patient's pulmonary function may be distinctly abnormal (reduction in vital capacity) despite a normal chest radiograph; however, when serial radiographic studies are available, some patients show a progressive loss of lung volume manifested as diaphragmatic elevation.[19, 22] Normal results on pulmonary function tests and chest radiographs also have been reported in cases of diffuse interstitial leukemic infiltration of the lungs. Parenchymal infiltration is commonly observed pathologically in patients who die of leukemia,[23, 24] but seldom radiographically; in fact, it has been estimated that infiltration with leukemic cells is sufficiently extensive to produce symptoms and disturb pulmonary function in less than 3% of cases.[24]

Significant pulmonary vascular disease may also be present without radiographic manifestations—for example, the extensive obstruction of the vasculature in thromboembolic disease and the pulmonary vasculopathy associated with connective tissue diseases.[25]

Diseases of the Airways

Many patients who have diseases of the conducting airways have normal chest radiographs. In fact, in simple chronic bronchitis characterized by a history of cough and expectoration, this is the rule rather than the exception. Although the majority of patients who experience acute asthmatic attacks show evidence of pulmonary overinflation on pulmonary function testing, radiographic evidence of its presence is seldom convincing except in children and adolescents who have early-onset asthma. However, the presence of overinflation during an attack can sometimes be appreciated by comparison with films obtained during remission. Using a radiographic technique, one group measured total lung capacity (TLC) in 10 asthmatic patients at the time of an acute attack, when the mean of measured values for forced expiratory volume in 1 second (FEV$_1$) was 1.44 ± 0.43 liters, and compared this with similar measurements obtained at the time of recovery (mean FEV$_1$, 2.76 ± 0.58);[26] in 9 patients, TLC decreased between exacerbation and recovery (mean values were 6.21 liters during exacerbation and 5.51 at recovery). A chest radiologist was able to detect the hyperinflation in most patients when comparing the acute and recovery radiographs but was unable to appreciate its presence on the exacerbation films alone.

About 10% of patients who have bronchiectasis fail to show evidence of the disease on standard chest radiographs.[27, 28] Patients who have emphysema, particularly advanced disease, have distinctly abnormal radiographs; however, patients who have mild to moderate disease may have completely normal films.[29] For example, in one study in which the accuracy of the radiologic diagnosis of emphysema was assessed on the basis of paper-mounted whole-lung sections made subsequent to autopsy, a correct diagnosis was made radiologically in only 41% of the patients who had moderately severe emphysema.[30]

Patients who have endobronchial or endotracheal tumors that only partly obstruct an airway can have normal chest radiographs, at least when films are exposed at full inspiration; this has been described in patients who have carcinoid tumor,[31] pulmonary carcinoma,[32–34] papillomatosis,[35, 36] or mesenchymal neoplasms.[37, 38] More commonly, the volume of lung parenchyma distal to the partial obstruction is smaller than normal; obviously, in such circumstances a radiograph exposed following full expiration will reveal air trapping distal to the partial obstruction. When the obstruction is in the trachea or a major bronchus, dyspnea and generalized wheezing may suggest a diagnosis of asthma. Lesions arising within the trachea or compressing it from outside should be suspected when wheezing (sometimes relieved by a change in position) is more pronounced during inspiration than expiration, when wheezing is accompanied by hemoptysis, or when the patient's symptoms fail to respond to the usual therapy for asthma.[37] A particularly difficult problem is presented by cases of pulmonary carcinoma in which the diagnosis is made cytologically but in which a lesion is not apparent either bronchoscopically or radiographically. This situation is discussed in greater detail in Chapter 31.

Pulmonary Venoarterial Shunts

The intrapulmonary form of shunting that occurs in patients who have cirrhosis can develop in the presence of a normal chest radiograph. Using a micropaque gelatin suspension, one group of investigators demonstrated severe dilation of small pulmonary arteries in 13 patients who had died of cirrhosis;[39] "spider nevi" were also detected on the pleura in 6 patients. In 1 patient, the shunts were sufficiently extensive to explain the hypoxemia detected during life. Eight of the 13 patients were considered to show parenchymal abnormalities radiologically; in 6 of these patients, these were described as small, rather ill-defined nodular shadows, and in the other 2 patients, as linear shadows. In all cases, the abnormalities were bilateral and predominant in the lower lobes.

Ventilation-perfusion mismatch caused by increased airway closure at the lung bases contributes to the hypoxemia in patients who have cirrhosis and hypoproteinemia.[40–43] Mismatch is also caused by impaired hypoxic vasoconstriction in some patients.[44] Studies in which quantitative perfusion scintigraphy has been employed have revealed indirect evidence for pulmonary arteriovenous communications that are too small to be detected angiographically.[45, 46] For example, in one investigation of three patients who had cirrhosis and moderate hypoxemia, the amount of intravenously injected macroaggregated albumin that traversed the pulmonary vasculature was much larger than in normal persons.[46] Associated abnormal vascular channels were considered to be responsible for the hypoxemia; chest radiographs were normal. A patient has also been described in whom arterial blood gases worsened as a result of the opening up of intrapulmonary shunts during periods of hepatic functional deterioration, but in whom improvement in clinical status occurred coincident with a reduction in shunt.[47]

Intrapulmonary right-to-left shunting also can be demonstrated by contrast echocardiography in patients who have cirrhosis.[48] Normally, when ultrasound contrast material (which contains microbubbles) is injected into the peripheral circulation, it is removed during the first pass through the pulmonary circulation, and no echogenic material reaches the left side of the heart; in patients who have intrapulmonary or extrapulmonary right-to-left shunt, bubbles reach the left heart and can be detected ultrasonographically.

Although the hypoxemia in patients who have cirrhosis is related primarily to intrapulmonary arteriovenous shunting through dilated peripheral pulmonary vessels, the response of this "shunt" to the breathing of 100% O$_2$ is greater than would be expected in a true anatomic shunt. It is probable that the shunt in these cases actually represents a unique form of diffusion impairment in which there is failure of equilibration between alveolar gas and capillary blood as a result of the large diameter of the vessels, the long distances for diffusion to occur, and a very rapid red blood cell transit time. Patients who have intrapulmonary right-to-left shunt may have lowered carbon monoxide diffusing capacity.[49]

The hypoxemia observed in patients who have hepatic cirrhosis may be more severe in the erect than in the recumbent position (orthodeoxia),[50] a phenomenon that is attributable to the increased blood flow through the lung bases, where most shunts are found. When orthodeoxia is severe, the patient may complain of increased dyspnea when in the erect position (platypnea).[51, 52] Most patients who have advanced cirrhosis present with symptoms and signs attributable to the liver disease; the hypoxemia and hypocapnia are rarely severe enough to cause symptoms or signs. Secondary polycythemia occurs occasionally and, without the benefit of blood gas analysis, can be confused with the erythrocytosis associated with hepatomas.[53]

In addition to patients who have cirrhosis, whose hypoxemia is caused by pulmonary arteriovenous shunts, there are some patients in whom blood is shunted from pulmonary artery to pulmonary vein during the postoperative period but whose chest radiographs are normal. The precise mechanism for the development of such shunting is unclear, but it may be caused by microatelectasis. When hypoxemia persists for several days after surgery, impairment of ventilation-perfusion ratios may be demonstrable.[54–56] Arteriovenous shunts (malformations) are also characteristic of Rendu-Osler-Weber disease (*see* page 655) and may be found in patients who have Fanconi's syndrome[57] or polysplenia syndrome associated with multiple cardiac anomalies;[58] small lesions may not be detectable radiographically.

Diseases of the Pleura

The chest radiograph may be normal in cases of acute pleuritis. However, pleurisy without an effusion (dry pleurisy) often is associated with diaphragmatic elevation and reduction in diaphragmatic excursion. As discussed in Chapter 21 (*see* page 563), effusions with a volume as large as 500 ml may not be visible on standard posteroanterior chest radiographs exposed with the patient in the erect position.[59] However, films exposed with the patient in the lateral decubitus position can reveal effusions with a volume of 100 ml or less, and special radiographic techniques may show as little as 10 to 15 ml, an amount that may be present even in healthy persons.[60, 61] Asbestos-associated pleural plaques may also be invisible on standard radiographs.[62]

ALVEOLAR HYPOVENTILATION

The term *alveolar hypoventilation* (ventilatory failure) is used to designate a deficiency in ventilation that is sufficient to raise the arterial level of carbon dioxide (Pa_{CO_2}) to greater than 45 mm Hg. The diagnosis cannot be made by clinical examination or by measurement of minute ventilation. In patients breathing room air, alveolar hypoventilation is necessarily accompanied by a degree of alveolar hypoxia and therefore arterial hypoxemia. Although regional underventilation can contribute to ventilation-perfusion mismatch and arterial hypoxemia without causing hypercapnia, the term *hypoventilation* should be reserved for a generalized decrease in ventilation that is characterized by the presence of hypercapnia.

Occasionally a marked decrease in alveolar ventilation can exist without an elevation in carbon dioxide tension (P_{CO_2}) when there is an additional method for removal of CO_2 from the blood. This situation has been described during renal hemodialysis: removal of CO_2 in the dialysate lowered mixed venous and alveolar P_{CO_2}, resulting in "hypoventilation" relative to metabolic CO_2 production despite a normal arterial P_{CO_2}.[63]

It is obvious that in circumstances in which ventilation-perfusion inequality results in regional underventilation and hypoxemia, an absence of hypercapnia indicates that overall ventilation is adequate. This occurs because ventilation to

certain areas of the lung is relatively increased to compensate for the regional CO_2 retention that occurs in areas of reduced ventilation. As discussed in Chapter 2 (*see* page 110), the shapes of the dissociation curves for CO_2 and O_2 explain the respiratory system's ability to compensate for regional hypercapnia and its inability to compensate for regional hypoxia: the relatively overventilated areas of lung cannot compensate for the underventilated areas with regard to O_2 because of the curvilinear nature of the O_2 dissociation curve.

Pulmonary diseases that cause ventilation-perfusion mismatch and intrapulmonary shunt resulting in hypoxemia and a normal or low arterial P_{CO_2} are discussed elsewhere in this book. Acute hypoxemic respiratory failure of this type is seen most commonly in the adult respiratory distress syndrome (ARDS), cardiogenic pulmonary edema, and acute bacterial pneumonia, whereas chronic hypoxemic respiratory failure occurs predominantly in interstitial granulomatous and fibrotic disorders. Respiratory failure associated with hypercapnia occurs in two broad groups of disorders: those of pulmonary origin (Table 79–1) and those of nonpulmonary origin (Table 79–2). The latter disorders are dealt with more extensively in this chapter, because they are frequently associated with a normal chest radiograph.

Disorders of the mechanisms that drive the chest bellows may result in either acute or chronic respiratory failure—pathophysiologic states that vary not only in their management but also in their clinical presentation. For purposes of clarity, these disorders are considered in two groupings: those that result from defective ventilatory control and those caused by an inadequate respiratory pump (see Table 79–2). Included in disorders of ventilatory control are disorders of cerebral and brainstem respiratory center functions and abnormalities of the efferent outputs from the upper motor neurons that drive the respiratory muscles and of the

Table 79–1. PULMONARY CAUSES OF VENTILATORY FAILURE WITH HYPERCAPNIA

UPPER AIRWAY OBSTRUCTION

Acute	Infection (pharyngitis, tonsillitis, epiglottitis, laryngotracheitis)
	Edema (irritant gases, angioneurotic edema)
	Retropharyngeal hemorrhage (trauma, postoperative, hemophilia, acute leukemia)
	Foreign bodies
Chronic	Postintubation stenosis (fibrosis, granulation tissue)
	Neoplasm (squamous cell carcinoma, adenoid cystic carcinoma)
	Vocal cord paralysis
	Hypertrophied tonsils and adenoids
	Macroglossia
	Micrognathia
	Obstructive sleep apnea

LOWER AIRWAY OBSTRUCTION

Acute	Infection (acute bronchiolitis)
	Edema (pulmonary venous hypertension, capillary leakage)
	Bronchospasm (asthma, anaphylactoid reactions)
Chronic	Chronic obstructive pulmonary disease
	Bronchiolitis
	Extensive idiopathic bronchiectasis
	Cystic fibrosis
	Familial dysautonomia

Table 79–2. NONPULMONARY CAUSES OF VENTILATORY FAILURE WITH HYPERCAPNIA

DISORDERS OF VENTILATORY CONTROL

CEREBRAL DYSFUNCTION

Infection (encephalitis), trauma, vascular accident
Status epilepticus
Narcotic and sedative overdose
Respiratory dyskinesia

RESPIRATORY CENTER DYSFUNCTION

Impaired brain stem controller
    Primary alveolar hypoventilation (Ondine's curse)
    Obesity hypoventilation syndrome
    Myxedema
    Metabolic alkalosis (compensatory)
    Sudden infant death syndrome
    Parkinson's syndrome
    Tetanus
Ablation of afferent and efferent spinal pathways
    Bilateral high cervical cordotomy
    Cervical spinal cord trauma
    Transverse myelitis
    Multiple sclerosis
    Parkinson's disease

PERIPHERAL RECEPTOR DYSFUNCTION

Carotid body destruction (bilateral carotid endarterectomy
    and carotid body resection for asthma)
Bilateral damage to afferent nerves (Arnold-Chiari syndrome
    with syringomyelia)
    Familial dysautonomia
    Diabetic neuropathy
    Tetanus

DISORDERS OF THE RESPIRATORY PUMP

NEUROMUSCULAR DISEASE

Anterior horn cells
    Poliomyelitis
    Amyotrophic lateral sclerosis
Peripheral nerves
    Landry-Guillain-Barré syndrome
    Acute intermittent porphyria
    Toxic dinoflagellate poisoning
        Neurotoxic shellfish poisoning (*Ptychodiscus brevis*)
        Paralytic shellfish poisoning
            (*Protogonyaulyx cantenella* and *P. tamarensis*)
        Ciguatera fish poisoning (*Gambierdiscus toxicus*)
    Puffer fish poisoning (tetrodotoxin)
Myoneural junction
    Myasthenia gravis
    Myasthenia-like syndromes (medications, particularly antibiotics,
        and neoplasms)
    Clostridium botulinum poisoning

Respiratory muscles
    Muscular dystrophies
    Acid maltase deficiency
    Nemaline myopathy
    Polymyositis
    Hypokalemia (in treatment of diabetes with insulin,
        renal tubular acidosis)
    Hypophosphatemia
    Hypermagnesemia
    Idiopathic rhabdomyolysis (myoglobinuria)

CHEST CAGE DISORDERS

Flail chest
Kyphoscoliosis
Thoracoplasty

---

afferent inputs into the central nervous system from peripheral receptors. Disorders of the respiratory pump include abnormalities of the anterior horn cells, the myoneural junction, the respiratory muscles, the phrenic and intercostal nerves that innervate those muscles, and the chest cage itself.

Chest radiographs are normal in the majority of patients in whom hypoventilation results from central nervous system or neuromuscular disease. In those instances in which hypoventilation is caused by respiratory muscle weakness or paralysis, the diaphragm is often elevated; however, this finding is frequently ignored on the supposition that the chest radiograph was exposed at a position of incomplete inspiration. Although the chest radiograph may be normal initially in patients who hypoventilate, the complications and consequences of prolonged alveolar underventilation may become apparent over time. Patients who hypoventilate, particularly those who have a raised diaphragm, are subject to the development of atelectasis and pneumonia;[64] in fact, such complications may be responsible for bringing the primary disease to the attention of the physician. In severe, prolonged states of hypoventilation, cor pulmonale also may develop; this may be reflected on the chest radiograph by diminution of the peripheral vasculature and enlargement of the cardiac silhouette.

Disorders of Ventilatory Control

A knowledge of normal ventilatory control is required in order to understand the various disorders of this system that result in alveolar hypoventilation. The subject is reviewed in greater detail in Chapter 9 (*see* page 235), and the interested reader is also directed to excellent reviews in the literature.[65–72] The main components of central ventilatory control and the neurologic inputs and outputs from the central nervous system are summarized here.

Central control of ventilation resides in two anatomically and functionally separate systems that subserve voluntary and automatic breathing. Neurons in the cerebral cortex control voluntary ventilation and can also influence brainstem output or can completely bypass it to accomplish behavior-related respiratory activities such as speech, defecation, micturition, and so on (Fig. 79–1). Automatic breathing originates from a highly complex agglomeration of intercon-

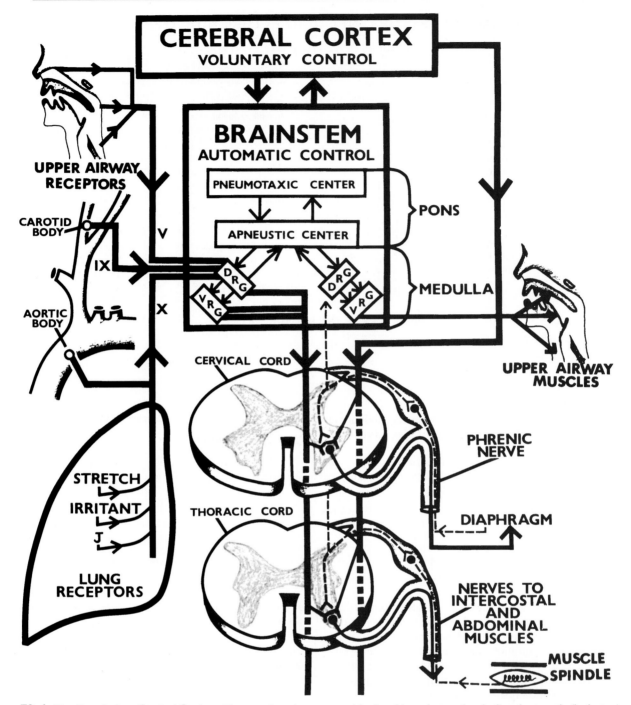

Figure 79–1. The Respiratory Control System. The central respiratory control is shared by voluntary (cerebral) and automatic (brainstem) centers. The efferent fibers from each run in distinct spinal cord pathways, as depicted on the left side of the coronally sectioned spinal cord (right side of drawing). A variety of interconnections exist between the cortex and the different components of the brainstem. Afferent fibers ascending the fifth (V), ninth (IX), and tenth (X) cranial nerves from upper airway receptors, peripheral chemoreceptors, and lung receptors connect with the ipsilateral dorsal respiratory group of neurons (DRG). In addition, afferents from Golgi tendon organs in the diaphragm and intercostal muscle spindles travel in the phrenic and intercostal nerves and reach the anterior horn cells as well as ascending to the DRG via the dorsal columns. Respiratory neurons in the DRG are connected with those in the ventral respiratory group (VRG) from which the descending neural output originates. The efferent fibers cross in the brainstem and supply the upper airway muscles via cranial nerves as well as descending in the cord to supply the diaphragm, intercostal, accessory, and expiratory muscles.

nected nerve cell groups situated in the brainstem. The most rostral of these centers is the pneumotaxic center (PNC) situated within the pons; the PNC is believed to be responsible for the fine-tuning of the respiratory pattern rather than for the generation of primary respiratory rhythm. Caudal to the PNC near the pontomedullary border lies the apneustic center (APC), the site of projection of the various inputs that can terminate an inspiration. Damage to this area inactivates the inspiratory cutoff switch and results in the phenomenon of apneusis (prolonged respiratory pause at end-inspiration). Transection of the brainstem between the medulla and pons does not abolish respiratory rhythmicity, and it is the present view that the medulla alone is capable of generating a primary respiratory pattern and that the PNC and the APC are modulators of that primary pattern.

Within the medulla, respiratory neurons are grouped into two distinct areas: the dorsal respiratory group (DRG), consisting almost entirely of inspiratory cells, and the ventral respiratory group (VRG), containing both inspiratory and expiratory cells. The DRG is the site of primary projection of numerous afferent fibers that constitute the afferent inputs into the respiratory center. These include afferents that originate in the upper airways, lungs, and peripheral chemoreceptors and travel in the cranial nerves, as well as afferents from the respiratory muscles themselves. The DRG is thought to be the primary site of rhythm generation; the axons of cells from this area descend in the contralateral spinal cord to innervate the diaphragm and inspiratory intercostals. The VRG does not appear to have primary respiratory rhythmicity or sensory input but receives input from the DRG and sends projections down the contralateral spinal cord to innervate the anterior horn cells of the cervical and thoracic segments of the cord; these in turn project to the intercostal inspiratory and expiratory muscles and the accessory muscles of inspiration. In addition, neurons from the DRG project to the lower motor neurons subserving the abdominal expiratory muscles and to the muscles of the larynx and upper airway that serve to maintain airway patency.

Sensory input, both chemical and neurogenic, plays a major role in the regulation of respiration. This originates in several sites, including the peripheral chemoreceptors located in the carotid and aortic bodies, the central chemoreceptors that are believed to lie near the ventrolateral surface of the medulla, receptors situated in the upper airways and lungs, and the muscle spindles and tendon organs that are located in the respiratory muscles themselves. The carotid and aortic bodies respond to increased arterial P_{CO_2} and decreased arterial oxygen tension (P_{O_2}). The pertinent stimulus for the central chemoreceptors is the hydrogen ion concentration of the brain's extracellular fluid. A variety of receptors in the nose, oropharynx, larynx, and tracheobronchial tree can influence the intensity of respiratory center neural output and the timing of respiration. Tracheobronchial receptors are subclassified into irritant, stretch, and J-receptors. The main striated muscle receptors are Golgi tendon organs and muscle spindles. In the diaphragm there are abundant Golgi tendon organs but only rare muscle spindles, the latter being more frequent in intercostal and accessory muscles. Finally, it has been suggested that splanchnic receptors in abdominal organs can also influence respiratory control.[73]

Axons from the automatic (involuntary) controller in the brainstem descend in the ventrolateral spinal white matter, whereas fibers involved in voluntary respiration originate in the cortex and travel separately in the dorsolateral columns of the spinal cord. Impulses from cortical and brainstem centers are integrated at the level of the spinal respiratory motor neurons in the anterior horns, the site of transmission of local spinal reflexes. A patient has been described who had partial transverse cervical myelitis and

paralysis of limb and trunk muscles; rhythmic respiratory movement was preserved, but the patient could not voluntarily alter his respiration.[74] The converse of this situation—impaired automatic control with maintenance of normal voluntary breathing—can occur following bilateral cordotomy performed for the relief of pain. This procedure interrupts the spinothalamic tracts and results in ablation of respiratory axons, including those that both ascend and descend in the ventrolateral spinal cord. In the resulting syndrome ("Ondine's curse"), the patient breathes relatively normally during the day but experiences long periods of apnea at night when respiratory control is automatic (*see* further on).

Various techniques have been devised to determine the output of the respiratory center, including measurement of ventilatory responses to alterations in inspired oxygen and CO_2 tension, added inspiratory and expiratory loads, and exercise (*see* page 416). Because a subject's lung mechanics can profoundly influence the ventilatory response to these challenges, a measurement of mouth occlusion pressure (P0.1) has been used as a more specific estimate of respiratory drive. Ultimately, electromyographic or electroneurographic recordings of diaphragmatic and phrenic activation provide the most accurate assessment of the output of the respiratory center.

Disorders of the Central Nervous System

Cerebral Dysfunction

Many disorders that affect cerebral function are associated with respiratory depression, especially during sleep.[75] In some of these disorders, the depression is a direct effect of cerebral dysfunction, whereas in others, it is secondary to the effects on the brainstem of increased intracranial pressure. Narcotic, analgesic, and sedative agents in prescribed amounts frequently produce hypoventilation and respiratory failure in patients who have underlying chronic pulmonary disease but only rarely have these effects in persons who have normal lungs; in the latter group, drug-induced hypoventilation usually occurs following suicide attempts in adults and following accidental ingestion in children. Drugs that have been associated with respiratory depression in adults include the barbiturates,[76, 77] glutethimide,[78] the phenothiazines and benzodiazepines,[77, 79–81] the tricyclic antidepressants,[82, 83] ethchlorvynol,[77, 84] diphenhydramine,[82, 85] and meprobamate.[77, 86]

Cerebral damage resulting from infection, trauma, or vascular accidents can cause hypoventilation, which usually follows an initial period of hyperventilation. In many patients, it is probable that increased intracranial pressure, caused at least partly by edema, plays a role in the hypoventilation. An unusual cerebrovascular cause of respiratory arrest is familial hemiplegic migraine; one case was reported in which microinfarcts were identified in the basal ganglia.[87]

Another group of conditions in which higher centers can influence respiration (but not necessarily cause respiratory depression) consists of the disorders associated with respiratory dyskinesia. Dyskinesia of the respiratory muscles is characterized by irregular contraction of inspiratory and expiratory muscles and simultaneous contraction of opposing muscles acting on the rib cage and upper airway. It occurs most often in patients who have neuroleptic-induced tardive dyskinesia in association with a generalized choreiform movement disorder.[88, 89] A polysomnographic study of one such patient disclosed a varying position of the rib cage and abdomen at end-expiration that indicated variable end-expiratory lung volume;[90] grunting sounds were evidently caused by simultaneous contraction of anterior abdominal wall muscles and partial closure of the laryngeal airway. During sleep, the respiratory pattern became normal, indicating that the origin of the impulses was in centers above the brainstem respiratory center. A similar ventilatory dyskinesia has been reported in Rett's syndrome, a disorder of girls that consists of autistic tendency, dementia, ataxia, and loss of purposeful hand movements.[91–94]

Primary Alveolar Hypoventilation

Alveolar hypoventilation that occurs predominantly as a result of an abnormality of central neurogenic control has been termed primary alveolar hypoventilation of the nonobese ("Ondine's curse"[95] or central sleep apnea[96–98]). Affected persons have normal or almost normal gas exchange and lung function when awake and breathing under voluntary ventilatory control but may experience respiratory failure and even death during sleep.[99, 100] The disorder can be caused by a specific congenital or hereditary defect in the respiratory center, or it can be acquired as a consequence of a variety of diseases that affect the central nervous system.

The characteristic physiologic feature is a decrease in the sensitivity of the central nervous system to CO_2 that results in alveolar hypoventilation, especially during sleep. A profound decrease in the ventilatory response to hypoxemia also has been seen in some patients.[101] Characteristically, patients who have Ondine's curse can voluntarily increase their ventilation and lower their $Paco_2$ to within the normal range. Although they experience no discomfort during inhalation of CO_2 or during prolonged breath-holding, they can experience a normal sensation of breathlessness during exercise,[102] even though their ventilation during exercise is somewhat attenuated.[103] The response of peripheral chemoreceptors to hypoxemia is normal, at least in those patients who hypoventilate only during sleep.[104] Because upper or lower airway obstruction and neuromuscular disorders first must be ruled out before the diagnosis is accepted, primary alveolar hypoventilation represents a diagnosis of exclusion. Suggested criteria include an arterial Pco_2 greater than 45 mm Hg, respiratory arrest or apnea during sleep, normal or near-normal tests of ventilatory capacity, and a marked decrease in the ventilatory response to CO_2.

Although upper airway obstruction is the pathophysiologic mechanism in the vast majority of patients who have sleep apnea, it is important to identify the occasional individual in whom central neurogenic hypoventilation is the cause, because the management is very different. In patients who have primary alveolar hypoventilation, the apneic episodes are usually of shorter duration and are associated with less bradycardia than in patients who have obstruction. In addition, patients who have primary alveolar hypoventilation complain more of insomnia and less of daytime hypersomnolence.[105]

As indicated, primary alveolar hypoventilation can be congenital or can present in adulthood. Familial forms have been described;[106–108] in some families, there is an increased risk for sudden infant death syndrome.[109] The congenital form becomes manifest within minutes or hours of birth in the form of cyanosis and respiratory acidosis necessitating prolonged mechanical ventilation.[110, 111] Two patients suffering from neonatal Ondine's curse have been reported in whom the level of the dopamine metabolite homovanillic acid was approximately 2.4 times higher than normal in the cerebrospinal fluid (CSF).[112] On the other hand, lower-than-normal levels of homovanillic acid in the CSF have been reported in families that have a neuropsychiatric disorder, inherited in autosomal dominant fashion, characterized by central hypoventilation and apnea.[113, 114] Some infants who have primary alveolar hypoventilation also show generalized hypotonia and hyporeflexia and abnormal brainstem evoked potentials in response to auditory stimuli.[115] Of interest, this last abnormality also has been observed in an alcoholic patient who had acquired Ondine's curse, presumably secondary to brainstem damage from excess alcohol.[116] Central hypoventilation can occur in association with Moebius' syndrome, which is characterized by bilateral cranial nerve palsies,[117] sometimes associated with deletions of chromosome 13[118] and calcification of the brainstem.[119]

In one family, central apnea was associated with subacute necrotizing encephalomyopathy (Leigh's disease);[106] autopsy showed that lesions were confined to the respiratory center of the lower brainstem. Leigh's disease also has been associated with the development of primary alveolar hypoventilation in adulthood.[120] In another family of patients who had central sleep apnea, concomitant findings included anosmia, color blindness, seizures, and cognitive dysfunction.[107] Primary alveolar hypoventilation can also occur in association with Leber's disease, a disorder with a sex-linked recessive inheritance pattern complicated by hereditary optic atrophy.[121]

In adults, central neurogenic hypoventilation occurs as often in association with another primary disease as it does in an isolated fashion. In one review of 31 patients, the syndrome was more common in men than in women, in a ratio of 5 to 1.[99] The patients' ages ranged from 20 to 50 years, and approximately 50% had a history of prior central nervous system disease, usually encephalitis, Parkinson's disease, syringomyelia, or neurosyphilis; the other 50% had no associated neurologic disorder.[99, 122–130] Hypoventilation may be the sole or principal manifestation in patients who have cerebrovascular disease[131] or brain tumors[132] that selectively involve the brainstem respiratory centers. Alveolar hypoventilation during sleep and wakefulness is also a sequela of western equine encephalitis[133, 134] and has been reported following radiation therapy for midline cerebellar hemangioblastoma,[135] following high percutaneous cordotomy for relief of chronic pain,[136] and transiently after bilateral carotid endarterectomy.[137] In the latter two situations, the apnea and hypoventilation are secondary to an interruption of afferent input into the respiratory center rather than to a disturbance of the respiratory center itself.

Primary alveolar hypoventilation also has been seen in association with Hirschsprung's disease[138, 139] and with total colonic aganglionosis (Zuelzer-Wilson syndrome), a rare congenital form of gut immotility related to Hirschsprung's disease.[140] According to one group of investigators, 16% of children who have congenital central hypoventilation are also affected by Hirschsprung's disease,[141] and approximately 2% of patients affected by Hirschsprung's disease also have central hypoventilation.[142] Acquired Ondine's curse has been reported in patients who have multiple sclerosis affecting specific regions of the medulla oblongata[143] and following cerebrovascular accidents that selectively involve the caudal brainstem.[144] Patients who have chronic congestive heart failure show a high frequency of central sleep apnea.[145]

There is a clinical spectrum of severity in patients who have primary alveolar hypoventilation. Hypoventilation occurs only at night in some patients, and arterial blood gas tensions become normal during waking hours. The hypoventilation persists throughout the day in others; as might be expected, these patients have the poorer prognosis.[146] In some patients, nocturnal oxygen therapy decreases the frequency of apneas and increases nocturnal ventilation, suggesting that hypoxic depression of ventilation may occur.[147, 148] In other patients, nocturnal oxygen alleviates the hypoxemia but also exacerbates hypercapnia; headache and lethargy can result.[150]

An unusual neurologic syndrome characterized by an abnormality of ventilatory control virtually opposite to primary alveolar hypoventilation has been described in three girls, who showed an irregular and inadequate minute ventilation when awake but normal ventilation during sleep.[151]

Obesity Hypoventilation Syndrome

The first description of the obesity hypoventilation syndrome probably can be ascribed to Felix Platter (1536–1614), who described a morbidly obese patient "who tended to fall asleep all the time: in the course of talking, even while eating."[152] A constellation of cyanosis, polycythemia, and obesity was described in 1936,[153] but it was not until 1956 that the syndrome became widely recognized as the "pickwickian syndrome"—so called because of the similarity of these patients in appearance and behavior to the fat boy Joe in the novel *Pickwick Papers* by Charles Dickens.[154]

Although various mechanisms have been proposed to explain the hypoventilation in obese persons, studies of breathing during sleep have allowed separation of these patients into those in whom the primary problem is obstructive sleep apnea and those in whom the problem appears to be primarily one of ventilatory control. Considerable confusion exists in the literature as to precisely what the term "obesity hypoventilation syndrome" means. Morbidly obese patients who have obstructive sleep apnea are more likely to have persistent hypoventilation, and such patients have been considered to have "sleep apnea/obesity hypoventilation syndrome."[155] Other patients who have sleep apnea without obesity have persistent hypoventilation and have been considered to have "sleep hypoventilation syndrome."[156] We think that "obesity hypoventilation syndrome" should be reserved for those cases in which the patient hypoventilates but does not fit the criteria for a diagnosis of obstructive sleep apnea. In some of these patients, there may be a primary hypothalamic defect that causes both obesity and hypoventilation. Alternatively, affected persons may have a ventilatory response to CO_2 and hypoxemia that is at the low end of the wide normal range; when challenged by the increased work of breathing associated with obesity, they

may hypoventilate in much the same way that so-called "blue bloaters" hypoventilate when faced with the increased work of breathing associated with chronic obstructive pulmonary disease (COPD).[96] Probably the commonest clinical setting in which the pickwickian syndrome is recognized is that in which obese persons have moderate air-flow obstruction and may or may not have obstructive sleep apnea. The term "pickwickian syndrome" has outlived its usefulness,[157] and it is now preferable to refer to patients as having obesity and obstructive sleep apnea or the obesity hypoventilation syndrome.

The interrelationships among obesity, obstructive sleep apnea, and depressed central respiratory drive are complex.[158] Although it is likely that differences in central drive to breathe are responsible for the hypoventilation, there is some evidence that obese patients who hypoventilate have a lower thoracic compliance, an increased work of breathing, an increased ratio of dead space ventilation to total ventilation (VD/VT), and decreased respiratory muscle efficiency compared with equally obese persons who do not hypoventilate.[159] Patients often have additional respiratory problems because of heavy smoking, asthma, or recurrent pulmonary thromboemboli. In many, it is probable that the combination of cigarette smoke–induced abnormalities of air flow and ventilation-perfusion matching plus the mechanical effects of obesity causes respiratory failure. Obese smokers have significant hypoxemia; nocturnal ventilation is decreased even in normal persons, and such a decrease has a greater effect on arterial Po_2 in obese smokers, because values for Pao_2 and O_2 saturation are on or close to the steep portion of the O_2 dissociation curve.

As discussed in Chapter 53 (*see* page 2059), obesity markedly increases the incidence of obstructive sleep apnea, probably because of narrowing of the oropharyngeal airway by increased fat deposition. In addition, obesity exerts profound effects on the static and dynamic mechanical properties of the respiratory system; by altering lung volumes, it influences ventilation-perfusion matching and arterial blood gas tensions. Despite the foregoing, the vast majority of patients who have morbid obesity do not suffer from obstructive sleep apnea or the obesity hypoventilation syndrome. For example, only 12% of patients who were undergoing gastric surgery for morbid obesity in one study had ventilatory failure.[160] The authors considered that one third of these patients had obesity hypoventilation syndrome alone, one third had obstructive sleep apnea alone, and the final third had a combination of the two conditions. In another investigation of 200 morbidly obese men whose average weight was 144 kg, only 8 were considered to fulfill the criteria for pickwickian syndrome.[161]

Chronic Mountain Sickness

Chronic mountain sickness (CMS), also called Monge's disease, is an unusual cause of chronic hypoventilation characterized by decreased ventilation in long-time residents of high-altitude regions, associated with polycythemia, headache, dizziness, loss of memory, fatigue, and, in the later stages of the disease, dyspnea and peripheral edema. The reason why only a small percentage of the population develops CMS is unknown.[162] Genetic factors appear to play a role; although CMS is seen in Tibet and the Andes, it rarely develops in Tibetan natives and is more often observed in the immigrant Han Chinese population, in whom it develops after an average residence of 15 years at altitude.[163, 164] Additional risk factors include older age, male gender, cigarette smoking, and abnormal lung function.[163, 165, 166] Although most high-altitude dwellers have depressed hypoxemic and hypercapnic ventilatory drives, those who develop CMS appear to represent a small subset who develop profound depression in ventilatory drive and perhaps an exaggerated erythropoietic response to hypoxemia.[166, 167]

Myxedema

Hypothyroidism can have a number of effects on the lung and respiratory system (*see* Chapter 68, page 2729). A decrease in central neurogenic drive to breathe can be a contributing factor in the hypoventilation sometimes observed in patients who have myxedema.[168–170] An additional factor in some patients is obstructive sleep apnea, which is not uncommon in hypothyroidism,[171–173] possibly as a result of narrowing of the upper airway by macroglossia secondary to deposition of mucopolysaccharides.[168] Patients who have hypothyroidism also demonstrate significant respiratory muscle weakness, which is ameliorated after thyroid replacement therapy.[169]

Coma is not uncommon in patients who have myxedema; when it occurs, it usually affects elderly, obese women.[174, 175] In one survey of 77 patients who developed coma, 60 were female, and nearly half were in the seventh decade of life;[174] hypoventilation appeared to be responsible for coma in one third of the cases. Because most patients who develop coma are obese, it has been suggested that the hypoventilation may be a consequence of the obesity *per se.* However, this conclusion has not been supported by the findings in studies of affected patients in whom blood gas values returned to normal with thyroid therapy despite little or no change in body weight.[176, 177]

Metabolic Alkalosis

Another cause of central respiratory depression that results in hypoventilation is metabolic alkalosis.[178] This occurs when CO_2 retention and an increase in serum bicarbonate follow repeated episodes of vomiting, as a result of either psychologic or organic causes.[179, 180] This combination also has been reported after gastric resection[181] and in association with Cushing's syndrome.[182] The hypoventilation in these patients represents a compensatory mechanism that permits a rise in serum bicarbonate, thereby enabling the acid-base balance to return toward normal.

Parkinson's Syndrome

Patients who have Parkinson's syndrome can suffer respiratory insufficiency for several reasons.[183, 184] In some affected persons, the hypoventilation and hypoxemia appear to be related to central hypoventilation.[185, 186] A familial syndrome also has been described in which patients present with mental depression that progresses to Parkinson's syndrome and primary alveolar hypoventilation.[187] The results of one study showed that patients who had classic idiopathic Parkinson's disease had little abnormality of respiration during sleep when compared with age- and sex-matched control patients, whereas those in whom the parkinsonism was associated with autonomic disturbance demonstrated disorganized respiration and frequent episodes of central and obstructive apnea.[188] However, before ventilatory respiratory failure can be ascribed to brainstem depression in patients who have Parkinson's syndrome, it is important to exclude respiratory muscle weakness.[189, 190] Patients with parkinsonism demonstrate decreased maximal expiratory flow and oscillatory fluctuations in expiratory flow that are believed to be related to tremor involving the upper airway[191] and expiratory muscles.[192] In one study, the results of pulmonary function tests suggested that subclinical upper airway obstruction and decreased effective muscle strength were responsible for pulmonary insufficiency in a significant number of patients.[193]

Respiratory failure in Parkinson's disease can also be caused by intrinsic pulmonary disease such as aspiration pneumonia and atelectasis, both of which are not infrequent complications of the condition. In a comprehensive pulmonary function study of 31 patients, obstructive ventilatory defects were identified in one third;[194] these had a history of chronic bronchitis and showed no functional improvement following therapy with 3,4-dihydroxyphenylalanine (L-dopa). However, because significant neurologic improvement was observed, it was concluded that the impairment of pulmonary function was not the result of the Parkinson's disease *per se.* In a similar study of 10 patients, a significant increase in maximal voluntary ventilation was observed following treatment with L-dopa, although there was no direct correlation between clinical and pulmonary functional improvement.[195]

Tetanus

The mechanism of the ventilatory failure that can accompany tetanus is unclear; however, it is probable that the severe, prolonged spasm of the respiratory musculature is capable of causing inadequate ventilation.[196] Tetanus toxin has been shown to cause blockade of inhibitory synapses at both the cortical[197, 198] and spinal cord[199] levels. The disease is frequently associated with symptoms and signs of autonomic dysfunction, including hypertension, tachycardia, bradycardia, cardiac arrhythmias, profuse sweating, pyrexia, increased urinary catecholamine excretion, and, in some cases, the development of hypotension, indicating that parasympathetic and sympathetic fibers may be affected.[200, 201] Therefore, it is possible that involvement of the afferent inputs to the respiratory center contributes to the respiratory failure. However, the remarkable improvement that occurs in patients who have severe tetanus after the administration of muscle-paralyzing agents and the institution of artificial ventilation[196, 202–204] indicates that muscle dysfunction plays a significant role causing respiratory failure. In one study, a case fatality rate of 44% was reduced to 15% after establishment of an intensive care unit in which all patients were managed with paralysis and assisted ventilation. In another study of 100 patients who were admitted to an intensive care unit, the disease was sufficiently severe to necessitate the institution of paralysis and assisted ventilation in 90.[205]

Tetanus is now more often found in "developing" countries in which hygiene is poor and there is increased likelihood of wound contamination on bare feet by animal feces containing *Clostridium tetani.*[206-208] In the United States, the incidence of tetanus has decreased considerably;[209] however, in certain large cities where drug addiction is a major problem, the disease has undergone a resurgence. Puncture wounds and lacerations acquired on the farm or in the garden are common sites of infection, although ulcers secondary to pressure (decubitus ulcers), venous stasis, and frostbite, tumors, and dental abscesses can also serve as nidi;[209] even an aspirated foreign body has been incriminated.[210] Patients who have mild tetanus experience trismus (inability to open the mouth) and hypertonicity of the chest wall and abdominal muscles; those who have moderate and severe disease also have tetanic spasms. Even patients who have mild disease manifest hypoxemia and hyperventilation associated with metabolic acidosis and a restrictive pattern of pulmonary function.[211, 212]

The mortality rate remains substantial—29% in one study[213]—despite modern supportive care. A common cause of death is cardiac arrest, often occurring during the second or third week of the illness; this complication can be caused by either increased catecholamine secretion or respiratory failure secondary to toxin-induced myopathy.[214]

Disorders of the Spinal Cord

Lesions of the cervical and thoracic segments of the spinal cord can interfere with both afferent and efferent spinal pathways to and from the respiratory center. An appreciation of the various syndromes that result from spinal cord damage is aided by knowledge of the spinal levels from which innervation of the various respiratory muscles originates. The diaphragm is innervated by the nerve roots from C3 to C5, which join to form the phrenic nerve, whereas parasternal and lateral external intercostal muscles are innervated by the nerve roots from T1 to T12 via the intercostal nerves. Of the accessory muscles, the scalenes are innervated by nerve roots from C4 to C8, while the sternocleidomastoid is innervated by cranial nerve XI and the cervical nerve roots C1 and C2. The expiratory muscles consist of the lateral internal intercostal muscles, which derive innervation from T1 to T12 via the intercostal nerves, and the rectus abdominis, external and internal obliques, and transversus abdominis, which are innervated by lumbar nerves originating from nerve roots T7 to L1.

Patients who suffer spinal cord injury at the level of C5 or lower have preserved diaphragmatic function but paralyzed intercostal muscles. In this circumstance, diaphragmatic contraction during inspiration results in exaggerated protrusion of the abdomen and indrawing of the sternum and lower ribs; on expiration the diaphragm relaxes and ascends, with the abdomen flattening and the lower chest expanding as a result of the elasticity of the rib cage.[215] This pattern, termed *paradoxical chest wall motion,* tends to decrease with time following the development of quadriplegia, presumably because the denervated intercostal muscles develop spasticity, or owing to some recovery of phrenic nerve function. As a result, pulmonary function tends to improve during the period of 6 to 12 months after the injury.[215a] In one study, serial measurements of lung volumes were obtained at 1, 3, and 5 weeks and at 3 and 5 months after spinal cord injury.[216] Patients whose lesions were at the C5 to C6 level showed

initial reductions in vital capacity to 30% of predicted, although over the ensuing 3 months this doubled to 60%; patients who had lesions at levels C4 and higher showed greater decreases in vital capacity. The investigators found that patients whose vital capacity was 25% of predicted or less tended to develop hypercapnia, whereas hypoxemia was common even in the absence of hypercapnia, presumably as a result of the patients' inability to take deep breaths and reverse microatelectasis.

Although hypoventilation after spinal cord injury is caused mainly by inspiratory muscle dysfunction, involvement of expiratory muscles is also important, because it interferes with effective clearance of pulmonary secretions. This was illustrated in one retrospective study in which 9 of 22 patients who had high cervical cord lesions died;[217] in the same study, none of an additional 22 patients died who were followed prospectively and in whom careful attention was given to tracheal toilet and the need for mechanical ventilation.

Although there is little doubt that the majority of patients die in the absence of ventilatory support when cervical cord lesions are above the origin of the phrenic motor neurons, a case has been described of a quadriplegic patient who had a spinal cord lesion at the C2 to C3 level whose breathing was totally dependent on neck muscles supplied by the upper two spinal nerves and cranial nerve XI.[218] He employed "glossopharyngeal breathing," a repetitive maneuver consisting of coordinated movements of the tongue, cheeks, and soft palate to pump a bolus of air into the lungs, using the glottis as a one-way check valve; this form of breathing resulted in a threefold increase in vital capacity.

As indicated previously, cervical cordotomy can interfere with respiratory control and result in sleep-induced apnea and even sudden death. This surgical procedure, which is used to relieve intractable pain, is accomplished by inserting a stainless steel needle electrode into the ventral quadrant of the cervical spinal cord and applying a radiofrequency current to the electrode. Lesions produced in this way are permanent, and in some cases both afferent and efferent respiratory axons are severed. The result is a reduction in vital capacity, maximal breathing capacity, minute ventilation, and tidal volume, particularly if the operation is bilateral. Although such findings can be attributed to section of efferent pathways to the phrenic nerve nuclei, there is evidence that respiratory control mechanisms are also disturbed, probably as a result of ablation of reticular formation spinal tracts.[219] The major clinical manifestations consist of hypoventilation, diminished CO_2 response, and irregular breathing. In one report of two patients, bilateral cervical cordotomy resulted in sleep-induced apnea, and O_2 induced sudden death.[220] Of 100 patients in whom bilateral percutaneous cervical cordotomy was performed for intractable pain associated with malignant disease, relief of pain was complete in 64 patients;[221] however, 6 patients died as a result of postoperative respiratory dysfunction. Similar physiologic dysfunction has been described in patients who have multiple sclerosis, presumably as a result of destruction of cervical spinal pathways or midline ventral medullary lesions.[222, 223] Unilateral cervical spinal cord injury can result in hemiplegia and unilateral paradoxical chest wall motion that mimics a flail chest.[224]

Disorders of the Peripheral Chemoreceptors

Peripheral chemoreceptors situated in the carotid bodies account for virtually all the hypoxic drive in humans.[225] Bilateral carotid endarterectomy[226] or removal of both carotid bodies (a "therapeutic procedure" that was once employed for relief of asthma[227, 228]) can abolish the compensatory hyperventilation that normally occurs when hypoxemia supervenes. Bilateral (but not unilateral) carotid body resection causes a decreased ventilatory response to exercise.[229] Sleep apnea also has been reported as a complication following bilateral excision of carotid body tumors.[230]

The syndromes of autonomic dysfunction represent a heterogeneous group of congenital and acquired disorders usually characterized by orthostatic hypotension, hypohidrosis, a relatively fixed heart rate, and bladder and sexual dysfunctions.[231] Patients who have such syndromes may have abnormalities of peripheral chemoreceptor and mechanoreceptor input to the respiratory center resulting in respiratory difficulty. For example, in one review of 297 of these patients, 5% had a history of respiratory arrest.[231] Children who have familial dysautonomia (Riley-Day syndrome) are relatively unresponsive to hypoxia and hypercapnia:[232, 233] in one investigation of 210 affected children, 66% were found to have "breath-holding attacks."[234] The breathing of hypoxic mixtures by patients who have familial dysautonomia results in an exaggerated fall in arterial oxygen saturation (SaO_2) compared with that in normal persons. Some workers consider this lack of ventilatory response to hypoxia to be the result of a defect in the carotid body.[232] Other investigators have observed a fleeting hyperventilation followed by profound hypoxia,[235] a phenomenon they attributed to an inordinate central depression secondary to reduced cerebral blood flow. Unlike normal persons, patients who have dysautonomia become hypotensive while hypoxic.

Diabetic patients who have severe autonomic neuropathy have been reported to experience "unexplained" cardiac arrest.[236, 237] Because this complication occurs after anesthesia, bronchopneumonia, or the administration of depressant drugs, it has been suggested that the chemoreceptors are unable to respond to hypoxia.[236] A number of investigators have demonstrated depressed ventilatory responses to hypoxia and hypercapnia in diabetic patients, especially those who have autonomic neuropathy.[238, 239] Despite these findings, a comparative study of eight diabetic patients who had severe autonomic neuropathy and eight age-matched diabetic patients without neuropathy disclosed no increase in the incidence of sleep-disordered breathing or apnea in the former.[240]

Patients who have Arnold-Chiari malformation and syringomyelia have been described in whom central respiratory failure was presumably caused by destruction of afferent pathways in the ninth cranial nerve.[241, 242] As discussed previously, tetanus toxin has been shown to cause a blockade of inhibitory synapses at both the cortical[197, 198] and spinal cord levels.[199] It is frequently associated with evidence of autonomic dysfunction, suggesting that interference with afferent input to the respiratory center may be a contributing factor to the respiratory depression.

Disorders of the Respiratory Pump

For descriptive purposes, it is useful, although somewhat arbitrary, to visualize the central ventilatory control as terminating in the anterior horn cells, where impulses that serve voluntary and automatic stimulation of breathing are integrated with spinal reflexes. According to this view, the respiratory pump includes not only the rib cage and muscles of respiration but also their electrical connections. Disturbances of the respiratory pump can thus result from disease of the anterior horn cells, the phrenic and intercostal nerves, the myoneuronal junctions, or the respiratory muscles themselves.

The respiratory muscles can be divided into three distinct groups having different mechanisms of action: the diaphragm, the intercostal and accessory muscles, and the abdominal muscles.[243, 244] Although these muscles are involved in both inspiration and expiration, only dysfunction of the inspiratory muscles causes significant ventilatory impairment. Expiration is largely passive, and expiratory flow limitation results from alteration in the mechanical properties of the lungs rather than from muscle failure. However, because the expiratory muscles are important for the generation of an effective cough, and an inadequate cough can result in retained secretions and pulmonary infection, expiratory muscle dysfunction can exacerbate respiratory failure in patients who have neuromuscular disease.

Respiratory muscles differ from other skeletal muscles in several respects: (1) they function continuously, (2) they are under both automatic and voluntary control, and (3) unlike most other skeletal muscles that must overcome inertial loads, they cope primarily with elastic and resistive loads. The diaphragm is the principal muscle of inspiration. It probably acts alone during quiet breathing, the intercostal and accessory muscles being recruited only when the demand for ventilation increases.[245] The abdominal muscles play an important role in augmenting ventilation when exertion increases oxygen requirements: contraction during expiration displaces the abdominal contents inward and upward, lengthens the diaphragmatic muscle, and decreases its radius, thus improving the efficiency of the diaphragm as a pressure generator on the subsequent inspiration.[243]

It is not necessary that respiratory muscle weakness be profound to provoke symptoms and signs. Disability from weakened respiratory muscles can be accentuated or precipitated by an increased load on the respiratory system, such as that occasioned by exercise or concomitant COPD. Respiratory muscles, like other skeletal muscles, may become fatigued. The mechanical aspects of respiratory muscle contraction and the factors that can cause such fatigue are discussed in some detail in Chapter 10 (*see* page 246). However, because fatigue is probably the final common pathway causing respiratory failure in patients who have neuromuscular and chest wall abnormalities, a brief review of respiratory muscle fatigue is warranted.

Respiratory Muscle Fatigue

Muscle fatigue is defined as the inability of a muscle to generate a predetermined force continuously. For the inspiratory muscles, force is assessed by measuring pressure generation, either for maximal inspiratory pressure at the mouth (giving an overall estimate of inspiratory muscle strength) or for transdiaphragmatic pressure (which provides a specific estimate of the force generated by the diaphragm). Respiratory muscle fatigue can be either central or peripheral. Central fatigue is characterized by a diminution in force generation that is greater during voluntary effort than during electrical stimulation. Peripheral fatigue is characterized by decreased force generation despite maximal stimulation and may be categorized as either high-frequency or low-frequency in type. High-frequency fatigue is a loss of force-generating ability at very high stimulation frequencies and is thought to be caused by impaired neuromuscular transmission; it is distinguished by a decrease in amplitude of electromyographically recorded muscle action potential. Low-frequency fatigue is a loss of force generation at low stimulation frequencies; it is thought to be caused by impaired excitation-contraction coupling and is not associated with a decrease in the size of the action potential. High-frequency fatigue is reversible within minutes, whereas the low-frequency variety can persist for hours or days. Factors that may be responsible for fatigue include depletion of nutrient stores in the muscle, accumulation of metabolic end products that inhibit or reduce muscular contraction, and actual damage to respiratory muscle fibers.

Ultimately, respiratory muscles fatigue when an imbalance exists between their energy demand and the energy supply. Adenosine triphosphate (ATP) is the basic fuel for muscular contraction. Respiratory muscles require oxygen and substrate to generate ATP. O_2 transport is directly related to blood flow and to the O_2 content of the arterial blood; substrate is derived from circulating glucose and free fatty acids and from substrate stores, largely in the form of glycogen.

The factors that determine the energy demand on a respiratory muscle are the work of breathing and the strength and endurance of the muscle; the strength is in turn affected by the length-tension relationship. As with all skeletal muscles, respiratory muscles display distinct length-tension behavior. There is a specific muscle length at which the overlap between actin and myosin filaments is optimal for the generation of pressure. When contracting at this length, the muscle is most efficient in terms of tension generation for a given consumption of ATP. At lengths shorter or longer than optimal, less tension can be generated, despite similar activation and similar levels of fuel consumption. Chronically, the respiratory muscles can adapt, so that optimal length occurs within the operating range of the muscle; however, any factor that acutely alters the resting length (such as lung hyperinflation) will have a profound effect on efficiency. Respiratory muscle strength is also decreased in patients who have neuromuscular disease and in those who are malnourished. Malnutrition causes a depletion of energy stores and can result in atrophy of muscle fibers.

Respiratory muscles will inevitably fatigue when they are forced to continuously generate greater than 40% to 50% of the maximal pressure of which they are capable.[246-248] The development of respiratory muscle fatigue in response to a load can be predicted by calculating the product of the pressure generated by the muscle as a percentage of the maximal capacity of that muscle and the fraction of the total respiratory cycle time devoted to inspiratory muscle effort. This parameter is known as the tension-time index (TTdi).[249, 250] The TTdi of the diaphragm is calculated by multiplying the ratio of the mean transdiaphragmatic pressure change during inspiration (ΔPdi) to the maximal transdiaphragmatic pressure achieved with voluntary contraction

(Pdi max) by the respiratory duty cycle expressed as the inspiratory time (TI) divided by the total respiratory cycle time (Ttot):

$$TTdi = \frac{\Delta Pdi}{Pdi\ max} \times \frac{TI}{Ttot}$$

When the tension-time index exceeds 0.15 for an appreciable length of time, respiratory muscle fatigue will inevitably occur. Examination of this relationship illustrates that respiratory muscle fatigue is more likely to occur (1) when ΔPdi is increased as a result of an increase in the work of breathing, (2) when Pdi max is decreased by the disorders that result in respiratory muscle weakness, or (3) when both factors are operative. Respiratory muscle fatigability is increased in the presence of respiratory acidosis[251] and hypoxemia.[252]

Although the diagnosis of respiratory muscle fatigue is ultimately made on the basis of a failure of pressure generation, a number of investigators have recommended the use of tests to predict the eventual development of fatigue prior to a decline in force generation. For example, examination of the frequency spectrum of the diaphragmatic or intercostal muscle electromyogram (EMG) signal shows a characteristic decrease in the ratio of high- to low-frequency impulses even before mechanical fatigue can be demonstrated;[253, 254] such a pattern can be detected using either esophageal or surface EMG signals.[255] A more practical approach to predicting fatigue is the measurement of the relaxation rate of respiratory muscles following contraction; because fatiguing skeletal muscle shows delayed relaxation, measurement of the rate of decline in the transdiaphragmatic pressure[256] or mouth pressure[257] (or both) can predict fatigue.

Clinical Manifestations of Respiratory Muscle Weakness

Patients who have respiratory failure secondary to neuromuscular abnormalities complain of anxiety, lethargy, headache, dyspnea, and (sometimes) a feeling of suffocation. When ventilation is severely restricted, confusion, coma, and death can ensue rapidly. Cyanosis may or may not be present, depending upon the degree of hypoventilation. It is important to remember that, in the presence of a normal hemoglobin concentration, hypoxemia can be detected clinically by a change in color of the nail beds and mucous membranes only when SaO_2 has dropped to 80% or less. Similarly, appreciation of the degree of alveolar ventilation clinically is unreliable except when apnea has occurred,[258] by which time the patient will be severely cyanotic.

Because the diaphragm is the principal muscle of inspiration, evidence of diaphragmatic weakness or paralysis on physical examination is important in identifying a neuromuscular cause for respiratory failure. When it contracts, the diaphragm not only pushes down on the abdominal viscera and displaces the abdominal wall outward but also lifts and expands the rib cage. The latter action results in an increase in the diameter of the chest in both its anteroposterior and lateral dimensions and is dependent on the acute angle of insertion of diaphragmatic muscle fibers into the ribs. The degree of thoracic expansion also depends on the abdominal pressure: If the abdominal muscles are contracted, descent of the diaphragm is restricted and rib cage movement is accentuated. At the end of a quiet expiration, the diaphragm is relaxed, and pleural pressure and abdominal pressure are almost equal. On inspiration, intrapleural pressure becomes more negative and abdominal pressure more positive, resulting in a transdiaphragmatic pressure difference (ΔPdi). When the abdominal muscles are relaxed, this increase in intra-abdominal pressure causes the abdominal wall to protrude (Fig. 79–2).

When one hemidiaphragm is paralyzed or weakened, paradoxical movement may be apparent (Fig. 79–3). The development of negative intrapleural pressure secondary to rib cage expansion and the normal descent of the nonparalyzed hemidiaphragm "suck" the paralyzed hemidiaphragm into the thoracic cavity. Although the resulting inward motion of the anterior abdominal wall on the paralyzed side

can be detected clinically, paradoxical motion is much more apparent on fluoroscopic examination; on inspiration, the paralyzed hemidiaphragm moves upward coincident with expansion of the rib cage and descent of the normal hemidiaphragm, a motion that can be appreciated to better advantage during "sniffing" by the patient.

When both hemidiaphragms are paralyzed, as in bilateral phrenic nerve palsy, or when a neuropathic or myopathic disorder causes bilateral diaphragmatic weakness, paradoxical abdominal wall motion is more apparent clinically. With each inspiratory effort of the external intercostal and accessory muscles of respiration, the rib cage expands, resulting in a decrease in intrapleural pressure and "sucking" of the diaphragm into the thorax—a most inefficient form of breathing (Fig. 79–4*A* to *D*). This upward movement of the

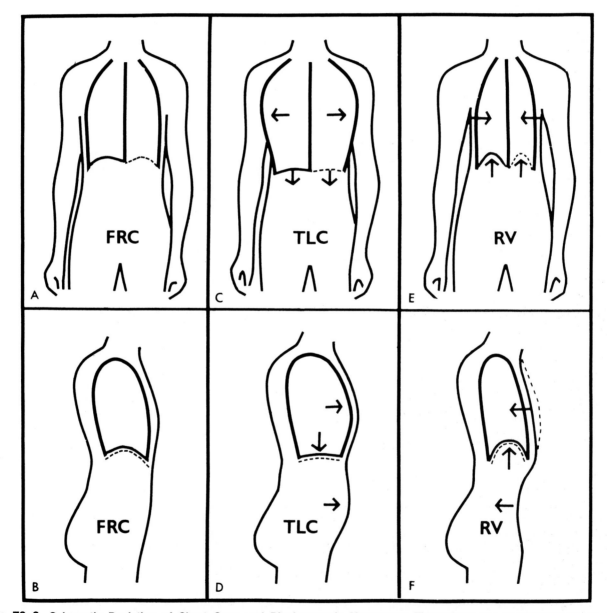

Figure 79–2. Schematic Depiction of Chest Cage and Diaphragmatic Movements Throughout the Respiratory Cycle: Normal. Anteroposterior *(A)* and lateral *(B)* views show the position of the chest wall and diaphragm at resting lung volume (FRC). At full inspiration *(C and D)*, the diaphragm contracts with resultant expansion of the chest cage, increase in intra-abdominal pressure, and a consequent protrusion of the abdominal wall. At full expiration *(E and F)*, abdominal muscle contraction causes a rise in intra-abdominal pressure and elevation of the relaxed diaphragm. FRC, functional residual capacity; TLC, total lung capacity; RV, residual volume.

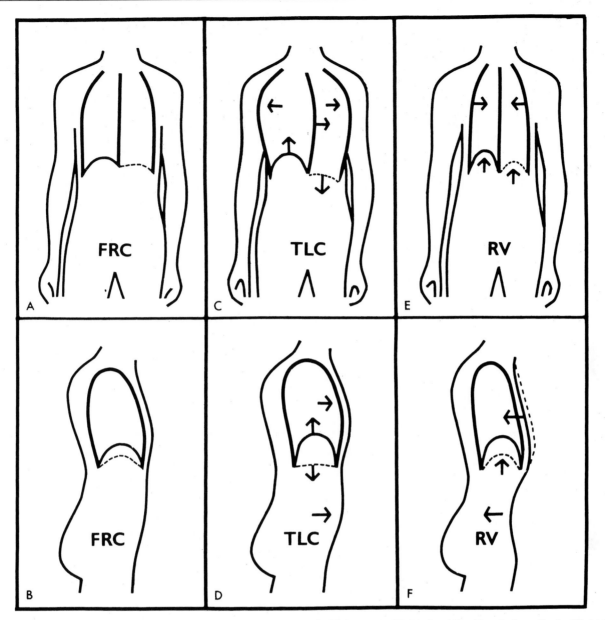

Figure 79–3. Schematic Depiction of Chest Cage and Diaphragmatic Movements Throughout the Respiratory Cycle: Right Hemidiaphragmatic Paralysis. At FRC *(A* and *B)*, the right hemidiaphragm is elevated. On full inspiration to TLC *(C* and *D)*, the left hemidiaphragm contracts and descends, whereas the flaccid right hemidiaphragm passively elevates in response to the more negative intrapleural pressure. On full expiration to RV *(E* and *F)*, a rise in intra-abdominal pressure evokes an even greater elevation of the paralyzed right hemidiaphragm. FRC, functional residual capacity; TLC, total lung capacity; RV, residual volume.

diaphragm results in an equal reduction of both abdominal and pleural pressures, so that the transdiaphragmatic pressure difference (ΔPdi) remains zero. The fall in abdominal pressure induces indrawing of the abdominal wall that is readily apparent clinically. In patients who have incipient diaphragmatic fatigue, paradoxical abdominal wall motion can develop during or after a period of increased respiratory muscle activity (e.g., when they are being "weaned" from ventilatory support).

The recruitment of abdominal expiratory muscles can mask paradoxical breathing and diaphragmatic weakness.[259] During expiration, the abdominal wall muscles may contract and force the flaccid diaphragm into the thoracic cavity; at the onset of inspiration, the sudden relaxation of these mus-

cles causes rapid diaphragmatic descent and apparent outward movement of the abdomen (Fig. 79–4E, F). Recruitment of expiratory abdominal muscles during tidal breathing can be detected by palpation of the anterior abdominal wall. Abdominal muscle contraction can restore an apparently normal pattern of movement to the anterior abdominal wall (Fig. 79–4G to J). This pattern of expiratory muscle recruitment may be responsible for the false-negative findings on fluoroscopic examination in some patients who have bilateral diaphragmatic paralysis or weakness.

Pulmonary Function Tests

Routine pulmonary function tests may suggest the possibility of respiratory neuromuscular disease. When the lung

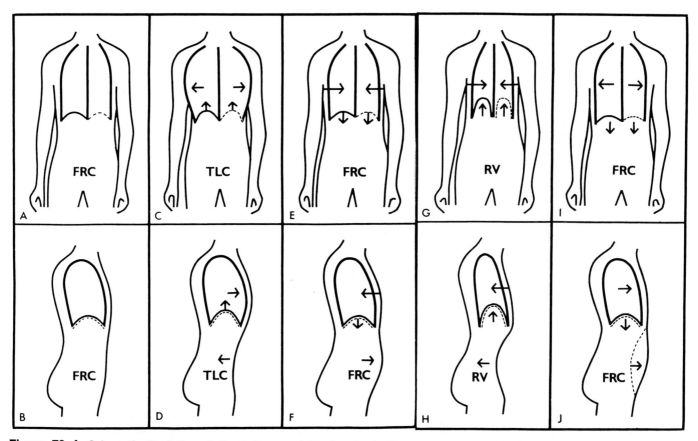

Figure 79–4. Schematic Depiction of Chest Cage and Diaphragmatic Movements Throughout the Respiratory Cycle: Bilateral Diaphragmatic Paralysis. On inspiration to TLC from FRC *(A to D)*, the increased negative intrapleural pressure "sucks" the diaphragm up and draws the abdominal wall in. On expiration to FRC *(E and F)*, the diaphragm descends and the abdomen protrudes. With a deeper expiration to RV accompanied by active contraction of the abdominal muscles *(G and H)*, the diaphragm rises. Subsequently, during the first part of inspiration to FRC *(I and J)*, abdominal muscle recoil is associated with descent of the flaccid diaphragm, creating the false impression of active contraction. FRC, functional residual capacity; TLC, total lung capacity; RV, residual volume.

parenchyma is normal and patient cooperation is complete, a decrease in TLC or an increase in residual volume (and thus a decrease in vital capacity) may indicate respiratory muscle weakness.[243] When vital capacity is reduced to 25% or less of that predicted, ventilatory failure is either present or imminent.[261] Decreased expiratory and inspiratory flow rates may also reflect neurogenic or myopathic disorders. Most laboratories include generation of flow-time or flow-volume curves as screening procedures; because expiratory flow early in the forced expiratory maneuver is effort-dependent and late flow is effort-independent, a disproportionate decrease in flow in the first part of the forced expiratory vital capacity breath suggests a neuromuscular defect.[262] Thus, a disproportionate reduction in FEV_1 relative to the mean forced expiratory flow during mid-FVC (FEF_{25-75}) should suggest the possibility of respiratory muscle weakness; however, it should be remembered that upper airway obstruction can produce a similar pattern (*see* page 2027). The characteristic expiratory and inspiratory flow-volume curve of patients who have global muscle weakness is an egg-shaped loop; there is a delay in achieving peak expiratory flow, and both maximal expiratory and inspiratory flow are reduced. The descending limb of the expiratory curve tends to be convex, because expiratory muscle weakness prevents the maintenance of flow below functional residual capacity.

Abnormalities of arterial blood gas tensions constitute a late finding in patients who have primary neuromuscular disease. Although patients may hyperventilate initially,[261] hyperventilation is inevitably succeeded by hypoventilation as the disease progresses. However, even severe hypoxemia and hypercapnia can be corrected in these patients by voluntary hyperventilation; this is a clear indication that measurements of static and dynamic lung volumes (i.e., flows and pressures that require maximal effort and hence cerebral cortical input) may not truly reflect the degree of dysfunction. In patients who have severe weakness or complete paralysis of the diaphragm, assumption of the supine posture causes further deterioration in gas exchange. The explanation for this lies in a change in gravitational forces: the weight of the abdominal organs displaces the flaccid diaphragm upward into the thoracic cavity, thus further reducing the effectiveness of the remaining inspiratory muscles.[263–265] In addition, a further drop in Pa_{O_2} and a rise in Pa_{CO_2} often occur during sleep, when breathing control is solely automatic.[265]

Impedance plethysmography or magnetometry measures the anteroposterior and lateral dimensions of the rib cage and abdomen simultaneously and separately during the respiratory cycle. Either method can be useful in documenting diaphragmatic weakness and paralysis. Normally, volume increases in both the abdominal and rib cage compartments during inspiration. When the diaphragm is nonfunctioning or weak, the diameter of the thorax increases, while that of the abdomen decreases during inspiration.[266]

The measurement of maximal inspiratory and expiratory pressures provides useful indices of respiratory muscle strength; this is a simple test, but its performance requires patient cooperation. Although there is a wide variation in inspiratory and expiratory pressures among normal persons, measurement is reasonably reproducible in any given subject. Serial measurement of inspiratory and expiratory pressures is a useful means of recognizing the development of respiratory muscle weakness or fatigue and of documenting recovery of respiratory muscle strength.[267] Measurement of the pressure-volume curve of the lung may suggest respiratory muscle weakness when lung volumes and pulmonary compliance are decreased, despite a normal or low maximal elastic recoil pressure.[268]

Perhaps the most specific method of identifying weakness or paralysis of the diaphragm is measurement of transdiaphragmatic pressure (Pdi). This is accomplished by recording pressures in balloons placed in both the esophagus (reflecting pleural pressure) and the stomach (reflecting abdominal pressure). As with maximal inspiratory and expiratory pressures, there is a wide range of normal values; however, those below 60 cm H_2O are indicative of diaphragmatic weakness. In the presence of complete diaphragmatic paralysis, Pdi does not change during maximal inspiratory effort against a closed airway or during full inspiration. As discussed in Chapter 77 (*see* page 2993), phrenic nerve function can be measured by recording the diaphragmatic muscle action potential with either esophageal[269] or surface[270] electrodes following transcutaneous stimulation of the phrenic nerve in the neck. A positive response in the presence of documented diaphragmatic paralysis indicates that the disorder is myopathic rather than neuropathic.[243]

Disorders of the Anterior Horn Cells

A variety of disorders of the anterior horn cells that subserve the respiratory muscles can result in acute or chronic respiratory failure. The most common of these disorders are poliomyelitis, which is now virtually abolished in North America, and amyotrophic lateral sclerosis. An infrequent hereditary and slowly progressive form of anterior horn cell degeneration, Kugelberg-Welander syndrome, can also manifest as respiratory muscle paralysis and ventilatory failure.[271]

Poliomyelitis

Although poliomyelitis associated with respiratory failure has been almost eradicated in "developed" countries by immunization, occasional cases are still seen, and affected patients can experience unexpected life-threatening hypoventilation.[272] Some patients develop a state of chronic hypoventilation,[273] which may result in secondary polycythemia.[274] Others develop ventilation-perfusion ($\dot{V}/\dot{Q}$) imbalance secondary to kyphoscoliosis and exhibit late-onset respiratory failure. In one follow-up study of 55 patients who had had poliomyelitis, 33 were found to manifest exertional dyspnea and frequent respiratory tract infections;[275] gross kyphoscoliosis (Cobb's angle >60 degrees) was present in 15 of these patients, and fluoroscopic evidence of unilateral diaphragmatic paralysis in 13. Poliomyelitis should be suspected as the cause of acute respiratory failure when symptoms of bulbar palsy are present in an unvaccinated person. Patients who have apparently recovered from polio may later develop a post-polio syndrome that can be associated with obstructive sleep apnea or hypoventilation, or both.[276]

Amyotrophic Lateral Sclerosis

Amyotrophic lateral sclerosis (motor neuron disease) can also result in ventilatory failure.[260, 277] Although respiratory muscle involvement develops in most patients after the diagnosis has been well established on the basis of peripheral muscle weakness, respiratory failure is occasionally the initial mode of presentation.[278–281] In addition to ventilatory failure caused by destruction of the anterior horn cells that innervate the inspiratory muscles, involvement of the neurons supplying the abdominal expiratory muscles and the muscles of the upper airway can result in abnormalities of expiratory flow. A characteristic flow-volume curve has been described in which expiratory flow is decreased and residual volume increased, a combination that occurs in patients who have predominant expiratory muscle weakness.[282] Selective paralysis of upper airway and oropharyngeal muscles can also influence maximal expiratory flow.[283]

As in many forms of neuromuscular disease that cause ventilatory failure, patients who have spinal cord degeneration may benefit from intermittent assisted ventilation, particularly at night; such assistance can stabilize or temporarily improve the respiratory status.[284] The exact mechanism by which mechanical ventilation improves interim lung function is uncertain; possibilities include the reversal of chronic respiratory muscle fatigue, a resetting of central chemoreceptors, and an improvement in pulmonary mechanics.

Disorders of the Peripheral Nerves

Landry-Guillain-Barré Syndrome

Acute polyneuritis (Landry-Guillain-Barré syndrome) is probably the most common neuromuscular disease to cause ventilatory failure.[285] It can be associated with either acute or subacute hypoventilation. Although in some respects it is a diagnosis of exclusion, an accepted clinical presentation includes symmetric ascending paralysis associated with a lack of cellular response in the CSF. Patients sometimes manifest evidence of autonomic dysfunction, including elevated blood pressure, tachycardia, cardiac arrhythmias, and episodes of pyrexia and hyperhidrosis.[285] The disease shows a striking predilection for patients less than 25 years of age; a second, smaller peak incidence occurs between the ages of 45 and 60 years. Cases tend to show a seasonal clustering, almost half the patients being afflicted during a 4-month period of late summer and autumn.[286] Males and females are equally affected.

The incidence of respiratory failure and the benefits that are achieved with mechanical ventilation have been examined in several large series.[287–290] Between 15%[287] and 60%[290] of patients develop sufficient respiratory muscle paralysis to require mechanical ventilation. In these patients, there is a slow but progressive improvement in respiratory muscle strength, although assisted ventilation may be required for several months;[291] two patients have been reported who received mechanical ventilation for 374 and 396 days, respectively, before being successfully "weaned."[288] The need for assisted ventilation should be assessed by repeated measurements of vital capacity or maximal inspiratory pressure.[292] Serial measurements of phrenic nerve conduction velocity may be a more sensitive method of assessing the severity of the disease and of predicting impending ventilatory failure.[293]

The use of plasmapheresis and intravenous immunoglobulins is effective in attenuating the severity of the neurologic manifestations and can prevent the use of mechanical ventilation in selected patients.[294] However, about 10% to 30% of patients still require mechanical ventilation, and 3% to 8% die as a result of largely avoidable complications.[295] Factors that are associated with an increased risk of the development of ventilatory failure include a short time interval between the preceding (and presumably precipitating) infection and the onset of weakness, cranial nerve involvement, and a CSF protein level greater than 800 mg/L.[294] The results of follow-up studies show that significant respiratory muscle weakness may persist despite symptomatic recovery.[296] Cantharidin poisoning can cause a "Guillain-Barré–like syndrome."[297]

Porphyria

The hepatic porphyrias—acute intermittent porphyria, porphyria variegata, and hereditary coproporphyria—are inborn errors of porphyrin metabolism inherited in an autosomal dominant fashion. They are characterized by increased excretion of porphyrins and the porphyrin precursors aminolevulinic acid (ALA) and porphobilinogen (PBG). The basic defect appears to be a partial block along the hemebiosynthetic pathway of the enzyme ALA-synthetase. A peripheral neuropathy is caused by the toxic effect of the accumulated porphyrin precursors ALA and PBG.[298] Some patients also manifest symptoms of bulbar involvement and experience difficulty in clearing bronchial secretions. The diagnosis is supported when it is learned that other members of the family are afflicted, and confirmation can be obtained by the discovery of porphyrin precursors, including ALA and PBG, in the urine.[298] Each form of porphyria can be associated with ascending paralysis and respiratory failure. Exacerbations of the disease may require prolonged mechanical ventilation.[299] Remissions may be followed by exacerbations that do not necessarily affect the respiratory musculature.

Fish and Shellfish Poisoning from Toxic Dinoflagellates

At least four different species of toxic dinoflagellates can cause shellfish and fish poisoning; the respiratory muscles can be involved in such poisoning by all species.[300] These microscopic unicellular sea algae are the cause of "red tide," a reddish discoloration of sea water resulting from an extremely high concentration of organisms. The four dinoflagellates that produce toxins for humans are *Ptychodiscus brevis (Gymnodinium breve), Protogonyaulyx cantenella, Protogonyaulyx tamarensis,* and *Gambierdiscus tox-*

icus. Three forms of poisoning occur, depending on the species involved.

Neurotoxic Shellfish Poisoning. This variety is caused by clams or oysters that have ingested *P. brevis* and concentrated its toxins (brevetoxins, the classic "red tide" toxins).[301] The syndrome is characterized by nausea, diarrhea, and abdominal pain and neurologic symptoms such as circumoral paresthesia; onset can range from a few minutes to 3 hours after ingestion of the clams or oysters. Paresthesia typically progresses to involve the pharynx, trunk, and extremities. Cerebellar symptoms, vertigo, incoordination, convulsions, bradycardia, and respiratory depression may develop. In addition to the problems associated with ingestion of the toxin, respiratory symptoms can also develop following inhalation of the toxin generated by whitecaps and breaking waves and liberated as an odorless aerosol. People exposed to the toxin on beaches can develop nonproductive cough, shortness of breath, lacrimation, sneezing, and rhinorrhea.[300, 302] *In vitro* studies have shown that the toxin of *P. brevis* contracts both animal[303] and human[304] airway smooth muscle.

Paralytic Shellfish Poisoning. The second major syndrome resulting from the toxins of unicellular sea algae is caused by the ingestion of mussels, clams, scallops, and oysters that have concentrated saxitoxin, the neurotoxin present in *P. cantenella* and *P. tamarensis.* The symptoms are very similar to those associated with the ingestion of brevetoxins and consist of circumoral paresthesia followed by cerebellar symptoms, dysphonia, dysphagia, and paralysis; the paralysis sometimes affects the respiratory muscles.[305, 306] The case mortality rate ranges from 3% to 23%.[300] The toxin responsible for paralytic shellfish poisoning has also been detected in starfish that prey on the shellfish.[306a]

Ciguatera Fish Poisoning. This form of algae-related neurotoxicity results from eating fish contaminated with toxins derived from *G. toxicus.* The toxin is concentrated in the flesh of large fish that feed on the plankton. Between 1970 and 1980, 418 cases were reported in the United States, mainly from Florida and Hawaii. These occurred in 94 outbreaks, and the mortality rate ranged from zero to as high as 20%.[307] Although the disease occurs primarily in the tropics, isolated cases in temperate climates have been reported in people who have eaten fish imported from tropical areas.[308]

Clinical manifestations usually develop within 12 hours of ingestion of the contaminated fish and include gastrointestinal symptoms, evidence of cerebellar dysfunction, sensory disturbances, and motor paralysis; the paralysis can develop up to 1 week after the onset of the illness. In one series of 33 patients, gastrointestinal symptoms developed in 91%, pain and weakness in 58%, and dysesthesias in 58%;[309] the dysesthesias lasted as long as 2 months. In another retrospective series of 129 patients from the Miami area, 39 displayed significant muscle weakness, but none required mechanical ventilation.[310] Muscle weakness can persist for long periods of time.[300, 311]

Other Neurotoxins

Poisoning from fish and shellfish can also occur from substances other than those derived from dinoflagellates. For example, an outbreak of poisoning related to the ingestion of mussels containing demoic acid was reported in Nova Scotia, Canada;[312] symptoms included memory loss, an increase in bronchial secretions, and neurologic impairment; respiratory failure developed in the patients who died.[312] Severe neuromuscular paralysis with rapid ventilatory failure also can occur after ingestion of puffer fish. The responsible neurotoxin, tetrodotoxin, blocks sodium channels in the peripheral nerves. In Japan, where puffer fish is considered a delicacy, specially trained chefs are entrusted with its preparation. The sushi masters who prepare the puffer fish do so in such a way that the effects of the neurotoxin are experienced without the risk of death. Ideally, the gourmand develops circumoral paresthesias but not ventilatory failure. Chefs who miscalculate lose out on any possibility of a tip! The case fatality rate when ventilatory failure occurs is approximately 50%.[313]

A variety of other animals can secrete poisons that affect peripheral nerve function and result in respiratory muscle paralysis and ventilatory failure. These include the blue-ringed octopus (*Hapalochlaena maculosa*),[314] the eastern coral snake (*Micrurus fulvius fulvius*),[315] the krait (*Bungarus*),[316] and the Philippine cobra (*Naja naja philippinensis*).[317] Ventilatory failure necessitating mechanical ventilation also has been reported following envenomation from the tick *Ixodes cornuatus*, which is widely distributed in Victoria, Tasmania, and New South Wales, Australia.[318] Although unusual, acute respiratory muscle paralysis and ventilatory failure can also occur following accidental or suicidal ingestion of organophosphate insecticide.[319]

Disorders of the Myoneural Junction

Conditions that cause impaired neuromuscular transmission at the myoneural junction with consequent acute or chronic hypoventilation include myasthenia gravis, myasthenia-like syndromes associated with neoplasms, the ingestion of various medications, and infection with or ingestion of toxins from *Clostridium botulinum*.

Myasthenia Gravis

The defect in myasthenia gravis is postsynaptic and is related to immunoglobulin G (IgG) autoantibodies that attach to and destroy acetylcholine receptors at the motor end plate.[320] Ventilatory failure is a frequent complication.[321] Exacerbations of respiratory muscle weakness and the development of respiratory failure can be precipitated by surgery, infection, or the parenteral administration of radiographic contrast media.[322, 323] Predictors of respiratory failure after thymectomy for myasthenia gravis include severe bulbar involvement, high preoperative cholinesterase inhibitor intake, the presence of a thymic tumor, and age greater than 50 years.[324]

Prior to the onset of hypoventilation, patients who have myasthenia and myasthenia-like syndromes usually manifest paresthesia, diplopia, dysphagia, ptosis, generalized weakness, and dyspnea. Rarely, respiratory failure is the presenting manifestation.[325, 326] In some cases, the diagnosis is evident only after a surgical procedure in which the effects of sedation and muscle relaxants cause a long period of inadequate ventilation postoperatively.[327] The administration of acetylcholinesterase inhibitors results in an immediate increase in respiratory muscle strength and lung volumes,[328, 329] although it can also cause a transient increase in airway resistance and a decrease in maximal expiratory flow, presumably because of an accentuation of cholinergic tone in the airway smooth muscle.[330] In one study, progressive decline of vital capacity was found to be a poor predictor of the eventual need for assisted ventilation, perhaps because of the episodic nature of the disorder.[331]

Patients who have myasthenia gravis generally respond to treatment with intravenous pyridostigmine or pyridostigmine plus corticosteroids.[332, 333] Those who do not respond to this more conservative therapy show a dramatic response to plasmapheresis[322, 324, 334] and immunosuppressive drug therapy—an improvement that has been shown to correlate with a fall in titers of serum antibody directed against the acetylcholine receptor.[335] Ventilatory failure usually necessitates mechanical support for days to weeks and sometimes for months; one patient has been reported in whom ventilatory support was maintained for 2 years![336]

Myasthenia-like syndromes such as Eaton-Lambert syndrome also occur in association with neoplasia, particularly small cell carcinoma of the lung.[337] The presence of neuronal antinuclear antibodies[337] and the response to plasmapheresis and immunosuppressive therapy[338] are consistent with an autoimmune pathogenesis (*see* page 1173).

More than a hundred drugs have been reported to impair muscle function by either inhibiting neural drive, causing peripheral neuropathy, blocking neuromuscular junctions, producing myopathy, or precipitating myasthenia gravis.[339] Myasthenia is particularly common after the administration of antibiotics and antiseizure medications. Examples of the former include the aminoglycosides[340, 341] such as streptomycin,[342] viomycin,[343] polymyxin B, and colistin (polymyxin E).[344, 345] Neuromuscular blockade caused by these agents has been seen in patients who have renal disease or myasthenia gravis.[344, 346] Aminogycosides are believed to produce a competitive blockade that may be reversed by neostigmine. By contrast, polymyxins produce a noncompetitive blockade that actually can be potentiated by neostigmine.[344] Ventilatory muscle depression can develop within 1 to 24 hours after the administration of these drugs. In most cases, the respiratory failure is of short duration, and spontaneous ventilation resumes within 24 hours.[344] The reaction can occur following administration intraperitoneally,[347] intrapleurally, or into pseudocyst cavities.[348] Respiratory depression can be very prolonged following the intraperitoneal administration of neomycin or streptomycin in patients who also have been treated with succinylcholine chloride as a muscle relaxant during abdominal surgery.[349]

Penicillamine administration has been associated with the development of myasthenia gravis;[350] this may be attributed erroneously to pre-existing lung disease.[351] In the few reported cases, anti-acetylcholine receptor and antistriational antibodies have been found in the serum. Myasthenia has been observed in patients receiving procainamide,[352] and the symptoms of myasthenia may be worsened by the superimposition of a steroid myopathy.[353]

The increasing use of nondepolarizing neuromuscular blocking agents in critically ill ventilated patients has been associated with reports of prolonged muscle weakness;[354] the incidence of this complication may be particularly frequent when the neuromuscular-blocking agents are combined with systemic corticosteroids.[355-357]

Organophosphate poisoning caused by the insecticides parathion and malathion results from inhibitition of acetylcholinesterase at nerve endings (see page 2584).[358, 359] Acetylcholine accumulates at cholinergic synapses, resulting in an initial stimulation and a later inhibition of synaptic transmission, with consequent paralysis of the respiratory muscles.

Clostridium botulinum Poisoning

Although *C. botulinum* types A and B are most often responsible for acute respiratory failure, the complication has also been documented with type E organisms following the ingestion of contaminated canned fish.[360, 361] The neurotoxin of botulism acts by causing a presynaptic blockade at the cholinergic neuromuscular junction.[362, 363] The disease can occur after ingestion of food contaminated with the toxin[364] or as a result of wound infection by the organism;[365] the latter is most often accidental but has been reported to occur in needle-track infections in chronic drug abusers.[366]

Peripheral muscle weakness and bulbar symptoms secondary to cranial nerve involvement usually appear within 18 to 36 hours after ingestion of contaminated food. Patients complain of blurred vision, weakness, dizziness, dysphonia, dysphagia, respiratory difficulty, and urinary retention. The pupils are dilated and nonreactive, and there is marked dryness of the mouth and tongue associated with muscle weakness.[360, 367] Ocular findings may be prominent and early features:[368] in one study of 59 patients, 98% developed a fourth cranial nerve palsy and 51% partial or complete third nerve palsy. The development of full-blown third nerve palsy was predictive of eventual ventilatory failure; 8 of the 9 patients who required mechanical support showed evidence of complete third nerve palsy, whereas only 1 patient who had ventilatory failure did not have pre-existing complete third nerve palsy. Ventilatory failure secondary to ventilatory muscle weakness occurs in 30% to 60% of affected patients and is the primary cause of mortality.[364, 369] The complication may be very prolonged, although there is usually slow and eventual complete recovery of muscle strength. Despite this, a number of patients continue to complain of fatigability and exertional dyspnea 1 to 2 years after the poisoning episode.[364, 369]

Disorders of the Respiratory Muscles

Muscular Dystrophies

The muscular dystrophies are inherited disorders characterized by progressive weakness of skeletal muscle. They are generally divided into several types. *Duchenne type muscular dystrophy* is a disorder with a sex-linked recessive inheritance pattern that begins in childhood. It is commonly associated with respiratory disease and in fact causes death from ventilatory failure in at least 80% of affected persons.[370] Respiratory involvement typically develops insidiously[371, 372] and, as with other forms of respiratory failure related to muscle weakness, is aggravated during sleep.[373, 374] As in other forms of respiratory failure related to neuromuscular

disease, intermittent ventilatory support can result in an improvement in lung function and a prolongation of useful life.[375] *Facioscapulohumeral dystrophy* is a disorder of autosomal dominant inheritance that begins in adolescence; a syndrome has been described in which the dystrophy is associated with sensorineural hearing loss, tortuosity of retinal arterioles, and an early onset and rapid progression of respiratory failure.[376]

Myotonic dystrophy, inherited in autosomal dominant fashion, can begin at any age. Ventilatory failure develops in approximately 10% of patients;[372, 377] the respiratory difficulties relate both to weakness and to an increase in impedance of the respiratory system secondary to the increased tone in the abdominal and chest wall muscles.[378, 379] The increased tone is caused by inappropriate electrical activity of the muscles during the respiratory cycle.[380] In one investigation of 17 patients who had progressive muscular dystrophy, 9 exhibited myotonia;[381] 12 of the 17 patients had dyspnea or other respiratory symptoms. Although impairment of vital capacity and maximal breathing capacity was more severe in the nonmyotonic patients, those who had myotonia had reduced minute ventilation, hypoxemia, hypercapnia, and pulmonary hypertension.

Acid Maltase Deficiency

Acid maltase deficiency is a disorder with a recessive inheritance pattern that is being recognized with increasing frequency as a cause of neuromuscular ventilatory failure.[382-384] It is caused by a deficiency of the enzyme acid maltase (acid alpha-glucosidase), which leads to an accumulation of glycogen in intracellular vacuoles of muscle and other tissues. The accumulation of glycogen in diaphragmatic muscle cells occurs predominantly in type I (slow twitch) fibers.[385]

The condition occurs in three forms depending on the age at onset: (1) an infantile form, in which patients usually die before the age of 2 years and in which hepatic and splenic enlargement is a prominent finding; (2) a childhood form, characterized by variable muscle and organ involvement and usually by slow progression to respiratory failure; and (3) an adult form, in which specific muscle groups can be involved and the course is even more insidiously progressive.[383] The phenotypic expression is dependent on specific mutatations in the alpha-glucosidase gene.[386] Ventilatory failure is an inevitable development in the majority of patients;[387, 388] in adults, it may be the presenting feature,[387-389] as in 3 of 10 and 4 of 9 patients described in two small series.[383, 390]

Nemaline Myopathy

Nemaline myopathy is a nonprogressive disorder that usually affects neonates and is associated with a relatively good prognosis;[391] however, there is also a rapidly progressive form of the disease that can prove fatal.[392] Although distinctly uncommon in adults, the disorder can present in this group as respiratory failure.[393-395] Some cases are associated with a monoclonal gammopathy.[396] The term *nemaline* derives from the formation in affected muscle cells of rodlike structures composed of nuclear material. Such nemaline bodies have also been reported in the muscles of human immunodeficiency virus (HIV)-infected patients who have generalized skeletal muscle myopathy.[397]

Myopathy in Connective Tissue Disease

Although pulmonary disease in polymyositis and dermatomyositis can be caused by aspiration of gastric contents secondary to pharyngeal muscle paralysis, some patients have sufficient involvement of the respiratory muscles to cause acute or chronic hypoventilation (*see* page 1465). Respiratory muscular dysfunction is sometimes not recognized because of the direction of undue attention to associated bronchiolitis or interstitial pulmonary disease; in such cases, withdrawal of corticosteroid therapy may uncover the underlying muscle weakness. Some patients who have bilateral diaphragmatic paralysis or myopathy appear to have an associated blunting of respiratory drive.[265, 398, 399] The cause of this blunting is not clear; however, there is evidence that it may result from a resetting of central sensitivity to CO_2 attributable to intermittent hypercapnia during sleep-induced hypoventilation.[265, 399]

Muscular weakness has been postulated as the mechanism that causes an apparent shrinking of the lungs in patients who have systemic lupus erythematosus (SLE).[400] In the "shrinking lung syndrome," serial chest radiographs reveal progressive loss of lung volume unassociated with other abnormalities of the lung parenchyma. Although it is clear that patients who have SLE often show a decrease in respiratory muscle strength,[401, 402] the pathogenesis of the weakness has not been established. Generalized neuropathic[403] and myopathic[404] processes are known to occur in patients who have SLE, and either process could involve the diaphragm. However, to date the "shrinking lung syndrome" has been observed mainly in patients who do not have generalized neuromuscular disease. Pulmonary involvement in SLE is discussed in detail in Chapter 39 (*see* page 1432).

Miscellaneous Myopathies

A number of rarer generalized disorders of skeletal muscle also can involve the respiratory muscles, including familial mixed congenital myopathy,[405] Pompe's disease,[406] multicore myopathy,[407] mitochondrial respiratory chain abnormalities,[408–410] and X-linked myotubular myopathy.[411]

Respiratory muscle weakness and resulting ventilatory failure have been reported in patients who have hyperthyroidism[411a] and in asthmatic patients following the parenteral administration of large doses of steroids.[412] Rhabdomyolysis (myoglobinuria) is another rare muscular disease that causes acute respiratory paralysis and hypoventilation.[413, 414] Although the cause of this condition is unknown in most cases, a 23-year-old woman has been described in whom it was associated with a deficiency of muscle carnitine and in whom treatment with *d,l*-carnitine was followed by dramatic improvement.[415]

Acute flaccid paralysis requiring mechanical ventilation has been reported in association with hypophosphatemia;[416, 417] this condition, whether caused by infection or the use of phosphate-binding antacids, can lead to worsening respiratory failure in patients who have COPD and in patients with respiratory failure of other causes who are difficult to wean from artificial respiration.[418] In one patient in whom respiratory failure was secondary to hypophosphatemia, monitoring of phosphocreatine and pH by nuclear magnetic resonance spectroscopy revealed defective muscle metabolism.[419] In another study of 22 patients with COPD and age- and sex-matched control subjects, the muscle phosphorus content of both respiratory and peripheral muscles as measured by spectrophotometric methods was significantly reduced in the COPD patient group;[420] the reduction was thought to be the result of reduced dietary phosphorus intake and abnormal renal phosphorus handling.

Hypokalemia related to familial periodic paralysis, diabetes, diabetic ketoacidosis,[421, 422] or renal tubular acidosis[423] rarely results in sufficient muscle weakness to cause respiratory failure. Severe hypermagnesemia caused by irrigation of the renal pelvis, chronic renal failure, or the ingestion of magnesium-containing antacids can also result in hypoventilation and respiratory failure.[424, 425] Progressive polyneuropathy and myopathy resulting in respiratory failure is the most common cause of death in patients who have the eosinophilia-myalgia syndrome.[426]

ALVEOLAR HYPERVENTILATION

Normally, alveolar ventilation is proportional to the metabolic requirements of the tissues. In response to fever, exertion, or thyrotoxicosis, the demand for O_2 at the tissue level increases, as does CO_2 production. Alveolar ventilation increases, but because the increase is appropriate, arterial P_{CO_2} remains within the normal range. Hyperventilation is ventilation in excess of that required to maintain Pa_{CO_2} between 35 and 40 mm Hg.

Assessment of the adequacy of ventilation requires either direct analysis of the P_{CO_2} in the blood or measurement of the mixed venous P_{CO_2} by the rebreathing technique. Every clinician who has experience in the management of respiratory disease and uses blood gas analysis is aware of the inaccuracy of the clinical appraisal of ventilation. This unreliability was aptly demonstrated in one study that involved students, house staff, and attending staff observing a normal person breathing at different tidal volumes and rates:[258] not only was the clinical estimate of ventilatory volume grossly inaccurate, but individual observers could not repeat their original estimates when the subjects breathed at the same tidal volume. Training and experience were of little help in the clinical assessment of the volume of ventilation. The results of this study also showed that gross degrees of overventilation could be recognized with greater accuracy than underventilation, but there was still a definite tendency to overestimate minute volume.

Hyperventilation that causes a reduction in Pa_{CO_2} to 35 mm Hg or less can result from both pulmonary and extrapulmonary causes.

Pulmonary Disease

Hyperventilation and hypocapnia may occur in patients who have asthma, pneumonia, pulmonary thromboembolism, or diffuse granulomatous or fibrotic interstitial disease. Hypocapnia is usually associated with hypoxemia; however, the Pa_{O_2} may be normal at rest and fall only during exercise in some patients who have diffuse pulmonary fibrosis. Although diffuse interstitial disease sometimes engenders dyspnea on exertion, overventilation at rest seldom causes symptoms by itself.

If the hyperventilation is of recent origin, bicarbonate levels remain relatively elevated in proportion to the Pa_{CO_2}; this is reflected in a lower hydrogen ion concentration (elevated pH). If overventilation is of longer duration, renal compensation for the lowered Pa_{CO_2} results in increased urinary excretion of bicarbonate and a lowered serum bicarbonate level; the hydrogen ion concentration is maintained within normal limits. In some patients who have COPD or asthma, the minute ventilation may be greatly increased over the estimated normal value; yet the Pa_{CO_2} may be normal or higher than normal because of severe $\dot{V}/\dot{Q}$ inequality.

Extrapulmonary Disorders

Central Nervous System Disorders

Central nervous system disorders that can cause hyperventilation include cerebrovascular accidents, trauma, meningitis, and encephalitis. The mechanism by which hyperventilation develops has not been established. Based on the results of a study of patients who had suffered a cerebral hemorrhage, it has been suggested that some breakdown product in the brain is responsible for a rise in hydrogen ion concentration in the CSF that directly stimulates the respiratory center.[427] Blood gas analysis in these patients may indicate respiratory alkalosis.

Cheyne-Stokes Breathing

Cheyne-Stokes respiration is a breathing pattern characterized by a cyclic fluctuation in ventilation in which periods of central apnea or hypopnea alternate with periods of hyperpnea in a gradual crescendo-decrescendo fashion.[428] Tidal volume increases progressively during the phase of hyperpnea and subsequently decreases without change in respiratory rate.[429] This cyclic form of breathing is caused by instability of the ventilatory control system, in which the circulation time, the sensitivity of the central ventilatory controller, and the damping characteristics of the O_2 and CO_2 stores play important roles.[430] Instability of the automatic control systems occurs when the activity of the controller is excessive, either because of a delay in the feedback signal or because the controller is too sensitive or responds to stimulation in a nonlinear fashion.[431] During Cheyne-Stokes respiration there is a paradoxical relationship between blood gas tensions and the level of ventilation because of the delay in feedback; the stage of hyperventilation is associated with a decreased Pa_{O_2} and increased Pa_{CO_2}, while during the apneic phase, Pa_{O_2} and pH are increased and Pa_{CO_2} is decreased.[432]

This form of periodic breathing occurs in patients who have left ventricular failure or impaired cerebrovascular circulation. In the former, the Cheyne-Stokes breathing occurs particularly during sleep and is a poor prognostic sign.[433] Although the respiratory centers of such patients are hypersensitive to CO_2,[434] the fluctuations that occur in mental state, the electroencephalogram, and neurologic signs proba-

bly result primarily from phasic alterations in cerebral circulation.[435] Periodic cardiac dysrhythmias have been noted to occur coincidentally and synchronously with fluctuations in ventilatory pattern.[436]

Psychogenic Hyperventilation

Most commonly, hyperventilation is of psychologic origin. The hyperventilation syndrome has been defined as "a syndrome characterized by a variety of somatic symptoms induced by physiologically inappropriate hyperventilation and usually reproduced in whole or in part by voluntary hyperventilation."[437] Psychogenic hyperventilation varies in degree and clinical presentation; affected patients range from those who complain of dyspnea at rest, and who require frequent deep respiratory efforts, to the hysterical patient who overbreathes to the extent of inducing coma or tetany. Occasionally, psychogenic hyperventilation is epidemic in type; for example, in one secondary school, it occurred in one third of 550 girls, 85 of whom required admission to the hospital.[438] Subsequent psychologic testing of these children revealed an increase in susceptibility to hysteria among those who had reacted the most dramatically.

The psychogenic hyperventilation syndrome has been closely related to a psychiatric condition termed *panic disorder* that is characterized by the sudden onset of extreme fear for which there is no known cause.[439] At least 50% of affected persons suffer from the hyperventilation syndrome, which can develop during the attack; in fact, attacks can be precipitated by voluntary hyperventilation.

The symptoms of psychogenic hyperventilation are primarily neurologic and cardiorespiratory. In one study of 78 patients, neurologic symptoms of giddiness or light-headedness were observed in 59%, paresthesias in 36%, loss of consciousness in 31%, and visual disturbances in 28%;[439] other symptoms included headache, ataxia, tremor, and tinnitus. The mechanism for these symptoms probably consists of both cerebral hypoxia and metabolic alkalosis. By producing hypocapnia, hyperventilation decreases cerebral blood flow and causes a shift of the O_2 dissociation curve to the left, decreasing unloading of O_2 at the tissue level.[440]

Dyspnea and palpitations are the most common cardiorespiratory symptoms, the former occurring in 53% and the latter in 33% of patients in the series just cited.[439] The majority of patients describe the shortness of breath as an inability to "get enough air down into the lungs"; some complain of a smothering feeling at night just before falling asleep or immediately on wakening.[441] They also complain of an inability to take a satisfying breath.[442] In one review of the records of 107 patients in whom the major diagnosis was hyperventilation syndrome of psychologic origin, dyspnea was usually noted at rest;[441] when it was associated with exertion, it characteristically occurred after rather than during effort. In the same report, the author described two types of pain: the first a sharp pain that was thought to be caused by distention of the stomach, and the second a dull, aching tightness in the chest; the latter sensation is the more common of the two and probably results from excessive use of the intercostal muscles.

Although the diagnosis of psychogenic hyperventilation is often readily made on the basis of its characteristic history, in some patients the symptoms may closely simulate those of organic disease. For example, one group of investigators described 19 patients who initially presented with focal neurologic symptoms, such as transient ischemic attacks, or with symptoms suggestive of multiple sclerosis or myasthenia gravis.[443] Hyperventilation can also precipitate migraine headaches[444] or seizure disorders.[445] Although most patients who experience numbness and tingling during periods of hyperventilation state that these sensations are bilateral, some describe them in only one extremity; in one study of 90 volunteers who hyperventilated for 3 to 5 minutes, 16% developed symptoms of unilateral numbness, tingling, weakness, pain, and muscle spasm, usually in an upper extremity.[446]

Spirometry may suggest the diagnosis of psychogenic hyperventilation when its presence is suspected on clinical grounds. The characteristic pattern is highly irregular breathing punctuated by deep inspiration. In the majority of patients, arterial blood gas analysis shows a reduction in $PaCO_2$, usually with a proportionate reduction in bicarbonate levels. The electrocardiogram may reveal depression of the ST segment and a reduction or inversion of the T waves in any or all leads.[441, 447, 448] Hyperventilation also may be associated with junctional tachycardia[448] and has been implicated in the production of angina as a result of coronary spasm.[449] When hyperventilation is severe, the electroencephalogram may record slowed activity.

Although hyperventilation is usually a benign disturbance readily reversible by suggestion or reassurance, in some patients the overbreathing can have serious consequences. For example, it is probable that maternal hyperventilation during labor can result in severe fetal hypoxia and metabolic acidosis.[450, 451] The critical level of PCO_2 in maternal arterial blood is estimated to be 15 to 17 mm Hg—a level unlikely to develop in most spontaneous deliveries, but one that could occur in hysterical patients or in women being maintained on artificial ventilation during cesarean section.[451]

Miscellaneous Causes

Hyperventilation in primary metabolic acidosis results from stimulation of the respiratory center and carotid bodies by an increase in hydrogen ion concentration. The major causes of this type of hyperventilation are the ketosis associated with uncontrolled diabetes and the metabolic acidosis of renal failure. Unlike in other disorders that cause hyperventilation, blood gas analysis reveals acidosis, the hydrogen ion concentration being increased and the bicarbonate level reduced; PaO_2 is within normal limits, and $PaCO_2$ is reduced. Many patients who overventilate as a result of central nervous system lesions or metabolic acidosis are semicomatose; the hyperventilation is obviously an inconsequential feature of a much more complex problem.

Hyperthyroid patients have been shown to have an increase in hypoxic and hypercarbic ventilatory drive[452] and may have an increase in minute ventilation at rest and during exercise.[453] The ingestion of salicylates in sufficiently large quantities to provoke hyperventilation usually occurs accidentally in children but is sometimes associated with suicidal attempts by young adults or abuse of prescribed medications by elderly persons.[454] Salicylates probably act by increasing the sensitivity of the respiratory center to the existing level of CO_2. The acid-base disorder usually consists of a mixed respiratory alkalosis and anion gap–type metabolic acidosis; occasionally, it is an uncomplicated respiratory alkalosis or a pure metabolic acidosis.[454] Salicylate intoxication in young persons is generally considered to be a benign condition associated with a low mortality; however, this is not the case in elderly people, in whom the clinical presentation is often confusing and may suggest cardiopulmonary disease or encephalopathy.[454] Permeability pulmonary edema (ARDS) is a frequent complication and is associated with a high mortality.

Occasionally, patients who have respiratory alkalosis caused by extrapulmonary organic disease develop lactic acidosis, presumably as a "compensatory" mechanism for the alkalotic state.[455–457] In one study, changes in the acid-base balance were measured in 20 patients who were hyperventilated while under anesthesia.[458] Serial arterial blood samples were drawn from 1 to 4 hours after initiation of hyperventilation; in the presence of respiratory alkalosis ($PaCO_2$ of 15 to 20 mm Hg), the hydrogen ion concentration rose, and both total fixed acid and blood lactic acid levels increased.

In patients in whom abnormal prolonged hyperventilation is the result of organic disease,[456, 457] "overcompensation" appears to occur, and the hydrogen ion concentration can actually exceed normal levels, with the patient presenting a picture of acidemia rather than alkalemia. The acidosis can be very difficult to control and can hasten death. Death also has been reported after voluntary hyperventilation in a patient who had chronic alveolar hypoventilation associated with a PaO_2 of 38 mm Hg and a $PaCO_2$ of 83 mm Hg;[459] when he was requested to hyperventilate, the pH rose from 7.39 to 7.63, and apnea and convulsions promptly ensued. Intensive therapy resulted in the patient's becoming alert once again, but apnea recurred and was followed by ventricular fibrillation and death.

EXTRAPULMONARY VENOARTERIAL SHUNTS

Oxygen transport to the tissues may be inadequate despite normal structure and function of the lung parenchyma, airways, and respiratory pump. In these circumstances, the hypoxemia is caused by shunting of venous blood into arterial channels, and blood gas analysis reveals a reduced PaO_2 and a normal or reduced $PaCO_2$. The most common cause of such shunting is congenital heart disease; although this is usually manifested radiographically by pulmonary pleonemia or hypertension (*see* page 664), the chest radiographs may also be normal. Shunting also may be the result of abnormal venoarterial communications associated with hepatic disease or intrapulmonary arteriovenous malformations (*see* page 655).

A form of extrapulmonary venoarterial shunting is found in some patients who have advanced cirrhosis. Such patients usually have normal chest radiographs, and evidence of shunting lies in the results of arterial blood gas analyses revealing mild to moderate hypoxemia and respiratory alkalosis.[460, 461] The lowered $PaCO_2$ is balanced by a proportional decrease in bicarbonate, indicating that a prolonged state of hyperventilation has resulted in compensation through renal excretion of bicarbonate. In one study of 34 patients who had cirrhosis and 20 healthy persons, the mean SaO_2 was 93.2% in the patients and 95.8% in the normal subjects;[462] the mean PaO_2 in 17 of the patients was 73 mm Hg, and in the control group, 95 mm Hg.

There is reason to believe that more than one mechanism is responsible for the hypoxemia associated with cirrhosis, the shunt being extrapulmonary in some patients and intrapulmonary in others. In the extrapulmonary form, blood from the portal system reaches the left side of the heart through anastomoses with pulmonary veins. This was believed to be the explanation in a patient in whom 40% of cardiac output was shunted from right to left and in whom careful pathologic examination of the lungs failed to reveal arteriovenous fistulas.[463] In one investigation of five patients who had cirrhosis, radioactive krypton was injected into the spleen in an attempt to determine the mechanism of hypoxemia;[464] definite portopulmonary anastomoses were apparent in only one case.

METHEMOGLOBINEMIA

Methemoglobin is hemoglobin in which the ferrous iron has been oxidized to the ferric form. Blood turns a chocolate-brown color when approximately 15% of hemoglobin is oxidized to methemoglobin; the result is "cyanosis" that is unresponsive to O_2 therapy.[465] Methemoglobinemia can result from exposure to drugs or chemicals that act by increasing the rate of hemoglobin oxidation or by exhausting the erythrocyte mechanisms that protect hemoglobin against oxidation.[466–468] It can also result from impairment of the capacity to reduce hemoglobin, on either an enzymatic or a chemical basis.

Acquired methemoglobinemia is most often caused by nitrates, which can be introduced into the body in several ways. The condition has been reported to follow the ingestion of well water containing a high concentration of nitrate;[469] a case has also been reported of a patient on renal dialysis who developed methemoglobinemia as a result of the use of nitrate-contaminated well water as the dialysate.[470] The disorder has also occurred following the use of topically applied nitrate in the treatment of burns,[471] following the ingestion of meat to which nitrates (saltpeter) have been applied as preservatives,[472] and as a result of absorption of nitrates through skin burned in a chemical explosion.[465] It can also result because of the use of Cetacaine[473] or other topical anesthetic containing prilocaine,[474] benzocaine,[475] or lidocaine.[476] Methemoglobinemia is also seen after therapy or accidental and suicidal overdosage with dapsone[477, 478] and with the use of vasodilating nitrates as aphrodisiacs.[479, 480] Clinically significant levels of methemoglobinemia are not reached during therapeutic administration of inhaled nitric oxide.[481, 482]

Two types of hereditary methemoglobinemia have been described. One form is related to a generalized abnormality of the nicotinamide adenine dinucleotide (NADH) cytochrome b_5 reductase enzyme; in this variant, the methemoglobinemia is associated with severe mental retardation and neurologic impairment.[466, 483] In the other form of disease, only the soluble form of the NADH enzyme, which is present in red blood cells, is affected, and cyanosis is the only consequence.[484]

Methemoglobinemia causes no alteration in the chest radiograph. Patients usually present with symptoms and signs related to tissue anoxia, including headache, nausea, dizziness, pounding pulse, and listlessness.[467] In most cases, there is a diffuse, persistent, grayish discoloration of the skin; however, this may not be obvious. The diagnosis may be suspected when pulse oximetry shows SaO_2 values that are inappropriately low for the measured PaO_2.[485, 486]

CARBON MONOXIDE POISONING

Carbon monoxide (CO) is an odorless, colorless gas that binds in a reversible manner with hemoglobin and has an affinity for the hemoglobin-binding site that is 200 times greater than that of O_2. The ensuing compound, carboxyhemoglobin (COHb), shifts the O_2 dissociation curve to the left and has a direct toxic effect on the cytochrome enzymes.[487, 488]

CO poisoning is the most frequent cause of poisoning death in the United States.[489] Acute poisoning most frequently results from inhalation of motor vehicle exhaust fumes in suicide attempts;[490, 491] less often, it occurs in association with defective heating and cooking systems[492] or the inappropriate use of such systems indoors.[493] Small epidemics of acute and chronic CO poisoning related to the use of such devices have been reported during severe winter storms and exceptionally cold winters.[493, 494]

Additional scenarios associated with unintentional CO poisoning include house fires,[495] indoor cooking with charcoal briquettes,[496, 497] travel in the back of a pickup truck,[498] and exposure to exhaust from systems obstructed by a heavy snowfall[499] or from a propane-powered fork lift,[500] gasoline-powered motors on recreational boats,[501] indoor skating rinks,[502] or mine explosions and the use of concrete saws and other devices indoors.[503] A more unusual source is the use of paint remover containing methylene chloride, which is converted to CO in the blood.[488, 504]

The deleterious effects of CO in humans appear to be attributable to two factors: (1) tissue hypoxia resulting from the formation of COHb, which reduces the O_2 transport capacity of the blood and causes a shift of the oxyhemoglobin dissociation curve to the left, thus curtailing the amount of O_2 available to the tissues; and (2) a direct cytotoxic effect.[505] Characteristically, clinical symptoms, which include headache, nausea and vomiting, and decreased manual dexterity, develop when carboxyhemoglobin saturation reaches 20%; unconsciousness and convulsions occur at about 50% to 60%, and death at about 80%.[487] Acute poisoning can cause death as a result of either cerebral anoxia[506] or the development of ARDS;[507] the pulmonary edema in the latter situation may be the result of a direct effect of CO on the permeability of the alveolocapillary membrane.[507] Generalized rhabdomyolysis and acute renal failure are occasional complications.[508] Severe CO poisoning can result in persistent derangements of pulmonary function[509, 510] and neuropsychiatric abnormalities,[511] including personality deterioration and memory impairment.[512]

Of possibly even greater significance than acute CO poisoning is the morbidity associated with long-term exposure to low concentrations of the gas. The blood COHb level in healthy nonsmoking persons is about 0.5%.[513] By contrast, the average COHb level of a person who smokes one pack of cigarettes a day is about 6%,[514] a figure that may rise to between 10% and 20% with heavy smoking.[513, 515] It is obvious that such persons will develop significant hypoxia, particularly if they live at high altitudes. The percentage of inspired CO may be increased in heavy traffic, because car exhausts contain between 1% and 7% CO;[516] it may also rise in closed breathing circuits during anesthesia or in closed air systems such as in submarines.[514] It has been shown that blood levels of COHb less than 2% may result in interference with time-duration discrimination, and that automobile drivers involved in accidents have higher levels of COHb than those in controls.[514] Low levels of CO increase myocardial ischemia and induce angina after less cardiac work than is required in control patients breathing room air.[517, 518]

Abnormalities occasionally may be detected on the chest radiograph in acute CO poisoning. In a study of 62 patients observed over a 2-year period, investigators observed abnormalities in 18 (30%).[519] The age range of the 14 males and 48 females was 1 to 84 years (mean, 30.8 ± 4.2 years). The most common radiographic abnormality, observed in 11 of the 18 patients, was a ground-glass opacity of homogeneous density occurring predominantly in the lung periphery. An air bronchogram was not identified, nor was there evidence of pulmonary venous hypertension. The abnormality was attributed to parenchymal interstitial edema,

probably caused by a combination of tissue hypoxia and a direct toxic effect of CO on the alveolocapillary membrane. The second most common change, observed in six cases, was a parahilar haze with peribronchial and perivascular cuffing caused by interstitial edema. In these cases, there was usually cardiac enlargement, suggesting the presence of myocardial damage. In some cases, the ground-glass appearance, parahilar haze, bronchial vascular cuffing, and cardiac enlargement coexisted in various combinations. Intra-alveolar edema was identified in three patients, all of whom had convincing evidence of cardiac enlargement. In this series, hyperbaric O_2 therapy at a pressure of 2 atmospheres was administered to all patients immediately after admission. Radiographic abnormalities cleared in most patients by 3 days and in all by 5 days; however, the presence of parahilar haze or intra-alveolar edema signified a poor overall prognosis despite radiographic resolution. Cases of acute pulmonary edema following CO intoxication have also been reported by other authors.[520, 521]

CO toxicity can be detected by measuring COHb levels. Pulse oximetry is unreliable in detecting O_2 saturation in CO-exposed patients, because it cannot distinguish between COHb and oxyhemoglobin.[522] In the presence of significant CO exposure, there may be a "pulse oximetry gap"; the difference between the pulse oximetry value for O_2 saturation and the true oxyhemoglobin saturation is approximately equal to the level of COHb.[522, 523]

REFERENCES

1. Brogdon BG, Kelsey CA, Moseley RD Jr: Factors affecting perception of pulmonary lesions. Radiol Clin North Am 21:633, 1983.
2. Austin JHM, Romney BM, Goldsmith LS: Missed bronchogenic carcinoma: Radiographic findings in 27 patients with a potentially resectable lesion evident in retrospect. Radiology 182:115, 1992.
3. Rigler LG: Roentgen examination of the chest. Its limitations in the diagnosis of disease. JAMA 142:773, 1950.
4. Worsley DF, Alavi A, Aronchick JM, et al: Chest radiographic findings in patients with acute pulmonary embolism: Observations from the PIOPED study. Radiology 189:133, 1993.
5. Liebow AA, Hales MR, Bloomer WE, et al: Studies on the lung after ligation of the pulmonary artery. II. Anatomical changes. Am J Pathol 26:177, 1950.
6. Steele JD, Buell P: Asymptomatic solitary pulmonary nodules. Host survival, tumor size, and growth rate. J Thorac Cardiovasc Surg 65:140, 1973.
7. Findling JW, Tyrrell JB: Occult ectopic secretion of corticotropin. Arch Intern Med 146:929, 1986.
8. Kwong JS, Carignan S, Kang E-Y, et al: Miliary tuberculosis: Diagnostic accuracy of chest radiography. Chest 110:339, 1996.
9. Müller NL, Kullnig P, Miller RR: The CT findings of pulmonary sarcoidosis: Analysis of 25 patients. Am J Roentgenol 152:1179, 1989.
10. Müller NL. Clinical value of high-resolution CT in chronic diffuse lung disease. Am J Roentgenol 157:1163, 1991.
11. Young RL, Krumholz RA, with the technical assistance of Harkleroad LE: A physiologic roentgenographic disparity in sarcoidosis. Dis Chest 50:81, 1966.
12. Snider GL, Doctor L: The mechanics of ventilation in sarcoidosis. Am Rev Respir Dis 89:897, 1964.
13. Adhikari PK, Bianchi F, Boushy SF, et al: Pulmonary function in scleroderma. Its relation to changes in the chest roentgenogram and the skin of the thorax. Am Rev Respir Dis 86:823, 1962.
14. Marshall R, Smellie H, Baylis JH, et al: Pulmonary function in sarcoidosis. Thorax 13:48, 1958.
15. Orens JB, Kazerooni EA, Martinez FJ, et al: The sensitivity of high-resolution CT in detecting idiopathic pulmonary fibrosis proved by open lung biopsy: A prospective study. Chest 108:109, 1995.
16. Remy-Jardin M, Remy J, Wallaert B, et al: Subacute and chronic bird breeder hypersensitivity pneumonitis: Sequential evaluation with CT and correlation with lung function tests and bronchoalveolar lavage. Radiology 189:111, 1993.
17. Wilson RJ, Rodnan GP, Robin ED: An early pulmonary physiologic abnormality in progressive systemic sclerosis (diffuse scleroderma). Am J Med 36:361, 1964.
18. Ritchie B: Pulmonary function in scleroderma. Thorax 19:28, 1964.
19. Huang CT, Lyons HA: Comparison of pulmonary function in patients with systemic lupus erythematosus, scleroderma and rheumatoid arthritis. Am Rev Respir Dis 93:865, 1966.
20. Remy-Jardin M, Remy J, Cortet B, et al: Lung changes in rheumatoid arthritis: CT findings. Radiology 193:375, 1994.
21. Bankier AA, Kiener HP, Wiesmayr MN, et al: Discreet lung involvement in systemic lupus erythematosus: CT assessment. Radiology 196:835, 1995.
22. Huang CT, Hennigar GR, Lyons HA: Pulmonary dysfunction in systemic lupus erythematosus. N Engl J Med 272:288, 1965.
23. Green RA, Nichols NJ: Pulmonary involvement in leukemia. Am Rev Respir Dis 80:833, 1959.
24. Resnick ME, Berkowitz RD, Rodman T: Diffuse interstitial leukemic infiltration of the lungs producing the alveolar-capillary block syndrome. Report of a case, with studies of pulmonary function. Am J Med 31:149, 1961.
25. Pace WR Jr, Decker JL, Martin CJ: Polymyositis: Report of two cases with pulmonary function studies suggestive of progressive systemic sclerosis. Am J Med Sci 245:322, 1963.
26. Blackie S, Al-Majed S, Staples C, et al: Changes in total lung capacity during acute spontaneous asthma. Am Rev Respir Dis 142:79, 1990.
27. Gudbjerg CE: Bronchiectasis: Radiological diagnosis and prognosis after operative treatment. Acta Radiol Suppl 143, 1957.
28. van der Bruggen-Bogaarts BAHA, van der Bruggen HMJG, van Waes PFGM, et al: Screening for bronchiectasis: A comparative study between chest radiography and high-resolution CT. Chest 109:608, 1996.
29. Thurlbeck WM, Henderson JA, Fraser RG, et al: Chronic obstructive lung disease. A comparison between clinical, roentgenologic, functional and morphological criteria in chronic bronchitis, emphysema, asthma and bronchiectasis. Medicine 49:81, 1970.
30. Thurlbeck WM, Simon G: Radiographic appearance of the chest in emphysema. Am J Roentgenol 130:429, 1978.
31. Weisel W, Lepley D Jr, Watson RR: Respiratory tract adenomas: A ten-year study. Ann Surg 154:898, 1961.
32. Woolner LB, Andersen HA, Bernatz PE: "Occult" carcinoma of the bronchus: A study of 15 cases of in situ or early invasive bronchogenic carcinoma. Dis Chest 37:278, 1960.
33. Melamed MR, Koss LG, Cliffton EE: Roentgenologically occult lung cancer diagnosed by cytology. Report of 12 cases. Cancer 16:1537, 1963.
34. Holman CW, Okinaka A: Occult carcinoma of the lung. J Thorac Cardiovasc Surg 47:466, 1964.
35. Singer DB, Greenberg SD, Harrison GM: Papillomatosis of the lung. Am Rev Respir Dis 94:777, 1966.
36. Greenfield H, Herman PG: Papillomatosis of the trachea and bronchi. Am J Roentgenol 89:45, 1963.
37. Sanders JS, Carnes VM: Leiomyoma of the trachea. Report of a case, with a note on the diagnosis of partial tracheal obstruction. N Engl J Med 264:277, 1961.
38. Spinka J, Zwetschke O: Tracheal lipoma simulating the picture of severe bronchial asthma. Cas Lek Cesk 101:395, 1962.
39. Berthelot P, Walker JG, Sherlocks S, et al: Arterial changes in the lungs in cirrhosis of the liver—lung spider nevi. N Engl J Med 274:291, 1966.
40. Furukawa T, Hara N, Yasumoto K, et al: Arterial hypoxemia in patients with hepatic cirrhosis. Am J Med Sci 287:10, 1984.
41. Krowka MJ, Cortese DA: Pulmonary aspects of chronic liver disease and liver transplantation. Mayo Clin Proc 60:407, 1985.
42. Sherlock S: The liver-lung interface. Semin Respir Med 9:247, 1988.
43. Mélot C, Naeije R, Dechamps P, et al: Pulmonary and extrapulmonary contributors to hypoxemia in liver cirrhosis. Am Rev Respir Dis 139:632, 1989.
44. Schaefer JW, Reeves JT: The lung and the liver. Chest 80:526, 1981.
45. Vergnon JM, De Bonadona JF, Riffat J, et al: Techniques for the exploration of pulmonary arteriovenous shunts in liver cirrhosis. Apropos of 2 cases. Rev Mal Respir 3:145, 1986.
46. Wolfe JD, Taskin DP, Holly FE, et al: Hypoxemia of cirrhosis. Detection of abnormal small pulmonary vascular channels by a quantitative radionuclide method. Am J Med 63:746, 1977.
47. Chen NS, Barnett CA, Farrer PA: Reversibility of intrapulmonary arteriovenous shunts in liver cirrhosis documented by serial radionuclide perfusion lung scans. Clin Nucl Med 9:279, 1984.
48. Shub C, Tajik AJ, Seward JB, et al: Detecting intrapulmonary right to left shunt with contrast echocardiography: Observations in a patient with diffuse pulmonary arteriovenous fistulas. Mayo Clin Proc 51:81, 1976.
49. Stanley MN, Woodgate DJ: Mottled chest radiograph and gas transfer defect in chronic liver disease. Thorax 27:315, 1972.
50. Robin ED, Horn B, Goris ML, et al: Detection, quantitation and pathophysiology of lung "spiders." Trans Assoc Am Physicians 88:202, 1975.
51. Robin ED, Laman D, Horn BR, et al: Platypnea related to orthodeoxia caused by true vascular shunts. N Engl J Med 294:941, 1976.
52. Kennedy TC, Knudson RJ: Exercise-aggravated hypoxemia and orthodeoxia in cirrhosis. Chest 72:305, 1977.
53. Brownstein MH, Ballard HS: Hepatoma associated with erythrocytosis. Report of eleven new cases. Am J Med 40:204, 1966.
54. Palmer KNV, Gardiner AJS, McGregor MH: Hypoxaemia after partial gastrectomy. Thorax 20:73, 1965.
55. Diament ML, Palmer KNV: Postoperative changes in gas tensions of arterial blood and in ventilatory function. Lancet 2:180, 1966.
56. Diament ML, Palmer KNV: Venous/arterial pulmonary shunting as the principal cause of postoperative hypoxemia. Lancet 1:15, 1967.
57. Taxman RM, Halloran MJ, Parker BM: Multiple pulmonary arteriovenous malformations in association with Fanconi's syndrome. Chest 64:118, 1973.
58. Papagiannis J, Kanter RJ, Effman EL, et al: Polysplenia with pulmonary arteriovenous malformations. Pediatr Cardiol 14:127, 1993.
59. Collins JD, Burwell D, Furmanski S, et al: Minimal detectable pleural effusions. Radiology 105:51, 1972.
60. Müller R, Löfstedt S: The reaction of the pleura in primary tuberculosis of the lungs. Acta Med Scand 122:105, 1945.
61. Hessen I: Roentgen examination of pleural fluid: A study of the localization of free effusion, the potentialities of diagnosing minimal quantities of fluid and its existence under physiological conditions. Acta Radiol Suppl 86:1, 1951.
62. Svenes KB, Borgersen A, Haaversen O, et al: Parietal pleural plaques: A comparison between autopsy and X-ray findings. Eur J Respir Dis 69:10, 1986.
63. Martin L: Hypoventilation without elevated carbon dioxide tension. Chest 77:720, 1980.
64. Wathen CG, Capewell SJ, Heath JP, et al: Recurrent lobar pneumonia associated with idiopathic Eaton-Lambert syndrome. Thorax 43:574, 1988.
65. Berger AJ, Mitchell RA, Feveringhaus JW: Regulation of respiration (first of three parts). N Engl J Med 297:92, 1977.
66. Berger AJ, Mitchell RA, Feveringhaus JW: Regulation of respiration (second of three parts). N Engl J Med 297:138, 1977.
67. Berger AJ, Mitchell RA, Feveringhaus JW: Regulation of respiration (third of three parts). N Engl J Med 297:194, 1977.
68. Hornbein TF, Lenfant C (eds): Regulation of Breathing, Parts 1 and 2. Lung Biology in Health and Disease. New York, Marcel Dekker, 1981.
69. Armand BL, Denavit-Sauvbié M, Champagnat J: Central control of breathing in mammals: Neuronal circuitry, membrane properties, and neurotransmitters. Physiol Rev 75:1, 1995.
70. Mateika JH, Duffin J: A review of the control of breathing during exercise. Eur J Appl Physiol 71:1, 1995.
71. Sant'Ambrogio G, Tsubone H, Sant'Ambrogio FB: Sensory information from the upper airway: Role in the control of breathing. Respir Physiol 102:1, 1995.
72. Henke KG, Badr MS, Skatrud JB, et al: Load compensation and respiratory muscle function during sleep. J Appl Physiol 72:1221, 1992.
73. Ford GT, Whitelaw WA, Rosenal TW, et al: Diaphragm function after upper-abdominal surgery in humans. Am Rev Respir Dis 127:431, 1983.
74. Newsom Davis J: Control of the muscles of respiration. *In* Widdicombe JB

(ed): Respiratory Physiology (MTP International Review of Science—Physiology Series: Vol 2). Baltimore, University Park Press, 1974, pp 221–245.

75. Guilleminault C, Stoohs R, Quera-Salva MA: Sleep-related obstructive and nonobstructive apneas and neurologic disorders. Neurology 42:53, 1992.

76. Spear PW, Protass LM: Barbiturate poisoning—an endemic disease. Five years' experience in a municipal hospital. Med Clin North Am 57:1471, 1973.

77. Jay SJ, Johanson WG Jr, Pierce AK: Respiratory complications of overdose with sedative drugs. Am Rev Respir Dis 112:591, 1975.

78. Hansen AR, Kennedy KA, Ambre JJ, et al: Glutethimide poisoning. A metabolite contributes to morbidity and mortality. N Engl J Med 292:250, 1975.

79. Clark TJH, Collins JV, Tong D: Respiratory depression caused by nitrazepam in patients with respiratory failure. Lancet 2:737, 1971.

80. Hall SC, Ovassapian A: Apnea after intravenous diazepam therapy. JAMA 238:1052, 1977.

81. Varma AJ, Fisher BK, Sarin MK: Diazepam-induced coma with bullae and eccrine sweat gland necrosis. Arch Intern Med 137:1207, 1977.

82. Matthew H, Proudfoot AT, Brown SS, et al: Acute poisoning: Organization and work-load of a treatment centre. BMJ 3:489, 1969.

83. Biggs JT, Spiker DG, Petit JM, et al: Tricyclic antidepressant overdose. Incidence of symptoms. JAMA 238:135, 1977.

84. Teehan BP, Maher JF, Carey JJH, et al: Acute etchlorvynol (Placidyl) intoxication. Ann Intern Med 72:875, 1970.

85. Management of unconscious poisoned patients. BMJ 2:647, 1969.

86. Maddock RK Jr, Bloomer HA: Meprobamate overdosage. Evaluation of its severity and methods of treatment. JAMA 201:123, 1967.

87. Neligan P, Harriman DGF, Pearce J: Respiratory arrest in familial hemiplegic migraine: A clinical and neuropathological study. BMJ 2:732, 1977.

88. Goswami U, Channabasavanna SM: On the lethality of acute respiratory component of tardive dyskinesia. Clin Neurol Neurosurg 87:99, 1985.

89. Chiang E, Pitts WM, Rodriguez-Garcia M: Respiratory dyskinesia: Review and case reports. J Clin Psychiatry 46:232, 1985.

90. Kuna ST, Awan R: The irregularly irregular pattern of respiratory dyskinesia. Chest 90:779, 1986.

91. Cirignotta F, Lugaresi E, Montagna P: Breathing impairment in Rett syndrome. Am J Med Genet 24(suppl 1):167, 1986.

92. Lugaresi E, Cirignotta F, Montagna P: Abnormal breathing in the Rett syndrome. Brain Develop 7:329, 1985.

93. Bradley TD, Day A, Hyland RH, et al: Chronic ventilatory failure caused by abnormal respiratory pattern generation during sleep. Am Rev Respir Dis 130:678, 1984.

94. Southall DP, Kerr AM, Tirosh E, et al: Hyperventilation in the awake state: Potentially treatable component of Rett syndrome. Arch Dis Child 63:1039, 1988.

95. Severinghaus JW, Mitchell RA: Ondine's curse—failure of respiratory center automaticity while awake. Clin Res 10:122, 1962.

96. Ahmad M, Cressman M, Tomashefski JF: Central alveolar hypoventilation syndromes. Arch Intern Med 140:29, 1980.

97. Guilleminault C, Robinson A: Central sleep apnea. Sleep Disord 14:611, 1996.

98. Thalhofer S, Dorow P: Central sleep apnea. Respiration 64:2, 1997.

99. Mellins RB, Balfour HH Jr, Turino GM, et al: Failure of automatic control of ventilation (Ondine's curse): Report of an infant born with this syndrome and review of the literature. Medicine 49:487, 1970.

100. Naughton J, Block R, Welch M: Central alveolar hypoventilation: A case report. Am Rev Respir Dis 103:557, 1971.

101. Farmer WC, Glenn WW, Gee JB: Alveolar hypoventilation syndrome. Studies of ventilatory control in patients selected for diaphragm pacing. Am J Med 64:39, 1978.

102. Shea SA, Andres LP, Shannon DC, et al: Respiratory sensations in subjects who lack a ventilatory response to CO_2. Respir Physiol 93:203, 1993.

103. Paton JY, Swaminathan S, Sargent CW, et al: Ventilatory response to exercise in children with congenital central hypoventilation syndrome. Am Rev Respir Dis 147:1185, 1993.

104. Gozal D, Marcus CL, Shoseyov D, Keens TG: Peripheral chemoreceptor function in children with the congenital central hypoventilation syndrome. J Appl Physiol 74:379, 1993.

105. Kryger MH: Central apnea. Arch Intern Med 142:1793, 1982.

106. Adickes ED, Buehler BA, Sanger WG: Familial lethal sleep apnea. Hum Genet 73:39, 1986.

107. Manon-Espaillat R, Gothe B, Adams N, et al: Familial "sleep apnea plus" syndrome: Report of a family. Neurology 38:190, 1988.

108. Kerbl R, Litscher H, Grubbauer HM, et al: Congenital central hypoventilation syndrome (Ondine's curse syndrome) in two siblings: Delayed diagnosis and successful noninvasive treatment. Eur J Pediatr 155:977, 1996.

109. Weese-Mayer DE, Silvestri JM, Marazita ML, Hoo JJ: Congenital central hypoventilation syndrome: Inheritance and relation to sudden infant death syndrome. Am J Med Genet 47:360, 1993.

110. Yasuma F, Nomura H, Sotobata I, et al: Congenital central alveolar hypoventilation (Ondine's curse): A case report and review of the literature. Eur J Pediatr 146:81, 1987.

111. Mather SJ: Ondine's curse and the anesthetist. Anaesthesia 42:394, 1987.

112. Hedner J, Hedner T, Breese GR, et al: Changes in cerebrospinal fluid homovanillic acid in children with Ondine's curse. Pediatr Pulmonol 3:131, 1987.

113. Perry TL, Wright JM, Berry K, et al: Dominantly inherited apathy, central hypoventilation, and Parkinson's syndrome: Clinical, biochemical, and neuropathologic studies of 2 new cases. Neurology 40:1882, 1990.

114. Kitamura J, Kubuki Y, Tsuruta K, et al: A new family with Joseph disease in

Japan. Homovanillic acid, magnetic resonance, and sleep apnea studies. Arch Neurol 46:425, 1989.

115. Beckerman R, Meltzer J, Sola A, et al: Brain-stem auditory response in Ondine's syndrome. Arch Neurol 43:698, 1986.

116. Long KJ, Allen N: Abnormal brain-stem auditory evoked potentials following Ondine's curse. Arch Neurol 41:1109, 1984.

117. Igarashi M, Rose DF, Storgion SA: Moebius syndrome and central respiratory dysfunction. Pediatr Neurol 16:237, 1997.

118. Slee JJ, Smart RD, Viljoen DL: Deletion of chromosome 13 in Moebius syndrome. J Med Genet 28:413, 1991.

119. Fujita I, Koyanagi T, Kukita J, et al: Moebius syndrome with central hypoventilation and brainstem calcification: A case report. Eur J Pediatr 150:582, 1991.

120. Cummiskey J, Guilleminault C, Davis R, et al: Automatic respiratory failure: Sleep studies and Leigh's disease (case report). Neurology 37:1876, 1987.

121. Hunter AR: Idiopathic alveolar hypoventilation in Leber's disease. Unusual sensitivity to mild analgesics and diazepam. Anaesthesia 39:781, 1984.

122. Paré JAP, Lowenstein L: Polycythemia associated with disturbed function of the respiratory center. Blood 2:1077, 1956.

123. Rodman R, Close HP: The primary hypoventilation syndrome. Am J Med 26:808, 1959.

124. Lawrence LT: Idiopathic hypoventilation, polycythemia, and cor pulmonale. Am Rev Respir Dis 80:575, 1959.

125. Rodman TR, Resnick ME, Berkowitz RD, et al: Alveolar hypoventilation due to involvement of the respiratory center by obscure disease of the central nervous system. Am J Med 32:208, 1962.

126. Tsitouris G, Fertakis A: Alveolar hypoventilation due to respiratory center dysfunction of unknown cause. Am J Med 39:173, 1965.

127. Grant JL, Arnold W Jr: Idiopathic hypoventilation. JAMA 194:119, 1965.

128. Richter T, West JR, Fishman AP: The syndrome of alveolar hypoventilation and diminished sensitivity of the respiratory center. N Engl J Med 256:1165, 1957.

129. Paine CJ, Hargrove MD Jr: Primary alveolar hypoventilation in a thin young woman. Chest 63:854, 1973.

130. Sukumalchantra Y, Tongmitr V, Tanphaichitr V, et al: Primary alveolar hypoventilation. A case report with hemodynamic study. Am Rev Respir Dis 98:1037, 1968.

131. Vingerhoets F, Bogousslavsky J: Respiratory dysfunction in stroke. Clin Chest Med 15:729, 1994.

132. Valente S, De Rosa M, Culla G, et al: An uncommon case of brainstem tumor with selective involvement of the respiratory centers. Chest 103:1909, 1993.

133. Cohn JE, Kuida H: Primary alveolar hypoventilation associated with western equine encephalitis. Ann Intern Med 56:633, 1962.

134. White DP, Miller F, Erickson RW: Sleep apnea and nocturnal hypoventilation after western equine encephalitis. Am Rev Respir Dis 127:132, 1983.

135. Udwadia ZF, Athale S, Misra VP: Radiation necrosis causing failure of automatic ventilation during sleep with central sleep apnea. Chest 92:567, 1987.

136. Polatty RC, Cooper KR: Respiratory failure after percutaneous cordotomy. South Med J 79:897, 1986.

137. Beamish D, Wildsmith JA: Ondine's curse after carotid endarterectomy. BMJ 2:1607, 1978.

138. Nakahara S, Yokomori K, Tamura K, et al: Hirschsprung's disease associated with Ondine's curse: A special subgroup? J Pediatr Surg 30:1481, 1995.

139. Verloes A, Elmer C, Lacombe D, et al: Ondine-Hirschsprung syndrome (Haddad syndrome). Eur J Pediatr 152:75, 1993.

140. O'Dell K, Staren E, Bassuk A: Total colonic aganglionosis (Zuelzer-Wilson syndrome) and congenital failure of automatic control of ventilation (Ondine's curse). J Pediatr Surg 22:1019, 1987.

141. Bolk S, Angrist M, Schwartz S, et al: Congenital central hypoventilation syndrome: Mutation analysis of the receptor tyrosine kinase RET. Am J Med Genet 63:603, 1996.

142. el-Halaby E, Coran AG: Hirschsprung's disease associated with Ondine's curse: Report of three cases and review of the literature. J Pediatr Surg 29:530, 1994.

143. Auer RN, Rowlands CG, Perry SF, Remmers JE: Multiple sclerosis with medullary plaques and fatal sleep apnea (Ondine's curse). Clin Neuropathol 15:101, 1996.

144. Bogousslavsky J, Khurana R, Deruaz JP, et al: Respiratory failure and unilateral caudal brainstem infarction. Ann Neurol 28:668, 1990.

145. Javaheri S. Central sleep apnea-hypopnea syndrome in heart failure: Prevalence, impact, and treatment. Sleep 19(Suppl):S229, 1996.

146. Bradley TD, McNicholas WT, Rutherford R, et al: Clinical and physiologic heterogeneity of the central sleep apnea syndrome. Am Rev Respir Dis 134:217, 1986.

147. Raetzo MA, Junod AF, Kryger MH: Effect of aminophylline and relief from hypoxia on central sleep apnoea due to medullary damage. Bull Eur Physiopathol Respir 23:171, 1987.

148. McNicholas WT, Carter JL, Rutherford R, et al: Beneficial effect of oxygen in primary alveolar hypoventilation with central sleep apnea. Am Rev Respir Dis 125:773, 1982.

149. Bubis MJ, Anthonisen NR: Primary alveolar hypoventilation treated by nocturnal administration of O_2. Am Rev Respir Dis 118:947, 1978.

150. Barlow PB, Bartlett D, Hauri P, et al: Idiopathic hypoventilation syndrome: Importance of preventing nocturnal hypoxemia and hypercapnia. Am Rev Respir Dis 121:141, 1980.

151. Lugaresi E, Cirignotta F, Rossi PG, et al: Infantile behavioural regression and respiratory impairment. Neuropediatrics 15:211, 1984.

152. Schiller J: A note on the pickwickian syndrome and Felix Platter (1536–1614). J Hist Med 40:66, 1985.

153. Kerr WJ, Lagen JB: The postural syndrome related to obesity leading to postural emphysema and cardiorespiratory failure. Ann Intern Med 10:569, 1936.

154. Burwell CS, Robin ED, Whaley RD, et al: Extreme obesity associated with alveolar hypoventilation—a pickwickian syndrome. Am J Med 21:811, 1956.

155. Ahmed Q, Chung-Park M, Tomashefski JF, Jr: Cardiopulmonary pathology in patients with sleep apnea/obesity hypoventilation syndrome. Hum Pathol 28:264, 1997.

156. The Chicago criteria for measurements, definitions and severity rating of sleep-disordered breathing in adults. Report of an American Sleep Disorders Association Task Force, in conjunction with The European Respiratory Society, The Australian Sleep Association, and the American Thoracic Society. (In press.)

157. Phillipson EA: Pickwickian, obesity-hypoventilation, or Fee-Fi-Fo-Fum syndrome? Am Rev Respir Dis 121:781, 1980.

158. Lopata M, Onal E: Mass loading, sleep apnea, and the pathogenesis of obesity hypoventilation. Am Rev Respir Dis 126:640, 1982.

159. Sugerman HJ: Pulmonary function in morbid obesity. Gastroenterol Clin North Am 16:225, 1987.

160. Sugerman HJ, Baron PL, Fairman RP, et al: Hemodynamic dysfunction in obesity hypoventilation syndrome and the effects of treatment with surgically induced weight loss. Ann Surg 207:604, 1988.

161. Drenick EJ, Baie GS, Seltzer F, et al: Excessive mortality and causes of death in morbidly obese men. JAMA 243:443, 1980.

162. Sun SF, Huang SY, Zhang JG, et al: Decreased ventilation and hypoxic ventilatory responsiveness are not reversed by naloxone in Lhasa residents with chronic mountain sickness. Am Rev Respir Dis 142:1294, 1990.

163. Pei SX, Chen XJ, Si Ren BZ, et al: Chronic mountain sickness in Tibet. Q J Med 71:555, 1989.

164. Curran LS, Zhuang J, Sun SF, Moore LG: Ventilation and hypoxic ventilatory responsiveness in Chinese-Tibetan residents at 3,658 m. J Appl Physiol 83:2098, 1997.

165. Leon-Velarde F, Arregui A, Vargas M, et al: Chronic mountain sickness and chronic lower respiratory tract disorders. Chest 106:151, 1994.

166. Monge CC, Arregui A, Leon-Velarde F: Pathophysiology and epidemiology of chronic mountain sickness. Int J Sports Med 13(Suppl):S79, 1992.

167. Klepper M, Barnard P, Eschenbacher W: A case of chronic mountain sickness diagnosed by routine pulmonary function tests. Chest 100:823, 1991.

168. Millman RP, Bevilacqua J, Peterson DD, et al: Central sleep apnea in hypothyroidism. Am Rev Respir Dis 127:504, 1983.

169. Weiner M, Chausow A, Szidon P: Reversible respiratory muscle weakness in hypothyroidism. Br J Dis Chest 80:391, 1986.

170. Ingar SH, Woebar KA: The thyroid gland. In Wilson JB, Foster DW (eds): Williams Textbook of Endocrinology. 7th ed. Philadelphia, WB Saunders, 1974, pp 95–232.

171. Skatrud J, Iber C, Ewart R, et al: Disordered breathing during sleep in hypothyroidism. Am Rev Respir Dis 124:325, 1981.

172. McNamara ME, Southwick SM, Fogel BS: Sleep apnea and hypothyroidism presenting as depression in two patients. J Clin Psychiatry 48:164, 1987.

173. Orr WC, Males JL, Imes NK: Myxedema and obstructive sleep apnea. Am J Med 70:1060, 1981.

174. Forester CF: Coma in myxedema. Report of a case and review of the world literature. Arch Intern Med 111:734, 1963.

175. Menendez CE, Rivlin RS: Thyrotoxic crisis and myxedema coma. Med Clin North Am 57:1463, 1973.

176. Massumi RA, Winnacker JJ: Severe depression of the respiratory center in myxedema. Am J Med 36:876, 1964.

177. Domm BM, Vassalo CL: Myxedema coma with respiratory failure. Am Rev Respir Dis 107:842, 1973.

178. Javaheri S, Kazemi H: Metabolic alkalosis and hypoventilation in humans. Am Rev Respir Dis 136:1011, 1987.

179. Lavie CJ, Crocker EF Jr, Key KJ, Ferguson TG: Marked hypochloremic metabolic alkalosis with severe compensatory hypoventilation. South Med J 79:1296, 1986.

180. Blank MJ, Lew SQ: Hypoventilation in a dialysis patient with severe metabolic alkalosis: Treatment by hemodialysis. Blood Purif 9:109, 1991.

181. Shear L, Brandman IS: Hypoxia and hypercapnia caused by respiratory compensation for metabolic alkalosis. Am Rev Respir Dis 107:836, 1973.

182. Tanaka M, Yano T, Ichikawa Y, Oizumi K: A case of Cushing's syndrome associated with chronic respiratory failure due to metabolic alkalosis. Intern Med 31:385, 1992.

183. Nugent CA, Harris HW, Cohn J, et al: Dyspnea as a symptom in Parkinson's syndrome. Am Rev Respir Dis 78:682, 1958.

184. Lilker ES, Woolf CR: Pulmonary function in Parkinson's syndrome: The effect of thalamotomy. Can Med Assoc J 99:752, 1968.

185. Fraser RS, Sproule BJ, Dvorkin J: Hypoventilation, cyanosis and polycythemia in a thin man. Can Med Assoc J 89:1178, 1963.

186. Garland T, Linderholm H: Hypoventilation syndrome in a case of chronic epidemic encephalitis. Acta Med Scand 162:333, 1958.

187. Darwish RY, Fairshter RD, Vaziri ND, et al: Hypoventilation in a case of nonfamilial Parkinson's disease. West J Med 143:383, 1985.

188. Apps MC, Sheaff PC, Ingram DA, et al: Respiration and sleep in Parkinson's disease. J Neurol Neurosurg Psychiatry 48:1240, 1985.

189. Sabate M, Gonzalez I, Ruperez F, Rodriguez M: Obstructive and restrictive pulmonary dysfunctions in Parkinson's disease. Neurolog Sci 138:114, 1996.

190. Tzelepis GE, McCool FD, Friedman JH, Hoppin FG Jr: Respiratory muscle dysfunction in Parkinson's disease. Am Rev Respir Dis 138:266, 1988.

191. Vincken WG, Gauthier FG, Dollfuss RE, et al: Involvement of upper airway muscles in extrapyramidal disorders: A cause of air flow limitation. N Engl J Med 311:438, 1984.

192. Estenne M, Hubert M, De Troyer A: Respiratory-muscle involvement in Parkinson's disease. N Engl J Med 311:1516, 1984.

193. Hovestadt A, Bogaard JM, Meerwaldt JD, et al: Pulmonary function in Parkinson's disease. J Neurol Neurosurg Psychiatry 52:329, 1989.

194. Obenour WH, Stevens PM, Cohen AA, et al: The causes of abnormal function in Parkinson's disease. Am Rev Respir Dis 105:382, 1972.

195. Langer H, Woolf CR: Changes in pulmonary function in Parkinson's syndrome after treatment with L-dopa. Am Rev Respir Dis 104:440, 1971.

196. Adams EB, Holloway R, Thambiran AK, et al: Usefulness of intermittent positive-pressure respiration in the treatment of tetanus. Lancet 2:1176, 1966.

197. Carrea R, Lanari A: Chronic effect of tetanus toxin applied locally to the cerebral cortex of the dog. Science 137:342, 1962.

198. Brooks VB, Asanuma H: Action of tetanus toxin in the cerebral cortex. Science 137:674, 1962.

199. Brooks VB, Curtis DR, Eccles JC: The action of tetanus toxin on the inhibition of motor-neurones. J Physiol 135:655, 1957.

200. Kerr JH, Corbett JL, Prys-Roberts C, et al: Involvement of the sympathetic nervous system in tetanus. Studies on 82 cases. Lancet 2:236, 1968.

201. Udwadia FE, Lall A, Udwadia ZF, et al: Tetanus and its complications: Intensive care and management experience in 150 Indian patients. Epidemiol Infect 99:675, 1987.

202. Lawrence JR, Sando MJW: Treatment of severe tetanus. BMJ 2:113, 1959.

203. Wessler S, Avioli LA: Therapeutic grand round—No. 10. Tetanus. JAMA 207:123, 1969.

204. Smythe PM, Bull AB: Treatment of tetanus: With special reference to tracheotomy. BMJ 2:732, 1961.

205. Edmonson RS, Flowers MW: Intensive care in tetanus: Management, complications, and mortality in 100 cases. BMJ 1:1401, 1979.

206. MacRae J: A new look at infectious diseases: Tetanus. BMJ 1:730, 1973.

207. Tetanus—Still here? (editorial). N Engl J Med 280:614, 1969.

208. Abhyankar NY, Bhambure NM, Kasekar SG, et al: Intensive respiratory care service—our eight-year experience. Indian J Chest Dis Allied Sci 34:65, 1992.

209. LaForce FM, Young LS, Bennett JV: Tetanus in the United States (1965–1966): Epidemiologic and clinical features. N Engl J Med 280:569, 1969.

210. Notcutt WG, Ashley D: Tetanus and inhalation of a foreign body. BMJ 2:1193, 1977.

211. Femi-Pearse D: Blood gas tensions, acid-base status, and spirometry in tetanus. Am Rev Respir Dis 110:390, 1974.

212. Femi-Pearse D, Afonja AO, Elegbeleye OO: Value of determination of oxygen consumption in tetanus. BMJ 1:74, 1976.

213. Chao CH, Yu KW, Liu CY, et al: Tetanus: 20 years of clinical experience. Chung Hua I Hsueh Tsa Chih [Chinese Medical Journal] 48:110, 1991.

214. Heurich AE, Brust JCM, Richter RW: Management of urban tetanus. Med Clin North Am 57:1373, 1973.

215. Sandor F: Diaphragmatic respiration: A sign of cervical cord lesion in the unconscious patient ("horizontal paradox"). BMJ 1:465, 1966.

215a. Loveridge B, Sanii R, Dubo HI: Breathing pattern adjustments during the first year following cervical spinal cord injury. Paraplegia 30:479, 1992.

216. Ledsome JR, Sharp JM: Pulmonary function in acute cervical cord injury. Am Rev Respir Dis 124:41, 1981.

217. McMichan JC, Michel L, Westbrook PR: Pulmonary dysfunction following traumatic quadriplegia. JAMA 243:528, 1980.

218. James WS, Minh V-D, Minteer MA, et al: Cervical accessory respiratory muscle function in a patient with a high cervical cord lesion. Chest 71:59, 1977.

219. Kuperman AS, Krieger AJ, Rosomoff HL: Respiratory function after cervical cordotomy. Chest 59:128, 1971.

220. Kuperman AS, Fernandez RB, Rosomoff HL: The potential hazard of oxygen after bilateral cordotomy. Chest 59:232, 1971.

221. Lahuerta J, Lipton S, Wells JC: Percutaneous cervical cordotomy: Results and complications in a recent series of 100 patients. Ann R Coll Surg Engl 67:41, 1985.

222. Rizvi SS, Ishikawa S, Faling LJ, et al: Defect in automatic respiration in a case of multiple sclerosis. Am J Med 56:433, 1974.

223. Yamamoto T, Imai T, Yamasaki M: Acute ventilatory failure in multiple sclerosis. J Neurol Sci 89:313, 1989.

224. Jaspar N, Kruger M, Ectors P, et al: Unilateral chest wall paradoxical motion mimicking a flail chest in a patient with hemilateral C7 spinal injury. Intensive Care Med 12:396, 1986.

225. Swanson GD, Whipp BJ, Kaufman RD, et al: Effect of hypercapnia on hypoxic ventilatory drive in carotid body–resected man. J Appl Physiol 45:971, 1978.

226. Wade JG, Larson CP Jr, Hickey RF, et al: Effect of carotid endarterectomy on carotid chemoreceptor and baroreceptor function in man. N Engl J Med 282:823, 1970.

227. Lugliani R, Whipp BJ, Seard C, et al: Effect of bilateral carotid-body resection on ventilatory control at rest and during exercise in man. N Engl J Med 285:1105, 1971.

228. Holton P, Wood JB: The effects of bilateral removal of the carotid bodies and denervation of the carotid sinuses in two human subjects. J Physiol (Lond) 181:365, 1965.

229. Honda Y, Myojo S, Hasegawa S, et al: Decreased exercise hyperpnea in patients with bilateral carotid chemoreceptor resection. J Appl Physiol 46:908, 1979.

230. Zikk D, Shanon E, Rapoport Y, et al: Sleep apnea following bilateral excision of carotid body tumors. Laryngoscope 93:1470, 1983.

231. Hines S, Houston M, Robertson D: The clinical spectrum of autonomic dysfunction. Am J Med 70:1091, 1981.
232. Bartels J, Mazzia VDB: Familial dysautonomia. JAMA 212:318, 1970.
233. Filler J, Smith AA, Stone S, et al: Respiratory control in familial dysautonomia. J Pediatr 66:509, 1965.
234. Brunt PW, McKusick VA: Familial dysautonomia: A report of genetic and clinical studies, with a review of the literature. Medicine 49:343, 1970.
235. Edelman NH, Cherniack NS, Lahiri S, et al: The effects of abnormal sympathetic nervous function upon the ventilatory response to hypoxia. J Clin Invest 49:1153, 1970.
236. Page MM, Watkins PJ: Cardiorespiratory arrest and diabetic autonomic neuropathy. Lancet 1:14, 1978.
237. Lloyd-Mostyn RH, Watkins PJ: Defective innervation of heart in diabetic autonomic neuropathy. BMJ 3:15, 1975.
238. Montserrat JM, Cochrane GM, Wolf C, et al: Ventilatory control in diabetes mellitus. Eur J Respir Dis 67:112, 1985.
239. Silverstein D, Michlin B, Sobel HJ, et al: Right ventricular failure in a patient with diabetic neuropathy (myopathy) and central alveolar hypoventilation. Respiration 44:460, 1983.
240. Catterall JR, Calverley PM, Ewing DJ, et al: Breathing, sleep, and diabetic autonomic neuropathy. Diabetes 33:1025, 1984.
241. Bokinsky GE, Hudson LD, Weil JV: Impaired peripheral chemosensitivity and acute respiratory failure in Arnold-Chiari malformation and syringomyelia. N Engl J Med 288:947, 1973.
242. Bullock R, Todd NV, Easton J, et al: Isolated central respiratory failure due to syringomyelia and Arnold-Chiari malformation. BMJ 297:1448, 1988.
243. Derenne JP, Macklem PT, Roussos CL: The respiratory muscles: Mechanics, control and pathophysiology. Part I. Am Rev Respir Dis 118:119, 1978.
244. Campbell EJM, Agostoni E, Newsom Davis J: The Respiratory Muscles: Mechanics and Neural Control. 2nd ed. Philadelphia, WB Saunders, 1970.
245. Loh L, Goldman M, Davis JN: The assessment of diaphragm function. Medicine 56:165, 1977.
246. Roussos C: The failing ventilatory pump. Lung 160:59, 1982.
247. Roussos C, Macklem PT: Diaphragmatic fatigue in man. J Appl Physiol 43:189, 1977.
248. Roussos C, Fixley M, Gross D, et al: Fatigue of inspiratory muscles and their synergic behavior. J Appl Physiol 46:897, 1979.
249. Bellemare F, Grassino A: Effect of pressure and timing of contraction on human diaphragm fatigue. J Appl Physiol 53:1190, 1982.
250. Bellemare F, Grassino A: Evaluation of human diaphragm fatigue. J Appl Physiol 53:1196, 1982.
251. Juan G, Calverley P, Talamo C, et al: Effect of carbon dioxide on diaphragmatic function in human beings. N Engl J Med 310:874, 1984.
252. Jardim J, Farkas G, Prefaut C, et al: The failing inspiratory muscles under normoxic and hypoxic conditions. Am Rev Respir Dis 124:274, 1981.
253. Cohen CA, Zagelbaum G, Gross E, et al: Clinical manifestations of inspiratory muscle fatigue. Am J Med 73:308, 1982.
254. Roussos C: Respiratory muscle fatigue in the hypercapnic patient. Bull Eur Physiopathol Respir 15:117, 1979.
255. Gross D, Grassino A, Ross WRD, et al: Electromyogram pattern of diaphragmatic fatigue. J Appl Physiol 46:1, 1979.
256. Esau SA, Bye PTP, Pardy RL: Changes in rate of relaxation of sniffs with diaphragmatic fatigue in humans. J Appl Physiol 55:731, 1983.
257. Levy RD, Esau SA, Bye PTP, et al: Relaxation rate of mouth pressure with sniffs at rest and with inspiratory muscle fatigue. Am Rev Respir Dis 130:38, 1984.
258. Mithoefer JC, Bossman OG, Thibault DW, et al: The clinical estimation of alveolar ventilation. Am Rev Respir Dis 98:868, 1968.
259. Grinman S, Whitelaw WA: Pattern of breathing in a case of generalized respiratory muscle weakness. Chest 84:770, 1983.
260. Miller A, Granada M: In-hospital mortality in the pickwickian syndrome. Am J Med 56:144, 1974.
261. Harrison BDW, Collins JV, Brown KGE, et al: Respiratory failure in neuromuscular disease. Thorax 26:579, 1971.
262. Goldstein RL, Hyde RW, Lapham LW, et al: Peripheral neuropathy presenting with respiratory insufficiency as the primary complaint. Problem of recognizing alveolar hypoventilation due to neuromuscular disorders. Am J Med 56:443, 1974.
263. Spitzer SA, Korczyn AD, Kalaci J: Transient bilateral diaphragmatic paralysis. Chest 64:355, 1973.
264. Sandham JD, Shaw DT, Guenter CA: Acute supine respiratory failure due to bilateral diaphragmatic paralysis. Chest 72:96, 1977.
265. Newsom Davis J, Goldman M, Loh L, et al: Diaphragm function and alveolar hypoventilation. Q J Med 45:87, 1976.
266. Konno K, Mead J: Measurement of the separate volume changes of rib cage and abdomen during breathing. J Appl Physiol 22:407, 1967.
267. Black LF, Hyatt RE: Maximal static respiratory pressures in generalized neuromuscular disease. Am Rev Respir Dis 103:641, 1971.
268. Gibson GJ, Pride NB, Davis JN, et al: Pulmonary mechanics in patients with respiratory muscle weakness. Am Rev Respir Dis 115:389, 1977.
269. Delhez L: Modalités chez l'homme normal de la réponse électrique des piliers du diaphragme à la stimulation électrique des nerfs phréniques par des chocs uniques. Arch Int Physiol 73:832, 1965.
270. Newsom Davis J: Phrenic nerve conduction in man. J Neurol Neurosurg Psychiatry 30:420, 1967.
271. Haas H, Johnson LR, Gill TH, et al: Diaphragm paralysis and ventilatory failure in chronic proximal spinal muscular atrophy. Am Rev Respir Dis 123:465, 1981.
272. Saxton GA Jr, Rayson GE, Moody E, et al: Alveolar-arterial gas tension relationships in acute anterior poliomyelitis. Am J Med 30:871, 1961.
273. Steinborn KE, Zimdahl WT, Loeser WD: Chronic cor pulmonale in the respiratory poliomyelitis patient. Arch Intern Med 110:249, 1962.
274. Cherniack RM, Ewart WB, Hildes JA: Polycythemia secondary to respiratory disturbances in poliomyelitis. Ann Intern Med 46:720, 1957.
275. Lane DJ, Hazleman B, Nichols PJR: Late onset respiratory failure in patients with previous poliomyelitis. Q J Med 43:551, 1974.
276. Hsu AA, Staats BA: "Postpolio" sequelae and sleep-related disordered breathing. Mayo Clin Proc 73:216, 1998.
277. Fromm GB, Wisdom PJ, Block AJ: Amyotrophic lateral sclerosis presenting with respiratory muscle paralysis and dependence on mechanical ventilation in two patients. Chest 71:612, 1977.
278. Mayrignac C, Poirier J, Degos JD: Amyotrophic lateral sclerosis presenting with respiratory insufficiency as the primary complaint. Clinicopathological study of a case. Eur Neurol 24:115, 1985.
279. Hill R, Martin J, Hakim A: Acute respiratory failure in motor neuron disease. Arch Neurol 40:30, 1983.
280. Parhad IM, Clark AW, Barron KD, et al: Diaphragmatic paralysis in motor neuron disease. Report of two cases and a review of the literature. Neurology 28:18, 1978.
281. Nightingale S, Bates D, Bateman DE, et al: Enigmatic dyspnoea: An unusual presentation of motor-neurone disease. Lancet 1:933, 1982.
282. Kreitzer SM, Saunders NA, Tyler HR, et al: Respiratory muscle function in amyotrophic lateral sclerosis. Am Rev Respir Dis 117:437, 1978.
283. Brach BB: Expiratory flow patterns in amyotrophic lateral sclerosis. Chest 75:648, 1979.
284. Braun SR, Sufit RL, Giovannoni R, et al: Intermittent negative pressure ventilation in the treatment of respiratory failure in progressive neuromuscular disease. Neurology 37:1874, 1987.
285. O'Donohue WJ, Baker JP, Bell GM, et al: Respiratory failure in neuromuscular diseae management in a respiratory intensive care unit. JAMA 235:733, 1976.
286. Dowling PC, Menonna JP, Cook SD: Guillain-Barré syndrome in greater New York–New Jersey. JAMA 238:317, 1977.
287. Gracey DR, McMichan JC, Divertie MB, et al: Respiratory failure in Guillain-Barré syndrome: A 6-year experience. Mayo Clin Proc 57:742, 1982.
288. Sunderrajan EV, Davenport J: The Guillain-Barré syndrome: Pulmonary-neurologic correlations. Medicine (Baltimore) 64:333, 1985.
289. Ropper AH, Kehne SM: Guillain-Barré syndrome: Management of respiratory failure. Neurology 35:1662, 1985.
290. Hu-Sheng W, Qi-Fen Y, Tian-Ci L, et al: The treatment of acute polyradiculoneuritis with respiratory paralysis. Brain Develop 10:147, 1988.
291. Chalmers RM, Howard RS, Wiles CM, et al: Respiratory insufficiency in neuronopathic and neuropathic disorders. Q J Med 89:469, 1996.
292. Chevrolet JC, Deleamont P: Repeated vital capacity measurements as predictive parameters for mechanical ventilation need and weaning success in the Guillain-Barré syndrome. Am Rev Respir Dis 144:814, 1991.
293. Gourie-Devi M, Ganapathy GR: Phrenic nerve conduction time in Guillain-Barré syndrome. J Neurol Neurosurg Psychiatry 48:245, 1985.
294. Rantala H, Uhari M, Cherry JD, Shields WD: Risk factors of respiratory failure in children with Guillain-Barré syndrome. Pediatr Neurol 13:289, 1995.
295. Teitelbaum JS, Borel CO: Respiratory dysfunction in Guillain-Barré syndrome. Clin Chest Med 15:705, 1994.
296. Borel CO, Tilford C, Nichols DG, et al: Diaphragmatic performance during recovery from acute ventilatory failure in Guillain-Barré syndrome and myasthenia gravis. Chest 99:444, 1991.
297. Zouvanis M, Feldman C, Smith C, et al: Renal and neuromuscular respiratory failure—is this a syndrome associated with cantharidin poisoning? S Afr Med J 84:814, 1994.
298. Becker DM, Kramer S: The neurological manifestations of porphyria: A review. Medicine 56:411, 1977.
299. Doll SG, Bower AG, Affeldt JW: Acute intermittent porphyria with respiratory paralysis. JAMA 168:1973, 1958.
300. Sakamoto Y, Lockey RF, Krzanowski JJ: Shellfish and fish poisoning related to the toxic dinoflagellates. South Med J 80:866, 1987.
301. Ellis S: Introduction to symposium: Brevetoxins: Chemistry and pharmacology of "red tide" toxins from *Ptychodiscus brevis* (formerly *Gymnodinium breve*). Toxicon 23:469, 1985.
302. Pierce RH: Red tide *(Ptychodiscus brevis)* toxin aerosols: A review. Toxicon 24:955, 1986.
303. Ishida Y, Shibata S: Brevetoxin-B of *Gymnodinium breve* toxin–induced contractions of smooth muscles due to the transmitter release from nerves. Pharmacology 31:237, 1985.
304. Shimoda T, Krzanowski J, Nelson R, et al: In vitro red tide toxin effects on human bronchial smooth muscle. J Allergy Clin Immunol 81:1187, 1988.
305. Hughes JM, Merson MH: Fish and shellfish poisoning. N Engl J Med 295:1117, 1976.
306. Paralytic shellfish poisoning. Laboratory Center for Disease Control, Ottawa, Ontario. Can Dis Wkly Rep 4:21, 1978.
306a. Asakawa M, Nishimura F, Miyazawa K, Noguchi T. Occurrence of paralytic shellfish poison in the starfish, *Asterias amurensis,* in Kure Bay, Hiroshima Prefecture, Japan. Toxicon 35:1081, 1997.
307. Morris JG: Ciguatera fish poisoning. JAMA 244:273, 1980.
308. Tatnall FM, Smith HG, Welsby PD, et al: Ciguatera poisoning. BMJ 281:948, 1980.

309. Morris JG, Lewin P, Hargrett NT, et al: Clinical features of ciguatera fish poisoning—a study of the disease in the United States Virgin Islands. Arch Intern Med 142:1090, 1982.

310. Lawrence DN, Enriquez MB, Lumish RM, et al: Ciguatera fish poisoning in Miami. JAMA 244:254, 1980.

311. Withers NW: Ciguatera fish poisoning. Annu Rev Med 33:97, 1982.

312. Gray C: Mussel mystery: "The more you know, the more you don't know." Can Med Assoc J 138:350, 1988.

313. Mills AR, Passmore R: Pelagic paralysis. Lancet 1:161, 1988.

314. Walker DG: Survival after severe envenomation by the blue-ringed octopus *(Hepalochlaena maculosa)*. Med J Aust 2:663, 1983.

315. Kitchens CS, Van Mierop LH: Envenomation by the Eastern coral snake *(Micrurus fulvius fulvius)*. A study of 39 victims. JAMA 258:1615, 1987.

316. Karalliedde LD, Sanmuganathan PS: Respiratory failure following envenomation. Anesthesia 43:753, 1988.

317. Watt G, Padre L, Tauzon L, et al: Bites of the Philippine cobra *(Naja naja philippinensis)*: Prominent neurotoxicity with minimal local signs. Am J Trop Med Hyg 39:306, 1988.

318. Tibballs J, Cooper SJ: Paralysis with *Ixodes cornuatus* envenomation. Med J Aust 145:37, 1986.

319. Rivett K, Potgieter PD: Diaphragmatic paralysis after organophosphate poisoning. S Afr Med J 72:881, 1987.

320. Drachman DB, Adams RN, Josifek LF, et al: Functional activities of autoantibodies to acetylcholine receptors and the clinical severity of myasthenia gravis. N Engl J Med 307:769, 1982.

321. Zulueta JJ, Fanburg BL. Respiratory dysfunction in myasthenia gravis. Clin Chest Med 15:683, 1994.

322. Dua PC: Respiratory failure in myasthenia gravis; use of plasmapheresis. Chest 85:721, 1984.

323. Chagnac Y, Hadani M, Goldhammer Y: Myasthenic crisis after intravenous administration of iodinated contrast agent. Neurology 35:1219, 1985.

324. Turani E, Szathmary I, Molnar J, Szobor A: Myasthenia gravis: Prognostic significance of clinical data in the prediction of post-thymectomy respiratory crises. Acta Chir Hung 33:353, 1992–93.

325. Mier A, Laroche C, Green M: Unsuspected myasthenia gravis presenting as respiratory failure. Thorax 45:422, 1990.

326. Dushay KM, Zibrak JD, Jensen WA: Myasthenia gravis presenting as isolated respiratory failure. Chest 97:232, 1990.

327. Suxamethonium apnoea (editorial). Lancet 1:246, 1973.

328. De Troyer A, Broestein S: Acute changes in respiratory mechanics after pyridostigmine injection in patients with myasthenia gravis. Am Rev Respir Dis 121:629, 1980.

329. Radwan L, Strugalska M, Koziorowski A: Changes in respiratory muscle function after neostigmine injection in patients with myasthenia gravis. Eur Respir J 1:119, 1988.

330. Shale DJ, Lane DJ, David CJF: Air-flow limitation in myasthenia gravis—the effect of acetylcholinesterase inhibitor therapy on air-flow limitation. Am Rev Respir Dis 128:618, 1983.

331. Rieder P, Louis M, Jolliet P, Chevrolet JC: The repeated measurement of vital capacity is a poor predictor of the need for mechanical ventilation in myasthenia. Intensive Care Med 21:663, 1995.

332. Newball HH, Brahim SA: Effects of alternate-day prednisone therapy on respiratory function in myasthenia gravis. Thorax 31:410, 1976.

333. Berrouschot J, Baumann I, Kalischewski P, et al: Therapy of myasthenia. Crit Care Med 25:1228, 1997.

334. Gracey DR, Howard FM, Divertie MB: Plasmapheresis in the treatment of ventilator-dependent myasthenia gravis patients. Report of four cases. Chest 85:739, 1984.

335. Dau PC, Lindstrom JM, Cassel CK, et al: Plasmapheresis and immunosuppressive drug therapy in myasthenia gravis. N Engl J Med 297:1134, 1977.

336. Selecky PA, Ziment I: Prolonged respiratory support for the treatment of intractable myasthenia gravis. Chest 65:207, 1974.

337. Dropcho EJ, Stanton C, Oh SJ: Neuronal antinuclear antibodies in a patient with Lambert-Eaton myasthenic syndrome and small-cell lung carcinoma. Neurology 39:249, 1989.

338. Lang B, Newsom Davis J, Wray D, et al: Autoimmune aetiology for myasthenic (Eaton-Lambert) syndrome. Lancet 2:224, 1981.

339. Aldrich TK, Prezant DJ: Adverse effects of drugs on the respiratory muscles. Clin Chest Med 11:177, 1990.

340. Pridgen JE: Respiratory arrest thought to be due to intraperitoneal neomycin. Surgery 40:571, 1956.

341. Ream CR: Respiratory and cardiac arrest after intravenous administration of kanamycin with reversal of toxic effects by neostigmine. Ann Intern Med 59:384, 1963.

342. Fisk GC: Respiratory paralysis after a large dose of streptomycin. Report of a case. BMJ 1:556, 1961.

343. Adamson RH, Marshall FN, Long JP: Neuromuscular blocking properties of various polypeptide antibiotics. Proc Soc Exp Biol Med 105:494, 1960.

344. Lindesmith LA, Baines D Jr, Bigelow DB, et al: Reversible respiratory paralysis associated with polymyxin therapy. Ann Intern Med 68:318, 1968.

345. Koch-Weser J, Sidel VW, Federman EB, et al: Adverse effects of sodium colistimethate. Manifestations and specific reaction rates during 317 courses of therapy. Ann Intern Med 72:857, 1970.

346. Antibiotic-induced myasthenia (editorial). JAMA 204:164, 1968.

347. Emery ERJ: Neuromuscular blocking properties of antibiotics as a cause of postoperative apnoea. Anaesthesia 18:57, 1963.

348. Davidson EW, Modell JH, Moya F, et al: Respiratory depression after antibiotic use in pleural and pseudocyst cavities. JAMA 196:456, 1966.

349. Foldes FF, Lunn JN, Benz HG: Prolonged respiratory depression caused by drug combinations. Muscle relaxants and intraperitoneal antibiotics as etiologic agents. JAMA 183:672, 1963.

350. Masters CL, Dawkins RL, Zilko PJ, et al: Penicillamine-associated myasthenia gravis, antiacetylcholine receptor and antistriational antibodies. Am J Med 63:689, 1977.

351. Adelman HM, Winters PR, Mahan CS, Wallach PM: D-Penicillamine-induced myasthenia gravis: Diagnosis obscured by coexisting chronic obstructive pulmonary disease. Am J Med Sci 309:191, 1995.

352. Godley PJ, Morton TA, Karboski JA, Tami JA: Procainamide-induced myasthenic crisis. Ther Drug Monit 12:411, 1990.

353. Vallet B, Fourrier F, Hurtevent JF, et al: Myasthenia gravis and steroid-induced myopathy of the respiratory muscles. Intensive Care Med 18:424, 1992.

354. Gooch JL: Prolonged paralysis after neuromuscular blockade. J Toxicol Clin Toxicol 33:419, 1995.

355. Waclawik AJ, Sufit RL, Beinlich BR, Schutta HS: Acute myopathy with selective degeneration of myosin filaments following status asthmaticus treated with methylprednisolone and vecuronium. Neuromuscul Disord 2:19, 1992.

356. Douglass JA, Tuxen DV, Horne M, et al: Myopathy in severe asthma. Am Rev Respir Dis 146:517, 1992.

357. Awadh N, Al-mane F, D'yachkova Y, et al: Myopathy following mechanical ventilation for acute severe asthma: The role of muscle relaxants and corticosteroids. Submitted for publication.

358. Namba T, Nolte CT, Jackrel J, et al: Poisoning due to organophosphate insecticides. Acute and chronic manifestations. Am J Med 50:475, 1971.

359. Hunter D: Devices for the protection of the worker against injury and disease. Part II. BMJ 1:506, 1950.

360. Koenig MG, Spickard A, Cardella MA, et al: Clinical and laboratory observations on type E botulism in man. Medicine 43:517, 1964.

361. Armstrong RW, Stenn F, Dowell VR Jr, et al: Type E botulism from home-canned gefilte fish. JAMA 210:303, 1969.

362. Kao I, Drachman DB, Price DL: Botulinum toxin: Mechanism of a presynaptic blockade. Science 193:1256, 1976.

363. Koenig MG, Drutz DJ, Mushlin AI, et al: Type B botulism in man. Am J Med 42:208, 1967.

364. Wilcox P, Andolfatto G, Fairbarn MS, et al: Long-term follow-up of symptoms, pulmonary function, respiratory muscle strength, and exercise performance after botulism. Am Rev Respir Dis 139:157, 1989.

365. Lewis SW, Pierson DJ, Cary JM, et al: Prolonged respiratory paralysis in wound botulism. Chest 75:59, 1979.

366. MacDonald KL, Rutherford GW, Friedman SM, et al: Botulism and botulism-like illness in chronic drug abusers. Ann Intern Med 102:616, 1985.

367. Whittaker RL, Gilbertson RB, Garrett AS: Botulism type E, report of eight simultaneous cases. Ann Intern Med 61:448, 1964.

368. Terranova W, Palumbo JN, Breman JG: Ocular findings in botulism type B. JAMA 241:475, 1979.

369. Schmidt-Nowara WW, Samet JM, Rosario PA: Early and late pulmonary complications of botulism. Arch Intern Med 143:451, 1983.

370. Begin R, Bureau M, Lupien L, et al: Control of breathing in Duchenne's muscular dystrophy. Am J Med 69:227, 1980.

371. McCormack WM, Spalter HF: Muscular dystrophy, alveolar hypoventilation, and papilledema. JAMA 197:957, 1966.

372. Gillam PMS, Heaf PJD, Kaufman L, et al: Respiration in dystrophia myotonica. Thorax 19:112, 1964.

373. Skatrud J, Iber C, McHugh W, et al: Determinants of hypoventilation during wakefulness and sleep in diaphragmatic paralysis. Am Rev Respir Dis 121:587, 1980.

374. Cirignotta F, Mondini S, Zucconi M, et al: Sleep-related breathing impairment in myotonic dystrophy. J Neurol 235:80, 1987.

375. Bach JR, O'Brien J, Krotenberg R, et al: Management of end stage respiratory failure in Duchenne muscular dystrophy. Muscle Nerve 10:177, 1987.

376. Yasukohchi S, Yagi Y, Akabane T, et al: Facioscapulohumeral dystrophy associated with sensorineural hearing loss, tortuosity of retinal arterioles, and an early onset and rapid progression of respiratory failure. Brain Develop 10:319, 1988.

377. Cannon PJ: The heart and lungs in myotonic muscular dystrophy. Am J Med 32:765, 1962.

378. Bégin R, Bureau MA, Lupien L: Control and modulation of respiration in Steinert's myotonic dystrophy. Am Rev Respir Dis 121:281, 1980.

379. Bégin R, Bureau MA, Lupien L, et al: Pathogenesis of respiratory insufficiency in myotonic dystrophy—the mechanical factors. Am Rev Respir Dis 125:312, 1982.

380. Jammes Y, Pouget J, Grimaud C, et al: Pulmonary function and electromyographic study of respiratory muscles in myotonic dystrophy. Muscle Nerve 8:586, 1985.

381. Kilburn KH, Eagan JT, Sieker HO, et al: Cardiopulmonary insufficiency in myotonic and progressive muscular dystrophy. N Engl J Med 261:1089, 1959.

382. Engel AG, Gomez MR, Seybold ME, et al: The spectrum and diagnosis of acid maltase deficiency. Neurology 23:95, 1973.

383. Rosenow EC, Engel AG: Acid maltase deficiency in adults presenting as respiratory failure. Am J Med 64:485, 1978.

384. Wokke JH, Ausems MG, van den Boogaard MJ, et al: Genotype-phenotype correlation in adult-onset acid maltase deficiency. Ann Neurol 38:450, 1995.

385. Papapetropoulos T, Paschalis C, Manda P: Myopathy due to juvenile acid maltase deficiency affecting exclusively the type I fibres. J Neurol Neurosurg Psychiatry 47:213, 1984.

386. Raben N, Nichols RC, Boerkoel C, Plotz P: Genetic defects in patients with glycogenosis type II (acid maltase deficiency). Muscle Nerve 3(Suppl):S70, 1995.
387. Lenders MB, Martin JJ, de Barsy T, et al: Acid maltase deficiency in adults. A study of five cases. Acta Neurol Belg 86:152, 1986.
388. Trend PS, Wiles CM, Spencer GT, et al: Acid maltase deficiency in adults. Diagnosis and management in five cases. Brain 108:845, 1985.
389. Moufarrej NA, Bertorini TE: Respiratory insufficiency in adult-type acid maltase deficiency. South Med J 86:560, 1993.
390. Keunen RW, Lambregts PC, Op de Coul AA, et al: Respiratory failure as initial symptom of acid maltase deficiency. J Neurol Neurosurg Psychiatry 47:549, 1984.
391. Banwell BL, Singh NC, Ramsay DA: Prolonged survival in neonatal nemaline rod myopathy. Pediatr Neurol 10:335, 1994.
392. Sasaki M, Takeda M, Kobayashi K, Nonaka I: Respiratory failure in nemaline myopathy. Pediatr Neurol 16:344, 1997.
393. Harati Y, Niakan E, Bloom K, et al: Adult onset of nemaline myopathy presenting as diaphragmatic paralysis. J Neurol Neurosurg Psychiatry 50:108, 1987.
394. Dodson RF, Crisp GO, Nicotra B, et al: Rod myopathy with extensive systemic and respiratory muscular involvement. Ultrastruct Pathol 5:129, 1983.
395. Falga-Tirado C, Perez-Peman P, Ordi-Ros J, et al: Adult onset of nemaline myopathy presenting as respiratory insufficiency. Respiration 62:353, 1995.
396. Eymard B, Brouet JC, Collin H, et al: Late-onset rod myopathy associated with monoclonal gammopathy. Neuromuscul Disord 3:557, 1993.
397. Miro O, Masanes F, Pedrol E, et al: A comparative study of the clinical and histological characteristics between classic nemaline myopathy and that associated with the human immunodeficiency virus. Med Clin (Barc) 105:500, 1995.
398. Bellamy D, Newsom Davis J, Hickey BP, et al: A case of primary alveolar hypoventilation associated with mild proximal myopathy. Am Rev Respir Dis 112:867, 1975.
399. Riley DJ, Santiago TV, Daniele RP, et al: Blunted respiratory drive in congenital myopathy. Am J Med 63:459, 1977.
400. Gibson GJ, Edmonds JP, Hughes GRV: Diaphragm function and lung involvement in systemic lupus erythematosus. Am J Med 63:926, 1977.
401. Wilcox PG, Stein HB, Clarke SD, et al: Phrenic nerve function in patients with diaphragmatic weakness and systemic lupus erythematosus. Chest 93:353, 1988.
402. Worth H, Grahn S, Lakomek HJ, et al: Lung function disturbances versus respiratory muscle fatigue in patients with systemic lupus erythematosus. Respiration 53:81, 1988.
403. Gibson T, Myers AR: Nervous system involvement in systemic lupus erythematosus. Ann Rheum Dis 35:398, 1976.
404. Isenberg DA, Snaith ML: Muscle disease in systemic lupus erythematosus: A study of its nature, frequency, and cause. J Rheumatol 8:917, 1981.
405. Reichmann H, Goebel HH, Schneider C, Toyka KV: Familial mixed congenital myopathy with rigid spine phenotype. Muscle Nerve 20:411, 1997.
406. Kim DG, Jung K, Lee MK, et al: A case of juvenile form Pompe's disease manifested as chronic alveolar hypoventilation. J Korean Med Sci 8:221, 1993.
407. Rimmer KP, Whitelaw WA: The respiratory muscles in multicore myopathy. Am Rev Respir Dis 148:227, 1993.
408. Mousson B, Collombet JM, Dumoulin R, et al: An abnormal exercise test response revealing a respiratory chain complex III deficiency. Acta Neurol Scand 91:488, 1995.
409. Naumann M, Reiners K, Gold R, et al: Mitochondrial dysfunction in adult-onset myopathies with structural abnormalities. Acta Neuropathol (Berl) 89:152, 1995.
410. Reichmann H, Schalke B, Seibel P, et al: Sarcoid myopathy and mitochondrial respiratory chain defects: Clinicopathological, biochemical and molecular biological analyses. Neuromuscul Disord 5:277, 1995.
411. Smolenicka Z, Laporte J, Hu L, et al: X-linked myotubular myopathy: Refinement of the critical gene region. Neuromuscul Disord 6:275, 1996.
411a. Brussel T, Matthay MA, Chernow B: Pulmonary manifestations of endocrine and metabolic disorders. Clin Chest Med 10:645, 1989.
412. Williams TJ, O'Hehir RE, Czarny D, et al: Acute myopathy in severe acute asthma treated with intravenously administered corticosteroids. Am Rev Respir Dis 137:460, 1988.
413. Berenson M, Yarvote P, Grace WJ: Idiopathic myoglobinuria with respiratory paralysis. Am Rev Respir Dis 94:956, 1966.
414. Taverner D, Zardawi IM, Walls J: Acute ventilatory failure and myoglobinuria. Neurology 34:369, 1984.
415. Prockop LD, Engel WK, Shug AL: Nearly fatal muscle carnitine deficiency with full recovery after replacement therapy. Neurology 33:1629, 1983.
416. Aubier M, Murcino D, Legocquic Y, et al: Effect of hypophosphatemia on diaphragmatic contractility in patients with acute respiratory failure. N Engl J Med 31:420, 1985.
417. Varsano S, Shapiro M, Taragan R, et al: Hypophosphatemia as a reversible cause of refractory ventilatory failure. Crit Care Med 11:908, 1983.
418. Fisher J, Magid N, Kallman C, et al: Respiratory illness and hypophosphatemia. Chest 83:504, 1983.
419. Lewis JF, Hodsman AB, Driedger AA, et al: Hypophosphatemia and respiratory failure: Prolonged abnormal energy metabolism demonstrated by nuclear magnetic resonance spectroscopy. Am J Med 83:1139, 1987.
420. Fiaccadori E, Coffrini E, Fracchia C, et al: Hypophosphatemia and phosphorus depletion in respiratory and peripheral muscles of patients with respiratory failure due to COPD. Chest 105:1392, 1994.
421. Fischer DS, Nichol BA: Intraventricular conduction defect and respiratory tract paralysis in diabetic ketoacidosis. Am J Med 35:123, 1963.
422. Dorin RI, Crapo LM: Hypokalemic respiratory arrest in diabetic ketoacidosis. JAMA 257:1517, 1987.
423. Hermann RA, Mead AW, Spritz N, et al: Hypopotassemia with respiratory paralysis. Case due to renal tubular acidosis. Arch Intern Med 108:925, 1961.
424. Jenny DB, Goris GB, Urwiller RD, et al: Hypermagnesemia following irrigation of renal pelvis. Cause of respiratory depression. JAMA 240:1378, 1978.
425. Ferdinandus J, Pederson JA, Whang R: Hypermagnesemia as a cause of refractory hypotension, respiratory depression, and coma. Arch Intern Med 141:669, 1981.
426. Swygert LA, Back EE, Auerbach SB, et al: Eosinophilia-myalgia syndrome: Mortality data from the US national surveillance system. J Rheumatol 20:1711, 1993.
427. Froman C, Smith AC: Hyperventilation associated with low pH of cerebrospinal fluid after intracranial haemorrhage. Lancet 1:780, 1966.
428. Lorenz R, Ito A: The definition of "Cheyne-Stokes rhythms." Acta Neurochir (Wien) 43:61, 1978.
429. Morse SR, Chandrasekhar AJ, Cugell DW: Cheyne-Stokes respiration redefined. Chest 66:345, 1974.
430. Cherniack NS, Longobardo GS: Cheyne-Stokes breathing: An instability in physiologic control. N Engl J Med 288:952, 1973.
431. Cherniack NS: Commentary: Abnormal breathing patterns, their mechanisms and clinical significance. JAMA 230:57, 1974.
432. Gotoh F, Meyer JS, Takagi Y: Cerebral venous and arterial blood gases during Cheyne-Stokes respiration. Am J Med 47:534, 1969.
433. Findley LJ, Zwillich CW, Ancoli-Israel S, et al: Cheyne-Stokes breathing during sleep in patients with left ventricular heart failure. South Med J 78:11, 1985.
434. Brown HW, Plum F: The neurologic basis of Cheyne-Stokes respiration. Am J Med 30:849, 1961.
435. Karp HR, Sieker HO, Heyman A: Cerebral circulation and function in Cheyne-Stokes respiration. Am J Med 30:861, 1961.
436. Findley LJ, Blackburn MR, Goldberger AL, et al: Apneas and oscillation of cardiac ectopy in Cheyne-Stokes breathing during sleep. Am Rev Respir Dis 130:937, 1984.
437. Lewis RA, Howell JBL: Definition of the hyperventilation syndrome. Bull Eur Physiopathol Respir 22:201, 1986.
438. Moss PD, McEvedy CP: An epidemic of overbreathing among schoolgirls. BMJ 2:1295, 1966.
439. Ley R: Panic disorder and agoraphobia: Fear of fear or fear of the symptoms produced by hyperventilation? J Behav Ther Exp Psychiat 18:305, 1987.
440. Nisam M, Albertson TE, Panacek E, et al: Effects of hyperventilation on conjunctival oxygen tension in humans. Crit Care Med 14:12, 1986.
441. Rice RL: Symptom patterns of the hyperventilation syndrome. Am J Med 8:691, 1950.
442. Bass C, Gardner WN: Respiratory and psychiatric abnormalities in chronic symptomatic hyperventilation. BMJ 290:1387, 1985.
443. Coyle PK, Sternman AP: Focal neurologic symptoms in panic attacks. Am J Psychiatry 143:648, 1986.
444. Blau JN, Dexter SL: Hyperventilation in migraine attacks. BMJ 280:1254, 1980.
445. Magarian GJ, Olney RK: Absence spells. Hyperventilation syndrome as a previously unrecognized cause. Am J Med 76:905, 1984.
446. Tavel ME: Hyperventilation syndrome with unilateral somatic symptoms. JAMA 187:301, 1964.
447. Aronson PR: Hyperventilation syndrome. A comparative study of the effects of tranquilizers and a sedative upon the electrocardiogram. Clin Pharmacol Ther 5:553, 1964.
448. Heckerling PS, Hanashiro PK: ST segment elevation in hyperventilation syndrome. Ann Emerg Med 14:1122, 1985.
449. Freeman LJ, Nixon PG: Are coronary artery spasm and progressive damage to the heart associated with the hyperventilation syndrome? BMJ 291:851, 1985.
450. Motoyama EK, Rivard G, Acheson F, et al: Adverse effect of maternal hyperventilation on the foetus. Lancet 1:286, 1966.
451. Annotations: Hyperventilation and foetal acidosis. Lancet 2:1401, 1966.
452. Zwillich CW, Matthay MA, Potts DE, et al: Thyrotoxicosis: Comparison of effects of thyroid ablation and beta-adrenergic ventilatory control. J Clin Endocrinol Metab 46:491, 1978.
453. Thurnheer R, Jenni R, Russi EW, et al: Hyperthyroidism and pulmonary hypertension. J Intern Med 242:185, 1997.
454. Anderson RJ, Potts DE, Gabow PA, et al: Unrecognized adult salicylate intoxication. Ann Intern Med 85:745, 1976.
455. Eichenholz A: Respiratory alkalosis. Arch Intern Med 116:699, 1965.
456. Huckabee WE: Abnormal resting blood lactate. II. Lactate acidosis. Am J Med 30:840, 1961.
457. Dossetor JB, Zborowski D, Dixon HB, et al: Hyperlactatemia due to hyperventilation: Use of CO inhalation. Ann N Y Acad Sci 119:1153, 1965.
458. Papadopoulos CN, Keats AS: The metabolic acidosis of hyperventilation produced by controlled respiration. Anesthesiology 20:156, 1959.
459. Bates JH, Adamson JS, Pierce JA: Death after voluntary hyperventilation. N Engl J Med 274:1371, 1966.
460. Rodman T, Sobel M, Close HP: Arterial oxygen unsaturation and the ventilation-perfusion defect of Laënnec's cirrhosis. N Engl J Med 263:73, 1960.
461. Heinemann HO, Emirgil C, Mijnssen JP: Hyperventilation and arterial hypoxemia in cirrhosis of the liver. Am J Med 28:239, 1960.
462. Abelmann WH, Kramer GE, Verstraeten JM, et al: Cirrhosis of the liver and decreased arterial oxygen saturation. Arch Intern Med 108:34, 1961.
463. Rodman T, Hurwitz JK, Paston BH, et al: Cyanosis clubbing and arterial oxygen unsaturation associated with Laënnec's cirrhosis. Am J Med Sci 238:534, 1959.
464. Shaldon S, Ceasar J, Chiandussi L, et al: The demonstration of porto-pulmonary

anastomoses in portal cirrhosis with the use of radioactive krypton (^{85}Kr). N Engl J Med 265:410, 1961.

465. Harris JC, Rumack BH, Peterson RG, et al: Methemoglobinemia resulting from absorption of nitrates. JAMA 242:2869, 1979.

466. Jaffé ER: Hereditary methemoglobinemias associated with abnormalities in the metabolism of erythrocytes. Am J Med 41:786, 1966.

467. Wetherhold JM, Linch AL, Charsha RC: Chemical cyanosis—causes, effects, prevention. Arch Environ Health 1:353, 1960.

468. Simmel ER: Methemoglobinemia due to aminosalicylic acid (PAS). Am Rev Respir Dis 85:105, 1962.

469. Comly HH: Cyanosis in infants caused by nitrates in well water. JAMA 129:112, 1945.

470. Carlson DJ, Shapiro FL: Methemoglobinemia from well water nitrates: A complication of home dialysis. Ann Intern Med 73:757, 1970.

471. Ternberg JL, Luce E: Methemoglobinemia: A complication of the silver nitrate treatment of burns. Surgery 63:328, 1968.

472. Kennedy N, Smith CP, McWhinney P: Faulty sausage production causing methaemoglobinaemia. Arch Dis Child 76:367, 1997.

473. Douglas WW, Fairbanks VF: Methemoglobinemia induced by a topical anesthetic spray (Cetacaine). Chest 71:587, 1977.

474. Dumont L, Mardirosoff C, Dumont C, et al: Methaemoglobinemia induced by a low dose of prilocaine during interscalenic block. Acta Anaesthesiol Belg 46:39, 1995.

475. Guertler AT, Pearce WA: A prospective evaluation of benzocaine-associated methemoglobinemia in human beings. Ann Emerg Med 24:626, 1994.

476. O'Donohue WJ, Moss LM, Angelillo VA: Acute methemoglobinemia induced by topical benzocaine and lidocaine. Arch Intern Med 140:1508, 1980.

477. McGoldrick MD, Bailie GR: Severe accidental dapsone overdose. Am J Emerg Med 13:414, 1995.

478. Plotkin JS, Buell JF, Njoku MJ, et al: Methemoglobinemia associated with dapsone treatment in solid organ transplant recipients: A two-case report and review. Liver Transplant Surg 3:149, 1997.

479. Machabert R, Testud F, Descotes J: Methaemoglobinaemia due to amyl nitrite inhalation: A case report. Hum Exp Toxicol 13:313, 1994.

480. Bradberry SM, Whittington RM, Parry DA, Vale JA: Fatal methemoglobinemia due to inhalation of isobutyl nitrite. J Toxicol Clin Toxicol 32:179, 1994.

481. Young JD, Dyar O, Xiong L, Howell S: Methaemoglobin production in normal adults inhaling low concentrations of nitric oxide. Intensive Care Med 20:581, 1994.

482. Dotsch J, Demirakca S, Hamm R, et al: Extracorporeal circulation increases nitric oxide–induced methemoglobinemia in vivo and in vitro. Crit Care Med 25:1153, 1997.

483. Vieira LM, Kaplan JC, Kahn A, Leroux A: Four new mutations in the NADH-cytochrome b5 reductase gene from patients with recessive congenital methemoglobinemia type II. Blood 85:2254, 1995.

484. Manabe J, Arya R, Sumimoto H, et al: Two novel mutations in the reduced nicotinamide adenine dinucleotide (NADH)-cytochrome b5 reductase gene of a patient with generalized type, hereditary methemoglobinemia. Blood 88:3208, 1996.

485. Chisholm DG, Stuart H: Congenital methaemoglobinaemia detected by preoperative pulse oximetry. Can J Anaesth 41:519, 1994.

486. Johnson PL: Pulse oximetry signals local anesthetic–induced methemoglobinemia. Anesth Prog 41:11, 1994.

487. Jackson DL, Menges H: Accidental carbon monoxide poisoning. JAMA 243:772, 1980.

488. Fisher J, Rubin KP: Occult carbon monoxide poisoning. Arch Intern Med 142:1270, 1982.

489. Hardy KR, Thom SR: Pathophysiology and treatment of carbon monoxide poisoning. J Toxicol Clin Toxicol 32:613, 1994.

490. Ostrom M, Thorson J, Eriksson A: Carbon monoxide suicide from car exhausts. Soc Sci Med 42:447, 1996.

491. Shelef M: Unanticipated benefits of automotive emission control: Reduction in fatalities by motor vehicle exhaust gas. Sci Total Environ 146–147:93, 1994.

492. Hopkinson JM, Pearce PJ, Oliver JS: Carbon monoxide poisoning mimicking gastroenteritis. BMJ 281:214, 1980.

493. Houck PM, Hampson NB: Epidemic carbon monoxide poisoning following a winter storm. J Emerg Med 15:469, 1997.

494. Wrenn K, Conners GP: Carbon monoxide poisoning during ice storms: A tale of two cities. J Emerg Med 15:465, 1997.

495. Walker AR: Emergency department management of house fire burns and carbon monoxide poisoning in children. Curr Opin Pediatr 8:239, 1996.

496. Hampson NB, Kramer CC, Dunford RG, Norkool DM: Carbon monoxide poisoning from indoor burning of charcoal briquets. JAMA 271:52, 1994.

497. Wilson EF, Rich TH, Messman HC: The hazardous hibachi. Carbon monoxide poisoning following use of charcoal. JAMA 221:405, 1972.

498. Hampson NB, Norkool DM: Carbon monoxide poisoning in children riding in the back of pickup trucks. JAMA 267:538, 1992.

499. Rao R, Touger M, Gennis P, et al: Epidemic of accidental carbon monoxide poisonings caused by snow-obstructed exhaust systems. Ann Emerg Med 29:290, 1997.

500. Ely EW, Moorehead B, Haponik EF: Warehouse workers' headache: Emergency evaluation and management of 30 patients with carbon monoxide poisoning. Am J Med 98:145, 1995.

501. Silvers SM, Hampson NB: Carbon monoxide poisoning among recreational boaters. JAMA 274:1614, 1995.

502. Carbon monoxide poisoning at an indoor ice arena and bingo hall—Seattle, 1996. MMWR Morb Mortal Wkly Rep 45:265, 1996.

503. Hawkes AP, McCammon JB, Hoffman RE: Indoor use of concrete saws and other gas-powered equipment. Analysis of reported carbon monoxide poisoning cases in Colorado. J Occup Environ Med 40:49, 1998.

504. Stewart RD, Hake CL: Paint-remover hazard. JAMA 235:398, 1976.

505. Thom SR, Xu YA, Ischiropoulos H: Vascular endothelial cells generate peroxynitrite in response to carbon monoxide exposure. Chem Res Toxicol 10:1023, 1997.

506. Swada Y, Takahashi M, Ohashi N, et al: Computerized tomography as an indication of long-term outcome after acute carbon monoxide poisoning. Lancet 1:783, 1980.

507. Fein A, Grossman RF, Gareth Jones J, et al: Carbon monoxide effect on alveolar epithelial permeability. Chest 78:726, 1980.

508. Florkowski CM, Rossi ML, Carey MP, et al: Rhabdomyolysis and acute renal failure following carbon monoxide poisoning: Two case reports with muscle histopathology and enzyme activities. J Toxicol Clin Toxicol 30:443, 1992.

509. Kolarzyk E: The effect of acute carbon monoxide poisoning on the respiratory system efficiency. I. Values of spirometric parameters in different degrees of poisoning. Int J Occup Med Environ Health 7:225, 1994.

510. Kolarzyk E: The effect of acute carbon monoxide poisoning on the respiratory system efficiency. II. Types of ventilatory disorder and dynamics of changes according to the severity of carbon monoxide poisoning. Int J Occup Med Environ Health 7:237, 1994.

511. Gorman DF, Clayton D, Gilligan JE, Webb RK: A longitudinal study of 100 consecutive admissions for carbon monoxide poisoning to the Royal Adelaide Hospital. Anaesth Intensive Care 20:311, 1992.

512. Smith JS, Brandon S: Morbidity from acute carbon monoxide poisoning. A three-year follow-up. BMJ 1:318, 1973.

513. Astrup P: Some physiological and pathological effects of moderate carbon monoxide exposure. BMJ 4:447, 1972.

514. Goldsmith JR, Landaw SA: Carbon monoxide in human health. Science 162:1352, 1968.

515. Cowie J, Sillett EW, Ball KP: Carbon-monoxide absorption by cigarette smokers who change to smoking cigars. Lancet 1:1033, 1973.

516. Carbon monoxide poisoning—A timely warning (editorial). N Engl J Med 278:849, 1968.

517. Aronow WS, Isbell MW: Carbon monoxide effect on exercise-induced angina pectoris. Ann Intern Med 79:392, 1973.

518. Anderson EW, Adelman RJ, Strauch JM, et al: Effect of low-level carbon monoxide exposure on onset and duration of angina pectoris. A study in ten patients with ischemic heart disease. Ann Intern Med 79:46, 1973.

519. Sone S, Higashihara T, Kotake T, et al: Pulmonary manifestations in acute carbon monoxide poisoning. Am J Roentgenol 120:865, 1974.

520. Kittredge RD: Pulmonary edema in acute carbon monoxide poisoning. Am J Roentgenol 113:680, 1971.

521. Fein A, Grossman RF, Jones JG, et al: Carbon monoxide effect on alveolar epithelial permeability. Chest 78:726, 1980.

522. Buckley RG, Aks SE, Eshom JL, et al: The pulse oximetry gap in carbon monoxide intoxication. Ann Emerg Med 24:252, 1994.

523. Bazeman WP, Myers RA, Barish RA: Confirmation of the pulse oximetry gap in carbon monoxide poisoning. Ann Emerg Med 30:608, 1997.

APPENDIX

Tables of Differential Diagnosis

Previous editions of this book included a number of tables in which various thoracic diseases were grouped according to specific radiographic patterns. Each of the tables summarized the findings for a variety of abnormalities, some common and some rare. The intent was to provide the reader with a rapid if somewhat simplistic means of developing a differential diagnosis based on a recognition of radiographic patterns. In fact, the format used in the tables is a somewhat formalized outline of how many physicians approach the differential diagnosis of thoracic disease in everyday practice and thus serves both educational and practical purposes.

A set of 17 such tables of differential diagnosis were developed for this edition, with the following modifications:

1. All reference to clinical and laboratory findings in specific diseases has been deleted. Although this is clearly somewhat artificial, and we by no means mean to imply that radiographic interpretation should be performed in the absence of clinical information, practical considerations related to complexity and uniformity of the tables required that these categories of information be omitted. In keeping with this decision, the tables concerned with pleural effusion that were included in previous editions have been omitted altogether, because a consideration of differential diagnosis in this situation usually necessitates the use of laboratory information.

2. Reference to the vast majority of uncommon or rare abnormalities has been deleted. Instead, we have attempted to include only those conditions that are likely to be encountered in the routine practice of most physicians. Again, this is somewhat artificial, in that certain diseases that are prevalent in some geographic regions (e.g., as a result of high ethnic prevalence or the presence of an endemic microorganism) may be omitted. However, the tables include those conditions that overall are most likely to be seen by the *majority* of chest physicians. An indication of the most common abnormalities within each radiographic category is indicated by bold type.

3. Reference to ancillary radiologic techniques, particularly HRCT, has been added where appropriate from a differential diagnostic point of view. This is particularly relevant in the consideration of reticular and small nodular opacities. A selection of HRCT depictions of disease processes has been included to illustrate the various CT patterns.

Table A–1

HOMOGENEOUS OPACITIES WITHOUT SEGMENTAL DISTRIBUTION

This table includes abnormalities that are unilateral or bilateral but focal rather than diffuse. The pattern is epitomized by acute air-space pneumonia caused by *Streptococcus pneumoniae*. Typically, the inflammation begins in the subpleural parenchyma and spreads centrifugally through collateral channels. Because segmental boundaries do not impede such spread, consolidation tends to be nonsegmental. An air bronchogram is almost invariably present and should not be misinterpreted as evidence of inhomogeneity. If the distribution of the disease is roughly segmental (as, for example, when acute air-space pneumonia fills a whole lobe), the presence of an air bronchogram should take precedence over apparent segmental distribution in suggesting the pathogenesis and therefore the underlying causative disorder.

The nonsegmental character of parenchymal consolidation relates largely to its pathogenesis. For example, the volume of lung affected by acute radiation pneumonitis corresponds roughly to the area irradiated, with little tendency to segmental or lobar distribution.

Table A-1

HOMOGENEOUS OPACITIES WITHOUT SEGMENTAL DISTRIBUTION

ETIOLOGY	LOSS OF VOLUME	ANATOMIC DISTRIBUTION	ADDITIONAL FINDINGS	COMMENTS
DEVELOPMENTAL				
Intralobar sequestration	0	Typically abuts the diaphragm; more common on the right	—	Diagnosis can be confirmed by CT, MR imaging, or angiography
INFECTIOUS				
Bacteria				
Streptococcus pneumoniae (Fig. A–1–1)	0 to +	**Dependent portions of upper and lower lobes; usually unilobar**	**Air bronchogram almost invariable; fairly sharply circumscribed margins, even where not abutting fissure; cavitation rare except with superimposed anaerobic infection**	**Confluent air-space consolidation begins in subpleural parenchyma and spreads centrifugally via inter- and intra-acinar channels; therefore, there is no tendency to segmental involvement.**
Klebsiella-Enterobacter-Serratia species	**Tendency to expansion of involved lung, although volume may be normal or even reduced**	**Upper lobe predilection; often multilobar**	**Cavitation common; air bronchogram almost invariable; pleural effusion may be present**	**Differs from pneumococcal pneumonia in propensity to cavitate and greater tendency to expand involved lung**
Mycobacterium tuberculosis: "primary"	0 to +	Slightly more frequent in upper lobes; no predilection for either anterior or posterior segments	Ipsilateral hilar or paratracheal lymph node enlargement almost invariable in children but in only about 30% of adults; pleural effusion in 10% of affected children (almost always associated with parenchymal disease) and in approximately one third of adults (often as the sole manifestation); cavitation and miliary spread rare	
Mycobacterium tuberculosis: "postprimary"	0 to +	Upper lobe predilection, predominantly posterior	Cavitation common; small nodules frequently identifiable elsewhere in lungs as a result of endobronchial spread; air bronchogram common	Acute tuberculous pneumonia. Infection may transgress interlobar fissures from one lobe to another or (occasionally) extend into chest wall (empyema necessitatis).
Legionella species	0 to +	Usually unilateral and unilobar when first seen, with tendency to multilobar and bilateral involvement with time; lower lobe predilection	Abscess formation uncommon except in immunocompromised patients; pleural effusion in 35–65% of cases	Consolidation may progress rapidly despite antibiotic therapy. Resolution is often prolonged.
Pseudomonas aeruginosa	0	Generalized or nonspecific	Pleural effusion common	Less common manifestation than homogeneous segmental consolidation (*see* Table A–2). The majority of infections are acquired in hospital.
Haemophilus influenzae	0	No lobar predilection	Effusion common	Uncommon presentation
Anaerobic bacteria	0	Posterior portion of upper or lower lobes	Tends to progress to lung abscess	

Table continued on following page

Table A–1

HOMOGENEOUS OPACITIES WITHOUT SEGMENTAL DISTRIBUTION *Continued*

ETIOLOGY	LOSS OF VOLUME	ANATOMIC DISTRIBUTION	ADDITIONAL FINDINGS	COMMENTS
Escherichia coli	0	Strong lower lobe bias, usually multilobar	Pleural effusion frequent; cavitation uncommon	
Actinomyces and *Nocardia* species	0	Lower lobe predilection, often bilateral	Cavitation common; pleural effusion and tendency for extension into chest wall (with or without rib destruction); may transgress interlobar fissures from one lobe to another	Radiographic patterns of these organisms are indistinguishable from each other.
Fungi				
Blastomyces dermatitidis (blastomycosis)	0	Upper lobe predilection in ratio of 3:2	Cavitation uncommon (15%); pleural effusion, chest wall involvement, and lymph node enlargement rare	
Histoplasma capsulatum (histoplasmosis)	0	No predilection	Hilar lymph node enlargement common; cavitation may occur	Nonsegmental pattern is considerably less common than inhomogeneous segmental disease.
Coccidioides immitis (coccidioidomycosis)	0	Lower lobe predilection	Hilar and paratracheal lymph node enlargement may be present; cavitation common	
Aspergillus species (invasive aspergillosis)	0	No predilection	Cavitation common	Can also result in segmental consolidation due to pulmonary infarction
Pneumocystis carinii	0	Generalized	Pleural effusion uncommon	
Cryptococcus neoformans (cryptococcosis)	0	Lower lung zones	Cavitation uncommon, as is node enlargement	Less common radiographic presentation than a discrete mass
Parasites				
Entamoeba histolytica (amebiasis)	0	Right lower lobe almost exclusively	Right pleural effusion very common; cavitation occurs in minority of cases	Liver abscesses common
Paragonimus westermani (paragonimiasis)	0	No predilection	Isolated nodular shadows, usually cavitary; pleural effusion may be present	
Ascaris lumbricoides (ascariasis)	0	Multilobar	—	Loeffler-type pattern suggested by fleeting nature of consolidation
Strongyloides stercoralis	0	Multilobar	—	Loeffler-type pattern

Category	Condition		Predilection	Radiographic Findings	Comments
IMMUNOLOGIC	Simple pulmonary eosinophilia (Fig. A–1–2)	0	Peripherally situated without lobar predilection	Foci of consolidation may be single or multiple, generally ill-defined and transitory or migratory in character; cavitation, pleural effusion, lymph node enlargement, and cardiomegaly absent	
	Chronic eosinophilic pneumonia (Fig. A–1–3)	0	Peripheral lung zones without lobar predilection	—	In contrast to simple pulmonary eosinophilia, lesions tend to remain unchanged for days or weeks.
	Drug reactions		Peripheral lung zones without lobar predilection	—	Resembles simple pulmonary eosinophilia
NEOPLASTIC	Hodgkin's disease (Fig. A–1–4)	0	No predilection	Almost invariably associated with hilar or mediastinal lymph node enlargement; pleural effusion in 30% of cases; air bronchogram almost invariable	Individual lesions may coalesce to form larger areas of homogeneous consolidation.
	Primary non-Hodgkin's lymphoma	0	No predilection	Often without associated hilar and mediastinal node enlargement; pleural effusion in about 10%; air bronchogram common	
	Secondary non-Hodgkin's lymphoma	0	No predilection	Hilar and mediastinal lymph node enlargement common; air bronchogram common	
	Bronchioloalveolar carcinoma (Fig. A–1–5)	0	No predilection	Air bronchogram almost invariable	
TRAUMATIC	Pulmonary parenchymal contusion	0 to +	Usually in lung directly deep to area traumatized, although it may develop as well or predominantly on the side opposite from the trauma due to contrecoup effect	Radiographic abnormalities almost invariably develop within 6 hours; pattern varies from irregular patchy areas of air-space consolidation to diffuse and extensive homogeneous consolidation	The most common pulmonary complication of blunt chest trauma
	Acute radiation pneumonitis	+ + to + + + +	The volume of lung affected generally but not always corresponds to the area irradiated	Air bronchogram almost invariable	
IDIOPATHIC	Bronchiolitis obliterans organizing pneumonia	0 to +	No predilection	—	CT often shows predominantly peribronchial or subpleural distribution.

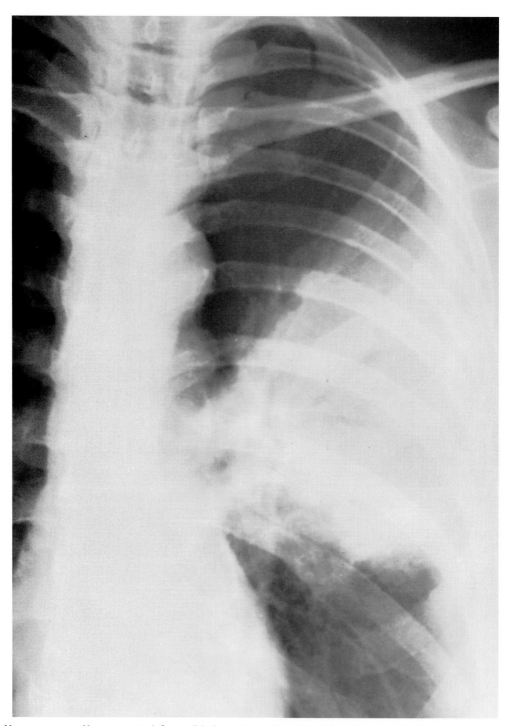

Figure A–1–1. Homogeneous Nonsegmental Consolidation: Acute Pneumococcal Pneumonia. A posteroanterior radiograph of the left hemithorax reveals consolidation of the axillary zone of the left upper lobe; the consolidation is homogeneous except for a well-defined air bronchogram. There is no loss of volume. The spreading margins are fairly sharply circumscribed despite the fact that they do not abut against a fissure. This pattern is virtually pathognomonic of acute air-space pneumonia, most commonly caused by *Streptococcus pneumoniae.*

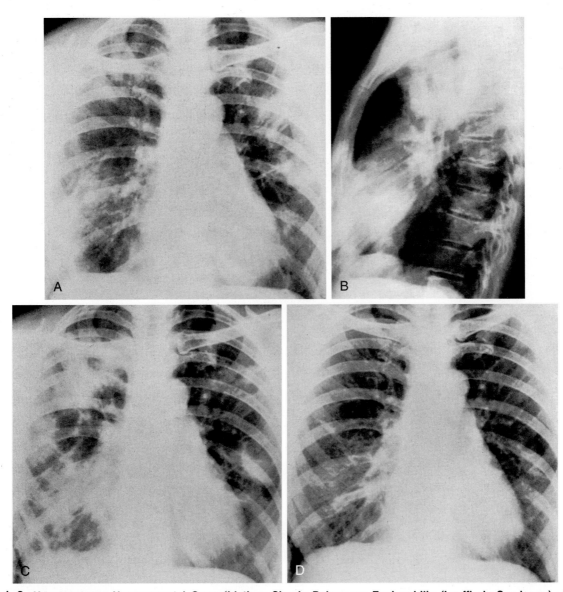

Figure A–1–2. Homogeneous Nonsegmental Consolidation: Simple Pulmonary Eosinophilia (Loeffler's Syndrome). A 61-year-old woman was admitted to the hospital for the first time with a 2-month history of anorexia, a 10-pound weight loss, afternoon fever, and mild cough productive of greenish phlegm occasionally flecked with blood; there was no history of allergies. On admission, posteroanterior *(A)* and lateral *(B)* chest radiographs revealed numerous shadows of homogeneous density in both lungs, occupying no precise segmental distribution; note particularly the broad shadow of increased density along the lower axillary zone of the right lung. At this time her total white cell count was 11,000/mm³ with 1,700 (15%) eosinophils. One week later *(C),* the anatomic distribution of the shadows had changed considerably, being more extensive in the right upper and both lower lobes and less extensive in the left upper lobe; at this time the total white cell count was 14,000/mm³ with 20% eosinophils. A diagnosis of Loeffler's syndrome was made, and the institution of corticosteroid therapy resulted in prompt remission of symptoms. One week later, the white cell count had returned to normal levels, the eosinophilia had disappeared, and the radiographic abnormalities had completely resolved *(D).*

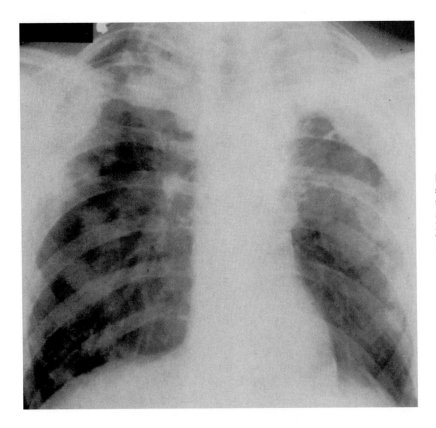

Figure A–1–3. Homogeneous Nonsegmental Consolidation: Chronic Eosinophilic Pneumonia. A posteroanterior chest radiograph reveals bilateral air-space consolidation, predominantly upper lobe in distribution; note the highly characteristic peripheral distribution of the disease. The patient was a middle-aged woman who presented with wheezing, cough, nocturnal fever, and blood eosinophilia.

Figure A–1–4. Homogeneous Nonsegmental Consolidation: Hodgkin's Disease. A posteroanterior chest radiograph reveals extensive consolidation of much of the right lung, particularly its lower two thirds: the consolidation possesses no clear-cut segmental distribution. An air bronchogram is present. There is little if any loss of volume. Patchy shadows of a similar nature can be identified in the lower portion of the left lung. The patient was a 27-year-old woman.

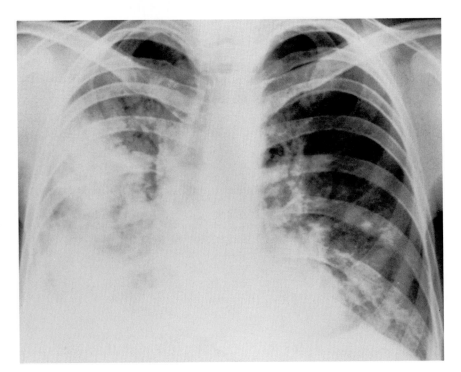

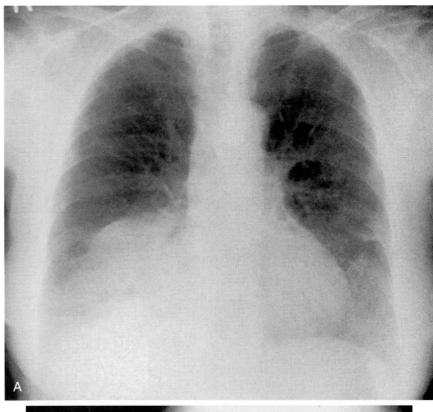

Figure A–1–5. Homogeneous Nonsegmental Consolidation: Bronchioloalveolar Carcinoma. Posteroanterior *(A)* and lateral *(B)* chest radiographs show bilateral nonsegmental air-space consolidation involving the middle lobe and parts of both lower lobes.

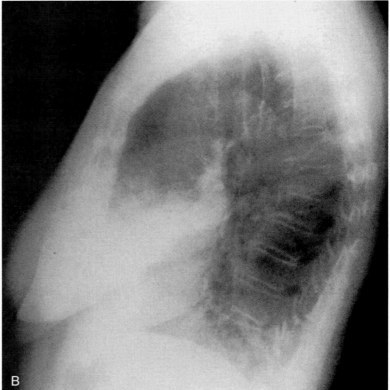

Table A–2
HOMOGENEOUS OPACITIES OF SEGMENTAL DISTRIBUTION

This pattern is caused most often by endobronchial obstructing lesions and reflects the presence of atelectasis with or without obstructive pneumonitis. Because the pathogenesis involves bronchial obstruction, the resultant shadow necessarily is of specific bronchopulmonary segmental distribution. An air bronchogram should be absent, except when the atelectasis is "adhesive" or "nonobstructive" in type or when therapy has relieved the obstruction, thereby permitting the entry of air into the involved segmental bronchi.

Acute confluent bronchopneumonia, commonly of staphylococcal etiology, also produces this pattern. The pathogenesis of bronchopneumonia implies a segmental distribution; the severity of the infection usually results in confluence of consolidation and consequent homogeneity. As in obstructive pneumonitis, an air bronchogram is seldom present.

Table A–2

HOMOGENEOUS OPACITIES OF SEGMENTAL DISTRIBUTION

	ETIOLOGY	LOSS OF VOLUME	ANATOMIC DISTRIBUTION	ADDITIONAL FINDINGS	COMMENTS
INFECTIOUS	**Bacteria**				
	Staphylococcus aureus (Fig. A–2–1)	0 to + +	No lobar predilection	**Abscess formation common; pleural effusion (empyema) common, particularly in children, with or without bronchopleural fistula (pyopneumothorax)**	**Air bronchogram exceptional; bilateral in over 60% of adults**
	Streptococcus pneumoniae		Predominantly lower lobes	Air bronchogram almost invariable; cavitation rare	True segmental distribution very uncommon, and only when whole lobe involved
	Streptococcus pyogenes *Klebsiella-Enterobacter-Serratia* *Haemophilus influenzae* *Pseudomonas aeruginosa*	0 to + +	Predominantly lower lobes	Pleural effusion common	Represents confluent bronchopneumonia
	Anaerobic organisms	0 to + +	Posterior segments of upper lobes and superior segment of lower lobes	Cavitation and empyema common	
	Mycobacterium tuberculosis	0 to + + + +	3:2 predominance of right lung over left	Associated paratracheal or hilar lymph node enlargement in the majority of patients	Atelectasis results from airway compression by enlarged lymph nodes or from endobronchial tuberculosis; traditionally considered a manifestation of primary disease.
	Fungi				
	Aspergillus species	0 to +	No predilection	—	Segmental consolidation in invasive disease may result from bronchopneumonia or from pulmonary infarction or hemorrhage secondary to pulmonary artery invasion. Segmental consolidation may also be seen in allergic bronchopulmonary aspergillosis.
	Viruses and Rickettsiae				
	Coxiella burnetii (Q fever)	0	Predominantly lower lobes	Pleural effusion occasionally seen; hilar lymph node enlargement rare	Extent of consolidation may range from one segment to a complete lobe.
NEOPLASTIC	Pulmonary carcinoma (Fig. A–2–2)	+ to + + + +	**The ratio of right to left lung is 3:2; similar ratio exists for upper to lower lobes**	**Enlarged lymph nodes may be present in the hilum and elsewhere; pleural effusion in 10–15% of cases**	**Distinction of the obstructing tumor and distal atelectasis/pneumonitis can usually be made using contrast-enhanced CT or MR imaging.**
	Carcinoid tumor	+ to + + + +	Tends to arise from lobar or segmental bronchi; no lobar predilection	Typical findings are those of atelectasis/obstructive pneumonitis; tumor may be identified on chest radiographs or by CT; lymph nodes usually normal in size	Most common radiographic manifestation of this neoplasm

Table continued on following page

Table A–2

HOMOGENEOUS OPACITIES OF SEGMENTAL DISTRIBUTION *Continued*

ETIOLOGY	LOSS OF VOLUME	ANATOMIC DISTRIBUTION	ADDITIONAL FINDINGS	COMMENTS
Mesenchymal neoplasms	+ to + + + +	No definite predilection	—	The more common method of presentation is as a solitary nodule. The tumors have a nonspecific appearance on CT scans except for lipomas, which have homogeneous fat density.
EMBOLIC				
Thromboembolism with infarction (Fig. A–2–3)	**0 to + +**	**Lower lobes, usually posteriorly but often nestled in the costophrenic sulcus; less than 10% in upper lobes; may be multiple**	**Infarcted area generally 3 to 5 cm in diameter but ranges from barely visible to 10 cm in diameter, and occasionally shows truncated cone appearance ("Hampton's hump"); ipsilateral hemidiaphragm frequently raised; increase in size and abrupt tapering of feeder artery is characteristic; pleural effusion is common; manifestations of postcapillary hypertension due to associated cardiac disease may be present**	
INHALATIONAL				
Aspiration of solid foreign bodies	+ to + + + +	Lower lobes most commonly affected, ratio of right to left being 2:1	The foreign body is opaque (e.g., a tooth) in approximately 10% of patients; foreign body easier to recognize on CT scan than on the radiograph	Segmental atelectasis or consolidation occurs in only 25% of cases, the remainder having air trapping on expiratory radiographs or CT scans.
Lipid pneumonia	0 to +	Generally dependent portions of lower and upper lobes	Radiologic pattern is air-space consolidation; segmental nature of the consolidation may be quite precise	CT, particularly HRCT, often allows a specific diagnosis by demonstrating the presence of fat.
TRAUMATIC				
Bronchial fracture	+ + to + + + +	One or more lobes or an entire lung	Pneumothorax, pneumomediastinum, and subcutaneous emphysema	Atelectasis develops as a result of displacement of fracture ends and is commonly a late development.
Postoperative adhesive atelectasis	+ to + + +	Left lower lobe predilection	Air bronchogram is common; the usual findings associated with postoperative thoracotomy, such as pleural effusion and diaphragmatic elevation	Occurs predominantly following cardiac surgery, particularly with use of extracorporeal circulation; inhomogeneous segmental opacification more common

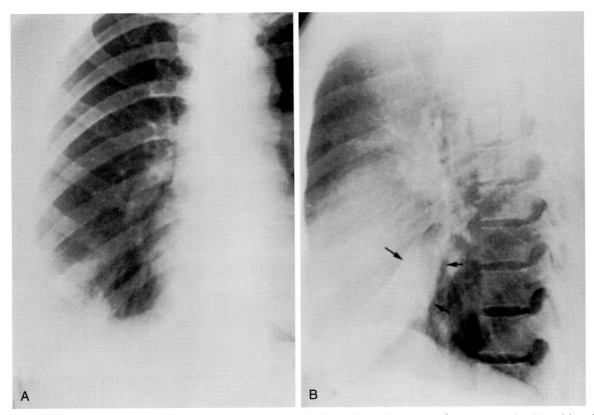

Figure A–2–1. Homogeneous Segmental Consolidation: Acute Confluent Bronchopneumonia. Posteroanterior *(A)* and lateral *(B)* chest radiographs of the right hemithorax reveal homogeneous consolidation confined to the precise anatomic distribution of the anterior basal bronchopulmonary segment of the right lower lobe. The consolidation occupies a triangular segment of lung, with its apex at the hilum and its base at the visceral pleura *(arrows* in *B).* There is no evidence of an air bronchogram. Sputum culture produced heavy growth of *Staphylococcus aureus;* complete radiographic resolution occurred in 10 days.

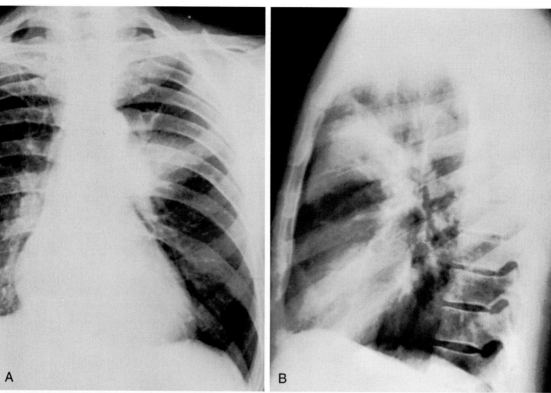

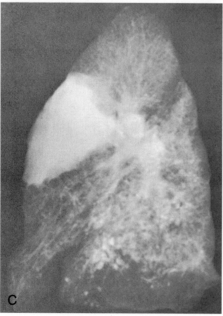

Figure A–2–2. Homogeneous Segmental Consolidation: Bronchogenic Carcinoma. A triangular shadow of homogeneous density is situated in the anterior portion of the left upper lobe, its base contiguous to the retrosternal pleura and its apex at the left hilum. The shadow is seen _en face_ in posteroanterior projection _(A)_ and in profile in lateral projection _(B)_. The absence of an air bronchogram indicates bronchial obstruction; the relatively minor degree of loss of volume denotes obstructive pneumonitis. Squamous cell carcinoma was identified in the anterior segmental bronchus of the left upper lobe. A lateral radiograph of the resected lung _(C)_ shows the sharp definition and precise segmental distribution of the shadow to excellent advantage.

Figure A–2–3. Homogeneous Segmental Consolidation: Pulmonary Infarct. Posteroanterior *(A)* and lateral *(B)* chest radiographs from a 40-year-old man reveal a fairly well circumscribed shadow of homogeneous density occupying the posterior basal segment of the right lower lobe. In lateral projection, the shadow has the shape of a truncated cone with its apex directed toward the hilum (Hampton's hump) *(arrows);* a small effusion can be identified. This combination of changes is highly suggestive of pulmonary thromboembolism with infarction.

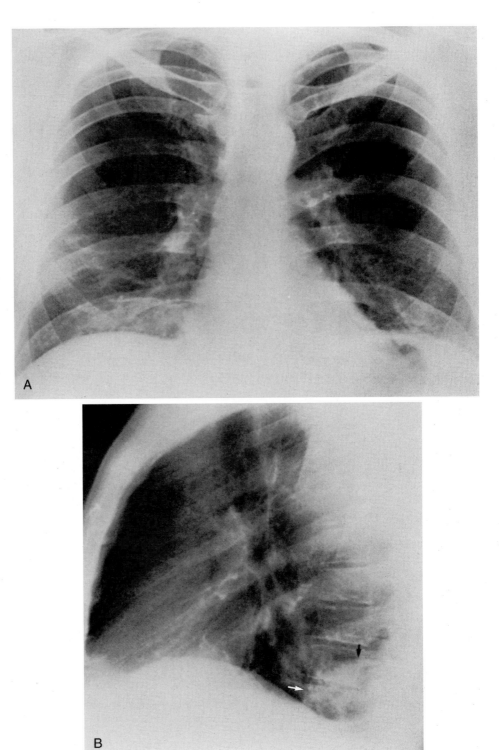

Table A–3

INHOMOGENEOUS OPACITIES WITHOUT SEGMENTAL DISTRIBUTION

Postprimary tuberculosis undoubtedly is the most common cause of this pattern—focal areas of parenchymal consolidation separated by zones of air-containing lung. Although tuberculosis commonly is localized to the apical and posterior regions of an upper lobe, it seldom is truly segmental; in other words, it does not tend to affect a pyramidal section of lung of which the apex is at the hilum and base at the visceral pleura. It must be emphasized that the presence of cavitation *in itself* should not be interpreted as a cause of inhomogeneity. For example, acute confluent bronchopneumonia, which typically produces homogeneous segmental consolidation, may cavitate and thus create a shadow of relative inhomogeneity; such disease clearly is different pathogenetically from postprimary tuberculosis, in which cavitation accentuates an already inhomogeneous pattern.

Table A–3

INHOMOGENEOUS OPACITIES WITHOUT SEGMENTAL DISTRIBUTION

	ETIOLOGY	LOSS OF VOLUME	ANATOMIC DISTRIBUTION	ADDITIONAL FINDINGS	COMMENTS
INFECTIOUS	**Bacteria** *Mycobacterium tuberculosis* (Fig. A–3–1)	0	**Apical and posterior segments of upper lobes (rarely anterior alone); superior segment of lower lobes**	**Cavitation common; effusion and lymph node enlargement relatively uncommon**	
	Klebsiella-Enterobacter-Serratia species	+ to +++	Predominantly upper lobes	May be associated with cavitation	The chronic phase of the disease; closely simulates tuberculosis
	Fungi *Histoplasma capsulatum*	0	Primary infection commonly in lower lobes	Hilar lymph node enlargement frequent; pleural effusion not common; cavitation may be present	Radiologically indistinguishable from tuberculosis
	Coccidioides immitis	0	Upper lobes	Densities may be "fleeting" in character and may leave behind thin-walled cavities	This is the acute pneumonic form of the disease.
	Blastomyces dermatitis	0	Upper lobe predominance in ratio of 3:2	Cavitation in 15% of cases; bone involvement in 25%, either by direct extension across pleura or by bloodstream; pleural effusion and lymph node enlargement rare	
	Viruses and Mycoplasma	0	Predominantly lower lobes	None	A specific segmental distribution may not be recognizable at certain stages of these acute pneumonias.
IMMUNOLOGIC	Simple pulmonary eosinophilia	0	Peripheral lung zones without upper or lower predilection	Consolidation generally ill-defined and transitory or migratory in character	Consolidation more characteristically homogeneous
TRAUMATIC	Acute or chronic radiation pneumonitis (Fig. A–3–2)	0 to +++	Generally corresponds to the area irradiated	Air bronchogram common	Acute radiation pneumonitis characteristically produces a homogeneous nonsegmental pattern (*see* Table A–1) but in some cases is inhomogeneous.

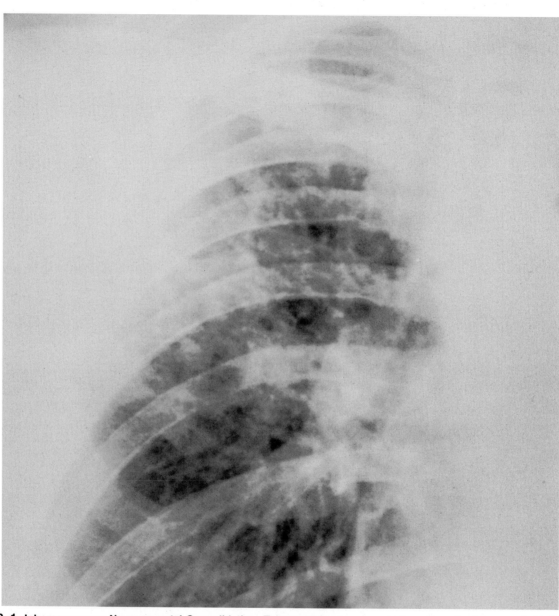

Figure A–3–1. Inhomogeneous Nonsegmental Consolidation: Tuberculosis. A posteroanterior radiograph of the upper half of the right lung demonstrates numerous patchy opacities separated by zones of air-containing lung. Both the posterior portion of the upper lobe and the superior portion of the lower lobe are affected, but involvement is not truly segmental. The patient was a 40-year-old man. *Mycobacterium tuberculosis* was cultured from the sputum. (Courtesy of Dr. J.F. Meakins, Montreal.)

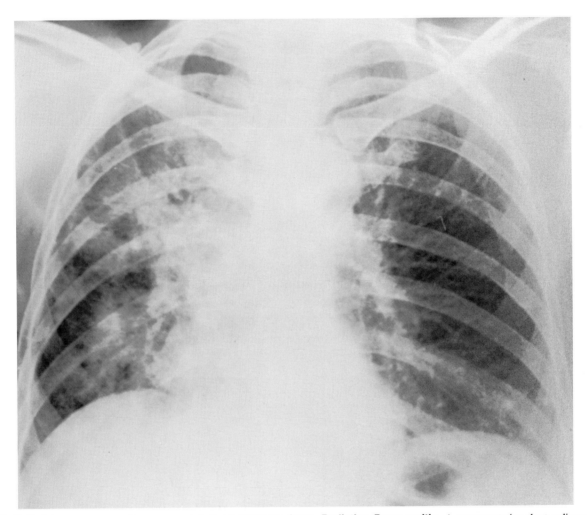

Figure A–3–2. Inhomogeneous Nonsegmental Consolidation: Acute Radiation Pneumonitis. A posteroanterior chest radiograph reveals extensive disease throughout the right lung, possessing a random distribution without confinement to specific segments; the central and mid-lung zones are affected more than the peripheral ones. An air bronchogram indicates that the process is chiefly one of air-space consolidation, although there is moderate loss of lung volume, as evidenced by mediastinal shift and right hemidiaphragmatic elevation. The patient was a 68-year-old woman seen approximately 2 months following a course of radiation therapy to the anterior mediastinal lymph nodes for metastatic carcinoma of the breast; complete radiographic resolution occurred in 6 months.

Table A–4

INHOMOGENEOUS OPACITIES WITH SEGMENTAL DISTRIBUTION

This pattern is characteristic of bronchopneumonia. The infection is propagated distally via the airways and thus invariably is of segmental distribution. The parenchymal changes consist of a combination of consolidation, atelectasis, and over-inflation, resulting in an inhomogeneous radiographic pattern. Bronchiectasis can produce the same appearance.

Table A–4

INHOMOGENEOUS OPACITIES WITH SEGMENTAL DISTRIBUTION

	ETIOLOGY	LOSS OF VOLUME	ANATOMIC DISTRIBUTION	ADDITIONAL FINDINGS	COMMENTS
INFECTIOUS	**Bacteria**				
	Mycobacterium tuberculosis: **"postprimary"**	**+ to + + +**	**Apical and posterior segments upper lobes; superior segment lower lobes**	**Frequently associated with tuberculous bronchiectasis and sometimes with cavitation**	**Chronic stage of the disease, usually fibrotic (but not necessarily inactive)**
	Staphylococcus aureus *Streptococcus pyogenes* *Haemophilus influenzae* *Streptococcus pneumoniae* *Klebsiella-Enterobacter-Serratia* species (Fig. A–4–1)	+ to + +	Predominantly lower lobes	Pleural effusion relatively common	On rare occasions, any of these organisms may give rise to an inhomogeneous segmental pattern.
	Fungi *Histoplasma capsulatum*	+ to + + +	Upper lobes	—	Indistinguishable in appearance from chronic postprimary tuberculosis
	Viruses and "Atypical Organisms" *Mycoplasma pneumoniae* *Chlamydia psittaci* *Chlamydia pneumoniae* Influenza virus Adenovirus	0	Predominantly lower lobes	Pleural effusion and lymph node enlargement uncommon	Characteristic reticular pattern with superimposed patchy areas of airspace consolidation
NEOPLASTIC	**Pulmonary carcinoma**	**0 to + + + +**	**Upper to lower lobe ratio 3:2**	**Lymph node enlargement and pleural effusion relatively common**	**Incomplete obstruction may permit visualization of air-containing structures within the obstructed segment.**
	Carcinoid tumor	0 to + + + +	No predilection	Lymph node enlargement rare	

Table continued on following page

3097

Table A–4
INHOMOGENEOUS OPACITIES WITH SEGMENTAL DISTRIBUTION *Continued*

ETIOLOGY	LOSS OF VOLUME	ANATOMIC DISTRIBUTION	ADDITIONAL FINDINGS	COMMENTS
THROMBOEMBOLIC Pulmonary thromboembolism	0 to + +	Lower lobes	**May be multiple; ipsilateral hemidiaphragm frequently elevated**	
INHALATIONAL Recurrent aspiration	+ to + + +	Posterior segments of lower or upper lobes; anatomic distribution may vary considerably on serial radiographs		The radiographic picture suggests "bronchopneumonia." Multiple segments may be involved. Bronchiectasis may develop in involved segments.
Aspiration of solid foreign bodies (Fig. A–4–2)	+ to + +	Most commonly lower lobes, the ratio of right to left being 2:1	Radiopaque foreign body visible on radiograph in approximately 10% of cases; foreign body easier to identify on CT scan than on radiograph	May be associated with bronchiectasis.
Lipid pneumonia	0 to +	Primarily dependent portions of upper and lower lobes	CT, particularly HRCT, often reveals the fatty nature of the opacity	A reticular pattern may develop as a result of the movement of oil (in macrophages) from the air spaces into the interstitial tissues.
AIRWAY DISEASE Bronchiectasis	+ to + + +	More frequent in lower lobes and right middle lobe. Multiple segments or lobes may be involved.	Saccular bronchiectasis may show fluid levels; compensatory overinflation may be present in unaffected lung	Diagnosis is readily confirmed by HRCT.

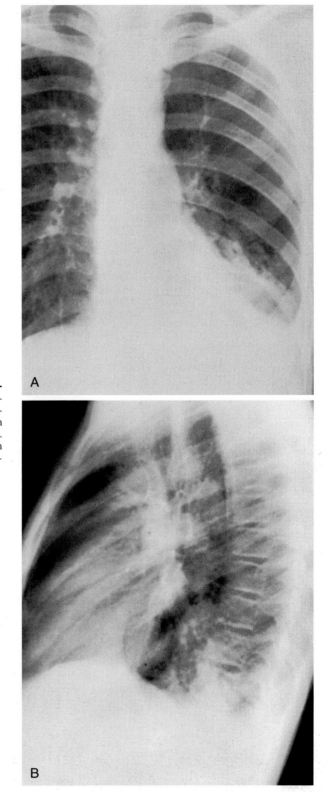

Figure A–4–1. Inhomogeneous Segmental Consolidation: Acute Bronchopneumonia. Posteroanterior *(A)* and lateral *(B)* radiographs of the left hemithorax show patchy inhomogeneous consolidation of the posterior and lateral bronchopulmonary segments of the left lower lobe. The affected lung is roughly conical in shape, with its apex at the hilum and its base at the diaphragmatic visceral pleura. There is some loss of volume, as evidenced by elevation of the left hemidiaphragm and shift of the mediastinum. Sputum culture revealed heavy growth of *Haemophilus influenzae.*

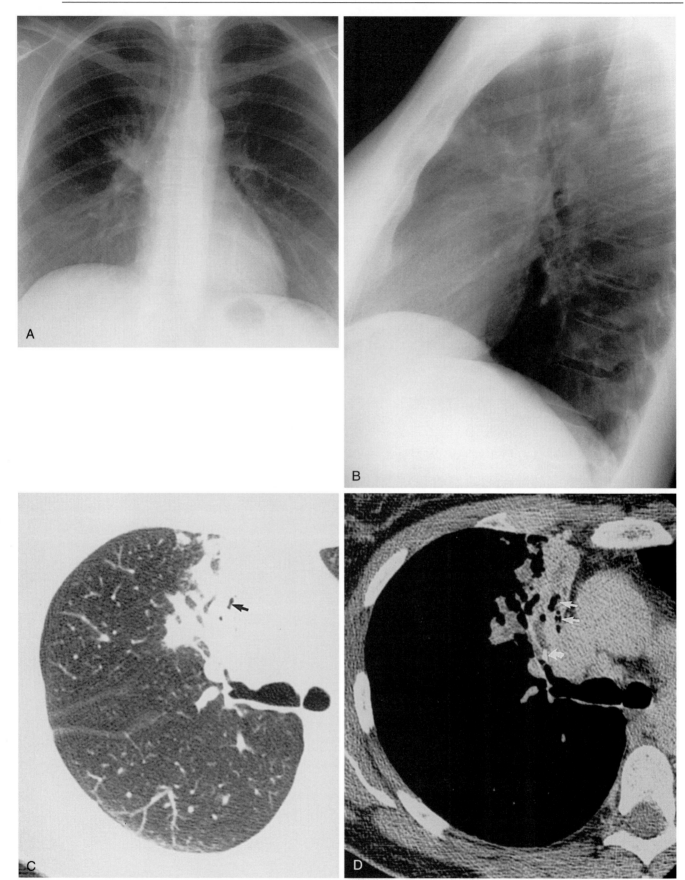

Figure A–4–2. Inhomogeneous Segmental Consolidation: Bronchiectasis Caused by Aspiration of a Popcorn Kernel. Posteroanterior *(A)* and lateral *(B)* chest radiographs from a 44-year-old woman demonstrate localized inhomogeneous consolidation and atelectasis involving the anterior segment of the right upper lobe. HRCT scans *C* and *D* demonstrate evidence of obstructive pneumonitis and bronchiectasis *(straight arrows)*. The localized area of high attenuation *(curved arrow)* within the bronchial lumen represents an aspirated popcorn kernel.

Table A–5
CYSTIC AND CAVITARY DISEASE

This pattern includes all forms of pulmonary disease characterized by circumscribed air-containing spaces with distinct walls, including cavitated pneumonia or carcinoma, blebs, bullae, and cystic bronchiectasis. Air-fluid levels may be present or absent; cavities may be single or multiple.

Table A–5

CYSTIC AND CAVITARY DISEASE

	ETIOLOGY	ANATOMIC DISTRIBUTION	CHARACTER OF WALL	ADDITIONAL FINDINGS	COMMENTS
INFECTIOUS	**Bacteria**				
	Staphylococcus aureus (Fig. A–5–1)	No lobar predilection	Tends to be thick with ragged inner lining	Empyema with or without bronchopleural fistula (pyopneumothorax) may occur	Cavitation most often complicates bronchopneumonia; occasionally (particularly in children) a pneumatocele is seen. Staphylococcal pyemia may lead to multiple cavitated nodules widely distributed throughout both lungs.
	Klebsiella-Enterobacter-Serratia species	Predominantly upper lobes	Tends to be thick with ragged inner lining	Pleural effusion (empyema) may be present; cavity rarely contains a mass of necrotic lung (acute lung gangrene)	Cavities are usually single but tend to be multilocular; multiple cavities may be present if pneumonia is multilobar.
	Pseudomonas aeruginosa Escherichia coli	Predominantly lower lobes	Highly variable	Empyema frequent	
	Streptococcus pneumoniae	Upper lobe predilection	Thick, with ragged inner lining	The cavity may contain a mass of necrotic lung—acute lung gangrene	A rare complication of fulminating pneumococcal pneumonia
	Anaerobic organisms	Posterior portion of both lungs	Tends to be thick with ragged inner lining	Cavities frequently multiple; empyema common	
	Mycobacterium species (Fig. A–5–2)	Apical and posterior regions of upper lobes and apical region of lower lobes	Tends to be of moderate thickness; inner lining generally smooth	Cavities may be multiple	
	Actinomyces species *Nocardia* species	Lower lobe predilection, bilateral	Generally thick-walled	Pleural effusion (empyema) is relatively common; extension into the chest wall with or without rib destruction is uncommon nowadays	

3102

Fungi

Organism	Location	Wall	Radiographic features	Comments
Pneumocystis carinii (Fig. A–5–3)	**Upper lobe predilection**	**Thin**	**Widespread ground-glass opacities often present; pneumothorax frequent**	**This complication of the infection occurs most commonly in patients who have the acquired immunodeficiency syndrome.**
Histoplasma capsulatum	Predominantly upper lobes	Variable	Cavities may be multiple	Radiographic features similar to those of postprimary tuberculosis
Coccidioides immitis	Predominantly upper lobes	Tends to be very thin-walled	These thin-walled cavities tend to occur in asymptomatic patients following "fleeting" pneumonitis	
Blastomyces dermatitidis	No predilection	Variable, but generally thick-walled	Cavitation occurs in about 15% of cases; pleural effusion and hilar lymph node enlargement very uncommon	
Cryptococcus neoformans	Predominantly lower lobes	Variable, but generally thick-walled	Cavitation occurs in about 15% of cases; pleural effusion and hilar lymph node enlargement very uncommon	
Aspergillus species	—	—	—	The angio-invasive form of the disease is often associated with cavitation and often results in an air crescent.

Parasites

Organism	Location	Wall	Radiographic features	Comments
Paragonimus westermani	No predilection	Characteristically thin, with local elevation or hump on inner lining	In addition to cystic lesions, there may be areas of consolidation and linear shadows	Relatively common in southeast Asia. CT scans may demonstrate an ovoid structure within the cysts representing the worm.
Echinococcus granulosus (hydatid cyst)	Lower lobe predilection	Air may dissect between ectocyst and endocyst, creating a halo, or contents of cyst may be expelled into bronchial tree, leaving a thin-walled cystic space	Irregularities of fluid layer caused by collapsed membranes (water-lily sign or sign of the camalote); hydropneumothorax occasionally	CT demonstrates water density cyst or water-lily sign.

Table continued on following page

Table A–5
CYSTIC AND CAVITARY DISEASE *Continued*

	ETIOLOGY	ANATOMIC DISTRIBUTION	CHARACTER OF WALL	ADDITIONAL FINDINGS	COMMENTS
IMMUNOLOGIC	Wegener's granulomatosis (Fig. A–5–4)	Widely distributed and bilateral, with no predilection for upper or lower lung zones	Usually thick, with irregular inner lining. In time, cavities may become thin-walled.	Cavities commonly multiple but all masses do not necessarily cavitate; areas of consolidation may be seen	Cavitation occurs eventually in one third to one half of patients. With treatment, cavitary lesions may disappear or heal with scar formation.
	Sarcoidosis	Upper lobe predominance	No typical characteristics	May contain fungus balls	"Cavities" usually represent ectatic bronchi.
NEOPLASTIC	**Pulmonary carcinoma** (Fig. A–5–5)	**Predilection for upper lobes, both lungs being affected equally**	**Tends to be thick, with an irregular, nodular inner lining (mural nodules)**		**Cavitation occurs in 5–10% of pulmonary carcinomas. The majority are squamous cell carcinoma (adenocarcinomas and large cell carcinomas cavitate occasionally, small cell carcinomas rarely).**
	Hematogeneous metastases	Cavitation occurs more frequently in upper than in lower lobe lesions	May be thin or thick	Cavitation may involve only a few of multiple nodules throughout the lungs, such nodules characteristically showing considerable variation in size	Occurs most frequently in squamous cell neoplasms
THROMBOEMBOLIC	Septic thromboembolism	Lower lobe predilection, predominantly posterior and lateral segments	Usually thin but may be thick, with shaggy inner lining	CT scans frequently demonstrate a vessel in close association with the nodules ("feeding vessel" sign)	Cavitation can also occur as a result of bacterial superinfection of a bland infarct.
AIRWAYS DISEASE	**Bullae** (Fig. A–5–6)	**Predilection for upper lobes**	**Smooth and thin**	**With infection, fluid levels may develop. In some cases, radiographic evidence of diffuse emphysema is present**	
	Cystic bronchiectasis (Fig. A–5–7)	Predilection for lower lobes	Smooth and thin or thick	Usually considerable loss of volume of affected segment or segments	"Cavities" represent severely dilated segmental bronchi; usually multiple and commonly with air-fluid levels
TRAUMATIC	Pulmonary parenchymal laceration (traumatic lung cyst)	Characteristically in the peripheral subpleural parenchyma immediately underlying the point of maximal injury	Typically thin	The cavities may be with or without air-fluid levels, single or multiple, unilocular or multilocular, and oval or spherical in shape	The presence of laceration may be masked by surrounding pulmonary contusion. In some bullet wounds of the lung, a central radiolucency may be observed along the course of the bullet track, simulating a cavity when viewed in the same direction as the wound.

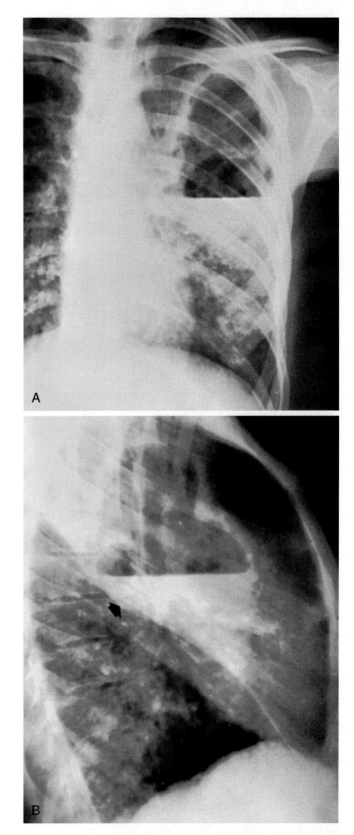

Figure A–5–1. Cavitary Disease: Acute Lung Abscess. Posteroanterior *(A)* and lateral *(B)* chest radiographs show a large cavity in the posterior portion of the left upper lobe, possessing a prominent air-fluid level. The cavity wall is of moderate thickness and possesses an irregular, shaggy inner lining. The major fissure is bowed posteriorly *(arrow* in *B)*. The patchy shadows in both lungs represent contrast medium from previous bronchography. The patient was a 24-year-old woman. Sputum culture revealed heavy growth of *Staphylococcus aureus.*

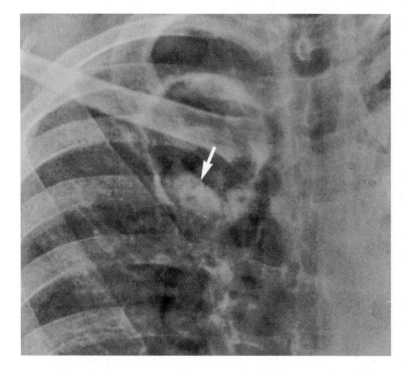

Figure A–5–2. Cavitary Disease: Chronic Tuberculous Cavity Containing a Fungus Ball. A posteroanterior radiograph of the upper half of the right lung reveals a thin-walled, irregular cavity in the paramediastinal zone. Situated within it is a smooth, oblong shadow of homogeneous density *(arrow)*, representing an aspergilloma.

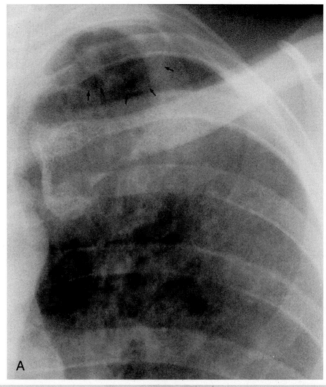

Figure A–5–3. Cyst Formation:
***Pneumocystis carinii* Pneumonia.** A
posteroanterior chest radiograph *(A)* of the
left upper lobe of a 28-year-old patient who
had the acquired immunodeficiency syndrome and *Pneumocystis carinii* pneumonia
shows thin-walled cysts *(arrows)* and
ground-glass opacities. An HRCT scan *(B)*
demonstrates bilateral areas of ground-glass
attenuation and thin-walled cystic lesions.
The findings are characteristic of *Pneumocystis carinii* pneumonia.

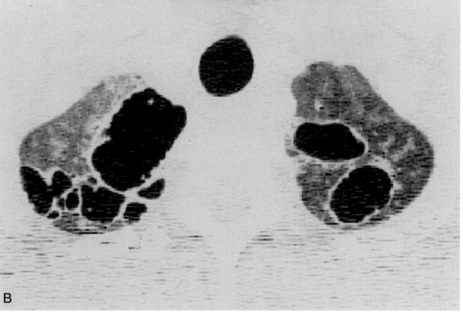

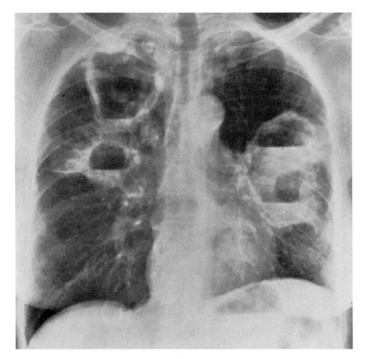

Figure A–5–4. Multiple Cavitated Nodules: Wegener's Granulomatosis. A posteroanterior radiograph demonstrates multiple, large, thick-walled cavities situated in both upper lobes. The patient was a 55-year-old woman.

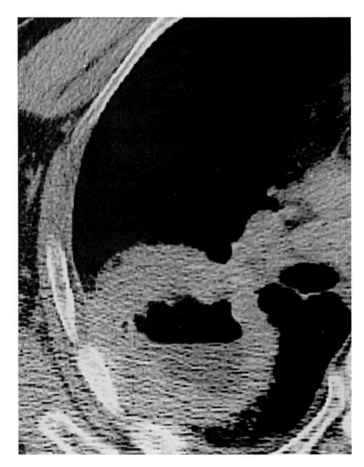

Figure A–5–5. Solitary Pulmonary Mass: Pulmonary Carcinoma. A CT scan demonstrates a 5-cm-diameter cavitated tumor that contains an air-fluid level. Findings suggestive of malignancy include the lesion's size and thick walls and the nodular contour of its inner wall. A squamous cell carcinoma was identified at surgery.

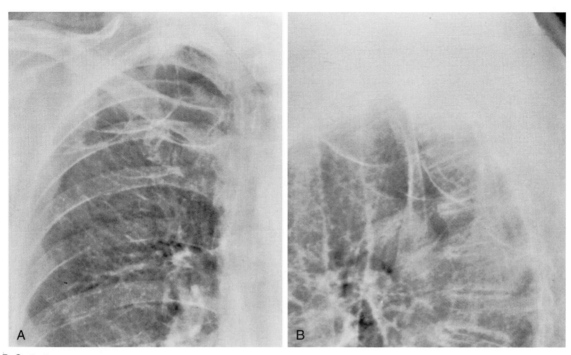

Figure A–5–6. Bullae. Radiographs of the upper half of the right lung in posteroanterior *(A)* and lateral *(B)* projections reveal several cystic spaces in the lung apex sharply separated from contiguous lung by curvilinear, hairline shadows.

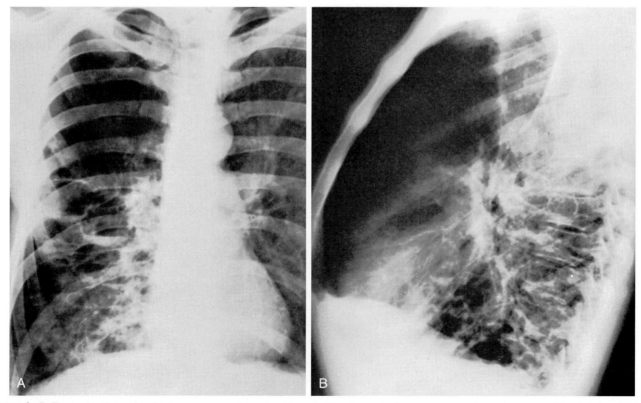

Figure A–5–7. Cystic Bronchiectasis. Posteroanterior *(A)* and lateral *(B)* radiographs demonstrate extensive replacement of the right lower lobe by multiple thin-walled cysts, many of which contain air-fluid levels.

Table A–6
SOLITARY PULMONARY NODULE

For the purposes of this table, the criteria for inclusion in this category are as follows:

1. The presence of a solitary radiographic shadow does not exceed 3 cm in its largest diameter.
2. The lesion is fairly discrete but not necessarily sharply defined.
3. It may have any contour (smooth, lobulated, spiculated, or umbilicated) or shape.
4. It may be calcified or cavitated.

5. Satellite lesions may be present.
6. The lesion is surrounded by air-containing lung or, if it is adjacent to the visceral pleural surface over the convexity of the thorax, at least two thirds of its circumference is contiguous to air-containing lung.

CT, particularly with the use of thin sections (1 to 3 mm collimation), is helpful in narrowing down the differential diagnosis. The presence of certain findings on CT may allow a specific diagnosis to be made.

Table A–6

SOLITARY PULMONARY NODULE

	ETIOLOGY	INCIDENCE	LOCATION	SHAPE	CALCIFICATION	CAVITATION	COMMENTS
DEVELOPMENTAL	Bronchogenic cyst	Uncommon	Lower lobe predilection, most commonly medial third	Round or oval, smooth, well defined	Rarely in wall	Yes, when communication occurs with bronchial tree	Cysts may have water density or soft tissue attenuation on CT scan.
	Pulmonary arteriovenous malformation (Fig. A–6–1)	Uncommon	More common in lower lobes	Round or oval, slightly lobulated, sharply defined	Occasionally, probably due to pheboliths	No	In two thirds of cases, lesions are solitary. Diagnosis by identification of feeding artery and draining vein can be readily made on spiral CT.
INFECTIOUS	**Bacteria**						
	Mycobacterium tuberculosis **(tuberculoma)** (Fig. A–6–2)	**Common**	**Predilection for upper lobes, the right more often than the left**	**Round or oval; 25% are lobulated**	**Frequent; readily identified on thin-section CT**	**Uncommon**	**"Satellite" lesions in 80%**
	Fungi						
	Histoplasma capsulatum (histoplasmoma)	Common in regions where the organism is endemic	More frequently in the lower than in the upper lobes	Round or oval; typically sharply circumscribed	Common, often central in location, thus producing a "target" appearance	Rare	"Satellite" lesions fairly common. Histoplasmomas may be multiple, varying considerably in size. Associated hilar lymph node calcification is common.
	Coccidioides immitis	Uncommon	Upper lobe predilection	Round or oval; typically sharply circumscribed	Occasionally	Common; may be thin- or thick-walled	
	Aspergillus species (fungus ball)	Uncommon	Upper lobe predilection	Round or oval	No	Invariably situated within a cavity	
	Parasites						
	Echinococcus (hydatid cyst)	Common in endemic areas	Lower lobe predilection, right more often than left	Almost always well circumscribed; tendency to bizarre, irregular shape	Very rare	Common	CT demonstrates water density cyst.

Table continued on following page

Table A–6

SOLITARY PULMONARY NODULE Continued

	ETIOLOGY	INCIDENCE	LOCATION	SHAPE	CALCIFICATION	CAVITATION	COMMENTS
NEOPLASTIC	**Pulmonary carcinoma** (Fig. A–6–3)	**Common**	**Upper to lower lobe ratio 3:2**	**Margins may be lobulated, smooth, or spiculated**	**Very rare on radiograph**	**Uncommon**	**Satellite lesions very uncommon**
	Carcinoid tumor	Uncommon	No lobar predilection	Round or oval, sharply defined, slightly lobulated	Rare on radiograph	Rare	
	Hamartoma (Fig. A–6–4)	Uncommon	No lobar predilection	Well defined; more often lobulated than smooth	Incidence varies widely in reported series but occurs in a minority of cases; "popcorn" configuration virtually diagnostic but rarely seen	No	Thin-section CT allows specific diagnosis in approximately 60% of cases by demonstrating localized areas of fat within the nodule.
	Hematogenous metastasis	Uncommon	Predominantly lower lobes	Smooth or slightly lobulated; tend to be well defined	Rare; almost only in osteogenic sarcoma or chondrosarcoma	Occasionally	
TRAUMATIC	Hematoma	Uncommon	Usually in a peripheral subpleural location	Oval or round, sharply defined, smooth	No	A hematoma occurs as a result of hemorrhage into a pulmonary parenchymal laceration or traumatic lung cyst—thus, an air-fluid level may be present as a result of communication with the bronchial tree	Generally undergo slow but progressive decrease in size, although they may persist for several months; may be multiple

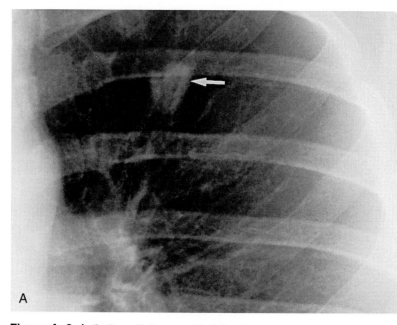

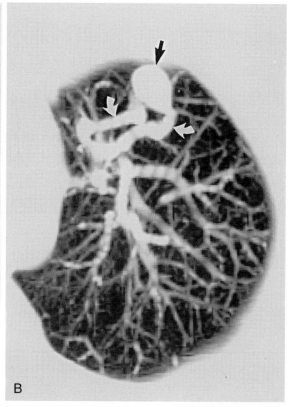

Figure A–6–1. Solitary Pulmonary Nodule: Arteriovenous Malformation.
A posteroanterior chest radiograph *(A)* of the left upper lung of a 33-year-old man
with Rendu-Osler-Weber disease demonstrates a slightly lobulated nodular opacity
(arrow). Maximal intensity projection (MIP) reconstruction obtained from a volumetric
5-mm-collimation spiral CT scan *(B)* demonstrates the malformation *(straight arrow)*
as well as the feeding artery and draining vein *(curved arrows)*.

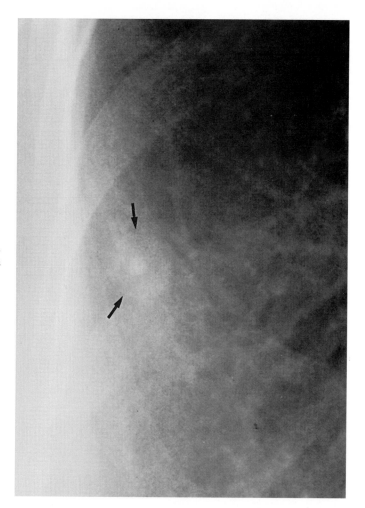

Figure A–6–2. Solitary Pulmonary Nodule: Tuberculoma. A posteroanterior chest radiograph of the right lung demonstrates a tuberculoma
(arrows) with a central nidus of calcification.

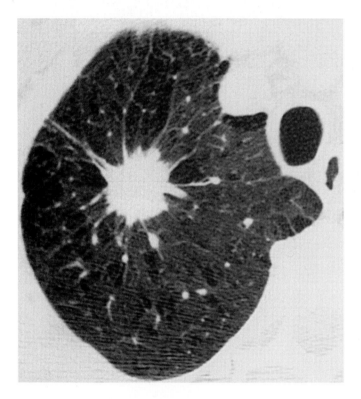

Figure A–6–3. Solitary Pulmonary Nodule: Pulmonary Carcinoma. An HRCT scan from a 62-year-old man demonstrates a 2.5-cm-diameter nodule in the right upper lobe. The nodule has multiple spicules radiating from the lesion into the surrounding parenchyma (corona radiata). The lesion was shown to be an adenocarcinoma at surgery.

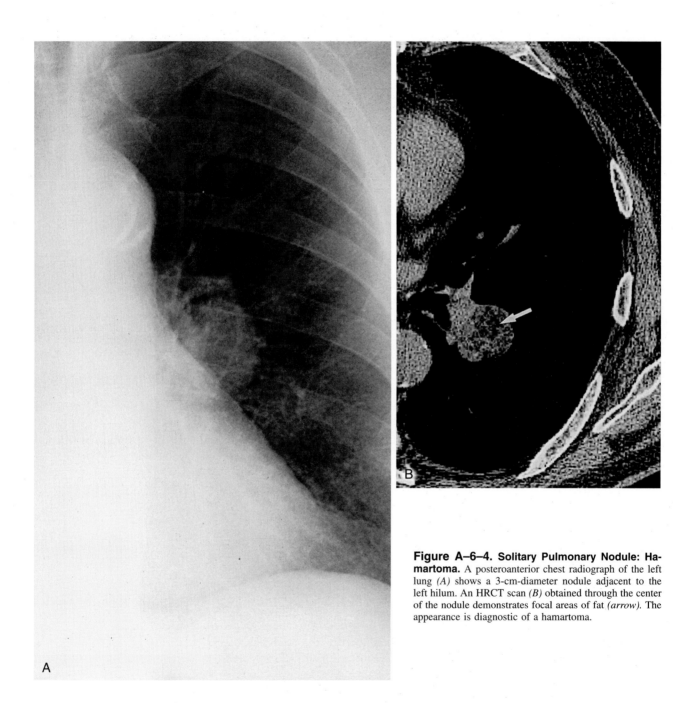

Figure A–6–4. Solitary Pulmonary Nodule: Hamartoma. A posteroanterior chest radiograph of the left lung *(A)* shows a 3-cm-diameter nodule adjacent to the left hilum. An HRCT scan *(B)* obtained through the center of the nodule demonstrates focal areas of fat *(arrow)*. The appearance is diagnostic of a hamartoma.

Table A–7
SOLITARY PULMONARY MASSES

The term *mass* refers to a lesion that measures more than 3 cm in diameter. For the purposes of this table, the general characteristics of such lesions are the same as for solitary nodules 3 cm or less in diameter.

Table A–7

SOLITARY PULMONARY MASSES

	ETIOLOGY	LOCATION	SHAPE	CALCIFICATION	CAVITATION	COMMENTS
DEVELOPMENTAL	Intralobar sequestration	Two thirds of cases left lower lobe; one third of cases right lower lobe; almost invariably contiguous to diaphragm in posterior bronchopulmonary segment	Round, oval, or triangular in shape and typically well defined	No	Cyst formation relatively common	Although cystic in nature, mass remains homogeneous until communication is established with contiguous lung as a result of infection. Lesion is supplied by systemic artery and drains via pulmonary veins.
INFECTIOUS	**Acute or chronic lung abscess caused by various bacteria**	**Predilection for posterior portions of upper or lower lobes**	**Tends to be round; somewhat ill-defined when acute but well defined when chronic**	**No**	**Common**	**Usually of staphylococcal or anaerobic etiology. The mass may remain unchanged for many weeks without perforation into bronchial tree.**
	Blastomyces dermatitidis	No lobar predominance	Margins tend to be ill-defined	No	Uncommon	Frequency of this manifestation varies widely in reported series; may simulate pulmonary carcinoma
	Echinococcus granulosus (hydatid cyst) (Fig. A–7–1)	Predilection for lower lobes, right more often than left	Sharply defined; tends to possess bizarre, irregular shape	Extremely rare	Common	Has homogeneous water density on CT
NEOPLASTIC	**Pulmonary carcinoma** (Fig. A–7–2)	**Upper to lower lobe ratio 3:2**	**Margins tend to be ill-defined, lobulated, or spiculated**	**Foci of calcification seen on CT in about 5% to 10% of large tumors**	**Relatively common**	
	Hematogenous metastasis	Predominantly lower lobes	Tends to be sharply defined, somewhat lobulated	Rare; almost exclusively restricted to metastatic osteogenic sarcoma or chondrosarcoma	Uncommon; predominantly in upper lobe lesions	Uncommon manifestation of metastatic disease

Table continued on following page

Table A–7

SOLITARY PULMONARY MASSES *Continued*

	ETIOLOGY	LOCATION	SHAPE	CALCIFICATION	CAVITATION	COMMENTS
INHALATIONAL	Lipid pneumonia	Dependent portions of upper and lower lobes (occasionally right middle lobe or lingula)	Well defined; often has shaggy outer margin	No	No	CT scan often allows specific diagnosis by demonstrating foci of fat attenuation.
	Silicosis (progressive massive fibrosis)	Initially in the periphery of the mid or upper lung zones; tendency over time to migrate toward the hilum	Tends to be broader in the sagittal plane than in the coronal; margins may be irregular and somewhat ill-defined, simulating pulmonary carcinoma	Foci of high attenuation may be apparent on HRCT scan	Sometimes	A background pattern of diffuse silicosis may be apparent; however, the more extensive the progressive massive fibrosis, the less the nodularity apparent in the remainder of the lungs. Compensatory overinflation or overt emphysema of remainder of lung is common. Hilar lymph node enlargement is usual and may be associated with "eggshell calcification."
	Coal workers' pneumoconiosis (progressive massive fibrosis)	Marked predilection for upper lobes, with tendency to originate in the periphery of the lung, migrating toward the hilum over a period of years	Similar to large opacities of silicosis	No	Sometimes	A background of diffuse nodular or reticulonodular shadows is usually evident, although incorporation of the individual foci into the conglomerate consolidation may render the nodular pattern inconspicuous. Compensatory overinflation or emphysema in lower lobes may be seen.
	Round atelectasis (most commonly associated with asbestos exposure) (Fig. A–7–3)	Lower zonal predominance; abuts localized area of pleural thickening	Round or oval	No	No	CT scan shows the mass abutting a thickened pleura; vessels and bronchi curve toward the periphery of the mass.
EMBOLIC	Intravenous talcosis (large opacities)	Upper lobe predominance; usually bilateral	Variable	Accumulation of talc results in increased attenuation similar to that of calcium on CT scan	No	Background pattern of general haziness and fine nodulation. Emphysema is commonly present.
TRAUMATIC	Pulmonary hematoma	Usually deep to point of maximum trauma	Sharply defined, round or oval	No	No	Resolution may take several months.

Figure A-7-1. Solitary Pulmonary Mass: Hydatid Cyst. A postero-anterior chest radiograph *(A)* of the left hemithorax demonstrates a smoothly marginated 6-cm-diameter mass in the lingula. A CT scan *(B)* demonstrates a thin-walled cyst that contains fluid with attenuation values similar to those of water (0 HU). The patient was a 51-year-old asymptomatic man who had hunted for many years in northern Canada.

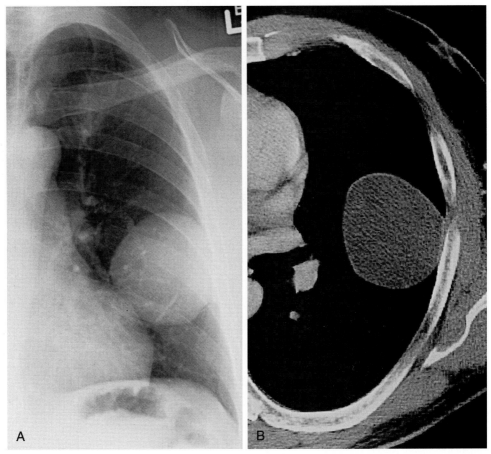

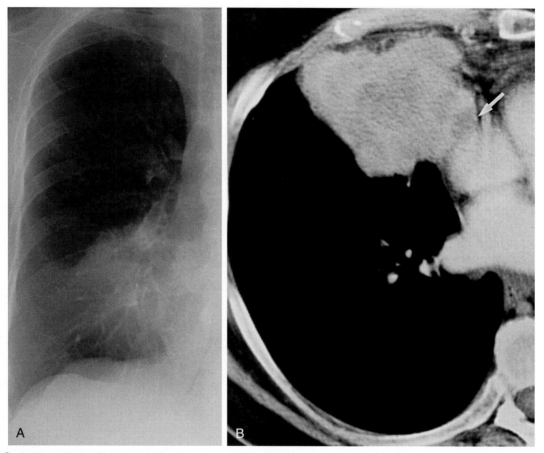

Figure A–7–2. Solitary Mass: Pulmonary Carcinoma. A posteroanterior chest radiograph *(A)* from a 62-year-old woman shows a large right middle lobe tumor abutting the heart. A contrast-enhanced CT scan *(B)* demonstrates the mass as well as associated focal thickening of the pericardium and localized mediastinal invasion *(arrow)*. The lesion was shown to be a resectable (T3) pulmonary carcinoma at surgery.

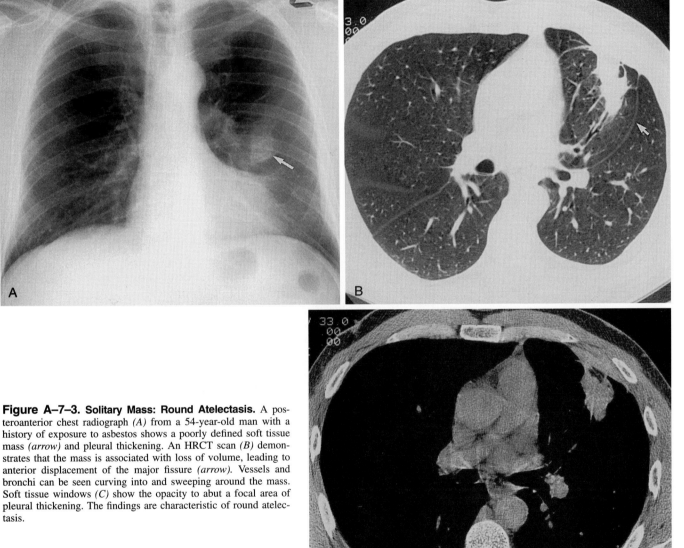

Figure A–7–3. Solitary Mass: Round Atelectasis. A posteroanterior chest radiograph *(A)* from a 54-year-old man with a history of exposure to asbestos shows a poorly defined soft tissue mass *(arrow)* and pleural thickening. An HRCT scan *(B)* demonstrates that the mass is associated with loss of volume, leading to anterior displacement of the major fissure *(arrow)*. Vessels and bronchi can be seen curving into and sweeping around the mass. Soft tissue windows *(C)* show the opacity to abut a focal area of pleural thickening. The findings are characteristic of round atelectasis.

Table A–8

MULTIPLE PULMONARY NODULES OR MASSES, WITH OR WITHOUT CAVITATION

The individual lesions generally possess the same characteristics as those described in Tables A–6 and A–7. Cavitation or calcification may be present or absent in some or all of the lesions.

Table A-8

MULTIPLE PULMONARY NODULES OR MASSES, WITH OR WITHOUT CAVITATION

	ETIOLOGY	LOCATION	SIZE AND SHAPE	CALCIFICATION	CAVITATION	GENERAL COMMENTS
DEVELOPMENTAL	Pulmonary arteriovenous malformation	Lower lobe predilection	One to several centimeters; round or oval, lobulated, well defined	No	No	Multiple in one third of all cases. Diagnosis by identification of feeding artery and draining vein can be made using spiral CT.
INFECTIOUS	Abscesses associated with bacteremia (Fig. A–8–1)	Generalized but more numerous in lower lobes	Usually 0.5 to 3 cm in diameter; typically round and well defined	No	Common, usually thick-walled	
	Invasive aspergillosis (Fig. A–8–2)	No predilection	Usually 0.5 to 3 cm in diameter	No	Common, typically with air crescent	HRCT scan frequently shows halo of ground-glass attenuation related to hemorrhage.
	Histoplasma capsulatum	No predilection	0.5 to 3.0 cm; round and sharply defined	Sometimes	No	May remain unchanged over many years or may undergo slow growth; seldom exceed 4 or 5 in number
	Paragonimus westermani	Lower lobe predilection, usually in the periphery	3 to 4 cm; well defined	Occasionally	Common	Multiple ring opacities or thin-walled cysts are characteristic.
IMMUNOLOGIC	Wegener's granulomatosis (Fig. A–8–3)	Widely distributed, bilateral, no predilection for upper or lower lung zones	0.5 to 10 cm; round, sharply defined	No	In one third to one half of patients; characteristically thick-walled, with irregular, shaggy inner lining	May be associated with focal areas of air-space consolidation
	Sarcoidosis	Widely distributed	Usually 0.5 to 3 cm in diameter	No	No	A rare manifestation of the disease
NEOPLASTIC	**Hematogenous metastases (Fig. A–8–4)**	**Predilection for lower lobes**	**0.5 to 10 cm or more in diameter; typically round and sharply defined**	**Rare, but if present, virtually diagnostic of osteogenic sarcoma or chondrosarcoma**	**In approximately 5% of cases, more frequently in upper lobes**	**Wide range in size of multiple nodules is highly suggestive of the diagnosis.**
	Non-Hodgkin's lymphoma	More numerous in lower lung zones	0.5 to 10 cm; round	No	Uncommon	Most often a manifestation of secondary lymphoma. Mediastinal and bronchopulmonary lymph node enlargement is associated in some cases.

Table continued on following page

Table A–8

MULTIPLE PULMONARY NODULES OR MASSES, WITH OR WITHOUT CAVITATION *Continued*

	ETIOLOGY	LOCATION	SIZE AND SHAPE	CALCIFICATION	CAVITATION	GENERAL COMMENTS
INHALATIONAL	Silicosis (progressive massive fibrosis) (Fig. A–8–5)	Predominantly upper lobes	Usually between 1 and 10 cm in diameter; lateral margin typically parallels chest wall ("angels' wings")	Foci of high attenuation may be apparent on HRCT scan	Sometimes	A background pattern of diffuse silicosis may be apparent; however, the more extensive the progressive massive fibrosis, the less the nodularity apparent in the remainder of the lungs. Compensatory overinflation or overt emphysema of remainder of lung is common. Hilar lymph node enlargement is usual and may be associated with "eggshell calcification."
	Coal workers' pneumoconiosis (progressive massive fibrosis)	Predominantly upper lobes	Usually between 1 and 10 cm	No	Sometimes	A background of diffuse nodular or reticulonodular shadows is usually evident, although incorporation of the individual foci into the conglomerate consolidation may render the nodular pattern inconspicuous. Compensatory overinflation or emphysema in lower lobes may be seen.
EMBOLIC	Septic thromboemboli	Lower lobe predilection	Highly variable; commonly 0.5 to 3 cm in diameter; round or wedge-shaped	No	Frequent, usually with thin walls	Nodules tend to be peripherally located and ill-defined on the radiograph. On CT scan, some of the nodules have a vessel leading into them ("feeding vessel" sign).
	Intravenous talcosis	Upper lobe predilection	Variable	Talc accumulation results in increased attenuation on CT scan	No	Background pattern of general haziness and fine nodulation. Emphysema is commonly present.
TRAUMATIC	Multiple hematomas	Unilateral or bilateral, generally in lung deep to maximal trauma	Highly variable; 0.5 to 10 cm in diameter; sharply defined	No	No	Generally undergo slow but progressive decrease in size and may persist for months. Initially, may be masked by surrounding pulmonary contusion.

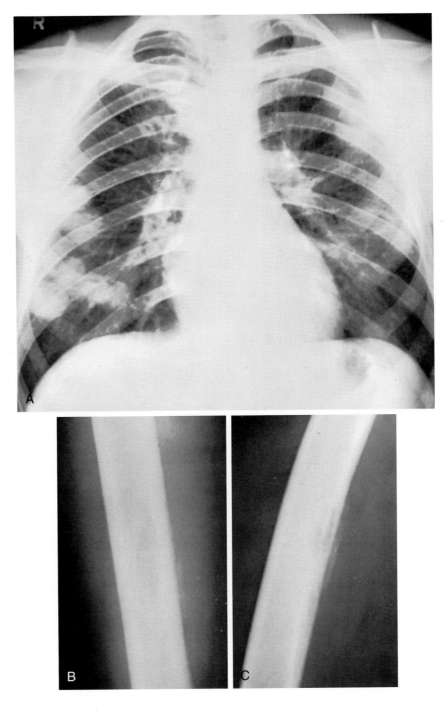

Figure A–8–1. Multiple Pulmonary Nodules: Bacteremic Abscesses. A posteroanterior chest radiograph from a 24-year-old man *(A)* reveals several sharply circumscribed nodules ranging from 2 to 3 cm in diameter situated predominantly in the right lower lobe and the left upper lobe. The nodules are homogeneous in density and show no evidence of cavitation (although cavitation eventually occurred in the majority). Anteroposterior *(B)* and lateral *(C)* views of the midshaft of the right femur show an irregular area of rarefaction in the cortex, associated with subperiosteal new bone formation along the posterior and medial aspects of the bone, consistent with osteomyelitis. *Staphylococcus aureus* was cultured from the sputum and from pus obtained from the thigh at incision and drainage.

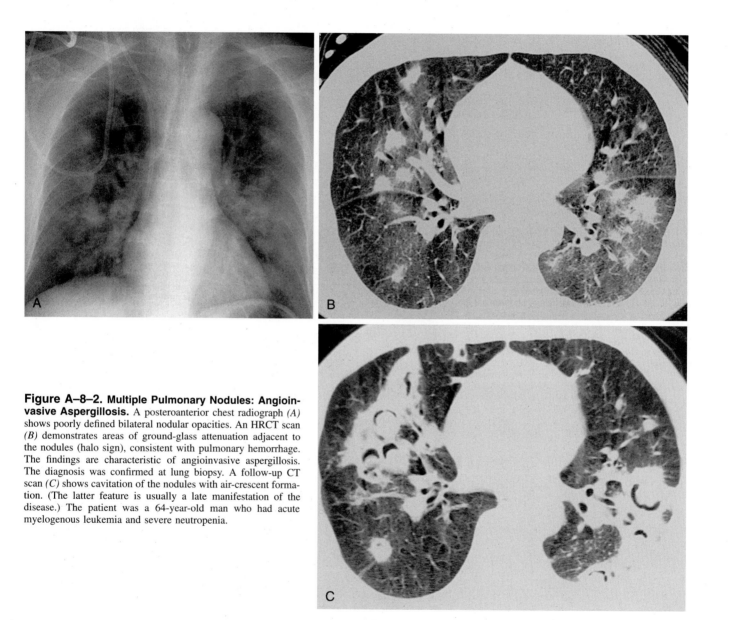

Figure A–8–2. Multiple Pulmonary Nodules: Angioinvasive Aspergillosis. A posteroanterior chest radiograph *(A)* shows poorly defined bilateral nodular opacities. An HRCT scan *(B)* demonstrates areas of ground-glass attenuation adjacent to the nodules (halo sign), consistent with pulmonary hemorrhage. The findings are characteristic of angioinvasive aspergillosis. The diagnosis was confirmed at lung biopsy. A follow-up CT scan *(C)* shows cavitation of the nodules with air-crescent formation. (The latter feature is usually a late manifestation of the disease.) The patient was a 64-year-old man who had acute myelogenous leukemia and severe neutropenia.

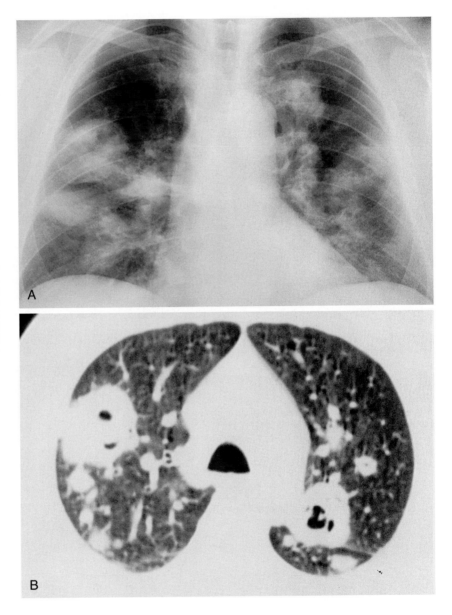

Figure A–8–3. Multiple Pulmonary Nodules and Masses: Wegener's Granulomatosis. A posteroanterior chest radiograph *(A)* and CT scan at the level of the upper lobes *(B)* demonstrate multiple bilateral nodules ranging from a few millimeters to 5 cm in diameter. The larger nodules are cavitated. The patient was a 54-year-old man, in whom the diagnosis of Wegener's granulomatosis was proved by open lung biopsy.

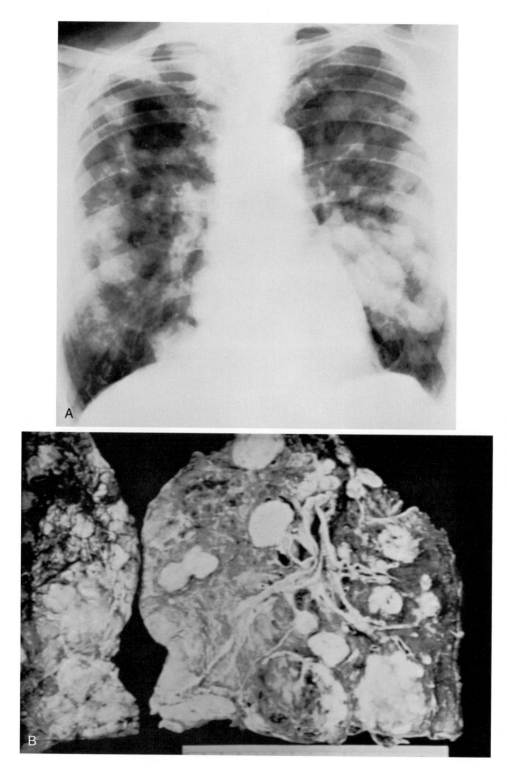

A

B

Figure A–8–4. Multiple Pulmonary Nodules: Hematogenous Metastases. A posteroanterior chest radiograph *(A)* reveals multiple, sharply circumscribed nodules scattered widely throughout both lungs; they range in diameter from 1 to 6 cm and are homogeneous in density and roughly spherical. A photograph of a cross-section of the lung removed at autopsy *(B)* shows the sharp definition and marked variation in size of the metastatic nodules; the large mass in the left lower lobe has undergone hemorrhagic necrosis. The primary tumor was a fibrosarcoma of the ilium.

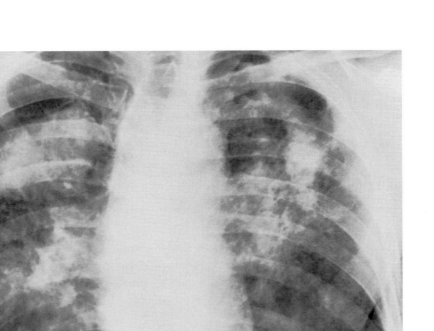

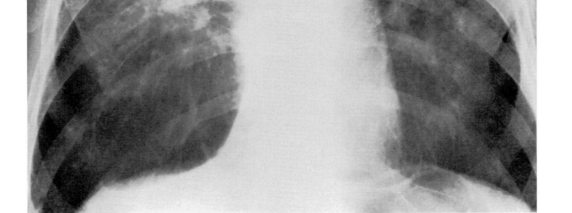

Figure A–8–5. Bilateral Pulmonary Masses: Silicosis with Progressive Massive Fibrosis. A posteroanterior radiograph from a 54-year-old foundry worker shows bilateral upper lobe masses due to conglomeration of silicotic nodules. The lung peripheral to the zones of progressive massive fibrosis shows evidence of emphysema.

Table A–9
DIFFUSE PULMONARY DISEASE WITH A PREDOMINANTLY AIR-SPACE PATTERN

"Diffuse" implies involvement of all lobes of both lungs. Although the disease necessarily is widespread, it need not affect all lung regions uniformly. For example, the lower lung zones may be involved to a greater or lesser degree than the upper, or the central and mid portions of the lungs may be more severely affected than the periphery ("bat's wing" distribution). Other abnormalities such as pleural effusion and cardiac enlargement may be present.

Table A–9
DIFFUSE PULMONARY DISEASE WITH A PREDOMINANTLY AIR-SPACE PATTERN

	ETIOLOGY	ANATOMIC DISTRIBUTION	ADDITIONAL FINDINGS	COMMENTS
INFECTIOUS	*Pneumocystis carinii* (Fig. A–9–1)	**Diffuse. May have upper or lower lobe predominance**	**Cyst formation and pneumothorax relatively common; pleural effusion uncommon**	
	Cytomegalovirus	Usually patchy; widespread consolidation uncommon	Commonly ground-glass, linear, or nodular opacities	
	Influenza virus	Diffuse		
IMMUNOLOGIC	Diffuse alveolar hemorrhage (Goodpasture's syndrome and small vessel vasculitis syndromes [including microscopic polyangitis and some cases of Wegener's granulomatosis and systemic lupus erythematosus])	Widespread but more prominent in perihilar areas and in mid-lung and lower lung zones.	Confluence of opacities may occur, in which circumstance an air bronchogram is seen	An air-space pattern is seen in relatively pure form in the early stages of these diseases; as the hemorrhage resolves, the pattern may become reticulonodular.
EDEMA	**Hydrostatic pulmonary edema** (Fig. A–9–2)	**Usually bilateral and symmetric; cortex of lung may be relatively spared (the "butterfly" pattern)**	**Associated findings typically include septal lines, pleural effusion, prominent upper lobe vessels, and cardiomegaly**	
	Permeability pulmonary edema (ARDS)	**Bilateral and symmetric**	**Septal lines, pleural effusions, prominent upper lobe vessels, and cardiomegaly typically absent**	**The pattern is similar regardless of etiology including trauma, sepsis, gastric acid aspiration, and drug toxicity. An identical pattern is seen in idiopathic disease (acute interstitial pneumonitis).**
INHALATIONAL	Water aspiration (near drowning)	Diffuse or patchy	Cardiac size is normal and signs of pulmonary venous hypertension are absent	
	Extrinsic allergic alveolitis	Diffuse; often mid and lower zone predominance	Poorly defined small nodules may be seen	HRCT typically shows diffuse ground-glass attenuation, mosaic attenuation, and centrilobular nodules.

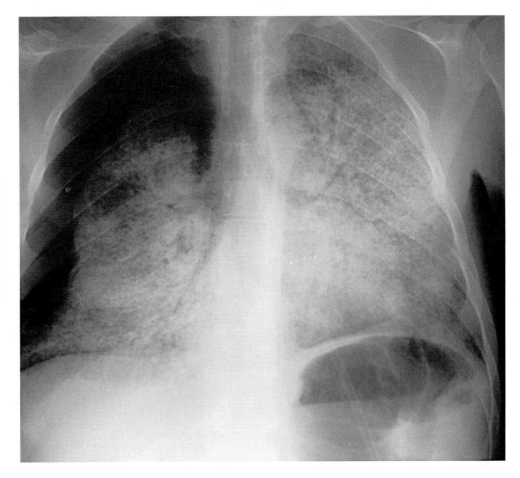

Figure A–9–1. Diffuse Air-Space Consolidation: *Pneumocystis carinii* **Pneumonia.** An anteroposterior chest radiograph demonstrates extensive areas of consolidation in both lungs associated with air bronchograms. Also note the presence of cysts, mainly in the right upper lobe, and a large right pneumothorax. The patient was a 31-year-old man who had the acquired immunodeficiency syndrome.

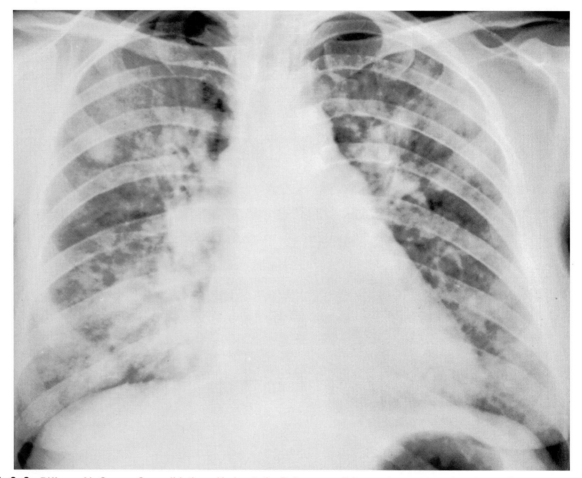

Figure A–9–2. Diffuse Air-Space Consolidation: Hydrostatic Pulmonary Edema. A posteroanterior chest radiograph reveals extensive involvement of both lungs by shadows having the typical characteristics of air-space consolidation. An air bronchogram is visualized, particularly in the right lung. The edema was secondary to mitral stenosis and completely resolved radiographically 48 hours later.

Table A–10
DIFFUSE PULMONARY DISEASE WITH A PREDOMINANTLY RETICULAR PATTERN

This pattern is characterized radiographically by the presence of linear opacities with a netlike appearance. It can be caused by superimposition of shadows resulting from smooth or irregularly thickened interlobular septa (septal lines), intralobular linear opacities, multiple small cystic spaces, or honeycombing. (Cystic air spaces or cysts are defined as thin-walled, circumscribed air-filled spaces; "honeycombing" refers to the presence of cystic spaces within areas of pulmonary fibrosis.) These various shadows may be difficult to distinguish from each other on the radiograph, but can be readily identified on HRCT scans.

Diffuse involvement connotes involvement of all lobes of both lungs, although the abnormalities are often more marked in some regions. In fact, the predominant distribution of abnormalities is often helpful in narrowing the differential diagnosis. Other abnormalities may be present that also help in differential diagnosis, including pleural effusion, pleural thickening, hilar and mediastinal lymph node enlargement, and cardiomegaly. HRCT is superior to radiography in the depiction of the pattern and distribution of parenchymal abnormalities, and in the assessment of pleural abnormalities and presence of lymph node enlargement, and therefore frequently provides helpful information.

Table A–10

DIFFUSE PULMONARY DISEASE WITH A PREDOMINANTLY RETICULAR PATTERN

	ETIOLOGY	ANATOMIC DISTRIBUTION	VOLUME OF THORAX	ADDITIONAL FINDINGS	COMMENTS
DEVELOPMENTAL	Pulmonary lymphangioleiomyomatosis and tuberous sclerosis	Generalized	Increased	Chylous pleural effusion and pneumothorax common; sclerotic (and sometimes lytic) lesions in bone	HRCT scans show characteristic pattern of thin-walled cysts throughout both lungs with relatively normal intervening parenchyma.
INFECTIOUS	Viruses	Generalized, uniform or asymmetric	Unaffected		
	Mycoplasma pneumoniae	Generalized, uniform or asymmetric	Unaffected	Kerley B lines in some cases	HRCT scans may show centrilobular nodules and branching linear opacities, which reflect the presence of bronchiolitis. Segmental consolidation is a more common manifestation.
	Pneumocystis carinii	**May have perihilar or upper lobe predominance**	**Unaffected**	**Cystic changes may be seen; no lymph node enlargement or pleural effusion**	**HRCT scans usually show extensive ground-glass attenuation. Less common findings include cystic changes, small nodules, or reticular pattern.**
IMMUNOLOGIC	Progressive systemic sclerosis	Generalized but more prominent in lung bases	Serial radiographs may reveal progressive loss of lung volume	Pleural effusion uncommon; pleural thickening seen on CT scan in up to 30% of patients; air-filled dilated esophagus may be seen	The HRCT findings include areas of ground-glass attenuation, a reticular pattern, and honeycombing involving mainly the subpleural lung regions.
	Rheumatoid disease (Fig. A–10–1)	Generalized but more prominent in lung bases	Serial radiographic studies may reveal progressive loss of lung volume	Pleural effusion, usually unilateral and small, relatively common; abnormalities of shoulder and sternoclavicular joints may be seen	Common HRCT findings include ground-glass attenuation, a reticular pattern, and honeycombing involving mainly the subpleural lung regions.
	Sarcoidosis (Fig. A–10–2)	**Usually upper lung zone predominance**	**Usually unaffected although fibrosis may be associated with emphysema and overinflation of less affected lung**	**Hilar and mediastinal lymph node enlargement often constitutes the earliest radiographic finding, with diffuse lung involvement developing subsequently (with or without disappearance) of the node enlargement); in approximately 25% of cases, the pulmonary changes exist alone**	**The pattern is usually reticulonodular in type, although ranging from purely nodular to purely reticular. In the approximately 20% of cases that progress to fibrosis, the pattern is coarsely reticular involving mainly the perihilar regions and upper lung zones. HRCT scans show a predominantly peribronchoarterial distribution of the abnormalities.**

	Distribution	Lung Volume	Additional Findings	Comments
Idiopathic pulmonary fibrosis (Figs. A–10–3 and A–10–4)	Predilection for lower lung zones in early stages; becomes more generalized and uniform as disease progresses	Sequential studies show progressive loss of lung volume	Hilar lymph node enlargement and pleural effusion do not occur; mild enlargement of mediastinal lymph nodes often evident on CT scans, particularly in patients who have extensive disease	In the early stage, the pattern is one of fine reticulation, predominantly in the lung bases; advanced disease is characterized by a generalized coarse reticular pattern with honeycombing. HRCT scans show areas of ground-glass attenuation, intralobular linear opacities, irregular thickening of interlobular septa, and honeycombing involving mainly the subpleural regions and lower lung zones.
Desquamative interstitial pneumonia	Generalized but often with lower lung zone predominance	Usually unaffected	The main radiologic finding usually consists of ground-glass opacities	HRCT scans show ground-glass attenuation, which may be diffuse or have a subpleural or lower lung zone predominance. Fibrosis is characteristically mild, although honeycombing can occur.
Nonspecific interstitial pneumonia	Diffuse but with a tendency to involve mainly lower lung zones	Unaffected	The predominant finding usually consists of ground-glass opacities and consolidation	
Langerhans' cell histiocytosis (Fig. A–10–5)	Diffuse but with a tendency for predominance of lesions in upper lung zones	Normal or increased	Hilar and mediastinal lymph node enlargement are exceedingly rare, as is pleural effusion; spontaneous pneumothorax in some cases	The radiologic pattern varies with the stage of the disease, beginning with nodular and progressing to reticulonodular and finally to a reticular pattern. HRCT scans demonstrate nodules and cystic spaces, often with bizarre shapes, throughout the upper and mid lung zones with relative sparing of the lung bases.
NEOPLASTIC				
Lymphangitic carcinomatosis	Commonly generalized but more prominent in the lower lung zones	Serial radiographs may reveal progressive reduction in volume	Hilar or mediastinal lymph node enlargement common; Kerley B lines frequent	HRCT scans demonstrate smooth or nodular thickening of interlobular septa and peribronchoarterial interstitium.
Secondary non-Hodgkin's lymphoma	Diffuse	Unaffected	Pleural effusion in about one third of cases; mediastinal and hilar lymph node enlargement may be inconspicuous or absent	The radiologic pattern simulates that of lymphangitic carcinomatosis.

Table continued on following page

Table A–10

DIFFUSE PULMONARY DISEASE WITH A PREDOMINANTLY RETICULAR PATTERN (Continued)

	ETIOLOGY	ANATOMIC DISTRIBUTION	VOLUME OF THORAX	ADDITIONAL FINDINGS	COMMENTS
EDEMA	**Hydrostatic pulmonary edema** (Fig. A–10–6)	**Diffuse but predominantly lower lung zones**	**May be reduced**		**Prominence of upper lobe vessels, septal lines, pleural effusions, and cardiomegaly common**
INHALATIONAL	Extrinsic allergic alveolitis (Fig. A–10–7)	Can be diffuse or random but often has mid or lower lung zone predominance	Unaffected except in patients with severe fibrosis	Ground-glass and small nodular opacities commonly seen	On HRCT scans, the fibrosis can have a random, predominantly peribronchial or, less commonly, predominantly subpleural distribution. Areas of ground-glass attenuation and centrilobular nodules are commonly present.
	Asbestosis (Fig. A–10–8)	Predominantly lower lung zones	Sequential studies may show progressive loss of lung volume	Associated pleural manifestations of asbestos exposure, consisting of plaque formation or general thickening with or without calcification; are evident in most cases	Most common HRCT findings include subpleural dotlike opacities due to peribronchiolar fibrosis, intralobular lines, irregular interlobular septal thickening, subpleural lines, and pleural plaques or diffuse pleural thickening.
AIRWAY DISEASE	Cystic fibrosis	Generalized, uniform	Considerable overinflation	May be associated with segmental areas of consolidation or atelectasis due to bronchopneumonia	The radiographic pattern is one of accentuation of the linear markings throughout the lungs, giving a coarse reticular appearance. HRCT scans demonstrate extensive bronchiectasis, often with upper lobe predominance.
DRUGS AND POISONS	Nitrofurantoin	Generalized	Unaffected	Pleural effusion and septal lines relatively common in the acute form	
	Amiodarone	Generalized	Unaffected		Accumulation of iodine in the drug within tissue results in characteristic high attenuation of the lung parenchyma and liver.
	Other drugs	Unaffected	Unaffected	None	

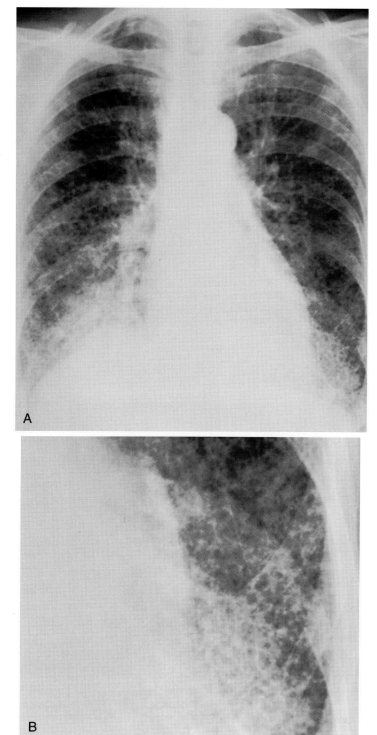

Figure A–10–1. Reticular Pattern: Interstitial Pulmonary Fibrosis (Rheumatoid Disease). A posteroanterior chest radiograph *(A)* reveals a diffuse reticular pattern throughout both lungs, more marked in the bases than elsewhere. The reticulation is "fine" in character. No other abnormalities are apparent. A magnified view of the lower portion of the left lung *(B)* reveals the pattern to better advantage. This pattern alone is not in any way diagnostic. The patient was a 68-year-old woman who had rheumatoid arthritis.

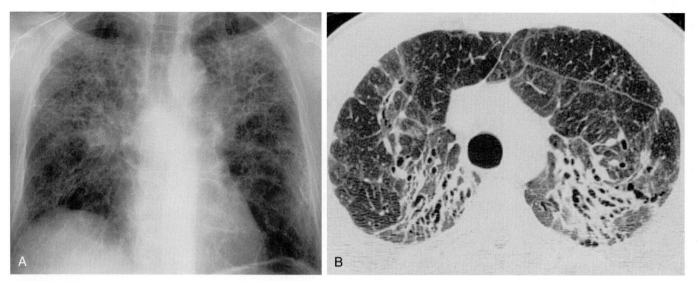

Figure A–10–2. Reticular Pattern: Sarcoidosis. A posteroanterior chest radiograph *(A)* and an HRCT scan *(B)* from a 36-year-old man who had sarcoidosis demonstrate a reticular pattern involving mainly the perihilar regions of the upper and mid-lung zones. The fibrosis is associated with superior retraction of the hila, best seen on the radiograph, and posterior displacement of the ectatic upper lobe bronchi, evident on the HRCT scan. Also present are thickening of interlobular septa, a few residual nodules, and focal areas of ground-glass attenuation.

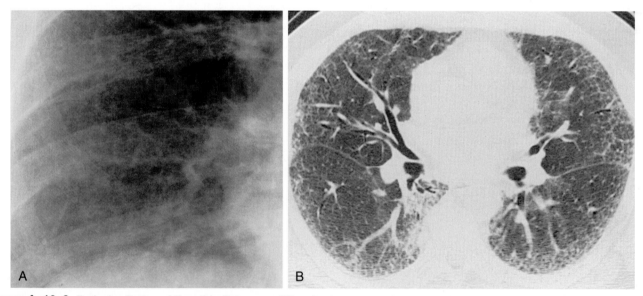

Figure A–10–3. Reticular Pattern: Idiopathic Pulmonary Fibrosis. A posteroanterior chest radiograph *(A)* of the right lower lung, in magnified view, reveals a fine reticular pattern. An HRCT scan *(B)* shows irregular lines of attenuation involving predominantly the subpleural lung regions. The reticular pattern on the scan is the result of irregular thickening of interlobular septa and the presence of intralobular lines. Areas of ground-glass attenuation involving mainly the subpleural lung regions are also present. The patient was a 66-year-old man.

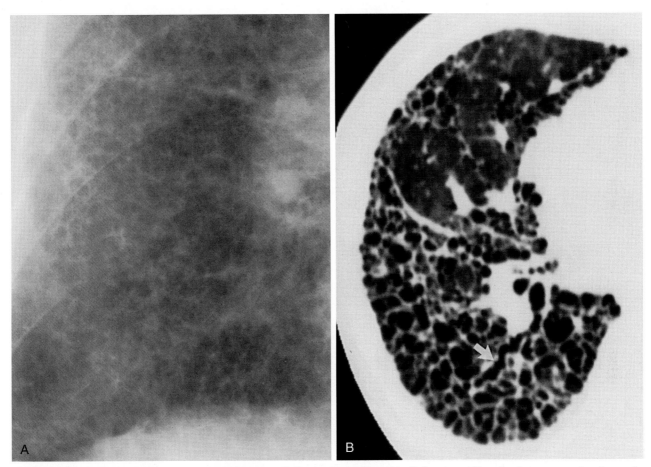

Figure A–10–4. Reticular Pattern Related to Honeycomb Formation: Idiopathic Pulmonary Fibrosis. A posteroanterior chest radiograph *(A)* of the right lower lung zone, in close-up view, demonstrates medium reticulation with 3- to 10-mm spaces between the reticular mesh. An HRCT scan *(B)* demonstrates honeycombing throughout the right lower lobe. Note associated dilation and distortion of the bronchi (traction bronchiectasis) *(arrow).* Although the honeycombing is diffuse in the right lower lobe, it demonstrates a subpleural predominance in the right middle lobe. This pattern and distribution are consistent with advanced disease. The diagnosis had been confirmed by open lung biopsy 4 years previously.

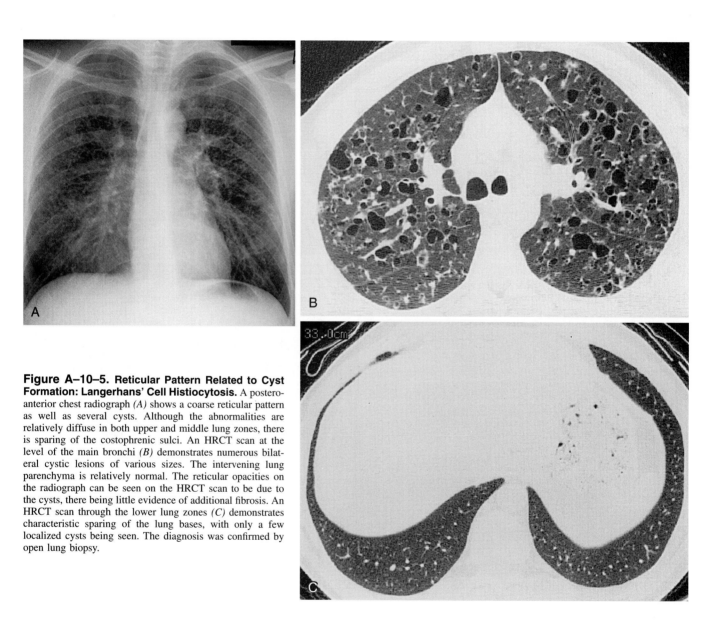

Figure A–10–5. Reticular Pattern Related to Cyst Formation: Langerhans' Cell Histiocytosis. A postero-anterior chest radiograph *(A)* shows a coarse reticular pattern as well as several cysts. Although the abnormalities are relatively diffuse in both upper and middle lung zones, there is sparing of the costophrenic sulci. An HRCT scan at the level of the main bronchi *(B)* demonstrates numerous bilateral cystic lesions of various sizes. The intervening lung parenchyma is relatively normal. The reticular opacities on the radiograph can be seen on the HRCT scan to be due to the cysts, there being little evidence of additional fibrosis. An HRCT scan through the lower lung zones *(C)* demonstrates characteristic sparing of the lung bases, with only a few localized cysts being seen. The diagnosis was confirmed by open lung biopsy.

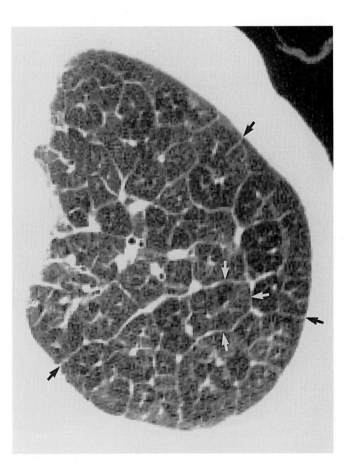

Figure A–10–6. Reticular Pattern: Interlobular Septal Thickening Secondary to Interstitial Pulmonary Edema. An HRCT scan targeted to the left upper lobe demonstrates thickened interlobular septa, identified as lines *(black arrows)* perpendicular to the pleura and extendng to it and, more centrally, as polygonal arcades *(white arrows)* outlining the secondary pulmonary lobules. The patient was a 77-year-old woman who had congestive heart failure.

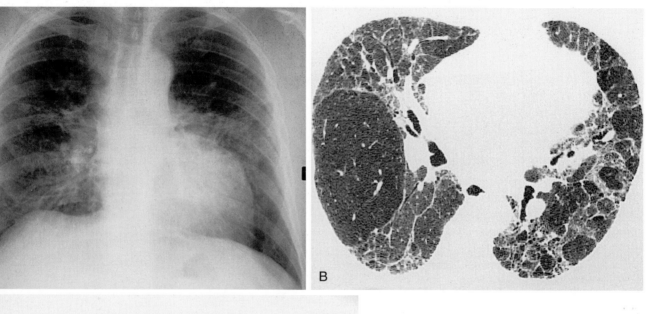

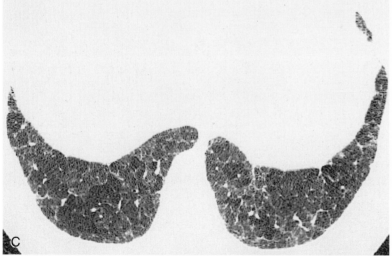

Figure A–10–7. Reticular Pattern: Extrinsic Allergic Alveolitis. A posteroanterior chest radiograph *(A)* demonstrates irregular linear opacities involving mainly the middle lung zones. An HRCT scan at the level of the right middle lobe bronchus *(B)* shows irregular linear opacities, irregular thickening of the interlobular septa, and architectural distortion indicating the presence of fibrosis. Also evident are extensive bilateral areas of ground-glass attenuation. An HRCT scan through the lung bases *(C)* shows relative sparing. The random distribution of the fibrosis and the relative sparing of the lung bases are suggestive of fibrosis resulting from chronic extrinsic allergic alveolitis. The diagnosis was confirmed by open lung biopsy.

Figure A–10–8. Reticular Pattern: Asbestosis.
An HRCT scan *(A)* demonstrates irregular thickening of
the interlobular septa *(straight arrows)* and intralobular
linear opacities *(curved arrows)* involving mainly the
subpleural lung regions. Subpleural areas of ground-glass
attenuation and distortion of lung architecture, particularly in the lingula, are also evident. Mediastinal windows
(B) demonstrate diffuse right pleural thickening and left
pleural plaques *(arrows)*. The patient was a 63-year-old
man who had worked for many years with automotive
brake linings.

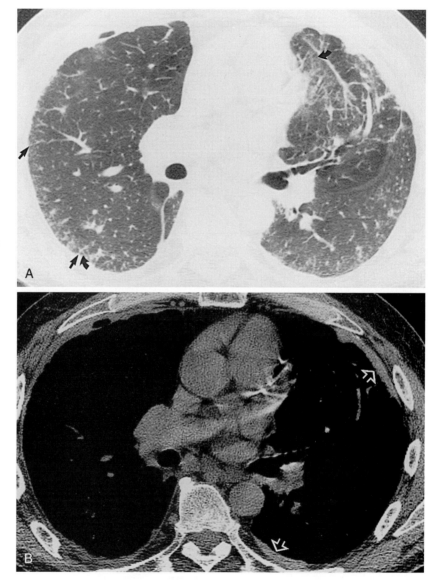

Table A–11

DIFFUSE PULMONARY DISEASE WITH A PREDOMINANTLY SMALL NODULAR PATTERN

This pattern is characterized radiographically by the presence of diffuse nodular opacities typically measuring less than 5 mm in diameter. The nodules may have well-defined margins, such as those in sarcoidosis or silicosis, or poorly defined margins, such as those in extrinsic allergic alveolitis.

HRCT is superior to the radiograph in depicting the nodules and in demonstrating their distribution within the lung parenchyma. Based on the distribution on HRCT, the nodules can be classified as having a predominantly centrilobular, perilymphatic, or random distribution. A centrilobular distribution is seen most commonly in extrinsic allergic alveolitis, endobronchial spread of tuberculosis, and bronchiolitis, particularly infectious bronchiolitis, panbronchiolitis, and respiratory bronchiolitis. A perilymphatic distribution, in which nodules are seen along the bronchovascular bundles, interlobular septa, and subpleural regions, is seen most commonly in sarcoidosis and lymphangitic carcinomatosis. A random distribution is seen most commonly in miliary tuberculosis and hematogenous metastases.

Table A-11

DIFFUSE PULMONARY DISEASE WITH A PREDOMINANTLY SMALL NODULAR PATTERN

	ETIOLOGY	RADIOGRAPHIC DISTRIBUTION	ADDITIONAL FINDINGS	COMMENTS
INFECTIOUS	**Viruses**	Generalized, uniform		Uncommon presentation; most often with CMV or varicella
	Bacteria			
	Mycobacterium tuberculosis (Figs. A–11–1, A–11–2)	**Generalized, uniform**	**Hilar and mediastinal lymph node enlargement may occur**	**Characteristic miliary pattern resulting from hematogenous dissemination. HRCT scans show random distribution of nodules.**
	Fungi	Generalized, uniform		Hilar node enlargement in some cases. Miliary pattern uncommon, often in immunocompromised patients. Causative organisms most often *Histoplasma capsulatum* and *Cryptococcus neoformans.* HRCT scans show random distribution of nodules.
IMMUNOLOGIC	Sarcoidosis (Fig. A–11–3)	**Generalized or upper lung zone predominance**	**Hilar and mediastinal lymph node enlargement in the vast majority of cases; a nodular pattern associated with bilateral symmetric hilar and paratracheal lymphadenopathy is highly suggestive of sarcoidosis**	**Majority of nodules have an irregular contour. HRCT scans show nodular thickening along the bronchial and perivascular interstitium, subpleural nodules, and, to a lesser extent, smooth or nodular thickening of interlobular septa.**
	Extrinsic allergic alveolitis (Fig. A–11–4)	Generalized or mid and lower lung zone predominance	—	HRCT scans frequently show areas of ground-glass attenuation and lobular areas of decreased attenuation and airtrapping. Poorly defined centrilobular nodules are characteristically seen in the subacute phase of the disease.
NEOPLASTIC	Bronchioloalveolar carcinoma	Diffuse	Pleural effusion in 10% of cases	Less common than a mixed air-space/nodular pattern. HRCT scans show a random distribution.
	Metastatic carcinoma	**Diffuse**		**The pattern is most commonly the result of metastatic thyroid carcinoma and pancreatic carcinoma. HRCT scans show a random distribution.**
EMBOLIC	Talcosis due to intravenous drug abuse	Diffuse	Pulmonary arterial hypertension and cor pulmonale in advanced cases	Creates a micronodular or ground-glass pattern that may progress to conglomerate masses similar to those seen in silicosis. HRCT scans show a random distribution and, in advanced cases, emphysema.
INHALATIONAL	**Coal workers' pneumoconiosis and silicosis** (Figs. A–11–5, A–11–6)	**Upper lung zone predominance, but distribution may be diffuse**	**Enlargement of hilar lymph nodes is common in silicosis; eggshell calcification may be seen**	**The radiographic pattern is typically nodular. Nodules tend to be less well defined in coal workers' pneumoconiosis than in silicosis. HRCT scans show centrilobular and subpleural predominance. Nodules are most numerous in the posterior half of upper lobes.**

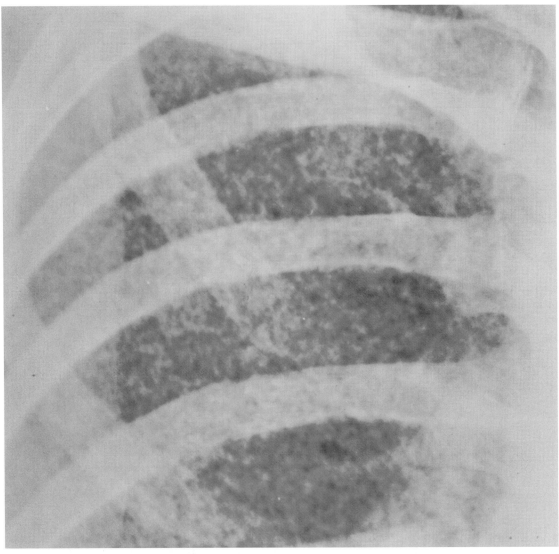

Figure A–11–1. Diffuse Nodular Pattern: Miliary Tuberculosis. A posteroanterior chest radiograph of the upper half of the right lung in magnified view shows multiple nodules of uniform size measuring approximately 2 mm in diameter. The shadows are quite discrete. (Courtesy of Dr. Romeo Ethier, Montreal Neurological Hospital.)

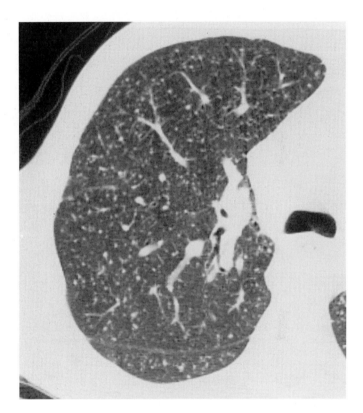

Figure A–11–2. Diffuse Nodular Pattern: Miliary Tuberculosis.
An HRCT scan targeted to the right lung demonstrates sharply defined nodules measuring 1 to 2 mm in diameter in a random distribution. The diagnosis of miliary tuberculosis was confirmed by lung biopsy.

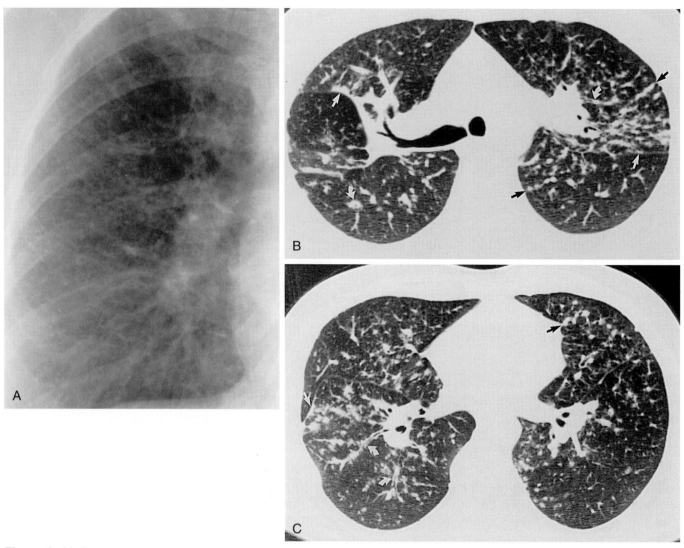

Figure A–11–3. Diffuse Nodular Pattern: Sarcoidosis. A posteroanterior chest radiograph *(A)* of the right lung demonstrates numerous nodules measuring approximately 3 mm in diameter. The nodules are most numerous in the middle and upper lung zones. HRCT scans at the level of the right upper lobe bronchus *(B)* and the inferior pulmonary veins *(C)* demonstrate that the nodules are located mainly along the bronchi *(curved white arrows)* and pulmonary vessels, in the subpleural lung regions, and along the interlobar fissures *(straight white arrows)*. Nodular thickening of interlobular septa *(black arrows)* is also evident. The patient was a 37-year-old man with biopsy-proven Stage 2 sarcoidosis.

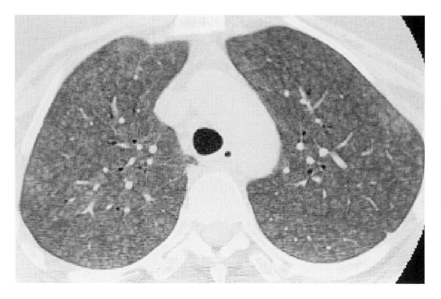

Figure A–11–4. Diffuse Nodular Pattern: Extrinsic Allergic Alveolitis. An HRCT scan demonstrates poorly defined small nodules throughout both lungs. Note that the nodules are a few millimeters away from the pleura and major vessels. This distribution is characteristic of centrilobular nodules, a finding observed in approximately 50% of patients with subacute extrinsic allergic alveolitis. The patient had pathologically proven bird-breeder's lung.

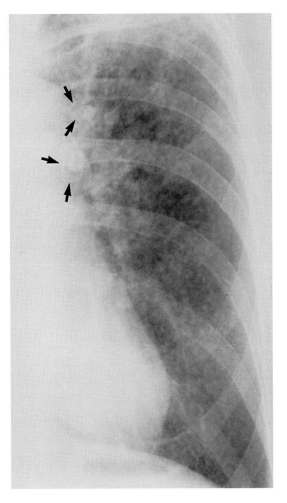

Figure A–11–5. Diffuse Nodular Pattern: Silicosis. A posteroanterior chest radiograph of the left lung of a patient who had silicosis demonstrates well-defined small nodules, most numerous in the upper lobes. Also note eggshell calcification of hilar and mediastinal nodes *(arrows)*, a finding that is highly suggestive of silicosis.

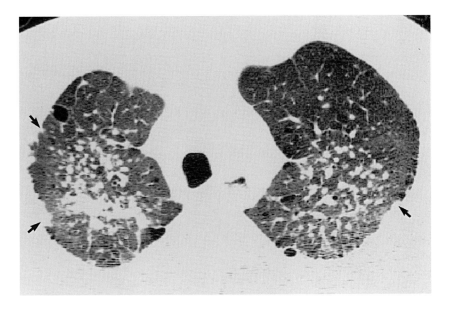

Figure A–11–6. Diffuse Nodular Pattern: Silicosis. An HRCT scan at the level of the upper lobes demonstrates sharply defined small nodules that are present mainly in the posterior half of the upper lobes and that have a predominantly centrilobular and subpleural *(arrows)* distribution. Early conglomeration is evident in the right upper lobe. Localized areas of low attenuation representing foci of emphysema are also apparent. The patient was a 58-year-old man.

Table A–12
GENERALIZED PULMONARY OLIGEMIA

This table includes all diseases in which there is reduction in the caliber of the pulmonary arterial tree throughout the lungs. Appreciation of such vascular change is a subjective process based on a thorough familiarity with the normal. Because reduction in the size of peripheral vessels constitutes the main criterion of diagnosis of all diseases in this category on the chest radiograph, differentiation depends upon secondary signs. The two ancillary signs of major importance are abnormal size and configuration of the central hilar vessels and general pulmonary overinflation. Three combinations of changes are possible:

1. Small peripheral vessels; no overinflation; normal or small hila. This combination indicates reduction in pulmonary blood flow from central causes and is virtually pathognomonic of cardiac disease, usually congenital.

2. Small peripheral vessels; no overinflation; enlarged hilar pulmonary arteries. This combination may result from peripheral or central causes (respectively, primary pulmonary arterial hypertension or massive pulmonary artery thromboembolism without infarction).

3. Small peripheral vessels; general pulmonary overinflation; normal or enlarged hilar pulmonary arteries. This combination is virtually pathognomonic of emphysema.

Depending on the suspected radiographic diagnosis, further evaluation can be performed using echocardiography, MR imaging, contrast-enhanced spiral CT, or HRCT. The first two procedures are particularly helpful in the assessment of congenital heart disease, while spiral CT is increasingly used in the assessment of patients suspected of having acute or chronic thromboembolism. HRCT provides close correlation with the pathologic extent of emphysema.

Table A–12

GENERALIZED PULMONARY OLIGEMIA

	ETIOLOGY	ADDITIONAL FINDINGS	COMMENTS
DEVELOPMENTAL	Congenital cardiac anomalies, including isolated pulmonic stenosis, Tetralogy of Fallot, absence of main pulmonary artery, persistent truncus arteriosus (type IV), and Ebstein's anomaly (Fig. A–12–1)	Cardiac enlargement present in some cases; no overinflation or air trapping; hila diminutive as a rule, permitting differentiation from primary pulmonary hypertension (exception is poststenotic dilation of main or left pulmonary artery in valvular pulmonic stenosis)	Pulmonary vascular pattern formed partly or wholly by hypertrophied bronchial circulation
IMMUNOLOGIC	Pulmonary hypertension associated with connective tissue disease, notably systemic lupus erythematosus, progressive systemic sclerosis, and the CREST syndrome	Indistinguishable from primary pulmonary hypertension; no overinflation	
EMBOLIC	Chronic thromboembolism with pulmonary hypertension	Main and hilar pulmonary arteries enlarged; lung volume normal or decreased	Definitive diagnosis can often be made using contrast-enhanced spiral CT or angiography. HRCT scans frequently show mosaic attenuation. Segmental artery–bronchial diameter ratio typically greater than 1.5. Ventilation-perfusion scan typically high probability.
CARDIOVASCULAR	Primary pulmonary hypertension	Main and hilar pulmonary arteries enlarged; peripheral vessels diminutive; absence of overinflation	Ventilation-perfusion scan typically low probability
AIRWAY DISEASE	**Emphysema** (Figs. A–12–2, A–12–3, A–12–4)	**Generalized overinflation serves to differentiate this disease from others characterized by diffuse oligemia; bullae may be present**	**The oligemia may be predominant in the upper lung zones or in one lung. Upper lung zone predominance is typical of centrilobular emphysema, while a lower zone predominance is typical of panacinar emphysema.**
	Obliterative bronchiolitis (Fig. A–12–5)	Hyperinflation and generalized or peripheral oligemia may be evident on the radiograph	HRCT scan shows mosaic pattern of attenuation at end-inspiration, air trapping at end-expiration, and, commonly, bronchial dilation.

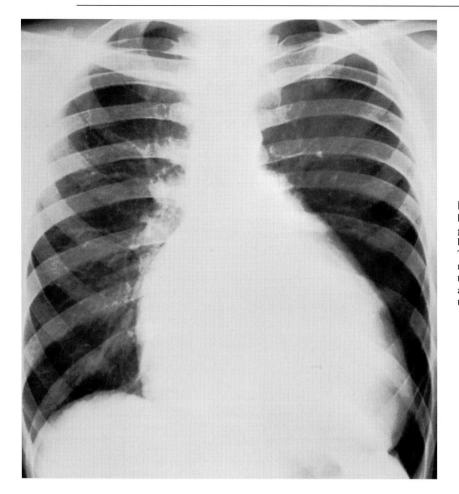

Figure A–12–1. General Pulmonary Oligemia: Ebstein's Anomaly. A posteroanterior chest radiograph reveals a markedly enlarged heart whose right border strongly suggests dilation of the right atrium. The hila are diminutive and the peripheral vessels narrow and attenuated. Pulmonary oligemia is uniform throughout both lungs. The patient was a 20-year-old asymptomatic man who was able to take part in sports; there was no cyanosis.

Figure A–12–2. General Pulmonary Oligemia: Emphysema. A posteroanterior radiograph reveals generalized reduction in the caliber of peripheral vessels throughout the lungs. Severe generalized pulmonary overinflation is present (note the low flattened configuration of the diaphragm). Cardiomegaly is absent, and the hilar pulmonary arteries are not enlarged; thus, despite the generalized oligemia, there is no evidence of pulmonary arterial hypertension.

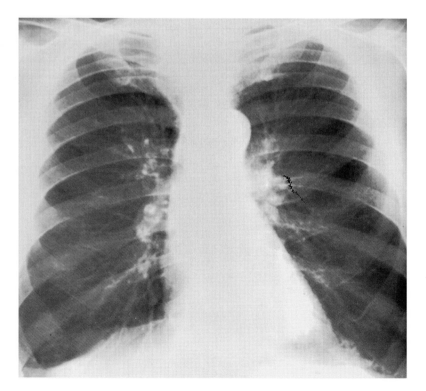

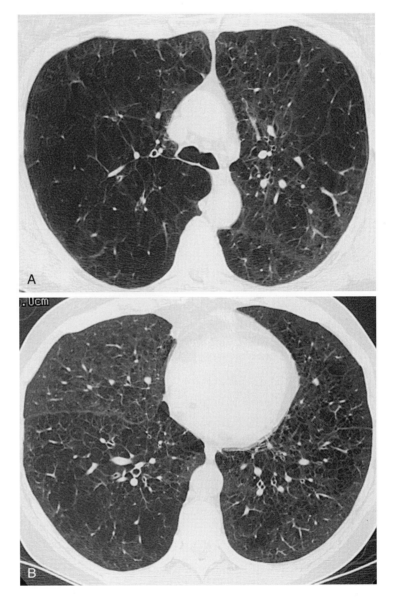

Figure A–12–3. Generalized Oligemia: Centrilobular Emphysema. An HRCT scan *(A)* shows areas of abnormally low attenuation throughout the upper lobes. An HRCT scan through the lower lung zones *(B)* shows less severe involvement. The patient was a 53-year-old smoker.

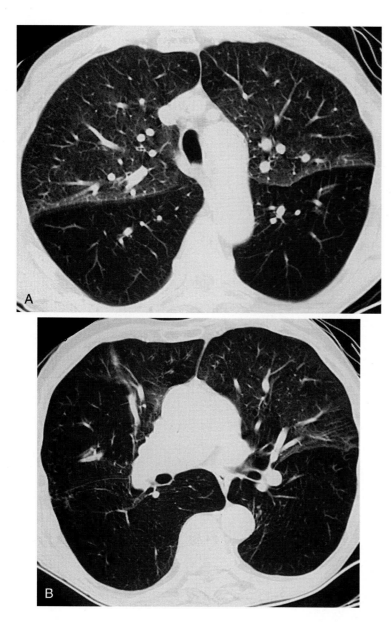

Figure A–12–4. Generalized Oligemia: Panlobular Emphysema. A CT scan at the level of the aortic arch *(A)* shows relatively normal upper lobes and oligemia of the superior segments of the lower lobes. A CT scan at a more caudad level *(B)* shows oligemia throughout the lower lobes, with less severe involvement of the right middle lobe and lingula. The patient was a 63-year-old man with panlobular emphysema secondary to intravenous drug abuse.

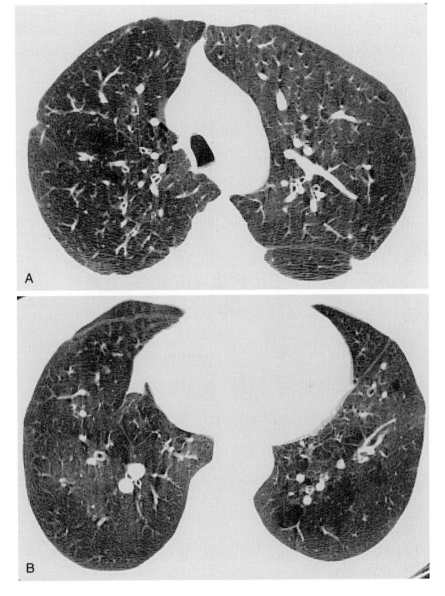

Figure A–12–5. Peripheral Oligemia: Oblitera-tive Bronchiolitis. HRCT scans (*A* and *B*) demonstrate areas of decreased attenuation and vascularity in a patchy distribution, mainly in the periphery of the lungs. Mild bronchial dilation and bronchial wall thickening are also evident. The patient was a 65-year-old woman who had obliterative bronchiolitis secondary to neuroendocrine cell hyperplasia. The diagnosis was confirmed at lung transplantation.

Table A–13
UNILATERAL, LOBAR, OR SEGMENTAL PULMONARY OLIGEMIA

The same three combinations of changes apply in this pattern as in general pulmonary oligemia:

1. Small peripheral vessels, no overinflation; normal or small hilum. This is epitomized by lobar or unilateral hyperlucent lung (Swyer-James syndrome).
2. Small peripheral vessels; no overinflation; enlarged hilar pulmonary arteries (or an enlarged hilum). This combination is almost invariably the result of unilateral pulmonary artery thromboembolism without infarction.
3. Small peripheral vessels; overinflation; normal hilar pulmonary arteries. This combination is typically seen in bronchial atresia and congenital lobar emphysema.

Table A–13

UNILATERAL, LOBAR, OR SEGMENTAL PULMONARY OLIGEMIA *Continued*

	ETIOLOGY	ADDITIONAL FINDINGS	COMMENTS
DEVELOPMENTAL	Hypogenetic lung syndrome	Anomalous vein forms "scimitar sign"	Associated anomalies include dextrocardia, mirror-image bronchial tree, and anomalous venous drainage of right lung to inferior vena cava. Right lung is supplied by systemic arteries, in part or wholly.
	Congenital bronchial atresia (Fig. A–13–1)	Almost invariably associated with a smooth, lobulated soft tissue opacity (inspissated mucus) distal to the point of atresia; most commonly affects the apicoposterior segment of the left upper lobe; affected bronchopulmonary segments are air-containing as a result of collateral ventilation	Diagnosis can be confirmed by CT.
	Congenital lobar emphysema (Fig. A–13–2)	Characterized by severe overinflation of a pulmonary lobe, most commonly the left upper or right middle lobe; air trapping is severe and results in marked enlargement of the lobe and contralateral displacement of the mediastinum	Occasionally first diagnosed in an adult patient
NEOPLASTIC	Pulmonary carcinoma	A mass is almost invariably identifiable; air trapping may be noted	A rare manifestation of pulmonary carcinoma. It may progress to a pattern of homogeneous segmental consolidation as a result of obstructive pneumonitis/atelectasis. Volume of affected parenchyma is usually smaller than normal at full inspiration.
	Carcinoid tumor (Fig. A–13–3)	Same as for pulmonary carcinoma	Same as for pulmonary carcinoma
EMBOLIC	**Thromboembolism without infarction**	**Almost invariably associated with obstruction of a major pulmonary artery; affected artery is characteristically widened and of sharper than normal definition; involved bronchopulmonary segments may show moderate loss of volume**	**Local oligemia resulting from thromboembolism constitutes Westermark's sign.**
INHALATIONAL	Foreign body aspiration	Lower lobe predominance; foreign body identifiable as an opaque shadow in some cases	Air trapping and local oligemia are more common manifestations of foreign body inhalation than are atelectasis or obstructive pneumonitis.
AIRWAY DISEASE	Emphysema	Affected regions are overinflated; attenuated vascular markings usually evident	
	Unilateral or lobar hyperlucent lung (Swyer-James syndrome) (Fig. A–13–4)	Oligemia characteristically involves a whole lung, producing unilateral radiolucency, but single lobes may be similarly affected; both hilar and peripheral vessels are diminutive; volume of affected lung at total lung capacity is normal or reduced, seldom if ever increased; air trapping on expiration is a *sine qua non* to the diagnosis, and permits differentiation from agenesis of a pulmonary artery	HRCT scans show decreased attenuation and vascularity of the involved lung, bronchiectasis, and air trapping.
	Bullae	**Sharply defined, air-containing spaces bounded by curvilinear, hairline shadows; vascular markings are absent; adjacent lung parenchyma is compressed; overinflation and air trapping are usual**	

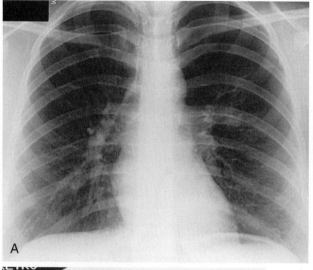

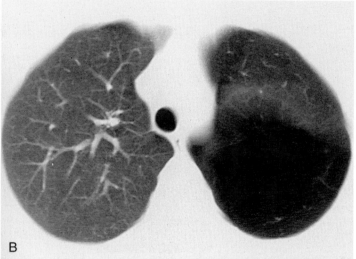

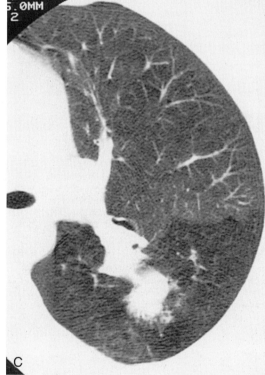

Figure A–13–1. Oligemia and Hyperinflation: Bronchial Atresia. A posteroanterior chest radiograph _(A)_ demonstrates marked lucency and decreased vascularity in
the left upper lobe. Also present is an ill-defined opacity near the left hilum. A
conventional 10-mm-collimation CT scan _(B)_ shows a marked decrease in attenuation
and vascularity in the region of the apical posterior segment of the left upper lobe. An
HRCT scan _(C)_ demonstrates focal opacity near the origin of the apicoposterior segmental bronchus and decreased attenuation of the adjacent lung.

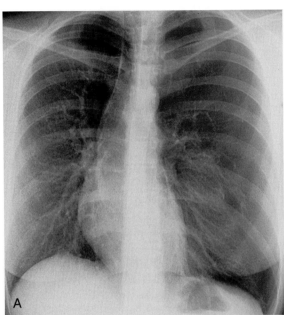

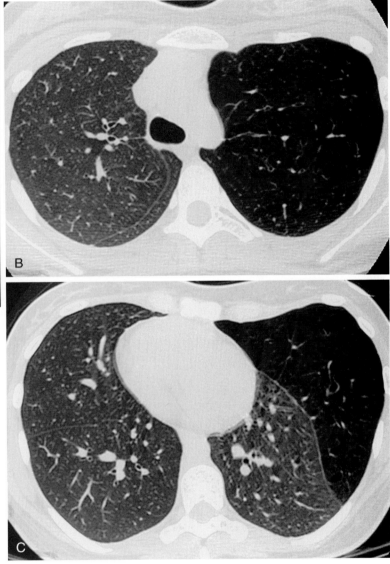

Figure A–13–2. Oligemia and Hyperinflation: Congenital Lobar Emphysema. A posteroanterior chest radiograph *(A)* reveals overinflation of the left upper lobe and lingula associated with a shift of the mediastinum to the right and mild compression of the left lower lobe. An HRCT scan at the level of the aortic arch *(B)* demonstrates increased volume and decreased attenuation and perfusion of the left upper lobe. An HRCT scan through the lower lung zones *(C)* shows overinflation of the lingula. The bronchi within the left upper lobe and lingula are dilated. The patient was a 21-year-old woman. (Courtesy of Dr. Marie-Pierre Cordeau, Department of Radiology, Hôtel-Dieu de Montréal.)

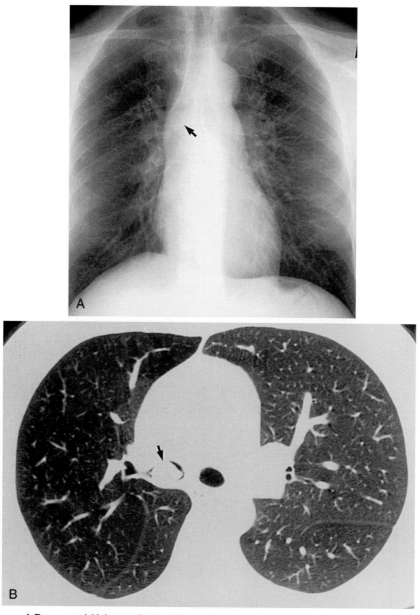

Figure A–13–3. Oligemia and Decreased Volume: Partly Obstructing Central Carcinoid Tumor. A posteroanterior chest radiograph *(A)* demonstrates decreased vascularity and slight decrease in size of the right lung. A tumor can be seen within the right main bronchus *(arrow)*. A CT scan *(B)* better demonstrates the marked decrease in vascularity of the right lung. Reflex vasoconstriction also resulted in decreased attenuation of the right lung compared with the left. The partly obstructing tumor *(arrow)* can be clearly seen in the right main bronchus. The diagnosis of typical carcinoid tumor was made at bronchoscopy and confirmed at surgery. The patient was a 48-year-old woman.

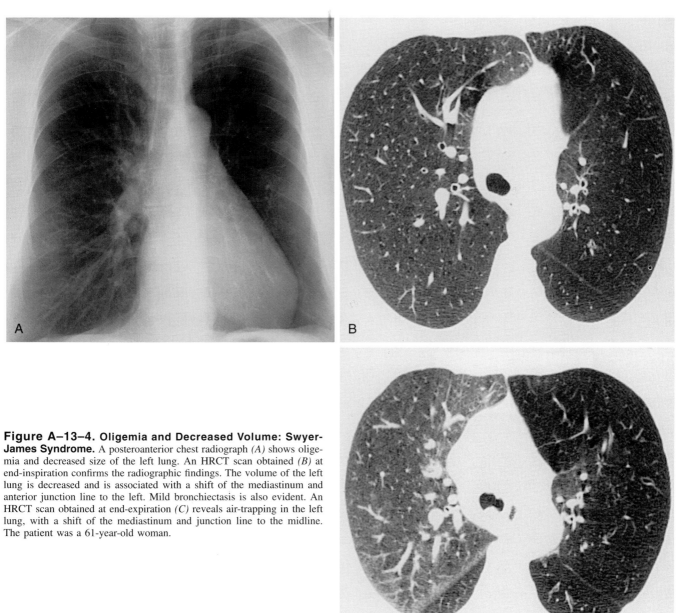

Figure A–13–4. Oligemia and Decreased Volume: Swyer-James Syndrome. A posteroanterior chest radiograph *(A)* shows oligemia and decreased size of the left lung. An HRCT scan obtained *(B)* at end-inspiration confirms the radiographic findings. The volume of the left lung is decreased and is associated with a shift of the mediastinum and anterior junction line to the left. Mild bronchiectasis is also evident. An HRCT scan obtained at end-expiration *(C)* reveals air-trapping in the left lung, with a shift of the mediastinum and junction line to the midline. The patient was a 61-year-old woman.

Table A–14

HILAR AND MEDIASTINAL LYMPH NODE ENLARGEMENT

This table includes abnormalities that produce lymph node enlargement within the thorax, either alone or in combination with other radiographic abnormalities. It includes only conditions in which evidence of lymph node enlargement is seen on the chest radiograph; diseases associated with mild mediastinal lymph node enlargement evident only on CT scans are not included.

Table A–14
HILAR AND MEDIASTINAL LYMPH NODE ENLARGEMENT

	ETIOLOGY	SYMMETRY	NODE GROUPS INVOLVED	ADDITIONAL FINDINGS	COMMENTS
INFECTIOUS	**Bacteria**				
	Mycobacterium tuberculosis: "primary" (Fig. A–14–1)	Unilateral in 80% of cases	Approximately 60% hilar and 40% combined hilar and mediastinal	Almost always associated with ipsilateral parenchymal disease	On contrast-enhanced CT scans, nodes often have low attenuation and may have rim enhancement. Nontuberculous mycobacterial infection may cause similar appearance in patients who have the acquired immunodeficiency syndrome.
	Fungi				
	Histoplasma capsulatum	Unilateral or bilateral	Hilar or mediastinal or both	Enlarged nodes may obstruct airways through extrinsic pressure, resulting in obstructive pneumonitis and atelectasis; usually associated with parenchymal disease	
	Coccidioides immitis	Unilateral or bilateral	Hilar or mediastinal or both	Node enlargement may occur with or without associated parenchymal disease	
	Viruses				
	Epstein-Barr virus	Bilateral symmetric	Predominantly hilar	Lungs usually clear	Splenomegaly may also be evident.
IMMUNOLOGIC	**Sarcoidosis** (Fig. A–14–2)	**Almost invariably symmetric, unilateral node enlargement occurring in only 1–3% of cases**	**Paratracheal, tracheobronchial, and bronchopulmonary groups. Paratracheal enlargement occasionally occurs without concomitant enlargement of hilar nodes**	**75–90% of patients show mediastinal and hilar lymph node enlargement; approximately 40% of these show diffuse parenchymal disease as well**	**75% of patients with hilar lymph node enlargement show complete resolution of the enlarged nodes. Symmetric appearance and diminution of lymph node size with onset of diffuse lung disease aid in differentiating sarcoidosis from lymphoma and tuberculosis.**

NEOPLASTIC				
Pulmonary carcinoma (Fig. A-14-3)	Usually unilateral	Hilar or mediastinal or both	Other manifestations of pulmonary carcinoma (e.g., lung nodule or mass, atelectasis/obstructive pneumonitis, or pleural effusion) usually evident; enlargement of mediastinal lymph nodes may be sole abnormality radiographically, a finding almost always indicating spread from a small cell carcinoma	
Hodgkin's disease	Typically bilateral but often asymmetric; unilateral node enlargement is very unusual	Most commonly involved are anterior mediastinal nodes, followed by paratracheal nodes	Pulmonary involvement occurs in less than 30% of patients and is almost invariably associated with mediastinal node enlargement; pleural effusion in approximately 30% of cases, usually in association with other intrathoracic manifestations	**Intrathoracic involvement occurs in 90% of patients at some stage of the disease, most commonly in the form of mediastinal lymph node enlargement; the latter is seen on the initial chest radiograph in approximately 50% of patients.**
Non-Hodgkin's lymphoma	Bilateral but asymmetric	Mediastinal nodes involved in most cases	Sometimes associated with pleuropulmonary involvement	**The most common intrathoracic manifestation of the disease**
Leukemia	Usually symmetric	Mediastinal and hilar	Both pleural effusion and parenchymal involvement may be associated	**The most common radiographic manifestation of leukemia within the thorax (25% of patients); a much more common manifestation of lymphocytic than of myelocytic leukemia**
Metastatic carcinoma (Fig. A-14-4)	Unilateral or bilateral	Hilar or mediastinal or both	Pulmonary nodules often seen	**Most commonly seen with breast and renal cell carcinoma and testicular tumors**
INHALATIONAL				
Silica exposure	Symmetric	Predominantly hilar	Eggshell calcification of hilar lymph nodes occurs in approximately 5% of cases and may also be observed in lymph nodes in the anterior and posterior mediastinum and in the thoracic wall; usually associated with a diffuse nodular pattern throughout both lungs	

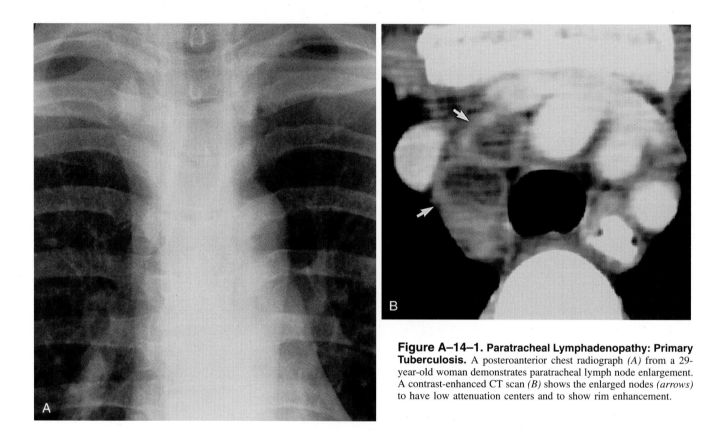

Figure A–14–1. Paratracheal Lymphadenopathy: Primary Tuberculosis. A posteroanterior chest radiograph *(A)* from a 29-year-old woman demonstrates paratracheal lymph node enlargement. A contrast-enhanced CT scan *(B)* shows the enlarged nodes *(arrows)* to have low attenuation centers and to show rim enhancement.

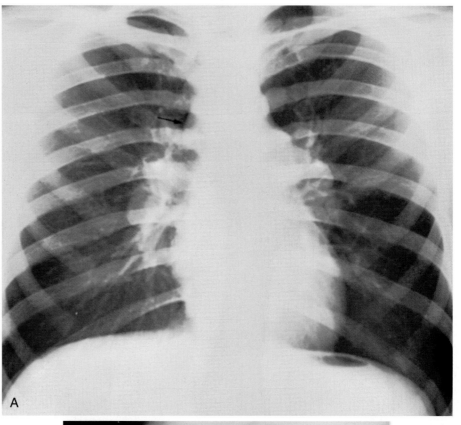

Figure A–14–2. Hilar and Mediastinal Lymph Node Enlargement: Sarcoidosis.
Posteroanterior *(A)* and lateral *(B)* chest radiographs reveal enlargement of both hilar shadows due to enlarged lymph nodes; the lobulated contour is particularly well demonstrated in lateral projection. Bilateral paratracheal and tracheobronchial lymph node enlargement is also present, the azygos lymph node being clearly visible in posteroanterior projection *(arrow)*. The lungs are clear.

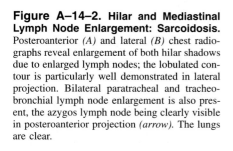

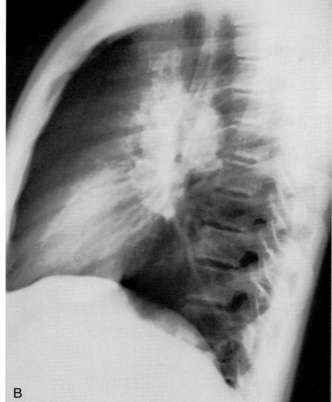

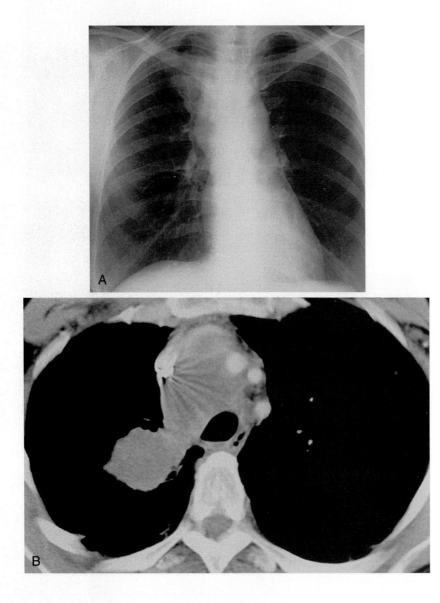

Figure A–14–3. Paratracheal Lymph Node Enlargement: Pulmonary Carcinoma. A posteroanterior chest radiograph *(A)* from a 47-year-old woman shows a poorly defined right upper lobe opacity and right paratracheal lymph node enlargement. A contrast-enhanced CT scan *(B)* shows right upper lobe tumor and extensive lymphadenopathy. Obliteration of the fat planes between the mediastinal nodes is highly suggestive of diffuse tumor infiltration. The tumor was shown to be large cell carcinoma.

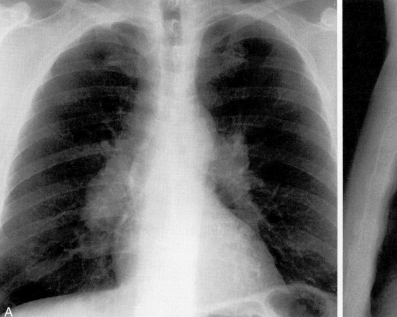

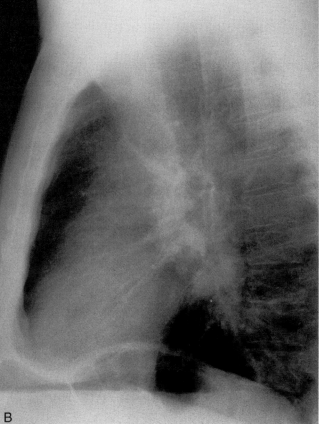

Figure A–14–4. Hilar and Mediastinal Lymph Node Enlargement: Metastatic Renal Cell Carcinoma. Posteroanterior *(A)* and lateral *(B)* chest radiographs from a patient recently diagnosed as having renal cell carcinoma demonstrate extensive paratracheal and bilateral hilar lymph node enlargement. Lymph node biopsy confirmed the diagnosis of metastatic renal cell carcinoma.

Table A–15

MEDIASTINAL MASSES SITUATED PREDOMINANTLY IN THE ANTERIOR COMPARTMENT

Anatomically, this mediastinal compartment is bounded anteriorly by the sternum and posteriorly by the pericardium, aorta, and brachiocephalic vessels. The anterior margin of the brachiocephalic vessels and the ascending aorta are often difficult to identify on the lateral chest radiograph; moreover, anterior mediastinal masses often project over the heart (middle mediastinum). Therefore, on the chest radiograph a mediastinal mass is considered to probably lie in the anterior compartment when it is situated in the region anterior to a line drawn along the anterior border of the trachea and the posterior border of the heart. It should be noted, however, that a mass that displaces the trachea laterally or posteriorly probably has a major middle mediastinal component.

CT and MR imaging allow visualization of the exact location of lesions, some assessment of their tissue composition, and identification of the specific structures from which they arise. With these techniques, it is therefore preferable to describe the exact location of the lesion and its relation to the adjacent structures rather than limiting the description to a particular mediastinal compartment.

Table A–15
ANTERIOR MEDIASTINAL MASSES

	ETIOLOGY	CONTOUR	ADDITIONAL FINDINGS	CT FINDINGS	COMMENTS
DEVELOPMENTAL	Mesothelial cyst (pericardial and pleuropericardial cysts) (Fig. A–15–1)	Usually round, oval, or "tear-drop" in appearance, with smooth margin	Variation in shape of cyst may occur on changing position of patient	Usually of homogeneous water density	
NEOPLASTIC	Thymolipoma	Smooth or lobulated	None	Pliable mass of predominantly fat attenuation originating from thymus	These tumors can grow very large; because of their fat content and soft consistency they tend to slump toward the diaphragm, leaving the upper mediastinum relatively clear.
	Thymic cysts	Smooth	None	Homogeneous fluid attenuation	
	Thymoma (Fig. A–15–2)	**Smooth or lobulated; well defined**	**Contains calcium in some cases**	**Homogeneous or heterogeneous attenuation; can contain cystic areas and calcification**	
	Thymic carcinoma	Irregular, poorly defined	Invasion of adjacent structures common at the time of diagnosis	Homogeneous or heterogeneous attenuation; frequent invasion of adjacent structures	Bulky masses ranging from 5 to 15 cm in diameter
	Germ cell neoplasms (Fig. A–15–3)	Smooth or lobulated, oval or round; may protrude to either side or bilaterally	Calcification, bone, teeth, or fat may be identified in teratomas	Mature cystic teratomas often contain areas of fat attenuation and may contain fluid and foci of calcification; malignant germ cell tumors may have homogeneous or heterogeneous soft tissue attenuation	
	Thyroid goiter and tumors	**Smooth or lobulated**	**Anterior lesions displace trachea posteriorly; middle mediastinal masses displace it laterally; posterior masses displace it anteriorly and the esophagus posteriorly; calcification fairly common**	**Lesion can be seen to arise from thyroid gland; goiters typically have high attenuation and marked enhancement with intravenous contrast; often with calcification; neoplasms may have homogeneous or heterogeneous soft tissue attenuation**	**Most commonly a nodular goiter; scintigraphy or CT sometimes diagnostic; biopsy often required when only a single nodule is evident**

Table continued on following page

Table A–15

ANTERIOR MEDIASTINAL MASSES Continued

	ETIOLOGY	CONTOUR	ADDITIONAL FINDINGS	CT FINDINGS	COMMENTS
	Non-Hodgkin's lymphoma and Hodgkin's disease (Fig. A–15–4)	**Symmetrically widened mediastinum or solitary or multiple lobulated masses**	**Pulmonary consolidation and pleural effusion in some cases**	**Mediastinal lymph node enlargement; may have homogeneous or heterogeneous attenuation and contain cystic areas**	
	Metastatic carcinoma		Phrenic nerve involvement may result in diaphragmatic paralysis; lobulated paratracheal or hilar lymph node enlargement common	Mediastinal lymph node enlargement	Primary usually pulmonary carcinoma
CARDIOVASCULAR	Aortic aneurysm	Fusiform or saccular	Calcification may be present in wall	CT and MR imaging are diagnostic	
TRAUMATIC	Mediastinal hemorrhage or hematoma	May be local or diffuse, commonly in upper mediastinum	Rarely, superior vena cava compression	Contrast-enhanced CT diagnostic for aortic dissection; angiography often required to diagnose traumatic tear of the aorta or great vessels	
MISCELLANEOUS CAUSES	Herniation through foramen of Morgagni	Round or oval; usually to right of pericardium	If mass is completely radiopaque, CT may differentiate hernia from epicardial fat or pericardial cyst	CT diagnostic; shows discontinuity of the diaphragm and herniation of omental fat and, less commonly, colon	

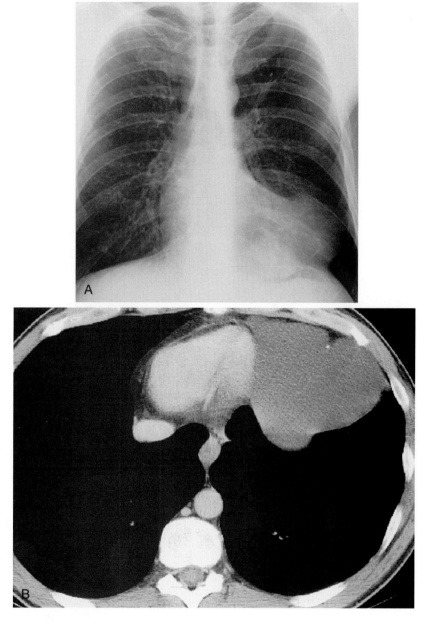

Figure A–15–1. Anterior Mediastinal Mass: Pericardial (Mesothelial) Cyst. A posteroanterior chest radiograph *(A)* from a 46-year-old man demonstrates a smoothly marginated increased opacity in the left cardiophrenic angle. The obscuration of the left heart border indicates the anterior location of the abnormality (silhouette sign). A contrast-enhanced CT scan *(B)* demonstrates a water-density cyst.

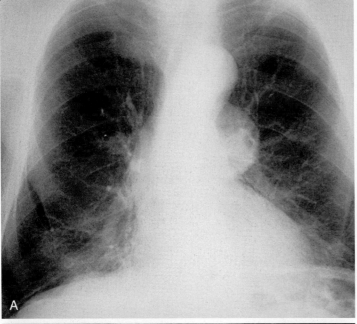

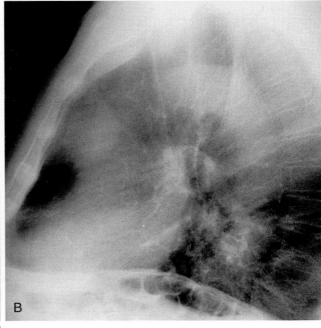

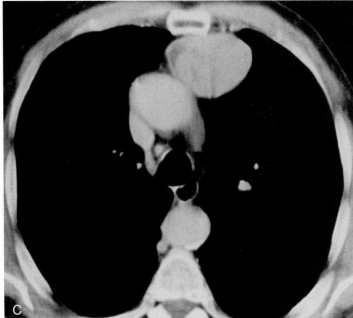

Figure A–15–2. Anterior Mediastinal Mass: Thymoma. Posteroanterior *(A)* and lateral *(B)* chest radiographs from a 75-year-old man demonstrate an anterior mediastinal mass. A contrast-enhanced CT scan *(C)* shows a smoothly marginated mass with slightly heterogeneous enhancement. The mass was confirmed at surgery to be a benign thymoma.

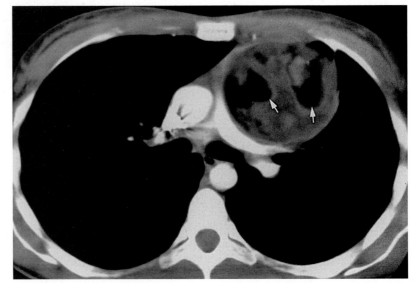

Figure A–15–3. Anterior Mediastinal Mass: Mature Cystic Teratoma. An intravenous contrast-enhanced CT scan in a 29-year-old woman demonstrates a heterogeneous anterior mediastinal mass, which contains areas of fat attenuation *(arrows)*. The diagnosis of teratoma was confirmed at surgery.

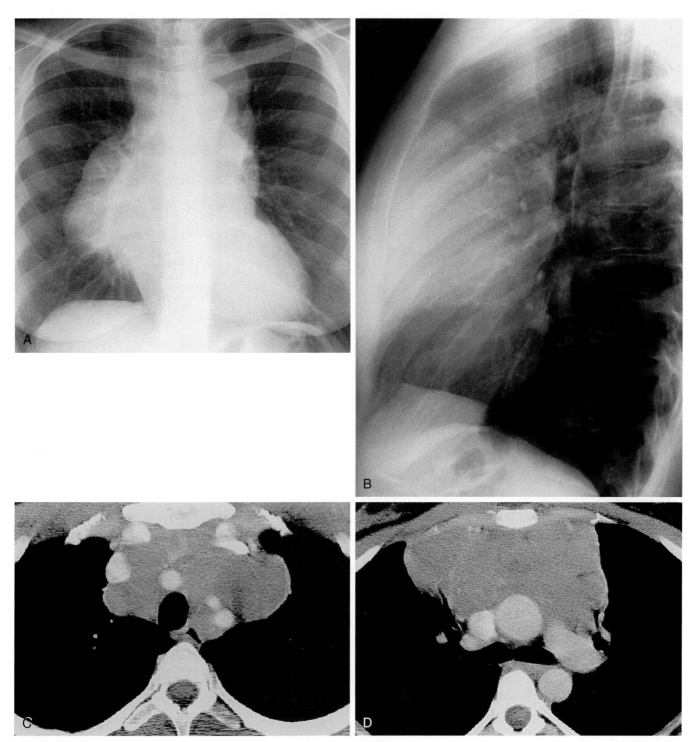

Figure A–15–4. Anterior Mediastinal Mass: Diffuse Large Cell Lymphoma. Posteroanterior *(A)* and lateral *(B)* chest radiographs reveal a large, lobulated anterior mediastinal mass. Note the absence of hilar lymphadenopathy, the interlobar arteries being clearly seen through the soft tissue masses ("hilum overlay" sign). Contrast-enhanced spiral CT scans *(C* and *D)* demonstrate diffuse enlargement of the anterior mediastinal and paratracheal lymph nodes with obliteration of the fat planes between the nodes. In spite of the extensive lymphadenopathy, there is no evidence of compression of the vascular structures. Mediastinoscopy revealed diffuse large cell lymphoma showing B-cell differentiation. The patient was a 31-year-old woman.

Table A-16

MEDIASTINAL MASSES SITUATED PREDOMINANTLY IN THE MIDDLE AND POSTERIOR COMPARTMENTS

Anatomically, the middle mediastinum contains the heart, the pericardium, the major vessels, the trachea and main bronchi, paratracheal and tracheobronchial lymph nodes, the phrenic nerves, and the upper portions of the vagus nerves. The posterior mediastinum contains the descending thoracic aorta, the esophagus, the thoracic duct, the lower portion of the vagus nerves, and the posterior group of mediastinal lymph nodes. Because the posterior limit of the mediastinum is formed by the anterior surface of the vertebral column, the paravertebral zones and posterior gutters are by definition excluded.

On the lateral chest radiograph it is not possible to reliably distinguish abnormalities located in the middle mediastinum from those in the posterior mediastinum. Therefore, these two compartments are considered together from the point of view of differential diagnosis. A lesion can be considered to probably lie in the middle or posterior compartment when it is located between a line drawn through the anterior aspect of the trachea and posterior aspect of the heart and a line drawn through the anterior margins of the vertebral bodies.

As with the anterior compartment, CT and MR imaging allow visualization of the exact location of the lesions, some assessment of their tissue composition, and identification of the structures from which they arise. Therefore, with these techniques, it is preferable to describe the exact location of the lesion and its relation to the adjacent structures rather than limiting the description to a particular mediastinal compartment.

Table A–16

MIDDLE/POSTERIOR MEDIASTINAL MASSES

ETIOLOGY	CONTOUR	ADDITIONAL FINDINGS	CT FINDINGS	COMMENTS
DEVELOPMENTAL				
Bronchogenic cyst (Fig. A–16–1)	Round or oval, well defined; contour may be affected by contact with more solid structures	May compress the tracheobronchial tree or esophagus; calcification rare	Approximately 50% of cysts have water density and 50% have soft tissue attenuation on CT scans	Cyst may be multilocular. Seldom communicates with tracheobronchial tree. MR imaging shows homogeneous high signal intensity on T2-weighted images.
Diverticula of the pharynx or esophagus	Cystlike structure in superior (pharyngeal) or inferior (esophageal) regions	Invariably communicate with pharynx or esophagus; may displace contiguous esophagus; aspiration pneumonia may develop from pharyngeal (Zenker's) diverticulum	Often have heterogeneous attenuation owing to the presence of air, food, and secretions	
INFECTIOUS				
Fibrosing mediastinitis	Lobulated, usually in right paramediastinal area	May show calcification; compression of major airway in some cases	May show compression of superior vena cava and collateral circulation; calcification highly suggestive of previous histoplasmosis or, less commonly, tuberculosis	—
Acute mediastinitis	Symmetric widening as a result of diffuse involvement or localized following abscess formation	May be air in mediastinum	Obliteration of fat planes; areas of low attenuation suggest abscess formation	
NEOPLASTIC				
Thyroid goiter and neoplasms	Smooth or lobulated	Anterior masses displace trachea posteriorly; middle mediastinal masses displace it laterally; and posterior mediastinal masses displace it anteriorly and the esophagus posteriorly; calcification fairly common	Lesion can be seen to arise from thyroid gland; goiters typically have high attenuation and marked enhancement with intravenous contrast; often with calcification; malignant tumors may have homogeneous or heterogeneous soft tissue attenuation	Most commonly a nodular goiter. Scintigraphy or CT is sometimes diagnostic. Biopsy is often required.
Primary tracheal neoplasms (Fig. A–16–2)	Smooth or lobulated	—	Airway narrowing and peritracheal tumor extension	Most commonly squamous cell carcinoma or adenoid cystic carcinoma
Soft tissue tumors and tumor-like conditions				
Lipomatosis	Smooth and symmetric; sometimes lobulated	Enlargement of pleuropericardial fat pads	Fatty infiltration of the mediastinum	CT diagnostic

Table continued on following page

Table A–16

MIDDLE/POSTERIOR MEDIASTINAL MASSES Continued

ETIOLOGY	CONTOUR	ADDITIONAL FINDINGS	CT FINDINGS	COMMENTS
Non-Hodgkin's lymphoma and Hodgkin's disease	Symmetrically widened mediastinum or solitary or multiple lobulated masses	Pulmonary consolidation and pleural effusion in some cases	Mediastinal lymph node enlargement; may have homogeneous or heterogeneous attenuation and contain cystic areas	Usually have associated anterior mediastinal component
Metastatic carcinoma	**Lobulated**	**Phrenic nerve involvement may result in diaphragmatic paralysis**	**Mediastinal lymph node enlargement**	**Primary usually pulmonary carcinoma**
Esophageal neoplasms	Smooth, rounded margin		Abnormalities can include focal esophageal thickening, extensive soft tissue infiltration, or, less commonly, a large focal mass	Usually carcinoma
CARDIOVASCULAR				
Aortic aneurysms (Figs. A–16–3, A–16–4, A–16–5)	**Fusiform or saccular**	**Calcification may be present in wall**	**CT and MR imaging are diagnostic**	
Buckling or aneurysm of the innominate artery	Smooth, lateral bulging, convex laterally from level of aortic arch upward	Tortuous thoracic aorta secondary to atherosclerosis may be evident	CT and MR imaging are diagnostic	Opacity typically courses cephalad and laterally from the level of aortic arch to the level of the clavicle.
Superior vena cava dilation	Smooth, extending from hilum along right paramediastinal border	Signs of underlying causative disorder, e.g., cardiac dilation, mediastinal mass	CT and MR imaging are diagnostic	Secondary to central pressure rise or to compression and obstruction
Azygos and hemiazygos dilation	Smooth, round or oval mass at tracheobronchial angle	Change in size with change in body position	CT and MR imaging are diagnostic	
Dilation of pulmonary artery	Smooth	Stenotic pulmonary valve or peripheral vascular attenuation in secondary types	CT and MR imaging are diagnostic	
TRAUMATIC				
Mediastinal hemorrhage or hematoma	May be local or diffuse, commonly in upper mediastinum	Other findings of trauma, e.g., rib fractures or pulmonary contusion, commonly seen	Contrast-enhanced CT diagnostic for aortic dissection; angiography often required to diagnose traumatic tear of the aorta or great vessels	
MISCELLANEOUS CAUSES				
Esophageal hiatus hernia	**Retrocardiac mass of variable size containing air; usually smooth**	**May contain one or more fluid levels; rarely completely opaque**	**CT diagnostic but seldom required**	**Usually contains omentum and stomach**
Megaesophagus (Fig. A–16–6)	Broad vertical opacity on the right side of the mediastinum	Air in lumen with fluid level at varying distance from diaphragm	CT diagnostic but seldom required	Usually the result of progressive systemic sclerosis or achalasia
Bochdalek hernia	Round or oval retrocardiac or paravertebral density; rarely bilateral		CT diagnostic; demonstrates discontinuity of diaphragm and herniation of omental fat and, less commonly in the adult, abdominal viscera	Focal defects in diaphragm leading to Bochdalek hernia in the adult increase in frequency with age; paravertebral location more common

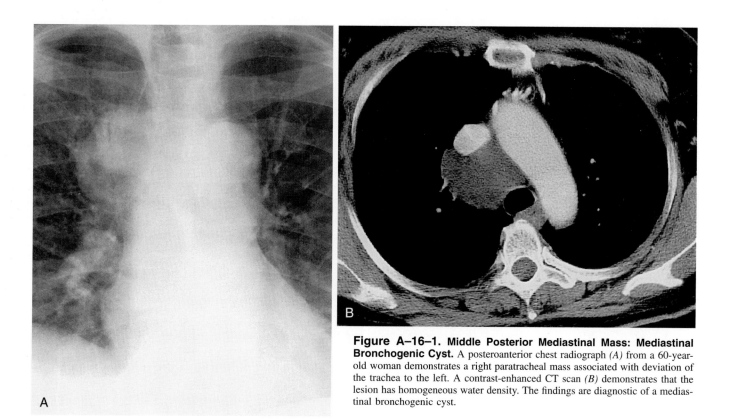

Figure A–16–1. Middle Posterior Mediastinal Mass: Mediastinal Bronchogenic Cyst. A posteroanterior chest radiograph *(A)* from a 60-year-old woman demonstrates a right paratracheal mass associated with deviation of the trachea to the left. A contrast-enhanced CT scan *(B)* demonstrates that the lesion has homogeneous water density. The findings are diagnostic of a mediastinal bronchogenic cyst.

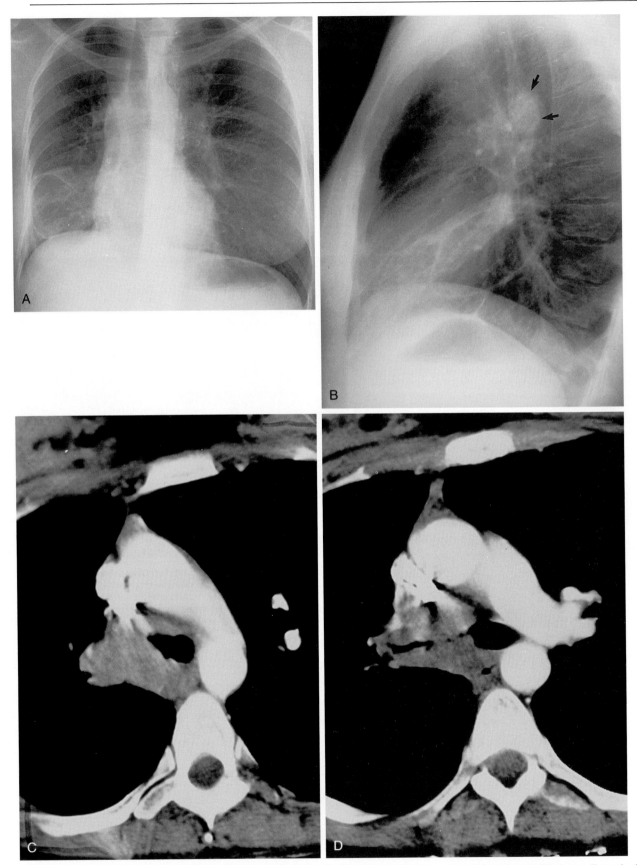

Figure A–16–2. Middle/Posterior Mediastinal Mass: Adenoid Cystic Carcinoma. Posteroanterior *(A)* and lateral *(B)* chest radiographs from a 27-year-old man demonstrate a mass posterior to the lower trachea *(arrows)*, associated with thickening of the posterior wall of the distal trachea and right bronchus. Also noted are areas of atelectasis in the right middle and lower lobes. Contrast-enhanced CT scans *(C* and *D)* demonstrate circumferential tumor at the level of the tracheal carina and the right main and right upper lobe bronchi, associated with narrowing of the airway lumen. Focal extension into the left main bronchus is evident.

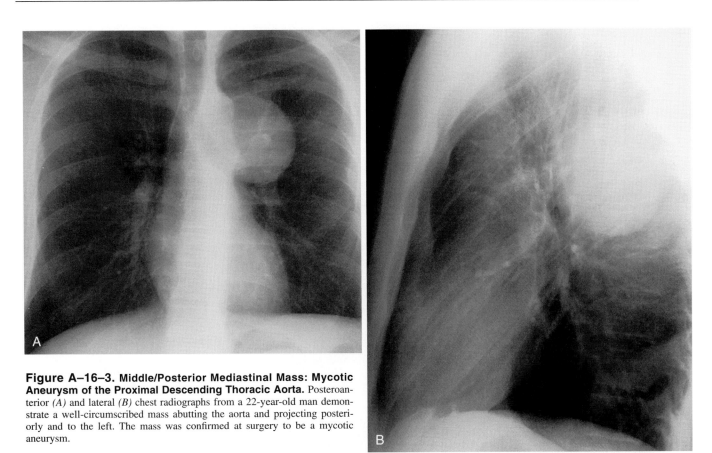

Figure A–16–3. Middle/Posterior Mediastinal Mass: Mycotic Aneurysm of the Proximal Descending Thoracic Aorta. Posteroanterior *(A)* and lateral *(B)* chest radiographs from a 22-year-old man demonstrate a well-circumscribed mass abutting the aorta and projecting posteriorly and to the left. The mass was confirmed at surgery to be a mycotic aneurysm.

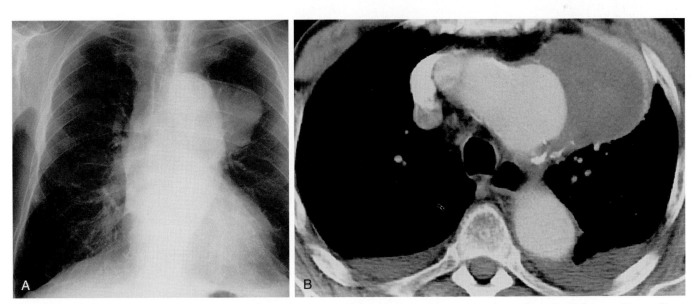

Figure A–16–4. Middle/Posterior Mediastinal Mass: Aneurysm of the Aorta. A posteroanterior chest radiograph *(A)* from an 87-year-old man demonstrates a homogeneous soft tissue opacity abutting the proximal descending thoracic aorta. A contrast-enhanced CT scan *(B)* shows a saccular aneurysm involving the proximal descending thoracic aorta and containing a large thrombus. Small bilateral pleural effusions are also evident. The aneurysm was shown to be secondary to atherosclerosis.

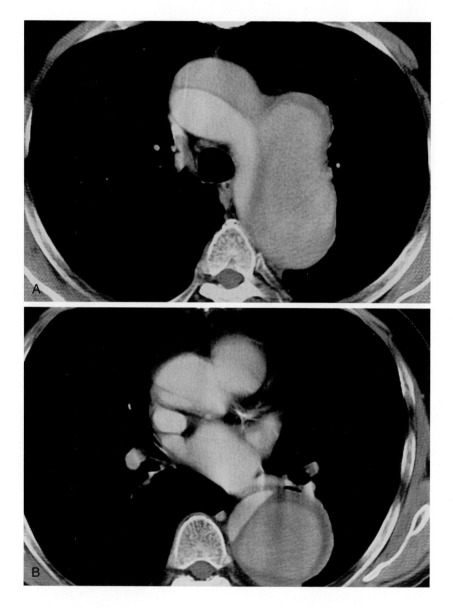

Figure A–16–5. Middle/Posterior Mediastinal Abnormality: Aortic Aneurysm with Dissection. A contrast-enhanced CT scan at the level of the aortic arch *(A)* demonstrates marked enhancement of the true aortic lumen and poor enhancement of the false lumen of the aortic dissection. Note the presence of a linear filling defect (intimal flap) separating the true from the false lumen. A CT scan at a more caudad level *(B)* shows that the dissection involves the ascending aorta (type A), which is of normal caliber, and the descending thoracic aorta, which shows aneurysmal dilation. The patient was a 57-year-old man who had systemic arterial hypertension.

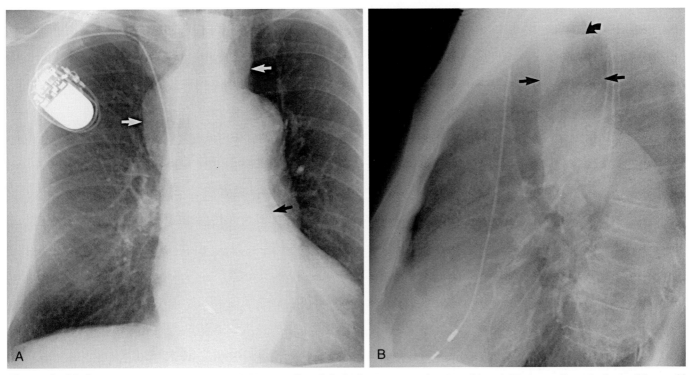

Figure A–16–6. Middle/Posterior Mediastinal Abnormality: Achalasia. Posteroanterior *(A)* and lateral *(B)* chest radiographs from a 74-year-old man demonstrate marked dilation of the esophagus *(straight arrows),* which contains an air-fluid level *(curved arrow)* and displaces the trachea anteriorly. The patient had long-standing achalasia.

Table A–17

MASSES SITUATED IN THE PARAVERTEBRAL REGION

The posterior limit of the mediastinum is formed by the anterior surface of the vertebral column. Although traditionally considered as "posterior mediastinal," masses located in the paravertebral zones and posterior gutters are thus not in the mediastinum and are better considered as a separate category. On the lateral chest radiograph, a mass can be considered to be located in the paravertebral region when it lies posterior to the anterior surface of the vertebral bodies. Associated abnormalities of the vertebrae are relatively common. CT and MR imaging allow assessment of the exact location of the lesion and of its soft tissue characteristics and therefore should be performed almost routinely.

Table A–17
PARAVERTEBRAL MASSES

	ETIOLOGY	CONTOUR	ADDITIONAL FINDINGS	CT FINDINGS	COMMENTS
DEVELOPMENTAL	Meningocele and meningomyelocele (Fig. A–17–1)	Sharply circumscribed, solitary or multiple, unilateral or bilateral	Frequently spine and rib deformities; no calcification	Communication with subarachnoid space; homogeneous water density	
INFECTIOUS	Suppurative or tuberculous spondylitis (Fig. A–17–2)	Smooth, fusiform mass	Erosion or destruction of vertebrae at level of paravertebral mass	Inhomogeneous paravertebral soft tissue; erosion or destruction of adjacent vertebrae	Most common in lower thoracic spine
NEOPLASTIC	**Neurogenic tumors (Fig. A–17–3)**	**Round or oval, well defined; rarely dumbbell-shaped**	**Usually unilateral; rib or vertebral erosion variable; rarely calcification in tumor**	**Can have homogeneous soft tissue attenuation (similar to or lower than that of chest wall muscles) or contain cystic areas; often show inhomogeneous contrast enhancement**	**Neurofibroma and neurilemoma most common**
	Bone and cartilage neoplasms	Round	Destruction of affected bone, often associated with soft tissue mass protruding into and compressing lung	CT or MR imaging used to assess tumor characteristics and extension into adjacent structures	
TRAUMATIC	Fracture of vertebra with hematoma	Smooth paravertebral swelling, usually bilateral	Vertebral and rib fractures	CT diagnostic	
MISCELLANEOUS CAUSES	**Bochdalek hernia (Fig. A–17–4)**	**Round or oval retrocardiac or paravertebral**		**CT diagnostic; demonstrates discontinuity of diaphragm and herniation of omental fat and, less commonly in the adult, abdominal viscera**	**Focal defects in diaphragm leading to Bochdalek hernia in the adult increase in frequency with age.**
	Extramedullary hematopoiesis (Fig. A–17–5)	Smooth or lobulated, usually bilateral	Spleen may be enlarged	Homogeneous soft tissue attenuation; fatty replacement can occur after resolution of the causative hemolytic disorder	

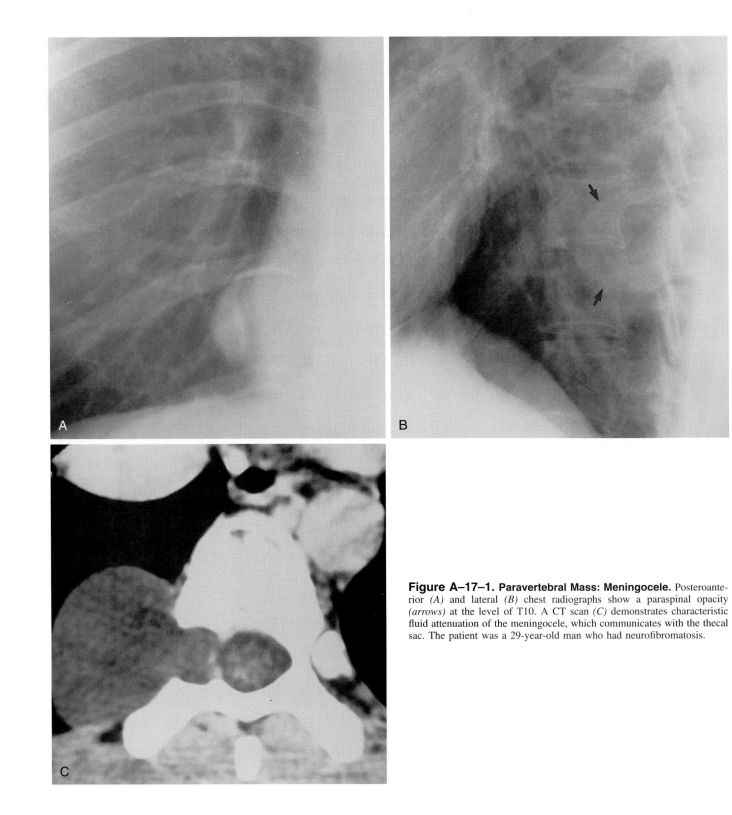

Figure A–17–1. Paravertebral Mass: Meningocele. Posteroanterior *(A)* and lateral *(B)* chest radiographs show a paraspinal opacity *(arrows)* at the level of T10. A CT scan *(C)* demonstrates characteristic fluid attenuation of the meningocele, which communicates with the thecal sac. The patient was a 29-year-old man who had neurofibromatosis.

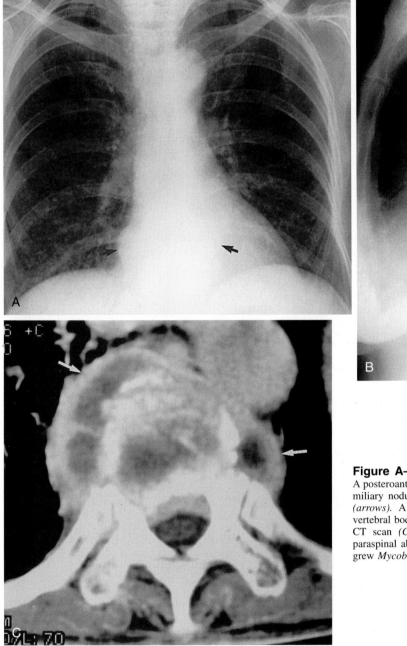

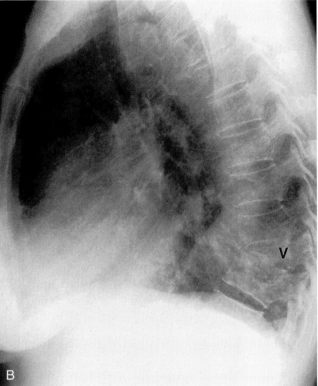

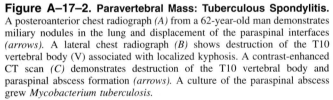

Figure A–17–2. Paravertebral Mass: Tuberculous Spondylitis.
A posteroanterior chest radiograph *(A)* from a 62-year-old man demonstrates miliary nodules in the lung and displacement of the paraspinal interfaces *(arrows)*. A lateral chest radiograph *(B)* shows destruction of the T10 vertebral body (V) associated with localized kyphosis. A contrast-enhanced CT scan *(C)* demonstrates destruction of the T10 vertebral body and paraspinal abscess formation *(arrows)*. A culture of the paraspinal abscess grew *Mycobacterium tuberculosis.*

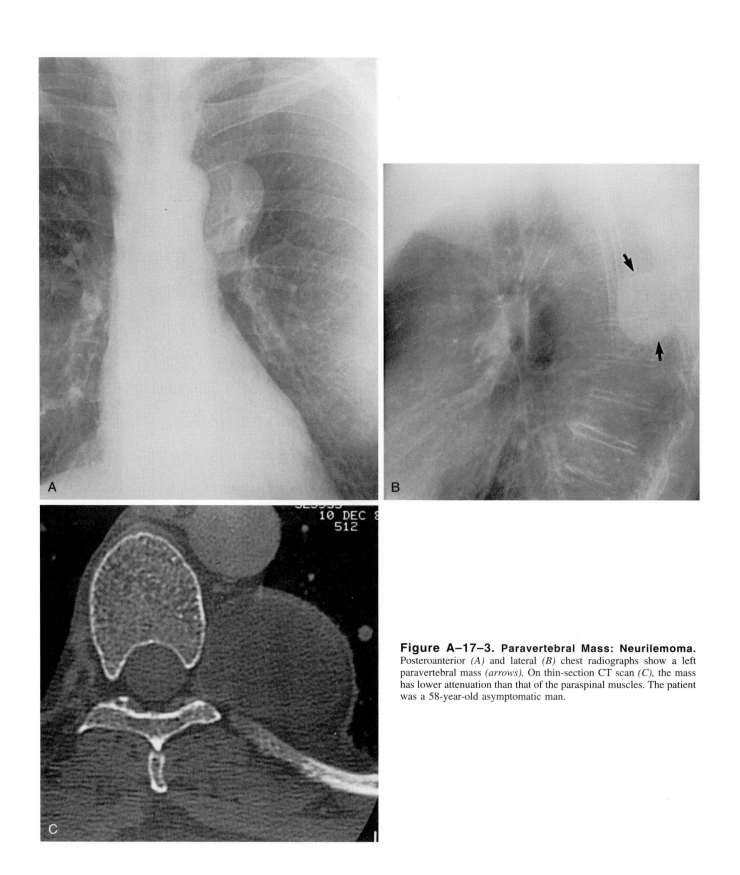

Figure A–17–3. Paravertebral Mass: Neurilemoma.
Posteroanterior *(A)* and lateral *(B)* chest radiographs show a left paravertebral mass *(arrows)*. On thin-section CT scan *(C)*, the mass has lower attenuation than that of the paraspinal muscles. The patient was a 58-year-old asymptomatic man.

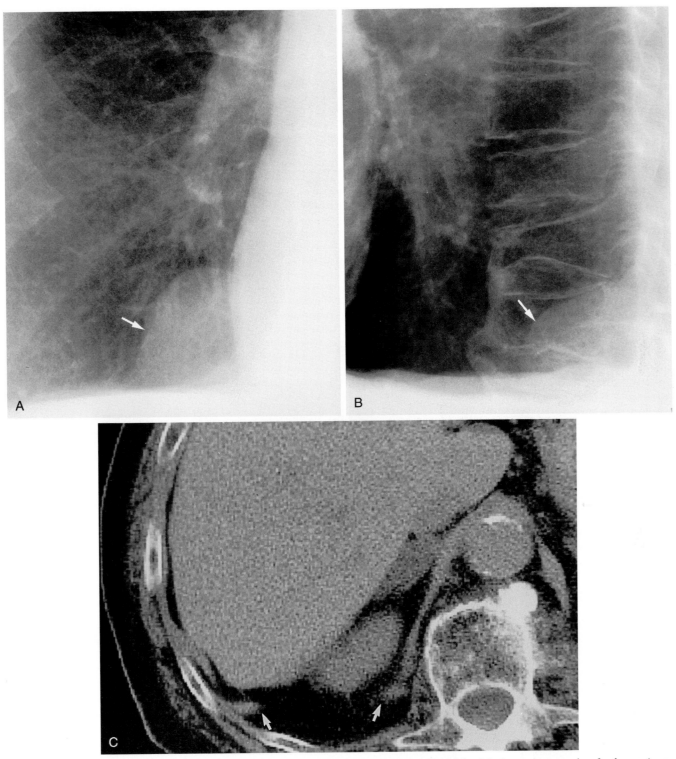

Figure A-17-4. Paravertebral Mass: Bochdalek Hernia. A posteroanterior radiograph *(A)* of the right lower chest reveals a focal mass *(arrow);* the lateral radiograph *(B)* shows it to be located posteriorly *(arrow).* The mass is of lesser opacity than that of the heart and soft tissues of the abdomen, consistent with a fatty composition. A CT scan of the right hemidiaphragm *(C)* reveals a defect *(arrows)* in its posterior aspect associated with herniation of omental fat. The patient was an 83-year-old woman; she had no symptoms related to the diaphragmatic defect. A radiograph obtained 5 years previously had been normal.

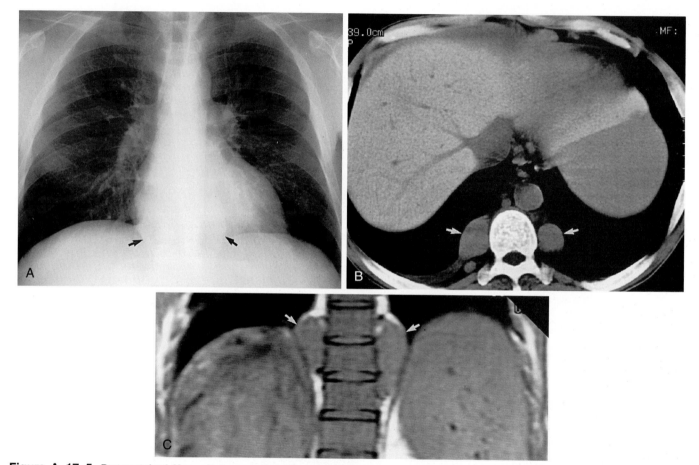

Figure A–17–5. Paravertebral Mass: Extramedullary Hematopoiesis. A posteroanterior chest radiograph *(A)* from a 39-year-old man shows displacement of the paravertebral interfaces *(arrows)*. A CT scan performed without intravenous contrast *(B)* shows paravertebral soft tissue masses *(arrows)*. Note the increased attenuation of the liver resulting from hemosiderosis. A coronal T1-weighted MR image *(C)* better demonstrates the extent of the extramedullary hematopoiesis *(arrows)*. The patient had β-thalassemia intermedia.

Index

Note: Page numbers in *italics* refer to illustrations; numbers followed by t indicate tables; numbers followed by n indicate notes.

Vol. 4 ISBN 0-7216-6198-X

90071

9 780721 661988